THE MERCK VETERINARY MANUAL

FIFTH EDITION

First Edition 1955
Second Edition 1961
Third Edition 1967
Fourth Edition 1973
Fifth Edition 1979

THE MERCK VETERINARY MANUAL is dedicated to
the Doctor of Veterinary Medicine and
to his colleagues and associates
in the animal sciences.

THE MERCK VETERINARY MANUAL

A HANDBOOK OF DIAGNOSIS
AND THERAPY FOR THE VETERINARIAN

FIFTH EDITION

EDITORIAL BOARD
Otto H. Siegmund, *Editor*
Clarence M. Fraser, *Associate Editor*
James Archibald
Douglas C. Blood
James A. Henderson
Paul M. Newberne
Glenn H. Snoeyenbos
Sir William L. Weipers
Consulting Editor
Richard A. Huebner
Assistant to the Editors
Lawrence S Soffer

Published by
MERCK & CO., INC.
RAHWAY, N.J., U.S.A.
1979

MERCK & CO., INC.
Rahway, New Jersey, U.S.A.

MSD AGVET
Rahway, N.J.

HUBBARD FARMS, INC.
Walpole, N.H.

MERCK SHARP & DOHME RESEARCH LABORATORIES
Rahway, N.J./West Point, Pa.

Research Farms

Springdale, Ark.
Hebron, Md.
Fulton, Mo.
North Branch, N.J.
Armidale, Australia
Hamilton, Australia
Ingleburn, Australia
Campinas, Brazil
Uruguaiana, Brazil
Hertford, England
Mantes-la-Julie, France
Lauterbach, Germany
Kyoto, Japan
Masterton, New Zealand
District of Pretoria, South Africa

Library of Congress Catalog Card Number 61-12679
ISBN Number 911910-52-2
ISSN Number 0076-6542

First Printing—October 1979
Second Printing—April 1980

Printed in the U. S. A.

FOREWORD

The original object set down for The Merck Veterinary Manual in 1955 was in essence a restatement of one first proposed in 1899. In that year, Merck's Manual for the Materia Medica was first published. It was the ancestor of The Merck Manual for physicians, which was later to serve as the model for the present volume. It reminded the reader that "memory is treacherous" and that reminders were necessary to make him "master of the situation and enable him to prescribe exactly what his judgment tells him is needed". Demands upon all members of the health professions are greater today than they were 80 years ago. The veterinarian must have ready to hand an extensive resource of accurate information; thus the obligation of The Merck Veterinary Manual is at once established: To afford a concise but authoritative reference for the veterinarian and his colleagues in the animal sciences.

More than 50 of the discussions in this edition are entirely new and at least 90% of the remainder extensively revised. By stringent editing, the text of the book itself has become only about 10% longer. The emphasis on diagnosis and treatment has been kept intact, but related discussion of altered physiologic states and the procedures that aid in the solving of medical problems has been enlarged where possible.

The development of the text of the 5th edition, as in each of the preceding volumes, is largely the product of an international group of more than 300 authors and reviewers. Their considerable effort lends the Manual the larger part of its quality. Also, in this edition we wish to express our indebtedness to the contributors to The Merck Veterinary Manual by listing them in the pages following. The guidance offered by the Editorial Board in the formative stages of the book must be acknowledged, as it refined the practical character of the text without affecting its scholarly integrity. In this connection, I must say, however inadequately, how grateful I am to our Consulting Editor, Richard Huebner, V.M.D., and manuscript editor, Margaret Nilsson, who made suggestions and contributions far beyond what obligation demanded. In the end, nothing the editors accomplished could have come to fruit but for the unselfish labor and proficiency of Barbara Sloan, Doreen Roth and Gertrude Friese. Their cheerful and skillful dispatch of intimidating workloads continued to surprise me throughout the preparation of the book.

The 5th edition of The Merck Veterinary Manual is divided into nine parts. These are listed in the Table of Contents on p. vii. Within these larger divisions, the many sections are arranged generally by systems; important bodies of discussions not so conveniently grouped are titled by subject, e.g., Infectious Diseases, Toxicology, Nutrition, etc., and so identified by the coded thumb index tabs. Each section is headed by its own table of contents. The red ℞ thumb index tab signals the prescription section. Many of the individual prescriptions are presented in traditional style which retains the advantage of transmitting in the smallest space all the necessary information regarding a given treatment. Such survivals have not interfered with the inclusion of the latest therapy accepted in general use for specific disorders. Whenever possible, generic names are used; when a proprietary name is given, information as to the nature and composition of the product is included. The prescriptions are numbered serially, and arranged into groups having similar pharmacologic activity and clinical indications. Recommendations as to drug usage, either singly or in particular combinations, are those of the various authors. The mention of a specific remedy does not imply editorial endorsement of such preparations over others of similar composition. Moreover, what is an approved treatment in one country may not be in another. The veterinarian should be aware of restrictions and warnings as they apply to his own situation. Careful attention to the manufacturer's instructions on the label will avoid difficulty with the regulations governing use of the product. In most cases, doses are given in metric measures; conversion tables are given in the pages immediately preceding the prescription section.

Completeness of coverage and convenience for the reader were the sole objectives in constructing the Index. The liberal use of cross-references provides several routes of access to important subjects. Care has been taken to assure accuracy of the scientific names and to conform the taxa to latest approved use. In most cases the 8th edition of Bergey's Manual of Determative Bacteriology has been used as the authority for microbial names. In some instances *de novo* nomenclature has been suggested by our authors. All scientific names for plants, fungi, and internal and external parasites have been examined for accuracy and acceptability by scientists in appropriate branches of the ARS-USDA. Organisms likely to be recognized better by older names (or by other names in foreign places) are identified by such names in parentheses, following the newer terms.

A few minutes spent reviewing the Guide for Readers on p. viii will help the reader consult the book to greater advantage.

O.H. Siegmund, Editor
Merck Sharp & Dohme Research Laboratories
Rahway, New Jersey, U.S.A.

CONTENTS

GUIDE FOR READERS

1. The Table of Contents on p. vii shows the title of each section of the Manual, and the corresponding thumb index abbreviation.
2. A list of chapter titles, with subtitles where necessary, is given at the beginning of each section.
3. In most instances, the first statement following a chapter title is a brief definition of the condition to be discussed. In some sections there are no definitions, e.g., Nutrition.
4. Prescriptions are grouped in a separate section (Part VIII) which follows the text of the book. Although grouped by action or indication, they are numbered serially and correspond with the numbers of the ℞ symbols in the text.
5. A number of abbreviations and symbols are used routinely as space savers throughout the text. These are listed on p. xxviii.
6. In the text, the names of proprietary drugs are capitalized; those in the prescription section are shown within quotation marks.
7. Each page heading indicates the last chapter title to be discussed on that page.
8. A large number of tables appear throughout the book, summarizing important data in readily assimilable form. A list of these tables, titled by subject matter, appears on pp. xxx to xxxii.
9. A useful miscellany of information is presented in Part VII, especially arranged for quick reference. This includes Diagnostic Procedures for the Office Laboratory, Routine Immunologic Procedures, and the Ready Reference Guides—Weights, Measures, Equivalents and Conversion Tables—on p. 1521.

CONTRIBUTORS

Melvin K. Abelseth, D.V.M., PH.D., *Director, Laboratories for Veterinary Science, Division of Laboratories and Research, New York State Department of Health, Albany, New York.*

O.R. Adams, D.V.M., M.S., *(Deceased), Professor, Department of Clinical Sciences, College of Veterinary Medicine and Biomedical Sciences, Colorado State University, Fort Collins, Colorado.*

H.E. Adler, D.V.M., PH.D., *Professor, Department of Epidemiology and Preventive Medicine, School of Veterinary Medicine, University of California, Davis, California.*

John E. Alexander, D.V.M., *Chairman, Department of Veterinary Clinical Medicine and Surgery, Washington State University, Pullman, Washington.*

T.J.L. Alexander, B.SC., M.V.SC., PH.D., *Department of Clinical Veterinary Medicine, University of Cambridge, Cambridge, England.*

H.E. Amstutz, B.S., D.V.M., DIPL. A.C.V.I.M., *Professor, Department of Large Animal Clinics, School of Veterinary Medicine, Purdue University, West Lafayette, Indiana.*

David E. Anderson, PH.D., *Professor of Biology, The University of Texas System Cancer Center, M.D. Anderson Hospital and Tumor Institute, Houston, Texas.*

Harry D. Anthony, D.V.M., *Director of Veterinary Diagnostic Laboratory, College of Veterinary Medicine, Kansas State University, Manhattan, Kansas.*

Max J. Appel, D.V.M., PH.D., *James A. Baker Institute for Animal Health, New York State College of Veterinary Medicine, Cornell University, Ithaca, New York.*

R.K. Archer, M.A., PH.D., SC.D., F.R.C.V.S., *Medical Research Council Laboratories, Woodmansterne Road, Carshalton, Surrey, England.*

James Armour, PH.D., *Professor, Faculty of Veterinary Medicine, University of Glasgow, Glasgow, Scotland.*

Arthur L. Aronson, D.V.M., PH.D., *Professor of Pharmacology, Department of Physiology, Biochemistry and Pharmacology, New York State College of Veterinary Medicine, Cornell University, Ithaca, New York.*

J.H. Arundel, M.V.SC., DIP. CHEM., *Reader in Veterinary Parasitology, Veterinary Clinical Centre, University of Melbourne, Werribee, Victoria, Australia.*

R.A. Bankowski, D.V.M., PH.D., *Professor, Veterinary Medicine, School of Veterinary Medicine, University of California, Davis, California.*

Ian K. Barker, D.V.M., PH.D., *Department of Pathology, Ontario Veterinary College, Guelph, Ontario, Canada.*

Richard M. Barlow, D.SC., D.V.M.&S., *Animal Diseases Research Association, Moredun Institute, Edinburgh, Scotland.*
Charles W. Beard, D.V.M., PH.D., *Laboratory Director, Southeast Poultry Research Laboratory, U.S. Department of Agriculture, 934 College Station Road, Athens, Georgia.*
Robert W. Bennett, *One Governor's Lane, Shelburne, Vermont.*
John Bentinck-Smith, D.V.M., *Professor of Clinical Pathology, New York State College of Veterinary Medicine, Cornell University, Ithaca, New York.*
Michael Bernstein, D.V.M., *Director of Clinics, Angell Memorial Animal Hospital, Boston, Masssachusetts.*
Everett D. Besch, D.V.M., *School of Veterinary Medicine, Louisiana State University, Baton Rouge, Louisiana.*
K.J. Betteridge, M.V.SC., PH.D., M.R.C.V.S., *Animal Pathology Division, Health of Animals Branch, Agriculture Canada, Animal Diseases Research Institute, Ottawa, Ontario, Canada.*
J.D. Bezuidenhout, B.V.SC., *Veterinary Research Institute, Onderstepoort, Republic of South Africa.*
Arthur A. Bickford, V.M.D., M.S., PH.D., *Extension Veterinarian, Veterinary Extension, Surge IV Complex, University of California, Davis, California.*
C. Bierschwal, D.V.M., M.S., *Professor and Chief, Theriogenology Section, Department of Veterinary Medicine and Surgery, College of Veterinary Medicine, University of Missouri-Columbia, Columbia, Missouri.*
R.D. Bigalke, B.V.SC., D.V.SC., *Onderstepoort, South Africa.*
Allen G. Binnington, D.V.M., M.SC., *Assistant Professor, Department of Clinical Studies, Ontario Veterinary College, University of Guelph, Guelph, Ontario, Canada.*
Wayne Binns, D.V.M., *Research Veterinarian (Retired), U.S. Department of Agriculture, Agricultural Research Service, Poisonous Plant Research Laboratory, Logan, Utah.*
William D. Black, D.V.M., PH.D., *Associate Professor, Department of Biomedical Sciences, Ontario Veterinary College, Guelph, Ontario, Canada.*
George T. Blackledge, D.V.M., M.S., *Professor of Small Animal Medicine, School of Veterinary Medicine, Tuskegee Institute, Tuskegee, Alabama.*
Joseph T. Blake, B.S., M.S., D.V.M., PH.D., *Professor of Veterinary Science, Utah State University, Logan, Utah.*
Rowan Blogg, B.V.SC., M.S., M.A.C.V.SC., DIPL., A.C.V.O., *Armidale, Victoria, Australia.*
D.C. Blood, M.V.SC., F.A.C.V.SC., *Professor of Veterinary Clinical Sciences, University of Melbourne, Princes Highway, Werribee, Victoria, Australia.*

J.C. Boray, D.V.M., C.V.SC., PH.D., D.V.M., HABIL, F.A.C.V.SC., *Research Director, Biotechnical Products, Ciba-Geigy Australia Limited, Research Centre, Kemps Creek, N.S.W., Australia.*

J. Gregg Boring, D.V.M., M.S., *Associate Professor, Chief, Radiology Section, Veterinary Medical Teaching Hospital, College of Veterinary Medicine, Mississippi State University, Mississippi State, Mississippi.*

William T.K. Bosu, D.V.M., PH.D., *Associate Professor, Section of Theriogenology, Department of Clinical Studies, Ontario Veterinary College, University of Guelph, Guelph, Ontario, Canada.*

Kenneth C. Bovee, D.V.M., M.MED.SC., *Professor of Medicine, School of Veterinary Medicine, University of Pennsylvania, Philadelphia, Pennsylvania.*

A.C. Brandenburg, D.V.M., M.SC., *Department of Clinical Studies, Ontario Veterinary College, Guelph, Ontario, Canada.*

John B. Brooksby, D.SC., PH.D., F.R.C.V.S., *Animal Virus Research Institute, Pirbright, Woking, Surrey, England.*

J.G. Brotherston, F.R.C.V.S., DIP. BACT., *Scientific Adviser, Department of Agriculture and Fisheries for Scotland, Chesser House, Gorgie Road, Edinburgh, Scotland.*

John F. Brown, D.V.M., PH.D., *Director of Scientific Affairs, Evsco/Vineland Pharmaceutical Corp., Vineland, New Jersey.*

John T. Bryans, PH.D., *Professor of Microbiology, Department of Veterinary Science, University of Kentucky, Lexington, Kentucky.*

William B. Buck, D.V.M., M.S., *College of Veterinary Medicine, University of Illinois, Urbana, Illinois.*

M.B. Buddle, B.V.SC., D.SC., F.A.C.V.SC., *Maoribank, Upper Hutt, New Zealand.*

G.L. Bullock, B.S., M.S., PH.D., *Research Bacteriologist, National Fish Health Laboratory, Kearneysville, West Virginia.*

B.R. Burmester, B.S., D.V.M., M.A., PH.D., *Collaborator, Regional Poultry Research Laboratory, Science and Education Administration, U.S. Department of Agriculture, East Lansing, Michigan.*

Mitchell Bush, D.V.M., *Head, Office of Animal Health, National Zoological Park, Smithsonian Institution, Washington, D.C.*

Robert J. Byrne, D.V.M., M.S., *Deputy Director, Extramural Activities Program, National Institute of Allergy and Infectious Diseases, National Institutes of Health, Bethesda, Maryland.*

James R. Campbell, PH.D., B.V.M.S., F.R.C.V.S, *Professor of Surgery, Royal (Dick) School of Veterinary Studies, Summerhall, Edinburgh, Scotland.*

Edward A. Carbrey, V.M.D., M.S., *National Veterinary Services Laboratories, Dayton Road, Ames, Iowa.*

William W. Carlton, D.V.M., PH.D., *Professor, Veterinary Pathology and Toxicology, Department of Veterinary Microbiology, School of Veterinary Medicine, Purdue University, West Lafayette, Indiana.*

Norman F. Cheville, D.V.M., M.S., PH.D., *National Animal Disease Center, Science and Education Administration, U.S. Department of Agriculture, Ames, Iowa.*

Bruce R. Christie, B.V.SC., M.S., PH.D., M.R.C.V.S., *Casa Las Chichiguas, Malibu, California.*

D.C. Church, B.S., M.S., PH.D., *Professor of Nutrition, Department of Animal Science, Oregon State University, Corvallis, Oregon.*

H.L. Chute, D.V.M., M.SC., D.V.SC., *Main Road, Orono, Maine.*

B.L. Clark, B.V.SC., DIP. BACT., *C.S.I.R.O., Division of Animal Health, Parkville, Victoria, Australia.*

E.G.C. Clarke, M.A., PH.D., D.SC., F.R.I.C., *(Deceased) Tilehurst, Reading, England.*

M.J. Clarkson, B.SC., M.V.SC., PH.D., *Professor, University of Liverpool, Department of Veterinary Preventive Medicine, Veterinary Field Station, Leahurst, Chester High Road, Neston, Wirral, England.*

T.R. Cline, PH.D., *Professor, Department of Animal Sciences, Purdue University, West Lafayette, Indiana.*

Gary L. Cockerell, D.V.M., PH.D., *Assistant Professor, Department of Pathology, New York State College of Veterinary Medicine, Cornell University, Ithaca, New York.*

Leroy Coggins, D.V.M., PH.D., *Professor, Department of Pathology, New York State College of Veterinary Medicine, Cornell University, Ithaca, New York.*

Bennett J. Cohen, D.V.M., PH.D., *Professor of Laboratory Animal Medicine, Director, Unit for Laboratory Animal Medicine, University of Michigan, Animal Research Facility, Ann Arbor, Michigan.*

Gabel H. Conner, D.V.M., PH.D., *Professor, University of Idaho, Veterinary Teaching Center, Caldwell, Idaho.*

W.R. Cook, PH.D., F.R.C.V.S., *Professor of Equine Medicine and Surgery, School of Veterinary Medicine, University of Illinois, Urbana, Illinois.*

James E. Corbin, B.S., M.S., PH.D., *Department of Animal Science, University of Illinois, Urbana, Illinois.*

Geoffrey S. Cottew, M.SC., *Principal Research Scientist, C.S.I.R.O., Division of Animal Health, Animal Health Research Laboratory, Parkville, Melbourne, Victoria, Australia.*

G.E. Cottral, D.V.M., M.S., *Research Veterinarian (Retired), Plum Island Animal Disease Center, U.S. Department of Agriculture; Senior Research Fellow, Australian National Animal Health Laboratory, C.S.I.R.O., Melbourne, Australia.*

M.S. Cover, V.M.D., *Director, Veterinary Services and Regulatory Division, Ralston Purina Laboratory, St. Louis, Missouri.*

J.E. Cox, B.SC., B.VET.MED., PH.D., M.R.C.V.S., *University of Liverpool Veterinary Field Station, Leahurst, Neston, Wirral, Merseyside, U.K.*

Robert A. Crandell, B.S., D.V.M., M.P.H., *Director, Laboratories of Veterinary Diagnostic Medicine, College of Veterinary Medicine, University of Illinois, Urbana, Illinois.*

R.A. Curtis, D.V.M., M.SC., *Professor, Department of Clinical Studies, Ontario Veterinary College, University of Guelph, Guelph, Ontario, Canada.*

Caroline M. Czarnecki, D.V.M., PH.D., *Professor, Department of Veterinary Biology, College of Veterinary Medicine, University of Minnesota, St. Paul, Minnesota.*

R.C.W. Daniel, B.V.SC., M.SC., PH.D., *Department of Veterinary Medicine, University of Queensland, St. Lucia, Australia.*

John W. Davis, D.V.M., PH.D., *Professor, Department of Veterinary Science, Virginia Polytechnic Institute and State University, Blacksburg, Virginia.*

Lloyd E. Davis, D.V.M., PH.D., *Professor of Clinical Pharmacology, College of Veterinary Medicine, University of Illinois, Urbana, Illinois.*

Richard B. Davis, D.V.M., M.S., *Professor of Avian Medicine, Poultry Disease Research Center, Athens, Georgia.*

Martin DeForest, D.V.M., *Department of Clinical Studies, University of Guelph, Guelph, Ontario, Canada.*

Dominic L. DeGiusti, PH.D., *Professor and Chairman, Department of Comparative Medicine, Wayne State University, Detroit, Michigan.*

Sherwin S. Desser, B.S., M.SC., PH.D., *Associate Professor, Department of Microbiology and Parasitology, Faculty of Medicine, University of Toronto, Toronto, Ontario, Canada.*

B.L. Deyoe, D.V.M., PH.D., *Research Leader, Brucellosis, National Animal Disease Center, Ames, Iowa.*

David C. Dodd, B.V.SC., M.A. (HON.), *Professor and Head, Department of Veterinary Pathology, College of Veterinary Medicine, Oklahoma State University, Stillwater, Oklahoma.*

W. Jean Dodds, D.V.M., *Research Director, Laboratories for Veterinary Science, Division of Laboratories and Research, New York State Department of Health, Albany, New York.*

Robert E. Dolphin, D.V.M., *Tacoma, Washington.*

C. Dow, B.V.M.S., M.R.C. (PATH), PH.D., *Veterinary Research Laboratory, Stormont, Belfast, Northern Ireland.*

R.S. Downey, D.V.M., M.SC., *Associate Professor, Department of Clinical Studies, Ontario Veterinary College, University of Guelph, Guelph, Ontario, Canada.*

R.O. Drummond, A.B., PH.D., *Director, U.S. Livestock Insects Laboratory, Agricultural Research, Science and Education Administration, U.S. Department of Agriculture, Kerrville, Texas.*

D.L. Dungworth, B.V.SC., PH.D., *Professor and Chairman, Department of Veterinary Pathology, School of Veterinary Medicine, University of California, Davis, California.*

J.R. Egerton, B.V.SC., DIP. BACT., M.A.C.V.SC., *Department of Veterinary Clinical Studies, University of Sydney, Sydney, Australia.*

K.C. Emerson, B.S., M.S., PH.D., *Collaborator, U.S. Department of Agriculture, Research Associate, Department of Entomology, Smithsonian Institution, Washington, D.C.*

Julius Fabricant, V.M.D., PH.D., *Professor of Avian Diseases and Microbiology, Department of Avian and Aquatic Animal Medicine, New York State College of Veterinary Medicine, Cornell University, Ithaca, New York.*

George C. Farnbach, V.M.D., PH.D., *Assistant Professor of Neurology, University of Pennsylvania, School of Veterinary Medicine, Philadelphia, Pennsylvania.*

R. Keith Farrell, D.V.M., *McCoy South, Washington State University, Pullman, Washington.*

W.B. Faull, B.SC., F.R.C.V.S., *Sr. Lecturer, Department of Veterinary Preventive Medicine, University of Liverpool, Leahurst, Neston, Wirral, U.K.*

Ronald Fayer, PH.D., *Animal Parasitology Institute, U.S. Department of Agriculture, Beltsville, Maryland.*

Peter J. Felsburg, V.M.D., PH.D., *School of Veterinary Medicine, University of Pennsylvania, Philadelphia, Pennsylvania.*

A.E. Ferguson, B.S.A., D.V.M., *Professor of Clinical Studies, Department of Clinical Studies, Ontario Veterinary College, University of Guelph, Guelph, Ontario, Canada.*

A.C. Field, M.V.SC., PH.D., *Animal Disease Research Association, Edinburgh, Scotland.*

Neal L. First, PH.D., *Professor, Department of Meat and Animal Science, University of Wisconsin, Madison, Wisconsin.*

E.W. Fisher, B.SC., D.V.M., PH.D., *Professor, University of Glasgow Veterinary Hospital, Bearsden Road, Bearsden, Glasgow, Scotland.*

Paul R. Fitzgerald, B.S., M.S., PH.D., *Professor, Department of Veterinary Pathology and Hygiene, College of Veterinary Medicine, University of Illinois, Urbana, Illinois.*

A.F. Fraser, M.V.SC., F.I. BIOL., *Department of Veterinary Clinical Studies, Western College of Veterinary Medicine, University of Saskatchewan, Saskatoon, Saskatchewan, Canada.*

Reino S. Freeman, B.S., M.A., PH.D., *Professor, Department of Microbiology and Parasitology, University of Toronto, Toronto, Ontario, Canada.*

Wayne M. Frerichs, D.V.M., PH.D., *Livestock Protozoan Diseases Laboratory, Animal Parasitology Institute, Beltsville Agricultural Research Center, U.S. Department of Agriculture, Beltsville, Maryland.*

Fredric L. Frye, D.V.M., M.S., *Clinical Professor of Medicine, School of Veterinary Medicine, University of California, Davis, California.*

Robert D. Furrow, D.V.M., *Beltsville, Maryland.*

Raymond J. Gagné, B.S., M.S., PH.D., *Research Entomologist, Insect Identification and Beneficial Insect Introduction Institute, U.S. Department of Agriculture, c/o U.S. National Museum, Washington, D.C.*

D.B. Galloway, B.V.SC., V.M.D., M.A.C.V.SC., M.V.SC., F.R.V.C.S., *University of Melbourne, Department of Veterinary Clinical Sciences, Princes Highway, Werribee, Victoria, Australia.*

Joseph H. Gans, V.M.D., PH.D., *Professor of Pharmacology, University of Vermont College of Medicine, Burlington, Vermont.*

Harold E. Garner, D.V.M., PH.D., *Professor, Department of Veterinary Medicine and Surgery, College of Veterinary Medicine, University of Missouri, Columbia, Missouri.*

Clive C. Gay, D.V.M., M.V.SC., M.A.C.V.SC., *Senior Lecturer, Department of Veterinary Clinical Studies, University of Melbourne, Werribee, Victoria, Australia.*

H. Gerber, DR. MED. VET., *Professor, Klinik für Nutztiere und Pferde, Universität Bern, Bern, Switzerland.*

Stanley Gershoff, B.A., M.SC., PH.D., *Director, Tufts University Nutrition Institute, Medford, Massachusetts.*

B.S. Gill, B.V.SC., M.V.SC., PH.D., F.N.A.SC., *Dean, College of Veterinary Science, Punjab Agricultural University, Ludhiana, India.*

Jerry R. Gillespie, B.S., D.V.M., PH.D., *Professor of Physiology, Department of Physiological Sciences, School of Veterinary Medicine, University of California, Davis, California.*

J.S. Gilmour, B.V.M.&S., F.R.C.V.S., *Animal Diseases Research Association, Moredun Institute, Edinburgh, Scotland.*

N.J.L. Gilmour, PH.D., B.V.M.S., M.R.C.V.S., *Animal Diseases Research Association, Moredun Institute, Edinburgh, Scotland.*

Daniel A. Gingerich, D.V.M., M.S., *Senior Research Clinician, Pitman-Moore, Inc., Washington Crossing, New Jersey.*

John R. Gorham, B.S., D.V.M., PH.D., *Research Leader, Science and Education Administration, U.S. Department of Agriculture, Washington State University, Pullman, Washington.*

I.M. Gourley, D.V.M., PH.D., *Professor of Veterinary Surgery, School of Veterinary Medicine, University of California, Davis, California.*

O.H. Graham, B.S., M.S., PH.D., *Research Entomologist, U.S. Livestock Insects Laboratory, Agricultural Research, Science and Education Administration, U.S. Department of Agriculture, Kerrville, Texas.*

Andrew S. Greig, D.V.M., PH.D., *Canada Department of Agriculture, Animal Diseases Research Institute, Ottawa, Ontario, Canada.*

W.B. Gross, D.V.M., PH.D., *Professor of Poultry Pathology, Department of Veterinary Science, Virginia Polytechnic Institute, Blacksburg, Virginia.*

Donald P. Gustafson, D.V.M., PH.D., *Professor of Virology, School of Veterinary Medicine, Purdue University, West Lafayette, Indiana.*

Robert E. Habel, D.V.M., M.SC., M.V.D., *Professor Emeritus, Department of Anatomy, College of Veterinary Medicine, Cornell University, Ithaca, New York.*

E.O. Haelterman, D.V.M., M.S., PH.D., *Professor of Microbiology, School of Veterinary Medicine, Purdue University, West Lafayette, Indiana.*

C.F. Hall, D.V.M., M.S., *Professor and Head, Department of Veterinary Microbiology and Parasitology, College of Veterinary Medicine, Texas A&M University, College Station, Texas.*

Richard F. Hall, D.V.M., *Extension Veterinarian and Research Professor, Veterinary Research Laboratory, Caldwell, Idaho.*

W.T.K. Hall, B.V.SC., M.A.C.V.SC., *Director of Pathology, Animal Research Institute, Yeerongpilly, Australia.*

Farouk Hamdy, D.V.M., PH.D., *Plum Island Animal Disease Center, U.S. Department of Agriculture, Greenport, New York.*

Lyle E. Hanson, D.V.M., PH.D., *Professor and Head of Department of Veterinary Pathology and Hygiene, College of Veterinary Medicine, University of Illinois, Urbana, Illinois.*

Robert P. Hanson, B.A., M.S., PH.D., *Professor, Department of Veterinary Science, University of Wisconsin, Madison, Wisconsin.*

James W. Hardin, PH.D., *Professor of Botany, Department of Botany, North Carolina State University, Raleigh, North Carolina.*

A.E. Harrop, M.R.C.V.S., *Senior Lecturer, Department of Animal Husbandry, Royal Veterinary College, (University of London), Boltons Park, Potters Bar, Hertfordshire, England.*

W.J. Hartley, M.V.SC., M.R.C.PATH., F.R.C.V.S., M.A.C.V.SC., *Reader, Department of Veterinary Clinical Studies, Sydney University, Camden, N.S.W., Australia.*

W.W. Hawkins, Jr., D.V.M., *Dillon, Montana.*

Don H. Helfer, D.V.M., M.S., *School of Veterinary Medicine, Oregon State University, Corvallis, Oregon.*

Wilson Henderson, D.V.M., *Vancouver, B.C., Canada.*

Mary A. Herron, D.V.M., PH.D., *Associate Professor, Biomedical Learning Resources Center, College of Veterinary Medicine, Texas A&M University, College Station, Texas.*

Charles P. Hibler, B.S., M.S., PH.D., *Professor, Department of Pathology, College of Veterinary Medicine and Biomedical Science, Colorado State University, Fort Collins, Colorado.*

F.W.G. Hill, PH.D., B.VET.MED., M.R.C.V.S., M.A.C.V.SC., *99 Station Parade, Harrogate, N. Yorkshire, England.*

B.F. Hoerlein, D.V.M., PH.D., *Professor and Head, Department of Small Animal Surgery and Medicine, School of Veterinary Medicine, Auburn University, Auburn, Alabama.*

Peter H. Holmes, B.V.M.S., PH.D., *University of Glasgow Veterinary School, Glasgow, Scotland.*

Cluff E. Hopla, B.S., M.S., PH.D., *Professor of Zoology/George Lynn Cross Research, University of Oklahoma, Department of Zoology, Norman, Oklahoma.*

F.D. Horney, D.V.M., *Professor, Department of Clinical Studies, University of Guelph, Guelph, Ontario, Canada.*

Aaron Horowitz, D.V.M., PH.D., J.D., *Dayton Veterinary Clinic, Dayton, Washington.*

James A. House, M.S., D.V.M., PH.D., *Veterinary Medical Officer, Plum Island Animal Disease Center, Greenport, New York.*

William T. Hubbert, B.S., D.V.M., M.P.H., PH.D., *Professor and Head, Department of Epidemiology and Community Health, School of Veterinary Medicine, Louisiana State University, Baton Rouge, Louisiana.*

J.M. Humburg, D.V.M., M.S., *Large Animal Clinic, School of Veterinary Medicine, Auburn University, Auburn, Alabama.*

Charles E. Hunt, D.V.M., PH.D., *Professor of Comparative Medicine and Nutrition Sciences, Department of Comparative Medicine, University of Alabama in Birmingham, University Station, Birmingham, Alabama.*

A.R. Hunter, B.V.M.S., DIP. A.H., *Senior Research Officer, Ministry of Agriculture, Food and Fisheries, Veterinary Laboratory, Eskgrove, Lasswade, Scotland.*

David L. Huxsoll, B.S., D.V.M., PH.D., *Commander, United States Army Medical Research Unit, Institute for Medical Research, Jalan Pahang, Kuala Lumpur, Malaysia.*

N.St.G. Hyslop, M.V.SC., D.T.V.M., F.R.C.V.S., *Head of Immunology, Animal Pathology Division, Health of Animals Branch, Agriculture Canada, Ottawa, Ontario, Canada.*

Oliphant F. Jackson, PH.D., M.R.C.V.S., *Royal Free Hospital, Pond Street, Hampstead, London, England.*

Lynn F. James, PH.D., *Poisonous Plant Research Laboratory, Agricultural Research, Science and Education Administration, U.S. Department of Agriculture, Logan, Utah.*

Oswald Jarrett, PH.D., B.V.M.S., *University of Glasgow, Veterinary School, Bearsden, Glasgow, Scotland.*

Alex Johnston, B.S.A., M.S., *Canada Department of Agriculture, Plant Service Section, Lethbridge, Alberta, Canada.*

Dudley E. Johnston, B.V.SC., M.V.SC., A.M., *Professor of Surgery, School of Veterinary Medicine, University of Pennsylvania, Philadelphia, Pennsylvania.*

I.B. Johnstone, D.V.M., M.SC., PH.D., *Assistant Professor, Department of Biomedical Sciences, Ontario Veterinary College, University of Guelph, Guelph, Ontario, Canada.*

Donald E. Kahn, D.V.M., PH.D., *Head, Virological Research, Biological Research Division, Pitman-Moore Inc., Washington Crossing, New Jersey.*

Lars H. Karstad, D.V.M., M.S., PH.D., *Wildlife Disease Section, Veterinary Research Laboratories, Kabete, Kenya.*

T.S. Kellerman, B.V.SC., *Toxicology Section, Onderstepoort Veterinary Research Institute, P.O. Onderstepoort, South Africa.*

John W. Kendrick, D.V.M., PH.D., *Professor, Department of Reproduction, School of Veterinary Medicine, University of California, Davis, California.*

Sam G. Kenzy, B.S., D.V.M., M.S., PH.D., *Professor Emeritus, Department of Veterinary Microbiology and Pathology, Washington State University, Pullman, Washington.*

Conrad J. Kercher, M.S., PH.D., *Professor of Animal Nutrition, Division of Animal Science, University of Wyoming, Laramie, Wyoming.*

Pattye A. Kessler, *Research Entomologist, Insect Identification and Beneficial Insect Introduction Institute, U.S. Department of Agriculture, Beltsville, Maryland.*

R. Kilgour, M.A., D. PHIL., *Ruakura Animal Research Station, Hamilton, New Zealand.*

Loren D. Kinter, D.V.M., M.S., *Professor of Veterinary Pathology, Veterinary Diagnostic Laboratory, University of Missouri, Columbia, Missouri.*

Hyram Kitchen, B.S., D.V.M., PH.D., *Department of Environmental Practice, College of Veterinary Medicine, University of Tennessee, Knoxville, Tennessee.*

Fred W. Knapp, B.S., M.S., PH.D., *Professor of Entomology, Department of Entomology, University of Kentucky, Lexington, Kentucky.*

S.E. Knapp, B.S., M.S., PH.D., *Dean of Undergraduate Studies, Oregon State University, Corvallis, Oregon.*

Lloyd Knutson, B.S., M.S., PH.D., *Insect Identification and Beneficial Insect Introduction Institute, U.S. Department of Agriculture, Beltsville, Maryland.*

E.M. Kohler, D.V.M., M.S., PH.D., *Professor and Chairman, Department of Veterinary Science, Ohio Agricultural Research and Development Center, Wooster, Ohio.*

L.D. Konyha, D.V.M., M.S., *Chief Staff Veterinarian, Animal and Plant Health Inspection Service, Veterinary Services, U.S. Department of Agriculture, Hyattsville, Maryland.*

Harold J. Kurtz, B.S., M.S., D.V.M., PH.D., *Professor of Pathology, Department of Veterinary Pathology, College of Veterinary Medicine, University of Minnesota, St. Paul, Minnesota.*

K.L. Kuttler, D.V.M., PH.D., *Associate Director, Institute of Tropical Veterinary Medicine, College of Veterinary Medicine, Texas A&M University, College Station, Texas.*

J.P. Lautenslager, D.V.M., M.SC., PH.D., *Veterinary Parasitologist, Veterinary Services Branch, Ontario Ministry of Agriculture and Food, Guelph, Ontario, Canada.*

Louis Leibovitz, B.S., V.M.D., *Professor, New York State College of Veterinary Medicine, Cornell University, Ithaca, New York.*

Jack C. Leighty, D.V.M., *Columbia, Maryland.*

H.W. Leipold, D.V.M., M.S., PH.D., *Professor, College of Veterinary Medicine, Kansas State University, Manhattan, Kansas.*

William L. Leoschke, B.A., M.S., PH.D., *Professor of Chemistry, Valparaiso University, Valparaiso, Indiana.*

A.W.D. Lepper, PH.D., B. VET. MED., *C.S.I.R.O. Animal Health Research Laboratory, Division of Animal Health, Parkville, Victoria, Australia.*

Norman D. Levine, B.S., PH.D., *Professor, College of Veterinary Medicine, University of Illinois, Urbana, Illinois.*

George E. Lewis, Jr., D.V.M., PH.D., *Veterinary Microbiologist, United States Army Medical Research Institute of Infectious Diseases, Fort Detrick, Frederick, Maryland.*

J. Ralph Lichtenfels, M.S., PH.D., *Agricultural Research, Northeastern Region, Science and Education Administration, U.S. Department of Agriculture, Beltsville, Maryland.*

William D. Lindquist, M.S., SC.D., *Professor of Veterinary Parasitology, College of Veterinary Medicine, Kansas State University, Manhattan, Kansas.*

R. P. Link, D.V.M., M.S., PH.D., *Urbana, Illinois.*

Robert M. Liptrap, D.V.M., M.V.SC., PH.D., *Professor of Biomedical Sciences, Ontario Veterinary College, University of Guelph, Guelph, Ontario, Canada.*

P.B. Little, D.V.M., M.S., PH.D., *Professor, Department of Pathology, University of Guelph, Guelph, Ontario, Canada.*

John E. Lloyd, B.S., PH.D., *Entomology Section, University of Wyoming, Laramie, Wyoming.*

L.C. Lloyd, B.V.SC., PH.D., M.A.C.V.SC., *C.S.I.R.O. Animal Health Research Laboratory, Parkville, Victoria, Australia.*

Franklin M. Loew, D.V.M., PH.D., *Chief, Laboratory Animal Medicine, Johns Hopkins University School of Medicine, Baltimore, Maryland.*

George J. Losos, D.V.M., M.V.SC., PH.D., *Veterinary Research Organization, Kikuyu, Kenya.*

Donald G. Low, D.V.M., PH.D., *School of Veterinary Medicine, University of California, Davis, Davis, California.*

Albert J. Luedke, B.S., D.V.M., M.S., *Arthropod-borne Animal Diseases Research Laboratory, Denver, Colorado.*

R.L. Lundvall, D.V.M., M.S., *Professor, Veterinary Clinical Sciences, Iowa State University, Ames, Iowa.*

Gordon K. Macleod, B.S.A., M.S., PH.D., *Professor, Department of Animal & Poultry Science, University of Guelph, Guelph, Ontario, Canada.*

Keith T. Maddy, D.V.M., M.P.H., *Staff Toxicologist, California Department of Food and Agriculture, Sacramento, California.*

Gary L. Mallo, D.V.M., M.S., *St. Charles Veterinary Clinic, St. Charles, Illinois.*

Charles E. Martin, D.V.M., M.S., *Department of Veterinary Medicine and Surgery, College of Veterinary Medicine, University of Missouri, Columbia, Missouri.*

Charles L. Martin, D.V.M., M.S., *Professor, Department of Small Animal Medicine, College of Veterinary Medicine, University of Georgia, Athens, Georgia.*

W.B. Martin, PH.D., M.R.C.V.S., D.V.S.M., *Director, Animal Diseases Research Association, Moredun Institute, Edinburgh, Scotland.*

Marcus M. Mason, D.V.M., *Shrewsbury, Massachusetts.*

T.A. Mason, B.V.SC., M.V.SC., M.R.C.V.S., M.A.C.V.SC., *Department of Veterinary Clinical Sciences, University of Melbourne, Princes Highway, Werribee, Victoria, Australia.*

Fred D. Maurer, B.S., D.V.M., PH.D., *Emeritus Director, Institute of Tropical Veterinary Medicine, Bryan, Texas.*

John McCaig, B.A., VET. M.B., M.R.C.V.S., *Paddock Wood, Kent, England.*

M.G. McCartney, B.S.A., M.S., PH.D., *Head, Department of Poultry Science, Chairman Poultry Division, University of Georgia, Athens, Georgia.*

G.L. McClymont, B.V.SC., PH.D., *Professor, University of New England, Armidale, N.S.W., Australia.*

Leslie E. McDonald, D.V.M., PH.D., *Professor, Physiology and Pharmacology, College of Veterinary Medicine, University of Georgia, Athens, Georgia.*

Donal B. McKeown, D.V.M., *Associate Professor, Department of Clinical Studies, Ontario Veterinary College, University of Guelph, Guelph, Ontario, Canada.*

D.G. McKercher, D.V.M., PH.D., M.A., *Professor of Virology, School of Veterinary Medicine, University of California, Davis, California.*

William Medway, B.S., D.V.M., PH.D., HON. M.A., *Department of Clinical Studies, School of Veterinary Medicine, University of Pennsylvania, Philadelphia, Pennsylvania.*

William P. Meleney, D.V.M., *Research Leader, Scabies and Mange Mite Research Unit, U.S. Livestock Insects Laboratory, Agricultural Research, Science and Education Administration, U.S. Department of Agriculture, Kerrville, Texas.*

Fred P. Meyer, B.A., M.S., PH.D., *Director, National Fishery Research Laboratory, U.S. Fish and Wildlife Service, LaCross, Wisconsin.*

William H. Miller, V.M.D., *School of Veterinary Medicine, University of Pennsylvania, Philadelphia, Pennsylvania.*

Frank J. Milne, D.V.M., DR. MED. VET., *Professor, Department of Clinical Studies, Ontario Veterinary College, University of Guelph, Guelph, Ontario, Canada.*

Peter H. Mortimer, B.V.SC., M.R.C.V.S., M.A., M.A.C.V.SC., *Ministry of Agriculture & Fisheries, Ruakura Agricultural Research Centre, Hamilton, New Zealand.*

Jacob E. Mosier, D.V.M., M.S., *Professor of Veterinary Medicine, Veterinary Medical Center, Kansas State University, Manhattan, Kansas.*

C.F.W. Muesebeck, B.S., *Honorary Research Associate, Department of Entomology, Smithsonian Institution, Washington, D.C.*

Paul A. Mullen, PH.D., B.SC., M.R.C.V.S., *The Union International Co., Ltd., Dewhurst House, London, England.*

M.D. Murray, B.SC., (VET. SC.), F.R.C.V.S., *McMaster Laboratory, C.S.I.R.O., Glebe, N.S.W., Australia.*

P.A. Neal, B.SC., B.V.SC., *University of Liverpool, Leahurst, Neston, Wirral, England.*

Frederick W. Oehme, B.S., D.V.M., M.S., DR. MED. VET., PH.D., *Professor of Toxicology, Medicine, and Physiology, Comparative Toxicology Laboratory, Kansas State University, Manhattan, Kansas.*

J.E. Oldfield, B.S., M.S., PH.D., *Head, Department of Animal Science, Oregon State University, Corvallis, Oregon.*

Duane E. Olsen, D.V.M., *Western Washington Research & Extension Center, Puyallup, Washington.*

Carl Olson, D.V.M., M.S., PH.D., *Professor, Veterinary Sciences, College of Agricultural and Life Sciences, University of Wisconsin, Madison, Wisconsin.*

Norman O. Olson, D.V.M., *Professor of Avian Pathology, West Virginia University, Division of Animal & Veterinary Sciences, Morgantown, West Virginia.*

B.I. Osburn, B.S., D.V.M., PH.D., *Professor, Department of Pathology, School of Veterinary Medicine, University of California, Davis, California.*

Edgar A. Ott, PH.D., *Associate Professor Animal Nutrition, Animal Science Department, University of Florida, Gainesville, Florida.*

Richard L. Ott, B.S., D.V.M., *Professor, Department of Veterinary Clinical Medicine and Surgery, College of Veterinary Medicine, Washington State University, Pullman, Washington.*

Gilbert F. Otto, SC. D., *Adjunct Professor of Zoology, University of Maryland, College Park, Maryland.*

Leslie A. Page, PH.D., *U.S. Department of Agriculture, Science and Education Administration, Agricultural Research, North Central Region, National Animal Disease Center, Ames, Iowa.*

N.C. Palmer, D.V.M., PH.D., *Veterinary Pathologist, Ontario Ministry of Agriculture and Food, Box 3612, Guelph, Ontario, Canada.*

Roger J. Panciera, D.V.M., M.S., PH.D., *College of Veterinary Medicine, Oklahoma State University, Stillwater, Oklahoma.*

W.M. Parker, D.V.M., DIP. MED., *Assistant Professor, Department of Clinical Studies, Ontario Veterinary College, Guelph, Ontario, Canada.*

R.R. Pascoe, M.V.SC., F.R.C.V.S., F.A.C.V.SC., *Oakey Veterinary Hospital, Oakey, Queensland, Australia.*

I.H. Pattison, F.R.C.V.S., *Newbury, Berkshire, England.*

Malcolm C. Peckham, D.V.M., *Professor of Avian Diseases, New York State College of Veterinary Medicine, Ithaca, New York.*

Niels C. Pedersen, D.V.M., PH.D., *Associate Professor, Department of Medicine, School of Veterinary Medicine, University of California, Davis, California.*

Paul W. Pennock, B.S., D.V.M., M.S., *Professor, Department of Clinical Studies, Ontario Veterinary College, Guelph, Ontario, Canada.*

R.H.C. Penny, D.V.SC., PH.D., F.R.C.V.S., M.A.C.V.SC., *Professor of Clinical Veterinary Medicine, Royal Veterinary College, Hawkshead House, Hawkshead Lane, North Mymms, Nr. Hatfield, Hertfordshire, England.*

T.W. Perry, B.ED., B.S., M.S., PH.D., *Professor of Animal Nutrition, Purdue University, Lilly Hall, West Lafayette, Indiana.*

John W. Pharr, D.V.M., M.S., DIPL. A.C.V.R., *Department of Clinical Studies, Western College of Veterinary Medicine, University of Saskatchewan, Saskatoon, Saskatchewan, Canada.*

B.W. Pickett, B.S., M.S., PH.D., *Director, Animal Reproduction Laboratory, Colorado State University, Fort Collins, Colorado.*

Allan C. Pier, D.V.M., PH.D., *Chief, Bacteriological and Mycological Research Laboratory, National Animal Disease Center, Agricultural Research, Science and Education Administration, U.S. Department of Agriculture, Ames, Iowa.*

Hugh M. Pirie, B.V.M.S., PH.D., M.R.C.PATH., *Reader Veterinary Pathology, Department of Veterinary Pathology, University of Glasgow Veterinary School, Bearsden Road, Glasgow, Scotland.*

John M. Preston, B.V.M.S., PH.D., M.R.C.V.S., *Merck Sharp & Dohme, Hoddesdon, England.*

O.M. Radostits, D.V.M., M.SC., *Professor of Veterinary Medicine, Department of Veterinary Clinical Studies, Western College of Veterinary Medicine, University of Saskatchewan, Saskatoon, Saskatchewan, Canada.*

B.A. Rasmusen, D.V.M., PH.D., *Professor of Animal Genetics, Department of Animal Science, University of Illinois, Urbana, Illinois.*

J.H. Reed, D.V.M., PH.D., *Diplomate ACVIM, Professor, Department of Clinical Studies, Ontario Veterinary College, University of Guelph, Guelph, Ontario, Canada.*

W. Malcolm Reid, B.S., M.S., PH.D., HON. D.SC., *Parasitologist, Department of Poultry Science, University of Georgia, Athens, Georgia.*

Keith R. Rhoades, D.V.M., PH.D., *Veterinary Medical Officer, National Animal Disease Center, U.S. Department of Agriculture, P.O. Box 70, Ames, Iowa.*

Craig Riddell, D.V.M., PH.D., *Department of Veterinary Pathology, Western College of Veterinary Medicine, University of Saskatchewan, Saskatoon, Saskatchewan, Canada.*

R.F. Riek, M.SC., D.V.SC., F.A.C.V.SC., *Professor, Dean, Faculty of Veterinary Science, Massey University, Palmerston North, New Zealand.*

Daniel H. Ringler, D.V.M., *Associate Professor, Laboratory Animal Medicine, University of Michigan, Ann Arbor, Michigan.*

David S. Roberts, D.V.SC., PH.D., *Head of Wellcome Vaccines Division, Burroughs Wellcome Company, Denver, Colorado.*

Ronald J. Roberts, PH.D., M.R.C.V.S., M.R.C.PATH., F.R.S.E., *Director, Unit of Aquatic Pathobiology, University of Stirling, Scotland.*

Stephen, J. Roberts, D.V.M., M.S., *Professor Emeritus, Woodstock, Vermont.*

T.J. Robinson, M.SC. (AGRIC.) PH.D., SC.D., *Department of Animal Husbandry, University of Sydney, Sydney, N.S.W., Australia.*

Peter D. Rossdale, M.A., F.R.C.V.S., *Beaufort Cottage Stables, High Street, Newmarket, Suffolk, England.*

Harry C. Rowsell, D.V.M., D.V.P.H., PH.D., *Professor, Department of Pathology, School of Medicine, University of Ottawa, Ottawa, Ontario, Canada.*

Michael D. Ruff, B.S., M.S., PH.D., *Beltsville Agricultural Research Center, Science and Education Administration, U.S. Department of Agriculture, Beltsville, Maryland.*

Dorsey A. Sanders, Sr., D.V.M., *Professor Emeritus, College of Veterinary Medicine, University of Florida, Gainesville, Florida.*

Vance L. Sanger, A.B., D.V.M., M.SC., *Department of Pathology, Michigan State University, East Lansing, Michigan.*

Christian H. Schettler, DR. MED. VET. HABIL., *Hagelshoek, Gildehaus, Germany.*

H.B. Schiefer, D.V.M., PH.D., *Professor of Veterinary Pathology, Western College of Veterinary Medicine, University of Saskatchewan, Saskatoon, Saskatchewan, Canada.*

Paul R. Schnurrenberger, D.V.M., M.P.H., *Professor of Public Health, Department of Microbiology, School of Veterinary Medicine, Auburn University, Auburn, Alabama.*

Kevin T. Schulz, D.V.M., *School of Veterinary Medicine, University of Pennsylvania, Philadelphia, Pennsylvania.*

Robert M. Schwartzman, V.M.D., M.P.H., PH.D., *Professor of Dermatology and Clinical Immunology, School of Veterinary Medicine, University of Pennsylvania, Philadelphia, Pennsylvania.*

Gordon R. Scott, B.SC., M.S., PH.D., *Centre for Tropical Veterinary Medicine, University of Edinburgh, Roslin, Midlothian, Scotland.*

M.L. Scott, PH.D., *Professor, Chairman, Department of Poultry Science, New York State College of Agriculture, Cornell University, Ithaca, New York.*

Patricia Pearl Scott, M.B.E., PH.D., F.I. BIOL., *Professor, Academic Department of Physiology, Royal Free Hospital School of Medicine, University of London, Pond Street, London, England.*

Ian E. Selman, B.V.M.S., PH.D., M.R.C.V.S., *Department of Veterinary Medicine, University of Glasgow Veterinary School, Bearsden Road, Bearsden, Glasgow, Scotland.*

Ben E. Sheffy, B.S., M.S., PH.D., *Caspary Professor of Nutrition, James A. Baker Institute for Animal Health, Cornell University, Ithaca, New York.*

Damon C. Shelton, PH.D., *Director, Laboratory Animal and Special Chows Research Department, Ralston Purina Company, St. Louis, Missouri.*

Bud Siemering, D.V.M., *Resident in Surgery, School of Veterinary Medicine, University of Pennsylvania, Philadelphia, Pennsylvania.*

Donald G. Simmons, D.V.M., PH.D., *Department of Veterinary Science, North Carolina State University, Raleigh, North Carolina.*

William L. Sippel, B.S., V.M.D., M.S., PH.D., *Texas Veterinary Medical Diagnostic Laboratory, College Station, Texas.*

S.J. Slinger, B.S.A., M.S.A., PH.D., *Professor of Nutrition, Department of Nutrition, University of Guelph, Guelph, Ontario, Canada.*

V. Sloss, DR. VET. MED., *University of Melbourne, Department of Veterinary Clinical Sciences, Princes Highway, Werribee, Victoria, Australia.*

Harry E. Smalley, D.V.M., *College Station, Texas.*

Robert L. Smiley, B.S., M.S., *Research Entomologist, Insect Identification and Beneficial Insect Introduction Institute, U.S. Department of Agriculture, Beltsville, Maryland.*

D.L.T. Smith, D.V.M., PH.D., *Professor of Pathology, Western College of Veterinary Medicine, University of Saskatchewan, Saskatoon, Saskatchewan, Canada.*

John M.B. Smith, PH.D., *University of Otago Medical School, Dunedin, New Zealand.*

Laura L. Smith, D.V.M., M.SC., *Assistant Professor, Ontario Veterinary College, University of Guelph, Guelph, Ontario, Canada.*

Sedgwick E. Smith, B.S., PH.D., *Professor Emeritus, Department of Animal Science, Morrison Hall, Cornell University, Ithaca, New York.*

S.F. Snieszko, PH.D., *National Fisheries Center, Leetown, Kearneysville, West Virginia.*

D.R. Snodgrass, B.V.M.&S., *Animal Diseases Research Association, Moredun Institute, Gilmerton Road, Edinburgh, Scotland.*

G.H. Snoeyenbos, D.V.M., *Professor of Veterinary Science, University of Massachusetts, Amherst, Massachusetts.*

W.A. Snowdon, B.V.SC., M.A.C.V.SC., *C.S.I.R.O., Division of Animal Health, Australian National Animal Health Laboratory, Melbourne, Victoria, Australia.*

W.H. Southcott, D.V.SC., *C.S.I.R.O., Division of Animal Health, Pastoral Research Laboratory, Armidale, N.S.W., Australia.*

Victor C. Speirs, M.V.SC., DR. MED. VET., M.A.C.V.SC., *University of Melbourne Veterinary Clinical Centre, Werribee, Victoria, Australia.*

W.T. Springer, D.V.M., PH.D., *Department of Veterinary Science, Louisiana State University, Baton Rouge, Louisiana.*

O.H.V. Stalheim, D.V.M., M.A., PH.D., *Veterinary Medical Officer, National Animal Disease Center, Agricultural Research Service, U.S. Department of Agriculture, Ames, Iowa.*

R.G. Stevenson, D.V.M., PH.D., D.V.S.M., *Director, Atlantic Area Laboratory, Agriculture Canada, Sackville, N.B., Canada.*

Robert Millard Stone, D.V.M., *Detroit, Michigan.*

J. Storz, D.V.M., PH.D., *Professor, Department of Microbiology, College of Veterinary Medicine and Biomedical Sciences, Colorado State University, Fort Collins, Colorado.*

Virginia P. Studdert, D.V.M., *Senior Lecturer in Veterinary Medicine, School of Veterinary Science, University of Melbourne, Werribee, Victoria, Australia.*

John D. Summers, B.S.A., M.S.A., PH.D., *Poultry Nutritionist, Department of Animal & Poultry Science, University of Guelph, Guelph, Ontario, Canada.*

William P. Switzer, D.V.M., M.S., PH.D., *Associate Dean for Research, College of Veterinary Medicine, Iowa State University, Ames, Iowa.*

D.J. Taylor, M.A., VET.M.B., PH.D., *Department of Veterinary Pathology, Glasgow Veterinary School, Glasgow, U.K.*

Bernard F. Trum, A.B., D.V.M., *Vice-President, Pathobiology, Inc., Marlborough, Massachusetts.*

R.B. Truscott, D.V.M., PH.D., *Research Scientist, Atlantic Area Laboratory, Animal Pathology Division, Health of Animals Branch, Canada Department of Agriculture, Sackville, N.B. Canada.*

James O. Tucker, B.S., M.S., D.V.M., *University Station, Laramie, Wyoming.*

David C. Tudor, B.S., V.M.D., *Cranbury, New Jersey. (Rutgers University–Retired).*

R.D. Turk, D.V.M., *Bryan, Texas.*

Donald W. Twohy, SC.D., *Associate Professor, Department of Microbiology and Public Health, Michigan State University, East Lansing, Michigan.*

Robert H. Udall, A.B., D.V.M., PH.D., *Department of Pathology, College of Veterinary Medicine and Biomedical Sciences, Colorado State University, Fort Collins, Colorado.*

Duane E. Ullrey, PH.D., *Professor of Comparative Nutrition, Department of Animal Husbandry, Michigan State University, East Lansing, Michigan.*

Norman R. Underdahl, B.A., M.S., *Professor of Veterinary Science, Department of Veterinary Science, University of Nebraska, Lincoln, Nebraska.*

V.E.O. Valli, D.V.M., M.SC., PH.D., *Professor of Pathology, Department of Pathology, Ontario Veterinary College, Guelph, Ontario, Canada.*

Louis van der Heide, D.V.M., PH.D., *Department of Pathobiology, University of Connecticut, Storrs, Connecticut.*

A.A. van Dreumel, D.V.M., M.SC., *Scientific Co-ordinator, Ontario Ministry of Agriculture & Food, Veterinary Services Laboratory, Guelph, Ontario, Canada.*

William C. Wagner, D.V.M., PH.D., *Professor and Head, Department of Veterinary Biosciences, College of Veterinary Medicine, University of Illinois, Urbana, Illinois.*

R.A. Ward, B.S., M.S., PH.D., *Research Associate, Department of Entomology, Smithsonian Institution, Washington, D.C.*

Richard G. Warner, PH.D., *Professor of Animal Nutrition, Department of Animal Science, Cornell University, Ithaca, New York.*

W.M. Wass, B.S., D.V.M., PH.D., *Professor and Head, Department of Veterinary Clinical Sciences, Iowa State University, Ames, Iowa.*

R.H. Wasserman, PH.D., *Department of Physical Biology/Section of Physiology, New York State College of Veterinary Medicine, Cornell University, Ithaca, New York.*

Steven H. Weisbroth, B.S., M.S., D.V.M., DIPL. A.C.L.A.M., *President, AnMed Laboratories, Inc., New Hyde Park, New York.*

K.E. Weiss, B.V.SC., *P.O. Onderstepoort, South Africa.*

Eric Wells, PH.D., D.T.V.M., *FAO Consultant, Edinburgh, Scotland.*

J.D. Wheat, D.V.M., *Professor of Veterinary Surgery, School of Veterinary Medicine, University of California, Davis, California.*

Charles K. Whitehair, D.V.M., M.S., PH.D., *Professor (Nutrition Pathology), Department of Pathology, Michigan State University, East Lansing, Michigan.*

Stephen R. Wightman, D.V.M., M.S., *Toxicology Division, Eli Lilly & Company, Greenfield, Indiana.*

Graham E. Wilcox, B.V.SC., PH.D., A.C.V.M., *School of Veterinary Studies, Murdoch University, Western Australia.*

J.K.H. Wilde, B.SC., M.SC., PH.D., A.R.C.S., *Bramleys, Barton St. David, Somerton, Somerset, England.*

J.S. Wilkinson, PH.D., B.SC., M.R.C.V.S., *Department of Veterinary Paraclinical Science, University of Melbourne, Werribee, Victoria, Australia.*

M.R. Wilson, B.V.SC., PH.D., *Professor, Clinical Research Building, Ontario Veterinary College, University of Guelph, Guelph, Ontario, Canada.*

Roland W. Winterfield, D.V.M., *Professor of Avian Diseases, School of Veterinary Medicine, Purdue University, West Lafayette, Indiana.*

Willis W. Wirth, B.S., M.S., PH.D., *Research Entomologist, Insect Identification and Beneficial Insect Introduction Institute, U.S. Department of Agriculture, c/o U.S. National Museum, Washington, D.C.*

G.A. Wobeser, B.S.A., M.SC., D.V.M., PH.D., *Professor, Department of Veterinary Pathology, Western College of Veterinary Pathology, University of Saskatchewan, Saskatoon, Saskatchewan, Canada.*

Kenneth E. Wolf, B.S., M.S., PH.D., *National Fish Health Research Laboratory, U.S. Fish and Wildlife Service, Kearneysville, West Virginia.*

Milton Wyman, D.V.M., M.SC., *Professor, Chief, Comparative Ophthalmology, Department of Veterinary Clinical Sciences, The Ohio State University, Columbus, Ohio.*

L.G. Young, B.S.A., M.S.A., PH.D., *Associate Professor, Department of Animal and Poultry Science, University of Guelph, Guelph, Ontario, Canada.*

ABBREVIATIONS AND SYMBOLS

āā	equal parts
b.i.d.	twice a day
BUN	blood urea nitrogen
C	Celcius (centigrade)
ca.	about
cal.	calories(s)
cm	centimeter(s)
CNS	central nervous system
cu	cubic
d	deci (10^{-1})
dL	deciliter
DNA	deoxyribonucleic acid
ECG	electrocardiograph
e.g.	for example
EPG	eggs per gram
et seq	and the following one(s)
f	femto (10^{-15})
ff	(immediately) following pages
F	Fahrenheit
FA	fluorescent antibody
fl	fluid
ft	foot, feet
gal.	gallon(s)
gm	gram(s)
Hgb	hemoglobin
ICU	international chick unit(s)
i.e.	that is
IM	intramuscular(ly)
in.	inch(es)
IP	intraperitoneal(ly)
IU	international unit(s)
IV	intravenous(ly)
Kcal	kilocalorie(s)
kg	kilogram(s)
kVp	kilovolt peak
L	liter(s)
lb	pound(s)
Lg. An.	large animals
m	meter(s)
M	molar
mA·s	milliampere(s) per second
Mcal	megacalorie(s)
mcg	microgram(s)
ME	metabolizable energy
mEq	milliequivalent(s)
mg	milligram(s)
min	minute(s)
ml	milliliter(s)
mm	millimeter(s)
mo	month(s)
mOsm	milliosmole(s)
N.B.	note well
NF	National Formulary
NRC	National Research Council
oz	ounce(s)
p./pp.	page/pages
ppm	part(s) per million
pt	pint(s)
q 4 h, etc.	every 4 hours, etc.
q.i.d.	four times daily
q.s. ad	quantity sufficient to make
qt	quart(s)
q.v.	which see
r	roentgen unit
RNA	ribonucleic acid
rpm	revolutions per minute
sec	second(s)
Sm. An.	small animal(s)
sp.	species (sing.)
spp.	species (pl.)
sq	square
subcut.	subcutaneous(ly)
tbsp	tablespoon(s)
TDN	total digestible nutrients
t.i.d.	three times a day
tsp	teaspoon(s)

u	unit(s)	°	degree(s)
USP	United States Pharmacopeia	μ	micron(s)
viz.	namely	μL	microliter
wk	week(s)	%	percent
wt	weight	℞	take
yr	year(s)	>	greater than
		<	less than
		~	approximately

TABLES

PART I
IMMUNOLOGIC DISEASES

IMMUNOPATHOLOGIC MECHANISMS

Normal immune responses are vital in protecting the host against invasion by foreign organisms, tissues and substances. Under certain circumstances, however, these usually protective responses can have a deleterious effect on the host; all such unfortunate responses are called allergies or hypersensitivities; **autoimmunity** is a special type of hypersensitivity, the chief feature of which is tissue injury caused by specific immunologic reaction of the host to its own tissues. There are 4 situations (Type I to IV) wherein the host's immune system damages its own tissues.

TYPE I REACTIONS
(Anaphylaxis)

These are caused by chemical substances released from basophils or mast cells. The substances include histamine, slow reacting substance of anaphylaxis, bradykinin, and eosinophil chemotaxis factor of anaphylaxis. The release of chemical mediators by mast cells is triggered when antigen (allergen) binds to specific antibody molecules (reagins) that are present on the mast-cell membrane.

Reaginic (or cytotropic) antibodies of man and animals are of the immunoglobulin E (IgE) class. These antibodies are also called homocytotropic because of their propensity to bind to mast cells and basophils. Many types of antigens are capable of inducing reaginic antibodies, including serums, hormones, enzymes, venoms, pollens, complex polysaccharides, iodinated X-ray contrast media, antibiotics and other drugs. Reaginic antibodies, while often detrimental, probably evolved as a specialized defense mechanism against parasitic infections. Unfortunately, certain individuals overreact to nonparasite antigens by producing high levels of reaginic antibodies. The genetic predisposition for producing high levels of reaginic antibody is a prerequisite for the allergic state. Susceptibility to this state is known as **atopy.**

The nature of the clinical disorder that occurs following the interaction of allergen and cell-bound IgE varies with the dose of allergen, the route by which the allergen enters the body, and the location of the IgE coated mast cells. Anaphylactic reactions may affect the respiratory system (bronchial spasms and laryngeal edema), gastrointestinal tract (nausea, cramps, vomiting, diarrhea), cardiovascular system (intestinal and hepatic vasodilitation), or skin (hives, urticaria, wheal and flare reaction).

TYPE II REACTIONS
(Antibody mediated cytotoxicity)

Cytotoxic reactions occur as a result of the binding of **IgG, IgM** or IgA antibodies to antigenic substances on the surface of body cells, or associated structures (myoneural receptors, intracellular cement substance, etc.). Complement also participates in the reaction. Many types of body cells can be damaged, but blood cells appear to be particularly susceptible to immune mediated lysis and phagocytosis.

It is still unclear why an animal produces "autoantibodies" that react against its own tissues. It is possible that mutant clones of autoantibody producing cells emerge in postnatal life. Such clones of cells are normally suppressed in the prenatal development of the immune system. In some "autoimmune" disorders there appears to be a deficiency of suppressor lymphocytes. Suppressor lymphocytes are important in the regulation of the normal immune response, and one of their functions might be to suppress autoantibody production. Some tissue antigens are hidden deep in the cell membrane or in other areas inaccessible to the host's lymphoid cells. Because of their sequestered nature, the host's immune system does not recognize them as "self" in embryonic development. If these antigens are unmasked or released during post-embryonic life, the host recognizes them as foreign and makes antibodies against them. This might explain the transitory appearance of autoantibodies to cell constituents following myocardial infarcts or liver disease in man. Cross-reacting antibodies may also damage host tissues. Certain microbial proteins and drugs are antigenically similar to host antigens or can react with and antigenically alter host proteins, e.g. streptococcal-M antigens that produce antibodies that cross-react with normal glomerular basement membrane. Neoplasms can elaborate embryonic antigens or neoantigens, which can stimulate cross-reacting antibodies. It is also possible for host cells to be damaged as a result of immunologic reactions occurring in other sites. Foreign substances (microbes or drugs) may enter the body and elicit antibodies against them. The antibodies combine with the foreign antigen, the first component of complement is bound to the complex, but for unexplained reasons the rest of the complement components are bound to normal host tissues. The host cells are then destroyed by complement mediated lysis or phagocytosis.

TYPE III REACTIONS
(Immune-complex disease)

These reactions occur as a result of the localization of antigen-antibody complexes in tissues, usually vessel walls. The prerequisites of such disease are a continuous source of circulating antigen, and a continuous production of antibody. When the level of circulating antigen and antibody reach critical concentrations, antigen-antibody complexes of intermediate size are produced. Smaller complexes are soluble and pass through the vessel walls, while larger complexes are removed by the reticuloendothelial system. Intermediate sized complexes have a tendency to pass through endothelial cell spaces, but become trapped around the basement membrane. Complement that is bound to the complexes chemotactically draws polymorphonuclear cells into the area, the complexes are ingested by these cells, and as a result the neutrophils release their lysosomal enzymes. This process damages the surrounding tissues.

There are a number of conditions that can lead to immune-complex disease: (1) Microbial infections—chronic, persistent, low-grade, viral, bacterial, fungal, protozoal or parasitic infections. (2) Malignancy—Neoplasms can have associated immune-complex disease. Lymphoreticular neoplasms are particularly prone to having associated immune-complex manifestations. (3) "Autoimmune" disorders—Immune-complex disease is an important part of systemic lupus erythematosus. (4) Drug reactions—Serum sickness is a classic example of an immune-complex disorder resulting from the therapeutic use of heterologous serum. (5) Idiopathic—In many cases the origin of the antigen, and therefore, the cause of the disease is not identifiable. Until a specific source of the antigen can be identified, the disease is called idiopathic.

Clinical manifestations of immune-complex disease are extremely variable. The **Arthus reaction** results from local formation of immune complexes; if the complexes are deposited mainly in the glomeruli, glomerulonephritis is the primary clinical presentation; synovitis is a result of synovial deposition; dermal eruptions result from the deposition of complexes in dermal vessels; and vasculitis results from the deposition of complexes in the walls of small arteries. Meningitis, myopathy, myelopathy, neuropathy or localized hemorrhages can be sequelae of immune-complex disease. In any given animal, signs of immune-complex disease can include any one of the above major organ systems, or a combination.

TYPE IV REACTIONS

(Cell-mediated immune reactions, Delayed hypersensitivity)

Of these, the most familiar example is the tuberculin reaction induced in the skin of sensitized individuals by the intradermal injection of a purified protein derivative of mycobacteria. The skin reaction occurs as a result of the interaction of sensitized thymus-derived lymphoctyes with the sensitizing antigen. The tissue reaction is a result of lymphokines elaborated by the sensitized lymphocytes. Lymphokines can be cytotoxic to specific target cells, activate macrophages to become cytotoxic, inhibit the movement of macrophages out of the area, and cause small lymphocytes to be transformed into large basophilic blast cells. This type of immunity is extremely effective in combating many macrobial infections, and is important in the destruction of some tumors; it is also important in the destruction of foreign-tissue grafts.

SPECIFIC DISEASE ENTITIES OF AN IMMUNOPATHOLOGIC NATURE

Specific disease entities of an immune basis have been best characterized in companion and laboratory animal species. Except for the relative frequencies of these various disorders between species, the clinical manifestations and treatment are similar regardless of the animal species.

DISEASES INVOLVING ANAPHYLACTIC REACTIONS

(Type I reactions, Atopic disease)

Type I reactions are either of systemic or localized nature. Injection of the sensitizing antigens (allergens) directly into the blood stream can result in anaphylactic shock or more focal reactions (hives, urticaria, facial conjunctival edema). If the sensitizing allergen enters through the mucous membranes or the skin, more localized reactions usually occur.

SYSTEMIC ANAPHYLAXIS

(Generalized Anaphylactic Reactions)

Anaphylactic shock occurs in sensitized animals following parenteral injections of vaccines or drugs, or after insect bites. Clinical signs occur seconds after the allergen enters the circulation. This latent period is the time required for allergen to bind to sensitized mast cells, and for vasoactive amines to be released. The clinical signs that occur depend somewhat on the primary target organs. In most domestic species there is a pronounced vasodilation of the intestinal and hepatic blood vessels. The result is pooling of blood in the intestines and liver with resultant shock and death. Clinical signs include colic, vomiting, diarrhea, hypersalivation, cyanosis and decreased perfusion of the skin and mucous membranes. In the guinea pig, and in individual animals of other species, bronchial constriction may be so severe that the animals die of asphyxia.

Urticarial reactions of the skin and subcut. tissue of the face **(angioedematous plaques)** and conjunctiva **(angioneurotic edema)** are less severe manifestations of a systemic allergic reaction. The reaction follows the injection of vaccines, administration of drugs, ingestion of certain foodstuffs or insect bites (*see* SWEET ITCH IN HORSES, p. 962 and DERMATITIS, p. 926). Urticarial reactions and **facial-conjunctival edema** occurs in most species of animals. The urticarial lesions or facial-conjunctival edema usually resolve within 24 hours if left untreated. These localized edematous lesions can be associated with mild signs of bronchial constriction, or portal-mesenteric vasodilatation. The reaction is seldom fatal in this form. *See also* URTICARIA, p. 949.

Milk allergy occurs occasionally in cows and less frequently in mares when delayed milking or rapid weaning increases intramammary pressure such that milk components, notably α-casein, gain access to the circulation; these "foreign" proteins induce a type I hypersensitivity with subsequent anaphylaxis. Usually recovery is prompt once the gland is emptied.

Anaphylactic shock is treated with an IV injection of epinephrine to counteract portal-mesenteric vasodilation and bronchial constriction. Ancillary support of blood pressure and respiration is often necessary. Because of the peracute onset of signs, antihistamines are of little benefit. Antihistamines are more effective in treating urticarial infections and facial-conjunctival edema.

Localized Anaphylactic Reactions

Allergic rhinitis, as manifested by serous nasal discharge and sneezing, is uncommon in animals when compared to man. It is often seasonal, correlating with the shedding of pollens. Nonseasonal rhinitis may be associated with exposure to allergens ubiquitous to the environment, such as molds, danders, bedding and feedstuffs. Chronic pulmonary emphysema, q.v., p. 921, in horses may be a sequela to low-grade respiratory allergies. A tentative diagnosis of allergic rhinitis can be made by identifying eosinophils in the nasal exudate, a favorable response to antihistamines, or by a disappearance of signs when the offending allergen is removed.

Chronic **allergic bronchitis** has been best characterized in the dog. The signs are a dry, harsh, honking type of cough that is easily precipitated by exertion or by pressure on the trachea. The disease may be seasonal or occur year-round. It is usually not associated with other signs of illness. The bronchial exudate is rich in eosinophils and is bacterially sterile. Chest radiographs are normal and there may or may not be a low-grade peripheral eosinophilia. The condition is treated with preparations containing bronchial dilators and expectorants (aminophylline and potassium iodide), which open up the air passages and aid in the removal of thick tenacious mucus that accumulates as a result of the condition. Glucocorticoids are dramatically effective, especially when their use can be limited to certain seasons or to low-dose, alternating day therapy. Avoidance of the particular allergen is not usually possible because the offending allergen(s) is only rarely identifiable.

Pulmonary infiltrates with eosinophilia (PIE syndrome) has been described in the dog. As the name implies, the disease is associated with diffuse inflammatory infiltrates in the lungs and a pronounced peripheral eosinophilia. Unlike the situation in allergic bronchitis, these animals are often dyspneic or tire easily with exercise. Diffuse interstitial pulmonary infiltrates are seen on radiographs and the bronchial exudate contains numerous eosinophils. There is a pronounced eosinophilia, and the serum globulins are frequently elevated. The specific offending allergen is usually not discovered. Glucocorticoids are the treatment of choice.

Allergic asthma is an uncommon condition among animals when compared with man. The symptomatology of the disease in animals is similar to that of man.

Allergic enteritis (food allergy) is a relatively common disease of animals, and has been best characterized in the dog. German shepherd dogs and toy poodles seem to be particularly predisposed. Although the allergic nature has not been definitely proven, the presence of peripheral eosinophilia, and the response to glucocorticoids or dietary control suggest strongly that it is of allergic origin. The condition is usually manifested by periodic vomiting, often only of bile or mucus. The stool is usually normal in volume and frequency, but varies from semiformed to watery in consistency. Except for an occasional animal that is excessively thin, there is often no other clinical sign of illness. The nature of the signs suggest that the stomach and proximal small intestine are most severely affected. **Allergic colitis** is much less common.

Allergic enteritis is treated with a strictly controlled diet. In the dog, this means foods that are low in protein and contain as few ingredients as possible. Fortunately, suitable commercial prescription diets are available. Where they are not available, a basic diet of rice, cottage cheese and mutton, supplemented with vitamins and minerals is a good starting diet. As the signs disappear additional foods can be introduced one at a time into the diet. Glucocorticoids at low daily, or every other day, doses can also provide excellent relief for dogs that cannot be controlled with changes in the diet. Allergic enteritis in the cat is treated by switching to diets that are high in natural meat protein, and lower in nonmeat protein and grains. As a result the nearer the cat's normal diet in nature, the more the disease will be controlled.

Atopic dermatitis is a pruritic, chronic dermatitis that occurs in many animal species, but has been most extensively studied in the dog. Animals with atopic dermatitis have a genetic predisposition that leads to excessive production of reaginic (IgE) antibodies. It has been estimated that about 10% of all dogs suffer from atopy, and in the case of some breeds, such as Dalmatians and terriers, the incidence is higher. Atopic dermatitis of animals is due to the inhaling of allergens (pollens, molds, danders, etc.) from the environment. Unlike man where the respiratory and conjunctival mucous membranes are the usual target tissues, in animals inhaled allergens frequently cause dermal reactions.

Clinical signs are seasonal, or fairly constant throughout the year. Reddening of the conjunctival membrane and sneezing (rhinitis) are uncommon manifestations. Atopic animals will often chew at their feet and axillae. Excessive sweating is especially noticeable in the hairless areas. The skin lesions are greatly increased in severity by licking, scratching and secondary bacterial infection.

Treatment consists of identifying the offending allergens by intradermal skin testing, and avoiding the allergens if possible. The "wheal and flare" reaction seen when the offending allergen is injected into the dermis is a focal manifestation of the allergic state. Hyposensitization is effective in about 60% of dogs with atopic dermatitis, and consists of injecting an appropriate amount of the offending allergen IM at monthly intervals until improvement is noted. If hyposensitization fails, or is not utilized, alternate day glucocorticoid therapy is beneficial. Antihistamines are of minimal effectiveness.

DISEASES INVOLVING CYTOTOXIC ANTIBODIES
(Type II reactions)
(*See also* IMMUNE MEDIATED ANEMIAS, p. 25.)

Autoimmune hemolytic anemia, q.v., pp. 11, 30 and **thrombocytopenia,** q.v., p. 36, are the 2 commonest type II reactions. They can be associated with systemic lupus erythematosus, q.v., p. 10, in the dog, or rarely with lymphoreticular malignancies in the dog, cat and horse. Drugs can also precipitate attacks of hemolytic anemia or thrombocytopenia. The clinical features of the resulting disease depend on the acuteness and severity of the anemia or thrombocytopenia. Acute hemolytic anemia is manifested by fever, malaise, fatigability, pallor of the mucous membranes, and in a proportion of cases, icterus and bilirubinuria. The blood picture is one of a regenerative anemia. Thrombocytopenia can be manifested by petechial and ecchymotic hemorrhages of the skin and mucous membranes, melena, epistaxis, or hematuria. Excessive capillary bleeding can lead to profound anemia. Although the hemolytic anemia and thrombocytopenia usually occur independently of each other, they can sometimes occur together.

Both conditions are usually treated with high-dose glucocorticoid therapy during the acute stage. Once the disease is in remission, low-dose alternating day glucocorticoid therapy is used for a period of 3 months or more. A small portion of affected animals respond poorly to glucocorticoids alone; these are treated with more potent immunosuppressive drugs such as cyclophosphamide or azathioprine, in addition to glucocorticoids.

Cold hemolytic disease has been recognized in the dog and horse. The disorder is often idiopathic, but can occur secondary to a chronic infection, collagen disease, or neoplastic process. Autoantibodies present can be agglutinating or nonagglutinating in nature and are directed against the red cell, causing a Type II reaction. The antibodies are not fully active at body temperature but rather reach peak pathogenicity at some lower temperature. Although signs are exacerbated by exposure to cold, they often occur without it. The animal presents with signs of a hemolytic disease; and in the agglutinating type, there may also be microcapillary stasis with subsequent acrocyanosis and necrosis of the nose, tips of the ears and tail, digits, scrotum and prepuce. Diagnosis is based on a reversible autoagglutination at a cool temperature. The direct Coomb's reaction is usually negative for IgG, frequently positive for C3, and usually positive for IgM if the reaction is carried out in the cold. The disease is frequently fatal. In the absence of precipitating disorders (e.g. infection, neoplasia), the disease is best controlled with high dosages of glucocorticoids used in combination with cyclophosphamide. Cyclophosphamide is withdrawn when the anemia disappears and cold agglutinins are not detected.

Pemphigus vulgaris, and the variant condition pemphigus foliaceus, are immunologic skin disorders involving cytotoxic antibodies directed against intracellular cement substances. Pemphigus vulgaris is relatively uncommon, and has been described in the dog. It is characterized by bullous lesions along the mucocutaneous junctions of the mouth, anus and vulva, and in the oral cavity. The skin is only mildly involved. Because the epidermis of animals is relatively thin when compared to man, the bullae rupture very rapidly and form erosions. Characteristic bullae, therefore, are very seldom seen. The bullae occur as a result of suprabasal acantholysis. Secondary bacterial infection often complicates the lesions, and if left untreated the disorder is often fatal.

Pemphigus foliaceus is much commoner and has been recognized in the dog, cat and horse. It is characterized clinically by erosions, ulcerations and thick encrustations of the skin and mucocutaneous junctions. The absence of lesions in the mouth and widespread thick, crusty nature of the skin lesions, tend to differentiate it from pemphigus vulgaris. Glucocorticoids in very high initial dosages are used to control the condition. Once the disease is under control, low-dose every-other-day therapy is used. More potent immunosuppressive drugs such as cyclophosphamide, azathioprine, or methotrexate are used with glucocorticoids in cases unresponsive to steroids.

Myasthenia gravis is a relatively uncommon disease of animals. It has been identified in the dog. The clinical manifestations of the disease mimic those produced by curare. Extreme muscle weakness is brought on by exercise. Administration of a short-acting anticholinesterase compound (endrophonium) will produce a dramatic increase in muscle strength. The etiology of the disease in man and dogs is thought to involve circulating antibodies to acetylcholine receptors.

Anticholinesterase compounds are used to counteract muscle weakness. The use of chronic immunosuppressive drug therapy needs to be investigated.

DISEASES INVOLVING IMMUNE COMPLEXES
(Type III reactions)

Immune complex disorders are among the commonest of the immunologic diseases. They are either idiopathic or of secondary origin.

Glomerulonephritis, q.v., p. 885, is caused by the deposition of antigen-antibody complexes in the subendothelial or subepithelial surface of the glomerular basement membrane. Over one-half of the cases of glomerulonephritis in animals are idiopathic, i.e. the origin of the antigen in the complexes is unknown. Secondary glomerulonephritis occurs as a side effect of chronic infectious, neoplastic, or immunologic disorders. Animals with idiopathic glomerulonephritis are usually presented with signs of renal disease, whereas secondary glomerulonephritis is often a relatively minor part of a more serious disease.

Renal amyloidosis (q.v., p. 886) has identical clinical and etiologic features. In this disorder dense deposits of amyloid are found in the glomerular basement membrane. This material consists in part of immunoglobulin light chains. Renal amyloidosis occurs in both idiopathic and secondary forms. Any disease condition where there is a marked increase in the production and catabolism of immunoglobulin can lead to amyloidosis. These disorders include chronic infections, neoplasia, or monoclonal gammopathies.

Systemic lupus erythematosus (SLE) is considered the prototype immune-complex disease of man. The condition is most frequently recognized in dogs, and is much less common in cats and large animal species. The clinical presentation of SLE in dogs is essentially the same as it is in man. The signs can be very diverse depending on the organ systems involved. Synovitis, dermal reactions, myositis, neuritis, myelopathy, glomerulonephritis and pleuritis are all manifestations of the vascular deposition of immune complexes in various organs. Autoimmune hemolytic anemia or thrombocytopenia may be the sole or an accompanying manifestation of the disease. In any given animal, multiple organ involvement may be present or clinical signs may be referable only to one organ system. Fever and lymphadenopathy may be an accompanying feature. German shepherd dogs, Britanny spaniels, pointers and retrievers, Doberman pinschers, Shetland sheepdogs, spitzes and toy poodles are breeds that are predisposed to the disorder.

SLE is characterized by the presence of antinuclear antibodies, which can be identified with nuclear antigens in the immune complexes. There is still considerable controversy over whether the antinuclear antibody is a primary or secondary feature of the illness. Antinuclear antibody is not pathogenic in itself, and a surprising number of cases of SLE in man and dogs do not have detectable circulating antinuclear antibodies. The current emphasis on research into the cause of SLE in both man and animals is on an infectious, possibly viral, etiology.

SLE can usually be treated with glucocorticoids. Glucocorticoids are used initially in high daily doses, and when remission occurs alternate-day low-dose therapy is used. Drug treatment should be continued for at least 2 to 3 months after all clinical signs have disappeared. Cyclophosphamide or azathioprine or both are used in combination with glucocorticoids in patients that are difficult to control with glucocorticoids alone.

Purpura hemorrhagica of the horse, q.v., p. 48, is analogous to nonthrombocytopenic purpura or Schönlein-Henoch purpura of man.

Anterior uveitis, q.v., p. 222, of animals often involves immune complex type reactions. A uveitis frequently occurs in the recovery stage of infectious canine hepatitis. This is due to the reaction of serum antibodies with uveal endothelial cells containing ICH virus. Similarly, periodic ophthalmia or anterior uveitis of horses can be associated with immunologic reactions to leptospira or *Onchocerca* organisms.

Canine rheumatoid arthritis (*see also* ARTHRITIS AND RELATED DISORDERS [SM. AN.], p. 567) is manifested initially as a shifting lameness with soft-tissue swelling around involved joints. Within a period of several weeks or months the disease localizes in particular joints, and characteristic radiographic changes develop. The earliest radiographic changes consist of soft-tissue swelling and a loss of trabecular bone density in the area of the joint. Lucent cyst-like areas are frequently seen in the subchrondral bone. The prominent lesion is a progressive erosion of cartilage and subchrondral bone in the area of synovial attachments. Associated with this process is a loss of articular cartilage and a collapse of a joint space. Angular deformities often occur, and luxation of the joint is a frequent sequela. Deformities occur most frequently in the carpal, tarsal and phalangeal joints, and less frequently in the elbow and stifle joints. Synovial fluid changes are indicative of an inflammatory synovitis, with elevated total cell count and a high proportion of neutrophils in the synovial fluid cell population.

Canine rheumatoid arthritis responds poorly to systemic glucocorticoids alone. Cyclophosphamide and azathioprine are frequently used with glucocorticoids to treat this disorder.

Idiopathic polyarthritis is a common disorder of dogs. It is termed idiopathic because there is no evidence of a primary chronic infectious disease process, serologic abnormalities of systemic lupus erythematosus are absent, and joint disease is often the sole manifestation. This condition occurs most commonly in large breeds of dogs, in particular, German shepherd dogs, Doberman pinschers, retrievers, spaniels and pointers. When seen in toy breeds, it most frequently occurs in toy poodles, Yorkshire terriers, and Chihuahuas, or mixes of these breeds.

Diagnosis is made by consideration of the clinical history of cyclic, antibiotic unresponsive fever, malaise and anorexia, superimposed on which is stiffness or lameness. Bony changes are not seen on radiographs. Synovial fluid is inflammatory in nature and sterile for microorganisms. The disease can usually be controlled with daily high dose glucocorticoids followed by low-dose alternating-day therapy to maintain the disease in remission. Treatment can usually be discontinued after 3 to 5 months. Dogs that do not respond well to such therapy are treated with more potent immunosuppressive drugs in addition to glucocorticoids.

DISEASES INVOLVING CELL-MEDIATED IMMUNITY
(Type IV reactions)

Granulomatous reactions to microorganisms such as mycobacteria, coccidioides, blastomyces, histoplasma, feline infectious peritonitis virus, etc., are examples of cell-mediated immune phenomena. Although cell-mediated immunity is extremely effective in controlling these types of infections in most individuals, for poorly understood reasons these same mechanisms are not entirely effective in others, and a granulomatous reaction occurs. **Lymphocytic choriomeningitis virus infection of mice** is another example of the deleterious effect of cell-mediated immunity on the host. The CNS damage occurs as a result of the interaction of thymus derived lymphocytes on virus infected cells. **Old-dog encephalitis** may also result from cell-mediated immune mechanisms directed against cells persistently infected with canine distemper virus.

Contact hypersensitivity is another manifestation of cell-mediated immunity. When certain chemical compounds are allowed to react with dermal proteins, new antigenic proteins are produced. The skin is damaged as a result of the host's cell-mediated immune response against these chemically altered dermal proteins. Examples of this reaction are poison oak and poison ivy reactions in man. It has been described in both dogs and horses, and usually occurs as a result of the animal contacting sensitizing chemicals incorporated in plastic food dishes, collars and in drug compounds placed on the skin.

Autoimmune thyroiditis has been recognized in the dog and is characterized by the destruction of the thyroid glands by an autoimmune process that has both humoral (type II) and cell-mediated components (type IV). Hypothyroidism may be the sole manifestation of the disease, or may be part of a more diffuse disease syndrome in which myopathy, polyarthritis, azotemia, hepatitis, hemolytic anemia, or Addison's disease may be present. Involvement of other organ systems probably reflect a more generalized autoimmune phenomenon such as SLE and in part may result from immune complex (type III) disease. Treatment is aimed at correcting the hypothyroidism and other concurrent problems. If the immune-complex disease is severe, immunosuppressive drug therapy may be required in addition to endocrine supplementation.

IMMUNE-DEFICIENCY DISEASES

Deficiencies in Phagocytosis: Phagocytosis is an essential feature of the host's immune system. Phagocytes are found underlying the mucous membranes and skin, and in the bloodstream, spleen, lymph nodes, meninges, synovial membrane, bone marrow, and around blood vessels throughout the body. Phagocytes are either in the tissue (histiocytes, synovial macrophages, Kupffer's cells, etc.), or in the blood (polymorphonuclear leukocytes, monocytes). Phagocytosis involves recognition by the phagocytes of foreign, noxious, or damaged materials, chemotaxis of the phagocyte to the material, adherence of the material to the phagocytes plasma membrane, incorporation of the material into a pinocytotic vesicle, formation of a phagosome, and activation of the lysosomal enzymes in the phagosome. Phagocytes have immunoglobulin and complement receptors on their surfaces that assist in the engulfment (opsonization) of foreign material coated with specific antibody (opsonins) or complement or both.

Deficiencies in the phagocytic process are often manifested by an increased susceptibility to bacterial infections of the skin, respiratory and gastrointestinal tract. These infections respond poorly to antibiotics. Phagocytic deficiencies are either congenital or acquired. Examples of acquired deficiencies of phagocytosis include disorders that lead to profound and chronic depressions of leukocytes. Feline leukemia virus infection, tropical canine pancytopenia, idiopathic granulocytopenias, drug induced granulocytopenias (anticancer drugs, estrogens, anticonvulsants, sulfonamides, etc.) and myeloproliferative disorders are a few conditions of animals that can have secondary infections as a life-threatening complication.

A cyclic decrease of all cellular elements, most notably the neutrophils, occurs in the peripheral blood, lowering the resistance of gray collie and collie crosses to infection (*see* CYCLIC NEUTROPENIA IN GRAY COLLIE DOGS, p. 81).

Congenital abnormalities that lead to impaired phagocytosis are well documented in people. Deficiencies of opsonins, complement factors, chemotactic abilities, myeloperoxidase, glucose-6-phosphate dehydrogenase, and lysosomal enzyme activation have all been recognized. To date they have not been described in animals. Chronic granulomatous disease has been recognized as an X-linked defect in some Irish setter dogs (canine granulocytopathy syndrome). In this disorder, neutrophils cannot destroy phagocytosed microorganisms.

Deficiencies in Immunoglobulins: Immunoglobulin deficiencies are either acquired or congenital. **Acquired deficiencies** occur in neonates that fail to get adequate maternal antibodies from their mothers (failure of passive transfer), or in older animals, from conditions that decrease active immunoglobulin synthesis. Failure of passive transfer of immunoglobulins occurs occasionally in all species of animals that have colostrum as the major source of maternal antibodies. It has been associated with clinical problems in calves and foals. Failure of passive transfer can occur when the young fail to nurse properly during the first several days of life, or when the mother's colostrum contains low levels of specific antibodies. Problems with the intestinal absorption of immunoglobulins in the milk can also theoretically occur. Immunoglobulin levels below 400 mg/dl in a post-nursing serum sample indicates a failure of passive transfer in the foal. Removing calves from their mothers too soon is a problem that frequently occurs in dairy herds. Foals or calves that fail to obtain adequate maternal antibodies often succumb to fatal bacterial or viral infections of the intestinal and respiratory tracts. *See also* DIARRHEA IN THE NEWBORN, pp. 172 to 180.

Acquired hypogammaglobulinemia of man is either idiopathic (essential) or secondary in nature. Essential hypogammaglobulinemia has not been described in animals, but undoubtedly it does occur. In man this condition is associated with a high number of circulating thymic derived lymphocytes that suppress antigen stimulated immunoglobulin synthesis by B-lymphocytes. In man the condition usually occurs after 15 to 35 years of age and is associated with an increased incidence of recurrent pyogenic infections.

Hypogammaglobulinemia of a clinical significance can be associated with any disorder that interferes with immunoglobulin synthesis. Tumors, such as plasma cell myelomas or lymphosarcomas that occasionally secrete large amounts of monoclonal antibody can be associated with profound deficiencies of beneficial antibodies. This may be because the tumor cells are competing for necessary substrate substances with normal immunoglobulin producing cells, or because of the presence of thymus-derived suppressor lymphocytes in the blood that inhibit normal immunoglobulin production. Animals with monoclonal antibody producing tumors can have severe problems with secondary infections. Some viral infections, in particular canine distemper, can damage the lymphoreticular system so badly that normal antibody production is virtually halted. Profound starvation or debilitating illness may have a depressive effect on humoral immunity probably because essential nutrients are unavailable to provide the substrates needed to make antibodies.

Congenital hypogammaglobulinemia has been recognized either by itself, or in combination with deficiencies in cell-mediated immunity (combined immunodeficiency—*see* below). Total immunoglobulin deficiencies have not been described in animals. Selective immunoglobulin deficiencies in IgG subclass synthesis have been seen in some breeds of cattle, and selective IgM deficiency has been described in horses. Selective deficiencies of IgA are relatively common in people (1:600 to 1:800), but have not been identified in animals. Selective immunoglobulin deficiencies may produce no clinical signs, such as in cattle with selective IgG subclass deficiencies, or may be associated with a higher incidence of respiratory, skin, and intestinal tract infections in the case of IgA or IgM deficiencies.

Transient hypogammaglobulinemia is a condition that has not been recognized in animals. In man, the condition is congenital in origin, and is manifested by a delay in the development of active immunity. Children with this problem frequently develop clinical signs of hypogammaglobulinemia (usually respiratory infections) around 6 months of age when their maternal antibody reaches very low level. After another 3 to 5 months they begin to produce immunoglobulins on their own.

Deficiencies in Cell-Mediated Immunity: Pure deficiencies in cell-mediated immunity are relatively rare in man, and have not yet been recognized in animals.

Combined Immunodeficiency Disease: An autosomal recessive type of this disease has been identified in Arab foals, and the condition has been reported in dogs. Affected animals are frequently asymptomatic during the first several months of life, but become progressively more susceptible to microbial infections after that time. Arab foals with the disorder frequently succumb to adenovirus pneumonia or other infections at around 2 months of age. The foals are persistently lymphopenic. Precolostral serum samples have no detectable IgM antibody. Following nursing, immunoglobulin levels will be normal, but there is a progressive decrease after that time compared to normal foals. At necropsy the thymus gland is difficult to identify and is architecturally abnormal. There is a pronounced depletion of lymphoid elements in lymph nodes, Peyer's patches and spleen.

Canine distemper virus infection can lead to severe combined immunodeficiency in dogs. Dogs with canine distemper virus infection often demonstrate a lymphopenia, a progressive decrease in serum globulin levels, and suffer from severe pulmonary and enteric infections. Activation of encysted toxoplasmosis infections, or dissemination of primary toxoplasmosis, can also occur in such immunologically compromised animals. Nocardiosis may also occur in puppies immunosuppressed by canine distemper virus infection.

In addition to congenital combined immunodeficiency syndrome, a number of other combined immunodeficient states have been recognized in man, but not yet recognized in animals. These include Nezelof's syndrome, immunodeficiency associated with ataxia-telangiectasia, the Wiskott-Aldrich syndrome, immunodeficiency with short-limbed dwarfism, and adenosine deaminase and nucleoside phosphorylase deficiencies.

Complement Deficiencies: Congenital deficiencies of complement components have not been described in any of the companion and food animal species, but have been recognized in some laboratory animals. Although complement is necessary for opsonization and neutrophil chemotaxis, humans or laboratory animals with these deficiencies do not always suffer from bacterial infections. Interestingly, a high rate of autoimmune disorders are linked to congenital complement deficiencies in man. C1q deficiency in man has been associated with X-linked hypogammoglobulinemia and with one case of SLE. C1r, C1s and C2 deficiencies of man are often associated with autoimmune disorders. Two types of C3 deficiency have been recognized in people, both of which were associated with a greater incidence of bacterial infections. Familial C5 deficiency in man has been associated with chronic bacterial infections of the skin and intestinal tract.

GAMMOPATHIES
(Immunoproliferative diseases)

These are characterized by greatly increased serum immunoglobulin levels. They are either polyclonal or monoclonal in nature. Polyclonal gammopathies involve an increase in all major immunoglobulin classes. Increased levels of all major immunoglobulin classes can occur anytime that there is a chronic antigenically stimulating disease.

Polyclonal gammopathies in animals are seen in chronic pyodermas, chronic bacterial or fungal infections, granulomatous diseases, abscessation, chronic parasitic infections, chronic rickettsial diseases such as tropical canine pancytopenia, chronic immunologic diseases such as systemic lupus erythematosus, rheumatoid arthritis and myositis, or with neoplasia. It can also be idiopathic in origin.

Monoclonal gammopathies are characterized by the presence in the serum of a homogeneous immunoglobulin protein. Monoclonal gammopathies are either benign, or they are associated with immunoglobulin secreting tumors. Benign monoclonal gammopathies are rare in animals, and are not associated with a demonstrable tumor or with clinical illness. In man, benign gammopathies may become overtly malignant at a later date.

Monoclonal antibody secreting tumors originate either from plasma cells (myeloma) or lymphoblasts (lymphosarcoma). Plasma cell myelomas can secrete intact proteins of any immunoglobulin class, or immunoglobulin subunits (light chains, or heavy chains). Myeloma proteins in the dog are usually either IgG or IgA types, and less commonly IgM. Myelomas of the IgA type are common in the Doberman pinscher breed. Monoclonal immunoglobulins produced by lymphosarcoma are often of the IgM class, regardless of the species.

Clinical signs of illness in animals depend on the location and severity of the primary neoplasm, and on the amount and type of immunoglobulin secreted. Plasma cell myelomas frequently develop in marrow cavities of flat bones of the skull, ribs and pelvis, and in the vertebrae. Pathologic fractures of diseased bone can lead to central nervous or spinal disorders, or pain and lameness. Lymphosarcomas frequently involve parenchymatous organs and clinical signs are therefore more diverse.

Clinical illness can result from the presence of the monoclonal protein itself. **Amyloidosis** can occur as a result of increased immunoglobulin catabolism. **Hyperviscosity syndrome,** especially with IgM or IgA monoclonal proteins, can occur if the protein levels in the blood are high. In this syndrome, plasma viscosity can be many times normal, which leads to profound vascular disturbances and bleeding diathesis. Mental depression, blindness and **neurologic manifestations** can occur as a result of hemorrhaging into the nervous system and retina. Some IgM monoclonal proteins act as cryoglobulins and aggregate *in vitro* and *in vivo* when the plasma is cooled. Animals with **cryoglobulinemia** will often develop gangrenous sloughs of the ear tips, eyelids, digits and tip of the tail, especially during cold weather. Some IgM monoclonal proteins behave as cold agglutinins and may cause hemolytic episodes, especially during cold weather. Finally, animals with monoclonal gammopathies may have greatly depressed levels of normal immunoglobulins and may, therefore, suffer from serious secondary infections.

Immunoglobulin secreting tumors are usually treated with glucocorticoids and alkylating drugs. Plasmapheresis may be needed to lower serum viscosity in animals with clinical signs of hyperviscosity syndrome. Antibiotics and globulin injections may be needed to help prevent secondary infections.

BLOOD, LYMPHATIC AND CARDIOVASCULAR SYSTEMS

ANEMIA

A disease characterized physiologically by insufficient circulating hemoglobin and clinically by reduced exercise tolerance and pale mucous membranes. It is due to decreased production or increased destruction of red cells. Therapy is determined by which of these latter 2 errors predominates. The polychromatic cell count or reticulocyte count is the most informative test to determine if anemia is hemolytic and responsive or hypoproliferative and unresponsive. Anemias are classified to provide a rational basis for treatment.

I. Anemia: Bone Marrow Hypofunction (**unresponsive**)
  A. Anemias due to reduction in red cell production.
     Nutritional anemia, stem-cell injury, myelophthisis.
  B. Anemias due to reduction in hemoglobin synthesis.
     Deficient iron, vitamin E or vitamin B_6
II. Anemia: Loss of Abnormal Red Cells (**responsive**)
  A. Red cells with deficient enzyme content. Heinz-body anemia. Pyruvate kinase deficiency in basenji dogs.
  B. Hemolytic anemia due to acquired defects of red cells.
     Immune mediated anemias: Isoimmune, Idiopathic and "Innocent bystander"; Hemolytic disease of the newborn.
  C. Hemolytic anemia due to intravascular fragmentation; vasculitis of small arteries.
III. Anemia: Loss of Normal Red Cells.
  A. Hemolysis of normal red cells (**responsive**)
     Splenomegaly, red cell parasitism, chemical or physical injury.
  B. Loss of normal red cells (**poorly responsive**).
     External or internal hemorrhage or parasitism.

The **laboratory diagnosis** of anemia is by determining levels of hemoglobin (Hgb), packed cell volume (PCV), and red cell count (RBC). The **characterization** of anemia is aided by the red cell indices, mean corpuscular volume (MCV), mean corpuscular hemoglobin (MCH) and mean corpuscular hemoglobin concentration (MCHC). As rubricytes (red cell precursors) mature in bone marrow their volume decreases as their hemoglobin content increases. Immature red cells released into the blood in responsive anemias will thus have a higher MCV. Very large red blood cells (macrocytes) with a high MCV may have a normal total Hgb or MCH although the percentage saturation or MCHC will be below normal. These large cells contain RNA and stain blue or are polychromatic. They mature in blood in 1 to 2 days by completion of Hgb synthesis and loss of their RNA and blue appearance. In a week they have lost sufficient membrane to become normal in size (MCV) and appearance (normocytic). Since polychromasia is short lived (1 to 2 days) and macrocytosis is long lived (7 to 10 days) the presence of polychromatic red cells is the most sensitive indicator of marrow production. Thus an anemic animal may develop marrow failure and have a peripheral picture of macrocytosis (previous response) but no polychromasia (unresponsive). Since the products of red cell destruction are required for new cells, an anemia with sustained reticulocytosis must presumably be hemolytic and not due to blood loss.

The quantitation of the marrow erythroid response is most accurate when blood is supravitally stained with new methylene blue and *reticulocytes* counted as a percentage of total red cells. Their absolute number should be determined so that the clinician has an answer that is independent of the degree of anemia; e.g. a normal dog has 6.5 million red cells and 1% reticulocytes or 65,000/μL of blood, an anemic dog has 2 million red cells and 3% reticulocytes or 60,000/μL of blood. Since both dogs have the same output, the effort of the anemic dog is poorly responsive. A good response is characterized by upwards of 300,000 reticulocytes/μL of blood (3 million red cells and 10%+ reticulocytes).

A simpler method of evaluating erythroid response is based on counting *polychromatic* red cells after Wright's or a similar routine stain is used. The mean number of polychromatic red cells is determined from 10 oil-immersion fields over the length of the blood film. A normal animal or unresponsive anemia will have 0 to 1 polychromatic red cells per field, mildly responsive anemias 5 per field, moderately responsive anemias 5 to 10 per field and highly responsive cases 10 to 20 per field. These determinations can be roughly converted to cells per μL by multiplying by 8000. Thus if there is a mean of 10 polychromatic red cells per field at 1000× total magnification there are approximately 80,000 per μL in the blood. Platelets may be enumerated in the same manner. This method will consistently underestimate the response as compared to the reticulocyte count.

The normal ranges of red cell values for some domestic species are given below:

Animal	PCV %	Hgb gm/dL	RBC $10^6/\mu$L	MCV fL	MCHC %	PPC gm/dL
Horse (Light breeds)	30–48	11–18	7–11	40–49	35–37	6–8
Horse (Heavy breeds)	25–45	8–14	6–9	37–52	32–38	6–8
Ox	25–45	8–15	5–10	30–56	28–36	6–8
Sheep	25–50	9–16	8–16	25–50	30–38	6–7.5
Goat	20–37	8–14	8–18	18–34	30–40	6–7.5
Pig	32–50	10–16	5–8	50–68	30–35	6–8
Dog	37–55	12–18	5–9	62–70	33–35	5.5–7.5
Cat	27–45	8–15	5–10	40–55	30–35	6–7.5
Rabbit	35–45	9–15	5–7	60–68	31–35	5–7
Chicken	30–40	9–13	3	127	29	3–5
Turkey	39	11	2	203	29	3–5

dL = deciliter = 100 ml = 1L × 10^{-1}.
μL = microliter = 1 cu mm = 1L × 10^{-6}.
fL = femtoliter = 1L × 10^{-15}.

Clinical Findings in Anemia: Certain signs are characteristic of anemia regardless of the cause or species. Generally, there is pallor of the mucous membranes, weakness, lethargy, reduced tolerance to exercise, loss of appetite, increased heart and respiratory rates and there may be a systolic murmur due to reduced blood viscosity. If the anemia is acute or hemorrhagic, or both, there may be hypotension and shock. Care should be exercised in the handling and examination of the anemic animal as excitement may cause collapse.

I. ANEMIAS OF BONE MARROW HYPOFUNCTION

A. Decreased Red Cell Production

NUTRITIONAL ANEMIA

These anemias are due to a reduction in red cell production as distinguished from a reduction in hemoglobin synthesis. Vitamin B_{12} and folic acid are required for DNA synthesis and in deficient animals there are reduced erythroid mitoses and hence a reduction in red cells. The disease in man is macrocytic and normochromic and characterized by ineffective erythropoiesis or abnormal cells that are not released into the circulation. No clear counterpart exists in animals; however, a deficiency of cobalt and thus of B_{12} occurs with a mild reduction in blood volume but not a marked drop in hemoglobin. Folic acid deficiency anemia in animals is mild and limited to animals with rapidly growing tumors. Anemia due to carbohydrate starvation is mild, while protein deficiency causes a more severe anemia with an accompanying drop in blood volume. The effects appear to be nonspecific and due to general debility and reduced activity. Recovery is slow and plasma proteins appear to be replaced prior to increased erythrogenesis. Thus, there may be an increase in plasma volume and a worsening of the anemia for a time even after improved diets are given.

Decreased red cell production is the prime cause of the anemia of chronic disease although some increase in hemolysis is usually present. The reasons for this type of anemia include toxemia of abscessation or uremia, lack of iron utilization and inadequate nutrition. In chronic diffuse liver disease, there is inadequate detoxification of normal metabolites and altered amino acid supply. These changes often result in the appearance of "target" red cells in the peripheral blood.

INJURY TO MARROW STEM CELLS

In **hypoplastic** and **aplastic anemias,** the shortage of red cells is not as critical as the lack of platelets and neutrophils. In total aplasia death occurs in 10 to 14 days due to hemorrhage and sepsis. Rarely there is an immune mediated red cell aplasia in which granulocytes and platelets are maintained; in these cases, the animals survive longer and benefit from blood transfusions (q.v., p. 45) and immunosuppression (℞ 152).

Damage to marrow stem cells is usually an individual idiosyncrasy and related to drug or toxic exposure. Chloramphenicol and cyclic hydrocarbons will very rarely cause marrow aplasia while body irradiation in the 200 to 500r range will regularly do so.

Bracken fern poisoning (q.v., p. 1015), in cattle, will cause a herd outbreak of marrow aplasia. The virus of panleukopenia (q.v., p. 330) causes aplasia and pancytopenia in Felidae, but death is due to agranulocytosis, dehydration and thrombocytopenia. Most cases of aplastic anemia are idiopathic. The disease should be confirmed by bone marrow aspiration biopsy. Treatment consists of a corticosteroid, such as prednisolone (℞ 152), methyltestosterone (℞ 191) or oxymethalone (℞ 663) and antibiotics.

MARROW DISPLACEMENT BY ABNORMAL CELLS (Myelophthisis)

Rarely an animal with chronic infection will develop myelofibrosis in which the specialized cells of the marrow are displaced by connective tissue. Much more common is the invasion of marrow by lymphoid tumors and less often by other types of tumors, either myelogenous in origin or metastatic sarcomas and carcinomas. In any case, the appearance of rubricytes in the peripheral blood in the absence of polychromasia, especially if the anemia is mild or absent, should alert the clinician that the cells may be displaced by tumor growth in the marrow cavity. A search should then be made for tumor cells in peripheral blood and bone marrow.

B. ANEMIAS OF DECREASED HEMOGLOBIN PRODUCTION

DEFICIENT HEME SYNTHESIS

These anemias are due to reductions in heme synthesis and therefore of hemoglobin as distinguished from the macrocytic anemias of reduced cellular multiplication. The result is a microcytic hypochromic anemia. The most important cause is **iron deficiency. Copper deficiency** may be **absolute** or **molybdenum-conditioned** (q.v., p. 975). Copper is required to recharge the ferroxidase enzyme system and deficiency blocks iron utilization resulting in an iron deficiency anemia which is hypochromic and microcytic. In absolute iron deficiency there will be no hemosiderin in bone marrow.

In copper deficiency anemias there will be adequate or abundant marrow hemosiderin but a low serum iron. Cobalt and copper are usually added to feeds via a salt block or supplement. All suckling animals are iron-deficient for a time, but only in swine is this deficiency regularly critical. Baby pigs should be given iron either parenterally (℞ 520) or orally (℞ 521) during the first week of life. Care should be exercised before iron is administered by either route to insure that the pigs are not vitamin-E deficient; any history of such deficiency (q.v., p. 597) in the herd, or previous evidence of iron toxicity is reason to delay iron administration until at least 24 hours after the administration of vitamin E. A persistent anemia in young pigs that has not responded to previous iron administration should invoke the same precaution. **Vitamin E** is required for the synthesis of heme and normally there is a large pool of heme present that scavenges any free iron resulting from oral or parental administration. Low levels of vitamin E, and therefore heme, allow free iron to circulate, resulting in peroxidation of cellular membranes and necrosis, particularly in the heart, liver and skeletal muscle (*see* IRON DEXTRAN TOXICITY IN BABY PIGS, p. 981).

Vitamin B_6 or pyridoxine deficiency reduces heme synthesis and causes anemia but the condition is not recognized clinically and is presumed to be rare.

DEFICIENT GLOBIN SYNTHESIS

The synthesis of the alpha and beta chains of globin which combine with heme to form hemoglobin is under genetic control. In animals, a globin deficiency has not been recognized, but anemia in some sheep causes a "switching" to alternate globin chains that form hemoglobin "C." This hemoglobin C releases oxygen more readily to the tissues than the normal hemoglobin, A or B; in this respect it is similar to fetal hemoglobin. This "switching" thus appears to be a protective mechanism which permits more efficient oxygen transport at low hemoglobin levels.

II. ANEMIA DUE TO LOSS OF ABNORMAL RED CELLS

A. Red Cells With Deficient Enzyme Content

Glucose 6-phosphate dehydrogenase (G6PD) deficiency: This enzyme is part of an intraerythrocytic metabolic chain that protects hemoglobin from oxidative denaturation. In the deficient cells, oxidants cause globin precipitation resulting in the formation of "Heinz bodies" and rapid cell lysis. Old red cells with a lower G6PD level are more susceptible to oxidative denaturation than are young red cells. Thus exposure to an oxidant drug such as phenothiazine, phenylhydrazine or primaquine causes selective hemolysis of older red cells. In man low G6PD levels are genetically transmitted deficiencies, while in animals the susceptibility to oxidant drugs occurs mainly in debilitated animals. Usually no treatment is required as the young population of red cells is spared. Blood transfusions should be considered if the PCV drops below 15%. The marrow is usually functional and spontaneous recovery rapid. A similar condition has been observed when test dogs were fed large quantities of onions, and anemias associated with feeding rape, kale, or turnips to herbivores also have a Heinz-body pathogenesis. G6PD or Heinz-body anemia can be diagnosed by incubating 0.1 ml of heparinized test and control blood in 100 mg% of acetylphenylhydrazine in 2 ml of buffer for 2 hours at 37°C. Test and control red cells are then stained with new methylene blue and examined microscopically for Heinz-body formation. Normal red cells should contain few Heinz bodies and G6PD-deficient red cells many.

Pyruvate kinase deficiency in basenji dogs is a genetically transmitted deficiency of the red cells similar to that reported in man. The disease is characterized by severe congenital anemia with marked polychromatic red cell response.

B. Hemolytic Anemia Due to Acquired Defects of Red Cells

IMMUNE MEDIATED ANEMIAS

See also DISEASES INVOLVING CYTOTOXIC ANTIBODIES, p. 8 and BLOOD GROUPS AND BLOOD TRANSFUSION, p. 41.

Red cells may become the target of antibodies that coat their surfaces and cause them to be removed from circulation by the reticuloendothelial (RE) system. This condition can be diagnosed with reagent antisera specific to the globulin of the species tested. Combination of the reagent antiglobulin with the globulin on the cell membranes constitutes a positive **Coombs' or antiglobulin test.**

The adsorption of virus to the red cells such as occurs in equine infectious anemia (q.v., p. 343) may cause a hemolytic crisis because of the attachment of antiviral antibody to the red-cell-bound virus. These cells are then destroyed by the RE cells in what is known as an "innocent bystander reaction." Similarly the adsorption of drugs to red cells will rarely induce an immune hemolysis in man; it seems likely that a similar reaction occurs in animals.

Isoimmune hemolytic anemia occurs naturally in the horse, rarely in the dog and in calves from vaccinated dams and in the pig. This is an acute anemia in which erythrocytes of the newborn are agglutinated or hemolyzed by specific isoantibodies produced in their dams.

HEMOLYTIC DISEASE OF NEWBORN FOALS

Affected foals are normal at birth but can absorb dangerous levels of isoantibodies through their alimentary tract for up to 36 hours thereafter if they obtain colostrum from their dams. Clinically recognizable neonatal isoerythrolysis rarely occurs in foals of primiparous mares and generally is not seen until a mare has had her third or fourth foal. Mares are isoimmunized naturally by focal placental breakdown allowing fetal-placental hemorrhage of incompatible foal blood into the maternal circulation. A fairly large fetal-placental hemorrhage may be required to initially isoimmunize a mare to a significant degree. Re-stimulation of the mare in subsequent pregnancies requires much less incompatible foal blood of the same type. Also, therapeutic agents such as blood transfusions and incompatible tissue vaccines may contribute to the problem. Neonatal isoerythrolysis can occur only when a foal and its sire possess a blood factor absent in the mare (often factor C, Q, E_2 or A_1). Certain stallions mated to sensitized mares will always sire susceptible foals because they are genetically homozygous for the offending blood factor. Other stallions (heterozygotes) will sire such foals only part of the time. Although neonatal erythrolysis may occur in foals of any breed it is more frequently seen in thoroughbreds and mules.

Clinical Findings: The severity of anemia varies considerably depending upon the amount and type of isoantibodies consumed. Hemolytic isoantibodies are the most damaging, and the highest titers exist in the first colostral milk, hence vigorous foals that nurse heartily soon after birth may be the most severely affected.

Signs of the disease may be manifested as early as 8 to as late as 120 hours post partum. They include lethargy, jaundice, dyspnea, pounding heart and, in severe cases, hemoglobinuria. The foals spend much of their time lying down and those severely affected often cannot stand. They nurse infrequently and only for short periods. The conjunctiva, sclera and mucous membranes become progressively icteric in seriously affected foals. Erythrocyte counts range from about 2,000,000 to 4,000,000/μL (2 to 4 $\times$ 10^{12}/L) and the erythrocytes tend to form rouleaux in their own plasma. Foals with erythrocyte counts of this level during the first 24 hours require treatment.

Diagnosis: This may be made on clinical grounds. A positive Coombs' test in the anemic foal is very strong presumptive evidence, and demonstration of specific antibody against foal red cells in maternal serum or colostrum is definitive. Except for anemia, icterus and sometimes hematuria, few lesions are regularly seen. Splenomegaly and generalized icterus are often seen in foals dying 24 to 48 hours post partum.

Prophylaxis: If the mare's serum shows a definite antibody titer (>1:2) near the end of gestation, or if a test of the mare's colostrum with the foal's cells at birth shows an antibody titer of >1:8, the disease may be avoided by taking the foal from its mother immediately at birth for 36 hours. The foal may be nursed by a normal foster mother or may be bottle-fed on colostrum from nonimmunized mares. Such colostrum can be frozen for this purpose. The mother of the foal should be milked in order to remove most of the colostrum. The foal may be safely returned to its mother at 36 hours of age. The disease can usually be prevented by mating mares that have already produced one or more affected foals to stallions whose red blood cells are not agglutinated or hemolyzed by isoantibodies present in the mare's serum. However, in such cases, serum antibody levels should be measured during late gestation to detect the possible appearance of new isoantibodies.

Treatment: For those foals that are not seriously affected, ordinary nursing care together with antibiotics (℞ 2, 63, 73) and restriction of exercise for the first week usually will result in recovery. Blood transfusion is the only known method of saving a severely anemic foal. The whole blood of either the dam or the sire cannot be used in transfusions since it contains the hemolytic antibody but the saline-washed erythrocytes of the mare are probably the treatment of choice. A compatible donor is difficult to find and should be selected for red blood cells that are not agglutinated or hemolyzed by the serum or colostrum of the mare, and whose serum contains no demonstrable isoagglutinins or isohemolysins of foal cells. The erythrocyte count of the foal should be maintained at 3,000,000 to 4,000,000/μL (3 to 4 $\times$ 10^{12}/L) or the PCV at least 15% until recovery. If the dam's erythrocytes are available, 2 or 3 washes in isotonic saline solution are essential. About 2 to 3 L of mare's blood will suffice. Alternatively, removal of 3 to 7 L of the foal's blood, replaced by 4 to 6 L of the donor's blood, will correct the anemia and temporarily relieve the signs. Additional transfusions may be necessary and supportive therapy is essential. Careful attention should be maintained to detect infection. Affected foals usually have a strong bone marrow response that is characterized by marked anisocytosis and spherocytosis of red cells on blood smears and an upward shift in the MCV from 45 to 50 to 55 fL. Polychromatic red cells are seldom found in peripheral blood and their absence should be recognized as a species characteristic and not marrow failure. Rubricytes will be seen in severe cases as well as occasional sideroleukocytes. An accompanying neutrophilic leukocytosis will be present. Leukocyte counts will increase to 15 to 25,000/μL (15 to 20 $\times$ 10^{12}/L) with steroid treatment, which should be accompanied by antibiotic therapy (℞ 2, 63, 73).

HEMOLYTIC DISEASE OF NEWBORN PIGS

Maternal sensitization may occur either by the use of a crystal violet inactivated hog cholera vaccine of blood origin or by natural transplacental sensitization. The spontaneous disease is primarily an isoimmune thrombocytopenia with lesser effects on the red cell system. The piglets are normal at birth and disease occurs after suckling. The isoantibodies are usually against the Ea, Ee, Gb and Kb red cell antigens.

The first signs are due to red cell and platelet destruction in the peripheral blood. The marrow is at first responsive and the disease is self correcting for the first week. As antibody continues to be absorbed there is depression of marrow precursors and the terminal petechiae are associated with decreased platelet production of marrow aplasia. The terminal anemia is due both to hemorrhage and hypoproliferation.

Clinical Findings: Signs occur between 1 and 4 days after birth and consist of pallor, inactivity, dyspnea and jaundice. These signs gradually subside. After 10 to 11 days multiple petechial hemorrhages occur over the ventral areas of the body and most piglets die at this time. The red cell count drops from a normal of 4.5 to 5.3 × $10^6/\mu L$ at birth to 1 to 3 × 10^6 at 4 days of age. As anemia develops, anisocytosis and polychromasia appear along with some circulating rubricytes. The MCV rises from a normal of 70 fL at birth to 100 to 120 fL at 7 to 14 days of age and returns to normal in survivors at 4 weeks of age. The neutrophils rise to 9 to 10,000/μL at 4 days when the red cells are lowest and then decline to normal at 3 to 4,000/μL. Platelets have a bimodal response and drop from 3 × $10^5/\mu L$ at birth to 1 × $10^5/\mu L$ at day one then rise to normal at the first week, followed by severe thrombocytopenia after 10 to 14 days. Pathologically the bone marrow is hypoplastic in piglets which die and megakaryocytes are absent. Red cells are Coombs' positive from day 1 to 7 and are negative by day 14.

Diagnosis: This is usually made on finding anemia, purpura and mild icterus in neonatal pigs. The anemia is initially hemolytic, macrocytic, normochromic and responsive and becomes hypoplastic. Confirmation is by demonstration of agglutination of sire and piglet red cells and platelets by dams serum and milk. Leptospirosis may be ruled out by demonstration of thrombocytopenia or by maternal titer.

Treatment and Prophylaxis: Treatment is usually not attempted; a substitute dam might be tried. Sows should not be rebred to the same sire after having affected litters.

HEMOLYTIC DISEASE OF NEWBORN CALVES

Spontaneous sensitization of cattle to fetal red cell antigens is rare or does not occur. Vaccines derived from blood and used for prevention of babesiosis and anaplasmosis may contain red cell antigens that immunize the dams. If the bull has the red cell antigens of the vaccine donor then the calves will share these antigens and may develop isoimmune hemolytic anemia when they receive colostrum. Gestation is normal. Antibody eluted from affected calf red cells has been shown to be an IgG and at least in some cases to be hemolytic. A single 2-ml dose of babesia vaccine within a few weeks of calving may result in neonatal isoerythrolysis and most fatal cases occur where dams have received 4 or 5 vaccinations over a period of a year. The Coombs' test is usually strongly positive. The antigens involved are usually the B, C, F-V and S-V systems. The presence of bovine J antigen on rabbit kidney cell line tissue cultures has been stated to be an alternative mechanism whereby a heterologous tissue culture vaccine might produce isoimmune anemia. Owners may note red urine in newborn calves and exacerbate the problem by revaccinating dams on suspicion of neonatal infection.

Clinical Findings: The disease may be mild or peracute with signs occurring 12 to 48 hours after birth. In peracute cases death may occur as early as 2 hours after signs of severe dyspnea and 12 to 16 hours after birth. Acute cases are characterized by depression, dyspnea and occasionally fever that develops 24 to 48 hours after birth. The calves continue to suck but weaken and have pallor that is masked in 1 to 2 days by mild to moderate jaundice. Death occurs at 4 to 5 days. Calves with mild cases show only dullness and reduced activity.

In peracute cases there is hemoglobinuria, hypofibrinogenemia and fibrin degradation products with rapid death, a large spongy spleen and hemoglobin discoloration of kidneys. There is an excess of blood-stained pleural fluid and the lungs are congested and edematous. In the acute form the PCV drops to 6 to 7% and there is often hemoglobinuria. The marrow is responsive but inadequate with 1 to 2% reticulocytes and up to 140 rubricytes per 100 leukocytes. The Coombs' test is positive and the dam's milk agglutinates the calf's red cells and hemolysis occurs if complement is added. In mild cases the PCV drops to 18% at a week after birth and rises to 30% at three weeks of age. The anemia is normochromic and macrocytic.

Diagnosis: This is usually made on clinical findings of a severe anemia in neonatal calves whose dams have been given a blood-origin vaccine. Confirmation is by agglutination of sire and calves red cells by colostrum and maternal serum.

Treatment: Blood transfusions usually are not done because of donor incompatability. A single transfusion from an unvaccinated cow may be used or transfusion of saline washed (3 times) packed dams red cells to raise PCV to 25%. Antibiotics (℞ 63) and steroids (℞ 152) may be helpful.

Prophylaxis: If the disease is suspected it can be predicted by determining if cows have a titer against the bull's red cells. When it is practical, colostrum from cows with no titer should be used until positive dams have been milked 24 to 48 hours.

IDIOPATHIC IMMUNE ANEMIA

Idiopathic immune anemia or hemolytic anemia (**IHA**) occurs in the cat, horse and dog and is qualitatively similar to the disease in man. The disease is called idiopathic until an inciting antigen, likely absorbed to the red cells, can be identified. IHA occurs in the dog as part of the uncommon syndrome of canine systemic lupus erythematosus along with thrombocytopenia and rheumatoid arthritis. (*See also* IMMUNE COMPLEX DISEASES, p. 11.) The usual form of IHA, i.e. unassociated with lupus, is not rare and is characterized by hemolytic crises with a very low PCV (< 10%), marked polychromasia, spherocytosis, severe rouleaux or red cell aggregations and frequently a positive direct Coombs' test.

In chronic cases, icterus will be present due to ischemic hepatic damage. If blood transfusions are to be given at all, they should be given only with great caution and after matching. Prednisone (℞ 152) in high doses of 50 to 100 mg daily for 2 to 3 days will usually result in a marked rise in the PCV and improved color and condition in the dog. The dosage of steroid should be decreased to half, or less, of the initial dose in 2 to 3 days and then to a maintenance dose of 5 to 10 mg daily which should be maintained for 6 weeks. Steroids may be required at high levels for 3 weeks to induce a rise in PCV. Splenectomy may be indicated if steroid therapy fails. Clinicians experienced with the use of cyclophosphamide (℞ 656) may use this drug if steroid therapy fails. The drug is myelotoxic and the leukocyte count must be monitored at least daily.

Most therapeutic failures result from steroid therapy being discontinued too soon after remission begins. Should a hemolytic crisis occur after a steroid-induced remission, even higher levels of steroid may be required to again bring the hemolysis under control. Dogs may develop signs resembling those of Cushing's disease (q.v., p. 200) during treatment of IHA, but return to normal as the treatment is decreased. Hematinics are usually not required, and iron should not be given.

The adsorption of the agent of equine infectious anemia (q.v., p. 343) to the horse red cells has been shown to result in a similar pathogenesis in this anemia. IHA probably occurs in other species but is unrecognized.

C. HEMOLYTIC ANEMIA DUE TO INTRAVASCULAR FRAGMENTATION

Diseases which cause vasculitis necessarily activate the clotting mechanism and cause **disseminated intravascular coagulation (DIC)** of some degree. The passage of red cells at high velocity through damaged arterioles results in fragmentation of red cells as they impinge on intraluminal strands of fibrin. The damaged cells are then removed by the RE system. This pathogenesis is referred to as a **microangiopathic hemolytic anemia (MHA).** It is characterized clinically by anemia with very marked poikilocytosis and reticulocytosis. MHA occurs in young calves with **hemolytic uremic syndrome (HUS)** where there is severe anemia, poikilocytosis, uremia, hemoglobinuria and collapse. MHA to a mild or severe degree occurs as a part of the pathogenesis of many other anemias where there is vasculitis, e.g. EIA, malignant catarrhal fever, chronic hog cholera, and in thrombotic purpuras. Anemia with marked poikilocytosis may occur in some parasitic diseases, especially where there is extensive somatic migration as in *Strongyloides* infection. In the non-anemic horse, especially with colic, the presence of a few highly distorted red cells is likely indicative of MHA due to parasitic vasculitis of the anterior mesenteric artery. MHA occurs in cases of malignancy, especially if there are cavernous and necrotic areas of tumor as in hemangiosarcomas.

III. ANEMIA DUE TO LOSS OF NORMAL RED CELLS

A. Hemolysis of Normal Red Cells

Hemolysis Due to Increased Reticuloendothelial Removal, Splenomegaly and Hypersplenism: Any condition which causes an enlargement of the spleen will result in increased erythrophagocytic activity in that organ. An enlarged spleen (**splenomegaly**) may occur as the result of hyperplasia due to chronic infection, autoimmune disease, or to splenic neoplasia. Diseases of the liver resulting in cirrhosis and portal hypertension will cause congestive splenomegaly. The stretching of the splenic reticulum in the enlarged spleen is a stimulus to both phagocytosis and fibroplasia. The enlarged spleen pools blood, where low glucose, low cholesterol and high pH results in a premature aging or "conditioning" or red cells, which causes them to become spherocytic and be removed from circulation. Splenomegaly then, for hemodynamic reasons alone, progresses to **hypersplenism,** which is defined as an enlarged spleen of any cause with marrow hyperplasia and decrease in one or more of the cellular elements of the blood. The clinical disease resulting from hypersplenism may be a thrombocytopenic purpura or hemolytic anemia or neutropenia or any combination of these. If immune factors are added to the congestive pathogenesis, then the disease is more severe. Splenectomy is usually curative. There is some danger of thrombotic disease in the immediate postoperative period (1 to 2 days) due to loss of splenic control on thrombocytosis. This complication is reflected clinically by cold extremities, particularly of the tips of the ears and tail in dogs. If these signs are marked, heparin should be administered IV at 0.5 to 1 mg/lb (1 to 2 mg/kg) body wt., repeated t.i.d. for 1 to 2 days or until signs of thrombosis subside.

Hemolytic Anemia Due to Red Cell Parasitism: Red cell parasitism may result in intravascular hemolysis of red cells with hemoglobinemia and hemoglobinuria as in babesiosis (q.v., p. 426). Alternatively, the parasites may be removed from the red cells by the spleen and the cells returned to the circulation, or the erythrocytes may be removed entirely and destroyed by the cells of the RE system. The latter pathogenesis occurs in hemobartonellosis of dogs and cats (q.v., p. 328), anaplasmosis in cattle (p. 416) and sheep (p. 416), eperythrozoonosis (p. 415) and malarial merozoites in mammals and birds. Ehrlichiosis in horses (q.v., p. 342), dogs (q.v., p. 338) and probably cattle, causes anemia with thrombocytopenic purpura due to platelet and leukocyte parasitism.

Trypanosomes are common in blood of cattle in North America, but are generally nonpathogenic. Rarely, a dog that has returned from South America will develop an acute hemolytic anemia with marked reticulocytosis and the presence of trypanosomes in the blood. Dogs which have been in the Mediterranean area may become infected with *Leishmania* spp. by arthropod vectors. There is epistaxis, but only mild anemia, and biopsy of bone marrow, lymph node or spleen will demonstrate the *Leishmania* organisms in RE cells.

In general, the marrow is hyperplastic in anemias due to red cell parasitism and there is a marked peripheral blood macrocytosis and reticulocytosis. If there is hemoglobinuria with iron and protein loss, recovery will be slower. The marrow in Ehrlichiosis is terminally hypoplastic. Diagnosis of the red cell parasitism is based on demonstrating the organism in the red cells; a wet mount and new methylene blue stain (q.v., p. 1473) is more efficient than examination of a dried-stained blood smear. Treatment and prevention must vary with the disease. The demonstration of *Hemobartonella* in an anemic cat without a marked polychromatic response is cause to look for an RE neoplasm which has lowered normal immunity. A positive Coombs' test has been demonstrated in some of the anemias of red cell parasitism.

Lysis of Normal Red Cells Due to the Action of Bacterial, Plant, Chemical or Physical Agents: Bacterial hemolysins: (*See* LEPTOSPIROSIS, p. 379, and BACILLARY HEMOGLOBINURIA, p. 399).

Bartonella bacilliformis causes a generally fatal hemolytic anemia in man, dogs and rodents. The disease is most likely to occur in splenectomized dogs. The disease **(Oroya fever)** can be diagnosed by demonstration of the intraerythrocytic organisms on stained blood smears. Chloramphenicol given IV at 5 to 10 mg/lb (11 to 22 mg/kg) daily for 3 to 5 days is the treatment of choice.

Plant hemolysins: Most of the plants that cause hemolytic anemia such as rape, kale, turnips and onions, do so because of depletion of the red cell enzyme glucose-6-phosphate dehydrogenase with

Heinz-body production, and these are discussed above (p. 24) under RED CELLS WITH DEFICIENT ENZYME CONTENT. Direct lysis of the red cell membrane can be caused by saponin from the waxy cuticle of plants, or by ricin from castor beans. Hemolysins are the toxic principles in most spider and snake venoms.

Chemical hemolysins: A wide range of chemical compounds may produce hemolysis and, in addition, an aplastic anemia. The agents most commonly involved with this latter form of anemia are the cyclic hydrocarbons such as benzene, toluene, acetanilide and phenacetin. Heavy metals such as lead and silver inhibit hemoglobin synthesis and arsenicals can cause hemolysis. Phenylhydrazine and other oxidant compounds produce Heinz bodies and hemolysis as described above (p. 24). Anemias of these causes should be treated symptomatically pending specific toxicologic diagnosis. Lead poisoning produces nervous signs without anemia. In dogs and man there may be basophilic stippling of red cells and showers of peripheral blood rubricytes and increased blood levels of lead.

Considerable quantities of copper may be accumulated gradually without apparent harm, but "chronic copper poisoning" (q.v., p. 977) results when any one of several "stresses" leads to a sudden release of stored copper, which causes acute hemolytic anemia in sheep, pigs and cattle. In sheep, the source of the copper is usually phytogenous, leading to high copper levels in the liver which may then be released by hepatic injury of any cause, such as mild pyrrolizidine alkaloid poisoning (q.v., p. 1048) or forced exercise. In pigs, copper may be included in rations as a growth stimulant. In marginally vitamin E-deficient pigs which develop hepatosis dietetica (q.v., p. 597) sufficient hepatic necrosis and release of stored copper may occur to cause a hemolytic crisis and icterus.

Excess molybdenum, usually phytogenous in origin, will inhibit the intermediary metabolism of copper and cause lameness, depigmentation of skin, diarrhea and hypoplastic anemia which is microcytic and hypochromic (*see* MOLYBDENOSIS, p. 975). Removal of molybdenum or increased dietary copper is indicated.

Physical agents causing hemolysis: Intravascular hemolysis will follow full thickness skin burns and can be expected if more than 20% of skin is affected. The excessive ingestion of cold water, especially in calves, may cause hemolysis, likely of osmotic origin, with anemia, dyspnea and hemoglobinuria. Occasionally an immune anemia may be triggered by exposure to cold (q.v., p. 9) if the offending antibody is of the cold agglutinin or IgM type.

B. Loss of Normal Red Cells

Loss Due to External Hemorrhage or External Parasitism: External hemorrhage may occur from wounds, uterine prolapse and lacerations or surgical trauma, especially dehorning and castration. In acute hemorrhage there is hypovolemia and hypotension with a normal PCV. In chronic hemorrhage there will be a low PCV usually with an unresponsive marrow due to iron loss. In acute bleeding, blood transfusions (q.v., p. 45) are indicated to replace blood volume and clotting factors. The marrow is usually responsive, and parenteral iron at 3.4 mg/gm of Hgb (estimated loss) and hematinics should be given. In anemias of chronic hemorrhage, transfusions are less likely to be required, especially if the animal is on its feet and bleeding has been stopped for 2 or more hours. Iron and hematinics should be given as above. Care should be taken in handling the anemic animal as stress may be fatal.

External parasitism may cause anemia, particularly in young animals. In general, bloodsucking insects such as Tabanidae, black flies and mosquitoes cause more irritation than blood loss. Calves occasionally become heavily infested with lice and become thin, weak and mildly to severely anemic. Kittens and puppies can become severely anemic due to a heavy louse infestation, and in endemic areas, bloodsucking ticks infect a wide variety of hosts. These anemias are primarily of blood loss and should be treated with iron (℞ 520) and application of insecticides (*see* TICK INFESTATION, p. 733). Cattle especially suffer marrow depression with heavy louse infestation, and recovery is slow.

Loss of Normal Red Cells Due to Internal Hemorrhage or Internal Parasitism: Internal hemorrhage may be acute or chronic and result from surgery, wounds, tumors or abscesses and enteric or urinary tract ulceration. Diagnosis is usually aided by aspiration of the chest, abdomen or subcutis. If generalized bleeding is present, blood should be drawn into a glass vial and the clotting time determined. Thrombocytopenia will cause purpura and poor clot retraction. If platelets are present in adequate numbers, as determined on a stained smear or by platelet count, then the prothrombin time should be determined. Prothrombin levels are low in warfarin or sweet clover poisoning (q.v., p. 1017) and hepatic failure. Clotting agents that act to raise blood calcium are generally not efficient and calcium gluconate can be given as easily. If the bleeding has been mild but very prolonged, iron deficiency should be suspected and treated as described above.

Internal Parasitism: (q.v., p. 671 et seq.): Profound anemia may be caused in young dogs and cats by hookworm infection. In severe cases with collapse, blood transfusions should precede anthelmintic treatment. Iron loss in enteric parasitism is not reabsorbed and in chronic cases there may be better response to parenteral iron (℞ 520) than to an anthelmintic. The marrow is usually productive if iron stores are not exhausted, and there will be a marked peripheral blood reticulocytosis occasionally with severe poikilocytosis. In sheep, acute haemonchosis may cause death due to anemia without debilitation. It should be noted that diarrhea will occur with most enteric parasitisms of the sheep except *Haemonchus*. In calves and yearling cattle, chronic *Ostertagia* infection will cause cachexia, an anemia with poor reticulocyte response and occasionally marked poikilocytosis. Iron may be given parenterally if there is severe anemia or if serum iron is low.

POLYCYTHEMIA

An excess in the number of circulating erythrocytes per unit volume of blood.

Relative Polycythemia: This results from a reduction in the fluid component of blood and is the commonest type of polycythemia found in domestic animals. The condition is called *hemoconcentration* or *apparent erythrocytosis* as the concentration of erythrocytes is increased but the total circulating volume of red blood cells is unchanged and the arterial oxygen tension is normal. It is a transient state due to shrinkage of the plasma volume and can result from shock, or dehydration following persistent vomiting or diarrhea, or insufficient fluid intake. Inadequate water intake in weakened anemic animals and hemoconcentration superimposed upon the anemia may mask the true state with apparently normal red cell, PCV and hemoglobin values. Excitement may induce a "stress polycythemia" in dogs and horses as a result of splenic contraction and the release of stored erythrocyte-rich blood into the general circulation. Severe pain may also induce splenic contraction.

Secondary Polycythemia: This is a compensatory increase in circulating erythrocytes in conditions of inefficient oxygenation. It is observed in animals raised at high altitudes or trained for racing, and in animals suffering from cardiac and pulmonary disease in which oxygenation is impaired (e.g. tetralogy of Fallot). Abnormal hemoglobins with increased oxygen affinity, and chemicals such as coal-tar derivatives and carbon monoxide may cause secondary polycythemia. Newborn mammals show this type of polycythemia temporarily. Both the total number and concentration of circulating red blood cells are increased due to the reduced arterial oxygen tension. Polycythemia associated with excessive erythropoietin production may occur with some renal lesions, e.g. renal carcinoma. In these cases arterial oxygen tension may be normal.

Polycythemia vera: This myeloproliferative condition, also known as *erythremia* or *true erythrocytosis*, is marked by persistent polycythemia due to excessive formation of erythroblasts in the bone marrow and is accompanied by an increased blood volume and viscosity, an enlarged spleen, cyanosis and sometimes leukocytosis and thrombocytosis. Arterial blood-oxygen saturation is normal This rare condition has been reported in the dog, cat and cow.

Treatment in the various polycythemias can only be directed towards correction of the causative mechanisms. Phlebotomy is warranted only in polycythemia vera, to provide temporary relief (10 to 20 ml/kg every 48 hours). Myelosuppressive agents such as cyclophosphamide have been suggested as an additional treatment for polycythemia vera.

CANINE THROMBOCYTOPENIC PURPURA (CTP)

Hemorrhagic disorders in dogs associated with severely reduced numbers of circulating platelets, usually the result of platelet destruction, utilization or sequestration exceeding the capacity of the bone marrow to replace these cells. Since platelets are essential for the initial formation of the hemostatic plug at sites of vascular injury, widely dispersed petechiae and ecchymosis in the skin and mucous membranes are observed clinically. Stress significantly enhances the bleeding tendency in thrombocytopenic states.

Etiology: The symptomatic form of CTP occurs when iatrogenic or other known causes are involved. Certain cytotoxic chemicals such as nitrogen mustard, busulfan, 6-mercaptopurine and cyclophosphamide will destroy platelet-producing megakaryocytes. Leukemias and aplastic anemia may also produce CTP. Infiltration of the bone marrow by leukemic or other malignant cells may compress the normal bone marrow elements, including megakaryocytes, and produce thrombocytopenia. In aplastic anemia the loss of normal marrow constituents often is not followed by replacement and a persistent thrombocytopenia results. In dogs, large doses of estrogens can be toxic to the bone marrow and may result in thrombocytopenia, leukopenia and progressive anemia.

Splenic enlargement due to a variety of causes including granulomatous inflammation, neoplasia and infarction, may be associated with CTP. The reduction in circulating platelet number is a result of an expanded platelet storage pool and increased sequestration within the spleen, and not a result of suppressed thrombogenesis.

A common cause of thrombocytopenia is **disseminated intravascular coagulation.** In this syndrome platelets are consumed in large numbers in the thrombotic process. A cyclic thrombocytopenia has been reported in association with cyclic neutropenia in collies (q.v., p. 81). Occasionally a moderate thrombocytopenia and a qualitative platelet defect may occur simultaneously (e.g. uremia, neoplasia).

Thrombocytopenias due to drug-induced antibody formation are recognized in man and no doubt occur in domestic animals. Drugs such as quinidine, quinine, digitoxin, chlorothiazides and some sulfonamides may provoke the formation of platelet antibodies in some individuals.

The idiopathic form of CTP can accompany certain autoimmune disorders such as autoimmune hemolytic anemia and systemic lupus erythematosus. In these diseases, dogs may develop antibodies against several of their own tissues, including blood platelets. Damage to platelets by antibodies leads to the excess sequestration of these cells by the reticuloendothelial system, particularly the spleen. A thrombocytopenia results despite normal or increased megakaryocyte activity in the bone marrow.

Thrombocytopenia following some viral infections may result from impaired platelet production due to invasion of megakaryocytes by the virus, destruction of circulating platelets by virus or sensitization of circulating platelets by viral antigen-antibody complexes.

Clinical Findings: Petechiae and ecchymosis appear suddenly on visible skin and mucous membranes. These may be accompanied by epistaxis, melena, hematuria, prolonged bleeding from sites of injury and excessive bruising or hematoma formation following routine clinical palpation. Pallor, weakness and edema may occur in cases where there is also a severe anemia.

Diagnosis: Direct platelet counts on fresh blood collected in EDTA will confirm a quantitative platelet defect. The platelet count often correlates poorly with the clinical hemorrhagic manifestations but bleeding is uncommon with platelet counts greater than $50 \times 10^9/L$. Platelet counts of less than $50 \times 10^9/L$ are strongly suggestive of CTP; they may drop to less than half this.

The peripheral blood smear will show a virtual absence of platelets; many abnormally large platelets may suggest an accelerated thrombogenesis. Other tests such as the whole-blood clotting time, the skin-bleeding time, clot retraction, and the prothrombin time may be of use in detecting and defining the thrombocytopenia. A positive direct Coomb's test associated with autoimmune hemolytic anemia and positive LE preparations with systemic lupus erythematosus support a diagnosis of idiopathic CTP. The idiopathic form of CTP may be confirmed by the detection of antiplatelet activity in the serum using the platelet factor-3 test.

Treatment: In dogs developing CTP after prolonged drug therapy or after short-term exposure to a new drug, an iatrogenic cause is a strong possibility; the suspected agent should be discontinued and the patient immediately given corticosteroids (e.g. prednisone, 1 to

3 mg/kg of body weight daily). Drug-induced CTP is usually readily reversed by removing the causative agent. CTP associated with malignancy or aplastic anemia is most difficult to treat, as control of the underlying cause may be impossible.

Remissions of idiopathic CTP can usually be achieved with corticosteroid therapy but relapses often occur after variable periods. Prednisolone is given at a daily dose of 1 to 3 mg/kg of body weight for 1 to 2 weeks, then maintenance doses of 2.5 to 5 mg/day are established and given for another 2 to 3 weeks. Splenectomy is recommended in some patients unresponsive to steroid therapy or in chronic recurrent cases.

Whole-blood transfusions are reserved for emergency use to correct severe anemia secondary to blood loss. To replenish platelets with transfusions, freshly collected whole blood or citrated platelet-rich plasma is required (*see* HEMOPHILIA AND OTHER HEMOSTATIC DISORDERS IN DOMESTIC ANIMALS, below).

HEMOPHILIA AND OTHER HEMOSTATIC DISORDERS IN DOMESTIC ANIMALS

Defects in hemostasis may be inherited or acquired. Normal hemostasis requires a normal vessel wall, normal levels of blood coagulation factors and adequate numbers of functional blood platelets. Platelets must adhere to the vessel wall at sites of disruption then stick to each other to form a hemostatic plug. This plug must then be strengthened by the incorporation of fibrin. A deficiency in vessel response, platelet activity or fibrin generation will lead to defective hemostasis.

Inherited Disorders: Inherited abnormalities of the vessel wall are not clearly defined in domestic animals. Connective tissue diseases such as the Ehlers-Danlos syndrome in mink and dogs may result in vascular purpura.

Many different types of inherited blood coagulation deficiencies have been reported in domestic animals. Most of these are single factor deficiencies or abnormalities, but multiple coagulation defects have been reported. The 2 hemophilias, A and B, are inherited as sex-linked traits and are commonly carried by the female and manifested clinically only in the male, except when hemophilic males are mated to carrier females. All other known inherited blood coagulation defects are transmitted as autosomal traits.

Several of the inherited blood coagulation defects that have been reported in domestic animals are: factor I (**fibrinogen**) deficiency in dogs and goats; factor VII (**proconvertin**) deficiency in beagle hounds and Alaskan malamutes; factor VIII deficiency (**classic hemophilia, hemophilia** A) in practically all breeds of dogs and in mongrels, standardbred and thoroughbred horses, and cats; factor IX deficiency (**Christmas disease, hemophilia B**) in Cairn terriers, black and tan coonhounds, St. Bernards, cocker spaniels, French bulldogs and Alaskan malamutes and in British shorthair cats; factor X (**Stuart factor**) deficiency in cocker spaniels; factor XI (**plasma thromboplastin antecedent**) deficiency in springer spaniels and Great Pyrenees, and in Holstein cattle; and factor XII (**Hageman factor**) deficiency in the cat. Marine mammals, birds and most reptiles are naturally lacking Hageman factor.

Von Willebrand's disease is an inherited defect reported in the German shepherd dog, miniature schnauzer, golden retriever, Scottish terrier and Doberman pinscher, in rabbits and in swine. This defect (similar to hemophilia A but inherited autosomally) is a combined blood coagulation/platelet function defect in which there is reduced plasma factor VIII procoagulant activity, as well as reduced or abnormal factor VIII antigenic (von Willebrand factor; factor VIII-related antigen) activity which is necessary for normal platelet and vascular functions.

Inherited platelet-function defects (hereditary thrombopathias) have been reported in otterhounds, basset hounds, Simmental cattle and fawn-hooded rats. Although the basic platelet defect differs, these disorders are manifested by increased bleeding tendencies due usually to platelets that react poorly or not at all to stimulation by collagen, adenosine diphosphate and thrombin, and thus fail to form an adequate hemostatic plug. These bleeding tendencies are often exacerbated by trauma or surgery. Transmission is as an autosomal trait.

Acquired Disorders: Acquired disorders of hemostasis may result from a number of diverse causes that affect specific components of the hemostatic mechanism, and are commoner in domestic animals than are the inherited defects. Vessel wall damage with accompanying petechiation occurs in such conditions as equine purpura hemorrhagica (q.v., p. 48) or in vessel wall hypoxias due to poor circulation or to anemia. Scurvy (vitamin C deficiency) in guinea pigs may result in vascular purpura.

Acquired blood coagulation disorders usually involve multiple factor deficiencies and may result from defective synthesis, excessive utilization or inhibition of one or more coagulation factors. Certain clotting factors in the circulating blood may be depressed by agents in the feed, by drugs, or by various diseases particularly those causing severe or moderate hepatic damage.

Warfarin or dicoumarol (*see* SWEET CLOVER POISONING, p. 1017) depresses the production of the vitamin K-dependent coagulation factors (factors II, VII, IX and X). Since the liver is a major site of coagulation factor synthesis, liver damage may result in defective blood coagulation. The low levels of clotting factors in the plasma of newborn animals may predispose to bleeding. Anaphylactic shock, intravenous hemolysis, excessive tissue necrosis (burns, neoplasia) or bacterial endotoxins can lead to activation of blood platelets and coagulation factors resulting in **disseminated intravascular coagulation** (DIC) and thromboembolism. Amniotic fluid contains potent thromboplastins that can be introduced into the maternal circulation during dystocias, leading to intravascular clotting. Besides depletion of coagulation factors, DIC results in the utilization of platelets, enhanced fibrinolytic activity, and the appearance of circulating fibrin degradation products (FDP), all of which contribute to the bleeding tendency that ensues.

Increased fibrinolytic activity has been recognized in dogs as a cause of excessive bleeding postoperatively or after trauma.

Inhibition of coagulation factors may be the result of antibodies directed against specific procoagulant proteins or due to interference (e.g. by heparin) with stages of the coagulation mechanism. The development of inhibitors has been reported with systemic lupus erythematosus and multiple myeloma in dogs.

Acquired thrombocytopenias can result from a variety of causes (*see* CANINE THROMBOCYTOPENIC PURPURA, p. 36) and the majority of these have an immunologic basis.

Acquired platelet function defects (acquired thrombopathias) are conditions in which platelet numbers may be normal but their function abnormal. Uremia results in reduced platelet adhesion, abnormal platelet aggregation to adenosine diphosphate and collagen, and a prolonged bleeding time.

Many drugs, such as aspirin, phenylbutazone, promazine derivatives and nitrofurantoin, interfere with normal platelet function and thus hemostatic plug formation. Other drugs that impair hemostasis include sulfonamides, penicillins, estrogens, phenothiazines, antihistamines, anti-inflammatory agents and plasma expanders. Qualitative platelet defects may also be associated with cirrhosis of the liver and leukemias. In some acquired platelet function defects, the platelet phospholipid (platelet factor 3) essential for normal blood coagulation is abnormal or is not released from the platelet.

Diagnosis: Depending on the nature of the hemostatic defect the commonest signs to be expected include persistent epistaxis or bleeding from the mouth or rectum, excessive bleeding after trauma or surgery, the appearance of hematomas, petechiation, recurrent shifting lameness or bleeding into body cavities.

Vessel wall abnormalities: Defects in the vessel wall are diagnosed by prolonged bleeding times in the absence of other defects in the hemostatic mechanism or obvious evidence of a ruptured aneurysm.

Blood coagulation abnormalities: Defects in the extrinsic coagulation mechanism can be detected using the one-stage prothrombin time (OSPT) test and the Russell's viper venom time (RVVT) test. Prothrombin deficiencies (warfarin, dicoumarol poisoning) produce a prolonged OSPT and RVVT. Uncomplicated factor VII deficiency produces a prolonged OSPT but normal RVVT.

Factors VIII, IX, XI and XII deficiencies can be detected by tests that measure the intrinsic coagulation mechanism, such as the whole blood clotting time in plain glass and siliconized glass, the thromboplastin generation time or the most commonly used, activated or nonactivated partial thromboplastin time. Screening tests such as the whole blood clotting time are relatively insensitive, however, and are prolonged only in the presence of severe or moderate defects. Specific assays for blood coagulation factors are necessary to determine the particular factor(s) that are deficient. The diagnosis of DIC is suggested by a mild to moderate thrombocytopenia with depletion of multiple clotting factors (particularly factors I, II, V and VIII); and evidence of increased fibrinolytic activity, particularly the presence of FDP. Many of the tests mentioned in this chapter are not usually conducted by the practitioner but can be done by veterinary or medical clinical laboratories. Advice should be sought regarding the laboratory samples and species-specific controls required as proper type, collection, and processing of the blood are critical.

Platelet abnormalities: An accurate platelet count should be done on fresh whole blood collected by clean venipuncture into EDTA or trisodium citrate anticoagulants, and not based solely on the indirect counting methods or observation of platelets in a stained smear. The whole blood clotting time, whole blood clot retraction and skin bleeding time are usually prolonged when the platelet count drops below 50,000 to 100,000/cu mm or 50 to 100 $\times$ 10^6/ml. In qualitative platelet defects, platelets and special tests such as the aggregation response of platelets to adenosine diphosphate, thrombin and collagen, and measures of platelet retention (adhesiveness) may be required. In qualitative platelet defects the skin bleeding time is prolonged but clot retraction varies from normal to delayed. Specific measurements of factor VIII procoagulant activity, factor VIII-related antigen and ristocetin-induced platelet aggregation are necessary for the definitive diagnosis of von Willebrand's disease.

Treatment: In external bleeding one can apply pressure bandages or applications of hemostatic sponge, topical thrombin (℞ 572) or epinephrine to help control hemorrhage. Lancing of superficial hematomas may result in hemorrhage that is difficult to control. To reduce the chance of sensitization to red-cell antigens and subsequent transfusion reactions, unmatched, untyped whole blood transfusions should be restricted to patients in which there is marked blood loss and signs of severe anemia.

In thrombocytopenia and thrombopathia, platelet-rich plasma

should be transfused where available equipment permits. Such plasma is obtained by slowly centrifuging freshly collected citrated blood in plastic containers (600 to 800 rpm or about 150× g for 8 to 10 min) or by more rapidly spinning the blood for a shorter period of time (1500 rpm or 300× g for 2 to 5 min).

In blood coagulation factor deficiencies, platelet-poor plasma (fresh citrated blood spun at 3,000 to 5,000 rpm or 700 to 1000× g for 15 to 20 min) may be used. Since many coagulation factors are labile (e.g. factor VIII), plasma should be prepared in sterile plastic containers and used as soon as possible. Alternatively most of the clotting factor activity of fresh plasma can be preserved for up to 12 months at −20° C or preferably at lower temperatures (−40 to −70° C) by freezing immediately after collection. Specific clotting factor concentrates are not yet commercially available for use in domestic animals.

Vitamin K_1 (℞ 574) is indicated in avitaminosis K, prothrombin-time abnormalities such as warfarin poisoning, and hepatic disease. It has little to no therapeutic value for other causes of bleeding. Ascorbic acid is useful for vascular purpuras and in some cases of liver disease. Steroids (℞ 147, 148, 154) are the medicaments of choice for thrombocytopenia and have also been used along with ACTH (℞ 136) to treat coagulation disorders and fibrinolytic states. Their efficacy in the latter 2 situations is questionable. Stilbestrol (℞ 166) may enhance capillary resistance but can have a paradoxic effect in certain species such as dogs by causing thrombocytopenia and thus increase bleeding.

Drugs known to interfere with platelet function are contraindicated or must be used with caution in animals with severe or moderate bleeding tendencies. The more commonly implicated drugs are mentioned on p. 40. Protamine sulfate (℞ 571) has been used to neutralize heparin in situations of heparin overdosage or heparinemia. Epsilon aminocaproic acid is useful to control primary fibrinolytic states but must be used with caution as it is contraindicated in cases of hyperfibrinolysis secondary to DIC. Heparin (℞ 675) in combination with antiplatelet drugs such as aspirin (℞ 613) and blood component replacement therapy, where indicated, is used to treat DIC.

Animals with severe hemostatic defects, particularly hemophiliacs, should receive drugs orally, subcut. or IV with a small gauge needle; IM injection may result in hematoma formation at the site of injection.

BLOOD GROUPS AND BLOOD TRANSFUSION

"Blood groups" as used here refers to genetically transmitted antigenic components of red-cell walls. Antigens believed to be products of allelic or closely linked genes are classified together in a blood-group system. Some of these systems are complex with many subgroups called **factors.** The blood-group systems are independent of each other and are transmitted, with few exceptions, as dominant characteristics. Each red-cell antigen is controlled by a pair of allelic genes, one of which is derived from each parent. Since the progeny of any mating can thus bear only those blood factors that were in either or both the parents, this forms the basis of **parentage exclusion testing** based on red-cell antigens. An individual will not have (iso) antibodies against any of the factors present on its own red cells but may have or be capable of developing antibodies against factors present on red cells of other individuals of the same or different species. In some species (man, sheep, cow, cat, pig and horse), so-called "naturally occurring" isoantibodies may occasionally be present in variable but significant titers. Only 20% of cats have naturally occurring isoagglutinins while less than 10% of randomly selected dogs have naturally occurring isoantibodies. Most isohemolysins in dogs are the result of previous blood transfusions. With random blood transfusion in the dog there is a 30% chance of isosensitization. In the horse, possibly in mink and rarely in swine, transplacental immunization of the female by fetal antigen inherited from the male, may occur. Isoimmunization may be the indirect result of some vaccinations, e.g. for anaplasmosis in cattle or viral enteritis in mink; the young are affected after ingesting antibodies with the colostrum. (*See also* IMMUNE MEDIATED ANEMIAS, p. 25.) The isoantibodies are globulins, usually of a gamma-G and -M type. They vary in their mode of action between species and against different factors within the same species. Most blood antibodies (to red-cell antigens) are agglutinins, but some are powerful hemolysins that fix complement (e.g. dog anti-A).

Blood Typing Tests: The sera used to identify blood groups are called typing reagents. These reagents are usually isoimmune but may be heteroimmune if produced in other species. Most blood-typing tests are carried out as saline hemagglutination systems but in some species such as cattle where the red cells do not aggregate readily, hemolysins are involved and complement is needed in the system. Simple direct agglutination tests in the horse may be unwise because of the tendency for horse erythrocytes to form rouleaux, giving false positive results. Other antibodies will act only in the serum or are enhanced by the addition of serum to the test system. Additional techniques such as treatment of red cells with papain, trypsin or dextran may be required to demonstrate specific red-cell antigens or serum antibodies. In these cases, the antibodies are termed "incomplete" as they will not cause agglutination in the usual saline hemagglutinating test. Although they attach to the red-cell antigen they are not able to make a direct connection between red cells. To detect an "incomplete" antibody on a red cell, a second antiserum is prepared (usually in rabbits) against the globulin of the species to be tested. This antiglobulin will then detect red cells that have an incomplete antibody bound to them by inducing agglutination (completing the bridge between red cells). This procedure is called the Coombs' test and is the basis for the diagnosis of autoimmune hemolytic anemia.

The Blood-Group Systems of Some Domestic Species: The table summarizes present knowledge on major blood groups in a number of species. In each case, the first character, a capital letter, is the name of the blood-group system. The figure immediately following, in parentheses, is the number of factors identified within each system. The genotypic alternatives exceed the number of factors because if only one factor is present per system, its presence or absence gives 2 alternatives.

SPECIES	SYSTEMS	FACTORS
Ox	12 reagents are isohemolysins	A(5), B(37), C(10), F-V(4), J(1), L(1), M(3), N(1), S(7), R-S(2), T(1), Z(2).
Sheep	7 reagents are isoagglutinins and lysins	A(3), B(52+), C(2), D(1), M(3), R-O(2), X(2).
Horse	9 reagents are isoagglutinins and lysins	A(4), C(1), D(6), K(1), P(3), Q(3), T(2), U(1), X(1).
Pig	16 reagents are iso- and heteroagglutinins	A(2), B(2), C(1), D(2), E(14), F(4), G(2), H(5), I(2), J(2), K(5), L(12), M(8), N(3), O(2), S(1).
Dog	7 reagents are isoagglutinins and lysins	A(2), B(1), C(1), D(1), F(1), Tr(1), He(1).
Cat	2 reagents are isoagglutinins	A(1), B(1).
Mink	5 reagents are isoagglutinins	A(3), C(1), D(1), E(1), G(1).

SPECIES	SYSTEMS	FACTORS
Rhesus monkey	6 reagents are isoagglutinins and lysins	G(4), H(2), I(2), J(1), K(1), L(1).
Rat	4 reagents are isoagglutinins	A(1), B(2), C-D(2), G(1).
Mouse (C57)	4 reagents are isoagglutinins	H_1(1), H_2(20), H_3(1), H_4(1).
Chicken	11	A(4), B(15), C(5), D(5), E(8), H(3), I(5), J(2), K(3), L(2), P(7).
Rabbit	5	Hb(2), Hc(2), He(1), Hg(3), Hh(1).

Applications of Blood-Group Typing: Blood-typing of bulls used in artificial breeding units is widely practiced. This procedure protects the pedigree of registered stock by allowing a "parentage exclusion" test. Since the dam is usually known, all blood factors in the calf that differ from hers must have been derived from the bull in question. All parentage testing is based on the principle of genetic exclusion by showing that an animal could not be the parent. Twin calves frequently have placental fusion that results in a mixing of blood types. If the calves are of opposite sex, the hormonal as well as blood stem-cell mixing usually results in a sterile or freemartin heifer and may, as well, cause sterility or reduced fertility in the male. An identical blood type indicates a 97% chance of placental fusion and sterility. The 3% discrepancy is the probability that calves of opposite sex would have inherited the same blood type. Parentage exclusion testing is now also being applied to swine, horses and dogs.

In a number of species, especially cattle and poultry, attempts to demonstrate that heritable traits in blood groups and serum proteins can be correlated with growth and production have been inconclusive. Blood groups may serve as markers for inheritance of certain biochemical characteristics, for example in sheep, the alleles of the "M" blood group that are inherited determine the potassium concentration in the red cells.

Blood Transfusion: In veterinary therapeutics the indications for blood transfusion are acute, and repeated transfusions are not often necessary. Consequently, an initial unmatched transfusion can generally be given to most species without serious risk. Repeated transfusions of the same unmatched blood are safe if given within 24 hours of the first transfusion. After 24 hours, significant titers of isoantibodies may have been produced so that repeated transfusions now lead to a serious reaction. Due to the diversity of blood groups in animal species, complete matching of donor and recipient blood is difficult; only an identical twin is a matched donor. For this reason, if blood is to be administered, an adequate volume should be given initially so that repeated transfusions are less likely to be required. Blood transfusions must be given with care as they have the potential of doing more harm than good. Whole blood transfusions are often the treatment of choice for severe hemorrhage; however many bleeding abnormalities can be more efficiently and safely treated by the administration of the required blood components, e.g. fresh or fresh-frozen plasma for prothrombin deficiencies.

The amount of blood to be given should be roughly calculated by considering the degree of anemia and the normal blood volume based on body weight. For practical purposes, a young calf or a thoroughbred horse will have 90 to 110 ml of blood per kg of body wt, dogs 80 to 100 ml/kg, cows 60 to 70 ml/kg and swine 40 to 60 ml/kg. The "tilt test" in man is a useful rule of thumb to estimate blood loss, and extrapolation to animals suggests that if inducing the animal to stand causes a sustained increased in pulse rate of 30 per minute there has been a 20 to 25% loss of blood volume. In acute hemorrhage, there will be a loss of blood volume and likely hypotension but no drop in packed-cell volume (PCV) for several hours until there has been a significant movement of fluid from the interstitial spaces into the vascular system. In these cases, dextran or plasma infusion may be sufficient to prevent shock. Acute loss of one third of the blood volume will cause shock, while a loss of one-third to two-thirds of the blood volume may be tolerated over a 24-hour period. If the bleeding has been of the latter type such as may follow dehorning or castration, whole blood is generally the treatment of choice. Species with a muscular contractile spleen (e.g. dog, horse) will tend to mask the degree of blood loss in acute hemorrhage for up to 12 hours. Great care should be exercised in restraining the severely anemic animal as forced exertion may be fatal.

In chronic anemias, the decision to give blood should be based on the marrow response and on the PCV. An animal with a PCV greater than 15 and a hemoglobin in excess of 5 gm need not be transfused if the drop in PCV was gradual and is arrested and if there is a strong peripheral reticulocytosis. Reticulocytes are not seen in the horse and evidence of increased marrow production should be based on an unward shift in the mean corpuscular volume (MCV), i.e. the presence of significant numbers of larger young cells. Large volumes of blood tend to delay erythropoiesis and thus hinder the recipient's response.

Blood for transfusion should be collected into a 3.8% citrate solution at the rate of 1 part anticoagulant to 9 parts blood. Suitable collecting bottles are 500-ml rubber-stoppered bottles containing 50 ml anticoagulant. The bottles are autoclaved, then the tops applied while the bottles are hot, which forms a vacuum on cooling. Commercial collection bottles containing acid citrate dextrose (ACD) should be used if blood is not to be used immediately. Even when stored at 4°C there is a progressive loss of red-cell enzyme in stored blood, which reduces the ability of these cells to carry oxygen. Therefore, fresh blood is most desirable for general use. All transfusions should be given slowly for the first 50 to 100 ml to check for signs of reaction (usually respiratory distress); blood should then be administered at 5 to 10 ml/min. Epinephrine should be available in case a reaction occurs.

Cross-matching of blood should always be carried out prior to blood transfusion in horses and in dogs if autoimmune hemolytic anemia is suspected. In the latter case, transfused cells will likely have a shortened life span and transfusion should only be considered if there is impending circulatory collapse and after glucocorticoids have been administered. The introduction of additional red cells may only increase the rate of red-cell destruction making the benefit of the transfusion transient and the hemolytic process worse. Massive hemolysis may be accompanied by abnormal bleeding due to disseminated intravascular coagulation. If typing is possible, canine blood for transfusion should be collected from A-negative donors (universal donors). Ideally this donor should also be Tr-negative.

Technique of Cross-Matching: 1. Collect anticoagulated blood and serum from donor and recipient. 2. Wash the red cells in 0.9% saline solution and prepare a 5 to 10% red-cell suspension. 3. Place equal volumes (2 drops) of donor's cells and recipient's serum in a test tube and mix (Major system). Mix recipient's cells with donor's serum in a second tube (Minor system). Mix donor's serum and cells and recipient's serum and cells and place in separate tubes for controls. 4. Leave tubes to incubate for 30 minutes then centrifuge for 1 minute at 1,000 rpm. The incubation should be done at room temperature, 4°C, and 37°C. 5. Examine tubes for hemolysis (slight hemolysis in dog cells is not specific). Shakes tubes against finger to resuspend cells; check for persistent red-cell agglutination. Transfer a drop of blood to a slide and check microscopically for agglutination. Significant hemolysis or agglutination in one or both of the cross matched tubes, but not in the controls, indicates incompatibility.

The above procedure can be simplified for use in detecting agglutinins by adding drops of the appropriate red cells and sera (minor and major crosses and controls) to glass slides, mixing with a rocking motion and examining for agglutination.

These slide and tube methods are adequate for detecting saline agglutinins but the antiglobulin test is required to detect incomplete antibodies.

EQUINE PURPURA HEMORRHAGICA

An acute, frequently fatal, noncontagious, apparently allergenic disease that is a clinical entity in the horse. The purpura is nonthrombocytopenic and as such, it differs from the idiopathic purpura of the dog and cow and from the isoimmune purpura of neonatal swine, but is similar to Henoch-Schönlein disease of man.

Etiology and Pathogenesis: The disease is a clinical syndrome that may have more than one cause. Characteristically it occurs as a sequela to upper respiratory *Streptococcus equi* ("Strangles") infection, following 1 to 3 weeks after the initial illness. Viruses are not felt to cause the disease directly but other pyogenic infections or bacterin injections (especially *S. equi*) may do so. The disease is likely a type of Arthus reaction and similar to "serum sickness." (*See* IMMUNE COMPLEX DISEASE, p. 10.) The pathogenesis is based upon antigen, presumably streptococcal protein, in continuous circulation. In recovery from the acute infection, antibody is produced that combines with the circulating antigen. Because initially the antigen is in excess, the immune aggregates formed are very small and therefore soluble, which allows them to continue in circulation. Complement is taken up by the antigen-antibody reaction and these soluble complexes cause vascular endothelial injury throughout the body with the resulting edema and purpura. Normally, antibody is in excess and the immune aggregates formed are large, insoluble and rapidly cleared from the circulation by the reticuloendothelial system without vascular injury.

Clinical Findings: Subcut. edema and petechiation of the visible mucous membranes of sudden onset are the characteristic signs. Urticarial wheals are often observed. The edema is most prominent around the head, eyes and lips. Dependent edema of the belly (1 to 3 in. thick) and legs is present. Edema is prominent in the viscera and is evidenced by pulmonary edema and occasionally diarrhea or colic due to hemorrhage and edema in the gut. There is neutrophilic leukocytosis with nearly normal platelet counts. Anemia occurs in severe cases, or hemoconcentration may occur if loss of plasma has exceeded loss of red cells. The blood clots normally and fibrinogen would be expected to remain at normal levels and complement levels should drop. Urine may be scanty and proteinuria has not been reported but should be expected. The disease lasts 1 to 2 weeks followed by recovery in about 50% of cases. Relapses are common as are secondary bacterial infections. Death may be rapid due to asphyxia, or due to anemia and toxemia of secondary infection in protracted cases.

Lesions: Marked edema is the most characteristic change while hemorrhages may be sparse or extensive. There may be edematous blockage of the airways of the head and patchy congestion and edema of both the respiratory and enteric canals. There is usually blood-tinged edema beneath the hepatic and renal capsules with some degree of ascites. There are commonly widely distributed focal lesions in skeletal muscles due to ischemia (pale) or hemorrhage (dark). Deep abscesses or pyogenic cellulitis due to the primary disease, often yielding *S. equi*, are frequently found.

Diagnosis: A history of recent pyogenic infection or immunization and the sudden appearance of angioneurotic edema and urticarial wheals that progress to extensive sharply demarcated dependent edema and edema of the head suggest the diagnosis. The purpura is usually more extensive than the petechiae of EIA (q.v., p. 343). In some cases, there may be no satisfactory history of precipitating disease.

Treatment: Since the disease is likely related to circulating bacterial protein, antibacterial therapy to clear the exciting antigen from the blood is indicated. Penicillin (℞ 63) with streptomycin (℞ 72), tetracycline (℞ 76), oxytetracycline (℞ 48) or triple sulfa (℞ 98) may be given. The antibiotics, but not the sulfas, may be given in dosage rates up to twice those indicated. Corticosteroids (℞ 142) may be indicated in those cases due to bacterin injections but must be accompanied by high levels of antibiotics. Tracheotomy may be necessary if asphyxia is imminent. Blood transfusion is indicated if the anemia is severe (hemoglobin < 5 gm and dropping). Bandaging of limbs is helpful and good nursing is indispensable.

LYMPHANGITIS OF HORSES

An inflammation of the lymph vessels and nodes, secondary to pyogenic cellulitis and usually affecting the pelvic limbs.

Etiology: This form of lymphangitis develops after infection by streptococci, less frequently by staphylococci or other pathogenic pyogens. Lack of regular exercise may be a contributing factor and the disease is observed more frequently in horses in good condition.

Clinical Findings: Signs develop one to several days after the infection becomes established. Commonly, systemic disturbance is observed with fever, anorexia, increased rate of pulse and respiration, leukocytosis, neutrophilia, increased sedimentation rate and slight icterus. Signs in the affected limb are those of a hot, spreading, painful, edematous swelling that may involve the entire limb. Severe lameness accompanies the swelling. Lymph ducts are visibly swollen, as are the regional lymph nodes. Exudation of serous fluid may occur at various areas, particularly at the hock and along the medial aspect of the thigh. Small vesicles or abscesses may develop in the skin, rupture and exude a serous or purulent fluid.

The course is acute or peracute. The swelling reaches maximal size in 2 to 4 days. If treatment is successful, the swelling gradually recedes over a period of days or weeks. Severe or untreated cases often become chronic with fibrosis and induration of the leg occurring. Recurrent attacks are not uncommon. Other conditions resembling this disease are ulcerative lymphangitis, North American blastomycosis, sporotrichosis, equine cryptococcosis, the early stages of purpura hemorrhagica and localized cellulitis of the area.

Treatment: Sulfonamides (℞ 96, 102) and antibiotics (℞ 63) are indicated and are most effective when used early in the course of the disease. Corticosteroids (℞ 142, 147, 154) may be useful but some danger attends their use unless the infection has been suppressed. Phenylbutazone (℞ 150) suppresses inflammation and pain. Diuretics, particularly furosemide (℞ 543), are of benefit in stimulating resorption of edematous fluids. Application of warm packs or warm water baths, especially along with a turbulator, will stimulate lymphatic and venous drainage and hasten the reduction of edema. Moderate exercise is indicated. Any vesicles or ulcers should be treated locally with antibiotic or antiseptic powders or ointments.

HEART DISEASE

Although heart disease is infrequently treated, except in the dog and cat, cardiac conditions often present diagnostic problems. Those aspects of cardiac disease that are of primary interest to clinicians are outlined in this chapter. Recommendations for therapy are limited to those conditions and species in which there has been substantial experience with treatment.

Examination and Diagnosis: A systematic examination is necessary in evaluating the state of the heart. The examination should include palpation of the cardiac region to detect thrills and cardiac displacement, prolonged careful auscultation in the standard areas of auscultation, percussion of the area of cardiac dullness, palpation of the arterial pulse and examination of the pulsations in the jugular vein. Roentgenologic examination of the cardiac silhouette for distortion and enlargement is an important diagnostic procedure in small animals. An electrocardiogram (ECG) should be obtained whenever feasible. In areas where heartworms may be encountered in the dog, the blood should be examined for microfilaria.

The first object of the examination should be to classify the animal with respect to the condition of its heart. Heart disease should be considered present only when a dependable sign is found, since many other conditions simulate true cardiac involvement.

In the dog, a diagnosis of heart disease should not be made unless at least one of the following dependable signs can be detected: (1) a Grade IV or greater systolic murmur (q.v., p. 52); (2) a Grade III systolic murmur in the absence of anemia; (3) a diastolic murmur; (4) a palpable precordial thrill; (5) generalized venous engorgement; (6) atrial fibrillation or flutter; (7) paroxysmal ventricular tachycardia; (8) atrial or ventricular extrasystoles consistently present and of frequent occurrence; (9) complete atrioventricular block; (10) left bundle branch block; (11) electrocardiographic right ventricular enlargement (*see* COR PULMONALE, p. 63) pattern; (12) roentgenologic evidence of gross heart enlargement, enlargement of one or more chambers, or pericardial effusion; (13) pronounced splitting of the second heart sound. Atrial fibrillation or flutter, complete atrioventricular block, pericardial friction rub, precordial thrills and generalized venous engorgement are reliable signs of cardiac disease in horses and in most other domestic species including the ox. Signs which are of controversial significance or questionable specificity include: infrequent ventricular extrasystoles, all arrhythmias and conduction disturbances disappearing after exercise, RS-T segment shifts, wandering pacemaker, diastolic murmur (a reliable sign in the dog), enlargement of the area of cardiac dullness. Diastolic and systolic murmurs are common in normal horses and in the absence of other signs cannot be considered reliable evidence of organic cardiac disease.

Since severe chronic or posthemorrhagic anemia can affect the heart unfavorably, one may consider this a sign of heart disease when the hemoglobin level is below 50% of normal.

The most common and obvious signs in animals with cardiac disease are: (1) systolic murmur, (2) dyspnea, (3) coughing, (4) pulmonary edema and ascites and (5) ease of fatigability or weakness, and, while highly suggestive of heart disease, a positive diagnosis should be made only after one or more of the dependable signs have been elicited, or other possibilities thoroughly eliminated. Rarely, in certain degenerative diseases of the myocardium, congestive heart failure may be present without abnormal heart sounds or diagnostic electrocardiographic changes.

HEART SOUNDS AND MURMURS

Normal heart sounds and variants: Four heart sounds are frequently audible in horses. The first (S_1) sound is associated with closure of the atrioventricular valves, the second (S_2) sound with closure of the semilunar valves and ventricular relaxation. The third (S_3) sound occurs in early diastole at the end of the period of rapid ventricular filling. The fourth (S_4) or atrial sound is related to atrial systole. While all these sounds may be heard, often only S_1 and S_2; S_1, S_2 and S_3; or S_4, S_1 and S_2 can be detected.

In **cattle** only S_1 and S_2 are ordinarily audible. Either S_3 or S_4 are sometimes heard, but less often than in horses. During the IV administration of calcium solutions in cattle with hypocalcemia, either S_4 or S_3 or both may be accentuated and become audible.

In the **dog**, only S_1 and S_2 are ordinarily heard. Inspiratory splitting of S_2 occurs, but the interval between the 2 components is usually too slight to be audible. Less commonly the first sound may be split.

The characteristics of heart sounds in other domestic mammals (e.g. goats, sheep, swine, cats) have received less study. In general only S_1 and S_2 are audible in these species.

Murmurs and other abnormal sounds: The following arbitrary classification of heart murmurs with respect to intensity is useful: Grade I—the murmur of lowest intensity that can be heard; Grade II—a faint murmur still audible after a few seconds auscultation; Grade III—a murmur that is immediately audible when auscultation begins; Grade IV—loudest murmur that is still inaudible when the stethoscope chest piece is just removed from the chest; Grade V—extremely loud murmur that can still be heard with the stethoscope just removed from the chest wall.

There are 2 general types of **systolic murmurs**, ejection and regurgitant. Ejection systolic murmurs are crescendo-decrescendo in intensity, with the greatest intensity during mid-systole. They are sometimes produced by stenosis of the semilunar valves, infundibular stenosis, dilation of the aorta or pulmonary artery or increased rate of flow through a semilunar valve orifice. Regurgitant systolic murmurs are pansystolic and frequently of constant intensity. They can be caused by mitral or tricuspid regurgitation, or by an interventricular septal defect. These abnormalities do not invariably produce murmurs that can be recognized as either ejection or regurgitant in type.

Diastolic murmurs fall in 3 general categories: (1) the arterial diastolic murmur of aortic and pulmonic insufficiency; (2) the passive atrioventricular diastolic murmur accompanying actual or relative atrioventricular valve stenosis; and (3) the atriosystolic or presystolic murmur associated with mitral or tricuspid stenosis.

Continuous or machinery murmurs may be present over arteriovenous fistulas as with patent ductus arteriosus (q.v., p. 71) that is present in animals at birth and is audible in foals, disappearing shortly after birth. This continuous murmur waxes and wanes in intensity with systole and diastole, being of greatest intensity during the second heart sound.

In horses, presystolic, early systolic and early diastolic murmurs are frequently audible in the absence of cardiovascular disease or anemia. The early systolic murmurs are most common and generally heard over the base of the heart (aortic and pulmonic auscultatory areas). A short, high-pitched, squeaking early diastolic murmur, greatest in intensity near the cardiac apex (mitral area), is not infrequently heard in healthy young horses.

Diastolic gallop rhythms: Triple, 3-beat or gallop rhythms resemble the cadence of a galloping horse. The "extra" sound is classified as an early diastolic (ventricular), presystolic (atrial) or summation gallop. These sounds represent abnormal accentuations of S_3 and S_4 in animals in which these sounds are normally inaudible. The early diastolic (ventricular gallop sound (exaggerated S_3) is associated, in the dog, with advanced myocardial disease and congestive heart failure. The presystolic (atrial) gallop sound (exaggerated S_4) becomes audible when the interval between atrial and ventricular systolic (P-R interval in the ECG) is prolonged. Summation gallop results from fusion of atrial and ventricular gallop sounds and may occur in congestive heart failure with tachycardia. All 3 of these gallop rhythms may be heard in normal horses and, rarely, in cattle. However, as in the smaller domestic species, they may have pathologic significance since accentuation of S_3 and S_4 in all species is favored by dilation of the heart.

Systolic click: Short, sharp, often transient sounds during systole are known to occur uncommonly in the dog and probably in other domestic species. They usually are single, but may be multiple; and may disappear completely in some cycles. Their clinical significance is uncertain, but they have been attributed to such extracardiac causes as tensing of the walls of a dilated aorta or pulmonary artery and pleuropericardial adhesions.

Splitting of the heart sounds: Audible splitting of either S_1 or S_2 may occur in the absence of other cardiac abnormality. S_1 may be markedly split when the contraction of the 2 ventricles is asynchronous, as in bundle branch block and certain ectopic ventricular beats.

S_2 may be split during inspiration in dogs and during either inspiration or expiration in horses. Abnormal splitting of S_2 is associated with pulmonary hypertension as in pulmonary emphysema of horses and heartworm infection of dogs. Other causes in dogs (and possibly in other species) include atrial septal defect, pulmonic stenosis, right bundle branch block, certain ventricular ectopic beats, aortic stenosis and left bundle branch block.

Triple rhythms: The various sounds that may produce triple rhythms may be summarized as follows: (a) physiologic: third heart sound in horses and cattle, fourth heart sound in horses and cattle, and summation gallop in horses during tachycardia; (b) abnormal: systolic click; (c) pathologic: diastolic ventricular gallop, diastolic atrial gallop, and diastolic summation gallop.

Splitting of S_1 or S_2 must be distinguished from triple rhythms in which 2 of the sounds are close together as in certain systolic clicks in dogs and when S_4 closely precedes S_1 in horses.

Synchronous diaphragmatic flutter: The diaphragm may contract synchronously with the heart to produce loud thumping noises on auscultation and usually visible contraction in the flank area. The syndrome results from stimulation of the phrenic nerve by atrial depolarization and occurs primarily where there is a marked electrolyte or acid-base imbalance. It is commonest in horses and occurs frequently in transit tetany (q.v., p. 518). It also occurs less commonly in association with gastrointestinal disease.

ARRHYTHMIAS

Disturbances in heart rate and rhythm arise when there is abnormality in the formation and propagation of the electrical impulse through the conducting system of the heart or when ectopic irritant foci discharge to assume pacemaker activity. They may occur from primary myocardial disease or secondary to increased or decreased myocardial irritability as the result of toxic, anoxic and drug effects or electrolyte imbalance. Arrhythmia may also occur as the result of normal variation in autonomic tone of the heart. Sinus arrhythmia in all species and second degree atrioventricular block in the horse may occur as normal physiologic variants. An electrocardiogram (ECG) is required for diagnosis and differentiation with most arrhythmias because antiarrhythmic therapy varies. Clinically the arrhythmias can be divided into those associated with relatively normal or slow heart rates and those associated with tachycardia. The former include sinus bradycardia, sinus arrest and sinoatrial block, atrioventricular block and premature contractions. In the horse, atrial fibrillation usually produces bradycardia whereas in other species it usually produces tachycardia. Fast heart rates occur with sinus tachycardia, atrial fibrillation and supraventricular and ventricular tachycardias. Pathologic tachycardias should always be suspected when the heart rate is elevated beyond that expected for the clinical condition of the animal.

Sinus bradycardia: This is a slow heart rate that may be normal in trained athletic animals at rest but also occurs in hypocalcemia and with syndromes of increased intracranial pressure in ruminants. Sinus arrhythmia may also be present—especially in the dog. Bradycardia may also occur with digitalis intoxication, hypoxia, hyperkalemia and adrenocortical insufficiency. Treatment is restricted to correction of the initiating cause.

Sinus arrhythmia: In this normal arrhythmia there is a variation in heart rhythm associated with variation in the intensity of vagal tone. The heart rate increases with inspiration and decreases with expiration. Sinus arrhythmia is most commonly detected in the normal resting dog. It is characterized by synchrony with respiration and by a normal and constant intensity of the heart sounds and arterial pulse. Sinus arrhythmia is abolished by influences that reduce vagal tone and increase heart rate such as excitement, exercise and the administration of atropine. Sinus arrhythmia may be associated with a wandering pacemaker and varying P-R interval on ECG recordings.

Sinus arrest and sinoatrial (S-A) block: In sinus arrest there is failure of generation of impulses at the S-A node, and with S-A block there is failure of propagation to the atrium. They cannot be clinically differentiated and are dealt with as a S-A block. The block may occur for one or more beats, there is no atrial or ventricular activity and consequently no heart sounds, arterial pulse or jugular pulsations. It may occur as the result of excessive vagal tone in all species, and reflex effects such as firm pressure on the eyeballs (oculocardiac reflex) and carotid sinus pressure may produce transient cardiac standstill in dogs. In the horse the occasional S-A block at resting heart rates and in the absence of P wave abnormality in the ECG can be considered a normal physiologic variant. Repetitive episodes involving consecutive beats and S-A block occurring at heart rates above resting normal, in all species is suggestive of myocardial disease. S-A block has been associated with syncope in Doberman pinschers and young boxers especially. If syncope is frequent, treatment with atropine (℞ 511) or isoproterenol (℞ 531) may be indicated.

Atrioventricular (A-V) block: There is impaired conduction between the atria and the ventricles. In first degree or incomplete A-V block the conduction time is increased and the diagnosis can only be made by demonstration of an increased P-R interval in the ECG. The occurrence of first degree heart block, in dogs and horses, is not necessarily indicative of myocardial disease. In second degree A-V block (incomplete block with dropped beats) occasional impulses fail to traverse the A-V node and atrial contraction is not followed by ventricular contraction. The block may occur at regular intervals or at random. During the block there is no first or second heart sound and no arterial pulse. In horses the sound associated with atrial contraction (S_4) is commonly heard and the occurrence of S_4 not followed by other heart sounds is diagnostic for second degree heart block. In all species, an atrial jugular wave may be observed during the block. Definitive diagnosis is by ECG. In third degree or complete heart block none of the impulses are conducted from the atria to the ventricles. The ventricular rhythm is established from an ectopic nodal or ventricular pacemaker that discharges at a slower rate than the S-A node and the atria and ventricles beat independently. The heart rate and pulse rate is regular but there is a pronounced bradycardia that is relatively unresponsive to factors such as exercise or excitement that usually increase heart rate. The difference between atrial and ventricular contraction rates produces variation in ventricular filling and some variation in the intensity of the first heart sound and arterial pulse amplitude. Periodically the atria contract when the ventricle is in systole resulting in cannon atrial waves in the jugular pulsations. In some animals the faster atrial contractions can be detected with a stethoscope.

The significance of the A-V block varies between species. Both first and second degree A-V block may be present without outward evidence of cardiac disease. First degree A-V block may result from excessive vagal tone and is generally not considered significant in the dog and horse unless other evidence of myocardial abnormality is present. In all species, second degree A-V block may be indicative of myocardial disease, and in the dog it is frequently the first indication of impending problems. However in the horse it occurs more commonly as the result of high vagal tone. It is detected at resting heart rates below 40 and like a S-A block may be induced or abolished by maneuvers that affect vagal tone. Complete A-V block is always abnormal in all species and its presence indicates a grave prognosis. It is frequently associated with syncopy especially with exercise or excitement and it generally results in cerebral damage from cerebral hypoxia due to the low cardiac output.

A-V block may be caused by primary myocardial disease or may be secondary to toxic, electrolytic or hypoxic influences on the myocardium. The treatment is primarily aimed at correcting the underlying cause. Complete heart block is usually associated with irreversible lesions. Antiarrhythmic therapy is generally restricted to animals with complete heart block and is aimed at increasing the slow heart rate using atropine (℞ 511) or isoproterenol (℞ 531). Drug therapy meets with limited success, and the only reliable treatment, when complete heart block is irreversible, is the installation of an electronic pacemaker. If A-V block develops during digitalis therapy, digitalis toxicity should be considered. Bundle branch block and the Wolff-Parkinson-White syndrome are rare conduction abnormalities. They have been observed in animals but can only be diagnosed by electrocardiography.

Premature beats: Premature beats or extrasystoles arise from irritant ectopic foci within the conducting tissue or myocardium. Atrial and ventricular extrasystoles may result from primary myocardial disease or occur secondary to toxic, anoxic or electrolyte effects on the heart. This arrhythmia is one of the more common irregularities observed in the presence of heart disease. Extrasystoles are always indicative of myocardial abnormality but there is some doubt of the clinical significance of the single extrasystole that is occasionally heard during examination in all species when there is no other evidence of heart disease. Occasional premature beats do not require specific antiarrhythmic therapy and treatment is directed at the correction of the underlying cause. Digitalis is indicated where extrasystoles are due to a failing myocardium. Tachycardias resulting from repetitive discharge may require specific antiarrhythmic therapy (℞ 538, 616). Digitalis toxicity should always be considered when extrasystoles develop during digitalis therapy.

Supraventricular tachycardias: The pacemaker activity may occur in the sinus node, atrium or atrioventricular node, and an ECG is required for differentiation. The heart rate and pulse rate are rapid but usually regular. **Sinus tachycardia** occurs normally with exercise or excitement but also occurs with fever, anemia, hyperthermia, toxemia, shock and other such influences that affect sinus activity. **Atrial and junctional tachycardias** occur in the presence of atrial myocardial disease. They are often paroxysmal in nature and characterized by periods of rapid, usually regular, contractions that start and stop suddenly. Syncope may occur. Frequently they are found in conjunction with premature atrial contractions and their most common association in the dog is with chronic mitral valvular fibrosis.

Supraventricular tachycardias may be terminated by factors that increase vagal tone such as carotid sinus pressure of the oculocardiac reflex. In refractory cases, the administration of vasopressors (℞ 535) or of propranolol (℞ 536) may be indicated. Digitalization is indicated where atrial hypertrophy or cardiac insufficiency is present.

Ventricular tachycardias: These arise from one or more ectopic pacemakers within the ventricular myocardium. When the discharge is considerably faster than that of the S-A node the ectopic pacemaker achieves dominance and the heart and pulse rate are fast but regular. When the ectopic pacemaker rate approximates that of the S-A node both pacemakers may influence the heart and there may be a gross irregularity in rhythm. There is marked variation in intensity of the heart sounds, of the apex beat and of the arterial pulse, and a pulse deficit may be present. Frequently the arrhythmia is paroxysmal. There are characteristic bizarre QRS complexes on the ECG. Ventricular tachycardias are evidence of serious myocardial disease. They occur with primary myocardial disease and are common in the terminal states of heart failure. They may also be induced by electrolyte imbalance and acute toxicities. There is usually severe dyspnea and weakness and syncope may be associated with paroxysmal attacks. Other signs of acute or chronic heart failure may be present. Ventricular tachycardias may progress to ventricular fibrillation and death. Intravenous lidocaine (℞ 616) may be used for immediate control of a life threatening tachyarrhythmia while blood levels of quinidine (℞ 538) are being established. Excitement of the patient should be avoided. In less severe situations oral quinidine alone may suffice. Other treatment is directed towards correction of the underlying cause (*see* MYOCARDIAL DISEASE, p. 63).

Atrial fibrillation: This is characterized by an irregular cardiac rhythm. Atrial depolarization and repolarization occur over numerous fronts and there is no coordinated atrial contraction. Stimulation of the A-V node occurs frequently but in a random fashion to result in a rapid and grossly irregular heart rate. The irregularity produces variation in the diastolic filling period between beats and consequently variation in the intensity of the heart sounds and the amplitude of the arterial pulse. With exceptionally short diastolic periods there is insufficient filling of the ventricles to produce an arterial pulse after ventricular contraction. At rapid heart rates this occurs sufficiently frequently to result in a pulse rate that is considerably lower than the heart rate (pulse deficit). Definitive diagnosis is by the ECG which shows P waves replaced by rapid f waves and an absolute irregularity in the R:R intervals. In dogs, atrial fibrillation is indicative of severe cardiovascular disease. It occurs in syndromes that produce atrial hypertrophy and is a common terminal finding in chronic mitral valve fibrosis. It also occurs in idiopathic cardiomyopathy and is more common in giant breeds. Dogs with atrial fibrillation seldom live longer than one year after the initial diagnosis. Treatment is with digitalis (℞ 526). The purpose is to reduce the heart rate to an acceptably efficient rate and to eliminate the pulse deficit if possible as well as to increase the efficiency of the myocardium. The maintenance dose needs to be adjusted according to the desired heart rate taking care to avoid toxicity. Conversion with quinidine is unlikely to meet with success and is seldom attempted. Electrical conversion is more successful but the long-term prognosis is poor due to the underlying and initiating cardiac disease.

In ruminants atrial fibrillation is frequently paroxysmal in association with alimentary tract disorders but it also may occur as a sequela to cor pulmonale or with cardiac disease.

In horses atrial fibrillation may occur in conjunction with other cardiac disease such as mitral insufficiency in which case it establishes as a tachyarrhythmia as in other species. It can also occur in the apparent absence of serious underlying cardiac disease and in horses with high vagal tone may establish as a bradycardia. There is gross irregularity of heart rhythm and variation in heart sound intensity and pulse amplitude but no pulse deficit. When the resting rate is between 26 and 48 beats/min there may be few signs of cardiac disability except with severe exercise. The heart rate will increase in response to moderate exercise. At very slow rates several seconds may elapse between some beats and there may be syncope. Atrial fibrillation occurs more commonly in draft and larger horses. It occurs in race horses in association with poor racing performance and may be paroxysmal. Atrial fibrillation with a low, resting heart rate is not incompatible with life but affected horses should not be used for riding. Conversion with quinidine (℞ 537) can be attempted and is often followed by a return to successful performance in racing animals. Greatest success occurs when conversion is attempted within a short period of the initial onset.

CARDIAC INSUFFICIENCY AND CARDIAC FAILURE

When cardiac or other disease results in a reduction in cardiac reserve the heart may be unable to meet the requirements of the body in all circumstances. When the reduction in reserve is such that the impairment of cardiac function only occurs under extremes of exercise a state of relative cardiac insufficiency exists. With increasing loss of reserve, increasing grades of severity occur and when the heart cannot fulfill its function in terms of the animal's day-to-day activity, cardiac failure exists. Cardiac insufficiency and failure may result from primary myocardial disease reducing the efficiency of myocardial function. It may also result from any factor that increases the work load on the heart and therefore decreases cardiac reserve. The common causes include diseases that produce a pressure load upon the heart such as stenosis of the outflow valves or pulmonary or systemic arterial hypertension and defects that result in an excess flow or volume load in the heart such as valvular insufficiency. Congenital cardiac or vascular defects with shunting of blood may also produce flow loads on areas of the heart. Less common causes of reduction of cardiac reserve and consequent cardiac insufficiency include disease producing disorders of filling such as pericardial effusions and stenosis of the atrioventricular valves, impairment of heart rate response in complete heart block, and reduction in artriovenous oxygen reserve in severe anemia. In all forms of chronic heart failure there is usually loss of coronary flow reserve resulting from cardiac hypertrophy or dilation. The failure of the heart to pump blood adequately results in an increase in end-diastolic volume and an increased venous pressure. Retention of sodium and water also occurs probably as a result of inadequate renal perfusion.

Clinically, cardiac failure can be recognized as left-sided, right-sided or generalized. As **left-sided failure** develops there is a decrease in exercise tolerance and dyspnea following exercise and excitement. Increased pulmonary venous pressure results initially in pulmonary and bronchial congestion. Coughing is a feature of the syndrome in dogs, occurring after exercise and especially at night. The cough is hacking and repetitive. Orthopnea with reluctance to lie down, restlessness at night and paroxysmal attacks of dyspnea are also common. With more severe failure pulmonary edema with severe dyspnea at rest and rales on auscultation will be evident.

Right-sided heart failure is manifest with systemic venous congestion. The jugular veins are engorged and support a column of blood much higher than normal and superficial veins are distended. The liver and spleen are enlarged and may be palpable in dogs. In cattle the liver may become palpable behind the right costal arch, and gross splenic and venous engorgement may be apparent on rectal examination in the horse. Fluid retention occurs in all species but the areas of occurrence vary. In dogs ascites is most common and usually occurs before the development of subcut. edema or hydrothorax or hydropericardium. In cats hydropericardium and hydrothorax are usually predominant.

In large animals subcut. dependent edema is more predominant. In cattle it occurs especially in the submandibular and brisket area, whereas in horses it tends to initiate in the preputial or mammary area. Ascites and hydrothorax also occur. Hydrothorax should be suspected when there is muffling of the heart and respiratory sounds in the ventral part of the thorax with a change in resonance on percussion. Hydropericardium produces muffling of the heart sounds and if severe will produce a defect in filling and low pulse pressure. Both may result in a low-amplitude ECG. The presence of ascites, hydrothorax or hydropericardium can be confirmed by radiography and by needle aspiration of fluid with subsequent fluid analysis. Disturbances in gastrointestinal function with diarrhea may also result from impaired venous drainage from the intestinal tract.

In generalized heart failure signs of both right- and left-sided failure occur.

The findings on auscultation vary depending on the initiating cause. Radiography is a considerable aid to diagnosis both in the detection of areas of cardiac hypertrophy or dilatation and in the detection of secondary changes such as pulmonary edema or hydropericardium. The ECG is of limited value except in the presence of arrhythmic heart disease where it is invaluable.

Treatment: A primary aim of therapy in congestive heart failure is to eliminate the edema. This may be done by decreasing the work of the heart (rest and restriction of exercise), reducing the sodium intake, increasing the sodium (and water) elimination through diuretics (℞ 542) and by bringing about cardiac compensation by means of digitalis glycosides (℞ 526).

In dogs, the diet may be regulated to decrease sodium intake. Suitable low-sodium diets are available commercially for dogs with congestive heart failure. In general, foods of animal origin contain much sodium and foods of vegetable origin contain little. Foods low in salt include fresh or frozen vegetables without salt, wheat-based cereals, polished and coated rice, dialyzed milk and soybean-oil meal. Meat, fish and poultry must be limited as should milk and milk-containing foods, although these foods often are tolerated as long as no salt is used in their preparation. Public water supplies usually do not contain much sodium, but well water may, and softened water nearly always is high in sodium. Distilled water is recommended if the sodium content of the water is unknown.

The use of diuretics to increase sodium (and water) elimination is important. In dogs, the most effective drugs are furosemide (℞ 543) and the chlorothiazide derivatives (℞ 542). Withdrawal of ascitic fluid by abdominocentesis is indicated only when the volume markedly interferes with breathing and then only to the extent necessary for comfort. Removal of ascitic fluid results in loss of protein, and the abdominal fluid will soon be replaced if cardiac compensation and diuresis are not brought about by appropriate medical therapy.

Digitalis glycosides slow the heart and increase the strength of myocardial contraction. While rest, sodium restriction and diuretics are useful adjuncts to the medical therapy of congestive heart failure, digitalis is always the primary therapeutic agent since it acts directly on the failing heart. Digitalization is seldom undertaken in animals other than the dog and cat. A number of digitalis glycosides are in current use, but evidence regarding their absorption, fate, and efficacy in various species is meager. The most complete studies have been made of the glycoside digoxin in the dog, and a desirable rate of absorption and excretion has been demonstrated. It is supplied in both oral and parenteral dosage forms (℞ 526).

Digitalization has been accomplished only when sufficient drug has been given to produce full therapeutic action. In general, the drug should be given until therapeutic levels are reached, as indicated by amelioration of the clinical signs of congestive heart failure, or until toxic signs become evident. The dosage calculated on a weight basis is effective in most animals, but the amount required to produce optimal effects in a given animal is not always predictable and the dosage must be governed by clinical results. Since most forms of heart disease in animals are chronic and progressive, digitalis therapy, once indicated, is usually continued indefinitely. Three methods of digitalization are employed, depending upon the urgency of therapy: They may be termed slow, rapid, and intensive digitalization.

Slow digitalization is used when signs of heart failure (right or left heart failure) develop gradually and are not severe. The animal is placed immediately on the oral maintenance dose without a prior loading dose. The incidence of toxic signs is low, and digitalization can usually be accomplished within 1 to 2 weeks. If no improvement is noted within 10 days, the dosage should be gradually increased.

Rapid digitalization is used when signs of congestive heart failure are more severe, and where close observation of the animal is possible during the process of digitalization. Using the oral form, the total digitalizing (loading) dose is calculated on the basis of body weight (℞ 526) and divided into 6 equal doses that are given at 8-hour intervals over a 48-hour period. The animal is then placed on a daily maintenance dose.

Intensive digitalization is used in extreme emergencies such as the acute pulmonary edema of severe left-heart failure. The loading dose is administered by the parenteral route (℞ 526). One-half of the calculated dose is given immediately by slow IV injection, followed by one-fourth of the dose in 6 hours and the final one-fourth dose 6 hours later. If a therapeutic effect is obtained, the animal may then be placed on the oral maintenance dose beginning 12 hours later. If a therapeutic effect does not occur, one-eighth of the calculated digitalizing dose is repeated at 6-hour intervals until a therapeutic effect is seen or evidence of toxicity occurs. A therapeutic effect is indicated by slowing of the heart rate, decreases in coughing and dyspnea in left-heart failure, a loss of ascitic fluid and subcut. edema in right-heart failure, and diuresis. In acute pulmonary edema bronchodilators (e.g. aminophylline, 10 mg/kg) may be useful.

Phlebotomy with the removal of 10 ml of blood per kilogram of body weight may prove life-saving in situations of acute terminal pulmonary edema but otherwise is seldom indicated.

Digitalis Toxicity: Since individual tolerance to digitalis glycosides varies widely, the patient should be observed carefully for signs of digitalis toxicity, particularly in the initial period of digitalization. Mild diarrhea is a common early sign of toxicity but does not necessitate discontinuation of the drug. Vomiting, depression, or the onset of cardiac arrhythmias, however, signal a need to discontinue digitalis therapy immediately. An increase in P-R interval and A-V block is the common arrhythmia developing with toxicity after oral therapy. Following rapid IV digitalization premature ventricular beats and multiple ventricular extrasystoles are more common. Rapid IV digitalization should always be monitored on the ECG. When toxicity occurs digitalis should be immediately withdrawn and 24 hours allowed for excretion of the drug and regression of toxic signs following which therapy can be reinstituted at a lower dosage level—usually 75% of that used before. Potassium deficiency will accentuate digitalis toxicity and concommitant diuretic therapy, steroid therapy or gastrointestinal disturbance may potentiate the hypokalaemia. Severe tachyarrhythmias associated with digitalis toxicity may require specific antiarrhythmic therapy (℞ 527, 616).

Acute heart failure occurs with ventricular fibrillation in electric shock and lightning stroke, in falling disease of cattle, nutritional cardiomyopathies and other myocardial diseases. Pathologic tachycardias both superventricular and ventricular in origin may lead to acute heart failure. Sudden pericardial tamponade occurs with atrial rupture in dogs and occasionally with traumatic pericarditis in cattle. Rupture of the chordae tendineae in dogs and the sinus of Valsalva in horses may produce acute heart failure. The acute failure of the heart to pump blood results in cerebral anoxia and acute massive pulmonary edema. Clinically the animal suddenly falls, it may thrash or bellow for a short period but rapidly loses consciousness. Death is accompanied by deep asphyxial gasps with an exaggerated inspiratory effort. Massive pulmonary congestion and edema are evident on postmortem examination.

Cor pulmonale is the name given to heart disease secondary to disordered pulmonary circulation. Pulmonary hypertension leads to right ventricular hypertrophy and dilation and in severe cases congestive heart failure may occur. Cor pulmonale may occur secondary to chronic pulmonary disease. It is common in goats following enzootic pneumonia and occurs in dogs most commonly in association with heartworm (*Dirofilaria immitus*). In cattle grazing at high altitudes pulmonary hypertension occurs in some individuals with consequent right-sided heart failure (*see* HIGH MOUNTAIN DISEASE, p. 525). Cor pulmonale also results from chronic obstructive lung disease or emphysema in horses. Cor pulmonale should be considered in the examination of any animal with respiratory disease and right-sided heart failure. Cardiac dilatation may be sufficient to result in tricuspid valve insufficiency.

THE PERICARDIUM AND ITS CONTENTS

The pericardium may be congenitally absent or only partially formed. Such abnormalities are usually of no clinical significance. Hydropericardium may occur in congestive heart failure and hydremia, e.g. in parasitism with associated anemia. Pericarditis with massive sanguineous effusion is a clinical entity which may occur in dogs. The clinical signs usually first noted by the owner are dyspnea, ease of fatigability and ascites. The diagnostic signs include muffled heart sounds, low electrocardiographic potentials and, on fluoroscopy, the cardiac silhouette is circular, greatly enlarged and cardiac pulsations cannot be easily discerned, or are absent. When the fluid is removed, it is found to resemble blood closely, but does not clot. It is bacteriologically sterile and its removal (in amounts up to 700 ml) results in dramatic alleviation of the clinical signs. The condition may recur, but it usually does not. Similar effusions are sometimes present owing to neoplasms within the pericardial sac (e.g. heart base tumors). In these cases removal of the fluid is merely palliative. Blood that clots may be withdrawn in cases of pericardial tamponade due to left atrial rupture or penetrating wounds. Pericarditis occurs in many infectious diseases in large animals but its occurrence is rarely detected. Clinical detection relies on muffling of heart sounds or the detection of pericardial friction rubs. If the pericardial effusion is marked there may be venous congestion and a poor pulse amplitude. Clinical pathologic examination of fluid aspirated from the pericardium is of great value in determining the cause. (*See also* TRAUMATIC RETICULOPERITONITIS, p. 138.)

THE MYOCARDIUM

Myocardial dysfunction may result from primary myocardial disease or may occur secondary to toxic influences or metabolic and electrolyte abnormalities. Degenerative changes may occur in lambs, calves and foals with white-muscle disease, in pigs with mulberry-heart disease and hepatosis dietetica, and in horses with paralytic myoglobinuria. They also occur in severe iron deficiency, copper deficiency and in toxicity associated with selenium, arsenic and injectable iron.

Myocarditis may accompany general bacterial, viral, parasitic and protozoal infections in all species. It is common in septicemic diseases and in pyemic infections in young animals. Significant myocarditis occurs with infection with encephalomyocarditis virus and with foot-and-mouth disease and blue-tongue virus in young animals. Myocarditis may also occur in equine infectious anemia, blackleg, hemorrhagic septicemia and pullorum disease.

Myocardial dysfunction is the cause of death in poisoning with sodium fluoroacetate (1080) and plants such as oleander, foxglove and phalaris. Myocardial dysfunction also occurs in acute toxemias, severe uremia, diabetic ketoacidosis, adrenocortical dysfunction and in other diseases with severe electrolyte imbalance, especially that involving potassium or calcium.

Myocardial infarction is rare in domestic animals, although occasionally observed on postmortem examination. In the dog, small foci of myocardial necrosis in various stages of resorption and scar formation are found in association with sclerotic narrowing of small intramyocardial arteries.

Many myocardial lesions, if extensive enough, will produce typical electrocardiographic changes, such as depression or elevation of the ST segment, depression of the T wave, increased duration of QRS, low voltage, abnormal notching of the QRS complex, and certain arrhythmias, such as atrial fibrillation, ventricular extrasystoles, paroxysmal ventricular tachycardia and atrioventricular block. Clinical diagnosis of myocarditis frequently is difficult or impossible in mild cases. The most frequent diagnostic signs of myocardial inflammation or degeneration are electrocardiographic changes listed above, tachycardia out of proportion to the increased temperature, arrhythmias and cardiac enlargement. Treatment is generally confined to correction or treatment of the initiating cause. Clinical chemistry may be an aid to diagnosis in electrolyte and metabolic disturbances. LDH isoenzymes may indicate myocardial damage. Where severe arrhythmia occurs specific antiarrhythmia therapy may be indicated (q.v., p. 54 et seq.).

Idiopathic cardiomyopathy characterized by multifocal areas of myocardial necrosis and fibrosis with mononuclear cell infiltration occurs in the dog and cat. The cause is still unknown although viral infections are suspect. In the dog it is most common in giant breeds and in males. The developing cardiomyopathy is generally not detected until signs of severe heart disease occur. There is usually atrial fibrillation or extrasystoles following left atrial hypertrophy. The onset is rapid and there is usually a history of a sudden onset of weight loss, exercise intolerance, dyspnea and abdominal distension. There is frequently a noticeable loss of muscling, especially along the back. Signs are associated with right- and left-sided congestive heart failure. There is frequently biventricular enlargement with dilatation of the valvular anulus to produce a pansystolic murmur of atrioventricular valve insufficiency. The prognosis is poor and affected dogs seldom live for more than a few months after onset. Treatment is with digitalis (℞ 526). Propranolol (℞ 536) may also be used where digitalis by itself is not fully effective in reducing the heart rate with atrial fibrillation.

In cats there is no age incidence but the disease is commoner in males. In young cats, endomyocarditis of unknown cause progresses to severe endomyocardial fibrosis in older cats with left ventricular hypertrophy, left atrial dilatation and finally cardiomegaly, with aortic and atrial thrombus formation. The disease is insidious and frequently no abnormality is observed until the onset of heart failure or embolic arterial occlusion. There may be a history of reduced appetite, lethargy, and dyspnea following exertion or of a mild and poorly defined lameness. Usually the cat is presented because of sudden onset of dyspnea or hind-leg locomotor difficulties or both. Dyspnea is both inspiratory and expiratory and results from left-sided heart failure. Pulmonary congestion, pulmonary edema and pleural effusion may be detected radiographically. The heart may be normal on auscultation but commonly there is a pansystolic murmur associated with dilation of the mitral valve anulus. An audible S_4 producing a gallop rhythm is frequently present. Radiographic and electrocardiographic examination show evidence of marked left atrial enlargement and sometimes left ventricular enlargement. Thromboembolic disease is common. Aortic occlusion if severe results in the sudden onset of posterior paresis or paralysis. There is severe pain with cold hind-limb extremities and tenseness of the gastrocnemius. The femoral pulse may be absent or variable between the hind limbs. Thromboembolism may involve other areas such as the renal arteries to produce renal infarcts or occasionally severe renal disease. The treatment of cardiomyopathy in cats is that for heart failure. Aortic emboli can be removed surgically but the value of doing so is debatable when compared to conservative medical therapy.

THE ENDOCARDIUM

Endocarditis, usually of bacterial origin, most commonly involves the endocardium of the valves. Mural endocarditis of the atria occurs in uremia in dogs, and acute mural endocarditis from other causes is occasionally seen postmortem but is rarely detected clinically. Valvular endocarditis usually requires a period of prolonged subclinical bacteremia to develop and is often secondary to conditions such as chronic pyemia, mastitis, metritis and prostatitis.

Streptococci, *Erysipelothrix rhusiopathiae* and *Corynebacterium pyogenes* are the organisms most commonly involved. In horses migrating strongyles may produce both mural and valvular endocarditis. The mitral, tricuspid and aortic valves may be affected in all species but rarely the pulmonary valve. In cattle the tricuspid valve is most frequently involved whereas in other species endocarditis of the aortic and mitral valve is more common. At all valves endocarditis results in insufficiency but occasionally stenosis and insufficiency occur together. Large vegetative lesions are common with endocarditis involving the atrioventricular valves. The clinical findings in endocarditis relate to those of chronic septicemia and embolism and to signs resulting primarily from the valvular abnormality. There is often a history of unthriftiness with periods of more severe malaise. The animal may be in poor condition with a rough coat. A low-grade fever is usually present but during more acute episodes high fever may occur. There may be evidence of chronic bacteremia and embolism. In cattle tenosynovitis and arthritis and evidence of renal infarction on urinalysis may be present. Signs relating to valvular damage depend upon the valve involved. With tricuspid valve insufficiency there is a loud pansystolic murmur most audible on the right side over the base of the heart.

There is usually a pronounced systolic jugular pulse and right-sided heart failure with generalized venous congestion may develop. Mitral valve endocarditis is associated with a pansystolic murmur most audible over the base of the heart on the left side and radiating dorsally. Signs of dyspnea and left-sided failure may develop. Aortic insufficiency produces a diastolic murmur most audible over the base of the heart on the left side. The arterial pulse has a high amplitude. Left-sided failure may develop. With acute bacterial endocarditis there is usually a pronounced leukocytosis. Blood culture should be attempted. The prognosis in endocarditis is poor especially where signs of congestive heart failure are present; it is rarely economic to treat this disease in farm animals. Prolonged antibacterial therapy is required to control the infection and where possible it should be based on sensitivity tests. Remission is common. Even when the infection is controlled there may be severe residual damage to the valve and continual treatment for cardiac insufficiency is usually necessary.

Chronic Valvular Fibrosis (Endocardiosis). Chronic fibrosis and nodular thickening of the atrioventricular valves with subsequent distortion and defective function is the commonest cause of cardiac disease in dogs. The mitral valve is usually more severely affected than the tricuspid valve and the lesion results in insufficiency. The cause is unknown. The onset of valvular fibrosis occurs relatively early in life and the associated systolic murmur may be detected incidentally during clinical examination for other reasons. In most cases the lesion produces no outward signs of abnormality until signs of cardiac insufficiency develop during middle age or later. The dog usually presents with a history of decreased exercise tolerance. There may be a history of coughing after exercise or excitement. Frequently there is a history of nocturnal coughing that keeps the owner awake. The cough is repetitive and hacking as if "something is caught in the throat." Less commonly abdominal distension, or acute pulmonary edema are the reasons for initial presentation. On examination there is a pansystolic murmur usually grade III or louder, associated with mitral or tricuspid insufficiency, or both, and associated signs of cardiac insufficiency. A third heart sound may be prominent in advanced cases. Radiographic evidence of left atrial and ventricular enlargement and pulmonary congestion or biventricular enlargement may be observed. There are no typical electrocardiographic changes but evidence of cardiac enlargement may be present. In advanced cases arrhythmias may be present. Left atrial enlargement and vascular lesions predispose to atrial premature beats which may progress to paroxysmal atrial tachycardia and atrial fibrillation. Ventricular premature beats occur at the advanced stages of heart failure. Untoward sequelae are left atrial rupture with pericardial tamponade and rupture of the chordae tendinae, both producing acute heart failure. Dogs with mild early cases may respond to salt restriction and diuretic therapy but digitalis is indicated for treatment and control in most cases (*see* CONGESTIVE HEART FAILURE, p. 59).

Chronic valvular fibrosis occurs much less commonly in other species but lesions on the atrioventricular valve occur in older horses and cattle to produce audible murmur and occasionally they result in clinical cardiac insufficiency.

Valvular blood cysts or hematomas are seen in up to 75% of young calves under 3 weeks of age. The atrioventricular valves are most commonly affected. These lesions are also seen in the young of other species and their significance is unknown.

Subendocardial hemorrhages are seen in septicemia and toxemia and are commonly observed in animals bled to death (e.g. slaughter by Jewish ritual).

CONGENITAL ANOMALIES OF THE CARDIOVASCULAR SYSTEM

In recent years, improved clinical methods and greater interest in heart disease have resulted in an increase in the number of cases of congenital heart disease recognized, especially in dogs. Certain of these can be corrected surgically. Those discussed below have been selected on the basis of their possible clinical significance in veterinary medicine and do not constitute a complete list.

I. Septal defects
  1. Interatrial septal defects
  2. Interventricular septal defects
II. Anomalies of the derivatives of the aortic arches
  1. Persistent ductus arteriosus
  2. Persistent right aortic arch
III. Pulmonic stenosis
IV. Aortic stenosis
V. Tetralogy of Fallot

In dogs the types of lesions seen, in approximate order of their frequency, are: patent ductus arteriosus, pulmonic stenosis, aortic stenosis, persistent right aortic arch, interventricular septal defect, atrial septal defect and tetralogy of Fallot. Cardiovascular malformations occur predominantly in purebred dogs, and certain specific anomalies are seen more often in certain breeds. This evidence, in addition to familial aggregations of affected dogs, indicates that genetic factors are of etiologic importance in that species. Genetic studies indicate that inheritance is complex (non-Mendelian). A prevalence rate as high as 0.7% of admissions has been recorded for dogs. The prevalence rate of congenital cardiac defects in cats is much lower. Malformations of the mitral-valve complex, dysplasia of the tricuspid valve, ventricular septal defect, aortic stenosis including supravalvular stenosis, persistent common atrioventricular canal, patent ductus arteriosus and tetralogy of Fallot are among the commonest defects in cats. In horses and cattle ventricular septal defects appear oftener than atrial septal defects; patent ductus arteriosus and tetralogy of Fallot also occur. Aortic stenosis has a heritable basis in pigs.

In mild conditions, such as small interatrial and interventricular septal defects and patent ductus arteriosus, the animals may reach an advanced age without outward signs of heart disease. When the condition is more serious, the newborn animal may show weakness, dyspnea, cyanosis and retarded growth. The most severely affected animals die in the early postnatal period. If the condition is not obvious soon after birth, signs of congestive heart failure may ensue at a later time, usually before maturity, but occasionally as late as at 5 to 7 years of age. The signs of congestive heart failure in a young or middle-aged animal suggests the possibility of an underlying congenital heart defect.

In some instances the early recognition of congenital heart disease may enable the pet owner to reclaim his investment, or the livestock producer to avoid attempting to raise an animal that is destined to die at an early age. Essentially complete surgical correction of certain defects, notably patent ductus arteriosus, pulmonic stenosis and persistent right aortic arch, is possible without extensive special equipment. Where equipment for extracorporeal circulation or hypothermia is available, correction of other malformations may be attempted.

Signs of congestive heart failure (systemic venous congestion, hepatomegaly, ascites, pulmonary congestion and edema) may occur when the underlying congenital malformation severely impairs cardiac function. Animals with such signs may show dramatic improvement when treated with rest, low-sodium diets, cardiac glycosides and diuretics. Unless the underlying defect is surgically corrected, the response is usually temporary and death eventually results from irreversible congestive heart failure.

In the dog, clinical criteria for the common malformations discussed here are well enough developed that a definitive diagnosis can often be made on the basis of physical, roentgenographic and electrocardiographic signs. When surgical correction is contemplated, or when more complex anomalies are encountered, it is often desirable to perform additional confirmatory studies such as angiocardiography and cardiac catheterization. The clinical features of specific congenital malformations in species other than the dog are not well known, and in them, an accurate diagnosis more often depends on such special studies.

SEPTAL DEFECTS

Atrial Septal Defects

The foramen ovale is an oblique opening in the interatrial septum normally allowing flow from the right atrium to the left atrium during intrauterine life. At birth, this opening is forced closed by the increase in left atrial pressure, which occurs at the onset of breathing. Anatomic closure of the foramen ovale occurs due to fibrosis during the postnatal period, and the foramen cannot reopen. This anatomic closure is complete within a week after birth in the dog, but may not be complete for some months in horses and cattle. Failure of the normal fibrotic reaction to occur results in a probe-patent foramen ovale. Although this may be considered to be an anatomic defect, it causes no functional abnormalities as long as left atrial pressure exceeds right atrial pressure. This "one way valve" may be reopened and allow right to left shunting of blood if right atrial pressure becomes abnormally elevated.

True atrial septal defects are consistently present openings in the interatrial septum. Defects of the septum secundum type are commonest and occur in the thin portion of the interatrial septum occupied by the foramen ovale. Septum primum atrial septal defects are situated low in the interatrial septum and usually involve the atrioventricular valves as well.

Functional Pathology: In the presence of a large atrial septal defect, blood passes from the left to the right atrium through the septal defect. This additional blood must be pumped as an extra load by the right side of the heart and in time causes a dilatation and hypertrophy of this portion of the heart. As a result of the greatly increased blood flow through the pulmonary system, pulmonary hypertension may ensue, followed by congestive heart failure. Usually, there is no shunting of unoxygenated blood into the systemic circulation. However, a slight cyanosis may appear indicating a reversed flow of blood from right to left atrium, particularly where pulmonary hypertension and congestive heart failure are present, or when a coexisting lesion such as pulmonic stenosis causes an increase in right atrial pressure.

Clinical Findings: A small patent foramen ovale may be present without producing detectable clinical signs. In large septal defects, dyspnea, palpitation and cyanosis may be observed. Usually, a harsh systolic murmur is noticed over the base of the heart. The second heart sound is increased in amplitude and may be split. The right ventricle and pulmonary outflow tract are enlarged. Increased pulmonary vascular markings may be evident in the thoracic radiographs.

Treatment: The atrial well technique may be used for surgical correction in dogs. Repair under direct vision is facilitated by heart-lung bypass.

INTERVENTRICULAR SEPTAL DEFECTS

These range in size from small openings of little functional importance to almost complete absence of the septum. Most of these defects occur in the upper membranous part of the interventricular septum. They may be combined with other congenital anomalies, such as patent ductus arteriosus, interatrial septal defects, pulmonic and aortic stenosis.

Functional Pathology: Small, interventricular septal defects transmit blood from the left to right ventricle with considerable force. However, the amount of blood passing through a small opening has little or no effect upon the general circulation.

In the presence of a large defect without pulmonic stenosis, direction of the shunt depends upon the relative resistance to flow through the intrapulmonary vascular bed as compared with that of the systemic vascular bed. In young animals, the resistance in the intrapulmonary vascular bed is lower than the resistance in the systemic circulation and the shunt is entirely from left to right. As a consequence, the load of the right ventricle is increased and leads to hypertrophy and dilatation of the right ventricle and pulmonary artery. Subsequently, the resistance to pulmonary blood flow may rise due to obliterative changes in the pulmonary vascular bed. In the earlier stages, when the pulmonary resistance reaches the level of the systemic resistance, there may be intermittent shunting in either direction, right-to-left or left-to-right, but later, when the pulmonary resistance has risen above the systemic level, the right-to-left shunt predominates and cyanosis usually appears.

Clinical Findings: An uncomplicated small septal defect often does not result in outward signs of heart disease. The physical signs, however, are usually distinctive and appear in the form of a holocystic, rather harsh murmur, frequently accompanied by a distinct thrill. The murmur and thrill are usually most pronounced in the right second to fourth intercostal spaces near the sternal margin. While the lesion itself may have little functional effect, there is the potential hazard of subacute bacterial endocarditis, which may develop along the margins of the septal defect. This complication has been reported most commonly in cattle. Radiographic evidence of right ventricular enlargement and increased pulmonary blood flow is present in defects of moderate to large size. Animals with a large septal defect and extensive occlusive lesions in the intrapulmonary vascular bed have pulmonary hypertension and a right-to-left shunt. They are cyanotic and show all the associated features of cyanotic congenital heart disease, such as fatigability, anorexia, weakness and dyspnea.

Treatment: The surgical correction of interventricular septal defect requires extracorporeal circulation or deep hypothermia. The defect is usually patched with a nonreactive plastic material. Small defects in which functional changes are minimal may not appreciably shorten life if left untreated, but there is an increased risk of bacterial endocarditis.

ANOMALIES OF THE DERIVATIVES OF THE AORTIC ARCHES

Among the embryonic aortic arches that persist in the normal mammal are the right and left third, the left fourth, and portions of the right and left sixth arches. The third pair of arches give rise to the carotid arteries. The left fourth remains as the definitive arch of the aorta, while the sixth arches give rise to the pulmonary artery, its branches, and the ductus arteriosus.

Persistent Ductus Arteriosus

During fetal life, an important communication exists between the aorta and the pulmonary artery. This connection is formed by the left sixth aortic arch and is known as the ductus arteriosus. Failure of the ductus arteriosus to close shortly after birth leads to an anomaly that is known as a persistent or patent ductus arteriosus. It is one of the commonest clinically recognized congenital cardiovascular anomalies of the dog. It may be combined with other cardiac anomalies. It is inherited as a polygenic defect in miniature and toy poodles.

Functional Pathology: Due to the existence of higher pressure in the aorta than in the pulmonary artery, a part of the arterial blood is pumped during the systole through the patent duct into the pulmonary system (left-to-right shunt). If pulmonary resistance remains low, there is increased flow through the lungs, left heart and ascending aorta, which constitute the path of the shunt. These structures dilate in response to the increased volume of blood they receive. If pulmonary vascular resistance is high, right ventricular hypertrophy and pulmonary hypertension are present, and a right-to-left shunt may occur through the ductus, sending venous blood to the descending aorta.

Clinical Findings: The so-called "machinery" murmur (*see* p. 52) is present during systole and diastole in the left-to-right shunt. The pulse usually is typical, quickly and strongly distending the artery (water hammer pulse). Electrocardiographic evidence of left ventricular hypertrophy may be present and thoracic radiographs show left atrial and ventricular enlargement, increased pulmonary vascular markings and dilatation of the ascending aorta.

When pulmonary hypertension with a right-to-left shunt is present, the machinery murmur is usually absent, there is accentuation and splitting of the second heart sound, and electrocardiographic and radiographic evidence of right ventricular hypertrophy. Secondary polycythemia is usually present.

Treatment: Ligation or complete surgical division of the persistent ductus arteriosus is recommended.

Persistent Right Aortic Arch

A right aortic arch represents a common vascular anomaly in dogs, in which the right fourth embryonic aortic arch persists, displacing the esophagus and trachea to the left. The trachea and esophagus are incarcerated in a vascular ring formed by the arch of the aorta on the right side, the pulmonary artery below, the base of the heart ventrally and the ligamentum arteriosum (or ductus arteriosus) dorsally and to the left.

Persistent right aortic arch is hereditary in the German shepherd dog. This anomaly has also been reported in cattle, horses and cats. Other anomalies of the aortic arch system may also result in vascular rings that partially or completely encircle the esophagus and trachea.

Functional Pathology: The vascular ring that encircles the esophagus and trachea may compress these organs with resultant dysphagia and regurgitation. A part of the esophagus cranial to the constriction is usually considerably dilated.

Clinical Findings: The clinical signs include dysphagia, regurgitation of food, and a reducible swelling in the caudoventral cervical region, owing to the dilated esophagus. The typical sign of regurgitation of solid food usually appears when puppies are 3 to 9 weeks old, although it may begin shortly after birth. Occasionally, the condition is discovered incidentally on postmortem examination. A barium swallow reveals dilatation of the esophagus cranial to the heart base.

Treatment: Relief of the constriction of the esophagus and trachea is obtained by surgical division of the ligamentum arteriosum (or ductus arteriosus). Some degree of dilatation of the precardiac esophagus usually remains after section of the vascular ring.

PULMONIC STENOSIS

In the dog, both valvular and subvalvular pulmonic stenosis have been described. In the former, the stenosis involves the valves only, while in the latter, the narrowing is in the outflow tract of the right ventricle below the pulmonic valve. Valvular pulmonic stenosis has been shown to be hereditary in beagles.

Functional Pathology: The primary functional disturbance is interference with emptying of the right ventricle. Right ventricular systolic pressure is elevated and there is right ventricular hypertrophy. The pulmonary arterial pressure is low or normal. Poststenotic dilatation of the pulmonary artery may occur, producing in advanced cases a rounded enlargement of the vessel resembling an aneurysm (poststenotic dilatation).

Clinical Findings: A harsh, crescendo-decrescendo systolic murmur, frequently accompanied by a thrill, is usually present with its point of maximal intensity located at the third or fourth left intercostal space, slightly below a horizontal line drawn through the point of the shoulder (pulmonic area). The cardiac silhouette shows enlargement of the right ventricular and atrial borders and poststenotic dilatation of the pulmonary artery may be visible. Electrocardiographically, there is usually marked deviation of the mean electrical axis to the right producing an ECG typical of right ventricular enlargement. It is impossible to differentiate between high subvalvular and valvular stenosis without the aid of angiocardiography.

Treatment: Pulmonary valvotomy is recommended for valvular stenosis. In the subvalvular type the infundibular ring is resected.

AORTIC STENOSIS

In the dog and pig, stenosis of the outflow tract of the left ventricle is a fairly common congenital cardiac lesion. It has been reported chiefly in boxers and German shepherd dogs, and has been shown to occur in familial aggregations in these 2 breeds, and in Newfoundlands. Little is known regarding its prevalence in other species. In most instances, the valves are not primarily involved, the narrowing occurring below them in the form of a fibrous ring (fibrous subaortic stenosis).

Functional Pathology: The chief disturbance is obstruction to emptying of the left ventricle with resultant left ventricular hypertrophy. There is often poststenotic dilatation of the ascending aorta.

Clinical Findings: In the dog, the systolic murmur of aortic stenosis is ordinarily located in the third or fourth left intercostal space and right second to third intercostal space. It may be well transmitted to the neck. Fainting and sudden death are not uncommon with this defect. Electrocardiographic evidence of left ventricular hypertrophy may be present, and arrhythmias and conduction disturbances are frequent. Radiographically, left ventricular enlargement and poststenotic dilatation of the aorta are prominent signs. Treatment is surgical.

TETRALOGY OF FALLOT

This complex malformation consists of pulmonic stenosis, usually of the subvalvular type, and ventricular septal defect with overriding aorta. Right ventricular hypertrophy is present. Tetralogy of Fallot has been reported a number of times in dogs, cattle, horses and cats. It is inherited in the keeshond breed.

Functional Pathology: The combination of pulmonic stenosis and ventricular septal defect is functionally similar to that of a large interventricular septal defect and pulmonary hypertension. Owing to the obstruction to outflow from the right ventricle, ventricular systolic pressure is elevated, resulting in a right-to-left shunt through the ventricular septal defect. The aorta, which partially overrides the septal defect, receives blood from both ventricles, while pulmonary blood flow is diminished. Mixing of arterial and venous blood results in cyanosis.

Clinical Findings: Cyanosis is usually present from birth, and is worsened by exercise, precipitating dyspnea, and often collapse. Polycythemia may be present, owing to chronic hypoxemia. Despite the marked disability that accompanies this defect, dogs have been known to live for a number of years before dying from congestive heart failure or embolic phenomena.

A loud, harsh systolic murmur is usually heard best in the pulmonic area and right second to third intercostal space, near the sternal margin. A thrill may be palpated in these areas. Right ventricular hypertrophy is indicated by marked right axis deviation in the ECG, accompanied by large S waves in the left precordial leads. Thoracic radiographs reveal right heart enlargement with normal diminished pulmonary vascular markings. The ascending aorta is usually dilated.

Treatment: The creation of an artificial ductus arteriosus (Blalock-Taussig shunt) may increase pulmonary blood flow and alleviate the cyanosis to some degree. Complete correction by relief of the pulmonary stenosis and closure of the ventricular septal defect is preferable, but requires open heart surgery.

THROMBOSIS, EMBOLISM, ANEURYSM

A **thrombus** is a blood clot still at its site of origin and accordingly may be classified as venous, arterial or cardiac (valvular or mural). Venous thrombosis is uncommon in animals. Thrombosis of the jugular veins or anterior vena cava can occur in large animals following IV administration of irritant drugs such as phenylbutazone or calcium salts. Thrombosis of the posterior vena cava occurs in association with hepatic abscessation. In dogs, heartworm disease may lead to venous and posterior vena caval thrombosis. Pulmonary embolism is a major secondary effect. Cardiac thrombi are usually associated with endocarditis. All or part of a thrombus may break off and be carried downstream as an **embolus** that lodges distally at a point of narrowing. An **aneurysm** is a saccular or cylindrical dilation due to weakness of a blood vessel wall. Aneurysms may form at the site of degenerative or inflammatory changes or because of partial rupture of the vessel wall. These changes may disrupt the endothelium as well, and cause overlying thrombus formation with subsequent formation of emboli. Although aneurysm, thrombosis and formation of emboli may be recognized simultaneously, distinct clinical syndromes involving mainly one or the other of these aspects are recognized in certain species.

The most common type of aneurysm occurs in the anterior mesenteric artery of horses as a result of arteritis caused by *Strongylus vulgaris* larval migration. Similar changes in the aorta and iliac arteries cause iliac thrombosis in some horses. Aneurysm of the thoracic aorta occurs in some dogs with esophageal granulomas caused by *Spirocera lupi*. Nonparasitic aneurysms are seen occasionally in all species. Rupture of dissecting aortic aneurysms (q.v., p. 1145) may cause significant losses in rapidly growing young turkeys.

Clinical Findings and Diagnosis: Aneurysms ordinarily do not cause clinical signs unless hemorrhage occurs or an associated thrombus develops. Except for aortic rupture in turkeys (with sudden death) and hemorrhage associated with guttural pouch mycosis in horses, spontaneous aneurysmal hemorrhage is rare and clinical signs usually are related to thrombosis. The signs vary according to the size and location of the thrombus and whether formation of emboli occurs. In some horses with verminous aneurysm and thrombosis, emboli become detached and partially or completely occlude terminal branches of the mesenteric arteries. Affected intestinal segments show changes ranging from passive congestion to hemorrhagic infarction. Clinical manifestations are those of colic, constipation or diarrhea. The colic is usually recurrent and attacks may be severe and prolonged. Paracentesis is an aid to diagnosis.

Aneurysms of the abdominal aorta and its branches may be felt by rectal examination as hard or elastic pulsating swellings. Fremitus may be present. In the case of excessive thrombus formation, the pulse distally may be delayed and have a slow rate of rise in pressure or may be absent.

Verminous thrombosis with or without aneurysm of the terminal aorta and proximal iliac arteries produces a characteristic syndrome in horses. Although they are normal at rest, graded exercise brings about an increasing severity of weakness of the hindlegs with unilateral or bilateral lameness, muscle tremor and sweating. Severely affected animals cannot endure exercise, they become lame and then fall or lie down. Following a short rest period, the signs disappear and the animal seems normal. Subnormal temperature of the affected limbs may be detectable along with decreased or absent arterial pulsations and delayed and diminished venous filling in the affected limbs.

A different syndrome occurs in cats as a result of aortic embolism. In most instances a primary cardiac disorder is present such as endocarditis or myocarditis with associated thrombus formation. When all or part of the thrombus breaks off, it lodges distally in the arterial system. Most often this occurs at the terminal aorta and typically there is sudden onset of posterior paralysis, severe pain and muscle spasm at rest. The hind limbs are cool, rectal temperature is subnormal and femoral pulses are absent. Apparently, vasospasm or other factors must play a significant role since ligation of the caudal aorta does not reproduce the syndrome.

In unclear cases or those in which surgery is contemplated, angiocardiography is helpful in confirming the diagnosis of aneurysm, thrombosis or embolism, and in providing an assessment of collateral circulation.

Thrombosis of the anterior vena cava will produce bilateral jugular engorgement without a jugular pulse. Edema of the submandibular area and brisket may occur. Thrombosis of the posterior vena cava produces a syndrome of respiratory distress due to pulmonary embolism and secondary pulmonary abscessation, with coughing, hyperpnea and occasionally severe anemia due to pulmonary hemorrhage.

Treatment: Surgical repair of certain types of aneurysm in a major vessel is technically feasible, but special experience is required. If the aneurysm is more distally located and there is adequate collateral circulation, the affected segment can be reached following appropriate ligations.

In horses an aneurysm rarely ruptures and the chief concern is with thrombosis and formation of emboli. The arteries commonly involved are not readily approachable from a surgical standpoint. Antibacterial treatment and anthelmintic dosing to kill the migrating larvae (℞ 264) is of considerable value in therapy. The most rational approach in the horse is the prevention and control of strongylosis (q.v., p. 695).

Aortic emboli in cats may be removed surgically; however, recurrent formation of emboli is common and most authorities recommend therapy only. This includes mainly fluid therapy to maintain hydration and blood pressure. Thrombolytic and anticoagulant drugs have not been sufficiently evaluated in cats or horses to justify therapeutic recommendations.

DEHYDRATION—FLUID AND ELECTROLYTE IMBALANCE

The term dehydration is usually used to describe a deficit of both water and electrolytes in the body. The exact physiologic nature of the water and electrolyte disorder in an individual animal is difficult to assess without extensive laboratory testing. The veterinarian can, however, rely on prior knowledge of the type of body fluid disturbance likely to be caused by a particular syndrome and take remedial measures accordingly, even without the benefit of laboratory tests.

Pure dehydration may arise either from a deficit of water intake, an increase in insensible losses, or a combination of both. A deficit of water intake often occurs in drought conditions, through neglect in stall-fed animals, or associated with disease conditions in which animals cannot drink. Increases in insensible losses often occur with fever, during heat stress, and in severe respiratory disease. The deficit of water is shared by all body compartments but efforts are made to maintain circulating volume at the expense of intracellular water which becomes more hypertonic. Intracellular hypertonicity may lead to a variety of adverse effects in the body such as respiratory paralysis if CNS cells are involved and marked decreases in the production of saliva in herbivores. Decreased salivation causes a reduction in food intake, thus adding nutritional deficit, but has the effect of prolonging life by sharply reducing overall fluid loss. The only clinical sign attributable only to dehydration is loss of elasticity of the skin.

Deficits of water plus electrolytes, particularly sodium deficits, are more immediately threatening to the survival of the animal, because sodium is the principle solute responsible for maintenance of plasma osmotic pressure and circulating volume. During starvation, the kidney can usually successfully conserve sodium and thus maintain circulating volume, but when excessive net losses of water and electrolytes occur, a more immediately life threatening form of dehydration occurs.

Vomiting causes excessive losses of water and electrolytes and may lead to life-threatening dehydration. If the vomiting is caused by high intestinal obstruction, losses of hydrochloric acid may lead to hypochloremic metabolic alkalosis in addition to losses of sodium and water. Metabolic acidosis is the more usual sequela to vomiting in the dog and cat, however, presumably because of decreased renal function that may be either the primary cause of vomiting or the result of the dehydration itself. High intestinal obstruction in ruminants often leads to dehydration and hypochloremic metabolic alkalosis because abomasal secretion accumulates in the forestomachs, a situation analogous to vomiting in monogastric species.

Diarrhea is another major cause of excessive water and electrolyte loss in animals. In addition to losses of sodium and water, bicarbonate is also lost in diarrheic feces and metabolic acidosis may result. Animals with functionally mature kidneys can compensate for seemingly large losses of water and electrolytes during diarrhea so long as a reasonably normal intake is maintained. If intake of water and food is in any way restricted, however, water and electrolyte dehydration rapidly ensues. Grain overload (q.v., p. 143) in cattle is an example of a condition characterized by severe dehydration due to the combined effects of complete anorexia (restricted intake) and severe diarrhea and accumulation of fluid in the static rumen (excessive loss). The dehydration may be further exacerbated if fever is a part of the clinical picture since excessive insensible losses are superimposed on water and electrolyte losses through diarrheic feces.

Renal losses of water and electrolytes can also lead to dehydration. During the polyuric phase of nephritis, sodium is lost with the excess urine output. This may lead to dehydration if vomiting occurs concurrently. In diabetes mellitus the osmotic polyuria due to the renal loss of glucose may cause significant water and electrolyte dehydration.

Treatment: Therapy for water deficits or water and electrolyte deficits can be either immediately life saving or supportive. Accurate diagnosis of the disease condition is essential since efforts must be made to interrupt the processes causing the excessive loss or deficient intake of fluids. If the process causing the loss is not amenable to therapy, fluid and electrolyte therapy may merely prolong survival. In conditions of water deprivation, particularly in ruminants, fluid administration is often in itself beneficial in promoting appetite and initiating recovery.

Before initiating fluid therapy consideration must be given to the composition, quantity and routes of losses of fluids in the patient and to the quantity and type of fluid and the route of administration most appropriate for the particular situation. The fluids that may be administered include plain water for oral administration, 5% glucose to provide water without electrolytes parenterally, isotonic (0.9%) saline solution, and a variety of formulations of electrolytes designed to correct specific imbalances.

The volumes of fluid to be administered must be adequate. The usual intake of a normal, healthy animal is approximately 40 mg/kg body wt per 24 hours. Any animal in which fluid and electrolyte deficits have arisen requires this minimal amount for normal hydration plus an increment for excessive losses. This increment in most instances can only be estimated. Up to 70 ml/kg (7% of body wt) may be administered over a 24-hour period.

The oral route of replacement should be chosen whenever this is permitted by the condition of the animal. If the route of loss is oral (vomiting), it is obvious that replacement by this route is contraindicated. Except in terminal uremia, the nephritic dog can be rehydrated orally with isotonic saline solutions. Newborn calves and pigs with diarrhea absorb orally administered isotonic solutions containing sodium and glucose or amino acids.

The IV route of administration is indicated in life-threatening situations (severe vomiting, diarrhea, impending circulatory failure). Rapid IV administration can, however, lead to congestion in the lungs, particularly in respiratory disease. Subcut. or IP administration can also be used effectively if circulation is adequate to ensure absorption.

SHOCK

A term used to describe a state of collapse characterized by an acute and progressive failure of blood flow to body tissues.

Etiology: The specific etiology of shock is unknown, but it occurs following many forms of serious stress, including severe trauma, cardiac failure, massive hemorrhage, burns, anesthesia, overwhelming infections, intestinal obstruction, anemia, dehydration, anaphylaxis and intoxication.

In the less severe forms of shock, the body compensates adequately by accelerating the heart and constricting peripheral vessels (both reflexly), thus preserving the "peripheral resistance" and blood flow to vital organs. When the shock is more severe, this compensation begins to fail and a vicious cycle appears. The poor circulation deprives the heart, the vasoconstrictor center and the vasoconstrictor smooth muscles of the necessary blood, hence the heart weakens, the peripheral vessels dilate, the blood flow is diminished, venous return to the heart declines, cardiac output is lowered still further and the body's ability to maintain its normal pH is reduced. As this sequence proceeds, a point is reached where, if treatment is delayed, the shock becomes irreversible and death soon follows. A number of explanations, on both nervous or humoral grounds, have been advanced for this syndrome; inapparent or underlying infection is doubtless important.

Clinical Findings: While the signs are variable depending on the cause, they include: apathy, prostration, rapid thready pulse, rapid respiration, thirst, low temperature and blood pressure, oliguria and hemoconcentration (except in hemorrhage).

Treatment: The prime goals in treatment are to restore blood volume and pressure, and to remove toxic factors particularly from bacteria. This can best be accomplished by infusions with colloids and buffered multiple electrolyte solutions (e.g. ℞ 588). In severe hemorrhage, the colloid should be in the form of blood; in other types of shock, plasma can be used. Plasma substitutes (e.g. gelatin, dextrans) may be used when neither blood nor plasma is available, but not as effectively, and some undesirable reactions have been seen, particularly interference with platelet activity.

It is generally recommended in the treatment of shock that buffered multiple electrolyte solution should form the bulk of the infused fluid—at least 3 parts electrolyte solution to one part blood. In severe hemorrhage, multiple electrolyte solution (MES) should be given rapidly in large volumes: up to 100 ml/kg can be given in 1 to 2 hours. The rate and amount can be monitored by central venous pressure and urine output. In other forms of shock, MES is given to correct any deficit (an amount equivalent to 5% to 10% of body wt is sufficient in mild to severe dehydration), and to supply normal maintenance requirements (40 to 60 ml/kg/day). Newer MES products containing gluconate and acetate as bicarbonate precursors are preferred to lactated Ringer's solution. The following additional measures should be taken: (1) Hemorrhage, if present, should be controlled. (2) Pain should be relieved, not only for the relief of the patient, but because it may aggravate the shock. Morphine (℞ 619) or meperidine (℞ 617) given IV are the most useful drugs for this purpose. (3) Antibiotics are of value in all cases of shock and should be given at once. The appropriate antibiotic to treat any infection that is present should be given, or a broad-spectrum antibiotic such as ampicillin may be used. (4) The corticosteroids (hydrocortisone, prednisone, dexamethasone) and ACTH are often helpful since they have the ability to combat stress (q.v., p. 603). In acute shock states, corticosteroids can be given early, in large doses, IV. (5) Oxygen therapy is useful. (6) Vasoconstrictor drugs, epinephrine (℞ 530), levarterenol (℞ 532), or pentylenetetrazole (℞ 665) should be given only when shock is characterized by vasodilation (as from spinal anesthesia). In other forms of shock, vessels are, in any case, constricted reflexly, and they then become weakened from anoxia; therefore, these drugs are contraindicated. (7) Vasodilator drugs such as phenoxybenzamine or chlorpromazine can be used cautiously to increase peripheral blood flow. Fluid therapy must be adequate and vigorous before these drugs can be used. (8) The body temperature should be maintained but not raised. "Keeping the patient warm" can be overdone to a point where it encourages vasodilation and thus operates to accentuate the shock syndrome. (9) Acidosis is an important feature of shock and should be combated. Mild to moderate acidosis is corrected by bicarbonate precursors in MES. Severe acidosis requires additional bicarbonate; 2 mEq/kg of sodium bicarbonate should be given IV, and up to 4 mEq/kg can be given over 24 hours.

Animals that require treatment for shock should be observed carefully for some time following apparent recovery, since serious relapses may occur.

CYCLIC NEUTROPENIA IN GRAY COLLIE DOGS

(Gray collie syndrome, Silver collie syndrome, Periodic myelodysplasia)

A rare and apparently heritable hematologic disease, characterized by cyclical recurrence of severe neutropenia, often associated with increased susceptibility to infection. Its heritability appears to be linked to coat color as it has been reported only in the gray collie, but whether all the lethal effects associated with this coat color can be attributed to the one disease is still to be determined.

Affected dogs are usually noted from 6 weeks to 6 months of age, and unless they are raised under close medical supervision, few live a full year. Both sexes are affected. Such dogs are smaller than their litter mates and commonly suffer repeated infections. During the 1- or 2-day neutropenic phases, which occur at about 10-day intervals, there is fever, anorexia, depression, weakness, arthralgia and sometimes gingivitis with shallow ulcers near the base of the teeth. During an episode the total white blood cell count may range from 5,000 to 7,000 cells/cu mm; no band neutrophils are seen and the total neutrophils may range from 38 to 500 cells/cu mm. Other signs include severe bilateral conjunctivitis and keratitis, vomiting and diarrhea, and commonly a terminal suppurative bronchopneumonia and pleuritis. Bone marrow biopsies indicate that there is a maturation defect early in the neutrophilic series.

Symptomatic and supportive therapy may extend the lives of such dogs, but obviously they should not be used for breeding purposes.

DIGESTIVE SYSTEM

APPETITE

Food intake: Appetite is determined by complex reflex mechanisms and is variable depending essentially on the caloric requirements of the individual, normal function of the hypothalamus and the quality, digestibility, energy content and palatabilily of the ration. The increased requirements of late pregnancy, lactation and repetitive muscular work result in increased food consumption. The food intake and productivity of grazing animals will vary according to the pasture plant species, its stage of growth and quality. The composition and the physical form of prepared rations have a marked influence on food intake (*see* nutrition section). There is considerable individual variation with respect to food intake. Many animals, fed to appetite, will overeat and become obese. This tendency is marked in certain individuals that are voracious or greedy. Others, although apparently healthy, are poor feeders and just maintain body condition under similar circumstances.

For economic reasons certain classes of farm livestock are kept under conditions of restricted food intake. When such animals are fed in groups, individual variations in appetite and in speed of food consumption coupled with the effect of dominance can result in marked variations in food consumption between members of the group. This variation can lead to problems associated either with excessive food intake, such as fermentation diarrhea in individual calves suckling "cafeteria" style, or to problems associated with severe food restriction, such as reproductive failure in individual sows group-fed on restricted rations during pregnancy.

Palatability: Palatability has a recognized, although ill-defined, effect on appetite. Certain feed constituents are more palatable than others and rations consequently vary in palatability. Substances such as molasses in livestock feeds and sucrose in piglet creep feeds are incorporated in an attempt to increase palatability. Moldy feeds generally cause a temporary reduction in appetite in all species, and the provision of frequent small amounts of fresh creep feed to piglets induces greater consumption in areas where hot and humid conditions may lead to rapid feed deterioration. There is undoubtedly a difference in palatability between various pastures and this may be sufficient to severely reduce food intake. This is one cause of the weaner "ill-thrift" syndrome that occurs in lambs grazing certain pasture species in the autumn months in the Southern Hemisphere.

Overindulgent pet owners sometimes encourage selective appetite in dogs and cats by catering to or developing their taste for certain foods. Frequently this can lead to gross nutritional imbalance and to deficiency disease such as osteodystrophia fibrosa in animals fed solely on lean meat and heart, and to osteodystrophies associated with excess vitamin A in adult cats fed solely on liver. If a conventional diet is offered, these animals may exhibit psychic anorexia. This can sometimes be overcome by withholding food for a day or 2 until true hunger develops.

Decrease or loss of appetite (inappetence; anorexia): A temporary decrease in appetite may result from fear, excitement, violent exercise or even scarcely apparent changes in the character of the diet. More prolonged inappetence can result from emotional disturbance such as that caused by the housing or yarding of pastured sheep—especially hill-breeds of sheep. Cats may refuse to eat for long periods when confined away from their home environment.

Voluntary restriction of food intake occurs during lactation in sows that were fed to appetite during pregnancy. Considerable weight loss may result. A voluntary restriction in food intake of fat ewes occurs in the terminal part of pregnancy and may initiate pregnancy toxemia.

Impairment of food intake may occur without loss of appetite. Local inflammatory lesions or wounds of the lips or oral structures, pharynx or esophagus may result in a lowered food intake because of pain during eating. Similarly, diseases that impair food intake either through their effect on nervous control (botulism, tetanus) or through their effect on muscles controlling these functions (white muscle disease) will produce a similar syndrome.

A degree of inappetence varying to frank anorexia is present with most disease states. The degree to which it is manifest, the speed of its onset and the selectivity of its loss are of some value in differential diagnosis. Inappetence may occur in such diverse conditions as specific amino acid or B-vitamin deficiencies and chronic infectious disease. A severe degree of inappetence is usually present with hepatic or renal disease and with any condition in which there is alimentary tract stasis, severe pain, high fever, toxemia or septicemia, and dementia or stupor.

Increased appetite (polyphagia): Increased appetite and thirst are seen in pancreatic fibrosis and diabetes mellitus in the dog although emaciation gradually develops. An increased appetite is sometimes seen in chronic malabsorptive states and may accompany certain pituitary tumors and hypothalamic dysfunctions. Helminth infections are said to be accompanied by increased food intake; however, inappetence is generally present in animals showing frank clinical signs of parasitism. An increase in appetite occurs following recovery from any disease in which inappetence has been manifest although this may be transient in remittent conditions such as equine infectious anemia. An increase in food intake above the normal occurs following periods of starvation or severe food restriction. Animals gaining access to palatable feeds, especially animals on restricted food intake, will grossly overfeed, and this may be followed by severe digestive disturbances such as rumen overload in the cow and acute gastric impaction in the horse.

Perverted or depraved appetite (pica): A craving for substances not ordinarily considered as food. The several species vary in their predilection for foreign material. Cattle ingest cloth, leather, pieces of metal, wood, stones and carcass material such as bone and hide. They may also lick larger objects and the sides of buildings. Horses may ingest dirt or sand or chew bones. The tendency for them to chew wooden objects is often merely a vice. Sheep may ingest dirt, bones and frequently wool; puppies frequently swallow sticks, bones, feces and grass, and adult dogs may acquire the vice of ingesting foreign objects. Such activities predispose to traumatic lesions within the mouth, alimentary tract obstruction and sand colics, botulism and poisoning with substances such as lead.

Pica most commonly is due to nutritional deficiency. It is classically associated with phosphorus deficiency; however, in all species it may occur with deficiency of protein, fiber, minerals and vitamins or salt. Boredom, especially in stabled animals, may lead to excessive licking and chewing, and on occasion apparent simple curiosity may result in the ingestion of foreign material. Pica may also accompany gastritis, pancreatic disease, rabies and gingivitis associated with teething. Psychic disturbances in pigs, dogs and cats may result in the savaging and even the ingestion of the newborn by the dam. Animals may show addiction to certain poisonous plants such as Darling pea and locoweed.

Treatment: A careful clinical examination and survey of the diet history is necessary to determine the cause of the altered appetite and to distinguish between the temporary alterations due to the nature of the food, environment, or the physiologic and psychic state of the animal, and those changes due to disease. It is essential that the cause of the altered appetite be determined since in most cases the appetite will not return to normal until the cause is corrected.

If the loss of appetite is complete, IV feeding with dextrose and protein hydrolysates or oral force feeding or both may be necessary. Liquids or semi-liquids can be pumped through a stomach tube in dogs, horses, cattle, sheep and swine. Cats may be intubated with a No. 8 or 10 soft rubber catheter. Care must be taken to avoid aspiration pneumonia, especially in recumbent animals.

During the convalescent period the return of appetite can often be hastened by offering highly palatable feeds. The administration of B-vitamins parenterally, or orally in the form of brewers' yeast, is occasionally beneficial in stimulating the appetite (℞ 623). Corticosteroids effectively increase the appetite in some cases and anabolic steroids are used by some for this purpose in dogs and in horses. Various substances such as strychnine, organic arsenicals and vitamins have traditionally been used to stimulate appetite, however their efficacy is open to some doubt. Rumen inoculation (q.v., p. 1506) may be useful in cattle where rumen atony is a factor in anorexia or where the administration of oral antibiotics has resulted in disturbances of the rumen flora.

In cases of pica the nutritional deficiency must be identified and corrected.

DENTAL DEVELOPMENT

One of the many criteria that should be considered in the estimation of age is the appearance of the teeth, but tooth development is subject to variation and dogmatic statements on the age of any individual animal should be avoided. The ages given in the tables of tooth eruption and wear are averages, which will be valid for most animals, but may be quite erroneous for any individual. The most valuable criterion is eruption, when the tooth breaks through the gum. To make use of this sign, one must know the deciduous and permanent dental formulas, the table of eruption and the difference in appearance between deciduous and permanent teeth.

DENTAL FORMULAS

	Deciduous	Permanent
Horse	$2\left(\text{Di}\frac{3}{3}\,\text{Dc}\frac{0}{0}\,\text{Dp}\frac{3}{3}\right) = 24$	$2\left(\text{I}\frac{3}{3}\,\text{C}\frac{1}{1}\,\text{P}\frac{3-4}{3}\,\text{M}\frac{3}{3}\right) = 40\text{-}42$
Ox Sheep Goat	$2\left(\text{Di}\frac{0}{3}\,\text{Dc}\frac{0}{1}\,\text{Dp}\frac{3}{3}\right) = 20$	$2\left(\text{I}\frac{0}{3}\,\text{C}\frac{0}{1}\,\text{P}\frac{3}{3}\,\text{M}\frac{3}{3}\right) = 32$
Swine	$2\left(\text{Di}\frac{3}{3}\,\text{Dc}\frac{1}{1}\,\text{Dp}\frac{3}{3}\right) = 28$	$2\left(\text{I}\frac{3}{3}\,\text{C}\frac{1}{1}\,\text{P}\frac{4}{4}\,\text{M}\frac{3}{3}\right) = 44$
Dog	$2\left(\text{Di}\frac{3}{3}\,\text{Dc}\frac{1}{1}\,\text{Dp}\frac{3}{3}\right) = 28$	$2\left(\text{I}\frac{3}{3}\,\text{C}\frac{1}{1}\,\text{P}\frac{4}{4}\,\text{M}\frac{2}{3}\right) = 42$
Cat	$2\left(\text{Di}\frac{3}{3}\,\text{Dc}\frac{1}{1}\,\text{Dp}\frac{3}{2}\right) = 26$	$2\left(\text{I}\frac{3}{3}\,\text{C}\frac{1}{1}\,\text{P}\frac{3}{2}\,\text{M}\frac{1}{1}\right) = 30$

Deciduous incisor teeth are distinctly smaller than those of the permanent set. In the horse, the deciduous incisor teeth have a distinct neck and lack the prominent central groove of the labial surface of the permanent incisor dentition.

ESTIMATION OF AGE BY THE WEAR OF THE TEETH

Horse: After eruption, it takes about 6 months for the tooth to grow out far enough to be in wear. When the entire occlusal (table) surface is in wear, the outer and inner enamel rings are completely separated by yellow dentin and the tooth is said to be level. Evidence derived from the eruption and leveling of the teeth should be given more weight than the signs given below.

The disappearance of the black cavity or cup in the infundibulum is much used in the estimation of age. It is not wholly reliable because it depends on the depth of the enamel infundibulum and the amount of cement in the bottom, both of which are variable. The cups are supposed to disappear from lower I 1, I 2, and I 3 at 6, 7 and 8 years, but this sign should be evaluated with the leveling of the teeth. For example, if the cup is gone from I 1, but I 3 is not yet in wear, the age probably is less than 5 years. The cups in the upper incisors are of little use in age estimation.

After the cup has disappeared, the bottom of the infundibulum remains, first as a long oval containing cement, then as a small round spot of enamel near the lingual side of the tooth. The enamel spot remains in the majority of horses through the 16th year.

The dental star is the darker dentin that fills the pulp cavity as the tooth wears. It appears first at 8 years as a dark-yellow transverse line in the dentin on the labial side of the infundibulum of I 1. As the enamel spot recedes toward the lingual side, the dental star becomes oval and moves to the middle of the occlusal surface. It reaches this position in all the lower incisors at 13. At 15, the dental stars are round. The star should not be confused with the enamel spot, which wears more slowly than the dentin and, therefore, remains elevated.

The shape of the occlusal surface changes as the tooth is worn down. At first, it is a long oval with the long diameter transverse. Then the lingual side becomes much more strongly curved, the 2 diameters become equal and the tooth is said to be round. At a later stage, the tooth is triangular with the apex toward the tongue. Finally, the tooth appears compressed from side to side with the long diameter sagittal. This final stage has been called biangular. The transitional forms are hard to classify and I 3 does not follow the pattern very closely. Consequently, the times of change given in the literature vary with the investigator. It is agreed that I 1 and I 2 become round at 9 and 10, and triangular by 16 and 17.

The so-called 7-year hook is the result of the failure of the lower I 3 to wear all of the occlusal surface of the upper I 3. An overhang is left at the back of the upper tooth. This hook is supposed to appear at 7, wear off at 9 and appear again at 11.

Galvayne's groove is a longitudinal groove in the labial surface of upper I 3. It is located midway in the length of the tooth so that at first it is concealed in the alveolus, then gradually emerges from under the gum as the tooth grows out, and finally disappears as the ungrooved proximal part of the tooth comes into view. The cement in the groove remains as a dark line, while that on the rest of the tooth is worn off to expose the white enamel. According to Galvayne, the groove appears at the gum line at 10, extends halfway down the tooth at 15, reaches the occlusal surface at 20 and disappears by 30. The groove is of little value as a single indicator of age. If it is present, the horse probably is over 10. The length of the groove or the absence of it can only be used in conjunction with other signs.

There are 3 other general indications of age. The angle formed by the upper and lower incisors, when the teeth are viewed in profile, becomes more acute with age. From the front, they are seen to diverge from the median plane in a young horse and to converge in an old one. The arcade of the incisors, when seen from the occlusal surface, is a half-circle in the young horse and a straight line in the old.

The more useful signs are arranged chronologically in the following list:

5 YEARS: I 1 and I 2 level, labial border of I 3 in wear.
6 YEARS: Cup gone from I 1.
7 YEARS: All lower incisors level. Cup gone from I 2. Hook in upper I 3. Cement has worn off, changing the color from yellow to bluish white.
8 YEARS: Dental star appears in I 1. Cup gone from I 3.
9 YEARS: I 1 round.
10 YEARS: I 2 round. The distal end of Galvayne's groove emerges from the gum on upper I 3.
13 YEARS: The enamel spot is small and round in the lower incisors. The dental stars are in the middle of the table surfaces.
15 YEARS: Dental stars round, dark and distinct. Galvayne's groove halfway down.
16 YEARS: I 1 triangular.
17 YEARS: I 2 triangular. Enamel spots gone from lower incisors.

Ox: As in the horse, the signs of wear are much less reliable than eruption for the estimation of age.

5 YEARS: All incisors are in wear. The occlusal surface of I 1 is beginning to become level; that is, the ridges on the lingual surface of the tooth are wearing out and the corresponding border of the occlusal surface is becoming a smooth curve instead of a zigzag line.
6 YEARS: I 1 is leveled and the neck has emerged from the gum.
7 YEARS: I 2 is leveled and the neck is visible.
8 YEARS: I 3 is leveled and the neck is visible. I 4 may be level.
9 YEARS: C is leveled and the neck is visible.

Dog: The data given below were found reliable in about 90% of large dogs. Small dogs and dogs with undershot or overshot jaws give misleading results.

1½ YEARS: Cusps worn off lower I 1.
2½ YEARS: Cusps worn off lower I 2.
3½ YEARS: Cusps worn off upper I 1.
4½ YEARS: Cusps worn off upper I 2.
5 YEARS: Cusps of lower I 3 slightly worn. Occlusal surface of lower I 1 and I 2 rectangular. Slight wear of canines.
6 YEARS: Cusps worn off lower I 3. Canines worn blunt. Lower canine shows impression of upper I 3.
7 YEARS: Lower I 1 worn down to root so that occlusal surface is elliptical with the long axis sagittal.
8 YEARS: Occlusal surface of lower I 1 is inclined forward.
10 YEARS: Lower I 2 and upper I 1 have elliptical occlusal surfaces.
12 YEARS: Incisors begin to fall out.

LARGE-ANIMAL DENTISTRY

Of the large domestic animals, the horse is most frequently affected by dental irregularities and disease. In other species lesions

ERUPTION OF THE TEETH

	Horse	Ox	Sheep, Goat	Swine	Dog	Cat
Di 1	Birth to 1 week	Before birth	Birth to 1 week	2-4 weeks	4-5 weeks	2-3 weeks
Di 2	4-6 weeks	Before birth	1-2 weeks	6-12 weeks	4-5 weeks	3-4 weeks
Di 3	6-9 months	Birth to 1 week	2-3 weeks	Before birth	5-6 weeks	3-4 weeks
I 1	2½ years	1½-2 years	1-1½ years	1 year	2-5 months	3½-4 months
I 2	3½ years	2-2½ years	1½-2 years	16-20 months	2-5 months	3½-4 months
I 3	4½ years	3 years	2½-3 years	8-10 months	4-5 months	4-4½ months
Dc	Does not erupt	*Birth to 2 weeks	*3-4 weeks	Before birth	3-4 weeks	3-4 weeks
C	4-5 years	*3½-4 years	*3-4 years	6-10 months	5-6 months	5 months
Dp 2	Birth to 2 weeks	Birth to 3 weeks	Birth to 4 weeks	5-7 weeks	4-6 weeks	Upper: 2 months Lower: none
Dp 3	Birth to 2 weeks	Birth to 3 weeks	Birth to 4 weeks	1-4 weeks	4-6 weeks	4-5 weeks
Dp 4	Birth to 2 weeks	Birth to 3 weeks	Birth to 4 weeks	1-4 weeks	6-8 weeks	4-6 weeks
P 1	5-6 months (wolf tooth)	None	None	5 months	4-5 months	None
P 2	2½ years	2-2½ years	1½-2 years	12-15 months	5-6 months	Upper: 4½-5 mo. Lower: none
P 3	3 years	1½-2½ years	1½-2 years	12-15 months	5-6 months	5-6 months
P 4	4 years	2½-3 years	1½-2 years	12-15 months	4-5 months	5-6 months
M 1	9-12 months	5-6 months	3-5 months	4-6 months	5-6 months	4-5 months
M 2	2 years	1-1½ years	9-12 months	8-12 months	6-7 months	None
M 3	3½-4 years	2-2½ years	1½-2 years	18-20 months	6-7 months	None

* The canine tooth of domestic ruminants has commonly been accounted a fourth incisor.

can and do occur as follows: In **sheep** the 2 main problems are: a) dental attrition (rapid and excessive wear of the teeth) and b) alveolar periostitis. The former condition is most commonly encountered in sheep raised on semi-arid or sandy areas. It may also occur in calcium-deficient pastures. The signs are those of inefficient prehension and mastication leading to poor feed utilization and unthriftiness, especially in ewes 5 years of age or older. Farm-fed sheep have a productive life about 2 years longer than that of range-fed animals. Other than the incorporation of 10% ground limestone into the diet, little can be done to alter the progress of the condition. The cause and signs of ovine alveolar periostitis are basically the same as described for the horse. In **pigs** dental disease is usually secondary to some condition such as mandibular abscess. Treatment is usually uneconomic and the affected animal is marketed. The primary cause of dental problems in **cattle** is usually actinomycosis (q.v., p. 442), which leads to alveolar periostitis and slackening and loss of the affected molar teeth.

Signs of Dental Disease: This section is devoted mainly to a consideration of equine dentistry, although in many cases the remarks also apply to cattle and to a lesser extent, sheep.

Foreign bodies may occasionally become wedged between the dental arcades or lodged in the soft tissues of the mouth cavity, causing irritation, discomfort and excessive salivation. Examination of the oral cavity reveals their presence and dictates the method of removal. *The possible presence of rabies should be kept in mind.*

Dental troubles affect the rate of mastication. During the chewing process, the horse may stop for a few moments, then start again. Sometimes the head is held to one side as if the animal were in pain. Occasionally "quidding," in which the horse picks up its food, forms it into a bolus and then lets it fall from the mouth after partially chewing it, is seen. The semi-chewed mass, instead of being dropped, may become packed between the teeth and cheeks. In some instances, to avoid using a painful tooth, a horse may bolt its food, with indigestion and colic as a frequent result. Unmasticated grain may be noticed in the feces; however, this sign may indicate nothing more than a greedy feeder. Other signs include: excessive salivation; blood-tinged mucus from the mouth, usually caused by sharp teeth lacerating the buccal mucosa; fetid breath; swelling of the face or jaw; lack of desire to eat any hard grain; loss of condition; and loss of coat luster.

CONGENITAL IRREGULARITIES OR ABNORMALITIES IN DEVELOPMENT

Abnormal number of teeth: It is rare to encounter a reduction in the number of teeth in the horse. Supernumerary teeth occasionally are encountered in the incisor or molar regions. Only if they cause mechanical interference with mastication or are irritated by the presence of the bit, is surgical removal indicated. For the same reason the removal of wolf teeth is recommended. They may require periodic rasping or trimming to prevent damage to neighboring soft tissues.

Irregularities of development or shedding of the teeth: The eruption of temporary teeth may cause trouble that is transitory. Sometimes the temporary teeth are shed prematurely leaving a depression of the gum surrounded by an inflamed margin. They may cause a temporary loss of condition resulting from the discomfort of eating. In the case of the premolar teeth, the root of the temporary tooth may be absorbed, but the crown persists as a covering or "cap" to the erupting permanent tooth; these caps are readily removed with forceps, if they have not separated spontaneously.

Abnormalities in position and direction of individual teeth: This condition may be encountered in the incisor region. Some of these teeth may be rotated on the long axis, or may overlap adjacent teeth.

Imperfect apposition of the teeth: (a) **Parrot mouth** (overshot jaw), where the upper jaw overhangs the lower jaw, results in imperfect apposition of the teeth of the upper and lower incisors. (b) **Sow mouth** (undershot jaw, prominent chin, bulldog jaw) is the opposite of parrot mouth; it is less common in horses. If a foal is badly affected, sucking is an impossibility. Treatment, where feasible, in both parrot and sow mouth consists of rasping or shearing the offending points and projections. It should be noted that it is possible for the molar arcades to have anterior and posterior projections without parrot or sow mouth.

Ectopic teeth: The best example of this is the dentigerous cyst or so called temporal odontoma, which most commonly is located in the mastoid process of the petrous temporal bone and is recognized by the presence of a discharging sinus along the edge of the pinna. The only treatment is surgical removal of the teratomatous mass of dental tissue and the associated secretory membrane.

IRREGULARITIES OF WEAR

Irregularities are common in the molar teeth of mature or old horses.

Sharp teeth: This is the commonest dental "disease" in the horse and is characterized by the presence of sharp edges or points on the cheek teeth. The outer or buccal margin of the upper arcade and the inner or lingual margin of the lower arcade are affected. In severe cases, lacerations are seen on the buccal and lingual mucosa. Treatment consists of rasping or cutting the long projections. The aim is to remove the offending edges only.

Shear mouth: This can be considered an extreme form of sharp teeth with an exaggerated obliquity of the molar tables. It usually is seen in old horses and may involve 2 or more opposing teeth but may be encountered in all arcades. Treatment is not very satisfactory, but rasping or shearing is necessary in an attempt to restore as near normal alignment as possible.

Wave mouth: Due to uneven wear of the teeth, a wave-like condition occurs on the molar arcades. Treatment is not very successful despite the removal of the offending wave.

Step mouth (step-formed tables): In this condition, there is a sudden variation in the height of adjacent molars. It may be caused by the loss or extraction of a tooth from the opposite arcade, or a fracture through the mandible. Clinical signs are the same as those caused by dental trouble in general. Cutters are necessary to remove the elongations. The float should be used after shearing affected teeth.

Smooth mouth: In this condition, the tables become smooth either through the crown being worn down to the root or through a defect in the tooth substance. Clinical signs are not of pain or inability to masticate, but the results of improper mastication, e.g. colic attacks and general unthriftiness. It is most commonly seen in the older horse, but may occur in young animals. Treatment is unsatisfactory. Feeding mashes or chopped feed will allow time for the different dental tissues to become uneven in wear, but the condition probably will recur.

ALTERATIONS IN THE SUBSTANCE OF THE TEETH

Fractures or fissures of the teeth: The incisors sometimes are affected as a result of trauma sustained in accidents. In the case of the cheek teeth, fracture usually is caused by the horse closing the jaws on some unexpected hard substance, such as a stone or piece of metal. Cows rarely fracture a molar tooth in this way since the object is swallowed immediately after being picked up. The fourth cheek tooth, which bears the brunt of the chewing process, is most commonly affected. If the fracture extends to the root, alveolar periostitis will result.

Treatment consists of removing any obvious spicules and smoothing the remaining roughened edge. If the fracture involves the root, the tooth must be extracted.

ALVEOLAR PERIOSTITIS

(Periodontal disease, Pyorrhea alveolaris)

Chronic ossifying alveolar periostitis (odontoma, pseudo-odontoma): This is characterized by the formation of an exostosis at the root of the affected tooth. The swelling is slow to develop and greatly hinders the extraction of the affected tooth. The cause is believed to be low-grade infection of the alveolar periosteum leading to a periostitis and osteitis with subsequent new bone formation over the root of the involved tooth. Removal of the affected tooth is indicated only if the condition is causing trouble.

Purulent or acute suppurative alveolar periostitis: In this condition, the periosteum usually is thickened and extremely vascular. Erosion of the tooth follows and, if any of the last 3 or 4 upper molars are involved, maxillary sinusitis usually results. In the lower jaw, osteomyelitis and a dental fistula may follow. Anything that leads to exposure of the alveolus may give rise to the disease, e.g. separation of the gum from the crown, lodgement of food between the teeth, caries, fissures or fractures of the teeth, also wearing of the teeth down to the level of the gum as sometimes occurs in old horses. The condition affects the cheek teeth and only rarely the incisor teeth, in which case it usually is secondary to compound fracture involving the alveolus or injury to the interalveolar space. The most commonly involved teeth are the fourth and third molars in that order. In cattle, actinomycosis of the jaws predisposes to the condition; it should be considered whenever loose cheek teeth are encountered in cattle.

Very often, the first sign is a purulent, unilateral nasal discharge if the affected tooth has its roots in the maxillary sinus. The pus is fetid and the smell is characteristic of necrotic bone. Other signs, as mentioned under signs of dental trouble, are evident. In the lower jaw there usually is an enlargement of the mandible over the root of the affected tooth. The gum around the tooth is inflamed and recedes from the crown. Pus also may be evident in and around the socket. There may be displacement of the affected tooth by virtue of the compression of the jaws. In the upper jaw, the tooth is displaced laterally, while in the lower jaw, it is displaced medially. Sometimes, the formation of a dental fistula occurs. When alveolar periostitis is suspected, every tooth and also the entire gum region should be examined with meticulous care. Radiographs are often necessary for an accurate diagnosis. In uncooperative or fractious animals, such examination should be carried out with the horse in recumbency. The affected tooth should be removed.

DENTAL FISTULA

A dental fistula connects the root of a tooth and the exterior, the dental maxillary sinus, or the nasal cavity. Causes are alveolar periostitis or external injury with secondary infection. In the former case, the disease spreads from the tooth outwards, while in the latter, the condition originates at the site of trauma and by a process of osteomyelitis extends to the tooth root. Removal of the affected tooth is indicated.

DISEASES AND CONDITIONS OF THE MOUTH (LG. AN.)

CONTUSIONS AND WOUNDS OF THE LIPS AND CHEEKS

In large animals, wounds of the lips and cheeks are most commonly encountered in the horse as a result of falls, kicks, inhumane bits, bites, or tears from projecting objects. The vascularity of the region means rapid healing as a rule, except when a penetrating wound gives rise to a fistula. Treatment is routine. When a laceration involves the border of the lip, suturing should commence at that border to obtain the best cosmetic effect. If penetrating wounds are encountered, deep sutures must be placed in addition to those approximating the skin edges.

LAMPAS
(Palatitis)

A hardening and swelling of the mucous membrane of the hard palate just behind the upper incisor arcade in horses. In young horses, it is largely associated with the change from temporary to permanent dentition. In older horses, it is more in the nature of a passive congestion of the region. Examination of the mouth shows that the most anterior rugae of the hard palate extend below the level of the adjacent incisor teeth, causing pain when the horse attempts to eat. The affected region is hard and swollen.

The animal should be placed on a laxative diet of soft feed such as a bran mash. The old horse with this condition should be fed from a manger or rack rather than from the ground. Recovery in a young horse is generally spontaneous and uneventful but the condition may persist for extended periods in the old horse.

CLEFT PALATE

This condition is occasionally found in newborn animals of all species. The sole cause was long thought to be hereditary but recent evidence indicates that ingestion of toxic agents by the pregnant female and viral infections during pregnancy are also causes. The initial sign is milk dripping from the nostrils when the newborn animal attempts to nurse. Respiratory infections due to inhalation of food commonly occur. Visual inspection of the mouth readily reveals the cleft palate. Attempts to surgically correct the condition are open to question because of ethical considerations and poor results. It commonly occurs simultaneously with other defects such as arthrogryposis.

STOMATITIS CAUSED BY TRAUMA OR CHEMICAL IRRITANTS

There are many specific diseases in which stomatitis is a prominent sign. This discussion is of nonspecific inflammation of the mucosa of the oral cavity caused by trauma or chemical irritants. The commonest causes of traumatic injury are awns of barley, foxtail, porcupine grass and spear grass, and feeding on plants infested with hairy caterpillars. Chemical stomatitis arises most commonly from oral contact with irritant drugs such as leg blisters. Consumption of plants of the crowfoot family, especially those containing anemenol (buttercups, crocus, pasque flower, cowslips) and prolonged medication with mercurials, arsenicals and iodides also result in stomatitis.

Examination of the oral cavity and tongue reveals local or generalized areas of acute inflammation. In chemically induced stomatitis the buccal mucosa may be edematous and coated with a catarrhal exudate. The regional lymph nodes may be enlarged.

The first clinical sign of disease is excessive frothy salivation, or in the case of plant awns, a reluctance to permit manual examination of the mouth cavity. Animals often exhibit evidence of irritation of the mouth, i.e. stand with their mouths open, loll their tongues or chew with their heads turned sideways. They soon develop difficulty in eating. Usually, the breath has a putrid or sweetish odor. Actinobacillosis (wooden tongue), foot-and-mouth disease, bovine malignant catarrh and bovine viral diarrhea must be considered in differential diagnosis in cattle. Epidemic diseases such as bluetongue in ruminants and swine vesicular disease must be taken into consideration.

Most animals make rapid and uneventful recoveries when the cause is removed. Treatment is necessary only in severe cases. If there is marked inflammation treatment with a broad-spectrum antibiotic is advisable. Mild antiseptics such as a solution of 0.5% hydrogen peroxide, 5% sodium bicarbonate and 1 to 3% potassium chlorate used as a mouthwash may hasten recovery.

"MYCOTIC" STOMATITIS

A distinctive stomatitis of cattle that commonly occurs at 6- to 10-year intervals in the late summer and early fall in Southern and Western U.S.A. For many years it was believed to be solely an allergic reaction to fungi that infect pasture grasses in late summer and fall but of recent years serologic and virus isolation findings have provided conclusive evidence that many cases are caused by the virus that produces bluetongue in domestic and wild ruminants (q.v., p. 253).

Clinical Findings: The chief clinical signs are inflammation of the mucous membranes of the mouth, superficial erosions of the epidermis, and lameness. Stomatitis and epidermal exfoliation generally are more marked in older animals and lameness less marked, while in younger animals, lameness is most pronounced and stomatitis less severe. The first sign is frothy salivation. Shortly, small erosions or ulcers can be detected on the mucosa of the lips, dental pad and anterior margins of the tongue. Within a few days, these lesions become covered with accumulations of necrotic tissue. Usually in about a week, extensive necrosis of the mucosa of the anterior part of the oral cavity and tongue has occurred. In most cases, only the anterior portion of the oral cavity is affected, but in severe cases necrosis of the entire oral cavity, tongue and muzzle occurs. The breath is fetid.

Lameness, apparently caused by laminitis, occurs early in the course of the disease. Affected animals lie most of the time and are extremely reluctant to rise. Severely lame animals generally walk on their heels, with a stiff gait; a few walk on their toes with a stilted gait. In many herds, lameness is the only sign of disease in young animals. Marked edema above the hoof occurs in many young animals. A bluish sensitive line above the coronary band, similar to that described in cases of bluetongue, occurs in some cases. Some degree of lameness usually persists for 2 to 3 weeks. Many older animals with marked oral involvement exhibit little or no lameness during the entire clinical course.

Exfoliation of the epidermis of the teats, udder and perineal region sometimes occurs. Some animals have nasal discharges. Severely affected animals have profuse diarrhea with much mucus and blood in the feces.

The course varies greatly, but, in extreme cases, recovery usually takes place in 1 to 3 weeks. The herd morbidity rate usually is low (5 to 20%) and the few fatalities observed result from secondary bacterial infection.

Lesions: The only striking pathologic changes, other than the necrotic stomatitis and epidermal exfoliation, are hyperemia, hemorrhage and necrosis of the alimentary canal extending from the omasum to the rectum.

Treatment: No specific treatment is available. Antihistamine drugs may give temporary relief. The use of very mild oral antiseptics helps to remove the necrotic debris and hasten healing. Strong mouthwashes should be avoided. Antiseptic ointments may be used to hasten healing of the teat lesions, which cause much discomfort to milking cows. Affected animals should be removed from pasture and fed a soft diet made into a slop or gruel.

PHLEGMONOUS STOMATITIS AND CELLULITIS

An acute, deep-seated, diffuse, rapidly spreading inflammation of the oral mucosa, pharynx and surrounding structures, including the subcut. tissue. It occurs sporadically in cattle of all types and endemically in some of the intensive dairying areas of the Midwestern U.S.A. The cause is not completely understood, but hemolytic streptococci or coliform organisms usually can be isolated early in the disease. In cases of moderate duration a common isolate is *Fusobacterium necrophorum (Sphaerophorus necrophorus)*.

The onset of clinical signs is sudden. An animal may progress from normal to near death in 24 hours. The first sign is excessive, watery salivation, usually associated with excessive lacrimation. These changes are accompanied by a febrile reaction, with a temperature of 105 to 107°F (40.5 to 41.5°C) and an increase in pulse and respiratory rates. The animal usually refuses to eat or drink. There is marked swelling of the tissues of the face, around the mouth and nostrils and in the intermandibular space. The affected tissues are painful and edematous. Breath is foul and large sheets of superficial oral epithelium peel off. A severe toxemia with weakness is characteristic. Large pockets of fluid may form in the mandibular region and along the trachea.

Some of the milder cases recover spontaneously, but the more severely affected animals usually die unless treated.

Treatment: Sulfonamides (e.g. ℞ 96, 102) administered IV during the acute phases of the disease, may be effective in controlling the infection. The "potentiated sulfonamides," where they are available, are superior. Oral therapy may be employed when the patient is again able to swallow. Penicillin (℞ 63) is less effective. Injection of part of the dose of penicillin into the diseased tissue is recommended.

PAPULAR STOMATITIS OF CATTLE

This mild disease of cattle from 1 month to 2 years of age is caused by a virus, and up to 100% of a susceptible herd may become affected. Lesions occur on the muzzle, inside the nostrils and on the buccal mucosa, and consist of reddish raised papules measuring 0.5 to 1 cm in diameter which appear active for about a week and then regress. Evidence of the healed lesion may be present for several weeks. There is no systemic disturbance; the disease is important chiefly because of the confusion it may cause in the clinical diagnosis of the several forms of stomatitis of cattle.

SMALL-ANIMAL DENTISTRY AND DENTAL EMERGENCIES

CONGENITAL ABNORMALITIES OF THE MOUTH

CLEFTS

Clefts are the commonest congenital abnormality involving the lips of small animals. The mode of transmission is unclear; they are probably hereditary although maternal nutritional deficiencies, stresses and drug or chemical exposures, and mechanical interference with the fetus are factors. **Cheiloschisis** (harelip) is due to failure of the processes making up the jaws and face during embryonic development. Cleft of the lower lip is rare and usually occurs in the median line. Clefts of the upper lip, usually at the junction of the premaxilla and maxilla, may be unilateral or bilateral, incomplete or complete, and are often associated with clefts of the alveolar process and palate. **Palatoschisis** (palate cleft) may appear in the palate alone or may extend from the lip through the alveolar part of the upper jaw into the palate. It is an aberrant development of embryonic processes of the upper jaw. Palatal clefts may be associated with other less obvious abnormalities. Often, their presence is revealed by regurgitation of milk through the nose in small, undernourished puppies. If untreated, the animals usually die from starvation or secondary infection of the nasopharynx or middle ear.

Treatment: The patient should be carefully examined for more serious congenital defects. Surgical correction is effective only if the defect is not too large and, if undertaken, it should be performed during the first few days or weeks of life, before the patient's general health is influenced by the defect. Lip clefts cause marked difficulty in nursing, requiring hand-feeding until the correction is completed. Correction of palate clefts is much more difficult and usually not as satisfactory. Euthanasia is advisable in animals with gross defects, and those treated successfully should not be used for breeding.

ABNORMALITIES IN THE DEVELOPMENT OF TEETH

Imperfect development of the deciduous teeth, usually deviation from the normal in number and placement, occurs most commonly in brachycephalic breeds. Supernumerary teeth are usually unilateral and, most often in the upper jaw. The number of cheek teeth is occasionally reduced especially in the brachycephalic breeds.

Deviated placement usually results from crowding in the dental arch. Failure to shed the deciduous teeth may affect normal eruption and placement especially of the lower canine teeth. The upper third premolar is the first tooth to rotate in the short-muzzled dog. Later, all upper premolars may rotate. The molar teeth are seldom affected. Anomalous placement of teeth is commoner in the upper dental arch. Teeth abnormally placed owing to an aberrant development of the tooth germ occur occasionally in all breeds. No special treatment is required unless malocclusion exists whereupon the offending tooth should be extracted or repositioned.

DENTAL CARIES

Dental decay is uncommon in small animals, possibly because

their diets largely are free of readily fermentable carbohydrates. In dogs, decay is usually seen on the table surfaces or on the necks of the molar teeth. In cats, erosion of the enamel is sometimes seen on the buccal surface of the molars and premolars, just below the gingival margin. Superficially, the teeth appear normal. Affected cats stand over their food and salivate, but hesitate to chew or to eat. Seriously affected teeth should be filled or extracted.

DENTOALVEOLAR ABSCESS

An acute or chronic inflammation and infection of the apex of a tooth, the periodontal membrane and the periapical alveolar bone, usually originating in the dental pulp. Such abscesses may be caused by injury to the tooth or by infection from the root canal resulting from pulpitis or suppurative pericementitis.

Clinical Findings: Acute alveolar abscesses are seldom diagnosed in small animals. The animal is usually presented with a history of reluctance to eat. A local swelling, frequently fluctuating, may be seen, but the tooth itself appears sound. A parulis, or gum-boil, may be near the involved tooth; at other times the infection may extend into the surrounding bone causing pain without visible evidence of abscessation.

In chronic abscesses, there is local inflammation of the gums near the affected tooth and soreness due to destruction of cortical bone over the apex of the tooth. Most commonly, the upper fourth premolar tooth in the dog develops an abscess at its root discharging intermittently through a fistula into the mouth (alveolar fistula). It may extend as the sinus develops into a fistula and ruptures on the face below the eye (maxillary fistula). The owner usually seeks aid for this obvious draining fistula.

Diagnosis: Chronic dentoalveolar abscess should be differentiated from chronic suppurative pericementitis wherein a pus pocket alongside the root of the tooth is followed by detachment of the periodontal membrane from the cement. Radiographs of the suspect tooth are valuable. A dentoalveolar abscess with an alveolar fistula causes fetid, purulent saliva. An animal's reluctance to chew food and a reddened gingiva around a slightly painful tooth should suggest a chronic dentoalveolar abscess, although the tooth may appear sound and no discharge be evident. An intermittently draining fistula below the eye on the affected side is pathognomonic.

Treatment: If a fluctuant swelling is present near the affected tooth, ventral drainage coupled with parenteral penicillin (℞ 63) is sometimes successful. General anesthesia is necessary and endotracheal intubation desirable to prevent aspiration of foreign materials during surgery and to maintain a patent airway.

With a maxillary fistula, continuity should be established between the fistulous tract and the alveolus of the extracted tooth. Granulation tissue and necrotic bone should be removed by curettage. The tract is flushed daily with benzalkonium chloride solution (℞ 423) until the infection is controlled. Penicillin (℞ 63) or other systemic antibiotics (℞ 27, 56) should be administered for several days. The mouth should be flushed several times daily with salt solution (℞ 453), sodium bicarbonate solution (℞ 455) or benzalkonium chloride solution (℞ 423). A soft diet is recommended.

PERIODONTAL DISEASE

(Periodontitis, Pyorrhea alveolaris)

An acute or chronic inflammation of the periodontal membrane characterized, in severe cases, by resorption of the alveolar bone, loosening of the teeth and often atrophy of the gums. It may be local, involving only one tooth, but is usually generalized.

Etiology: Periodontal disease begins with bacterial infection of the gingiva. Mechanical irritation from calculus with concurrent infection is common. Brachycephalic dogs with faulty occlusion may be predisposed by irregularities in form and position of the teeth causing food impactions. Lack of masticatory exercise causing functional insufficiency of the jaws may contribute to periodontal disturbance and subsequent disease. Atrophy of the supporting tissues of a tooth after loss of its antagonist may lead to food impaction and periodontal disease. Improper feeding and systemic conditions such as diabetes mellitus, low-calcium intake, hyperparathyroidism, and chronic nephritis also may result in periodontal disease.

Clinical Findings: The usual signs are hesitant mastication, excess salivation and occasionally inappetence. Early in the disease, tapping or probing the affected teeth with a tartar scraper causes pain, which lessens as the tooth loosens. As the condition progresses, slight pressure on the tooth or gum causes small amounts of pus to exude from pockets around the tooth. Foul-smelling breath is a constant sign.

Lesions: The teeth are usually encrusted with calculus that is soft when first deposited, but soon becomes quite hard. Accumulated calculus extends downward toward the gum, causing progressive irritation. The gums become congested and swollen and bleed readily; forced from the neck of the tooth, the gum margin becomes inflamed. If the calculus is not removed, food material lodges between the edge of the calculus and the gum and putrefies, causing secondary infection around the neck of the tooth. Foul-smelling pus forms and the tooth loosens in its socket, leading to loss of part or all of the tissue of the alveolar process, periodontal membrane and surrounding gum.

Patients with chronic systemic conditions, particularly chronic nephritis, show a slow-forming dental deposit, which leads to a foul-smelling, low-grade inflammation of the gums, favoring periodontal disease. Periodontal disease of the incisor teeth is common in toy breeds with low-calcium or improper calcium-phosphorus intake.

Treatment: General anesthesia is recommended. All tartar, including that below the gum line, should be removed from the affected teeth; seriously loosened or diseased teeth should be extracted. Following removal of large calculus accumulations, involved teeth are usually somewhat loose. Many will regain their normal attachment with treatment.

After scaling, polishing and necessary extractions, the gums should be flushed with saline solution and painted with tincture of iodine (℞ 441) or zinc chloride solution (℞ 462). If the gums are hypertrophied, the excess tissue should be removed by electrocautery. After surgery, administration of broad-spectrum antibiotics (℞ 56, 66) is indicated. Liquid or soft diets should be provided for several days until the gums have had adequate time to heal. Supportive therapy, including high dosages of injectable vitamin B complex, seems helpful in hastening recovery and preventing recurrence. Daily irrigation of the gum margins (℞ 423, 453) aids in preventing food and debris accumulation until the gums are healed. To prevent recurrence, early tartar accumulations should be removed periodically. Owners should be encouraged to feed solid foods and to provide large bones or hard rubber toys for gum and tooth exercise.

GINGIVITIS

An acute or chronic inflammation of the gums, characterized by congestion and swelling.

Etiology: Gingivitis may be caused by local irritation, by spread of infection from the other areas of the mouth, or may be secondary to systemic disease. The commonest local cause is dental calculus; others are physical trauma, foreign bodies, dental caries and irritation from broken teeth. Most diseases of the mouth cause some degree of gingivitis by direct extension of the infection. Among the most prominent general conditions causing gingivitis are hypovitaminosis B, uremia and leptospirosis. Cats develop severe gingivitis secondary to most chronic debilitating diseases.

Clinical Findings and Diagnosis: Because gingivitis often is secondary to systemic conditions, a thorough physical examination should seek the primary disease. Simple inflammatory gingivitis produces a narrow band of bright-red, inflamed gingival tissue surrounding the neck of a tooth. There may be edema with swelling of the papillae. The gums are tender and bleed easily. If untreated, the gums become more swollen, ulcerated and finally hypertrophied.

Usually, the patient shows little discomfort. Atrophic gingivitis is usually encountered in older patients or in those with chronic gingivitis.

Treatment: Local causes, such as calculus deposits, bacterial plaque or dental caries, are eliminated. In systemic diseases supportive therapy must be employed. Hypertrophied gums may be excised if the lesions are not extensive. Flushing with benzalkonium chloride (℞ 423) or salt solution should be employed, regardless of the cause.

EPULIS

(Fibromatosis gingivae, Fibromatous epulis, Ossifying fibroma, Gingival hyperplasia)

A benign, irregular fibrous hyperplasia of the gums, usually originating in the region of the alveoli and involving much of the gum margin. It is a relatively insensitive, vascular, tough, fibrous connective tissue structure, with an irregular surface covered with epithelium. The growths usually have a broad base of attachment, are the color of the normal gum and may grow large enough to cover completely the buccal and labial surfaces of the teeth. Apparently, predisposition to these growths exists among certain brachycephalic breeds in which the condition is termed gingival hyperplasia or familial gingival hypertrophy.

Epulis sometimes refers to giant-cell epulis or tumor of the gum of the dog. This tumor is usually single and characterized histologically by bizarre forms and giant cells. Histopathologic examination is encouraged to assure proper diagnosis, treatment and prognosis.

Epulis is commonest in older dogs, which are usually asymptomatic, although hair, food and debris may collect between the growth and the dental arcade causing irritation and halitosis.

Treatment: Treatment is unnecessary unless growths interfere with mastication. If removal is necessary, electrosurgical techniques are most satisfactory. The mouth should be rinsed with benzalkonium chloride solution (℞ 423) for several days following surgery.

HEMORRHAGE FROM THE MOUTH

Etiology: Oral bleeding may follow acute trauma, extraction of diseased teeth or occur as secondary hemorrhage from a previous disease involving the oral mucosa, gingiva or periodontium. It may be spontaneous and prolonged when associated with hemophilia, diabetes mellitus, blood dyscrasias or infection. Trauma is the most common cause. Accidental biting of the tongue or lips is uncommon, but does occur during convulsions. More common is the biting of a tumor in the mouth with subsequent bleeding. Bleeding may occur from ulcers in severe stomatitis or glossitis. Slight hemorrhage occasionally is encountered when the deciduous teeth are shed.

Clinical Findings: Hemorrhage ranging from blood-stained saliva to profuse venous or arterial bleeding is the obvious sign. With foreign bodies or injuries to the mouth, the animal shows obvious discomfort and annoyance by pawing and rubbing its muzzle. Larger foreign objects and wounds are evident on examination, but smaller ones may be difficult to locate in a bleeding, uncooperative patient. Anesthesia is sometimes needed. Very small wounds may cause profuse bleeding, if they are in a highly vascular area. The constant movement of the tongue over the wound often prevents normal clotting, causing the bleeding to persist.

Treatment: A cold pack held in place for a few minutes will usually control the hemorrhage from a small wound. All foreign bodies must be carefully removed; small ones (e.g. porcupine quills) are easily overlooked. If bleeding is profuse, the damaged vessels must be isolated and ligated. Large lacerations of the mucosa should be sutured; smaller wounds heal rapidly without repair. Gelfoam (℞ 567) or gauze soaked in 1:1,000 epinephrine should be used as packs over areas of persistent oozing hemorrhage. Systemic aids to coagulation may be used, but are not always successful.

For gross laceration or fracture, broad-spectrum antibiotics such as tetracyclines (℞ 56) should be given prophylactically. Injection of vitamin K (℞ 570) is effective in cases where bleeding is due to liver disease, bishydroxycoumarin poisoning or specific vitamin K deficiency. Rarely blood transfusions may be required to promote clotting and replace the blood loss.

POSTEXTRACTION PAIN AND SWELLING

The pain and swelling that occasionally follow extraction are usually due to operative trauma or to infection in the alveolus when several large, well-rooted or infected teeth are removed. The pain and swelling after operative trauma rarely persists more than 2 or 3 days. Infection appears from one to several days following extraction and is characterized by reluctance to eat, resistance to oral examination, depression and fever. Examination of the mouth reveals swelling and sometimes suppuration.

Flushing the mouth with benzalkonium chloride solution (℞ 423) or with warm saline solution will keep the mouth relatively clean and prevent accumulation of foreign material in the alveolus. Liquid or soft diets should be given until the gums are healed. If infection exists, a systemic antibiotic (℞ 27, 56, 63) or sulfonamides (℞ 90) should be given. Sedatives are seldom needed.

TOOTH LUXATION AND FRACTURE

Animals employ their teeth for apprehending food, gnawing, tearing, biting, fighting and carrying objects, thus the risk of tooth injury is continual.

Luxation of the teeth ranges from mere loosening of the alveolus to complete avulsion. Luxation usually results from fighting, automobile accidents, or accidental catching of the teeth in fences and cage doors. The teeth are occasionally driven into the nasal cavity, lip, cheek or tongue. If completely avulsed, they may be swallowed.

Luxation usually establishes a compound wound. Soft tissue is lacerated, alveolar bone is fractured and hemorrhage is usually present. The complete wound must be treated.

Totally or partially dislocated teeth are removed. Detached bone or soft tissue should also be removed and the area treated as for a typical extraction. If a dislocated tooth is especially important it may be replaced in the alveolus and fixed with wire to an adjacent tooth. These teeth usually become reattached to the alveolus and remain functional, but they must be watched carefully and removed if diseased. A systemic antibiotic (℞ 56, 63) or a sulfonamide (℞ 88) should be given.

Fractured teeth, not uncommon in dogs and cats, usually result from fights or automobile accidents. Puppies may chew on hard objects and fracture their teeth. An animal with a fractured tooth acts hungry but hesitates to eat. Some animals cannot retain saliva. Teeth with partially missing crowns are often discovered during routine examination of the mouth. If the dog shows no sensitivity and the pulp is not exposed, the fractured tooth may remain indefinitely without causing trouble. Frequently, the lateral surface of a molar splits away, allowing tartar to accumulate and resulting in periodontal disease.

If the pulp cavity is exposed, or if the fractured tooth is sensitive to pressure, heat or cold, a root-canal procedure or an extraction should be considered. Usually, the owner is advised of the presence of the fractured tooth and instructed to return the patient if the discomfort continues.

Mandibular fractures may result from difficulty encountered upon extraction of the canine teeth or larger molars. This is a particular danger in older dogs when the mandible itself is fragile and the alveolar attachments have become ossified, making tooth extraction difficult. Such fractures are repaired by wiring, pinning or other forms of immobilization.

DISEASES AND CONDITIONS OF THE MOUTH (SM. AN.)

CHEILITIS

An acute or chronic inflammation of the lips or lip folds.

Etiology: Wounds of varying severity are the commonest lip lesions in small animals. Dogs occasionally chew sharp objects such as recently emptied tin cans, inflicting slight or severe lip wounds, and fight wounds are common. Thorns, awns, burrs and fishhooks may imbed in the lips and cause marked irritation or severe wounds.

Infections of the lips may be secondary to wounds or foreign bodies, but more commonly are associated with infections elsewhere on the body or in the mouth. Direct extension of severe dental disease or stomatitis can produce cheilitis. Licking areas of bacterial dermatitis or infected wounds may spread the infection to the lips and lip folds. Severe external otitis, especially in long-eared dogs, may extend to the commissures of the lips. Local or generalized bacterial skin infections in small pups often cause infection of the lips and other parts of the face.

Other causes are hypovitaminosis B, allergic reactions, demodectic and occasionally sarcoptic mange, eczema and other skin disorders and paralysis of the lips due to facial nerve damage. The heavy folds present at the mucocutaneous border of spaniels or St. Bernards may predispose to infections of these areas.

Clinical Findings and Diagnosis: Animals with cheilitis usually scratch or rub at their lips, have a foul breath, and occasionally salivate excessively or have anorexia. With chronic infection of the lip margins or folds, the hair in these areas is discolored, moist and matted with a thick, yellowish or brown, malodorous discharge overlying hyperemic and sometimes ulcerated skin. Acute allergic reactions cause the lips to become edematous.

Dogs with a clotting defect may show diffuse swelling of both lips due to hemorrhage. This swelling may resemble that of allergic reactions, thus petechiae and ecchymoses in the skin and visible mucous membranes of other parts should be sought. Hypovitaminosis B can cause slightly reddened, dry, crusty lesions with visible cracks in the skin at the lip commissure, ulceration and necrosis of the tongue and gums. Cheilitis due to extension of infection from the mouth or from other body areas is usually easily detected because of the primary lesion.

Treatment: Wounds of the lips should be thoroughly cleaned, sutured if necessary and treated as if infected. Dental cleaning and improved oral hygiene may prove essential. A systemic antibiotic (℞ 63) should be administered for several days.

Infectious cheilitis which has spread from a lesion elsewhere usually improves with treatment of the primary lesion, but local treatment may also be necessary. With severe infection, hair should be completely clipped from the lesion and the area gently cleaned with a germicidal detergent (℞ 439), dried well and an antibiotic ointment (℞ 429) applied several times daily. Before each ointment application, the lesions may be rinsed with aqueous benzalkonium chloride solution (℞ 423).

Ulcerations and infections involving the skin folds at the mucocutaneous border of the lips are best handled by surgical extirpation. Mild cauterization with 5 to 10% silver nitrate solution is an acceptable alternative method but recurrence is common.

EOSINOPHILIC GRANULOMA OF CATS
(Rodent ulcer)

An inflammatory lesion of unknown origin characterized microscopically by ulceration of the surface epithelium, an underlying zone of necrosis and leukocytic infiltration, and a deeper layer containing large numbers of eosinophils. It usually involves the anterior upper lip, but may also be seen on the lower lip, tongue, soft palate, pharyngeal wall and other areas of the oral mucosa.

Clinical Findings: The early lesion is a small plaque on the lip margin. It increases in size gradually and may involve the lip up to the nose. The enlarging lesion assumes a typical brown, dry appearance and its edges roll over, giving the lip a characteristic scooped-out appearance. The lesions may spread, apparently by licking, to the skin on the inner surface of the thigh, popliteal region or ventral abdomen. The cat constantly licks the affected parts, which otherwise seem to have little adverse effect. Ulcers elsewhere in the mouth may cause some difficulty in mastication and deglutition. Frequently there is an associated peripheral eosinophilia.

Treatment: No treatment is entirely satisfactory. Some cats respond dramatically to systemic, intralesional or topical corticosteroid therapy (℞ 149, 152). Oral administration of megesterol (℞ 189) has been recommended. Removal of the lesion by electrosurgical techniques or surgical excision, repeated chemical cautery and radiation therapy have all been used with varying degrees of success. The latter mathods usually leave a deformed lip.

STOMATITIS

An inflammation of the mouth, which may be a primary oral disease or secondary to systemic disease. The inflammation may be localized or diffuse. The nature and severity of the lesions vary greatly. Glossitis (q.v., p. 113) and gingivitis (q.v., p. 105) are localized forms of stomatitis.

Etiology: Inflammatory lesions of the mouth may arise from infectious diseases, deficiency diseases, trauma or burns. Fusospirochetosis (q.v., p. 110) is perhaps the commonest infectious stomatitis in the dog. Feline rhinotracheitis and canine leptospirosis are frequently accompanied by ulcerative stomatitis. Inflammation and secondary infection of the mouth often are seen with such systemic conditions as malnutrition, avitaminosis B, anemia and uremia. Local factors include dental calculus, foreign bodies and thermal, chemical or electrical burns.

Clinical Findings: Signs vary widely with the type and extent of inflammation. Complete or partial anorexia, especially in cats, and excessive salivation when attempting to eat are common. The oral mucosa is reddened and hyperemic. The epithelium desquamates easily. The animal may paw at its painful mouth, and resents any attempt to examine it. The breath is malodorous. In more serious infections, a thick, brown, foul discharge is sometimes accompanied by bleeding. The animal frequently shows increased thirst. Regional lymph nodes may be swollen and tender.

Treatment: The cause should be eliminated. Broken or diseased teeth should be extracted, tartar scaled from the remaining teeth and any foreign bodies removed. Oral discharges should be cultured, direct smears made and sensitivity tests performed. Systemic infections, and other diseases, e.g. vitamin deficiencies or anemia, should be appropriately treated concurrently with symptomatic treatment of the stomatitis. Fusospirochetal disease requires vigorous local treatment and administration of penicillin (℞ 63), penicillin and streptomycin (℞ 66) or tetracycline (℞ 79) and injectable vitamin B complex should be initiated promptly and continued for at least a week. Antimicrobial agents as polymyxin B, chloramphenicol and neomycin and gentamicin sulfate are utilized depending on the infectious agent present. Debridement of necrotic tissue promotes more rapid healing when followed by thorough oral irrigation with mouthwashes, such as potassium permanganate solution (℞ 450), salt solution (℞ 453) or benzalkonium chloride solution (℞ 423). Small, painful ulcers may be cauterized with 5% silver nitrate (℞ 643). In gangrenous stomatitis, debridement or surgical excision of the lesions should be employed if the animal can be anesthetized safely. High doses of vitamin C and the B complex vitamins seem to hasten recovery. Animals that are unable or unwilling to eat should be given lactated Ringer's solution (℞ 588) or saline-dextrose parenterally (℞ 592) to prevent dehydration. Frequent offerings of appealing liquids and, later, semisolid foods will encourage eating.

Ulceromembranous Stomatitis

(Fusospirochetosis, Vincent's infection, Vincent's angina, Trenchmouth)

Fusiform bacilli and spirochetes, normal inhabitants of the mouth, cause this disease after some predisposing factor decreases the resistance of the oral mucosa. It frequently accompanies or follows other infections or deficiency diseases. It is commonest in cats on a restricted diet and in conjunction with chronic debilitating diseases. It appears first as reddening and swelling of the gingival margins, which are painful and bleed easily, and progresses to ulceration and necrosis of the gingivo-alveolar tissues with the formation of pseudomembranes. Extension to other areas of the oral mucosa is common. A characteristic offensive odor accompanies the escape of brown, purulent, slimy saliva, which stains the muzzle and forelegs. The infection may spread to the lower respiratory tract causing pneumonia. Spirochetal sinusitis, secondary to mouth infection, has been seen in cats. Stained smears of the oral exudate revealing large numbers of the organisms confirm the diagnosis.

Treatment: *See* p. 111.

Gangrenous Stomatitis

Gangrenous stomatitis is characterized by rapid and massive destruction of tissue. It occurs most frequently in avitaminosis B or as a sequela to Vincent's disease. It is also seen in advanced cases of uremia, especially those associated with subacute leptospirosis. The tip and free borders of the tongue are affected most commonly; the gum margin adjacent to the molars and premolars may also be involved and, sometimes, the condition extends throughout the mouth. It is usually accompanied by marked prostration and toxemia.

Treatment: *See* p. 111.

Ulcerative Stomatitis

Ulcerative stomatitis in cats and dogs is usually associated with systemic disease and is frequently pseudomembranous. Superficial destructive changes in the oral mucosa are marked. Cats infected with calicivirus or feline viral rhinotracheitis may have numerous rapidly developing, shallow ulcers on the tongue and palate and occasionally on the gums and buccal mucosa.

Ulcerative stomatitis may also occur in cats as a primary entity. Ulceration usually starts at the tip of the tongue, with reddening and loss of papillae. Progressively, the mucosa is lost and a pseudomembrane may form. An increased flow of saliva that is initially clear may become discolored, blood-stained and fetid as the disease progresses.

In dogs, ulcerative stomatitis is seen during the course of any severe systemic disease, or as a complication of catarrhal stomatitis. Debilitated or cachectic animals frequently exhibit oral ulceration; it may also accompany prolonged chronic disease, as nephritis with uremia, or occur as a sign of avitaminosis B. In these conditions it usually precedes gangrenous or ulceromembranous stomatitis.

Traumatic ulcers of the mouth occur from irregular, fractured or diseased teeth. Erosions of the buccal mucosa may result from abrasion caused by excessive accumulations of tartar or contact with infected tartar. These lesions are usually superficial with only circumscribed loss of epithelium, but they may develop into ulcers with loss of deeper tissues.

Treatment: *See* p. 111.

Follicular Stomatitis

A severe and prolonged form of stomatitis, with marked local tissue changes and prominent constitutional disturbances. It may be associated with a severe generalized disease, such as distemper, or with malnutrition or unsanitary environmental conditions. The mucous membrane shows vesicles that ulcerate showing shallow, well-defined, grayish yellow, denuded surfaces. Cats may develop a marked lesion on the mucous membrane at the angles of the upper and lower jaw which sometimes progresses to severe stomatitis and scarring. Affected cats will approach food with evident hunger then wail and paw at their face when they attempt to eat.

Mycotic Stomatitis

A specific type of ulcerative stomatitis in dogs and cats caused by *Candida albicans*, characterized by the appearance of ulcers and soft, white to gray, slightly elevated patches on the oral mucosa. The lesional periphery is usually reddened and the surface covered with a whitish tenacious membrane. The lesions may coalesce as the disease progresses. Similar lesions usually occur simultaneously in the pharynx and on the anal mucosa. The infection occurs most often in young animals following prolonged treatment with a broad-spectrum antibiotic. Tentative diagnosis may be confirmed by culture of the material from the lesion.

Treatment: An aqueous solution of gentian violet (℞ 438) or nystatin ointment (℞ 369) is effective locally if lesions are few. When the lesions are widespread, the oral administration of nystatin (℞ 368) along with topical application of nystatin solutions is advised. Concurrent use of specific systemic antibiotics may be necessary if secondary bacterial infection is involved.

GLOSSITIS

An acute or chronic inflammation of the tongue. The inflammation may be due to a primary disease of the tongue, viral infection, or secondary to disease elsewhere. Local causes include irritation from excessive tartar on the lingual surfaces of the molar teeth, penetrating foreign bodies, bite wounds, rubber bands, thread or string looped about or under the tongue, burns and insect stings. Other more generalized processes, including both infectious and metabolic diseases also may cause tongue lesions.

Clinical Findings: Excessive salivation and a reluctance to eat are common signs, but the cause may go undiscovered unless the mouth is examined closely. Irritation originating in the dental arcade causes reddening, swelling and occasionally ulceration of the edge of the tongue. A thread, string, or rubber band looped under the tongue may cause no inflammation of its dorsum but the frenum is painful, shows acute or chronic irritation and frequently is severed by the foreign body. Porcupine quills and plant awns may become imbedded so deeply that they are not palpable. Insect stings cause an acute, massive, edematous swelling of the tongue.

In long-standing cases with an ulcerative or gangrenous glossitis, there is a thick, brown, foul-smelling discharge and occasionally bleeding. The animal usually resists any attempt to examine its mouth.

Treatment: Foreign bodies, broken or diseased teeth should be removed, under anesthesia, if necessary. Infectious glossitis (usually ulcerative or gangrenous) should be treated with a systemic antibiotic such as penicillin (℞ 63) or penicillin with streptomycin (℞ 66), in conjunction with high dosages of injectable B-complex vitamins. Mouthwashes, such as benzalkonium chloride solution (℞ 423) and other antiseptics (℞ 450, 462) should be used to flush the mouth several times daily. A bland diet and parenterally administered fluids (℞ 584, 592) may be necessary. Acute glossitis due to insect stings may require emergency treatment including tracheal intubation or tracheotomy if the respiratory distress is severe. Infections of epinephrine (℞ 530) or antihistamines will aid in reducing the tissue swelling. Severe cases may require placement of a pharyngostomy tube.

If the glossitis is secondary to another condition, the primary disease should be treated. The tongue tissues heal rapidly after irritation and infection have been eliminated.

MOUTH BURNS

Burns involving any or all of the structures of the mouth are not uncommon. They range in severity from mild injury with only temporary discomfort to destructive lesions with loss of tissue, scar formation and contraction with subsequent deformity. The causes are general and not always due to prehension (*see* BURNS, p. 782 and ELECTRIC SHOCK, p. 780).

The inciting incident may have been observed, providing a history. Although hungry, the patient hesitates to eat or drink, salivates excessively and resents handling of its mouth or face. In untreated cases with marked tissue destruction, there is danger of a secondary ulcerative or gangrenous stomatitis.

Animals showing a reddened oral mucosa without tissue defects require no specific treatment other than a soft or liquid diet until the area has healed. If tissue damage is extensive, frequent flushing with isotonic saline solution keeps the burned areas free of necrotic debris and food particles, hastening healing. If the burn causes loss of tissue, the area should be cleaned and debrided under anesthesia. The risk of secondary infection should be minimized with antibiotic therapy (℞ 27, 56, 63) for several days. Local treatment is of little value.

CANINE ORAL PAPILLOMATOSIS

A benign canine neoplastic disease characterized by the occurrence of single or, more frequently, multiple papillomas on the oral mucous membranes. It is caused by a virus that infects only dogs, produces lesions in or around the mouth and is commonest in young animals (*see* PAPILLOMATOSIS, p. 250). Signs occur only when the warts interfere with eating. Occasionally, if the warts are very numerous, the dog may bite them when chewing and they may then become infected. The papillomas may regress spontaneously within a few weeks. If removal is necessary, it is best accomplished using electrosurgical techniques. The use of commercial or autogenous wart vaccines sometimes effects a cure.

PARALYSIS OF THE TONGUE
(Glossoplegia)

A partial or complete loss of function of the tongue that may be peripheral or central in origin. In the former, rough manipulation and excessive pulling on the tongue during dental examination may be the cause. Glossoplegia of central origin may accompany or follow such conditions as strangles, upper respiratory infection, meningitis, botulism, equine encephalomyelitis, moldy-corn disease or cerebral abscess. In the unilateral case, the tongue is deviated toward the nonaffected side. In the bilateral case, the tongue is limp and often protrudes through the relaxed jaws. In mild cases of either central or peripheral origin, a weakness in the muscle power of the tongue is often evident.

Careful nursing, with particular attention to feeding, will aid those cases where spontaneous recovery is likely. Where the condition persists beyond 6 weeks, likelihood of return to normal function is slight.

TONSILLITIS

Etiology: Tonsillitis is a common clinical problem in the dog and rare in the cat. In the dog, it may occur either as a primary disease or secondary to infections in the mouth, pharynx or nasal passages. Chronic tonsillitis may occur in brachycephalic dogs, in association with the elongation and hypertrophy of the soft palate and chronic pharyngitis so often found in these breeds.

Hemolytic streptococci and coliforms are the pathogenic bacteria most often cultured from diseased tonsils. Plant fibers or other foreign bodies which lodge in the tonsillar fossa may produce a localized unilateral inflammation or a peritonsillar abscess. Other physical and chemical agents listed under pharyngitis (q.v., p. 117) may also affect the tonsils.

Clinical Findings and Diagnosis: The earliest signs are fever, listlessness, salivation, inappetence and dysphagia. The mandibular lymph nodes may be enlarged. Frequently there is a short, soft cough that is followed by retching and the expulsion of small amounts of mucus. Swallowing movements, chewing grass or pawing at the base of ears are signs that may appear as the throat becomes sore. Tonsillar enlargement will range from almost inapparent to a size sufficient to cause mechanical difficulty in swallowing. A mucoid exudate containing leukocytes, epithelial cells and bacteria may surround the tonsil. The tonsillar tissue may be edematous and obviously reddened with small necrotic foci or plaques, and will protrude from the crypt in severe cases.

Repeated attacks may lead to chronicity. When this condition exists, the affected dog will be subject to occasional exacerbations of acute signs, generally poor health and lowered resistance to disease. Nephritis with lumbar tenderness may occur subsequent to tonsillitis. Chronic inflammation will result in a "muddy" tonsil with only slight enlargement. Inflammation of the palatine tonsil may be accompanied by a similar inflammation of the pharyngeal tonsil. Since inflammation of the tonsils may be a sign of generalized or regional infection, the diagnosis of primary tonsillitis should be made only after the existence of any underlying disease has been eliminated by a thorough physical examination. Neoplastic tonsillar enlargement should not be confused with tonsillitis.

Treatment: Prompt systemic administration of antibiotics is indicated for bacterial tonsillitis. The most effective and economical antibiotic, in most cases, is penicillin (℞ 63). It should be given for 10 days. Sulfonamide (℞ 96, 102), or tetracycline (℞ 76) therapy is effective. Swabbing the tonsils and tonsillar crypts with 2% aqueous iodine solution is beneficial. A soft, palatable diet is recommended for a few days until the dysphagia disappears. The parenteral administration of fluids is required for those animals that are unable to take food by mouth.

Surgical removal of the tonsils during a remission of the disease is recommended for animals with recurrent attacks.

PHARYNGITIS

Inflammation of the pharyngeal mucosa.

Etiology: Pharyngitis usually is infectious and frequently associated with inflammation of adjacent tissues. Retropharyngeal and subparotid lymph nodes may be inflamed or abscessed. Pharyngitis often accompanies systemic infectious diseases, especially respiratory infections, or is the result of extension from adjacent infections such as rhinitis. Pharyngeal lymphoid hyperplasia, probably initiated by viral infection or possibly by air pollutants, has become the commonest cause of upper airway obstruction in the racehorse. It often becomes chronic and is then characterized by nodules containing masses of lymphocytes on walls and roof of the pharynx. It improves with rest but often recurs with training. Trauma to the pharynx may result from foreign bodies or unskilled use of instruments, e.g. balling guns. Inhalation or ingestion of drugs and chemicals may cause intense irritation. Thermal irritation of the pharynx occurs in the dog as a result of ingesting hot food or liquids. Elongation of the soft palate or eversion of the lateral ventricles in brachycephalic dogs can cause respiratory distress and nasal regurgitation, with resulting pharyngitis and tonsillitis.

Clinical Findings and Diagnosis: Slow, deliberate ingestion of food or anorexia may be the first sign. If pain is great, the animal also may refuse to drink. Palpation of the pharynx shows increased sensitivity. There may be swelling of the submaxillary, retropharyngeal and pharyngeal lymph nodes and the tonsils often are enlarged and inflamed. If there is an accompanying laryngitis, a suppressed cough can be elicited by pressure on the pharynx. If pain causes resistance to opening of the mouth, examination can be facilitated with general anesthesia. Inability to swallow may cause drooling; retching and coughing are common and the possibility of aspiration pneumonia should be considered.

Infection in the pharynx is characterized by fever, bilateral purulent nasal discharge and stiffness of the neck. *Pharyngeal paralysis* (see below) *may be a sign of rabies.*

Pharyngeal lymphoid hyperplasia causes impaired breathing and distress with exercise, edema of soft palate, pharyngeal recess and epiglottis, coughing, and serous nasal discharge of varying degree.

Prognosis: The course of primary pharyngitis usually is favorable, although the condition occasionally is fatal, due to edema of the pharynx and subsequent asphyxia. The prognosis is less favorable if the process results in formation of diphtheritic membranes and ulcers.

Treatment: Treatment is similar to that of tonsillitis (q.v., p. 116). If the condition has been caused by mechanical trauma (foreign bodies), local application of Mandl's solution (℞ 641), after removal of the offending object, is usually effective. The affected animal should receive soft or liquid foods that can be swallowed easily. Supplementary IV feeding may be necessary during the acute stage.

Large animals should be given sulfonamides (℞ 96, 102) or antibiotics (℞ 63, 73) parenterally. Lymphoid hyperplasia is treated by rest, topical pharyngeal sprays (℞ 433), systemic antibiotics, corticosteroids, and in some instances local chemical or thermocautery of the nodules. In the horse, where swelling and exudates may cause distressing dyspnea, steam vapors with cresol (℞ 419) are helpful and may avoid the need for tracheotomy; abscessed lymph nodes are common and should be given appropriate surgical treatment. The cough may be relieved by applying syrupy expectorants on the tongue (℞ 416). It is unwise to attempt restraint and oral medication because of the danger of causing fatal asphyxiation.

Small animals with systemic signs should be given sulfonamides (℞ 96, 102) or preferably antibiotics (℞ 27, 50, 56, 63, 73). Local treatment with astringent and antiseptic solutions containing iodine (℞ 442), tannic acid and glycerin (℞ 644) or silver nitrate (℞ 642) is helpful in overcoming the inflammation. In chronic pharyngitis, local application of Lugol's solution is helpful. Diphtheritic membranes may be carefully removed and the underlying tissues treated locally. Elongated soft palate or everted lateral ventricles can be corrected surgically.

PHARYNGEAL PARALYSIS

A disorder of central or peripheral origin that most frequently occurs as a sign of encephalitis and is of special clinical significance in rabies in cattle and dogs. It is also an important sign in encephalomyelitis. It is seen in many intoxications (e.g. botulism), probably some fungus poisonings, as well as with the general paralysis of parturient paresis. Peripheral paralysis is infrequent and may result from injury to the glossopharyngeal nerve, pressure from tumors or abscesses, or injury from fracture of the floor of the cranium. Pharyngeal paralysis in the horse due to *Aspergillus* infection and erosion of the guttural pouch wall (*see* below) is relatively common.

Clinical Findings: The animal suddenly loses its ability to swallow, food particles and saliva drop from the mouth and nose, and gurgling sounds emanate from the pharynx. If the interior of the pharynx is palpated, no muscular contractions are produced. Such animals die from aspiration pneumonia or exhaustion. The signs of pharyngeal paralysis of central origin are partially or completely masked by others of the fundamental disease. A ready diagnosis of the fundamental disease often results in the pharyngeal paralysis being ignored.

Diagnosis: Probing with the stomach tube suffices to differentiate between peripheral paralysis and esophageal obstruction. Foreign bodies in the mouth of the horse may lead to error in diagnosis. Corn cobs and sticks may become wedged between the upper arcades of the cheek teeth. Of great significance is the frequency with which signs of pharyngeal paralysis dominate the clinical picture in rabies in dogs and cattle. It is of primary importance to determine whether the paralysis is of central or pheripheral origin.

The prognosis is always guarded. When of central origin, it depends upon the fundamental process; when peripheral, upon the possibility of removing the cause. There is always the danger of aspiration pneumonia.

Treatment: There is no treatment for the local paralysis other than efforts to remove the cause of peripheral paralysis and none should be attempted before making a complete examination. In peripheral paralysis, or that present in equine encephalomyelitis, the patient should be fed and watered through a stomach tube. Control of the concomitant dehydration may be lifesaving.

INFECTION OF THE GUTTURAL POUCHES

A sepsis of the guttural pouches of Equidae, usually resulting as an extension of a pharyngitis, q.v., p. 117.

Etiology: Bacteria (commonly *Streptococcus* or rarely *Pasteurella*) or fungi (*Aspergillus*) are the usual organisms associated with the disease, although herpesvirus or myxovirus infections have not been eliminated as inciting causes. The condition usually results from an extension of a pharyngitis into the eustachian tube or rupture of an abscess of retro- or suprapharyngeal lymph nodes.

Clinical Findings: The condition may be acute or chronic. Intermittent mucopurulent nasal discharge, especially when the animal lowers its head, is the commonest clinical finding. Swelling or displacement of the parotid gland often is present. Pyrexia, epistaxis, dysphagia, abnormal head posture, respiratory abnormalities, ocular changes and facial paralysis are strongly suggestive of the condition, although no feature has been reliably consistent.

Diagnosis: This is made by the clinical signs and confirmed by examination of the pharynx with an endoscope, or by radiographs showing the fluid line in the guttural pouch.

Treatment: Catheterization and irrigation of the pouches with antibiotics (℞ 70) combined with parenteral antibiotic therapy has been effective in many cases. Iodides given orally are frequently effective. Surgical drainage via Viborg's triangle may be needed for chronic or unresponsive infections.

The animal with **guttural pouch mycosis,** particularly when associated with epistaxis or evidence of cranial nerve damage, indicates a poor prognosis, but local treatment with enzymes followed by an antifungal may be successful. With the horse anesthetized and in dorsal recumbency, 250,000 u of trypsin in 30 ml saline solution is placed in the infected pouch via a Foley catheter and held there for 10 minutes. This is followed by a 15-minute application of 30 ml of nystatin (Mycostatin oral suspension).

Prompt control of pharyngitis will reduce the incidence of guttural pouch infection.

SALIVARY DISORDERS (SM. AN.)

PTYALISM

Hypersecretion of saliva characterized by profuse driveling.

Etiology: Ptyalism may result from: (1) drugs or poisons, such as bismuth, mercury, organophosphates, arsenic, and contact with toads; (2) local irritation or inflammation as from stomatitis, glossitis (especially in cats), pyorrhea, teething, foreign bodies in the buccal cavity, neoplasms, injuries and other mucosal defects; (3) infectious diseases, such as rabies, the nervous form of distemper, or other convulsive disorders; (4) disturbances of the nervous system, such as motion sickness or hysteria; (5) reflex stimulation from irritation of the esophagus or stomach, as in gastritis; (6) sublingual salivary cyst; (7) abscesses and other inflammatory conditions of the salivary glands; (8) tonsillitis; (9) administration of medicine in some species (particularly cats); (10) conditioned or natural reflex response to fear, to fondling (in some cats) or in anticipation of food. Rarely, ptyalism is a result of salivary gland involvement.

Pseudoptyalism is the dribbling of saliva due to difficulty in swallowing. It usually results from paresis of the lips, tongue or pharynx, dislocation or fracture of the jaw, or from any inability to swallow or open and close the mouth.

Clinical Findings: Driveling is the only conspicuous sign of ptyalism. *Eliminate the possibility of rabies before examination.* With some poisons (e.g. mercury), the salivary gland may become enlarged and painful and the saliva may be irritating.

In pseudoptyalism, there is drooping of the lower jaw, tongue-lolling or drooping of the lips, depending on the location and extent of paralysis or degree of mechanical interference.

Treatment: The underlying cause, local or systemic, should be determined and treated. In poisoning with mercury or arsenic, emetics and a gastric lavage should be given if the poison has been recently ingested. BAL (℞ 628) is effective soon after poisoning or, alternatively, sodium thiosulfate (℞ 637). Atropine (℞ 511) and pralidoxime chloride (PAM, ℞ 635) are indicated for organophosphate poisoning. Further access to the poison should be prevented.

Where inflammation or irritation is the cause, the mouth should be cleansed and foreign bodies, dental calculus or diseased teeth removed.

In nervous and reflex disturbances, sedatives, antimotion-sickness drugs or tranquilizers are helpful. If necessary, atropine sulfate (℞ 511) may be given to suppress salivation until the cause is determined.

Pseudoptyalism as a sign of acute eosinophilic myositis (q.v., p. 598) can usually be corrected by the administration of systemic corticosteroids. With chronic fibrosing myositis, general anesthesia usually is required to open the mouth.

APTYALISM

Diminished or arrested secretion of saliva.

Etiology: Aptyalism may result from the use of certain drugs (atropine or belladonna), from extreme dehydration of pyrexia, or during an animal's recovery from certain anesthetics (e.g. sodium pentobarbital). It may appear limitedly in severe diarrhea, nephritis, diabetes or other conditions in which elimination of water from the body is increased through other channels. Occasionally, a decreased secretion of saliva is due to disease of the salivary gland.

Treatment: Mouthwashes (℞ 453, 455) relieve the discomfort that results from aptyalism. Fluids (℞ 584, 592) should be administered systemically in acute fever and dehydration. Pilocarpine (℞ 667) may stimulate salivary secretion temporarily. Determination and treatment of any underlying cause is of primary importance.

SALIVARY CYST

An accumulation of saliva in the duct or in the tissue around the duct or gland. While any of the salivary glands may be affected, the condition is commoner in the sublingual and mandibular glands. A sublingual duct cyst is designated a ranula.

Etiology: Salivary cysts are caused by traumatic or inflammatory rupture of the duct of the sublingual, mandibular or parotid salivary gland. Because the duct of the mandibular salivary gland and the major duct of the sublingual salivary gland frequently empty through a common opening, these glands often are involved simultaneously.

Clinical Findings: The first sign is a noninflammatory fluctuant mass under the tongue, in the submaxillary region or ventral to the ear. Sometimes when pressure is applied to the cyst, a viscid, odorless, gray or brownish fluid may exude from the ducts at one or both sides of the ventral surface of the tongue, or opposite the upper fourth premolar, depending upon the glands involved. The dog may salivate profusely from acute discomfort. The cyst may interfere mechanically with eating and drinking.

Diagnosis: A cyst is detectable as a fluctuant swelling without inflammation or fever. This swelling must be differentiated from abscesses, tumors and other retention cysts of the neck. A cyst and a fluctuant abscess, with its inflammatory characteristics, may be differentiated further by tapping the swelling and examining the fluid. A tumor is usually firmer and slower growing than a cyst. Differentiation of mandibular and parotid salivary cysts from retention cysts, (e.g. thyroglossal-duct cysts and branchial-cleft cysts in the neck region) depends mainly on careful observation of the anatomic location of the cyst. Sialography, helpful in the differentiation, is sometimes difficult to perform satisfactorily in the dog or cat.

Treatment: Surgical intervention is the only effective treatment. Ranulas usually respond to liberal incision of the cyst wall, removal of its contents and cautery of its inner lining with tincture of ferric chloride or silver nitrate (℞ 643). Recurrent sublingual cysts may be treated by establishing a permanent draining fistula from the cyst into the floor of the mouth under the base of the tongue. Removal of the affected salivary gland and drainage of the cyst is most effective.

SALIVARY GLAND INFLAMMATION OR ABSCESS

Acute or chronic inflammation of a salivary gland or its duct may result in an abscess of the affected gland.

Etiology: The condition is usually due to trauma, commonly from penetrating wounds such as bites, or infection of the salivary gland or of the neighboring structures.

Clinical Findings and Diagnosis: A diffuse or localized swelling appears suddenly in the area of the salivary gland associated with signs of local inflammation and pyrexia. Salivation, anorexia and dysphagia due to the pain and swelling are frequent. Rupture of the abscess discharges pus into the surrounding tissue or the mouth. Such abscesses must be differentiated from salivary cysts and the various retention cysts. Rupture through the skin may cause formation of a salivary fistula. Swelling of the parotid gland is most prominent below the ear, swelling of the mandibular gland at the angle of the jaw and swelling of the zygomatic gland just caudal to the eye. Zygomatic gland involvement results in divergent strabismus of the affected eye, exophthalmus and swelling of the membrana nictitans, the temporal area, and the oral tissues immediately posterior to the last molar tooth.

Abscesses of the zygomatic and parotid glands are acutely painful. The animal holds its head rigidly and resents examination of the swelling or opening of its mouth.

Treatment: Moderately swollen mild infections may respond to systemic antibiotics or chemotherapy (℞ 27, 56, 63, 80, 90). More advanced nonlocalized infections may benefit from the application of hot packs to the inflamed region several times daily.

Early injection of antibiotics into the nonlocalized lesion is occasionally successful. A developed abscess should be drained through the overlying skin or, in the zygomatic gland, drained posteriorly and laterally to the last cheek tooth within the oral cavity.

In a large abscess cavity, cautery of the inner lining with tincture of ferric chloride or silver nitrate (℞ 643) hastens healing. A drain may be placed in the abscess cavity for 48 hours, or it may be flushed with saline daily until healing iy complete. Penicillin (℞ 63), sulfonamides (℞ 90), or a broad-spectrum antibiotic (℞ 27, 56, 80) should be given for 4 or 5 days following drainage. Recurrence suggests surgical removal of the affected gland.

SALIVARY FISTULA

A fistulous tract discharging saliva into the mouth, into the skin in the anteroventral region of the neck or over the parotid gland. Common causes are wounds that penetrate the gland or spontaneous rupture of gland abscesses. The constant flow of saliva prevents healing and a fistula develops.

Diagnosis and Treatment: History of injury in the gland area, location of the fistula and the nature of the discharge are characteristic. A salivary fistula must be differentiated from a draining sinus in the neck region from a penetrating foreign body, or from sinuses arising from congenital defects.

Complete surgical removal of the gland and fistulous tract is the only satisfactory treatment.

CYSTS AND SINUSES OF THE NECK DUE TO DEVELOPMENTAL ANOMALIES

These imperfections of fetal development are important in their differentiation from salivary gland infection, salivary cysts and salivary fistulas.

Thyroglossal-duct cyst develops from postnatal persistence of the early embryonic thyroglossal duct. Quite rare, this cyst is always single and found in the middle of the neck, usually at the level of the hyoid bone and larynx. It is smoothly rounded with a well-defined border, anchored to the hyoid bone and deep tissues. Unless infection is superimposed, it is seldom attached to the skin. Not tender, it contains clear fluid.

Branchial (or lateral cervical) cyst develops from branchial apparatus malformation, usually of the second branchial cleft. Unilateral or bilateral, branchial cysts occupy a lateral position in the upper neck and usually are only very slightly mobile. Their size varies considerably and an individual cyst may change size periodically as its contents escape through a small opening into the throat or through a small cutaneous fistula (branchial or lateral cervical fistula).

Surgical removal of the cyst is required.

DISEASES OF THE ESOPHAGUS (SM. AN.)

ESOPHAGITIS

Primary esophagitis is rare but secondary esophagitis may develop in small animals from foreign bodies in the esophagus, wounds, prolonged vomiting, or with severe gastritis. It is commonly associated with achalasia, megaesophagus and cardiospasm. It may develop after cardioplasty or from irritation caused by instruments or drugs, ingestion of caustic materials, neoplasms and parasitic *Spirocerca lupi* (q.v., p. 707).

Dysphagia, drooling and hematemesis are the primary signs. Violent retching and vomiting occur with the necrosis produced by caustic or corrosive agents. Food is refused or regurgitated soon after swallowing.

Lesions, varying with the cause, may be catarrhal, ulcerative or necrotic. Foreign bodies may lacerate or puncture the esophageal wall. Stenosis occasionally follows the healing of extensive lesions. Contrast radiography with fluoroscopy is essential to diagnosis. Esophagoscopy allows direct observation of the esophageal wall and accurate appraisal of the lesions.

Meperidine (℞ 617) will control pain during the acute stages. Small quantities of soft, bland diet should be offered frequently.

Antibiotics (℞ 66) are administered both therapeutically and prophylactically. If not contraindicated by the presence of infection, steroid therapy (℞ 142, 147, 154) may aid in counteracting inflammation.

FOREIGN BODIES IN THE ESOPHAGUS

Foreign bodies, e.g. bones, needles and fishhooks, usually lodge between the thoracic inlet and the base of the heart or between the base and the esophageal hiatus of the diaphragm.

Clinical Findings: Salivation, retching and extension of the neck are constant signs of cervical foreign bodies. A complete obstruction causes immediate regurgitation after food or water intake. Partial obstruction permits the passage and retention only of fluids; solid food is regurgitated. The signs depend upon the location and composition of the foreign body, the degree and duration of esophageal obstruction. Anorexia and weight loss may be predominant signs where the obstruction has been persistent.

With small, sharp, nonobstructive objects the outstanding sign is dysphagia resulting from esophagitis. Perforation of the cervical esophagus may result in local abscessation or, in the thoracic portion, extensive pleuritis and empyema. Radiography will demonstrate many foreign bodies. A nonradiopaque object may necessitate the use of a barium suspension or air contrast. Esophagoscopy, an important diagnostic procedure, permits direct examination of both the foreign body and the esophageal wall. Large masses in the cervical portion of the esophagus occasionally can be localized by external palpation.

Treatment: An object in the upper esophagus sometimes may be grasped with forceps and removed. For those in the posterior esophagus, gastric forceps may be usful. An esophagoscope may be passed down to the obstruction then, with long alligator forceps, the foreign body is grasped, withdrawn into the esophagoscope and removed. All manipulations must be effected cautiously to avoid puncture or laceration of the esophageal wall. Foreign bodies, particularly those sharp-edged, should never be pushed down the esophagus.

Surgery may be indicated by the location and size of the foreign body. Either presternal or intrathoracic esophagotomy, or gastrotomy and withdrawal of the object through the cardia into the stomach for removal, is appropriate.

DILATATION OF THE ESOPHAGUS

Esophageal dilatation, a generalized or regional increase in the caliber of the esophagus, may follow food retention from: (1) constrictive tissue bands originating from persistent right aortic arch or from the ligamentum arteriosum associated with the aorta, pulmonary artery and base of the heart; (2a) congenital paralysis of peristalsis in the thoracic esophagus, or (2b) similar paralysis in older dogs, considered to be a neuromuscular dysfunction from exogenous or metabolic toxins; (3) achalasia, where the terminal esophagus fails to dilate as food approaches the cardia, resulting from degeneration in the neural plexus or from cardiospasm.

Secondary dilatation of the cervical esophagus usually follows thoracic esophageal dilatation unless its cause is removed.

Clinical Findings: The cardinal signs are dysphagia, regurgitation and progressive loss of condition. Initially, regurgitation occurs immediately after swallowing; as the condition progresses and the esophagus becomes enlarged, regurgitation is delayed. The puppy with congenital dilatation characteristically suckles normally but regurgitates solid food. In advanced cases, pulmonary disease may follow aspiration of fluid from the esophagus, particularly if the animal is confined and often recumbent. Pressure applied to the abdomen may cause ballooning at the thoracic inlet. Radiography may reveal extreme dilatation and elongation of the entire esophagus, dilatation of that portion anterior to the base of the heart, or dilatation of the thoracic esophagus with a cone-shaped obstruction at the cardia.

Treatment: Where the cause is cardiospasm, mechanical dilatation by placement of bougies in the cardia may alter the contractile strength of the sphincter, allowing the esophagus to empty. Surgical correction by extramucosal esophagocardiomyotomy offers the better opportunity for satisfactory recovery.

With congenital or acquired paralysis, a semiliquid diet is given frequently in small portions. Dry dog food fed in small portions at 2-hour intervals may enhance the secondary peristaltic activity of the esophagus. Feeding the dog from an elevated dish, requiring it to eat while standing on its hind legs, allows gravity to help food pass into the stomach. Supportive therapy with vitamin B complex should be routine. Bethanechol chloride (℞ 655) is sometimes beneficial to increase gastric tone and motility.

ESOPHAGEAL STENOSIS

A narrowing of the lumen from pathologic changes in the esophageal wall may follow trauma, postsurgical scars, or tumors of the wall. Esophageal tumors rarely cause stenosis but the high incidence of esophageal sarcoma in animals harboring *Spirocerca lupi* (q.v., p. 707) requires consideration in areas where this parasite is prevalent.

Clinical Findings: Signs are similar, in general, to those occurring with foreign bodies. Contrast radiography may show dilatation or a diverticulum of the esophagus anterior to the stricture. Small doses of contrast material must be followed immediately by radiography to demonstrate stenosis of the cervical esophagus.

Treatment: When surgical intervention is undesirable, animals may be maintained on a liquid or semiliquid diet offered frequently in small amounts. Periodic use of mechanical devices to dilate the affected area may be attempted.

DISEASES OF THE ESOPHAGUS (LG. AN.)

CHOKE

An obstruction of the esophagus by food masses or foreign bodies.

Etiology: Horses choke most frequently on greedily eaten dry grains, and less often on ears of corn, potatoes or a bolus of hay, and occasionally on medicinal boluses. Choke in horses often occurs secondarily to stenosis or diverticulosis, as well as from inflammation of the esophagus. Ruminants usually choke on solid objects, such as apples, pears, beets, plums, potatoes, turnips or ears of corn. On rare occasions cattle choke on foreign objects obtained in the feed. In large animals, obstruction occurs most frequently in the cervical and less often in the thoracic portion of the esophagus.

Clinical Findings: Horse: The affected horse exhibits anxiety, an arched neck and retching. Salivation is profuse and food and saliva are regurgitated through the nostrils. Coughing is pronounced and the animal may paw at the ground, get up and down and show other signs of distress. Milk runs from the nostrils of nursing foals attempting to swallow, and this sign must be differentiated from that caused by cleft palate. After an hour or so, the forced or spasmodic efforts at swallowing become less frequent and the animal may become quiet.

Cattle: Bloat (q.v., p. 145) and salivation are characteristic signs. The degree of tympany varies with the completeness of esophageal closure and the length of time that it has existed. Chewing movements, protrusion of the tongue, extension of the head and neck, dyspnea, grunting and coughing are also seen.

Diagnosis: The diagnosis is made from the history and the prominent signs. An object causing obstruction in the cervical esophagus may be located by external palpation and passage of a stomach tube. Diagnosis of thoracic obstructions may be confirmed by the careful passage of a stomach tube.

Treatment: Horses: Obstructions from grain and hay tend to resolve spontaneously as the bolus is softened by saliva. The course may be a few hours to several days, however, and there is a risk of pressure necrosis or esophagitis resulting ultimately in a stenosis with dilation or diverticulum. Inhalation pneumonia may occur. Hasty procedures are to be avoided. Controlling the pain with sedatives, confining the animal and allowing it access to water, but not to food, may result in spontaneous recovery. Passage of a stomach tube to the obstruction and repeated pumping and siphoning may relieve grain choke. Pentazocine (℞ 620), xylazine (℞ 554), or methampyrone (℞ 618) to control the pain and the spasms, is the primary medication required. Tranquilization is often helpful (℞ 374, 383). In some cases, solid thoracic obstructions may be gently pushed into the stomach with a large stomach tube or probang, if the patient is tractable or anesthetized.

Cattle: Relief of tympany is the first consideration and in acute bloat the rumen should be trocarized promptly. Solid objects in the cervical portion of the esophagus may be massaged upward and removed through a mouth speculum, or a No. 9 steel wire may be made into a loop, passed through the mouth speculum until beyond the object and then slowly withdrawn. When other methods fail, a probang may be tried. Stiff stomach tubes of large caliber work well for this purpose. The disadvantage of this method is the risk of tissue damage and subsequent esophagitis. In a choke near the diaphragm, a rumenotomy may be performed to remove the object.

Esophagotomy may be elected in cervical choke in either species but should be resorted to only when usual methods of treatment fail; often it is followed by an esophageal fistula, which requires several months to heal, if it heals at all.

ESOPHAGEAL STENOSIS

Etiology: Stenosis may be caused by cicatricial tissue or by compression. Cicatricial tissue in the horse may follow esophageal obstruction that damages the wall, or irritation to the wall from rough handling in attempts to remove the obstruction. Aged horses may develop a stenosis of the terminal portion of the esophagus due to fibrosis of the muscular wall. On rare occasions, caustic chemicals may cause esophagitis and subsequent scarring. Compression of the esophagus occurs occasionally in cattle with lymphosarcoma and from adhesions and traumatic reticulitis near the esophageal hiatus. Compression of the esophagus by a persistent right aortic arch (q.v., p. 72) has also been reported. In sheep, compression from caseous lymphadenitis involving the mediastinal lymph nodes is a rare cause. In horses, stenosis is often accompanied by a diverticulum, or the diverticulum may cause stenosis.

Clinical Findings: Stenosis in horses results in repeated choke. Repeated obstruction leads to weakened walls and eventual dilatation or diverticulum. The clinical signs described in the section on choke occur intermittently. Water is swallowed with no difficulty. Animals chronically affected tend to remain thin.

Cattle with this condition tend to be chronic bloaters and may show a tendency to choke.

Diagnosis: Habitual choke in large animals suggests stenosis and esophageal diverticulum. The passage of a fairly large stomach tube will reveal the narrowing. It is sometimes advisable to use tubes of gradually increasing diameter to determine the degree of stenosis. Radiography after barium by mouth may be used in cervical choke to ascertain the area involved.

Treatment: Feeding on thin mashes and fine-cut hay will help to prevent obstruction, but this procedure is only palliative and so tedious that the patient is usually put down. If the primary cause is a diverticulum it may be possible to correct it surgically.

ESOPHAGEAL DIVERTICULUM (DILATATION)

This condition assumes its greatest importance in the horse. It most often occurs secondarily to stenosis and thus may be indirectly associated with esophagitis or chronic choke. Most diverticula are found in the low cervical and thoracic portions of the esophagus. The important signs are usually seen after feeding and are similar to those of choke.

The diagnosis is based on the history and clinical signs. Some cases of cervical dilation may be palpated and even observed by visual examination. Radiography following the administration of barium has been used in diagnosis. Surgical exposure of the diverticulum and careful apposition of the esophageal musculature without penetrating the esophageal mucosa is the only effective treatment.

ESOPHAGITIS

Esophagitis is rarely diagnosed as a clinical entity in large animals. It may occur occasionally in horses where it is due most often to trauma from foreign bodies or the injudicious use of stomach tubes. Irritating chemicals may infrequently be involved. In cattle the condition may be secondary to infectious diseases such as viral diarrhea, infectious bovine rhinotracheitis or malignant catarrhal fever.

In severe cases, dysphagia, salivation, spasms of the esophageal and cervical musculature, vomiting and extension of the head and neck may be seen.

Withholding feed and water for 2 days often relieves the condition. Electrolytes, methampyrone (℞ 618) and corticosteroids should be administered as supportive therapy and to control spasms. Water is then given and if this is tolerated, moistened mashes may be tried. Sulfonamides or antibiotics should be used to control infection.

SPASM OF THE ESOPHAGUS

(Esophagism)

A condition occurring in horses, most commonly in the young. Although the exact etiology is unknown, the condition has been observed in nursing foals when they begin to take solid food; in young animals convalescing from debilitating acute infections; in horses with acute esophagitis such as that induced by the breaking of a capsule containing some irritant drug; following the use of a stomach tube which may have injured the mucosa; and following the injection of large doses of morphine. Esophagism may also occur during routine stomach tube passage and in tetanus.

Clinical signs resemble those of esophageal obstruction, but do not necessarily have any relation to the intake of food. Sometimes they are brought on by drinking cold water.

There is contraction of the muscles of the neck, pulling the chin down and backward. Some animals make convulsive efforts to vomit, placing the feet under the body and extending the head. Frothy saliva is discharged from the mouth and nostrils and coughing is frequent. Periods of spasm may occur several times a day, or only at intervals of several days. Sometimes there is interference with the passage of a stomach tube. The spasms are symptomatic and cease once the primary cause is removed. Atropine (℞ 511) seems to control the spasms. Severe spasm may be relieved by morphine (℞ 619), or by use of spasmolytic agents such as dipyrone (℞ 513). Tranquilizers (℞ 374, 554) may control signs in nervous individuals.

GASTRITIS

(Gastric catarrh)

Acute or chronic inflammation of the gastric mucous membrane, often associated with enteritis. The term **gastroenteritis** is used to describe inflammation of both stomach and intestinal mucosa. The condition is common in all species of domestic animals. In this discussion gastritis includes rumenitis. (*See* p. 138, *et seq.*)

GASTRITIS IN LARGE ANIMALS

Etiology: Gastritis without involvement of other areas of the alimentary tract is rare. Primary gastritis in all species may be caused by the ingestion of caustic or irritating chemicals but it is usually accompanied by some degree of stomatitis and enteritis. Gastric disturbance with varying degrees of gastritis may follow overeating, sudden changes in diet or ingestion of feeds that are too hot, frozen, moldy or spoiled, the ingestion of sand or foreign bodies and crib-biting with wind-sucking in horses. Chemical rumenitis may occur with grain overload in cattle (q.v., p. 143) and is frequently followed by a fungal or bacterial rumenitis. Calves incorrectly fed may develop rumenitis when milk spills into the rumen and putrefies. Abomasal ulceration and abomasitis are common in young calves and often appear associated with the ingestion of straw or other poorly digestible roughage and with hair balls. In all species gastrointestinal parasitic infections are a common cause of gastritis.

Abomasal ulcers occur in braxy and in pasteurellosis in sheep, and gastric venous infarction is common in acute septicemic and toxemic disease in swine. Gastritis is common in the erosive and vesicular virus diseases of ruminants and occurs in conjunction with many enteric infections in all species.

Clinical Findings: The clinical syndrome is indistinct and varies with the cause. In the **horse**, chronic gastritis and milder forms of gastritis are manifest by unthriftiness and periodic bouts of subacute abdominal pain. Laminitis may accompany or follow gastric disturbance. The feces may be dark and tarry if gastric hemorrhage has occurred. The temperature and pulse rate are usually within the normal range. *Habronema* ulceration may be clinically inapparent. More acute attacks and those following overeating are generally the result of gastric dilatation and pyloric spasm. The temperature is usually elevated and the pulse is fast and weak. Severe pain is usually manifest; the horse sweats profusely and violent episodes of severe colic may occur. Retching movements are common and the horse may vomit. Gastric rupture is a possible sequela. Between these episodes, subacute abdominal pain is manifest and the horse may assume a sitting-dog position.

In **pigs**, vomiting is the cardinal sign of gastritis, with depression, inappetence and evidence of abdominal pain.

In **ruminants**, abomasitis is manifest by depression, inappetence and a fall in production. The temperature and pulse rate are usually mildly elevated and rumination is depressed. Occasionally a pain response may be elicited by percussion over the abomasum. Acute rumen overload produces a characteristic syndrome (q.v., p. 143). Abomasal ulceration in calves may produce a syndrome of unthriftiness but is usually clinically inapparent unless perforation sufficient to produce local peritonitis occurs. Putrefactive rumenitis in calves is manifest by depression, toxemia and diarrhea. The passage of a stomach tube allows the escape of foul-smelling gas and examination of material aspirated may facilitate diagnosis in all species.

Most parasitic infections of the stomach produce a protein-losing gastropathy with unthriftiness and diarrhea without evidence of abdominal pain. However, hemonchosis may be manifest purely as a severe anemia without diarrhea, and hyostrongylosis in adult pigs may simply produce a syndrome of chronic wasting.

Treatment: First and most important is to remove the cause. The animal should be placed on a restricted diet of easily digested food, such as bran gruels or mashes, and green feed or fine hay. If the condition is due to spoiled or irritating feeds, evacuation of the gastrointestinal tract with a mild laxative, such as mineral oil (℞ 505) is indicated. If infection is suspected, enteric sulfonamides (℞ 85, 94) or antibiotics (e.g. ampicillin 2 to 6 mg/lb [4 to 12 mg/kg] body wt. orally) should be administered. To provide protection to the irritated gastric mucosa, protective agents, such as kaolin (℞ 495) or bismuth subnitrate (℞ 491) may be given. In acute gastritis in horses, meperidine (℞ 617) and spasmolytics (℞ 514) are indicated. The passage of a stomach tube may allow relief of gas or of fluid distension. Gastric lavage with isotonic saline solution should be attempted in cases of chemical gastritis and where impaction has occurred. Intravenous fluid therapy and other measures to combat shock (q.v., p. 79) should be initiated. With severe impactions or overload in horses and ruminants, gastrotomy with removal of the food mass is indicated. Following cessation of the signs, the animal should be returned slowly to normal diet. In cattle, gastritis often results in disturbance of the normal rumen flora. Ruman inoculation (q.v., p. 1506) with fresh rumen contents is of considerable aid in hastening recovery in such cases. With putrefactive rumenitis in calves gastric lavage is indicated. Penicillin is given by mouth and the calf is taken off milk for a 24-hour period. An equal volume of electrolyte solution (℞ 575) is fed during this period and the full milk intake is restored gradually over a further period of 48 hours by increasing the milk and decreasing the electrolyte proportions in the fluid fed.

(For treatment of parasitic gastritis *see* parasitology section.)

GASTRITIS IN SMALL ANIMALS

A low-grade inflammation with shallow erosions of the gastric mucosa caused by overeating, ingestion of spoiled food, ingestion of indigestible material particularly in the growing animal (bones, hair, paper, toys) or the administration of irritant drugs (aspirin). Gastritis is also associated with infectious diseases, such as distemper, viral hepatitis, leptospirosis, acute pancreatitis, pyelonephritis, chronic renal failure and gastrointestinal parasites. Ingestion of caustics, arsenic, mercury, lead, thallium or phenol may produce acute corrosive gastritis.

Subacute gastritis occurs when acute gastritis has been improperly treated or when chronic ingestion of irritant materials continues. Chronic vomiting may also be present in gastric neoplasia, or in eosinophilic gastritis.

Clinical Findings: Vomiting, depression and abdominal pain are the cardinal signs: Animals may exhibit excessive thirst but vomiting occurs with the ingestion of water or at any time if there is extensive damage to the mucosa. If corrosive agents have caused the gastritis, the vomitus may contain blood and shreds of gastric mucosa. Food may be refused or animals may exhibit a depraved appetite (licking concrete, chewing dirt). Pain may be manifested by restlessness and objection to palpation of the anterior abdomen. Animals may assume a crouched position or stretch out on a cool surface. When the gastritis is severe there is often an accompanying enteritis. Subacute gastritis is manifested by continued vomiting and signs of weight loss, dehydration and electrolyte imbalance.

Diagnosis: The diagnosis is based on a history of the dietary habits of the animal, the ingestion of foreign or caustic materials and the clinical signs. Gastric radiography may reveal the presence of opaque foreign bodies while the use of a moderate amount of contrast medium in the stomach may facilitate the visualization of nonopaque foreign bodies. Abnormalities in position or contour of the stomach may also be demonstrated. Since it is difficult to visualize ulcers and neoplasms, it may be necessary to distend the stomach with contrast media or use a double-contrast technique. Hypertrophy of the gastric rugae is not a constant radiographic finding.

Treatment: In acute gastritis all food should be withheld for at least 24 hours. Water intake should be controlled by giving the animal ice cubes to lick only if the vomiting is persistent. If enteritis is present, parenteral fluid therapy must be instituted to offset dehydration and electrolyte imbalance. Ringer's solution (℞ 589) is indicated in diseases of the upper digestive tract. Other parenteral fluids such as isotonic saline solution, 5% dextrose in saline solution, and amino acid solutions may be used.

Phenobarbital (℞ 552) is given as a sedative and to reduce gastrointestinal hypermotility and secretions. Meperidine (℞ 617) may be used in cases of corrosive gastritis where there is evidence of pain. Chlorpromazine (℞ 377), or atropine sulfate (℞ 511) may be administered to inhibit vomiting. In cases where ingestion of a poison has been established, an emetic such as apomorphine (℞ 481) is administered soon after ingestion unless the substance swallowed is corrosive in nature. In cases of poisoning the antidote should be administered immediately or gastric lavage or gastrointestinal lavage with a 2% solution of sodium bicarbonate may be employed to remove the irritant foreign material from the stomach. Gastric sedatives such as bismuth subnitrate with kaolin (℞ 491), kaolin and pectin (℞ 495), or dihydrostreptomycin, kaolin and pectin (℞ 36) should be given in small frequent doses.

After the first 24 hours, broth, soup or boiled milk may be given. The following day a bland diet consisting of Pablum and milk, oatmeal, soft-boiled eggs, cooked rice and milk puddings can be instituted. This diet should be fed in small amounts 3 or 4 times daily and gradually modified until the animal returns to a normal diet. Polyvitamin therapy is a useful adjunct in the treatment of gastritis.

Palliative treatment may be required for gastritis secondary to a systemic disease (℞ 488) until specific therapy for the underlying condition becomes effective.

GASTRIC DILATATION (SM. AN.)

(Gastric torsion)

A distension of the stomach caused by the accumulation of gastric secretions, food or gases.

Etiology: Gastric dilatation in dogs occurs in several forms with vastly different clinical pictures. In one form, there is a compensatory enlargement of the stomach over a longer period because of an increased food intake. Etiologic factors in this category include parasitism, inadequate diet and pancreatic insufficiency. A second, much more acute form, occurs as a sudden episode in which there is an acute distension of the stomach with gastric secretions, food and gas. Acute gastric dilatation occurs most frequently in the large, deep-chested breeds, and various studies have noted a slightly higher incidence in males. Torsion is generally considered to be a sequela to dilatation.

There is probably no single cause. The various factors suggested have included trauma, gastric neoplasms, vomiting, parturition, pica, overeating and abdominal surgery. The rapid production of a quantity of gas in the stomach and the inability of the animal to get rid of it cause the dilatation. Bacterial fermentation has been shown to be an important factor in the pathogenesis of acute dilatation.

Gastric torsion has been linked to lengthening of the supporting gastric ligaments, a pendulous, food-filled stomach or an atonic stomach.

Clinical Findings: Acute gastric dilatation, with or without torsion, produces a characteristic clinical picture in which the animal initially shows signs of abdominal pain and then rapidly develops abdominal distension, excessive salivation, retching, dyspnea, peripheral circulatory collapse and shock.

Lesions: In chronic cases, a marked increased in abdominal size is the only abnormality. In acute gastric dilatation, the stomach wall is distended, hyperemic and very thin. When torsion of the stomach occurs, the organ rotates upon the attachments to its lesser curvature. The spleen becomes distended from occlusion of its vascular structures. Gastric changes include hemorrhage and necrosis of the gastric mucosa.

Diagnosis: When the condition is due to parasitism, pancreatic dysfunction or inadequate diet, the diagnosis will be adequately supported by history and the physical signs. Gastric torsion and acute gastric dilatation produce identical clinical pictures, and cannot be differentiated with certainty. If a tube can be passed into the stomach, it is safe to assume that severe torsion does not exist. However, it is sometimes impossible to pass a stomach tube in an uncomplicated acute dilatation. Laparotomy may be required for a positive diagnosis. Radiographs may show displacement of the pylorus when torsion is present, but may stress an already acutely ill animal.

Treatment: The treatment of secondary gastric dilatation consists of treating the primary condition. Simple overloading of the stomach is treated by inducing emesis with apomorphine (℞ 481).

Acute gastric dilatation is an emergency. If initial efforts to relieve the tympany by passing a stomach tube fail, the gas must be released through a large-gauge hypodermic needle inserted through the abdominal wall into the distended stomach. Meperidine (℞ 617) may be administered to combat pain, but should be used with caution. If release of the gas does not bring about immediate and marked improvement, a laparotomy should be performed promptly, and the stomach completely evacuated and examined carefully for possible rotation. Gastropexy may be necessary.

Animals that show signs of shock should be given IV corticosteroids (℞ 140), and lactated Ringer's solution (℞ 588) to which has been added up to 5 mEq/kg of bicarbonate. This should be given within the first 2 hours if possible. Antibiotics and oxygen are highly beneficial. Dogs that survive the acute attack should be starved for 24 hours, placed on a liquid diet for at least 3 days and then placed on a schedule of at least 3 meals a day and given bland foods similar to those described under the treatment of acute gastritis (q.v., p. 133). The use of a pharyngostomy tube for 4 to 5 days may be useful. Tube gastrostomy is sometimes used. Since the condition tends to recur, owners should be advised to take preventive measures, such as multiple daily feedings, diet change, withholding water for an hour after eating, and prohibiting feed and excess water after vigorous exercise until the dog has relaxed.

GASTRIC FOREIGN BODIES (SM. AN.)

Etiology: Young dogs and cats may swallow such foreign objects as rubber balls, stones, bones, women's stockings, fishhooks and needles. Cats often swallow large amounts of hair, which may form a mass in the stomach or intestines. A depraved appetite, such as that associated with rabies, pancreatic disease, avitaminosis, or mineral deficiency, frequently causes animals to ingest foreign substances. Some dogs develop a vice of swallowing stones, but, as a rule, these animals show few clinical signs of ill-health.

Clinical Findings: The signs produced by gastric foreign bodies are extremely variable; many produce no clinical signs and may remain undetected for long periods. In such cases there may be a history of intermittent vomiting after the ingestion of solid food. Affected animals often show a gradual loss of condition.

Large, rough foreign bodies produce a more violent reaction and affected animals show signs of gastritis (q.v., p. 132). Sharp and irritating objects may lacerate the mucous membrane and cause hematemesis, or rarely perforation. A characteristic and suggestive sign is vomiting.

Hair balls in the stomach of cats can cause occasional episodes of retching, vomiting and inappetence, and loss of condition, or sometimes a change in behavior in which the cat cries frequently for food, eats ravenously when it is offered, but loses interest after a few mouthfuls.

Diagnosis: A tentative diagnosis can usually be made from the history and physical examination. To confirm, the recommended procedure is to make a survey film to check for the presence of radiopaque objects; if this is negative, further roentgenographs may be necessary following the administration of a radiopaque mixture.

Treatment: Apomorphine (℞ 481) may be given to cause the expulsion of small, smooth objects. However, vomiting should not be induced if the foreign body is of such size or shape that it could injure the esophagus. Small objects can sometimes be removed with forceps through a gastroscope. Small sharp objects, such as needles, pins or tacks, often can be made to pass safely through the intestinal tract by feeding small balls of absorbent cotton that have been mixed with meat or bread soaked in milk, or packed into gelatin capsules. Methylcellulose (℞ 508) or agar compounds are useful in providing bulk. Hair balls in cats are usually passed with the feces after the administration of one or more doses of petrolatum. Many gastric foreign bodies can be removed only by a gastrotomy.

GASTROINTESTINAL ULCERS

In the dog, gastric ulceration is most commonly associated with either tumors of the stomach or hemorrhagic gastritis due to severe uremia. Gastric ulcers assume major importance in swine, and abomasal ulcers in mature cattle and young calves appear to be increasing in importance. Ulcers appear to be associated with feeding practices, the stress of high production and confinement rearing. (*See* ULCERATION OF THE ABOMASUM, p. 151.) Gastric ulcers are a cause of sudden death in foals. Duodenal ulcers occur rarely, perhaps less rarely in swine than in other species.

ESOPHAGOGASTRIC ULCERS IN SWINE

Esophagogastric ulcers affect the pars esophagea in swine and cause sporadic cases of acute gastric hemorrhage or unthriftiness due to chronic ulceration.

Etiology: The cause of the disease is unknown. It is commonest in confined growing pigs (45 to 90 kg) fed finely ground rations that may be deficient in fiber, and also in pigs fed large quantities of skimmed milk or whey. Also, the stress of confinement rearing is thought to promote hyperacidity which may contribute to the development of the lesion. A combination of confinement rearing, stress due to transportation, deprivation of feed, crowding and mixing with unfamiliar pigs results in a significant increase in the incidence of gastric ulcers in rapidly growing pigs. The disease may be inapparent in a group of rapidly growing feeder pigs or young breeding gilts until some anxiety, tension or physical stress precipitates the acute illness. This is particularly significant in pigs gathered for slaughter at abattoirs.

Clinical Findings: Gastric ulcers occur in swine of all ages but are commonest in rapidly growing feeder pigs. In the acute form, hemorrhage results in anorexia, weakness, anemia, black tarry feces and death in hours or days. In the chronic form, unthriftiness, black tarry feces and anemia are characteristic but the pig may survive for several weeks. The subclinical form, although symptomless, may result in affected pigs not reaching maturity at the expected time. In these the ulcer usually heals and a scar remains. In some herds up to 90% of the feeder pigs may be affected while in other herds it occurs only sporadically. Based on abattoir studies, the incidence of ulcers may be quite high in feeder pigs which have appeared thrifty and have grown normally; clinical disease apparently occurs only following hemorrhage of the ulcer.

Lesions: The typical terminal lesion is found in the wall of the stomach near the esophageal opening in an area that normally is a white, glistening, nonglandular, rectangular patch of squamous epithelium. It is common to find a crater 1 or 2 in. or more in diameter encompassing the esophagus. The crater appears as a cream or gray punched-out area and may contain blood clots or debris. In acute hemorrhage the stomach and upper small intestine will contain dark blood. Earlier the lesions are characterized by hyperkeratosis and parakeratosis of the squamous epithelium about the esophageal opening into the stomach. Later, the proliferative lesion erodes to form the ulcer. The healed ulcer appears as a stellate scar.

Diagnosis and Treatment: The appearance of 1 or 2 listless, anemic pigs in a pen, showing anorexia, loss of weight, reluctance to move, the passage of dark feces and sometimes labored breathing, or the sudden death of an apparently healthy pig is suggestive of gastric ulceration. There is no known effective treatment. Increasing the fiber content of the diet to 7% and the feeding of meal rather than pellets may be of value. The reduction of stressful conditions such as crowding may minimize the incidence. Growing pigs should not be moved from one pen to another but rather raised in the same pen until marketing.

TRAUMATIC RETICULOPERITONITIS

(Traumatic gastritis, "Hardware disease")

A disease of cattle resulting from perforation of the reticulum, and sometimes the rumen, by a sharp object. The condition is under almost constant consideration in the differential diagnosis of diseases of the digestive system in cattle because of the similarity of its signs to those of other such diseases. It is commonest in mature dairy cattle and in beef cattle less than 3 years of age. Occasionally, cases have been reported in other species of ruminants.

Foreign objects are common in the stomach of cattle because they lack discrimination against hard materials in the feed and incompletely masticate feed at the time of ingestion. The disease is common where silage and hay are made from fields containing old rusting fences and baling wire, or from areas where buildings have recently been constructed, burned or torn down.

Etiology: Swallowed metallic objects, such as nails or pieces of wire fall directly into the reticulum or fall into the rumen and are subsequently carried over the ruminoreticular fold into the lower anterior part of the reticulum. As the exit of this organ, the reticulo-omasal orifice, is elevated above the floor, retention of heavy objects in the reticulum is favored. The honeycomb-like reticular mucosa acts as a trap for sharp objects. Contractions of the reticulum promote penetration of the wall by the metallic object. The volume of the gravid uterus in late pregnancy and straining during parturition or mating are additional factors that may initiate this process.

The foreign object may pierce the wall of the reticulum and its overlying peritoneum resulting in contamination of the peritoneal cavity. A localized peritonitis follows, frequently resulting in adhesions, or a more severe and widespread peritonitis may occur. The object may penetrate the diaphragm and enter the thoracic cavity (causing pleuritis and sometimes pneumonitis) and the pericardial sac (causing pericarditis, sometimes followed by myocarditis, endocarditis and septicemia). Occasionally, other organs, e.g. liver, spleen, may be pierced and infected because the object takes a different course.

Clinical Findings: The initial attack is characterized by sudden onset, with anorexia and a sharp fall in production in lactating cows. The animal may exhibit an arched back, an anxious expression, a reluctance to move and an uneasy, careful gait. Forced sudden movements and the acts of defecation, urination and lying down may be accompanied by groaning. A grunt may be elicited by percussing in the area of the xiphoid, or by elevating this area firmly and then releasing rapidly, or by pinching the back. The grunt may be detected by placing the detector of the stethoscope over the trachea. Tremor of the triceps and abduction of the elbow may be observed. The pulse rate may be slightly elevated and respiratory movements tend to be shallow and accelerated and are sometimes accompanied by an expiratory grunt. Rectal temperature is often elevated by 1 or 2°F (0.5 to 1°C). A pulse rate of over 90 and a temperature over 104°F (40°C) usually indicate serious complications such as pleuritis, pericarditis or diffuse peritonitis. In these complications toxemia and depression are much more severe. Pleuritis may be unilateral or bilateral and is manifest by fast shallow respiration, muffling of lung sounds and the variable presence of pleuritic friction rubs. Thoracocentesis may allow the drainage of several liters of fluid. Traumatic pericarditis is usually manifest by muffling of the heart sounds with a variable presence of a pericardial friction rub and occasionally the presence of gas and fluid sounds on auscultation. Jugular engorgement with a pronounced atrial jugular pulse is present early in the course and congestive heart failure (q.v., p. 59) is a frequent sequela. In the presence of these complications the prognosis is grave.

Diagnosis: In early cases traumatic gastritis is not always readily distinguishable from peritonitis or indigestion arising from other causes. White blood cell counts usually indicate leukocytosis due to neutrophilia with a variable shift to the left. A history of sudden onset, fever and evidence of pain are not characteristic of ketosis or indigestion due to most other causes. The rapid, labored breathing accompanied by rales that are characteristic of pneumonia are not present. Abomasal displacement may be differentiated by history and on auscultation in many cases; it usually occurs after parturition, has a slower clinical onset, is afebrile and accompanied by ketonuria, and percussion in the xiphoid area is unlikely to cause "grunting."

Other syndromes that can be differentiated are abomasal torsion and dilatation, omasal impaction, lymphosarcoma involving the gastrointestinal tract and pyelonephritis. More difficulty may be expected with peritonitis arising from other causes, e.g. trauma, abomasal ulcer, intestinal obstruction. Careful evaluation of the history may help rule these out. Electronic metal detectors are used as diagnostic aids but many healthy cattle carry metal objects in their reticulum.

Cattle that come to notice late in the course of the disease and have not recovered spontaneously may be classified into one of 2 general types, acute and chronic. The acute cases usually present signs of acute peritonitis, pericarditis or septicemia. Chronic cases are recurrent and present a real challenge to the diagnostician and may involve vagus indigestion or diaphragmatic hernia (q.v., pp. 589 and 142).

Prophylaxis and Treatment: Avoiding the use of baling wire, magnetizing the bins used to prepare and store feed, and keeping the animals away from sites of new construction or removal of old buildings or fences are examples of steps that can be taken. As an additional precautionary measure bar magnets may be administered orally, preferably after fasting for 18 to 24 hours. Permanent magnets 2½ to 3 in. long and ½ to 1 in. in diameter (6 to 7 cm by 1.3 to 2.5 cm), either cylindrical or with a grooved surface, or magnets in plastic cages, are commonly used. Such a magnet usually remains in the reticulum and holds any ferromagnetic objects on its surface.

Treatment of the typical case seen early in its course may be surgical or medical. Either approach seems to improve the chances of recovery from about 60% in untreated cases to 80 to 90%. The surgical approach involves rumenotomy with manual removal of the object or objects if they can be reached. Medical treatment involves antibacterial therapy to control the peritonitis combined with administration of a magnet to prevent recurrence. Penicillin plus dihydrostreptomycin (℞ 66) or sulfonamides (℞ 102) are, in general, used for 3 days. Antibiotics may also be given IP. Affected animals should be kept immobilized for 1 to 2 weeks and placed on an inclined plane to help limit further anterior progress for the foreign object. Feed intake should be reduced and, if a laxative seems to be indicated, a mild one such as magnesium hydroxide (℞ 504) is preferred. Use of metal detectors to aid diagnosis and flexible magnetic metal retrievers introduced orally or through an incision in the flank to aid in removal of the objects or magnets is practiced by some.

More advanced cases, those with obvious secondary complications or that do not respond to initial therapeutic measures should be evaluated from an economic viewpoint.

DIGESTIVE DISORDERS OF THE RUMEN

RUMINAL PARAKERATOSIS

A noninfectious, noncontagious disease of sheep and cattle, characterized by hardening and enlargement of papillae of the rumen. The disease is caused by fattening on finely ground or pelleted feed and occurs commonly in feedlot cattle and lambs, in which it is observed at the time of slaughter. The incidence may be high in fattened animals.

Many of the papillae are enlarged and hardened and several may adhere together to form bundles. The papillae of the anterior ventral sac are commonly affected. In cattle, the roof of the dorsal sac may show multiple foci of parakeratosis, each focus being 2 to 3 sq cm in area. In sheep, abnormal papillae may be visible and palpable through the wall of the intact rumen. Microscopically, affected papillae contain excessive layers of keratinized epithelial cells, particles of food and bacteria. The rumens of affected cattle are difficult to clean in the preparation of tripe. The abnormal epithelium, by interfering with absorption, may reduce efficiency of feed utilization and rate of gain.

Ruminal parakeratosis may be prevented by fattening animals on rations that contain unground ingredients in the proportion of one part of roughage to 3 parts of concentrate. At present the necessity and economics of prevention are unknown.

"SIMPLE" INDIGESTION

(Mild dietary indigestion)

A minor disturbance in gastrointestinal function usually associated with a change of feed or overfeeding.

Etiology: Almost any factor that can cause a minor alteration in the environment of the rumen may cause simple indigestion. It is common in dairy cattle that suddenly eat excessive quantities of a highly palatable feed such as corn or grass silage, or root crops and their tops. A sudden change in feed, the use of spoiled or frozen feeds, the introduction of urea to a ration, turning cattle onto a lush cereal-grain pasture, and parturient cows eating their placentas can all result in simple indigestion. A degree of simple indigestion is common in feedlot cattle being introduced to a high-level grain ration.

Clinical Findings: The clinical signs depend upon the type of animal affected and the cause of the disorder. Dairy cattle with simple indigestion due to silage overfeeding are anorectic and milk production drops moderately. The rumen is usually full, firm and doughy; the primary contractions are absent but secondary contractions may be present. Temperature, pulse and respiration are normal. The feces are normal-to-firm in consistency but reduced in amount. Spontaneous recovery usually occurs in 24 to 48 hours.

Simple indigestion due to excessive feeding of grain results in anorexia and rumen stasis; the rumen is not necessarily full and may contain excessive quantities of fluid. The feces are usually soft and foul smelling. The affected animal is bright and alert and usually begins to eat within 24 hours. The result of a more severe upset from the same cause is described under grain overload (q.v., p. 143).

Diagnosis: This is based largely on the elimination of other possibilities and a history of a change in the nature or amount of the diet. The systemic reaction and painful responses to percussion seen in traumatic reticuloperitonitis are not observed. The absence of ketonuria, and the history, help eliminate ketosis from consideration. Displaced abomasum can usually be eliminated by auscultation. Vagus indigestion and abomasal torsions become more readily detectable as they progress because they have a longer course, but initial differentiation may be difficult. Rumen overload is distinguishable by its greater severity and the pronounced fall in the pH of the rumen contents.

Treatment: Treatment should be aimed at correcting the suspected dietary factors. Spontaneous recovery is usual. Administration of 5 to 10 gal. (20 to 40L) of warm water or saline via a stomach tube, followed by vigorous kneading of the rumen, may aid in restoring rumen function. Magnesium hydroxide (℞ 504) given orally, seems to be useful when excessive amounts of high-energy feeds have been ingested. If too much feed containing urea or large amounts of protein has been ingested, acetic acid or vinegar may be administered orally. If the activity of the ruminal microbes is reduced, administration of 1 to 2 gal. (4 to 8 L) of ruminal fluid from a healthy cow will help.

VAGUS INDIGESTION

A group of related clinical syndromes of cattle caused by vagal nerve injury as a result of the lesions of traumatic reticuloperitonitis (q.v., p. 138) and other less common suppurative lesions. In some cases vagal nerve injury cannot be demonstrated. Damage to the tension receptors, situated in the right wall of the reticulum, which reflexly control vagal activity, may explain such cases. It is most common in late pregnancy but can occur in nonpregnant cattle. It is characterized by inappetence and eventually anorexia, progressive distension of the abdomen, varying degrees of dehydration, scant feces and progressive loss of weight. Onset is insidious and most cattle have been ill for several days or weeks when first seen by the veterinarian. The temperature is usually normal, the heart rate may be slower than normal in the early stages but later ranges from 84 to 110 per minute. The rumen is usually distended with fluid and may be atonic or hypermotile. This can be confirmed by rectal examination except in cases of advanced pregnancy when palpation of the organ is precluded by the presence of the distended uterus. Auscultation of the left flank often reveals resonant sounds similar to those heard in cases of left abomasal displacement. The abomasum may be impacted and palpable externally through the abdominal wall behind the right costal arch or by rectal examination as a large firm doughy mass lying on the right side of the ventral floor of the abdomen. The rectum is usually empty except for sticky mucus. Most affected cattle die from secondary starvation, dehydration, acid-base and electrolyte imbalances.

Treatment: Response to treatment is unsatisfactory. Valuable cows that are near parturition (1 to 2 weeks) can be maintained on continuous IV fluid therapy using balanced electrolytes (℞ 579) and glucose. Rumenotomy provides only temporary relief and the use of cathartics, stomach and intestinal stimulants and lubricating substances has been disappointing. Fluid therapy and rumen lavage with a large-bore stomach tube are indicated. Parturition may be induced in pregnancies over 8 months (*see* INDUCED ABORTION, p. 834).

GRAIN OVERLOAD

(D-Lactic acidosis, Carbohydrate engorgement, Rumen impaction)

An acute disease of ruminants characterized by indigestion, rumen stasis, dehydration, acidosis, toxemia, incoordination, collapse and, frequently, death.

Etiology: The cause is excessive ingestion of feeds rich in starch or sugars, e.g. cereal grains, corn, fruits, root crops or high-energy prepared feeds. These favor the proliferation of gram-positive bacteria in the rumen whose end-production of fermentation is L- and D-lactic acid. The rumen pH falls to 4.0 to 4.5, destroying the protozoa, cellulolytic organisms and lactate-utilizing organisms as well as impairing rumen motility. Superimposition of lactic acid and its salt, lactate, on the existing solutes in the rumen liquid causes a substantial rise in osmotic pressure which draws fluid into the rumen causing dehydration. Mammals metabolize L-lactic acid more rapidly than D-lactic acid, the absorption of which leads to a more severe and protracted acidosis than an equivalent absorption of L-lactic acid. Progressive acidosis and dehydration may lead to the death of the animal in 1 to 3 days. In protracted cases hypochloremic alkalosis may follow the acidotic phase.

Clinical Findings: About 8 to 12 hours after feeding, the animals may show anorexia, signs of indigestion and irritability progressing to dullness. The rumen may be distended and show reduced motility. Progressive signs include atony of the rumen with increasingly fluid contents, increased pulse and respiration rates, variable rectal temperature, sunken eyes, loss of dermal elasticity, incoordination, collapse and coma. The feces are usually soft and malodorous; they may have a grayish color and small volume in severe cases; other animals develop a profuse diarrhea. Death may ensue within one to several days. Some animals show lameness that may be attributable to laminitis. Animals that survive the acute phase but develop fungal rumenitis remain anorectic, become cachectic and die within 2 weeks.

Diagnosis: The rumen contents have a low pH (4.0 to 4.8 would be considered diagnostic). The hematocrit may be greatly elevated (40 to 50), blood pH and bicarbonate values are extremely low and blood lactate is very high. History of deliberate or accidental exposure to an excess of a high-energy feed relatively low in protein or a sudden change in conditions in a feedlot help establish the correct diagnosis.

Treatment: Mortality is high in severely affected animals unless vigorous therapeutic procedures are initiated early. Emergency slaughter should be considered when many cattle are severely affected (recumbent and in shock). Treatment of the severe form necessitates rumenotomy with removal of all ingesta, washing out the rumen and replacing the contents with ingesta taken from healthy cattle.

Alternatively the rumen can be emptied, using a large stomach tube (1 in. diameter, 10 ft. long [2.5 cm x 3m]), and irrigating the rumen 15 to 20 times. The rumen is filled using water from an ordinary water hose connected to the stomach tube and then allowed to empty by gravity flow. Fluid therapy using balanced electrolytes (℞ 579) is necessary to correct the acid-base imbalance and dehydration, and to restore renal function. If balanced electrolytes are unavailable, a saline-sodium bicarbonate mixture (℞ 590) may be used. In severe cases, 5% sodium bicarbonate may be given IV at the rate of 2.5 to 5 qt/1,000 lb (2 to 4 L/400 kg) body weight and followed by isotonic sodium bicarbonate (1.3%). Less severely affected animals may be treated with oral antacids to control rumen pH (℞ 504) and supportive IV fluid therapy (℞ 579, 590). Many other treatments have been recommended but none is as beneficial as the combination of emptying the rumen either by rumenotomy or by lavage and the parenteral administration of antacids and fluids. During the convalescent period, which may last 2 to 4 days, cattle should be given good-quality hay with no grain.

BLOAT IN RUMINANTS

(Tympanites, Tympany, Hoven, Meteorism)

An excessive accumulation of gas in the first 2 compartments (rumen and reticulum) of the ruminant stomach. Mild distension is of little consequence clinically, but if it persists it reduces food intake and milk production. Severe bloat causes great discomfort and is frequently (and sometimes rapidly) fatal.

Bloat occurs in all domestic ruminants, but is common only in cattle. It is particularly important in Australia, New Zealand and wherever year-round grazing is practiced. In the U.S.A. and Great Britain, it occurs most commonly on newly developed, highly productive pastures and is an important deterrent to the development and utilization of such pastures. It rarely occurs in sheep, but is of economic importance in this species in restricted areas in the Western U.S.A.

Although pasture bloat may occur at any time, the incidence is higher in wet summers on clover-dominant pastures that are growing rapidly. Bloat occurs less often in animals on dry feed but it can be a significant cause of loss in feedlots.

Etiology: Bloat may be classified as primary or secondary. Solid objects, such as corn cobs, turnips, apples, potatoes and peaches, commonly lodge in the esophagus and, by preventing eructation, cause secondary bloat. External pressure on the esophagus by enlarged mediastinal lymph nodes; interference with cardial innervation, as in vagus indigestion and diaphragmatic hernia; and sporadic cases of bloat in young calves are further examples of causes of secondary bloat.

Primary bloat is by far the more important. In animals at pasture or on dry feed, it is caused by the interaction of a number of sometimes rather obscure factors that combine to reduce the ratio of gas eliminated by eructation to gas produced by fermentation. Overproduction of gas *per se* is not the important factor; most authorities agree that bloat is caused by a failure in the eructation mechanism rather than by excessive consumption of a dangerous material or lack of rumen motility.

The primary cause of pasture bloat appears to be a change in the composition of certain pasture plants, facilitating the development of a stable foam that in turn prevents eructation. Lush pastures, particularly those dominated by rapidly growing leguminous plants, most commonly induce serious bloating, but such pastures are not always hazardous nor are other types always safe. Some animal factors including individual susceptibility, the volume and composition of saliva, and possibly habituation, may influence the hazard of bloat on a given pasture, but if serious losses due to bloat are to be prevented, it is necessary to control the undesirable changes in plant composition. Alternatively, or as an interim measure, it is necessary to prevent the development of frothing by chemical or physical means. Feedlot bloat may be frothy or of the free-gas type. Its cause is uncertain but there is much evidence that excessive slime formation can cause retention of gases entrapped in the resulting froth.

Clinical Findings: The first sign is a distension of the left side, which may become so severe that the area of the left paralumbar fossa protrudes above the normal top line. Distension on the right side is lateral in direction. Breathing may become labored and, in some cases, there is profuse salivation. Grazing usually ceases when intraruminal pressure becomes moderately high, i.e. between 10 and 30 mm of Hg, or when the left side feels firm during the relaxed phase of the rumen motility cycle. Rumen motility can usually be detected until the condition of the animal is critical, although its effectiveness in clearing the cardia is obviously reduced. Eructation usually continues, but with decreased frequency and the amount of gas expelled is apparently reduced as the intraruminal pressure increases. When tympany becomes severe, eructation may eventually cease. At this point the visible mucous membranes become cyanotic and the gait staggering; the animal may vomit, respiration is labored and eventually collapse occurs. Death usually ensues within a few minutes after the animal falls to the ground. Bloating and death may occur within 30 to 40 minutes after the cow has entered the pasture. Usually, however, several hours pass between the beginning of pasture grazing and fatal termination. The clinical signs in secondary (obstructive) bloat do not differ materially from those of the primary (nonobstructive) forms, but eructation may be entirely absent in cases of choke. The causes of death in bloat are not known, although interference with respiration and gross visceral distension are probably important factors.

Diagnosis: The presence of the clinical signs is sufficient for diagnosis. To distinguish from early cases of tetanus, which often have ruminal tympany, it is necessary to look for prolapse of the third eyelid and other signs. Tympany is maintained after death but is not diagnostic in itself; the frothiness does not persist. At necropsy, the most significant findings are congestion and hemorrhage of the tissues of the cranial parts of the body with pallor and ischemia of the caudal parts. These changes are the result of occlusion of the caudal vena cava, which causes blood to be shunted to the cranial parts of the body.

Prophylaxis: The prevention of bloat may be attempted by carefully controlled management practices, but these are subject to many inexplicable failures and only guarded recommendations can be made: (1) maintaining pastures that do not exceed 50% legumes; (2) practicing strip-grazing that compels close or whole-plant grazing; (3) feeding at least 10 lb (5 kg) per head of dry, scabrous hay each day, before permitting the gazing of legume-rich pastures, or overnight-feeding of Sudan hay; (4) administering antifoaming agents such as nontoxic oils and poloxalene.

The prophylactic administration of either nonionic surfactants such as poloxalene or nontoxic oils or fats has been found to be generally effective, provided they are given regularly and in sufficient quantity. The oil or fat, usually emulsified with water, may be sprayed on strip-grazed pasture at the rate of 2 to 4 oz (60 to 120 ml) per cow daily. If grazing is uncontrolled, the material may be dosed orally, painted on the flanks where the cow can lick it, administered mixed with hay, especially to beef cattle, or mixed with the drinking water to make a 2% emulsion if an adequate intake is ensured. The selection of the oil or fat to be used depends largely on cost, although freedom from milk-tainting substances and depression of fat-soluble vitamin availability should be considered. In general, peanut oil and tallow are most favored. Poloxalene is administered in feed or mineral licks or blocks at the rate of 10 to 20 gm daily. Silicones and household detergents have been suggested as useful antifoaming agents, but are most unreliable.

The ruminal implantation of a slow-release device containing antifrothing agents is undergoing extensive field trials in Australia. Enzymatic activity in the rumen can be reduced by the feeding of an enzyme inhibitor (alkyl arylsulfonate) applied to a floating matrix (vermiculite) and coated (cellulose) for slow release in the rumen. When fed with grain this built-up compound is capable of greatly reducing legume bloat. Although none of the above methods are highly effective against feedlot bloat, they are used and, particularly the administration of oil, recommended for trial. Since bloat in feedlot cattle is often caused by insufficient roughage in the ration, increasing the amount may prevent bloating. The effect is enhanced if all grain is only coarse ground.

Treatment: Intraruminal pressure should be reduced as quickly as possible. This may be done by passing a large stomach tube, which is then manipulated in order to encounter gas pockets. In foamy bloat, the stomach tube method is usually disappointing, but it may have diagnostic value in determining the foaming characteristics of the ingesta. Sometimes, trocarization of the rumen through the left paralumbar fossa is justified. The cannula should be left in place until the danger is past. If the animal is in critical condition or has collapsed, rumenotomy should be performed at once.

Defoaming agents should be given immediately. The more useful compounds are vegetable oils, such as peanut oil, corn oil and soybean oil. Doses of 4 to 8 oz (120 to 240 ml) are probably sufficient, but in practice it is usual to administer at least 1 pint (0.5 L). Cream is quite effective in an emergency. Cresol (30 ml), turpentine (30 to 60 ml), formaldehyde solution (15 to 30 ml) and other so-called antiferments have little effect on gas formation. They are probably no more effective than the vegetable oils and may have undesirable side effects, such as the production of off-flavors in milk. The drug or defoaming agent may be given by drench, but, because of the danger of aspiration, administration by stomach tube or, in extreme cases, through a cannula entering the rumen through the paralumbar fossa is preferred.

ABOMASAL DISORDERS

LEFT DISPLACEMENT OF THE ABOMASUM

A disease of high-producing, heavily fed dairy cattle, usually near parturition, in which the abomasum is displaced to the left of the rumen. It is rarely seen in steers, calves, bulls and sheep.

Etiology: The basic cause is believed to be a reduction in abomasal tone. This could result from a variety of factors most of which are operative particularly at or about the time of parturition. The most important of these are heavy feeding of grain and silages just before and after calving. Some displacements occur following hypocalcemia, ketosis and toxemias due to metritis, mastitis, etc. but these appear to be of minor significance, as are mechanical factors associated with the act of parturition, and hereditary predisposition. It has been suggested that diminution in the size of the rumen due to a low-roughage diet creates a potential space beneath the ventral ruminal sac, and it is by this route that the atonic abomasum moves passively to the left side of the abdomen. Then, due to the absence of peristaltic movements, gas accumulates in the abomasum, causing it to move upwards on the left of the rumen. In addition, increased amounts of volatile fatty acids may be present in the abomasum of cows receiving large amounts of grain which would also allow the abomasum to move about more readily.

Clinical Findings and Diagnosis: The severity of clinical signs varies greatly depending on how long the abomasum has been displaced. Typically there is intermittent anorexia with marked preference for hay or grass rather than grain, weight loss and diminished milk yield. Feces are usually scant, pasty and mucus-covered, but diarrhea may occur. Rumen movements are decreased and may not be noted if the rumen is pushed too far medially. A fullness in the left flank may be noted. A constant sign is a mildly positive urine-ketone reaction, usually secondary to the reduced food intake.

A diagnosis can usually be made by auscultation over the last 3 ribs about halfway down the cow's left side, where occasional resonant splashing or gurgling sounds may be heard. In cases in which these sounds are particularly infrequent they can be elicited by vigorous ballottement low in the left flank. Alternatively, percussion and simultaneous auscultation over the last 2 or 3 ribs on the left gives rise to a clear resonant "pinging" sound. Since the abomasum can slip back and forth from a normal position to displacement, repeated examinations over several days may be required to establish a diagnosis.

Treatment: The simplest method of handling a displaced abomasum consists of rolling the cow on her back and massaging the anterior part of the abdomen from left to right for a few minutes. When the cow is let up she will often start eating at once. However, few cows respond permanently to this technique and in most cases surgery is required. A variety of operations are described, most of which are technically simple and have a high rate of success.

Prevention: Incidence can be reduced by decreasing the amount of grain and silages fed to cows before calving and by feeding greater amounts of long hay. The amount of grain should be gradually increased after calving to meet the requirements of milk production.

RIGHT DISPLACEMENT AND TORSION OF THE ABOMASUM

A condition in which the abomasum becomes progressively distended and sometimes undergoes torsion while occupying a position to the right of the midline. Insofar as the basic cause is abomasal atony, it shares a common etiology with left displacement. That the organ does not displace to the left in this condition is thought to be due to local anatomic factors such as the size of the rumen and the tightness of omental attachments.

Clinical Findings and Diagnosis: A history of recent parturition is commonly encountered but not as frequently as in left displacement. During the phase of distension, the appetite is depressed, the milk yield lowered and feces reduced in quantity. The pulse rate progressively increases. Distension of the right flank develops and high-pitched resonant sounds can be heard on auscultation and ballottement of the right flank. Surgical intervention at this point will usually prevent abomasal torsion and the prognosis is good provided that abomasal atony has not developed from prolonged dilations.

Torsion of the abomasum causes signs of acute abdominal pain, increased pulse rate (90 to 160/min), subnormal temperature and depression. The feces are usually scanty but there may be diarrhea. The distended abomasum can usually be palpated on the right posterior aspect of the abdomen by rectal examination.

Progressive dehydration is prominent. Death usually occurs within 1 or 2 days. Traumatic gastritis, intestinal accident, displaced abomasum, abomasal ulcers, abomasal impaction, torsion of the cecum and vagus indigestion all should be considered in the differential diagnoses at various stages. The acute onset and rapid progression of the condition usually allows a diagnosis to be made.

Treatment: An incision is made through the right paralumbar fossa and the abomasum drained. The torsion, if present, is corrected manually after releasing gas and removing contents. If the abomasum contracts promptly, it is considered a good prognostic sign, but in most cases this does not happen and mortality is high. Large volumes of electrolyte solution are indicated to counter the severe dehydration which is a constant feature.

Preventive measures are similar to those listed for the prevention of left displacement of the abomasum.

IMPACTION OF THE ABOMASUM

This gastric upset occurs in calves and lambs that ingest indigestible fibrous material such as hair, wool or rags. The impacted mass often contains putrefying, casein curds. It also occurs in ewes fed on grain stubble containing morning glory, and adult cattle and sheep fed poor-quality fibrous feed. Pregnant animals wintered on chopped straw without supplement are most commonly affected. Affected calves and lambs become unthrifty and may develop distended abdomens with excessive fluid detectable in the rumen or abomasum. The feces tend to be soft and discolored and may contain traces of fibrous material. These young animals frequently respond to abomasotomy with removal of the obstructing mass and supportive therapy.

Adult ruminants impacted with fibrous feed show anorexia, very scanty, tenacious, malodorous feces and right flank distension, initially without systemic involvement. They become weak, dehydrated and recumbent. In advanced pregnancy the uterus may force the impacted abomasum anteriorly making it less accessible to palpation. Many cases of vagus indigestion are complicated by impaction of the abomasum, and this in turn is often a sequela to traumatic gastritis. The prognosis is unfavorable regardless of the cause. Such animals may be sent to slaughter if their condition has not deteriorated too greatly and they have not received drugs causing tissue residues.

Prevention is based on proper feeding and management of calves and lambs and the routine administration of magnets to cattle to prevent the traumatic gastritis which can lead to vagus indigestion. Impaction of the abomasum with poor quality fibrous feeds can be prevented by feeding a high-protein supplement to encourage the digestion of chopped straw, etc.

ULCERATION OF THE ABOMASUM

Superficial abomasal ulceration occurs in such diseases as bovine viral diarrhea and malignant catarrhal fever; in nursing beef calves, often with marked licking of the haircoat; commonly in calves at weaning time, and rarely with lymphomatosis. Chronic ulcers occur occasionally in feedlot and dairy cattle. They are commonly associated with displacement or other causes of abomasal atony and may be a result of the stress of heavy production.

Many affected animals are asymptomatic and the ulcers heal spontaneously. Others show vague signs of anorexia and loss of condition, sometimes with black tarry feces and intermittent signs of abdominal pain. Displacement, atony or both may be present. Occasionally a major vessel is eroded and acute, even rapidly fatal hemorrhage into the lumen of the abomasum follows. In other cases, complete perforation of the abomasal wall leads to rapidly fatal peritonitis. In chronic cases, signs may be limited to unthriftiness, with vague and inconstant signs of abdominal pain.

Definite ante mortem diagnosis is difficult without a laparotomy but the presence of black tarry feces, which can be shown by laboratory tests to contain blood, along with the other clinical signs usually allows a tentative diagnosis to be made. The multiple and superficial nature of many of the ulcers makes surgical excision difficult but removal of hairballs in calves may be helpful. Many cases go undiagnosed and are detected only at necropsy. Surgical treatment of chronic ulcers has been reported. Medical treatment with protective and astringent preparations given over a 7- to 10-day period is useful in cattle with superficial ulcerations.

Since not all the etiologic factors are known, prevention is difficult. Management practices designed to reduced stresses and gradual increases in feed over 3- to 4-weeks, especially when putting cattle onto high-concentrate rations, may help to reduce the incidence of abomasal ulcers.

EDEMA DISEASE OF SWINE

(Colibacillary enterotoxemia, Stomach edema, Gut edema)

An acute disease of 4- to 14-week-old pigs, usually associated with weaning or some management change, and characterized clinically by paresis and subcut. edema.

Etiology: Edema disease results from the rapid proliferation of specific serotypes of hemolytic *Escherichia coli* in the upper small intestine with elaboration of toxin. Sudden changes of diet predispose to such proliferations. The disease occurs commonly 1 to 2 weeks after weaning. Following absorption, the toxin causes increased vascular permeability and neurologic disturbances. The etiology of edema disease is similar to that of acute postweaning enteritis (q.v., p. 153), and the 2 syndromes sometimes occur together.

Clinical Findings: Unexpected death, usually of the largest pig in the group, may be the first event noticed. Eyelid edema, pitting edema of the forehead and ataxia constitute the first clinical signs. The amount of edema is variable and the ataxia progressive. Flaccid paralysis develops terminally. Pupillary dilatation and voice changes also occur. The disease is sporadic. The morbidity may be high in affected groups but the herd incidence is usually low. Most affected pigs die.

Lesions: Edema in variable amounts and generalized degenerative arteriopathy are characteristic. Common sites of clear gelatinous fluid accumulation include the subcut. tissues of the forehead, the eyelids, the submucosa of the cecum and cardial gland region of the stomach and the mesentery of the spiral colon.

Diagnosis: The sudden onset of typical neurologic signs and edema in pigs of 4 to 14 weeks of age following several days after a management change indicates edema disease. The isolation and serologic identification of almost pure hemolytic *E. coli* from the anterior part of the small intestine immediately following death helps to confirm the diagnosis. Diseases that may be confused with edema disease include: mulberry-heart disease; salt poisoning; perirenal edema and nephropathy associated with pigweed (*Amaranthus*), lamb's quarters (*Chenopodium*) or fungal toxins in moldy feeds; acute ulceration of the esophageal cardia; Teschen disease; pseudorabies and arsenic poisoning.

Prophylaxis and Treatment: Treatment is largely impracticable.

Prophylaxis is aimed at reducing factors believed to predispose to the proliferation of *E. coli,* and at avoiding sudden changes in management. Feeding antibiotics during the critical period may help to reduce the incidence of the disease.

COLIBACILLOSIS OF WEANED PIGS

(Enteritis in feeder pigs)

A disease associated with almost pure infections of enteropathogenic *Escherichia coli* and characterized by a range of syndromes. The prevalent serotypes of *E. coli* may include those associated with edema disease (q.v., p. 152) and rarely cases of both diseases occur together in the same outbreak. Most outbreaks are in recently weaned, fast-growing pigs but older pigs may be affected. The disease is often associated with stress from crowding, mixing, abnormal environmental temperatures and sudden dietary change.

Clinical Findings: The clinical signs include depression, anorexia, slight fever (105°F [40.5°C]), dehydration and a brownish or grayish watery diarrhea containing no mucus or blood. Bluish discoloration of the extremities and venter may be seen in moribund animals. Occasionally deaths occur with little or no warning, or diarrhea may persist for several days with no deaths in the affected group. Morbidity may be high in the age group at risk.

Lesions: Postmortem findings include dehydration, a stomach filled with feed, reddening of the small intestinal wall and fluid contents. The large intestinal lining may also be mildly inflamed but there is no excess mucus present and the mesenteric lymph nodes are not inflamed. The remainder of the carcass appears normal. Histologically, there is a catarrhal enteritis of the small intestine.

Diagnosis: The disease must be distinguished from salmonellosis (q.v., p. 299), TGE (q.v., p. 293) and swine dysentery (q.v., p. 297). The history of the outbreak may suggest edema disease but the clinical signs and lesions usually permit differentiation. A pure culture of enteropathogenic *E. coli* can be obtained from the anterior small intestine of untreated animals and confirms the diagnosis.

Treatment and Control: Feed intake should be restricted at once and gradually restored to normal over several days. All pigs in an affected group should be treated promptly by medication of the drinking water with one of the following: neomycin, apramycin, streptomycin, spectinomycin, chlortetracycline, tetracycline, oxytetracycline, ampicillin, amoxycillin, trimethoprim, nitrofurazone.

Severely affected individuals may be given parenteral treatment with streptomycin, spectinomycin, ampicillin, a tetracycline or trimethoprim with a sulfonamide. All should be given strictly according to manufacturer's recommendations; failure to respond to treatment should be followed by sensitivity testing of enteropathogenic *E. coli* isolates and reconsideration of the diagnosis.

Post-weaning colibacillosis may be prevented by husbandry measures that reduce stress, by restriction of feed after weaning, mixing or dietary change and by medication of the feed with one of the drugs listed over the period of stress. Parenteral vaccination with killed *E. coli* vaccines may be prophylactic if carried out prior to the period of risk. The injection of hyperimmune serum to *E. coli* may also protect animals at risk. Oral vaccination using killed *E. coli* "O" antigens incorporated in suckler, creep and weaner rations to 55 lb (25 kg) liveweight may also protect. Vaccines prepared from serotypes current on a farm perform best.

ENTERITIS (SM. AN.)

An acute or chronic inflammation of the mucous membrane of the small intestine. Enteritis can exist as an isolated disease involving only the small intestine, or more commonly as part of a more generalized process involving the stomach or the colon. It is common to use "enteritis" as a general term which includes both **gastroenteritis** and **enterocolitis**; however, the 3 conditions should be clinically differentiated to insure proper therapy. (*See also* pp. 304 to 306.)

Etiology: The causes of enteritis are essentially the same as those listed for gastritis. This condition is an outstanding feature of certain infectious diseases, such as distemper, panleukopenia, leptospirosis, "salmon poisoning" and toxoplasmosis, and is manifested to a lesser degree in many other systemic diseases. It is frequently seen in animals harboring helminths or coccidia. Other protozoan parasites, such as *Giardia*, *Trichomonas*, *Entamoeba* and *Balantidium* play a somewhat less sharply defined role in enteritis. The ingestion of decaying or contaminated food, sprays or poison baits, irritating medications and foreign bodies are all causes of acute gastroenteritis. An allergic response to a specific food may produce edema of the intestinal wall and signs of inflammation. Certain heavy metal poisonings produce enteritis.

The role of bacteria in the production of enteritis of dogs and cats is not clear. Although *Proteus* sp. is often suggested as the cause of enteric disease, *Salmonella* spp. are the only organisms that are generally accepted as enteric pathogens. *Escherichia coli* and *Vibrio* sp. are perhaps responsible for acute enteritis. The role of virus infection in enteritis has not been fully elucidated.

Clinical Findings: Diarrhea is the outstanding sign of enteritis. This is accompanied by vomiting when the condition involves the anterior portion of the duodenum and the stomach, and by tenesmus when it extends for any distance into the colon. Severe, localized lesions of any part of the small intestine sometimes cause vomiting. The feces are liquid and foul-smelling, and may be dark green or black as a result of bleeding high in the small intestine, or blood-streaked from hemorrhage originating in the lower portions. The temperature may be elevated if the cause is infectious.

The abdomen is tense in acute cases and the animal evinces pain when it is palpated. The dog may lie with its legs outstretched and its abdomen pressed against the cool floor, or may assume a "praying attitude" with the elbows and sternum on the floor and the hindquarters elevated.

Initially, intestinal motility is increased and abdominal auscultation reveals borborygmi. Subsequently, some animals develop a reflex atony which enhances the accumulation of gas. Dehydration, electrolyte depletion and acidosis are the most dangerous complications of prolonged cases. Chronic cases may develop in which the lesions are so slight that they produce no signs other than recurrent diarrhea and slight loss of condition.

Lesions: The lesions seen in enteritis range from a mild hyperemia and edema to extensive necrotic changes.

Diagnosis: The diagnosis of enteritis is readily made from the signs and history, but establishment of the cause may require extensive laboratory work. Radiographic studies utilizing both plain films and barium contrast techniques are valuable in determining the type and extent of the lesions. The feces should be examined grossly and microscopically for the presence of parasites and protozoa. They also may be cultured to check for the presence of pathogenic bacteria. Urinalysis and hematologic studies sometimes yield pertinent information which, when combined with results of the other tests and the physical findings, aids in the establishment of a specific diagnosis.

Treatment: All food should be withheld for the first 24 hours. Thirst is minimized by offering 1 or 2 ice cubes to lick. Vomiting can be controlled with an anticholinergic and tranquilizer (prochlorperpazine and isopropamide), or by central inhibition of the vomiting reflex with chlorpromazine (℞ 377) or metoclopramide (℞ 485). An attempt should be made to offset dehydration and electrolyte imbalance by the parenteral administration of fluids. The choice of the solution to be used depends upon how much vomiting has accompanied the diarrhea. Lactated Ringer's solution (℞ 588), or isotonic saline solution (0.9%), alone or with 5% dextrose and amino acids, is frequently used.

Meperidine (℞ 617) is given to relieve pain. Simple diarrhea is controlled by preparations such as bismuth subcarbonate (℞ 491), belladonna (℞ 512), kaolin and pectin mixtures (℞ 495), tannic acid (℞ 499), charcoal (℞ 493), aluminum hydroxide gel (℞ 489) and atropine preparations (℞ 496).

If bacterial pathogens are incriminated, a suitable antibacterial agent should be administered, e.g. phthalylsulfathiazole (℞ 85), dihydrostreptomycin (℞ 36), chlortetracycline (℞ 27) or neomycin (℞ 46). These agents may be given separately or in combination with the antidiarrheic agents.

After the first 24 hours have elapsed, a bland diet consisting of soups, broths, Pablum, rice, boiled milk, soft-boiled eggs and small portions of lean meat should be instituted. This diet is gradually adjusted until regular feeding is achieved once again.

Hemorrhage as a result of *Ancylostoma caninum* is handled by using a suitable vermifuge and treating the concurrent anemia. Blood transfusions are given to animals with low levels of hemoglobin. In less advanced cases, treatment with hematinics is adequate.

Enteritis that accompanies infectious diseases or uremia is handled by treating the primary disease and using the foregoing methods for control of the enteritis. The outcome of poisoning with heavy metals may be favorable if an early diagnosis has been made and treatment with a specific antidote is instituted. Parenteral fluid therapy (℞ 588) and antidiarrheic agents should be used.

SMALL INTESTINAL OBSTRUCTION (SM. AN.)

Etiology: Partial or complete obstruction of the small bowel can be caused by indigestible foreign material, masses of parasites, postoperative adhesions, neoplasia, granulomas and abscesses. In addition, volvulus, intussusception and hernial incarceration can cause complete obstruction of the small intestine and occlusion of its vascular integrity. Intestinal rupture, peritonitis and endotoxic shock are complications of small bowel obstruction.

Mesenteric **volvulus** is rare in small animals. **Intussusception** is more frequent, particularly in the young animal suffering severe enteritis or a heavy parasite infection. It occurs commonly in the jejunum or proximal ileum, and less often at the ileocecal junction. Animals with paralysis or stasis of a segment of small bowel, caused by local or generalized peritonitis, enteritis, pancreatitis or postoperatively following laparotomy, may exhibit signs of intestinal obstruction.

Clinical Findings: The signs of complete duodenal obstruction are nausea, vomiting of bile, abdominal pain, anorexia, dehydration, depression and weakness. Electrolyte and water loss is rapid.

Obstruction in the distal small bowel may be tolerated longer than proximal obstruction. The vomitus is feces-like and the onset of dehydration and weakness may be delayed. Abdominal distension develops slowly. Gas and fluid-filled loops of bowel or a tender abdominal mass may be palpated. Frequently the foreign object can be outlined or the typical firm "sausage shaped" intussusception palpated.

Partial intestinal obstruction causes prolonged or intermittent signs similar to distal small bowel obstruction. The animal exhibits reduced food and water intake and chronic weight loss yet remains alert. The feces are fluid, bloody and putrid. Transient response to previous antibiotic therapy may have been noted.

Diagnosis: A history of chewing foreign objects, signs of anorexia, vomiting and dehydration, and palpation of dilated gut loops or the foreign objects are sufficient to suggest intestinal obstruction. If abdominal tenderness prevents palpation, sufficient relaxation may be achieved by the administration of meperidine (℞ 617). Normal peristaltic sounds cannot be auscultated but borborygmi can be heard in the dilated loops of gut. Radiographically the presence of radiopaque foreign objects, empty loops of gut dilated with gas, or gas-capped fluid at different levels of the dilated intestine are seen anterior to the obstruction. The increased soft-tissue density of the intussusception may be seen on abdominal radiographs. Radiolucent foreign bodies may be demonstrated by barium studies.

Treatment: Intestinal obstruction is a surgical emergency. Medical treatment includes meperidine (℞ 617) to relieve pain and the IV administration of fluids and electrolytes prior to and during surgery. If blood-gas and pH data are not available a balanced electrolyte solution (℞ 580) should be administered with broad-spectrum antibiotics IV. Where circulatory shock coexists, whole blood or plasma may be needed. Postoperatively the use of antibiotics and fluids should continue. After 1 to 3 days the oral intake of fluids and a bland low-residue diet are gradually introduced. Return to a regular diet can begin in 5 to 7 days.

COLON IMPACTION—CONSTIPATION (SM. AN.)

Etiology: Chronic impaction of the colon can result from mechanical obstruction such as perineal hernia, rectal diverticulum or tumors of the colon. External compression of the colon by malalignment of healed pelvic fractures, an enlarged prostate gland or neoplasia of the pelvic or abdominal cavity may inhibit propulsion of feces. Infected anal sacs, perianal fistula, anal fibrosis or occlusion of the anus with matted hair and feces may also prevent defecation. Segmental paralysis of the colon due to congenital nerve dysfunction occurs in young animals causing obstipation, e.g. Manx cats. Suppression of the defecation reflex can occur in older hospitalized animals, in paralyzed dogs and cats or in healthy animals when relatively indigestible material such as hair and bones has been eaten.

Clinical Findings: In chronic constipation frequent unsuccessful painful attempts to defecate are noted, and any fecal material passed is hard, brittle and occasionally streaked with fresh blood. The animal is otherwise in good physical condition. If constipation is obstinate the animal becomes thin, weak, depressed, dehydrated and may vomit occasionally. A watery brown putrid diarrhea may be passed as fluid passes around the hardened fecal mass. Digital examination of the rectum is resented. The firm fecal obstruction can be palpated in the rectum or through the abdominal wall.

Diagnosis: A history of difficult, painful or infrequent passage of feces and palpation of the impacted fecal mass in the colon is pathognomonic. Plain abdominal radiographs will reveal the distended colon. Proctoscopic examination or a barium enema following removal of the fecalith may be necessary to visualize obstructive masses or strictures.

Treatment and Control: For simple constipation an enema of warm tap water or small quantities of mineral oil, or glycerine suppositories are effective. In debilitated animals, IV administration of electrolyte solution (℞ 580) prior to manipulation is imperative. Gentle digital breaking of the mass may be needed or, in more severe cases, judicious manipulation of the impaction with forceps is required. Daily removal of portions of a stubborn impaction will allow medical treatment of the debilitated animal between manipulations. Retention enemas should not be used in obstipation since osmotic diffusion of fluids and electrolytes into the colon can cause circulatory imbalance and death.

When the impaction has been relieved, the feeding of excessive bone should be avoided. Oral mucilose flakes (℞ 506) or bran, surfactant laxatives (℞ 509) or lubricants such as mineral oil or more palatable commercial petrolatum-vitamin preparations are helpful when administered routinely. When obstructive masses exist in the colon, surgical removal is indicated.

ACUTE INTESTINAL OBSTRUCTIONS (LG. AN.)

INTUSSUSCEPTION

The invagination or "telescoping" of a portion of the intestine into an adjacent portion.

Etiology and Occurrence: The mechanical causes of intussusception are irregular or excessive peristaltic movements. Enteritis, intestinal parasites, errors in diet, and tumors of the bowel are possible exciting causes. Intussusception occurs most frequently in cattle and is not infrequent in sheep. It is less common in swine and horses. The commonest site is the ileocecal junction with the ileum invaginated into the colon. Agonal invaginations of the intestine are not uncommon in all species.

Clinical Findings: The signs in horses resemble those of volvulus, and differentiation of these conditions may only be accomplished by rectal examination or exploratory laparotomy. In the horse, the evacuation of dark, blood-tinged feces is less common than in other species. Paracentesis of the abdomen may yield blood-tinged peritoneal fluid.

In cattle the signs are rapid in onset and are those of abdominal pain (kicking at the abdomen, treading and stretching). Anorexia is complete. Bowel evacuations are scanty, contain dark, tarry, bloody material and may consist of masses of mucus mixed with dark blood.

Lesions: The invaginating portion forms a thickened ring enclosing the invaginated part and its mesentery. Compression of the veins results and a bluish red or purple color soon develops. In true intussusception, the opposed serous surfaces separate with difficulty, if at all, which helps to differentiate it from agonal invaginations.

Diagnosis: A definite diagnosis can be established by locating the intussusception on rectal palpation in the horse and cow. Distension of the small intestine with gas and fluid always occurs. In advanced stages, an abdominal peritoneal tap behind the sternum will yield abnormal peritoneal fluid. Early laparotomy is indicated in suspected cases.

Treatment: Laparotomy is performed and the intussusception may be reduced by extrusion or "pushing out" of the intussuscepted part. It is inadvisable to pull at an intussusception. If manual reduction is impossible or if necrosis of the bowel has occurred, the affected portion should be resected and the normal ends anastomosed. In the horse, ileocecal intussusception is difficult to reduce and end-to-side anastomosis into an accessible portion of the cecum is the most successful treatment.

INTESTINAL TORSION AND VOLVULUS

Volvulus is an intestinal obstruction due to a twisting of the bowel on its mesenteric axis; **torsion** is a twisting of the bowel on its own or long axis. Volvulus may also be due to a loop of intestine strangulating another section of intestine. Volvulus is commonest in the small intestine, and torsion in the large intestine and cecum.

Etiology: Volvulus and torsion are most likely to occur following events such as strenuous exercise, rolling, jumping and sudden bodily movements. Although reported in all species, these conditions occur most frequently in the horse. Larval strongyle migration is believed to play a prominent role in volvulus and other colics of the horse. Torsions of the abomasum and cecum occur occasionally in ruminants. Torsion of the cecum and displacement of the large intestine occur in the horse.

Clinical Findings: In volvulus of horses, the onset is sudden with signs of acute abdominal pain. The animal may kick at the abdomen, paw, stretch, sink almost to the ground and show other typical signs of colic. Conjunctival congestion becomes marked and diffuse. The pulse gradually increases in rate and becomes weak or thready. A pulse rate greater than 90 a minute indicates a critical condition. Initially the temperature may be elevated (103 to 104°F [39.5 to 40°C]), but it falls to subnormal in the terminal stages. Anorexia is complete; bowel evacuations are suppressed or scanty. Tenesmus is frequent. Peristalsis is slight or absent. Tympany may be noted in the small intestine, and twisting of the mesentery can often be determined by rectal examination. The course is short—a few hours to 48 hours. Terminally, the colic attacks give way to severe depression, the pulse becomes extremely fast and weak, and death ensues.

Signs of cecal torsion in cattle are similar to those of torsion of the abomasum (q.v., p. 149) except that they develop more slowly and diagnosis is almost always possible by rectal palpation. The markedly distended cecum can be palpated at the pelvic inlet or even in the pelvis. It is also possible to percuss the distended organ through the right paralumbar fossa.

In torsion in horses, the clinical signs are usually less acute than in volvulus. This is because the rotation of the colon is usually less than 360°, and the obstruction of the blood supply is usually incomplete. The actual torsion may not be within reach, but one can usually determine that there is a displacement by rectal palpation. Pathogenesis of torsion is similar to volvulus but takes longer to develop.

Lesions: Following displacement of a part of the gut, the outflow of venous blood is obstructed, while the thicker-walled arteries continue to supply some blood. The affected portion thus becomes dark red, the wall is thickened and the mucous membrane is red, swollen and may be necrotic. Gas accumulates, distending the lumen of the occluded bowel. Serohemorrhagic fluid is present in the abdominal cavity; focal or generalized peritonitis is present; rupture of the intestine may occur.

Diagnosis: A definite diagnosis can be made only by rectal palpation or, if this is impossible, by exploratory laparotomy. Tapping caudally to the xiphoid cartilage will yield an abnormal peritoneal fluid.

Treatment: Surgical correction with manual reduction undertaken early in the course of the disease is more likely to be successful than rolling and attempts at manual reduction per rectum. It is the preferred treatment in all species. General anesthesia with halothane gas and oxygen is the safest anesthetic in the horse. A standing operation with local anesthesia is preferred in the cow. The right paralumbar fossa is the preferred surgical site in the cow while the ventral paramedian site is preferred in the horse. After accumulated gas is released, the involved viscus can usually be rotated to its normal position. In some cases, completely emptying the distended cecum greatly facilitates repositioning. An abdominal support bandage and treatment after surgery with IV fluids (lactated Ringer's and sodium bicarbonate) and antibiotic therapy are recommended. Prognosis in cases of volvulus is uniformly poor, regardless of treatment, and recoveries are uncommon, unless only small portions of the small intestine are involved and early successful anastomosis can be done.

IMPACTION OF THE LARGE INTESTINE IN HORSES

Impaction usually occurs in the small colon and the transverse colon. It also may occur in the large colon, especially in the area of the pelvic flexure. Feed containing a large amount of coarse fiber (e.g. straw, cornstalks, alfalfa hay, mesquite beans) is the usual cause. A contributing factor is the lack of water intake in cold weather.

Clinical Findings: The onset of signs occurs after obstruction is complete. Distension of the large colon with gas causes acute abdominal pain. The usual signs described for colic are seen along with progressive congestion of the conjunctival mucous membranes (indicating toxicity). The pulse gradually increases in rate; above 90 per minute, the condition is critical. The temperature may be elevated in some cases. Rupture of the large colon may occur in the violent stages of colic, in which case there is sudden change in signs, to trembling and cold sweat. Rupture of the bowel terminates in death in a few hours.

Diagnosis: The diagnosis usually hinges on the lack of passage of fecal material, a dry sticky rectum, and the palpation of the impaction by rectal examination. Acute gas distension of the colon will be present cephalad from the impacted mass. If rupture has occurred, it may be possible to feel fecal contents on the surface of the bowel.

Treatment: Medical treatment will meet with variable success. Mineral oil and magnesium sulfate are popular laxatives. Dioctyl calcium sulfosuccinate is also used to penetrate the impacted mass. Antiferments and oral antibiotics such as neomycin are helpful to prevent gas formation. When it is obvious that medical relief is not to be obtained, or if the horse is acutely ill, left-flank laparotomy under local infiltration anesthesia is indicated. This approach is adequate for impactions in the transverse colon, pelvic flexure and small colon. The impacted mass is carefully massaged until it is broken down. A midline approach under halothane anesthesia is used in all cases that are doubtful for a left flank approach.

INTESTINAL FOREIGN BODY
(Enterolith)

In the horse, the commonest location for an enterolith is at the narrowing of the lumen in the transverse colon. These foreign bodies usually develop in the right or left dorsal or ventral colons and are mineralized masses that start with a nucleus such as a piece of metal. Concentric layers of mineral are built up around the foreign body, and eventually, through peristaltic action, the object may be pushed to the transverse colon and be too large to pass. Signs are then those of acute abdominal obstruction from impaction. The foreign body may be confused with an impaction, but the treatments are identical. In most cases enterotomy will be necessary to remove the foreign body. Other foreign bodies causing occlusion at the transverse colon include nylon fibers from tires used as feeders, and carpeting materials used anywhere accessible to the horse.

Penetrating foreign bodies in the horse: Rarely a horse will have a penetration of the small intestine or stomach by a sharp foreign body, causing signs of acute peritonitis. The metal may puncture adjacent organs and signs vary from case to case. In general, the signs are those of acute abdominal pain, high temperature, and rise in white blood cell count. Peritoneal tap will reveal an abnormal fluid containing a large number of segmented neutrophils. These penetrations usually result in death.

Foreign body penetration in cattle (*see* p. 138).

INTESTINAL INCARCERATION

An occlusion of the intestinal lumen by pressure from the serosal surface.

Etiology: A loop of intestine may pass through a rent in the mesentery, an opening in the peritoneum (hernia), or it may be strangulated by the stem of a pedunculated tumor or other fibrous cords or bands, such as adhesions. Scrotal hernia of bulls is one of the commonest causes of incarceration in cattle. Adhesions causing partial or complete incarceration may occur following laparotomy incisions in all species. They are, however, commoner following midline laparotomy incisions, especially in horses. The changes that occur in a strangulated portion of the bowel are similar to those of volvulus and torsion.

Clinical Findings: The general signs in the horse are similar to those of torsion. In cattle, they resemble those of intussusception, although the abdominal pain may be more marked and there may be complete retention of feces.

Diagnosis and Treatment: Diagnosis is confirmed by rectal examination or exploratory laparotomy. Laparotomy is almost always necessary for reduction since manipulation per rectum is rarely successful.

MUSCULAR HYPERTROPHY WITH STENOSIS OF THE ILEUM

A chronic hyperplastic disease of the ileum of unknown etiology has been reported in pigs, horses, cats and children. It occurs most frequently in pigs in which it has been described as the muscular type of **regional** or **terminal ileitis** (Crohn's disease). [*See also* INTESTINAL ADENOMATOSIS, p. 185.]

The disease appears to be a congenital neurogenic imbalance resulting in hyperplasia of the muscularis with an increased thickness of the wall. It may be familial in Yorkshire pigs and in man, where several siblings may be affected. No anatomic abnormalities have been demonstrated in the ileocecal opening that could have resulted in stenosis with secondary work-hypertrophy of the wall. Affected animals may exhibit signs of bowel stenosis, but often nothing is noted until the terminal stage of perforation and peritonitis. Pigs with hypertrophic ileal stenosis appear healthy and thrive normally as long as they are on a predominantly liquid diet. When dry-feed consumption increases, which usually happens at approximately 2 months of age, masses of dry, partly digested food lodge in the diseased ileum. The stasis results in necrosis of the intestinal wall with subsequent perforation, peritonitis and death.

The primary histologic lesion is a diffuse hyperplasia and hypertrophy of both circular and longitudinal layers of the muscularis affecting the terminal 1 to 3 feet of the small intestines. Due to the increase in size of the muscularis, the lumen is reduced in size, and the affected intestine becomes thick and inelastic, resembling a rubber hose. The mucosa and submucosa of the affected section are essentially normal, showing only changes attributable to stasis.

In horses, the pathology is identical to that in the pig. The signs are of an insidious onset of low-grade abdominal pain which gets progressively worse over a course of several weeks or even months. Complete intestinal obstruction is rare unless animals are neglected. The wall of the small intestine may be hypertrophied over a considerable length and the thickened and dilated intestine can be palpated per rectum, this being the most valuable diagnostic sign. Food intake is progressively reduced.

The most successful treatment in horses is to by-pass the diseased terminal ileum and the ileocecal valve by either creating a side-to-side anastomosis of healthy small intestine into cecum or by transecting the small intestine cranial to the lesion and performing an end-to-side anastomosis into the cecum. The distal ileum is oversewn securely.

COLITIS (SM. AN.)

Etiology: Acute inflammation of the colon can be caused by parasites (*Trichuris vulpis*), protozoa (*Entamoeba histolytica*), or bacterial infection following the ingestion of garbage or irritating foreign material, or associated with small intestinal disease. Chronic colitis occurs as a clinical entity in the boxer dog. Protozoa (*Balantidium coli*), food allergies, idiopathic and autoimmune causes have been incriminated in other breeds. In the dog, psychogenic spastic colitis may be induced by various environmental stresses. Feline colitis can be caused by intestinal parasitism, toxoplasma, tumor infiltration or associated with infectious feline peritonitis.

Clinical Findings: In acute cases the animal may vomit and hemorrhagic mucoid diarrhea or dysentery will cause dehydration and occasionally anemia. In chronic cases the onset is slow. Frequent attempts to pass scant, watery, blood-streaked, mucoid, putrid stools will occur. Insidious weight loss and an unthrifty appearance exist despite food intake. Vomiting is infrequent. In spastic colitis, fecal blood is uncommon, the stool may be intermittently mucoid or soft and the frequent passage of flatus is noted. On physical examination in chronic cases, the colon is thick walled, rubbery and the lumen is narrow. Large, firm mesenteric lymph nodes can be palpated through the abdomen.

Diagnosis: The history of large bowel disease is characterized by bloody mucoid feces and tenesmus. Either fecal flotation for parasite ova or fresh direct saline smears for protozoa may have to be performed repeatedly. Fecal cultures should be taken where salmonellosis is suspected, e.g. in acute colitis. Proctoscopic examination under general anesthesia following a mild warm water enema is imperative. In chronic colitis the mucosa is hyperemic, edematous and occasionally granular. The colon wall is fibrotic and fails to distend with air. Mucosal ulcers and hemorrhages are visible under the thick mucous coating of the colon wall. A barium enema will show the mucosal ulceration and narrowed lumen. Mucosal biopsy is necessary for a diagnosis except in spastic colitis. Provocative testing by altering dietary constituents may be a useful diagnostic test in "allergic" colitis.

Treatment: If mucosal changes are severe the prognosis is poor. Glycobiarsol is effective therapy for whipworm colitis. In protozoal infections metronidazole is used for treatment in conjunction with supportive IV fluid therapy, broad-spectrum antibiotics (℞ 5) and if anemia is present, whole-blood transfusions.

General colitis therapy includes a low-bulk diet of boiled lean meat, gelatin, eggs, cottage cheese and cooked cereal. Commercial low-residue diets are also available. Antispasmodics (℞ 524) are indicated and protectant preparations containing kaolin and pectin (℞ 495) that may be combined with antibiotics provide temporary control of the diarrhea. The use of soluble sulfonamides (℞ 86) or broad-spectrum antibiotics may control the disease. Systemic alternate-day corticosteroids (℞ 151) or topical hydrocortisone in a retention enema may be beneficial. In hyperactive dogs, sedation (℞ 376) may reduce bouts of stress colitis.

COLIC IN HORSES

A syndrome caused by diseases of the alimentary tract and characterized by subacute or acute pain. It may be confused with pain in other organs, e.g. hepatitis and urethral obstruction, and with other diseases such as laminitis, lactation and transit tetany, tetanus and peritonitis.

Etiology: Acute colic with severe pain may be caused by: engorgement with grain resulting in acute gastric dilation; impaction of the ileocecal valve due usually to feeding of finely chopped indigestible roughage; intestinal accidents including torsion, strangulation, intussusception and diaphragmatic hernia; enteritis, especially that caused by the ingestion of sand; hemorrhage into the intestinal wall as occurs in purpura hemorrhagica and anthrax; and the accumulation of gas due to the ingestion of lush green feed. A recently recognized colic is impaction of the small colon with foreign material, e.g. plastic coating from fence-wire, halter shanks or women's stockings.

Subacute colic includes the 2 common forms of the disease, **impaction of the cecum or colon** with undigested fiber, and **spasmodic colic** due to increased gut motility usually following periods of excitement, unusual activity and long cold drinks. Colic may also be recurrent or chronic. This may be due to a deficiency of blood supply caused by a verminous aneurysm; adhesions (due to migration of *Strongylus vulgaris* larvae), or impaction caused by poor teeth; indigestible roughage in the diet; phytobezoars and enteroliths; overfeeding; old age and debility; and feeding too large amounts too infrequently.

Clinical Findings: The clinical signs in colic are much the same irrespective of the cause, varying only in their severity. Restlessness is manifested by pawing, kicking at the belly, getting up and lying down and rolling. Looking at the flank is a common sign and affected horses lie down carefully and get up slowly, often adopting a dog-sitting posture. Other abnormal postures, including the adoption of a sawhorse attitude and lying on the back, may also occur.

The pain observed is usually intermittent, especially in the early stages, with longer intervals between bouts in subacute cases and being almost continuous in acute cases. In the most severe cases there is profuse, patchy sweating, "sobbing" respiration, signs of shock including a rapid pulse (100/minute) of small amplitude and a clammy skin. The horse's movements are so violent that it may do itself much physical injury within a short time.

Auscultation of the abdomen is helpful in diagnosis. In flatulent colic, apart from the distended abdomen, there are high-pitched "gassy pings"; in spasmodic colic there are loud gut sounds or borborygmi; and in impaction the normal sounds are decreased or absent. A rectal examination is essential in diagnosis. Gaseous distention of intestinal loops is characteristic of flatulent colic; in cases of verminous aneurysm the enlarged, obstructed vessel may be palpable and slack, distended loops of intestine can be found, and in spasmodic colic no abnormalities are detectable. A cylindrical mass in the terminal part of the ileum high up in the right flank is diagnostic of impaction of the ileocecal valve. Small intestinal accidents are characterized by fluid-filled loops of gut of appropriate size. Cecal and colic impactions are readily palpable. Hernias into the inguinal canal are best palpated per rectum, as the intestine may not protrude as far as the scrotum.

Passage of a nasal tube may result in the expulsion of large quantities of evil-smelling, green-stained fluid. This usually results from an obstruction of the intestine at any level from the pylorus to the ileocecal valve. Projectile vomiting of similar material may occur and is usually a terminal event causing rupture of the distended stomach. Paracentesis of the abdomen is nowadays a common method of examination in the horse when severe colic is apparent. Biochemical tests that disclose the degree of dehydration are also commonly carried out because of the severity of fluid loss and shock.

Treatment: Acute and chronic intestinal obstruction may need surgical relief. A verminous aneurysm does not respond to any known treatment but colic due to intestinal disease produced by the aneurysm or thrombus may respond to therapy with massive doses of an appropriate anthelmintic. Acutely ill horses suffering shock and dehydration require supportive therapy with alkaline IV infusions in large quantities. The relief of pain is of paramount importance to avoid self-injury. Meperidine (1 to 2 mg/lb [2 to 4.5 mg/kg] body wt by subcut. injection) or chloral hydrate (15 to 30 gm by stomach tube) are best. Tranquilizers are helpful in mild colic attacks (e.g. ℞ 374, 385). For impaction, mineral oil (℞ 505) is best, and in sand colic, magnesium sulfate (℞ 517) is recommended. In both diseases these treatments may be followed 12 to 24 hours later by an injection of carbachol (℞ 501). The latter treatments may be contraindicated in old or debilitated horses. In cases of spasmodic colic, atropine sulfate, ¼ to ½ grain (15 to 30 mg) is effective quickly when injected subcut. Aminopromazine, 10 to 30 ml of 3% solution, or methampyrone or dipyrone (℞ 513) are recommended for the same purpose. These drugs are antispasmodics and tend to reduce peristalsis.

In all cases, attention should be given to preventing a recurrence of the disease by providing dental attention, advice on feeding and exercise, and effective parasite control.

DIARRHEA IN WEANED AND ADULT HORSES

The causes of diarrhea in horses are poorly understood and in many cases diarrheal disease in this species must be treated symptomatically. The 2 commonest diseases producing acute diarrhea are colitis-X and salmonellosis. Chronic diarrhea may be associated with a number of diseases.

COLITIS-X

Colitis-X is characterized by the sudden onset of profuse watery diarrhea and rapid development of hypovolemic shock. It is usually a sporadic disease but on occasion may affect several horses within a group. All ages other than foals are affected, the disease occurring most commonly in 2- to 5-year-olds. The cause is unknown but it may be associated with endotoxic shock. Many, but not all, affected horses have a history of stress or upper respiratory infection 1 to 3 weeks prior to the onset, which has lead to the postulation that the disease is associated with adrenal corticoid exhaustion.

Clinical Findings: Onset is sudden. The diarrhea is copious, watery and mucoid, and may be bloodstained. In the initial stages of the disease it is passed frequently and with no effort. Affected horses show depression and mild abdominal discomfort. The temperature may be initially elevated but frequently by the time the animal is first examined it is normal or even subnormal. The heart rate is usually 80 to 100 at first examination but increases to 120 or greater as the disease progresses. Tachyarrhythmias are common. From the early stages there is evidence of extreme hypovolemic shock with cold extremities, an impalpable arterial pulse, poor capillary and jugular refill time, and marked hypotension. Skin elasticity is not markedly changed and is a poor guide to the extent of dehydration and shock in colitis-X. Death may occur within 3 hours of the onset or, in less acute cases, within 24 to 48 hours. Most horses remain standing until the terminal stage. At necropsy there is pronounced edema and hemorrhage in the wall of the large colon and cecum, with fluid and bloodstained intestinal contents.

Diagnosis: Colitis-X is the most likely cause of severe diarrhea where the onset is sudden and unexpected with rapid development of hypovolemic shock. Typically the packed cell volume exceeds 65% at the initial examination even though this may be only shortly after the onset of diarrhea. Conditions such as acute intestinal obstruction or acute arterial occlusion caused by *Strongylus vulgaris* larvae may produce severe and sudden shock but diarrhea is not a feature and these conditions are easily differentiated from colitis-X on rectal examination and abdominal paracentesis. Salmonellosis (q.v., p. 169) produces the greatest difficulty in differential diagnosis. Its onset is usually less sudden and the feces are more offensively odorous and contain mucosal shreds and blood. In colitis-X the white cell count is frequently normal although there may be neutropenia, whereas in salmonellosis there is usually marked neutropenia in the early stages of the disease with a pronounced left shift.

Another condition that may produce acute diarrhea in horses is a heavy intestinal infection with *Clostridium perfringens* (**intestinal clostridiosis**). Overdosing with dioctyl sodium sulfosuccinate may also produce acute diarrhea and death. A syndrome of diarrhea (possibly salmonellosis) that is frequently fatal may follow the IV administration of large doses of tetracyclines. A similar syndrome with death in 3 to 5 days may occur when routine doses of tetracyclines are given parenterally to horses following surgery.

Diarrhea associated with *Corynebacterium equi* infection is largely restricted to foals under 9 months of age. It may occur in the terminal phase of the more typical pneumonic syndrome or may occur without clinical evidence of respiratory disease. The onset is sudden with pyrexia and marked depression and the feces are very fluid. Commonly peritonitis is demonstrable by abdominal paracentesis and the organism can be cultured from the peritoneal fluid. There is marked leukocytosis.

Occasionally peritonitis from other infections may be accompanied by diarrhea. Uremia can cause acute diarrhea in horses and nephrosis should always be considered with diarrhea of unknown cause in this species. Excessive ingestion of sand may also be associated with diarrhea.

Treatment: The treatment of colitis-X is expensive, time consuming and frequently unrewarding. Fluids (℞ 588, 590) equivalent to at least 10% and preferably 15% of body weight (40 to 60 L/400-kg horse) should be administered IV using an indwelling catheter. One-third to one-half of this volume may be administered as rapidly as possible and thereafter the remainder is given more slowly to effect as judged by improvement in jugular venous filling, capillary refill and return of normal blood pressure. A massive dose of IV corticosteroids (℞ 141) is frequently given as part of the therapy. Antihistamines (℞ 560) and broad-spectrum antibiotics are frequently also administered but their value has not been fully ascertained. The value of pressor agents as an aid in treatment of colitis-X has not been determined.

SALMONELLOSIS

Salmonellosis (q.v., p. 299) may produce acute diarrhea in adult horses. The disease most commonly occurs sporadically without apparent predisposing cause but it also occurs 2 to 4 days following stress—especially surgical stress—and can become a problem in horse clinics. Worming, overtraining, hot weather, close stocking, yarding or transport of groups of horses, and food deprivation may also initiate infection. The onset is sudden with severe depression, anorexia, neutropenia and frequently marked abdominal pain. The feces are very fluid, foul smelling, bloodstained and usually contain mucosal elements. There is a rapid fall in condition with severe dehydration, acidosis and hyponatremia. Death commonly occurs during the first 2 to 5 days or the disease may result in chronic persistent diarrhea. Diagnosis and differentiation from other causes of diarrhea frequently rely on isolation of the organism, which can be difficult, and on laboratory tests. An odor of decay and the presence of mucosal shreds in the feces, in conjunction with a profound neutropenia with a degenerative left shift, a pronounced hyponatremia and hypoproteinemia are highly suggestive of salmonellosis.

Treatment: IV fluid and electrolyte replacement as described for colitis-X (q.v., p. 169) is essential. The dehydration is usually less severe and fluid replacement level between 5 to 10% of body weight may be sufficient but each case should be approached individually. Where there is pronounced hyponatremia the specific sodium deficit should be corrected with hypertonic sodium chloride and sodium bicarbonate solutions. Parenterally administered antibiotics are indicated in acute salmonellosis. Chloramphenicol (℞ 16) is frequently used but high doses of ampicillin (℞ 2) may be more effective. Oral antibiotics should be avoided. Orally administered serum (2 L daily, with 120 gm $NaHCO_3$) may be of value. General supportive treatment as in any diarrheal disease should be given.

CHRONIC DIARRHEA IN HORSES

Chronic diarrhea may occur with malabsorptive states resulting from chronic enteritis, extensive villous atrophy or infiltrative lesions that impair nutrient absorption in the intestinal tract. This may occur in horses with granulomatous enteritis, severe parasitic damage to the intestine, following any acute enteritis such as salmonellosis, and with intestinal lymphosarcoma and other gastrointestinal neoplasms. With these syndromes there is a history of weight loss and progressive emaciation despite normal or even increased food intake. In the case of granulomatous enteritis and lymphosarcoma, thickened intestines with enlargement of the mesenteric lymph nodes may be detected on rectal examination. Differential diagnosis is aided by the examination of peritoneal fluid obtained by abdominal paracentesis and by rectal and intestinal biopsy. Malabsorptive states may be demonstrated by absorption-function tests (q.v., p. 182). These conditions are almost invariably refractory to treatment and fatal.

Chronic liver disease may be accompanied by diarrhea in which the feces are soft and watery. There is usually a progressive fall in body condition. Jaundice may not be evident but there is a decreased sulfobromophthalein clearance (T ½ greater than 5 min), low serum albumen and increased prothrombin time.

A heavy patent parasitic infection may be accompanied with intermittent diarrhea. There is a history of weight loss and of periods where the feces resemble cow's feces in consistency. Anemia is present and there is a high fecal egg count. The condition responds well to anthelmintic therapy (*see* PARASITIC DISEASES, p. 671 et seq.). Migrating strongyle larvae may cause considerable vascular damage with impairment of intestinal function, and there is unthriftiness, a history of intermittent abdominal pain and passage of soft or fluid feces. In severe cases impaired absorption may be demonstrable by absorption-function tests. On rectal examination, arteritis may be detected in the anterior mesenteric artery and in the arteries supplying the intestine, especially the large bowel. Serum β-globulins are elevated and eosinophilia and increased numbers of eosinophils in peritoneal fluid are common. Fecal egg counts may be normal. Treatment is with high doses of thiabendazole (℞ 264).

Allergy to components of feed is believed to produce chronic diarrhea and can be determined by removing the offending material from the diet.

A syndrome of unknown etiology occurs predominantly in young mature horses. There is frequently a history of minor stress 3 to 14 days prior to onset, commonly antibiotic treatment of traumatic wounds, upper respiratory infection or adverse reaction to administered drugs. The onset of diarrhea is usually not accompanied by signs of systemic illness and the feces vary from soft porridge to cow-patlike in consistency. The appetite is maintained, there is weight loss during the initial period but subsequently the animal maintains a lowered condition despite persistence of diarrhea for weeks or months. Laboratory tests, absorption tests and biopsy reveal no abnormality. There is usually a marked reduction in fecal protozoa and often large numbers of *Trichomonas equi* can be demonstrated; however, this is believed to be effect and not cause. A deficiency in immunologic response has been demonstrated in some horses.

Treatment: In the absence of an etiologic diagnosis, treatment is symptomatic. Initially parenteral fluid and electrolyte replacement may be necessary but in most cases electrolytes placed in the drinking water (℞ 575) are sufficient. Variations in appetite for individual foodstuffs should be catered to as diarrhea will become more severe during periods of inappetence. Tincture of opium (30 to 80 ml orally daily for 1 to 3 days—where it is available for this use) effectively controls the diarrhea but scouring may return when treatment is discontinued. (Caution: Do not use opium in horses with liver disease.) Intestinal absorbants (℞ 495) may be of some value. Several treatment methods have been proposed but response varies. Repopulation of the enteric flora can be attempted using 4 to 8 liters of a gauze filtrate of fresh normal feces given by stomach tube. Iodochlorhydroxyquin (℞ 598) is effective in some cases but relapse can occur on withdrawal of therapy. Oral antibiotics are generally contraindicated and ineffective but IV ampicillin (℞ 2) may be used. Recent treatments for which success has been claimed include oral administration of 1 liter of fresh horse serum on 3 consecutive days and, where parasitic arteritis is suspected, 6% dextran 70 (℞ 576) as a thrombolytic agent. Because of the possibility of parasitic arteritis inducing this syndrome a high dose of thiabendazole

(℞ 264) should be given in all cases. Affected horses may recover spontaneously with time.

EQUINE GRASS SICKNESS

A disease of unknown etiology, attributable to a toxic disorder of the autonomic nervous system and usually fatal. All the Equidae are susceptible. The disease has been reported from Northern Europe and Australia. The Japanese literature contains reports of possibly related conditions, and one suspected outbreak has been seen in the U.S.A. Grass sickness has a peak incidence in 3- to 8-year-old animals and a peak occurrence in spring. However, it may occur at any age, and has been seen occasionally in housed stock without access to grass.

Clinical Findings: Acute, subacute and chronic forms are recognized. Acutely ill animals live for only 4 to 48 hours and those with subacute cases for about 6 days. Chronic cases continue for several weeks and the horses occasionally survive. The disease is afebrile and characterized by profound depression, restlessness, patchy sweating and fine muscular tremors over the shoulders and flanks. There is stasis of the alimentary tract; difficulty in swallowing leads to drooling, and stomach contents may be discharged via the nares. The pulse is soft and very rapid. In acute and subacute cases the rectum contains dark, hard, dry feces often coated with blood-flecked mucus. In the chronic form, dehydration is progressive.

At necropsy of acute and subacute cases the stomach is distended with evil-smelling green fluid, the colon is impacted and the spleen enlarged. In chronic cases the entire gastrointestinal tract is often contracted and virtually empty. Histologically there is degeneration of neurones in the alimentary mural plexuses, the vertebral and prevertebral ganglia and the autonomic centers of the CNS. Axonal dystrophy is also described in ganglia.

Treatment: The prognosis is poor. Evacuation of the stomach and rectum, parenteral replacement of fluid, and administration of massive doses of multivitamins may afford symptomatic relief. In the suspected outbreak in the U.S.A., subcut. administration of 10 ml of a 1:1000 neostigmine solution, given 3 times daily, was reported to produce dramatic improvement and several complete recoveries.

DIARRHEA OF NEWBORN ANIMALS

(Enteric disease of neonates [0 to 14 days])

General Considerations: An animal at birth is transferred from the protective sterile environment of the uterus to an environment containing a multiplicity of microorganisms some of which are definitely pathogenic; more are pathogenic only when the natural host defenses are reduced. There are 3 main portals of entry of these microorganisms into the newborn: (a) **The Umbilicus:** Entry through and production of disease via the umbilicus requires unsanitary birth conditions, presence of pathogens, misguided manipulation of the umbilical cord and possibly low transfer of maternal immunity. (b) **The Respiratory Tract:** Apart from inhalation pneumonia (a management problem) respiratory disease is uncommon in the neonatal period, possibly because of transferred maternal immunity. Other factors that may protect against respiratory disease in the early neonatal period are the unique defense mechanisms of the lung such as ciliary action and scavenging macrophages. (c) **The Alimentary Tract:** This provides the maximal portal of entry of microorganisms into the neonatal body since they can contaminate and be ingested together with the necessary food intake. Moreover any alimentary disturbance in the young can cause digestive upset, which appears to facilitate the activities of microorganisms in the gut. Milk substitutes, in particular badly constituted or formulated ones, appear to function in this manner.

In the great majority of instances, adequate immunity in the newborn will prevent a disturbance being prolonged or fatal. For all species of domestic animal and most exotic species this requires maximal transfer of maternal immunity via the colostrum. When this does not take place, death is highly probable from enteric disease. Thus enteric disease is a problem in the orphan animal or in animals subjected to management regimes preventing or limiting transfer of immunity. These statements assume that the dam has encountered the potentially lethal microorganisms and has developed an immunity. This is in general true or can be arranged by maternal vaccination.

ENTERIC DISEASE OF NEWBORN CALVES

Diarrhea in the newborn can be produced by slight alimentary upset but it requires the intervention of microorganisms in immune-deficient neonates for the upset to become fatal. Immune deficiency is the most important contributing factor but a heavily contaminated environment and poor or unsuitable feeding also contribute to the mortality.

Many microorganisms have been implicated in the several disease syndromes, either singly or in combination. These include *Escherichia coli*, salmonellae, *Pseudomonas* sp. and *Proteus* sp., chlamydiae, the virus of IBR, bovine viral diarrhea virus, corona and rotavirus particles. Viruses, particularly the corona and rotaviruses, can be found in many samples of diarrheic feces but by themselves in gnotobiotic calves (highly susceptible and immune deficient) cause only transient nonfatal diarrhea; probably they require *E. coli* for the full expression of their pathogenicity.

The protective role of immune globulins fully implicates microorganisms in the disease syndromes. For certain microorganisms, antibodies within the immune globulin class IgM prevent systemic invasion of the body from the gut; IgG antibodies protect against absorbed endotoxin; while IgA antibodies either prevent adherence of lethal microorganisms to the gut wall or in some way inhibit their multiplication within the gut.

The syndromes may be distinct and can be described, given names and acted against prophylactically even if the full etiology is unknown.

Colibacillosis

Although 3 syndromes are attributed to *E. coli*, it is useful to consider them separately.

Colisepticemia occurs in the first week of life and because of the development of endogenous immunity (IgM) in the calf is rare after this age. Sudden death may be reported but close observation reveals prior dullness and depression. Usually calves are depressed, anorectic, febrile and recumbent. They rapidly become moribund and die within 48 hours, usually much earlier. Diarrhea can be a feature but is not profuse. Other clinical features that may be noted are tachycardia, weak pulse and wetness around the mouth, presumably from slightly excessive salivation.

Postmortem lesions are characteristic of septicemia with petechiation on spleen, kidney and heart and an enlarged spleen. There is increased synovial fluid in the joints and meningeal congestion. *E. coli* can be isolated in pure culture from spleen, kidney and heart blood.

Therapy is usually unsuccessful.

Prophylactic use of antibiotics (℞ 51) immediately at birth is on occasion of value. However since the condition arises from extreme deficiency of maternal immune globulins, the best prophylaxis is to improve colostral absorption (*see* p. 177). If this is not possible, 1 L of blood from a cow other than the dam may be administered IV or IP.

Enteric colibacillosis is the traditional "white scour" of calves. It usually occurs during the first 2 weeks of life and terminates in death in 4 or 5 days if not satisfactorily treated. Initially appetite is good but as the feces become progressively more fluid the appetite decreases. Finally the calf is emaciated and dehydrated with sunken eyes and the hind quarters stained with fluid feces. At this terminal stage, temperature is subnormal, respiration may be hyperpneic from acidosis, and the heart can be slow or even arrhythmic. This final hopeless state may be avoided with adequate nursing and proper treatment. A proportion of survivors develop a chronic diarrhea.

Postmortem examination of fatal cases reveals a dehydrated, emaciated carcass with a fluid-filled gut but little else of significance.

Therapy may be intermittently successful. A variety of antibiotics (℞ 46, 51, 56) have been used, but their success is limited by the development of infectious drug resistance. Electrolyte mixtures (℞ 590) given orally or parenterally are useful if given in time. In some therapeutic regimes, milk is withheld while water and electrolyte mixtures (℞ 590) are used to maintain hydration.

Prophylaxis has been attempted using antibiotics (℞ 51) and chemotherapeutic agents, but as in colisepticemia this is again a condition of suboptimal absorption of globulins from colostrum; the obvious prophylaxis is to promote maximal absorption of maternal immune globulins (*see* p. 177).

Enterotoxic colibacillosis is a condition very similar to enteric colibacillosis and caused by a limited number of enteropathogenic serotypes. These serotypes, rare in field outbreaks, elaborate an enterotoxin causing fluid transfer from the body into the small intestine. Diarrhea similar to enteric colibacillosis occurs earlier (in the first week of life) and is shorter in duration to death (3 days). Rarely, death occurs without diarrhea. The postmortem lesions are similar also but in addition ecchymotic hemorrhages are found in the heart, on the spleen and on the serosae.

Therapy with antibiotics (℞ 6, 46, 56) has the same limitations as in other forms of infectious enteric disease in the calf but fluid and electrolytes are of value (℞ 590). Although type-specific antibodies may not be present, maximal absorption of colostral maternal antibodies is the effective prophylactic (*see* p. 177). A higher level of nonspecific immune globulins is required for protection than in other forms of colibacillosis.

Salmonellosis

Although salmonellae can infect older cattle, most cases occur in the newborn calf. (*See also* SALMONELLOSIS, p. 299.) The clinical picture in the newborn is determined by the level of transferred maternal immunity (as in colibacillosis) and the virulence of the specific salmonellae. Calves are dull, fevered and usually anorectic. There can be systemic invasion giving septicemia and also diarrhea, which can vary from increased amounts of pasty-to-fluid yellow, brown or dysenteric feces, characteristically with a fetid odor. Weight loss is marked. At necropsy there is some petechiation and the intestine is more congested than in colibacillosis. Salmonellae can be isolated from the tissues.

Therapy is usually unsuccessful. Prophylaxis depends on preventing contact with the causative organisms. Vaccination is of no value in this age of calf and vaccination of pregnant cows has usually given little protection because salmonellae are poor antigens.

Other Bacterial Diarrheas

On occasion *Pseudomonas* sp. and *Proteus* sp. have been the major fecal isolates in diarrhea in neonatal calves. It is uncertain at present if these are facultative pathogens requiring also enteroviruses. The clinical and pathologic picture is very similar to those of enteric colibacillosis (q.v., p. 174) but the course is somewhat shorter to a fatal outcome and the feces may be green or may have a sweetish odor. Therapy is not likely to be successful. Prophylaxis is again to arrange the maximal transfer of colostral immune globulins and breaking the chain of disease by preventing exposure to causative organisms.

Chlamydia have been implicated but their role in calf diarrhea remains unclear.

Viral Diarrheas of Neonatal Calves

The specific viruses of IBR and bovine viral diarrhea have been implicated in diarrhea in neonates but specific detailed clinical descriptions are lacking. Rotavirus and coronavirus particles appear to require *E. coli* to produce a lethal condition, which clinically is indistinguishable from enteric colibacillosis, and their roles are not yet clearly defined.

Therapy for Newborn Animals With Diarrhea

This is based on 3 things: replacement of fluid and electrolytes; antibacterials for pathogens; and, in severe cases, provision of antibodies. Since it is usually considered advisable to withhold milk, the antibodies are supplied by giving the calf 1 L of blood from the dam or any mature animal other than the dam. It should be given IV. The blood should be collected aseptically into citrate solution (handy proprietary packs are available) and given immediately.

Antibiotic (℞ 6, 46, 51, 56) or other antibacterial therapy has limited but definite value only if the etiologic pathogen is sensitive to the drug used.

Fluid replacement may be effected with proprietary solution, isotonic saline solution (9 gm NaCl in 1 L water) or saline-bicarbonate mixture (℞ 590). One of these should be given IV, beginning with 1 L over 2 hours and to a total equal to 10% of the body weight in 24 hours. Electrolyte solutions may also be given orally but initially, especially in severe cases, the IV route is preferable. *See also* FLUID AND ELECTROLYTE THERAPY, p. 77.

Colostrum and the Calf

A direct relationship exists: The greater the amount of immune globulins absorbed, the better are the chances of survival of the calf over the neonatal period, in particular with reference to enteric disease and regardless of the challenging organisms.

Factors Affecting Absorption: 1) Time of first suckling. Absorption from the calf gut decreases from the time of birth and is insignificant after 12 hours. The optimal time for absorption is under 6 hours. 2) **Quantity of colostrum ingested.** The greater the amount ingested the greater is the amount absorbed. Calves ingest significantly more when sucking than if fed in other ways. Circumstances can arise where calves do not get colostrum at the first meal, e.g. the dam has severe mastitis or does not come into lactation. Where cows are tied the calf can suckle the wrong cow. 3) **Quality of colostrum.** The quality (immune-globulin content) can vary considerably in healthy cows but this appears to be relatively unimportant compared to early ingestion of even poor quality colostrum. 4) **Vigor of cow and calf.** Cows exhausted by prolonged calving can be recumbent and the calf unable to suckle, as may be calves born weak. 5) **Maternal effects.** (a) A small proportion of heifers do not allow suckling. (b) The calf seeks the teats at the highest point of the underbelly and, in old beef cows and high-yielding dairy cows with pendulous udders, the calf may not find or be delayed in finding the teats and hence in feeding. (c) Teats may be too large for the calf to suck. (d) In some way, leaving the calf with its dam for the first 12 hours enhances absorption of immune globulins (mothering effect). 6) **Other factors.** Stress from the presence of other animals or excessive interference by strangers (to the cow) inhibit absorption. Other stress factors may play a part.

Management to Ensure Optimal Immune Globulin Absorption
(Under Intensive Conditions)

The ideal is the natural state; a cow free to calve outside selects an area away from other cattle. If confinement is necessary, the following outline should be followed: Provide a loose box 5 x 4 m (15 x 12 ft) closed on 3 sides with the front wall 1.5 m (5 ft) high with entrance door of the same height. Feed and water at the front. Ensure loose box is clean with fresh bedding. Place cow in box at least 24 hours before calving. Have cow looked after by an attendant she knows and keep others away. Observe cow and calf at calving and see if calf suckles in first 6 hours. If not, hold calf on to cow to feed (for at least 20 minutes). Leave cow with calf for 12 or preferably 24 hours after birth.

There are tests, specifically the zinc sulfate turbidity test and the refractometer measurement of absorbed immune globulins, which are used to estimate the blood level of globulins and thus to assess the success of management procedures designed to promote calf health. However, the details of these tests are beyond the scope of the Manual.

Vaccination of pregnant cows with *E. coli* and salmonella bacterin has given variable results. Corona and rotavirus vaccines have been highly effective in herds in which these viruses were the cause of diarrhea. Bacterins have not been effective when given to calves.

ENTERIC DISEASE OF NEWBORN LAMBS

Colibacillosis in the lamb is similar to the disease in the calf (q.v., p. 174). Possibly cold, inclement weather at birth may inhibit the lamb from feeding. There appears to be some evidence that good nutrition of the dam is of importance during pregnancy to ensure mammary development and hence the availability of immune globulins.

Lamb dysentery (q.v., p. 402) is a condition occurring usually in lambs in the first week of life but occasionally in the second or third week. The specific cause is *Clostridium perfringens* Type B.

Other enteric infections of lambs: It is possible that specific enteric pathogens such as salmonellae could cause diarrhea in lambs similar to salmonella enteritis of calves. However, the circumstances in which the lambs would meet the salmonellae would at the same time lead to the infection of susceptible ewes (after lambing) so that the epidemiologic picture would be of a diarrheic syndrome in all ages of sheep.

As in human infants, calves and piglets, rotavirus is being implicated in diarrheas in newborn lambs. Although these viruses can be isolated from a proportion of lambs with diarrhea and can cause diarrhea in gnotobiotic lambs, their exact role has still to be elucidated. They may facilitate the activities of so-called facultative pathogens by producing damage in the gut wall. What does appear to be certain is that transferred colostral immunity is protective; moreover, antibody in milk (as in the piglet) prevents adherence of the virus in the gut.

ENTERIC DISEASE OF NEWBORN FOALS

The foal is similar to the calf and the lamb in requiring colostral immunity for survival over the neonatal period. Conditions must be arranged for transfer to take place as soon after birth as possible under optimum conditions such as quiet undisturbed foaling conditions with helpers, if necessary, that are known to the mare. If the foal is weak and unwilling or unable to suckle it should be aided. In circumstances where the dam has no colostrum, parenteral administration of her blood to the foal may assist survival.

The foal, like other neonates, suffers from enteric disease in the first 10 days of life but differs in that a greater spectrum of organisms have been implicated including salmonellae, *Proteus* sp., *Shigella* sp. and *E. coli* in septicemic and enteric syndromes.

Septicemia occurs in the first week of life. There is progressive dullness and anorexia; frequently there is a fever and the joints become involved. Diagnosis is based on clinical signs and isolation of organisms from tissue and joints. Antibiotics, parenterally, (℞ 6,

51) are useful in treatment. Prophylaxis requires clean, hygienic foaling conditions and ensuring the maximal transfer of immune globulins.

Enteric diarrheic disease occurs towards the end of first week or earlier if part of a septicemia. The clinical signs are dullness, fever, anorexia, listlessness and profuse diarrhea, which is fetid if salmonellae are involved. Lesions are insignificant; isolation of incriminated organisms may be possible. Antibiotics (℞ 6, 46) and parenteral hydration (℞ 590) may be lifesaving. Clean hygienic surroundings at foaling and ensuring maximal transfer of maternal immune globulins as soon as possible after birth (certainly within 6 hours) are the basis of successful prophylaxis.

ENTERIC DISEASE OF NEWBORN PIGS

Three etiologic agents have been implicated: 2 are of major importance, *Escherichia coli* and TGE virus (q.v., p. 293); the third, *Clostridium perfringens* Type C, gives a more distinctive syndrome (q.v., p. 402).

Colibacillosis in the piglet: It appears that a limited number of serotypes of *E. coli* are responsible. Transferred maternal immunity is protective but if the dams do not have immunity against a specific serotype, an explosive outbreak can occur affecting the progeny of all ages of dams. Later in the outbreak the condition can settle down to affect only the progeny of gilts. Affected piglets are dull, cold and comatose. There may or may not be diarrhea with yellow-to-watery feces. With diarrhea the piglets are depressed, fail to feed and rapidly become dehydrated. At necropsy the carcass is emaciated and the gut contents fluid. Diagnosis is usually on clinical and epidemiologic grounds (*see* TGE, p. 293). Laboratory examinations may be utilized to serotype *E. coli*.

Antibiotics (℞ 6, 51) or chemotherapeutics (after sensitivity testing) and fluid therapy may be useful (℞ 590). For prophylaxis, ensure that the infection load is reduced by improvement of environmental hygiene, and ensure that the dam has adequate immunity by constant exposure to the pathogens present. This latter constitutes no problem for the sow but for the gilt may necessitate mixing sow feces in the feed.

An inactivated *E. coli* vaccine may be given to sows or gilts once at any time between breeding and 5 weeks before farrowing and a second time 3 weeks before farrowing. Piglets are given the same vaccine at 4 days and 10 to 14 days of age.

ENTERIC DISEASE OF THE NEWBORN PUPPY AND KITTEN

The kitten and puppy obtain a proportion of their transferred maternal immunity transplacentally and because of this and because of the management of pups and kittens, neonatal enteric disease does not constitute a problem except in the orphan. In this exceptional circumstance, antibiotics (℞ 6, 51) and chemotherapeutic agents should be given prophylactically and therapeutically.

MALABSORPTION SYNDROMES

Malabsorption syndromes occur when defective intestinal absorption of either a nutrient or electrolytes and fluid leads to clinical manifestations, usually chronic in nature. They are most commonly encountered in dogs, and less frequently in horses, and in both species may be associated with a concomitant protein loss. Malabsorption as a mechanism in specific diseases of these or other species (e.g. TGE in pigs), will not be considered here. An outline classification of pathogenetic mechanisms associated with maldigestion or malabsorption in dogs is presented in Table 1.

TABLE 1. CLASSIFICATION OF PATHOGENIC MECHANISMS POSSIBLY UNDERLYING MALDIGESTIVE OR MALABSORPTIVE SYNDROMES IN DOGS

1. Maldigestion: a. pancreatic exocrine insufficiency: pancreatic degenerative atrophy; subacute relapsing pancreatic necrosis; or obstruction of pancreatic duct—e.g. neoplasm.
   b. reduced intestinal bile salt concentration (rarely diagnosed): cholestasis or precipitation of bile salts as by neomycin, calcium carbonate.
   c. congenital or acquired mucosal enzyme deficiency: lactase deficiency.
2. Malabsorption: a. inadequate absorptive surface: iatrogenic (intestinal resection); or villous atrophy—often associated with inflammatory cell (eosinophil, neutrophil, histiocyte) infiltration, or lymphosarcoma.
   b. lymphatic obstruction (fat malabsorption): lymphangiectasis.
3. Protein-losing enteropathy: a. enteritis: acute or chronic inflammatory infiltrates, associated with transient or extensive epithelial permeability.
   b. erosive or ulcerative disease: inflammatory or neoplastic.
   c. lymphatic obstruction: lymphangiectasis or neoplasia.
   d. portal hypertension: congestive heart failure or hepatic fibrosis.

Animals with these problems may exhibit signs of diarrhea, cachexia or deficiency disease, or isolated findings that are not suggestive of a diagnosis of malabsorption. The pathophysiologic basis for possible presenting signs is summarized in Table 2 on page 181.

The diagnosis of malabsorptive disorders is aimed at implicating or identifying the presence of one or more of the underlying processes listed in Table 1. Many of the tests used may indicate abnormal digestion or absorption, but few suggest a specific diagnosis. Consequently it may be necessary to employ a combination of methods to reach a conclusion.

Tests useful in the identification of maldigestion (pancreatic exocrine insufficiency), malabsorption and protein-losing enteropathy and which are feasible in some practice settings are summarized in

TABLE 2. PATHOPHYSIOLOGIC BASIS FOR PRESENTING SIGNS OF MALABSORPTION SYNDROMES

Signs	Pathophysiology
Weight loss and malnutrition Increased appetite	Low calorie and amino acid intake from impaired absorption of fat, carbohydrate and proteins. Possible associated gastrointestinal plasma-protein loss.
Diarrhea	Excess load of solute and fluid in the colon may exceed its absorptive capacity; bile acids, fatty acids and colitis may cause decreased colonic absorption of sodium and water.
Bulky, frothy, voluminous stools	Excess fat and gas content in feces due to bacterial hydrolysis of malabsorbed carbohydrate.
Weakness	Anemia; electrolyte depletion; cachexia.
Edema	Hypoproteinemia due to protein depletion, from impaired amino acid absorption or excess protein loss from gut.
Anemia	Impaired absorption of iron and Vitamin B_{12}; loss of plasma transferrin and bound iron if enteric protein-loss occurs.
Bleeding problems	Vitamin K malabsorption, hypoprothrombinemia.
Skin problems	Causes uncertain.

Table 3 on pages 182 and 183. Comments on each follow. (*See also* DIAGNOSTIC PROCEDURES FOR THE OFFICE LABORATORY, p. 1465.)

Fecal Fat: A qualitative examination of feces for neutral fats and undigested muscle fibers may help differentiate between maldigestive and malabsorptive disorders. The most reliable test for steatorrhea is the quantitative determination of 24-hr fecal fat excretion using a chemical method available in clinical laboratories. Normal dogs have a coefficient of fat absorption (fat intake in gm/day minus fecal fat excretion in gm/day divided by fat intake) of greater than 95%. Fecal fat excretion may be normal in some malabsorptive states.

Fecal trypsin: The detection of fecal trypsin in any quantity by use of subjective tests indicates normal pancreatic exocrine function. Repeated absence suggests pancreatic exocrine insufficiency. Subjective tests may be done using gelatin or unexposed X-ray film as substrates, and quantitative tests using azocasein proteins may be available in clinical laboratories.

Carbohydrate Absorption Tests

Starch Absorption: Dog—3 gm/kg body wt soluble starch; **Horse**—2.5 gm/kg body wt of corn starch, as a 20% solution given orally. Under normal circumstances glucose evolved by hydrolysis of starch produces a transient elevation in plasma glucose concentration. A flat curve in the dog implies deficiency of pancreatic amylase. A flat curve in the horse implies mucosal malabsorption.

TABLE 3. TESTS USEFUL IN THE DIFFERENTIAL DIAGNOSIS OF MALABSORPTIVE DISORDERS
(To use the table, see text, p. 181 ff.)

Test	Normal Value	Findings in: Maldigestion (pancreatic exocrine insuff.)	Findings in: Malabsorption	Findings in: Protein-losing
Fecal fat (dog)				
Qualitative neutral fat	Present	Greatly increased	Normal	na
Quantitative total fat	> 95% coefficient of fat absorption	40-80%	80-90% (may be normal)	na
Fecal muscle fibers (dog)	Few	Many	Few	na
Fecal trypsin (dog)	Present 7-179 azocasein units	Negative or low	Normal or high	na
Starch absorption				
(dog)	∽ 50 mg% elevation in plasma glucose 1.5-2 hr after dosing	Flat curve	Not known	na
(horse)		Unknown	Flat curve	na
Oral D-xylose absorption				
(dog)	> 45 mg% plasma conc. 90 min after dosing	Normal	Flat curve	na
(horse)	> 30 mg% plasma curve 90 min after dosing	Normal	Flat curve	na
Oral glucose tolerance test				
(dog)	∽ 50 mg% elevation in plasma glucose conc. resting level 2 hr after dosing	Diabetic curve if pancreatic endocrine mass diminished	Often flat curve	na
(horse)		Unknown	Flat curve	na

Hemoglobin and/or serum iron concentration (dog)	Hgb: 12-18 gm/100 ml	Normal	Frequently reduced	na
Plasma albumin (dog)	3.57 mg/100 ml	Normal	May be reduced	May be reduced
(horse)	3.25 gm/100 ml	Normal	May be reduced	May be reduced
[51]Cr-labelled protein excretion (dog, horse)	Controls must be used	na	Normal	Increased
Biopsy—intestine		Normal	Diagnostic for morphologic changes	Diagnostic for morphologic changes

> = greater than
∽ = approximately
na = not applicable

D-Xylose absorption: Dog—0.5 gm/kg body wt orally as a 10% solution; **Horse—**2 gm/kg body wt orally as a 20% solution. Low plasma concentration following dosing, and resultant low urinary excretion imply reduced intestinal surface area.

Oral glucose tolerance test: Dog—2 gm/kg body wt orally as a 12.5% solution; **Horse—**1 gm/kg body wt orally as a 20% solution. This test is used in the horse instead of the D-xylose test for intestinal absorptive function since it is less costly. A "diabetic curve" in dogs may be consistent with destructive pancreatic disease producing both exocrine and endocrine insufficiency.

^{51}Cr-labelled protein excretion: This test is possible only in sophisticated settings with access to a γ-ray spectrometer. Rapid clearance of ^{51}Cr-labelled protein from plasma implies increased gastrointestinal loss, in the absence of renal glomerular disease. If feces uncontaminated by urine can be collected, the amount of the isotope appearing in the feces over several 24-hr periods can be calculated as a proportion of the dose administered, permitting a direct assessment of gastrointestinal loss. Normal controls must be used for comparison.

Small Intestine Biopsy: Biopsy of the small intestinal mucosa is essential in animals with suspected malabsorption or protein-losing enteropathy. Specific abnormalities in mucosal structure are associated with some of the conditions listed in Table 1, although nonspecific changes are often associated with these syndromes. The pathologist may be able to comment on prognosis, or possible etiology under some circumstances, and a follow-up biopsy may permit assessment of the response to therapy.

Therapy (dog): Pancreatic exocrine insufficiency must be treated by oral pancreatic enzyme replacement. Unprotected enzyme preparations may be inactivated by gastric acid. Although concomitant antacids or use of enteric coated products have been recommended, good results can be obtained by administering pancreatic enzyme granules in the food in increasing quantities to effect. Diets should be low in fat and starch and high in protein, in adequate quantities to maintain condition of the animal, and divided into several meals daily. Medium-chain triglycerides, e.g. coconut oil, may be a valuable alternate energy source in the diet. Fecal volume and consistency should improve, but body weight gains may be expected in only about half the cases. (*See also* PANCREATIC DISEASE IN THE DOG, p. 192.)

Undifferentiated malabsorption/protein-losing enteropathy responds to no specific therapy. The prognosis is grave in cases of lymphangiectasis, neoplastic infiltration and chronic granulomatous enteritis. If the syndrome is associated only with moderate inflammatory cell infiltration and villus atrophy, clinical improvement may recur. However, no critical evidence exists supporting the value of intestinal astringents and protectants, broad-spectrum antibiotics or corticosteroids in treatment. A low-residue diet with glucose and high-quality protein may be fed.

Lactase deficiency may produce milk intolerance in some dogs. Malabsorption screening tests are inconclusive. The diagnosis may be made by observing the effect on fecal consistency of excluding and reintroducing milk into the diet. Therapy involves removing milk and milk products, including cheese and chocolate, from the diet.

INTESTINAL ADENOMATOSIS OF PIGS

(Proliferative enteropathy of pigs)

A proliferative enteropathy (**regional ileitis**) of uncertain etiology occurring primarily in SPF pigs 2 to 6 weeks after weaning. *Campylobacter sputorum* subsp. *mucosalis* can be demonstrated in the intestines of affected pigs but its role is not established. Recovered animals appear to be immune; it is unclear whether there is a carrier state.

Clinical Findings: Unthriftiness and deaths increase insidiously and sporadically. Some pigs show mild to markedly hemorrhagic diarrhea, and may become anemic. Rarely there are abortions. Within a group, disease effects persist for approximately 4 weeks and affect successive weaner groups. If untreated, mortality may reach 10 to 20%. Less commonly the disease may occur as an outbreak, usually following some stress such as transportation.

The disease has a second peak of occurrence in replacement gilts at 6 to 10 months of age in herds where antibiotic growth promotants have been fed during the weaning and growing periods. The disease must be differentiated from swine dysentery, q.v., p. 297.

Lesions: Necropsy reveals crypt epithelial proliferation of the ileum, and variable portions of the jejunum, thickened intestinal mucosa with serosal edema and enlarged mesenteric lymph nodes. The line between affected and unaffected gut wall is sharply demarcated. In chronic cases mucosal polyps may appear. The disease can be confirmed histologically. Necrotic enteritis is a common sequela in weaner pigs.

Treatment and Control: Control is achievable with tylosin or nitrofurans (℞ 124) in the ration for 4 to 8 weeks after weaning; other antibacterials also are probably effective, but all should be accompanied by proper sanitation and maintenance of a closed herd.

Tylosin (℞ 82) is therapeutic unless the strain is resistant, in which case other antibacterials are indicated.

The **hemorrhagic bowel syndrome** appears to be related to intestinal adenomatosis. Pigs dying with hemorrhagic bowel syndrome and contemporaries apparently normal at the time of slaughter may show lesions of intestinal adenomatosis. The hemorrhagic syndrome may be an acute manifestation of adenomatosis or, perhaps, a secondary complication; it appears in replacement gilts, weaners and early growers as hemorrhagic diarrhea or as severe anemia from massive luminal hemorrhage. Up to 6% die suddenly.

At necropsy the skin is marble white. Luminal hemorrhage occurs from the ileum and adjacent jejunum occasionally to the proximal jejunum; these sites and the large bowel are filled with blood; the mucosa is thickened and velvet red but bleeding points are inapparent. The disease must be differentiated from esophagastric ulceration, acute swine dysentery and intestinal torsion.

Recovery is slow after therapy with corticosteroids (℞ 142), antihistamines (℞ 557), parenteral vitamin E and antibiotics.

DISEASES OF THE RECTUM AND ANUS

RECTAL DEVIATION

A condition of male dogs over 6 years of age usually seen in association with perineal hernia and concurrent relaxation of the structures of the pelvic diaphragm. The rectum is characteristically deviated laterally and feces become impacted within the flexure.

The outstanding sign is tenesmus. The perineum may bulge when the animal attempts to defecate. Digital examination will reveal pouching and lateral deviation of the rectum. Radiographs taken following a barium meal also will demonstrate the deviation.

Treatment consists of castration, which is usually followed by a return of normal tone to the pelvic diaphragm and a reduction in the extent of the rectal deviation. A low-residue, slightly laxative diet should be fed and daily enemas may be necessary. If the condition does not improve, more extensive surgery will be required.

RECTAL PROLAPSE

A complete eversion of the posterior portion of the rectum through the anus, usually characterized by the protrusion of a large cylindrical mass covered with a congested, inflamed and often hemorrhagic mucosa. The anterior part of the rectum or the posterior part of the colon may prolapse into the rectum and extend beyond the anus. This can be differentiated from true prolapse since it is possible to pass a probe some distance between the prolapsed mass and the anal sphincter. Anal prolapse is a partial prolapse in which the mucous membrane has moved posteriorly on the muscular coat to form a circular protrusion outside the anus.

Rectal prolapse is encountered most frequently in young, heavily parasitized animals that are depleted in protein, vitamins and fluids, and that have been consuming high-fiber rations. The resultant enteritis, diarrhea and tenesmus bring about the prolapse. It may occur in association with constipation, neoplasms, foreign bodies and lacerations in the rectum, and has been encountered in protracted dystocia and in old dogs suffering from prostatitis. The exciting cause is straining, such as occurs in cases of enteritis or during parturition, particularly where there is vaginal prolapse in the ewe and cow.

Rectal prolapse may occur in young animals that have a congenital weakness of the anal sphincter muscles. It appears to develop in Boston terrier puppies more often than in other breeds. Skunks are susceptible following surgical removal of the scent glands. It is common in young pigs, particularly those fed on large quantities of whey, and in young rams of certain breeds. Straining and prolapse of the rectum may be observed in bovine rabies.

Clinical Findings: Where the rectal mucosa alone is involved in the prolapse, the congested mucosa protrudes from the anus. This may occur only during defecation or when the animal is straining.

Where true prolapse occurs, the eversion of the rectum is complete and a cylindrical mass protrudes from the anus. Immediately after prolapse, the rectal mucosa is red and glistening. As the prolapse persists, the color deepens to dark red and may become almost black. Congestion of the prolapsed portion may proceed to ulceration and necrosis. Small amounts of liquid feces may be passed. Manipulation of the prolapse apparently causes little or no pain.

Treatment: Small animals: In cases of mucosal prolapse, reduction is effected by manipulation or with the aid of a bougie or soft paper cone. Application to the mucosa of cool astringent solutions such as 5% alum (℞ 639), 1% phenylephrine, or the instillation of a saturated sugar solution into the rectum will prevent recurrence in some cases. If the mucosal prolapse is persistent, or if a true rectal prolapse exists, it is best corrected by surgery such as purse-string suturing of the anus or colopexy.

Any underlying cause must be corrected and careful attention must be given to the diet and feeding schedule to prevent recurrence. Fluid therapy may have to be instituted to correct dehydration. For the first 24 to 48 hours, a liquid, low-residue diet should be fed. Milk should be avoided as it may precipitate further straining. Therapeutic diets, which are available commercially, may be indicated. Enemas of warmed olive or mineral oil at the rate of 60 to 90 ml morning and night, will produce soft evacuations. Applications of topical anesthetic agents, such as a dibucaine ointment (℞ 615), to the anal and rectal regions may prevent straining. In some cases, it will be advisable to administer a sedative such as phenobarbital (℞ 552).

Large Animals: Reduction and retention are indicated before marked necrosis of the bowel has occurred. Retention is accomplished with purse-string suturing. In the presence of marked necrosis, amputation or submucous resection of the prolapsed rectum should be performed.

ATRESIA

Uncomplicated anal atresia, in which the cloacal membrane persists, is a common defect wherein the closure is limited to the region of the anal outlet, and the anal depression and sphincter are normally developed. Not uncommonly, atresia ani in females is accompanied by a persistent communication between the rectum and vagina, producing a type of rectovaginal fistula (vulvovaginal anus).

Anal and rectal atresia involves the anus, and also a variable portion of the rectum, in which a segment consists of a strand of connective tissue lacking a normal lumen. In calves and foals, the patent gut may terminate in the region of the colon with no evidence of abnormality in the rectum or anus.

If unable to defecate, young animals show marked signs of distress manifested by tenesmus with grunting or whining depending on the species. Examination reveals the absence of the anal orifice in atresia ani and usually some degree of protrusion of the anal region caused by the collection of feces. Tenesmus, absence of feces, and distension of the abdomen are the most obvious signs observed in atresia coli. The anus and rectum appear normal, and the condition must be differentiated from meconium impaction. In atresia coli, even though the anus and rectum are normal, abdominal distension and the absence of feces are obvious. Radiographs, by showing the presence of gas in the rectum or the dilated blind end in the region of the colon, permit an estimation of the distance between the end of the rectum and the anus.

The only treatment is surgical. Colostomy or cecostomy may be considered in calves after insuring that other congenital or hereditary defects are not present.

PERIANAL FISTULA AND SINUS

Although the formation of infected tracts around the anus most commonly accompanies infection of the anal sacs, it may also be the result of minute fecaliths lodging in the pouches between the mucosal columns of the anal canal. The tracts run beneath the skin and into the perianal and pararectal tissue. Constipation, as evidenced by straining, may be a prominent sign before the fistula becomes obvious. Defecation is painful.

Topical and systemic administration of antibacterial agents as determined by the results of sensitivity testing may resolve the condition, but permanent relief is seldom achieved by this treatment. Complete healing is unlikely unless the infected tracts are completely excised.

ANAL FISSURE

A split in the mucosa of the anus, which may extend into the submucosa. Any laceration of the anal region may result in a fissure. The most common cause in dogs is the passage of pieces of bone or other hard or sharp objects in the feces. It may result from the passage of hard feces. In horses and cattle, mucosal lacerations may be inflicted during rectal examination. Care must be exercised to avoid perforation of the rectum during such examinations. Constipation is a prominent sign. The animal is reluctant to defecate because of pain. The feces usually are hard and small, and may have spots of blood on their surface. There may be tenesmus and the animal will resent examination of the anus. Diagnosis is made from the signs and inspection of the anal region.

Oral administration of mineral oil (℞ 505) or olive oil helps maintain soft feces. Topical treatment of the fissure may be attempted by the use of silver nitrate (℞ 643). If the fissure is deep, surgical repair is necessary. In cattle and horses, accidental perforation during rectal examination necessitates immediate surgery to reduce risk of peritonitis and death.

IMPACTION, SUPPURATION AND ABSCESSES OF THE ANAL SACS

Etiology: The 2 anal sacs open on either side of the anus near the junction of the mucous membrane and skin. The glandular lining produces a gray or brown, sebaceous secretion having an unpleasant odor. The sac ducts sometimes become occluded and the secretion accumulates. This leads to irritation that the dog attempts to relieve by rubbing its anus along the ground, an act known as "scooting." The sacs may subsequently become infected and abscessed.

Clinical Findings and Diagnosis: The first signs are "scooting" and frequent attempts to bite at the anal region. With infection, the characteristic gray-brown secretion is altered in color and consistency, usually becoming thin, yellow, foul-smelling and mixed with pus.

On examination, the anal region appears inflamed and swollen. If the ducts have been occluded for some time, a bulging of the skin is noted over the sacs. If the sacs are infected, abscessation may occur. Unless the owner of the animal is observant, these abscesses may rupture spontaneously, heal and again rupture with the ultimate formation of fistulous tracts leading from the anal sacs to the skin.

This condition results in painful defecation and ultimately in constipation.

Treatment: In uncomplicated occlusion of the ducts, simple pressure on the sacs is sufficient to dislodge the contents. This is best accomplished by introducing a gloved finger into the anal orifice and expressing the contents of the sac by pressing on the outside with the thumb.

Where infection has occurred, the sacs should be emptied and flushed with isotonic salt solution. Following this, a mixture of penicillin and streptomycin (℞ 38) or other suitable antibiotics, as determined by sensitivity tests, should be injected into the sacs. Mastitis preparations serve this purpose well. Treatment is repeated weekly until improvement is noted. For refractory or chronic cases in which fistulas have developed, surgical extirpation of the sacs is indicated.

RECTAL STRICTURE

The rectum may be injured by foreign objects (bone, needles, fishhooks) as they pass through the intestinal lumen, or by external factors (accidents, fights, maliciousness). Injured tissue adjacent to the intestinal wall may, in the process of healing, cause constriction of the lumen. An enlarged prostate gland may also result in a diminution of the size of the rectal lumen. Neoplasm is a rare cause. In cattle, narrowing of the lumen of the rectum may occur in abdominal fat necrosis. This is due to encircling fat depots undergoing necrosis and hardening. Since lesions are widespread, surgical intervention is not advised. Functional stricture, in the absence of any demonstrable organic lesion, has been described. Digital examination reveals only the pressure of muscle spasm producing an annular constriction within the rectum. Rectal strictures in swine may present a problem. Those that occur following surgery for rectal prolapse account for only a small percentage of cases. Recent investigation has incriminated **ulcerative proctocolitis,** probably caused by salmonellosis, as a precursor of rectal stricture.

If caused by cicatricial tissue, the stricture may be occasionally relieved by frequently passing bougies of increasing size. More usually, extensive surgical resection is necessary.

PERITONITIS

A local or general, acute or chronic inflammation of the peritoneal cavity.

Etiology: Peritonitis may result from bacterial contamination following surgical interventions, traumatic rupture of the stomach or intestine, or perforation of the abdominal wall. Rupture of a volvulus, an obstructed intestinal segment, a twisted stomach, an abscessed prostate, an infected uterus, or an incarcerated hernia can also contaminate the peritoneum. The greater omentum may adhere to the injured viscera, successfully localizing the peritonitis and resulting in abscess formation. A fibrinous exudate covers the peritoneum if generalized peritonitis ensues. Adhesions commonly occur between abdominal organs.

A variety of microbial agents may be found; *E. coli*, staphylococci, streptococci and *Nocardia* sp. are commonest. A viral form of peritonitis is seen in cats (q.v., p. 327). Chemical peritonitis results from the presence of blood, chyle, urine, bile or pancreatic juice released into the peritoneal cavity. Peritonitis is serious in all animals, particularly the horse.

Clinical Findings: Abdominal pain is severe and generalized; guarding of the abdomen is apparent and the animal walks with a stiff gait. The temperature is elevated. Anorexia is constant and in small animals, vomiting occurs. In horses, there are signs of severe colic, restlessness, groaning and intermittent episodes of lying down.

In cattle rumination ceases and milk production drops. In small animals, abdominal distension occurs and no feces are passed. Exudation into the peritoneal cavity causes abdominal enlargement. Fluid transudation into the abdominal cavity, the adynamic gut and subsequently venous stasis lead to hypotension and circulatory collapse. Toxemia and bacteremia contribute to the shock state. Icterus may be present in generalized bile peritonitis. When other diseases exist, e.g. intussusception, the animal additionally exhibits signs of the primary illness.

Diagnosis: The diagnosis is based on the signs of peritonitis and history of abdominal injury, previous surgery or signs of a primary disease. The leukocyte count is elevated and many immature forms appear. Abdominal paracentesis may yield peritoneal fluid containing ingesta, urine or bile. In time, the exudate becomes bloody, purulent or both. Cytologic examination and culture of the aspirated fluid is useful. Radiographically a "ground glass" appearance of the abdomen and loss of organ detail is characteristic. Gas- and fluid-filled loops of bowel may be evident. In some cases, free abdominal air may cap an abdominal fluid level when a viscus has ruptured.

Treatment: Broad-spectrum (℞ 5) antibacterial therapy should be instituted immediately, pending specific results. Electrolytes and fluids (℞ 580), plasma or whole blood are given IV to maintain adequate cardiac output. Surgical exploration of the abdomen is sometimes necessary if medical investigation fails to reveal the initiating cause. Repair of a ruptured viscus is essential, followed by peritoneal lavage with a soluble nonirritating antibiotic solution, e.g. streptomycin. Medical and postoperative management includes frequent peritoneal lavage with antibiotics. Since oral antibiotics may be poorly absorbed or vomited, parenteral therapy should continue. Pain can be controlled with meperidine. Food should be withheld until the clinical condition improves. Intravenous alimentation including vitamins may be given until oral liquids and gradually introduced solid foods are tolerated.

PANCREATIC DISEASE IN THE DOG

Disease of the pancreas occurs more commonly in the dog than in the other species of domesticated animals. The main syndromes are the result of acute pancreatitis, chronic relapsing pancreatitis, and its sequela, fibrosis. In addition, a syndrome characterized by malabsorption, q.v., p. 180, is recognized in young dogs but some argument exists as to whether the pathologic lesion is hypoplastic or atrophic. Carcinoma of the acinar pancreas is uncommon, but insidious and devastating in its manifestations. Functional islet cell adenocarcinomas are very rare and cause a syndrome characterized by convulsions due to hypoglycemia.

PANCREATITIS

Autoimmune mechanisms, metabolic abnormalities, vascular factors and obesity have been suggested but the cause(s) is not definitely known. The underlying lesion is one of necrosis, and many factors including trauma, nutritional deficiencies due to excess fat in the diet, infection, duct occlusion, reflux of bile or intestinal fluid into the gland and distension of the stomach with food have been associated with the disease. The common mechanism is probably ischemia leading to necrosis and release of activated proteolytic and lipolytic enzymes that digest the pancreas and surrounding tissue. Chronic relapsing pancreatitis is a continuance or a periodic recurrence of the necrosis. A proportion of chronic cases terminate in diabetes mellitus as a result of fibrosis of the gland.

Clinical Findings: Dogs that suffer from spontaneous pancreatitis tend to be middle-aged, inactive, obese house dogs that often eat fat, either from their masters' plates or from garbage containers. Working or athletic dogs are almost never affected, except on the rare occasions when pancreatic necrosis is a complication of abdominal surgery or trauma. In acute cases there is vomiting and marked abdominal pain, followed in some cases by shock. Hypoglycemia due to sudden release of insulin and hypocalcemia due to calcium combining with fat in the peritoneal cavity are possible complications. The feces usually contain some blood. Jaundice is an unusual complication that occurs when the common bile duct is occluded by the inflammatory reaction or digested by the enzymes released during the attack.

The chronic relapsing form of pancreatitis is characterized by repeated mild attacks of vomiting and abdominal pain of only a few days' duration. Discovery of the true cause of such attacks may come months or years later when a particularly severe attack warrants sufficient investigation to identify the disease. More commonly the problem is recognized after voluminous orange- or clay-colored, rancid-smelling, frequent stools containing undigested food are present. The appetite may be ravenous owing to the malabsorption and, in some cases, the concurrent diabetes mellitus. The pancreas is reduced to a fibrotic cord. Chronic pancreatitis also occurs in the domestic cat.

Diagnosis: The clinical diagnosis of acute pancreatitis may be suggested by abdominal pain, hyperlipemia, and elevated amylase or lipase concentration in the serum. Leukocytosis, hemoconcentration, elevated BUN and the presence of protein and casts in the urine may also occur. The disease may be confused with acute renal failure or intestinal obstruction but the acute pain tends to rule out the former and radiography will rule out the latter. Chronic pancreatitis is confirmed by an absence of trypsin and the presence of fat and undigested meat fibers in the feces (*see* PANCREATIC FUNCTION TESTS, p. 1477 and MALABSORPTION SYNDROMES, p. 180). Amylase and lipase concentrations are not elevated in the serum of animals with fibrosis of the pancreas. Fat absorption tests are particularly useful.

Treatment: The most important aspect of the treatment of acute pancreatitis is initiation of vigorous therapy aimed at combating pain with analgesics such as meperidine (℞ 617), and shock with electrolyte solutions designed to restore the decreased blood volume, blood pressure and renal function. Propantheline bromide (℞ 515) or atropine sulfate (℞ 511), which have an inhibitory effect on pancreatic secretion, may limit the extension of inflammation in milder cases. Penicillin (℞ 65) and streptomycin (℞ 34) or one of the tetracyclines are given to combat secondary infection of necrotic tissue. Parenteral feeding and good nursing care are essential. Oral feeding should be avoided to minimize pancreatic secretions. Heparin may be used to minimize the danger of thrombosis and intravascular coagulation.

In chronic pancreatitis, replacement therapy must be given for the duration of the animal's life. Three daily feedings of a high-protein, high-carbohydrate, low-fat diet are recommended. Pancreatin granules (℞ 518) are mixed with each meal in a dosage level sufficient to keep the feces normal. This may require as much as 15 gm per day. Absorption of fat is enhanced by the administration of an emulsifying agent, polysorbate 80 (℞ 519), with the meals. Choline (℞ 624) may be added to the diet for its lipotropic effect, but generally these latter 2 agents are unnecessary for long-term replacement therapy. Tablets of pancreatin should not be used as they are generally passed through the dog's digestive tract intact. The prognosis is good and management is not difficult as long as diabetes is absent. When the endocrine function is also lost, insulin therapy must be used; for these the prognosis is poor.

PANCREATIC HYPOPLASIA

This disease is also called juvenile atrophy of the pancreas and it is seen in young dogs, usually before 2 years of age. The pancreas is small, thin and lace-like in form. Affected dogs lose weight in spite of having a ravenous appetite. Coprophagy is often noted. They do not vomit or suffer abdominal pain. The stools become soft, unformed and voluminous, may take on a putty-like consistency and are passed frequently. Undigested food may be seen in the feces and the hair of the tail and perineal region may become oily because of the excess fat in the feces. Diabetes mellitus is very rare in conjunction with this disease.

The diagnosis is confirmed by the absence of trypsin in the feces and the presence of fat and undigested meat fibers. It must not be confused with intestinal malabsorption (q.v., p. 180) where trypsin will be present in the feces. Laparotomy may be necessary to make a positive diagnosis. Treatment is as for chronic pancreatitis without diabetes mellitus.

Pancreatic Neoplasms: (*See* NEOPLASMS OF SMALL ANIMALS, p. 612).

DISEASES OF THE LIVER, BILIARY TRACT AND GALLBLADDER

The liver is one of the organs whose function it is to guard the internal environment of the body. The diagnosis and treatment of liver disease is often difficult. Considerable damage may be present before obvious clinical signs are apparent. The clinical silence of liver injury largely stems from 3 important hepatic characteristics: a high degree of reserve functional capacity, a complex and multiple functional activity, and an unusual ability to regenerate.

Hepatic functions: The functions of the liver are more numerous than those of any other organ of the body; the main ones can be grouped most conveniently into 5 categories: circulatory, excretory, metabolic, defensive and hemopoietic. The degree to which any of these functions are impaired, or if any one is more seriously affected than another, will depend upon the particular qualities and quantity of the hepatotoxin present. Secondary damage seems to follow frequently from primary causes such as septicemia and intestinal obstruction. If the primary cause of these lesions can be treated successfully liver damage is reversible and does not play a significant role in the clinical picture.

Clinical Findings and Diagnostic Aids: In primary hepatic disease, the clinical signs are caused solely by the lesions in the liver, while in secondary involvement the syndrome may include signs unrelated to the hepatic lesions. Any diffuse disease will, to some extent, interfere with hepatic function. Signs of hepatic dysfunction for all species will include some of the following: anorexia, vomiting, constipation or diarrhea, discolored feces, pain on percussion of the hepatic area, hepatomegaly, icterus, discolored urine, edema, emaciation, photosensitization, interference with blood clotting, anemia of rapid onset, and nervous signs. The diagnosis of liver dysfunction based on clinical examination requires confirmation. Further evidence will be provided by measurements of total serum proteins particularly albumen and prothrombin, blood glucose, bile pigments, rate of dye clearance, the activity of enzymes in serum, and possibly the concentration of ketone bodies in plasma and also photodynamic substances. Liver biopsy to examine hepatic tissue morphology is sometimes valuable also.

Lesions: Few animals die of liver disease but many die with it. There may be virtually no macroscopic evidence of liver disease or the changes may be gross, the changes may involve size, shape, color, texture and continuity and may be due to inflammation, degeneration, trauma, may be congenital, nutritional, vascular or neoplastic.

Inflammation: A purulent hepatitis is the commonest, particularly in cattle, and occurs mainly in the form of liver abscesses. Pyogenic organisms may be carried to the liver via the portal system, along the bile tree, by lymph drainage, and with parasitic larvae. Necrobacillosis of the liver is caused by *Fusobacterium necrophorum* (particularly in cattle) and also by other specific infectious processes, fowl cholera, glanders, tuberculosis and salmonellosis (in which the infection persists in the gallbladder of adult cattle but not in calves). In cattle it occurs frequently as a sequela to rumen acidosis (q.v., p. 143). Penetrating foreign body abscesses are generally single (*See* TRAUMATIC RETICULOPERITONITIS, p. 138). In other cases hematogenous spread occurs by the portal vein, or in the newborn, the umbilical vessels. A sequela to hepatic abscessation in cattle can be a thrombosis of the posterior vena cava causing sudden death.

Tuberculous lesions of the liver are most frequent in pigs, cattle and fowls, the infection spreading always by the hematogenous route. Glanders lesions may be present in the liver of horses.

Actinomyces infection of the liver may arise from penetration of the liver by a foreign body from the reticulum. Infectious necrotic hepatitis (INH, q.v., p. 401) is an acute toxemia of sheep, cattle and pigs. Bacillary hemoglobinuria (q.v., p. 399), producing an acute toxemia of cattle and sheep, may occur in a similar manner to INH, but fluke burrowing is not always involved. Serum hepatitis of horses, following the injection of serum or vaccination, may cause a severe or fatal reaction in 42 to 60 days after vaccination though death may occur in 6 to 24 hours after onset of signs. Viral hepatitis occurs in dogs and fowl (*See* POULTRY DISEASES, p. 1055 et seq.). Diffuse interstitial hepatitis following parasitic infection may affect the liver as a whole, or individual lobes. Parasitic agents involved include *Cysticercus tenuicollis* and liver fluke. *Leishmania* produces hyperplasia of the liver cells. Hepatic distomatosis (either *Fasciola hepatica* or *Dicrocoelium dendriticum*) affects cattle, sheep and goats, but the severest lesion is found in sheep. Increased plasma activity of hepatic enzymes will be present, but only during the migration phrase. Low serum albumin concentrations are recorded as colonization of the liver proceeds. Inflammation, if severe enough, is followed by necrosis.

Intralobular and central lobular **necrosis** are frequently caused by hypoxia and are likely to develop in diseases that are associated with a rapid and intense hemolysis such as is seen in piroplasmosis, puerperal hemoglobinuria of cattle, hemolytic disease in foals and piglets, and acute or chronic copper poisoning and babesiasis in dogs. However, piglet anemia and equine infectious anemia and vascular disorders will also cause necrosis.

Chemical and infective toxins with a primary effect on liver cells include: dietary factors (deficiency of animal protein and therefore of sulfur containing amino acids, vitamin E deficiency); pyrrolizidine alkaloids (q.v., p. 1048); toxins of ascarids and ancylostomes, and from infectious and pyogenic diseases such as pericarditis, endometritis, leptospirosis, chronic hog cholera, chronic metabolic disturbances and viral abortion. Sufficiently severe damage will induce hepatocerebral disease. The repair of severely necrotic tissue is by **cirrhosis,** which occurs when there is much damage to the mesenchyme with a loss of liver tissue; scar formation results, giving postnecrotic scarring. Biliary fibrosis is the natural response to inflammation of the connective tissue in the portal triad. The actual causes are many and often unknown. In general, plant toxins, toxic infections and parasitic infestations are responsible. Toxins from *Senecio* spp. and *Crotalaria* spp. are frequently responsible for generalized fibrosis in cattle and sheep. The degree of cirrhosis present may be established from BSP clearance and from examination of biopsy samples. Cirrhosis stimulated by the presence of a parasite depends very much on how the parasite develops. Many parasite larvae pass along the portal vein to the liver where they track through the tissue on their way to their final destination. Others pass from the abdominal cavity to the liver. Parasites most commonly responsible for these conditions are liver fluke, *Cysticercus tenuicollis* and *C. pisiformis*. Interstitial foci are frequently seen in the livers of young pigs 3 weeks to 3 months old, when *Ascaris lumbricoides* are responsible.

Degeneration: Prolonged pressure on the liver tissue always results in atrophy, which may be localized or generalized due to internal or external occurrence, e.g. tumors, parasitic cysts, tuberculosis, actinomycosis and abscesses in the liver or neighboring organs. In the developmental stages of many tapeworms the oncospheres burrow through the intestinal wall to eventually reach the portal vein and enter the liver, where some may develop, e.g. *Cysticercus tenuicollis* and *Echinococcus* sp. Depending upon their size, the cysts produce varying degrees of compression, pressure atrophy and hypoxia of the liver tissue, ultimately compressing bile ducts and hepatic veins. Clinical signs are usually found only with heavy infestation. Toxic liver atrophy of pigs up to 6 months old is of uncertain etiology, but vitamin E and sulfur-containing amino acid deficiencies are thought to be involved. Similar lesions due to plant toxins are found in other animals causing conditions such as hepatocerebral disease in horses.

Amyloidosis is not a common condition among domestic animals, being seen most frequently in horses maintained for hyperimmune serum production. Amyloid is a protein complex, the product of an antigen antibody reaction, and is deposited in subendothelial locations. It is a sequela to chronic suppurative disorders such as glanders, peritonitis, pleurisy, strangles and tuberculosis. **Pathologic deposition of fat** is seen frequently in the liver. **Fatty degeneration** may be the result of reduced oxidation of lipid within the hepatic cell, loss of lipolytic function of liver cell due to reduced carried protein synthesis or increased mobilization from the periphery. Poisons such as antimony, arsenic, phosphorus compounds, carbon tetrachloride and chloroform, and plants such as lupins, vetches and fungi can be responsible. However fat deposition can be a normal response to either a diet or physiologic status. Pregnancy toxemia in sheep may be associated with extreme fatty infiltration and later degeneration with functional liver damage present.

Icterus has 3 possible origins: hemolytic, hepatocellular and obstructive. Failure to excrete bilirubin rapidly enough results in accumulation first within the liver and then eventually regurgitation of bilirubin from the hepatic cell. Reflux can also result from an obstruction to the biliary outflow. There are numerous causes of each category. Massive hemolysis will effect liver function by increasing the need for excretion and by overloading the normal pathways. Specifically the causes are multiple: bacteria, viruses and toxins will all produce jaundice. Leptospira, eperythrozoonosis, piroplasmosis and hemolytic disease of the newborn are all associated with jaundice.

Vascular conditions: Changes may result in hepatic overload. Congestion of the liver occurs to a varying extent whenever cardiac incompetence exists. In general, it is associated with disease conditions of the mitral and tricuspid valves, diseases of the myocardium and of the pericardium (causes include foreign body penetration, pericarditis, tuberculosis), chronic pulmonary disease, and enlarged lymph nodes. A chronic form, found particularly in cattle and pigs, develops when there is an obstruction to the outflow of blood from the hepatic veins, then either a part or the whole of the liver may become involved.

Tumors: Tumors, primary or secondary, are not common in farm animals, but are more frequent in dogs, and may include the bile ducts.

Gallbladder and Bile Ducts: Changes in the lumen diameter by compression may occur, whereas dilation can be produced by gallstones, parasites (ascarids) or foreign bodies. Prolonged retention of bile, a consequence of stenosis or intestinal inflammatory changes, is responsible indirectly for most cases of dilation. Gallstones are not common among domestic animals; when present, the clinical signs manifest are of colic and icterus. Inflammation of the biliary ducts (cholangitis) results from many different causes, which may include infections (e.g. canine hepatitis), parasites and foreign bodies. Spread usually occurs from the lumen of the intestine tracking into the biliary system, and includes *Salmonella* spp. and *E. coli* organisms. Perforation of the gallbladder causes bile peritonitis, which is very severe and frequently fatal.

Treatment: Treatment is aimed at removing the cause of the problem and then supporting the liver until it has recovered its function. If any agent can be called specific for liver injury it is glucose; this may be given orally or parenterally and is necessary to prevent the hypoglycemia that so often accompanies acute liver failure. Calcium should also be used to control guanidine toxicity.

Diet will depend upon the stage of the disease: high carbohydrate and fat (medium chain triglycerides) are advocated and a protein of high biologic value (except in incipient hepatic coma in which all protein must be avoided). Vitamin and mineral supplements may be valuable. Sterilization of the alimentary canal with antibiotic should be considered in coma. The patient should be rested, this reduces the pain induced in the hepatic capsule and promotes hepatic regeneration by allowing greater perfusion of the organ.

Veterinarians should be aware of the possible hazards of therapy with drugs that are processed by the liver. Treatment may be necessary for some of the sequelae of liver disease such as ascites. There is no consensus on the use of corticosteroids in acute hepatic disease.

ENDOCRINE SYSTEM

THE PITUITARY GLAND
(Hypophysis)

Pituitary hormones regulate cellular activity in their respective target organs, and malfunction of the pituitary results in an abnormal slowing down or speeding up in the rates at which the thyroid, adrenal cortex or gonads function.

Hormones secreted by the anterior lobe of the pituitary (**adenohypophysis**) are: somatotropin (STH or growth hormone); thyrotropin (TSH); adrenocorticotropin (ACTH); gonadotropins, which consist of the follicle-stimulating hormone (FSH) and luteinizing hormone (LH); and prolactin (lactogen). The hypothalamus produces specific neurohumoral agents (peptides) called releasing or inhibiting hormones, which regulate the synthesis and release of the adenohypophyseal hormones (protein). Gonadotropin releasing hormone (GnRH) has been synthesized and appears to be a promising agent to increase output of FSH and particularly LH.

Antidiuretic hormone (ADH, vasopressin) and oxytocin are octapeptides produced in the supraoptic and paraventricular nuclei of the hypothalamus and stored in the posterior lobe of the pituitary (**neurohypophysis**).

Most hypophyseal hormones are available in crude or partially purified form and some are synthesized. Anterior and posterior pituitary hormones are ineffective when given orally and must be injected.

Pituitary and hypothalamic disease may result from tumors, encephalitis, abscesses, local hemorrhage or injury. Pituitary tumors may be asymptomatic or produce increased or decreased function.

Anterior-lobe disorders: STH: Overproduction leads to gigantism in the young or to acromegaly with coarse features and thickened skin in the adult. Underproduction in the immature animal results in dwarfism. No practical therapy for over- or underproduction of STH is available.

TSH: Hypothyroidism due to TSH deficiency presents a clinical appearance identical to primary hypothyroidism and can be differentiated by measuring the thyroid response to injection of thyrotropin.

ACTH: Overproduction due to a pituitary tumor results in secondary hyperplasia of the adrenal cortices with an increased output of adrenocortical hormones yielding a clinical entity known as **canine Cushing's disease.** Hyperadrenocorticalism without a pituitary tumor presents a similar clinical picture and is called **canine Cushing's syndrome.** Signs include polydipsia, polyuria and increased appetite followed some months later by alopecia and pendulous abdomen. Adrenalectomy relieves the signs but careful pre- and postsurgical therapy must be given including mineralocorticoid (deoxycorticosterone acetate, DOCA, ℞ 139), glucocorticoid (℞ 138) and dietary salt.

Deficiency of ACTH as primary disorder is rare but may be observed in panhypopituitarism (*see* below). More commonly seen is a deficiency following intensive glucocorticoid therapy. Gradual reduction in dosage is recommended for prevention. ACTH (℞ 137) administration may be helpful.

Prolactin: Abnormalities in production have not been identified in domestic animals.

Gonadotropins (FSH and LH): Deficiency is rarely diagnosed in the dog but is observed in specific reproductive disorders in many farm animals.

Panhypopituitarism: Insufficiency of all anterior pituitary hormones is probably commoner in the dog than the specific deficiencies described above. Adrenal cortical, thyroidal and possibly gonadal function should be evaluated and replacement therapy with target gland hormones instituted.

Posterior-lobe effects: ADH helps maintain serum osmolality by reducing fluid loss as urine. Greater than physiologic levels of ADH can also elevate blood pressure.

Oxytocin causes contractions of the myometrium and is occasionally used in hastening normal parturition in small animals if the cervix is dilated (℞ 193). Manual delivery or cesarean section are preferred in large animals since oxytocin can induce uterine rupture.

Oxytocin regulates the contractility of the myoepithelial "basket cells" around the alveoli of the udder. Nursing produces a neural impulse that travels via the hypothalamus to the posterior lobe of the pituitary gland which instantly responds by releasing oxytocin. This hormone is carried by the bloodstream to the udder where it causes milk let-down. Injection of oxytocin produces the same effect and can also make available the "residual" milk which cannot normally be obtained by milking. Similarly, manipulation of genitalia causes release of oxytocin resulting in uterine contractions to aid in sperm transport. Because of the participation of the nervous system in this process, lactating females are very sensitive to disturbances or environmental stresses, which may as easily prevent release of oxytocin as proper stimuli enhance it. Oxytocin (℞ 193) can be used to correct agalactia in some postparturient sows, and milk let-down in cows and bitches can be augmented.

Adiposogenital syndrome: This condition is characterized by extreme obesity together with hypoplasia of the gonads. The animal has voracious appetite and signs of lethargy, sleepiness, sensitivity to cold and often polydipsia and polyuria. It is caused by neoplastic or destructive lesions involving the hypothalamus and posterior lobe.

DIABETES INSIPIDUS

A disorder of the hypothalamic-neurohypophyseal axis with chronic manifestations, characterized by the excretion of excessive quantities of very dilute but otherwise normal urine and associated with a severe polydipsia.

Etiology: Diabetes insipidus results from a deficiency in secretion or release of antidiuretic hormone, which controls the rate of water resorption in the distal convoluted tubules and collecting ducts of the kidney. Normal function is dependent on the integrity of the neurohypophyseal system which includes primarily the supraoptic and to some extent the paraventricular nuclei and their axon tracts, which extend into the posterior lobe. Injury to any part of this system may result in diabetes insipidus. It is occasionally seen in horses and cats, but most often in dogs.

Affected animals may be separated into 2 main groups. In the idiopathic group, no pathologic organic changes are demonstrable and the cause is unknown. The so-called symptomatic group comprises a number of pathologic conditions. The commonest lesion in dogs is a tumor of the neurohypophysis or of the adjacent intracranial structures. However, any intracranial space-occupying lesion that compresses or invades these structures can cause diabetes insipidus. Other causes are metastasis of a tumor to the pituitary or hypothalamus, abscess formation in this region, fracture of the base of the skull and basilar meningitis.

Clinical Findings: The condition is seen more often in older dogs of either sex. The onset usually is insidious, with progressively increasing polydipsia and polyuria if it is due to a tumor; it may be more sudden when due to trauma or meningitis. Enormous quantities of fluid are ingested and excreted: up to 5 liters a day in the dog and 100 liters in the horse. The urine is water-clear, of low specific gravity (1.002 to 1.006 in dogs) and contains no albumin. Urine osmolality varies between 50 and 200 mOsm/L of water. Housebroken dogs, if confined, are in constant distress as they seek access to the outdoors.

Diagnosis: Diagnosis depends on proof of chronic polydipsia and polyuria, with the production of urine of a constant or slightly fluctuating low specific gravity. Incontinence and increased frequency should, therefore, be distinguished from increased urinary volume. Since tumors of the neurohypophysis may frequently involve the adjacent adenohypophysis and the hypothalamus, diabetes insipidus, obesity and gonadal atrophy frequently coexist. In horses, in which diabetes insipidus is usually due to a tumor of the pars intermedia, there is concurrent somnolence and muscle weakness.

Diabetes insipidus should be distinguished from other disorders causing increased urinary volume. Diabetes mellitus is characterized by glycosuria, high specific gravity of urine (1.035 to 1.060 in dogs) with a darker color ranging from yellow to amber. In compensated chronic nephritis, polyuria may be present, but to a lesser extent, and with a higher specific gravity (1.010 to 1.020 in dogs). Albumin and casts are often present. Diagnosis of diabetes insipidus may be confirmed by parenteral injection of vasopressin (℞ 205). A temporary disappearance of polyuria and polydipsia for 6 to 24 hours should occur compared to the inability to concentrate urine following water deprivation.

Treatment: The control of diabetes insipidus requires the parenteral use of antidiuretic hormones usually as vasopressin tannate in oil (℞ 205), the dose being adjusted to the individual case. The effects are only palliative and temporary after each injection. Dietary restriction of urinary solutes, salt and protein, may help reduce urine output.

THE THYROID GLAND

The thyroid gland, under control of the hypothalamic-pituitary axis, secretes tetraiodothyronine (**thyroxine**) and **triiodothyronine,** which affect or coordinate many body functions by influencing tissue oxidation (metabolism). In domestic animals the effects are most apparent in growth, reproduction, and egg and milk production. The thyroid hormones are combined with a large protein to form thyroglobulin, which is stored in the follicular colloid of the thyroid gland. For practical therapeutic purposes, L-thyroxine is considered to be the active thyroid hormone. In some species, triiodothyronine has been isolated from the thyroid and blood and may be the metabolically active hormone at the tissue level.

In domestic animals, most disorders of the thyroid are characterized by the underproduction of thyroxine. The 2 common causes of hypothyroidism are iodine deficiency and inherited low production of thyrotropic hormone. Hyperthyroidism is occasionally observed in domestic animals. The parafollicular cells of the mammalian thyroid secrete the hormone calcitonin (q.v., p. 206) in response to high plasma calcium levels.

HYPOTHYROIDISM

Hypothyroidism, which includes goiter, cretinism and myxedema, may be the result of inadequate iodine intake. In some geographic areas the natural feedstuffs and water are deficient in iodine, and a reliable supplementary source of iodine, such as stabilized salt, must be fed. Hypothyroidism may also result from the presence of goitrogenic substances in feeds or the administration of synthetic goitrogens. Their effect is to alter the synthesis, release, or effect at the tissue level of the thyroid hormone. Raw soybeans, cabbage, rape, turnips, many other natural foods and some drugs have been shown to contain goitrogens. Hypothyroidism can also be the result of inborn errors of metabolism due to a simple autosomal recessive gene. Cases of congenital hypothyroidism have been reported in sheep, and piglets (barker syndrome) and suspected in cattle.

SIMPLE GOITER
(Colloid goiter, Endemic goiter)

A diffuse, symmetrical compensatory enlargement of the thyroid gland with clinical or subclinical hypothyroidism. The Great Lakes

Basin, the Rocky Mountains, the Northern Great Plains and upper Mississippi Valley, and the Pacific Coast regions of North America should be regarded as wholly or partially deficient in iodine. In other parts of the world, mountainous and inland areas distant from the sea should be regarded as potentially iodine-deficient.

Clinical Findings: Simple goiter due to iodine deficiency is most commonly observed in newborn pigs and lambs, is less common in foals and calves, and may occur in any mammal. The glands usually are at least twice the normal size, soft and dark red. Severely deficient, goitrous pigs and lambs may be dead or weak at birth. The neck is usually grossly enlarged and the skin and other tissues may be thick, flabby and edematous. Pigs, calves and lambs may be partially hairless or woolless, but extreme goiter may exist in the presence of the normal amount of hair or wool. Iodine deficiency in the pregnant mare may result in the birth of goitrous foals. Many foals from severely iodine-deficient dams are weak at birth, unable to suckle and may die. Goiter was common in dogs in iodine-deficient areas prior to the widespread use of iodized salt in human diets and the inclusion of trace minerals in prepared pet foods. Goiter has been reported in cats, but is regarded as rare.

The pregnant female appears to have an increased iodine requirement. Any deficiency, however, is more commonly manifested by the newborn. Microscopic examination of the thyroid may be necessary to detect subclinical goiter. Gross thyroid enlargement of any animal in the so-called goiter areas, in conjunction with a lack of dietary iodine supplementation, is strong evidence of simple goiter.

Prophylaxis and Treatment: Prophylaxis is more effective than treatment. The use of stabilized iodized salt (containing at least 0.007% iodine) is recommended in all areas known or suspected to be iodine deficient. Treatment does not seem to improve the chance of survival of severely affected newborn animals. The use of iodized salt in goitrous animals, if they do survive, will result in restoration of normal thyroid function. Specific iodine therapy may be employed (℞ 600, 606).

GOITROGEN-INDUCED HYPOTHYROIDISM

The feeding of raw soybeans, especially in the absence of adequate iodine intake, may produce simple goiter. Present methods of processing, which include heating the meal, destroy the natural goitrogen which soybeans contain. Although goiter has been produced in laboratory animals with natural plant goitrogens, it is not likely to occur in animals receiving adequate iodine. The compounds in plants responsible for goitrogenic activity are thiocyanates, thioglycosides and perchlorates. The *Brassica* group of plants contain a substance, goitrin, which is the active goitrogen.

CRETINISM

Extreme hypothyroidism in the newborn or young animal resulting from a deficiency of the thyroid hormones due to iodine deficiency, inherited enzyme defects, or deficiency of thyroid stimulating hormone. The immature animal fails to grow, has irreversible CNS dysfunction, mental dullness, dry brittle coat, thick skin, scaliness, dermatitis, lethargy and obesity. Thyroid preparations (℞ 203) may be tried in animals diagnosed as cretinous, but usually euthanasia is advisable. Iodine is of little value in cases of congenital hypothyroidism or pituitary involvement.

MYXEDEMA

A reaction to an insufficiency of thyroid hormones in the adult, characterized by lethargy and sensitivity to cold. Cutaneous thickening and edema, especially of the head and limbs are seen in the dog. This puffiness of the skin does not give the staining reaction typical of true myxedema. Body weight may be normal or increased, although appetite is reduced.

In farm animals, signs are less likely to occur. Although conclusive evidence is lacking, excessive fattening and reduction in signs of sexual behavior in both sexes may occur. In cows, reduced milk production and "silent heat" may be a result of hypothyroidism caused by high environmental temperatures.

An unequivocal diagnosis of hypothyroidism would require objective measurement of thyroid function, such as reduced radioactive iodine uptake, T_3 resin sponge uptake test, or serum thyroxine assay. In older dogs, obesity, lethargy, dryness of the skin and loss of hair are sometimes attributed to hypothyroidism. The administration of thyroxine (℞ 203) may alleviate these signs.

HYPERTHYROIDISM

Excessive secretion of the thyroid hormone, resulting in signs due to an increased metabolic rate. In the dog these are associated with a functional thyroid tumor.

Clinical Findings: The first sign of hyperthyroidism, whether spontaneous or induced, is weight loss accompanied by increased appetite. The animal is restless and nervous; heart and respiratory rates are increased and the metabolic rate is elevated. Blood cholesterol is reduced and glycosuria and creatinuria may occur. Polydipsia and polyuria may be present in some cases due to the diuretic effect of thyroid hormones. Increased gastrointestinal motility with diarrhea is occasionally seen.

Except possibly in the dog, hyperthyroidism does not often appear spontaneously in animals. The condition is sometimes reported as a cause of poor fattening in steers.

The discovery that thyroxine or thyroactive substances, such as desiccated thyroid and thyroprotein, influence milk production, growth rate, reproduction and, in chickens, egg production and feathering, has led to considerable experimental use of these materials. Thyroid hormone administration during the decline phase of milk production in cattle has been shown to increase both milk and butterfat production. Since the metabolic rate is increased by thyroid therapy, feed intake must be increased if body weight and a high level of lactation are to be maintained. The requirements of certain vitamins, particularly vitamin A and the B-vitamins, are increased. Excessive weight loss that cannot be corrected by feeding, extreme nervousness, higher incidence of injuries and excessive cardiac and respiratory rates are undesirable side effects that may occur and thus limit the use of thyroid preparations for increased production.

Treatment: Spontaneous hyperthyroidism can be dealt with surgically or medically. Complete thyroidectomy, when the tumor is bilateral, is followed by hypothyroidism which in turn must be corrected by thyroid administration. Partial thyroidectomy may correct hyperthyroidism, but the thyroid remnants may undergo further hypertrophy and thus re-establish hyperthyroidism.

Thiouracil and its derivatives depress thyroid activity. In dogs, 0.1 to 0.2 gm of thiouracil daily will usually reduce thyroxine secretion. Blood hemoglobin and red and white cell counts should be made before and during therapy since goitrogens may produce anemia, agranulocytosis, fever and skin reactions. Dosage must be determined by giving to effect.

THE PARATHYROID GLANDS

The parathyroid glands secrete **parathormone** (PTH) which elevates plasma calcium levels and enhances the renal excretion of phosphate. PTH maintains ionized calcium concentrations in extracellular fluid by bone resorption, gastrointestinal absorption of calcium in the presence of vitamin D and reduction in urinary calcium excretion. Calcium homeostasis is also regulated by **calcitonin** (CT). CT is secreted by the parafollicular cells of the thyroid in mammals and by ultimobranchial tissue in avian and other submammalian species. Calcitonin functions to prevent excessively high levels of blood calcium. Secretion of both PTH and CT are regulated by alterations in calcium levels.

Primary hyperparathyroidism has been recognized as a clinical entity in the dog. It is usually due to an adenoma of the parathyroid that leads to hyperplasia and overproduction of PTH. Hypercalcemia may be intermittent and clinical signs show considerable variability. The excessive PTH release may lead to demineralization of bones even leading to fractures and bone deformities. Treatment is limited to surgical attempts to remove sufficient hyperactive tissue to reduce the level of hormone production to normal limits.

Secondary hyperparathyroidism is secondary to (1) chronic renal disease or (2) chronic imbalance in the nutritional calcium-phosphorus intake (*see* NUTRITIONAL HYPERPARATHYROIDISM, p. 577 and INTERSTITIAL NEPHRITIS, pp. 881 and 886).

Secondary hyperparathyroidism (renal) of dogs is due to chronic renal dysfunction, which leads to phosphate retention with a reciprocal fall in serum calcium. During progressive development of renal lesions the altered calcium:phosphate ratio leads to excessive PTH secretion due to the low serum calcium values. This causes demineralization of bone. Clinical signs such as a slow, stiff gait and tenderness of the jaw reflect the decreased density seen in radiographs of the metaphyseal region of long bones and the lamina dura around the teeth. Nutritional secondary hyperparathyroidism occurs in animals fed an excess of phosphorus in proportion to calcium and results from excessive parathyroid activity with bone calcium resorption.

In puerperal tetany (q.v., p. 519) blood calcium levels are usually low and this has been attributed to temporary hypoparathyroidism relative to the sudden demand for calcium in lactating bitches or queens. Parathyroid insufficiency does not appear to be the primary cause of parturient paresis, (q.v., p. 513) although there is a parathyroid involvement in the calcium homeostatic upset. The role of calcitonin is uncertain at present.

THE THYMUS

The thymus gland is essential for the development and maintenance of immunological competence. It is large in the newborn but atrophies with the approach of sexual maturity. This diminution in size is attributed, in part, to gonadal steroids. Steroids of the adrenal cortex can also inhibit the thymus, a condition that may be observed following severe stress due to injury or infection. The thymus is believed to be the source of one or more blood-borne factors that induce differentiation of lymphoid cells so that they are able to participate in immune reactions. It may also be a source of immunologically competent cells that migrate to lymph nodes and spleen. Along with other lymphoid tissue, the thymus can be involved in the pathology associated with bovine lymphosarcoma.

DIABETES MELLITUS

A chronic disorder of carbohydrate metabolism due to insulin deficiency. Diabetes is probably the commonest endocrine disorder in the dog, and a mild form is occasionally diagnosed in other domestic animals.

Etiology: In most cases, the insulin-producing cells of the islet tissue of the pancreas have been damaged. The cause is known in only a small percentage of cases. In the dog, this damage is occasionally associated with disease of the pancreatic parenchyma, such as chronic pancreatitis or pancreatic atrophy or fibrosis. Previous infection may play a part in the onset of this condition. Most cases of diabetes mellitus occur in dogs over 5 years of age. It is about 5 times more frequent in female dogs.

Clinical Findings: Usually, the disease is fairly well-advanced when first seen, although latent diabetes may be detected in routine laboratory procedures. The onset is insidious, but the owner may have noticed increased thirst and urination or sudden loss of weight concurrently with increased appetite. The main signs are polyuria, polydipsia, polyphagia, weakness and emaciation. In advanced cases, an acetone odor may be detected on the breath. Acidosis with persistent vomiting occurs in severe cases, especially in dogs. The terminal episode is diabetic coma. Secondary signs are sometimes present in the form of corneal opacity or ulcer and cataract. If the pancreatic parenchyma has been damaged, digestive disorders paralleling those of pancreatitis may be present.

Diagnosis: Diabetes mellitus may be diagnosed by finding a fasting hyperglycemia, glycosuria and often a ketonemia in patients showing typical clinical signs. The normal fasting values for blood sugar in the dog are from 75 to 100 mg/100 ml. In fasting animals, blood sugar levels above 120 mg/100 ml are diagnostic of diabetes mellitus. Values have been reported as high as 500 mg/100 ml. The specific gravity of the urine is usually increased (1.040 to 1.060). The disease can be differentiated from diabetes insipidus, which is rare, by the hyperglycemia and glycosuria, and the high specific gravity of the urine. Chronic nephritis with polyuria can be ruled out in the same way and also by the presence of albumin in the urine and an elevated urea-nitrogen content of the blood.

Treatment: Long-term success is dependent upon the understanding and cooperation of the owner. Mild disease is rare but may be controlled by change to a semidiabetic diet. A diet low in carbohydrates and high in protein has been advocated. Day-to-day consistency and small multiple feedings are important. If the diet does not control the disease, insulin should be given, either the protamine-zinc form (℞ 184), or NPH form (℞ 183), adjusting the dose until the disease is brought under control and the urine contains only a trace of sugar. Doses usually range from 5 to 50 units daily, depending on the severity of the disease and the size of the animal. The insulin should be given several hours prior to feeding. If excessive insulin results in hypoglycemia, 5 to 20 gm of glucose should be given orally or parenterally and the daily insulin dose reduced. In the rare cases of mild diabetes, one of the oral hypoglycemic sulfonylureas may be tried (℞ 158). Oral dosing greatly simplifies treatment and encourages owners to carry out home treatment. The sulfonylureas stimulate release of insulin, hence, functional tissue must be present.

In diabetic acidosis, the prognosis varies directly with the degree of ketoacidosis, vomiting and dehydration. These cases must be treated as medical emergencies. The primary objectives are to reduce the ketonemia and to replace electrolytes lost through vomiting. Crystalline zinc insulin (℞ 182) is indicated along with IV injections of glucose and electrolytes. This rapid acting insulin may be given in an initial dose of 10 to 50 units, one-half IM and one-half IV, and repeated at 6- to 8-hour intervals depending upon the dog's response.

When insulin therapy has been instituted, it is helpful to check the urine sugar and blood sugar levels at frequent intervals until such time as an adequate maintenance dose is determined. Progress examinations, 2 or 3 times yearly, should be carried out.

In diabetes, as in pancreatitis, there is a tendency for fat deposition to occur in the liver. This can be prevented by the addition of choline (℞ 624) to the diet. Pancreatin and bile salts may also be used.

THE ADRENAL GLANDS

The adrenal glands consist of 2 parts, the medulla and the cortex. Secretion of **epinephrine** and **norepinephrine** by the medulla under the direct control of the sympathetic nervous system constitutes the initial response of the animal to stresses such as disease, trauma, extreme temperatures and hemorrhage. Although sympathetic stimulation causes the release of both hormones, norepinephrine release increases during periods of hypotension, whereas epinephrine release increases when metabolic adjustments such as increased blood glucose levels are needed to meet emergencies. Both cause ACTH release by the pituitary via stimulation of the hypothalamus.

Although the adrenal cortex is known to synthesize some 50 steroids, only a few are significant. The **adrenal sex steroids**—androgens, estrogens and progesterone—are of little clinical importance except during hyperplasia of the adrenal cortex. The glucocorticoids, cortisol (hydrocortisone) and corticosterone, are concerned with intermediary metabolism of carbohydrates, proteins and fats.

They are released under the control of ACTH during periods of stress and constitute a secondary response to meet emergencies.

The **glucocorticoids** elevate blood-glucose levels by stimulating liver gluconeogenesis from body protein. They mobilize body fats and proteins and inhibit peripheral utilization of glucose. The glucocorticoids also exert a profound anti-inflammatory effect by suppressing the activity of fibroblasts and depressing vascularization and formation of granulation tissue.

The **mineralocorticoids,** aldosterone and desoxycorticosterone, aid in the maintenance of normal sodium and water levels in extracellular fluid and are essential for life. They cause increased sodium retention and potassium loss by the kidney tubules. The mineralocorticoids are released in response to low-sodium serum levels and hypotension. Excessive administration of mineralocorticoids can cause death due to potassium depletion. In cases of adrenal hyperplasia where surgical removal of both adrenals is required, the animal must be maintained on mineralocorticoid therapy, usually subcut. desoxycorticosterone pellets, and must receive additional dietary sodium.

Many **synthetic steroids** possessing enhanced glucocorticoid activity but lessened mineralocorticoid activity are now widely used in veterinary medicine. Most of these represent alteration of the cortisol molecule by unsaturation, fluorination, or methylation. Perhaps the greatest use of glucocorticoids in veterinary medicine is for their anti-inflammatory effects in chronic conditions such as conjunctivitis, arthritis, tendonitis, dermatitis and bursitis. Local application to the inflamed area is preferred whenever possible, although they can be administered parenterally. Dairy cattle with ketosis usually respond to the blood-glucose-elevating properties of the glucocorticoids, and their use is especially indicated when ketotic cows fail to respond or relapse after IV glucose. Massive doses of glucocorticoids are used to alleviate the signs of shock although their exact mechanism of action in this condition is unknown. Because of their anti-inflammatory properties, glucocorticoids should not be administered parenterally for infectious diseases unless accompanied by an appropriate antibiotic. Glucocorticoids are known to cause abortion and retained placenta, so they should not be administered to pregnant animals, especially during the last third of pregnancy. Glucocorticoid administration to sheep partially inhibits wool growth and causes tenderness of the fleece. Similar signs are seen during periods of stress in sheep, presumably due to hyperactivity of the adrenal cortex. (*See* ADRENOCORTICAL AND RELATED THERAPY, p. 603.)

Adrenocortical insufficiency is rare in most species but has been reported in the dog due to destruction of the adrenal cortices (primary) or to a deficiency of ACTH (secondary). Iatrogenic adrenocortical insufficiency may follow abrupt termination of glucocorticoid therapy. Secondary insufficiency involves glucocorticoids mainly and usually is a minor clinical problem. The primary form also involves mineralocorticoid deficiency that accounts for most of the signs. Hyponatremia and hyperkalemia lead to vomiting, anorexia, diarrhea and muscle weakness. Mineralocorticoids can be given with IV fluid therapy in severe cases, followed by oral or IM treatment. Subcut. implants of DOCA (℞ 139) are used for long-term maintenance.

Hyperadrenocorticism may result from excess ACTH secretion due to a pituitary tumor (Cushing's disease) or to adrenal hyperplasia (Cushing's syndrome). Middle aged, purebred dogs are chiefly affected. Excessive appetite, polydipsia and polyuria precede by several months other signs such as muscle atrophy, alopecia of the body and upper limbs and pendulous abdomen due to enlarged liver and muscle weakness. Poor wound healing and thinning of the skin are occasionally seen. Hypophysectomy with long-term thyroxine treatment or adrenalectomy with postoperative implants of DOCA are reported as successful forms of treatment. Adrenal hyperplasia in the dog can be suppressed by the administration of mitotane (℞ 662).

THE GONADS

CONTROL OF OVULATION AND CORPUS LUTEUM FUNCTION

Gonadotropin releasing hormone (GnRH), a single decapeptide of hypothalamic origin, reaches the anterior pituitary via the vascular pituitary portal system to enhance the production and release of **follicle stimulating hormone** (FSH) and **luteinizing hormone** (LH). FSH initiates ovarian follicular development while LH stimulates follicular estrogen production. **Estrogen** increases the sensitivity of the pituitary to GnRH. This causes an upsurge in the plasma LH level, which results in ovulation and conversion of the ruptured follicle into a progesterone secreting corpus luteum (CL). The estrogens also stimulate uterine development and cause behavioral heat. **Progesterone** stimulates secretory activity of the uterine glands. If pregnancy ensues, the CL is maintained and continues to produce progesterone. Without pregnancy, the CL remains for a fixed period characteristic of the species. In species such as the cow, sheep, pig and horse a uterine luteolytic substance, believed to be **prostaglandin $F_{2\alpha}$** ($PGF_{2\alpha}$), causes regression of the CL. Progesterone withdrawal facilitates hypothalamic GnRH production so that pituitary gonadotropins reinstate cyclic ovarian activity. Appropriate environmental conditions influence gonadotropin release through the hypothalamus in seasonal breeders such as the ewe and mare. The nervous stimulus involved in coitus-induced ovulators like the cat, rabbit, ferret and mink also acts via the hypothalamus.

Superovulation can be induced in cattle by the injection of pregnant mare serum gonadotropin (PMSG) at a dosage rate of 1600 to 2400 IU on day 16 (℞ 175). LH or human chorionic gonadotropin (HCG) may be injected to induce ovulation and thereby avoid the possibility of cystic ovaries. Such procedures are used to enhance the rate of twinning (2 to 4 ova) or to stimulate multiple ovulations (3 to 20 ova) for embryo transfer. In sheep, a single injection of 500 IU of PMSG, given at the end of the progestational phase or of a period of progesterone treatment in synchronized programs, may increase the twinning rate.

OVARIAN MALFUNCTION

Hyperestrinism: The excessive production of estrogen by abnormal ovaries, possibly with persistent follicles, follicular cysts, or a granulosa tumor (*see also* p. 623). The usual signs are an irregular estrous cycle, infertility, excessive or prolonged uterine bleeding and sometimes nymphomania. It is often accompanied by squamous vulvar hyperplasia. The changes in the uterus consist of reddening and thickening of the endometrium, with a roughened surface and glandular hyperplasia. In the dog and horse, alopecia (q.v., p. 947) and hyperpigmentation of the skin are also believed to be signs of hyperestrinism. This condition is rather frequently seen in bitches of middle age or older. Spaying is the recommended treatment.

Persistently elevated levels of estrogens that approximate those during the follicular phase of the cycle are often associated with **cystic follicles.** This condition, which is an important cause of infertility, is seen in swine and cattle. In cows, these lesions are often associated with prolonged heats at variable intervals and the gradual assumption of external features and behavior characteristic of the male (*see* CYSTIC OVARIAN DISEASE, p. 824). In cattle, plasma estrogen levels are persistently elevated (but within the normal range) unless luteinization with progesterone production has occurred.

Hypoestrinism: A lack of estrogens, or possibly a lack of response by the CNS to estrogens in the entire animal, is fairly common. Silent heat, or ovulation without behavioral heat, is often encountered in cattle. Thyroprotein (℞ 201) may enhance behavioral estrus in some cases. In sheep, the same may occur at the beginning or the end of the breeding season. The result of a single dose of gonadotropin out of the normal season is also an ovulation without heat. In these conditions, there is no vulvar swelling or mucus secretion.

Hypoestrinism develops as a normal consequence in the spayed animal. One effect of estrogens is to cause epiphyseal calcification of the long bones and thus an early cessation of skeletal growth. Early spaying prolongs the growth period and the spayed female usually has a larger frame than the unspayed female. The lack of sexual stimulation and restlessness enables the spayed female to fatten more readily, and the carcass quality is generally improved. In spayed bitches, urinary incontinence may occur, but this usually responds well to the administration of diethylstilbestrol (℞ 166). Spaying may cause some bitches to become obese.

Hypoprogesteronism is not a common or easily recognized clinical entity. Most animals have the required progesterone from the corpus luteum; in some species the placenta takes over progesterone production during the latter part of pregnancy. The times when hypoprogesteronism might be clinically evident are (1) when improper corpus luteum function occurs resulting in short cycles, and (2) after the time in some species when placental production of progesterone is required but is inadequate—resulting in interruption of pregnancy. This latter time varies with the species. The cow placenta never takes over entirely, the mare placenta may take over after 150 days.

Hyperprogesteronism may exist as a result of persistent corpora lutea, and can predispose to cystic glandular hyperplasia of the endometrium (*see* PYOMETRA, p. 872) in the bitch. The same syndrome is seen with the excessive use of exogenous progestins, or it may follow pseudocyesis (q.v., p. 876). Such a condition may occur in the cow as a result of persistent corpora lutea due to the absence of a luteolytic factor such as prostaglandin from the uterus. This lack of luteolytic factor from the uterus occurs normally during pregnancy, and in endometritis or in the presence of a foreign body such as a mummified fetus. Prostaglandin $F_{2\alpha}$ (℞ 169) or its analogue (℞ 161) may be used to terminate CL activity for controlled breeding and for cases of pyometra or mummified fetus in the cow. This drug is not luteolytic in the bitch.

Relation of sex hormones to infection of the genitalia: There is a definite relationship between the susceptibility to infection of the uterine endometrium and the reproductive stage in cows. Cows during the follicular phase are much more resistant to uterine infections than they are during the luteal phase. Pyometritis is more frequently observed in cows with a corpus luteum in the ovaries than in those with follicles. Cows are thought to be more resistant to infections while under the influence of exogenous estrogens or stilbesterol (℞ 166). Conversely, the injection of progesterone increases the susceptibility of cows to infections of the reproductive tract.

EXTRINSIC SOURCES OF ESTROGENS AND THEIR EFFECTS

In Australia, sheep fed upon pastures dominated by certain strains of subterranean clover sometimes develop a form of **hyperestrinism** exhibited in the ewe by infertility, uterine prolapse and dystocia arising from uterine inertia, and in the castrated male by metaplasia of the accessory sex glands. In some countries infertility syndromes in cattle have also been attributed to pasture estrogens. Growing vegetation, especially legumes, contain a variety of substances, including genistin, that are mild estrogens. They are not a serious problem in the U.S.A. at present. In fact, the beneficial effects of spring grass upon milk yield and fertility have been ascribed to these substances, though without conclusive evidence. However, the estrogen content of pelleted diets for laboratory animals, especially mice, should be carefully watched as an excess has caused breeding problems and misinterpretation of research findings as a consequence. In the past, stilbestrol residues in meat scraps have caused trouble in mink. Contamination of grains with some molds such as the *Fusarium* spp. may cause abortion and signs of estrogenism due to estrogenic mycotoxins, especially in pigs.

Estrogens and growth: In most mammals, estrogens cause ossification of the epiphyses of the long bones at puberty. Thus, they generally limit growth, but this effect has not been noted in ruminants. In some countries, oral administration of diethylstilbestrol is permitted in the feed during the later phases of fattening and can increase the efficiency of feed utilization by as much as 10% and the rate of growth is correspondingly accelerated. The carcass quality may sometimes be decreased slightly if this method of fattening is used in cattle. In wethers, stilbestrol feeding may predispose to the development of urinary calculi.

TESTICULAR ABNORMALITIES

Testicular hypoplasia can occur in all species. In primary cases, the testes do not develop properly at puberty due to prepubertal malnutrition or hereditary factors. They may respond to exogenous gonadotropin injection. Secondary cases have been observed in hypothyroidism or canine Cushing's syndrome. The concentration of spermatozoa is usually subnormal with poor motility and a greater number of immature cells seen. No reliable treatment is known. Slow breeding males with normal testes and semen may sometimes be induced to mate by injection of human chorionic gonadotropin (℞ 178). (Testosterone depresses pituitary function and can cause testicular degeneration; HCG is preferred since it allows some internal regulation.) Hypoplastic testes are more susceptible to degeneration than are normal testes.

Testicular degeneration is the commonest cause of male infertility in most domestic species because it can be caused in so many ways: heat, systemic illness, increased pressure as with a hematoma or ascites, local infection, e.g. *Brucella* sp., drugs such as butazolidin, malnutrition.

Cryptorchidism is observed in most domestic species and may be unilateral or bilateral (*see* CONGENITAL ANOMALIES OF THE

GENITOURINARY TRACT, p. 820). Although hormone production may approach normal levels, spermatozoa do not develop at intra-abdominal temperatures. As the defect may be genetic, hormonal therapy or surgical correction is not recommended.

Sertoli cell tumors are observed in the dog (*see* TUMORS OF THE TESTICLE, p. 621). Signs of feminization, loss of libido, gynecomastia, symmetrical alopecia and attraction of male dogs may be seen to a variable extent. **Interstitial cell tumors** and **seminomas** derived from the seminiferous tubules are occasionally observed but usually produce only local signs.

EYE AND EAR

VETERINARY OPHTHALMOLOGY

Physical Examination of the Eye

A tractable animal in a dark, quiet room or stall approached gently and calmly with minimal restraint will allow examination of its outer and inner eye. All anterior structures are examined with a binocular magnifying loupe and a small focal light source (pencil flashlight or otoscope). The inner eye and fundus are examined with an ophthalmoscope. Detailed evaluation of the cornea, lens and vitreous requires a biomicroscope. Important and commonly useful aids are sodium fluorescein-impregnated staining paper, warm isotonic saline solution for irrigation, 1% tropicamide solution for mydriasis and 0.5% proparacaine solution for topical anesthesia. Many other agents are available.

EYELIDS

Entropion

An inversion of the eyelid margins, unilateral or bilateral, more commonly of the lower lids. It may be an inherited defect in dogs (especially chows, bulldogs, golden retrievers, Kerry blue terriers, Labrador retrievers, St. Bernards, setters) and in lambs. It is infrequent in foals.

Entropion may be secondary to conjunctival, corneal or uveal disease which should be sought during examination. Margin inversion allows eyelashes to irritate the cornea causing pain, epiphora and photophobia, which may favor superimposed infection. If elimination of any identified primary cause and medical treatment are unavailing, lid position must be corrected surgically.

Ectropion

An eversion of the lower eyelid margin. It may be hereditary or secondary to injury to the eyelid or facial (7th cranial) nerve. It is common in dogs, especially spaniels, St. Bernards, basset hounds, chows, English bulldogs and bloodhounds. Signs are conjunctival and corneal inflammation and epiphora of severity varying with the degree of eversion; exudates accumulate in the conjunctival folds. Surgical correction is required.

Blepharitis

Inflammation of the eyelids, which may be an extension of conjunctival or corneal disease, a primary dermatitis, an allergic reaction or self-induced. Bacteria or mites may invade the tarsal (meibomian) glands and hair follicles at the lid margin causing an inflammatory response. Lids are red, swollen and partially denuded with pruritus and epiphora. Dried purulent matter may encrust the lid margins. Usually the conjunctiva is congested or inflamed.

When mites are the cause, 3% rotenone ointment may be applied topically, avoiding the eye, or the disease may be treated as a generalized mite infestation. Bacteria and the inflammatory changes may be reduced with antibiotics or antibiotics with steroids as ophthalmic preparations without topical anesthetics or as systemic treatment. Frequent gentle cleansing of the lid margins with a collyrium and 15-minute applications of warm, moist compresses 2 to 3 times daily are beneficial.

Prolapse of the Gland of the Third Eyelid

Inappropriately called harderian gland enlargement, this appears suddenly as a mound of red tissue at the medial canthus. Most often it occurs in young, growing dogs unilaterally with involvement of the second eye several weeks later. The medial canthus and lower lid are soiled by a serous or mucous discharge. Discomfort is minimal. Surgical excision of the prolapsed mass or of the entire gland is required.

Cilia

Trichiasis (misdirected cilia) usually connotes any periocular hair, including nose-fold and epicanthal hair, causing corneal or conjunctival irritation. Usually, topical treatment fails and surgical correction is required.

Distichiasis is a partial or complete second row of cilia emergent from the tarsal gland ducts in the lid margin. It is seen in very young dogs. Cocker spaniels are genetically predisposed, as are Pekingese, toy and miniature poodles, boxers, English bulldogs, golden retrievers, St. Bernards, Irish setters and others. Where corneal or conjunctival irritation exists the obviousness of distichiasis should not preclude a thorough examination for other contributing factors. Epilation or electrolysis under magnification may provide only temporary benefit. Surgical correction is required.

Ectopic cilia are aberrant hairs exiting through the palpebral conjunctiva toward the cornea. They are frequent in dogs, occasional in horses, rare in cats. These cilia cause corneal ulceration, which may improve transiently under conventional ulcer therapy. With magnification, examination of the palpebral surfaces reveals hair shafts (often 4 or 5) extending from a reddened follicle in the palpebral conjunctiva. Hairs should be removed by epilation or surgical excision and the ulcer treated routinely.

LACRIMAL APPARATUS

Dacrocystitis, inflammation of the lacrimal sac, causes conjunctivitis, chronically recurrent epiphora and medial canthal swelling. Gentle manual pressure over the swollen sac expresses exudate through the lacrimal punctum. Irrigation of the nasolacrimal apparatus with saline solution may restore normal drainage. Radiographic visualization may reveal foreign bodies or neoplasms. To combat bacterial infection, ophthalmic antibiotic with steroid drops should be used topically for 10 to 14 days. Chronic canine dacrocystitis refractive to medical therapy may respond to placement of an indwelling catheter in the nasolacrimal duct for 10 to 14 days with concomitant topical use of ophthalmic drops.

Atresia of the lacrimal puncta causes epiphora in dogs and cats. Atresia of a nasolacrimal duct's distal opening causes copious purulent discharge from the medial canthus. Corrective surgery is required.

CONJUNCTIVA

Subconjunctival hemorrhage may fill the subconjunctival space following trauma or accompanying systemic disease. If uncomplicated, discomfort apparently is slight and resorption occurs within 1 to 2 weeks. Early frequent application of ice packs may lessen the amount of hemorrhage. After 72 hours, warm compresses may aid in resolution. Bulky protective collars may be applied to thwart the animal's attempts to scratch or rub the affected eye. Intraocular structures should be examined with an ophthalmoscope for uveitis and retinal diseases that may follow trauma. Any underlying disorder should be treated appropriately.

Chemosis is edema of the palpebral and bulbar conjunctivae characterized by swelling which, if severe, may protrude beyond the palpebral fissure. Causes are trauma, allergy, insect bites or orbital disease. In cats, it commonly accompanies viral or bacterial conjunctivitides. Conjunctival cultures and cytology identify the cause. Chlamydial infections should be treated with specific antibiotics topically (℞ 390, 391, 414) and systemically; feline herpesvirus infection with 0.1% idoxuridine solution every 1 to 6 hours or 0.5% ointment every 4 to 12 hours.

Conjunctivitis, inflammation of the conjunctival surfaces which may be local or associated with systemic disease. Causes are: bacteria (*see* INFECTIOUS KERATOCONJUNCTIVITIS, p. 225), viruses, parasites, molds, chemicals or trauma. General characteristic signs are hyperemia, swelling and serous-to-purulent discharge. The duration and character of the exudate categorizes conjunctivitis as: (1) acute or chronic catarrhal, (2) acute or chronic purulent, (3) follicular or hyperplastic. Chlamydial and viral infections produce intracellular inclusion bodies demonstrable in exfoliative cell specimens, while allergic conjunctivitis produces plasma cells, lymphocytes and mast cells.

When conjunctivitis is acute and unilateral, foreign bodies are common causes; the inner surface of the third eyelid should be carefully examined. When both eyes are acutely and severely affected soaps, tick dips or other chemicals may have been misused. The threadlike nematode *Thelazia californiensis*, 25- to 400-mm long, may occur singly or in clumps in the conjunctival sac of dog, cat, sheep, deer, coyote and black bear. Affected animals aggravate the conjunctivitis by self-mutilation.

Infections may be treated at 2- to 3-hour intervals with antibiotic combinations until bacterial sensitivity determinations allow specific drug choice. Frequent re-evaluation is required to regulate or modify therapy. Foreign bodies and parasites should be removed immediately. Chemicals should be flushed away with large volumes of saline solution or tap water. Allergic reactions are treated with topical corticosteroid ophthalmic ointments.

Since chronic follicular conjunctivitis results from chronic irritation, the cause should be determined and treated specifically. The chronic inflammation may be made acute by mechanically abrading and rupturing the follicles or by cautiously touching them with copper sulfate without "burning" the conjunctival epithelium. The resulting acute inflammation then is treated with antibiotic-steroid combinations.

CORNEA

Degenerative pannus (Uberreiter's syndrome) comprises subepithelial proliferation, neovascularization with pigmentation. It occurs spontaneously in dogs, most frequently in German shepherd dogs. Although of unidentified etiology, it may be an immune-mediated reaction. Usually bilateral, pannus begins at the temporal limbus and extends centrally as a pigmented, pink or fleshy, broad peninsula with, occasionally, dystrophic margins. The third eyelid may be depigmented, its anterior surface thickened. Epiphora occurs, apparently with minimal pain.

Topical steroids or antibiotic-steroid ophthalmic combinations in adequate concentrations control the disease. Medication must be applied every 2 to 4 hours then reduced weekly to a control level. As initial therapy, subconjunctival steroids may be injected cautiously followed by continual topical medication. Superficial keratectomy and β-irradiation also are only palliative. Most important are continual clinical evaluation and client understanding.

Keratitis, nonspecific inflammation of the cornea, is common in dogs with prominent eyes. Superficial keratitis may accompany distichia, entropion (q.v., p. 217) or other influences irritating or abrasive to the corneal surface. Infectious agents may then invade the deeper corneal tissue. If the eyelids fail to cover the cornea completely (lagophthalmos) corneal drying and erosion result.

Keratitis sicca (keratoconjunctivitis sicca, KCS, "dry eye"), a destructive drying of the cornea from inadequate tear secretion, may result from primary disease or denervation of the lacrimal gland, systemic disease or drug toxicity. Tear replacement therapy topically (e.g. ℞ 399, 406) is effective when tear production is not entirely absent. A systemic lacrimomimetic (e.g. pilocarpine 2 to 4 mg daily) in solution on the feed, may stimulate tear production. Artificial tears, the most effective therapy, must be applied frequently, as often as hourly in severe disease, for maximum benefit. Antibiotics and, where ulceration is absent, steroids constitute supportive therapy. If medical treatment fails, the parotid duct may be transposed surgically.

Interstitial keratitis, inflammation of the substantia propria, appears as dense corneal clouding. It may be a primary ocular disease but often is associated with systemic disease, e.g. infectious canine hepatitis, malignant catarrhal fever, tuberculosis, listeriosis, aspergillosis, lymphosarcoma, coccidioidomycosis. The cornea may "blue" from the edema and cellular infiltration of uveitis, or from the increased intraocular pressure of acute congestive glaucoma. Pain, photophobia and serous discharge vary in extent. Neovascularization deep within the cornea appears as brush-like vessels adjacent to the limbus (perilimbal flush). The bulbar conjunctiva is congested. Therapy is directed at the cause. Specific antibiotics are topically applied.

Infectious keratoconjunctivitis (q.v., p. 225) is a specific disease of cattle, sheep and goats characterized by intense lacrimation, photophobia and corneal opacity progressing to ulceration.

Ulceration of the cornea produces cloudiness adjacent to the loss of surface continuity. The conjunctiva is congested. Initially signs are photophobia and a serous discharge, which becomes purulent. Within 3 to 5 days after deep corneal erosion the devitalized zone is surrounded by newly formed blood vessels. Ulcer healing requires 4 to 8 weeks, leaving small, dense, white scars. Corneal ulceration usually is visible grossly but tiny ulcers may be apparent only after fluorescein staining. If ulceration is not arrested the posterior limiting Descemet's membrane may prolapse (**descemetocele, keratocele**) with aqueous escape through the prolapsed tissues. Corrective surgery is required. Prolapse of the anterior uvea causes **staphyloma.** Rupture of Descemet's membrane with iridal or uveal prolapse results in adherent **leukoma,** a dense corneal scar with an incarcerated iris. Chronic corneal irritation from any cause results in corneal vascular infiltration and pigmentation (pigmentary keratitis, melanosis oculi or **pannus**).

With any form of keratitis the animal should be comfortably confined in a dark room or stall and ocular exudates should be washed away several times daily with warm isotonic saline solution. When an infectious disease is the cause appropriate antibiotic therapy should be applied. In anterior uveal involvement, therapeutic mydriasis and cycloplegia (℞ 386, 409, 415) restores normal vessel permeability, ameliorating hypotony, miosis and photophobia.

Severe **collagenase ulceration** ("melting ulcer") occurs with the liberation of collagenase by necrotic cells. Acetylcysteine, an anticollagenase drug, has not been approved for ocular use.

Corneal choristoma (dermoid), a benign skin-like elevated neoplasm near the limbus, is found in young, growing animals of all species. Hair may grow from the superficial lesion. Dermoids cause local discomfort, serous discharge and, rarely, corneal ulceration. Early surgical removal is required, with the resulting lesion treated as an uncomplicated corneal ulcer. In horses, dermoids may be hairless and deep penetrants of the entire cornea. The dermoid's depth must be carefully evaluated before surgery to avoid penetrating the cornea during its excision.

UVEA

(Iris, ciliary body and choroid, together)

Filarial uveitis: follows helminthic invasion of the globe in horses, dogs, cattle, sheep, camels, springbok, domestic and wild birds. Filariid worms of the genus *Setaria* and immature *Onchocerca cervicalis* lodge in the anterior chamber of horses, of the genera *Angiostrongylus* and *Dirofilaria* in that chamber of dogs. Usually the parasites' presence causes little disturbance in the host although severe uveitis can occur. The worms are removable surgically through a corneal puncture close to the limbus.

Iritis in all species seldom occurs without cyclitis and, less frequently, choroiditis. It may follow laceration or contusion of the globe or its penetration by foreign bodies. Affected animals show acute onset, depression, congestion of the bulbar conjunctiva, corneal haze and pain. Darkroom examination of the iris reveals edema, miosis, hypotony, photophobia, blepharospasm and epiphora; clumps of leukocytes may appear as a white precipitate, usually sterile, in the anterior chamber (hypopyon). Secondary glaucoma is a serious sequela. Complete or partial adhesion of the iris to the lens or cornea is a common complication resulting in ocular compromise.

As treatment, corticosteroids are employed topically and systemically (℞ 154). Mydriatics maintain pupillary dilatation, cycloplegics relieve ciliary muscle spasm. Analgesics (℞ 145, 554) relieve pain. Prostaglandin release, an inflammatory stimulus, may be inhibited by indomethacin, phenylbutazone and aspirin. Antibiotics combat existing infection.

Iridocyclitis may be caused by trauma or accompany systemic disease as leptospirosis, infectious canine hepatitis, malignant catarrhal fever, hog cholera, African swine fever, tuberculosis, equine viral arteritis, adenoviral pneumonia in foals, strangles, feline infectious peritonitis, sepsis, neoplasia and autoimmune reactions. (*See* PERIODIC OPHTHALMIA, p. 226.)

GLOBE

Glaucoma is increased intraocular pressure incompatible with continued health and function of the eye. It may be primary, secondary or congenital. Among dogs, wire-haired terriers, basset hounds, beagles, cocker spaniels, miniature and toy poodles and Norwegian elkhounds show a high incidence. The affected animal may be depressed or irritable. The globe is enlarged (**buphthalmos**) and stonelike upon palpation. The bulbar conjunctival and scleral vessels are congested, the cornea edematous. The pupil is dilated and fixed. Later there appear cupping of the optic disc and retinal atrophy.

Drug therapy is directed toward (1) reduction of aqueous production, (2) increased facility of outflow, (3) reduction of intraocular volume. Carbonic anhydrase inhibitors (℞ 393, 539) reduce aqueous production. Autonomic cholinergics (℞ 405), anticholinesterases (℞ 392, 394) and, paradoxically, the sympathomimetic epinephrine (℞ 395) reduce aqueous production and increase outflow. Hyperosmotics (℞ 397, 398) rapidly decrease intraocular volume by moving water osmotically from the vitreous (which is 98% water) into its surrounding vascular bed and are useful in emergencies. Lately timolol maleate, a β-adrenergic blocker, has shown promise as a useful agent.

Constant re-evaluation is necessary as response of absolute glaucoma to medical therapy usually is disappointing. If sight still is present, surgery may be helpful; iridencleisis or cyclodialysis may allow a new route for aqueous removal, cryosurgery may decrease production by preventing secretion. When the eye is enlarged, blind and painful, an intrascleral prosthesis or enucleation is advocated.

Secondary glaucoma may result from sequelae of inflammation or mechanical obstruction of aqueous flow. Therapy should be directed at the inciting cause and the antecedent disease.

LENS

Cataract is any opacity of the lens or its capsule. Cataracts may be congenital or sequelae of trauma. Almost every dog more than 8 years old shows some degree of increased lens density (nuclear sclerosis). Juvenile cataracts may be associated with diet and preventable or responsive to arginine supplementation of the ration. Many breeds show an increased incidence of inherited cataracts. Slit-lamp examination through a dilated pupil allows detection of subtle lens opacities. When the lens equator is clear, topical atropine every second or third day may produce mydriasis adequate for useful vision. If the lens is opaque and nonfunctional, its surgical removal in selected instances will return good ambulatory vision.

Lens luxation is not uncommon and, in some breeds, may be associated with secondary glaucoma. It is always accompanied by some loss of vision. Both eyes should be examined. **Lenticular subluxation** is recognizable by iridal tremulousness (iridodonesis) and depth variation in the anterior chamber. The lens may dislocate anteriorly or posteriorly. A lens luxated into the anterior chamber should be removed surgically.

OCULAR FUNDUS

Retinopathy may be congenital or inherited or it may follow systemic disease, head trauma, ocular disease or neoplasia. Any retinal disease reduces visual function but focal blind spots may be difficult to identify. Retinal hemorrhage, detachment, tears and tumors may be diagnosed by careful ophthalmoscopic examination through a well-dilated pupil.

Papilledema may be a complication of hypovitaminosis A, hypertension, orbital disease, idiopathic thrombocytopenic purpura, male-fern poisoning in cattle, hexachlorophene poisoning in sheep and calves, space-occupying brain lesions, and chorioretinitis.

Optic nerve atrophy, appearing as a pale, shrunken optic disc, may result from inflammation, trauma, degeneration (e.g. advanced progressive retinal atrophy) and increased intraocular pressure. Optic neuropathy may follow meningitis, toxoplasmosis, cryptococcosis, hog cholera, diabetes, male-fern poisoning in cattle, arsanilic acid poisoning in swine, or intracranial neoplasia.

Collie-eye anomaly is a congenital, recessively inherited ocular defect characterized by choroidal hypoplasia, absence of the tapetum, peripapillary coloboma, retinal vascular tortuousity, detached retina and intraocular hemorrhage. Eyes of affected collies may be small or more deeply set. Visual loss occurs in less than 1% but retinal detachment causes blindness.

Hemeralopia, day blindness, is inherited via a simple autosomal recessive gene in some families of Alaskan malamutes and, perhaps, poodles. At about 8 weeks of age affected puppies show a marked loss of vision in bright light, but apparently normal vision in reduced light indoors or at dawn or dusk. No ophthalmoscopically visible retinal lesions are apparent.

Progressive retinal atrophy (PRA) is inherited among many breeds, especially poodles and setters. Clinically, visual acuity is diminished first at dusk (nyctalopia), later in daylight. The disease progresses over months or years, always terminating in blindness. Retinal receptor cells show congenital abnormalities or gradual atrophy. Tapetal reflectivity increases, the size of retinal blood vessels reduces progressively to their resorption. The disc atrophies. Cortical cataracts frequently appear during the disease course, perhaps as concomitant but unassociated lesions.

Retinal dysplasia is an inherited defect in Bedlington and Sealyham terriers, Labrador retrievers, springer and cocker spaniels. Lesions appear as retinal folds, as changes similar to old chorioretinal scars and as complete retinal detachment. Blindness is not always a presenting sign.

ORBITAL CELLULITIS

Inflammation of the tissue surrounding the globe follows trauma, infection, foreign body penetration or zygomatic sialadenitis. Unilateral sudden onset shows red, swollen periorbital tissues causing globe protrusion (which may be confused with glaucoma). Conjunctival surfaces may bear purulent exudate. The cornea, dry and unprotected, is susceptible to additional injury. Hypotony is present. Anterior or panuveitis may occur. The animal resists opening its mouth and ocular movements are painful. Radiographs of the orbit should reveal any foreign bodies or bone erosion. The animal should be confined in darkened quarters. Warm compresses should be applied frequently, with topical antibiotic ointments and artificial tears to cover the cornea. Parenteral antibiotics and corticosteroids, analgesics (℞ 554) and, if necessary, additional sedation are indicated. Orbital abscesses must be drained surgically.

INFECTIOUS KERATOCONJUNCTIVITIS

(IBK, Pink-eye, Infectious ophthalmia)

Infectious diseases of cattle, sheep and goats which are characterized by blepharospasm, lacrimation, conjunctivitis and varying degrees of corneal opacity and ulceration. The diseases in the 3 species are different and distinct clinical syndromes, apparently caused by species-specific agents.

Etiology: In cattle, *Moraxella bovis* is probably the commonest cause although infectious bovine rhinotracheitis virus and other viral agents have been associated with IBK; it appears probable that all may cause clinical disease singly as well as concurrently. The disease in sheep is thought to be caused by *Mycoplasma, Rickettsia* or *Chlamydia.* In goats a *Rickettsia* is the suspected cause.

Clinical Findings: The disease is acute and tends to spread rapidly. One or both eyes may be affected. In **cattle,** dry, dusty environmental conditions, bright sunlight, feeding in tall grass, or the presence of large numbers of flies tend to predispose and exacerbate the disease. Young stock are most commonly affected, whereas in **sheep** it usually involves only adults and outbreaks often follow close herding at or about lambing. The initial signs are blepharospasm and excessive lacrimation; later there is a mucopurulent discharge from the eye. Conjunctivitis and varying degrees of keratitis are present and the animals may seek shade. Adult cows may develop a mild fever with a slightly depressed appetite and decreased milk production. The clinical course varies from a few days to several weeks.

Lesions: The lesions vary in severity. In cattle, a small ulcer or ulcers occur near the center of the cornea or less often close to the limbus without initial notable corneal discoloration. After a short time the ulcers are surrounded by an opaque ring of varying size due to corneal edema and leukocytic infiltration; vascularization of the cornea follows from the limbus to the ulcer; the opacity may then involve the entire cornea. Regression may occur in the early stages or the lesions may continue to progress. Continued active ulceration may cause rupture of the cornea. In sheep, mild cases show only scleral congestion and a ring of vascularization at the limbus. In more severe cases, vascularization and opacity extend across the cornea. Ulceration of the cornea is uncommon and is rarely more than superficial. In chronic cases, the corneal lesions either regress over a long period or the cornea is permanently scarred.

Diagnosis: Care must be taken to ensure that the lesions are not due to foreign bodies or parasites. In IBR virus infections, upper respiratory signs predominate and conjunctivitis is more common than keratitis. In bovine malignant catarrh, the keratitis resolves from the center of the cornea whereas in IBK the corneal lesions resolve from the limbus toward the center.

Prophylaxis and Treatment: **In cattle,** recovered animals appear to have a good immunity, although they may remain carriers. Vaccines prepared against agents known to infect the eye have not as yet proved reliable for the control of IBK. A number of antibiotics are effective against *Moraxella bovis* (penicillin, chloramphenicol, nitrofurazone and tetracycline) and are beneficial if treatment is initiated early. They may be administered either topically as solutions or ointments, or by subconjunctival injection; repeated ocular applications are necessary and affected animals should be placed in a shaded area. Response to treatment, even after severe corneal ulceration, may be achieved by subconjunctival injection of antibiotic and a tarsorrhaphy involving both the eyelids and nictitating membrane. The tarsorrhaphy is performed using an intermarginal suture of absorbable gut. Viral agents in cattle will not be affected by antibiotic therapy but such treatment will help to alleviate secondary bacterial infection. In **sheep,** antibiotics effective against *Mycoplasma* and *Chlamydia* (tetracycline, chloramphenicol) are recommended. Treatment is usually confined to those cases where there is obvious corneal involvement. Immunity is weak and relapses and recurrences common.

PERIODIC OPHTHALMIA

(Equine recurrent uveitis, Recurrent iridocyclitis, Moon blindness)

An intermittent recurrent ocular inflammatory disease of horses and mules that frequently terminates in blindness. The severity of the manifestations range from a severe acute syndrome to a virtually subclinical chronic syndrome. In its acute form it is characterized by lacrimation, blepharospasms, conjunctivitis, keratitis, photophobia, miosis, ciliary vascular injection, flare, hypopyon and hypotony. The duration of the initial attack is variable, lasting 7 to 14 days but sequelae may include synechiae, iris atrophy, loss of corpora nigra, cataracts and radial keratopathy. During acute attacks, systemic signs may include depression, anorexia and fever. Recurrence is common; however, the interval is extremely variable. Some think the active lesion never subsides but continues as a subclinical uveitis subject to exacerbation.

The posterior uvea is also involved although the anterior segment pathology frequently precludes examination of the ocular fundus. Chorioretinal lesions, when visible, include rounded, yellowish foci of variable sizes distributed throughout the visible fundus (focal choroiditis), pale, sharply demarcated, circumpapillary areas and optic atrophy. Histologically the inflammatory lesions consist of lymphocytes, eosinophils and plasma cells. Chorioretinal adhesions are common and papillitis or optic atrophy is also reported.

Each recurrent attack produces more ocular structural alterations which, when advanced, result in blindness. These advanced lesions include cataracts, optic atrophy, retinal detachment and phthisis bulbi.

Etiology: The etiology is undoubtedly multiple. Many causes have been advanced including *Leptospira* spp., onchocerciasis, parainfluenza 3 (PI_3) virus, equine influenza virus, bacteria, and nutritional deficiencies including riboflavin deficiency. It seems clear that various isolated causes may sensitize the eye and result in the clinical signs observed.

Ocular onchocerciases has been well described and the etiopathogenesis has been identified as ocular sensitivity to the dead larvae or their metabolic waste products. Experimentally *Leptospira pomona* has produced typical syndromes 1 to 3 years after injection.

Diagnosis: Diagnosis is primarily based on clinical signs or laboratory tests. Titers for the leptospirosis in excess of 1:100, elevated *Leptospira* titers in the aqueous, conjunctival biopsy for *Onchocerca* larvae, hemagglutination inhibiting antibody against PI_3 virus, physical examination and other clinical or laboratory tests may identify the specific cause. When possible specific therapy should be instituted for the identified cause; e.g. isolation of *Onchocerca* larvae by conjunctival biopsy would indicate oral treatment with diethylcarbamazine (DEC) at 2 mg daily for 21 days. During therapy with DEC the eyes are atropinized (℞ 386) and pretreated with 10 mg of steroid, subconjunctually (℞ 401). Therapy with DEC must be done with caution as exacerbations may be precipitated by the death of the microfilaria. Therapy is repeated every 6 months.

In addition to specific therapy, when active uveitis is present the therapeutic goal is to prevent or minimize ocular structural alteration. Therapy consists of anti-inflammatory drugs, decreasing predisposition to synechiae and decreasing ciliary spasms with mydriatics and cycloplegics, and applying antibiotics either specifically or prophylactically (the affected eye is vulnerable to infection).

Corticosteroids may be given systemically, subconjunctivally or topically. Topical therapy provides therapeutic levels only in the anterior uvea, and frequent medication is important. Compounding this is the difficulty in applying topical medicaments in a horse with a painful eye. A subpalpebral lavage tube may be implanted to facilitate topical therapy. Systemic prednisolone, 0.25 to 0.5 mg/lb (0.5 to 1 mg/kg) body wt (or its equivalent), is given twice the first day and twice daily thereafter in decreasing doses until clinical improvement is obtained. Topical prednisolone acetate suspension (℞ 407) penetrates the intact cornea most effectively but ointments may be retained longer with the accompanying epiphora. Therapy is at least 4 times a day. Subconjunctival depot steroid injections (℞ 396, 402, 410) may be used in the absence of a corneal ulcer when the animal is not tractable.

Antiprostaglandins have been beneficial in ocular disease and thus aspirin, indomethacin, phenylbutazone and flunixin meglumine help control inflammation and pain in affected animals. Some investigators recommend using aspirin continuously to control exacerbations but controlled studies are needed to prove their efficacy.

Topical mydriatics include atropine sulfate (℞ 386), 10% phenylephrine (℞ 404), and scopolamine (℞ 409) alone or with phenylephrine (℞ 404).

The prognosis is guarded and any signs of ocular sequelae to inflammation, either unilateral or bilateral, must be considered an unsoundness.

DISEASES OF THE EXTERNAL EAR

OTITIS EXTERNA

Otitis externa is common in the dog, the domestic cat, and the rabbit. It is uncommon in the larger domestic species.

Etiology: Trauma (sometimes as a result of faulty cleaning), the presence of excessive amounts of dirt, wax, hair, moisture or foreign objects such as plant seeds, anatomic abnormalities and new growths predispose the ear to infection with bacteria and fungi. Ear mites (*Otodectes cynotis*) are important. Hot humid weather is also associated with an increased incidence of the disease. Breeds with long hair and pendulous ears are frequently affected, but erect-eared breeds are by no means immune. Otitis is also a feature of allergic dermatitis.

The bacteria infecting the external ear are species of *Proteus*, *Pseudomonas*, *Staphylococcus*, *Streptococcus*, *Corynebacterium*, coliforms and diptheroids, but of these only the *Proteus* and *Pseudomonas* organisms are not found in normal ears. Pasteurellae are commonly incriminated in rabbits, rarely in other animals.

Aspergillus, *Penicillium*, and *Rhizopus* species of molds are found in both diseased and healthy ears. Yeasts (*Pityrosporum* and *Monilia*) are found both in diseased and healthy ears, however the *Pityrosporum* species are found more frequently in diseased ears and may be a primary infection.

Clinical Findings: Animals with otitis externa may hold the affected ear low (if one ear is involved), shake, scratch or rub the ear along surfaces causing abrasions and bleeding. Excessive head shaking sometimes results in hematoma formation in the pinna of the ear. Kittens with ear mites may be so agitated as to appear to be convulsing.

The external ear canal is inflamed, painful and may be ulcerated; the hair will be wet or sticky with the discharge and it will have an abnormal odor. With persistent or untreated otitis externa, the epithelium of the ear canal undergoes hypertrophy and becomes fibroplastic. In extreme cases the ear canal is completely blocked by hypertrophied tissue and hearing is impaired. The nature of the cerumen and the discharge is to some extent characteristic of the microorganisms present. A brownish black cerumen, resembling shoe polish in consistency, is often associated with staphylococcus and *Pityrosporum*, a crumbly yellow-brown cerumen with staphylococci or yeasts and *Proteus*. A pale-yellow to green, watery, suppurative and odorous discharge is associated with the presence of *Proteus* or *Pseudomonas* organisms, which are commonly present in chronically infected ears.

Diagnosis: The general diagnosis is obvious in most cases. The specific cause, i.e. the presence of foreign objects or ear mites, will be identified only if the ear is carefully examined with an otoscope both before and after cleaning. Cultures followed by sensitivity tests may be prerequisites to specific diagnosis and effective treatment.

Treatment: Not all cases of otitis externa respond well to treatment. In general, a high percentage of failures and re-treatments can be anticipated. Persistence is essential if the disease is to be cured or the chronic form of the disease prevented.

Acute Otitis Externa

Because of the pain, anesthesia or tranquilization may be necessary prior to inspection and treatment. The ear must be thoroughly examined with an otoscope and foreign objects removed with a small wire loop, an ear spoon or an alligator forceps small enough to pass through the speculum. Swabs of purulent exudate should be collected for culture and sensitivity testing. The presence of ulcers or ear mites should be noted as well as the condition of the ear drum. If the epithelium is intensely inflamed, probing and swabbing should be avoided in order to prevent further injury of the ear canal. The ear should be cleaned by flushing away the debris and exudate using warm saline solution or water with a germicidal detergent, and the canal dried as gently as possible. An antibiotic-corticosteroid lotion or ointment should be applied to the ear canal (℞ 465, 472, 480). If the epithelium is raw and acutely inflamed a thin layer of protective astringent lotion or ointment (℞ 473, 474) can be applied. Antibiotics (℞ 22, 66) should be administered systemically for 4 to 5 days if the ear drum is acutely inflamed or if the animal has a fever. Analgesics or tranquilizers may be necessary. The antibiotic-steroid local treatment should be continued for one week. If antibiotic sensitivity testing is done, then the appropriate antibiotic must be used for the local and systemic treatment. The animal should be examined after 48 hours to ensure that treatment has been effective, then at weekly intervals until the inflammation has subsided. During this time small ulcers in the ear canal should be painted with an astringent solution (℞ 464). Taping the ears over the head may be of value in pendant-eared dogs.

Chronic Otitis Externa

The discharge from the ears should be cultured and a sensitivity test done. The ears should be thoroughly cleaned by gentle flushing with a germicidal-detergent solution. Heavy material may be flushed from the canal by use of a dental waterpick or a stream of sterile saline solution from a bulb-tipped 17-gauge needle. If the discharge is particularly waxy, a cerumenolytic agent (℞ 467) may be more useful. Excessive hair should be clipped from the ears. If indicated it may be an advantage to use a solution of antibiotic rather than an ointment for the first 48 hours of treatment. Such preparations must be used frequently (every 2 hours) in order to maintain a high concentration of antibiotic within the ear canal. Subsequently, an ointment containing the antibiotic can be used.

As with acute otitis, astringent solutions (℞ 464) should be painted sparingly on locally ulcerated or irritated areas of epithelium. Antibiotic-steroid combinations (℞ 465, 472, 480) may be useful to reduce pain and swelling as well as to control infection. The weekly use of these agents may be necessary to control chronic infections, especially in allergy susceptible dogs.

Surgical treatment may become necessary if therapy has failed or the disease has been neglected.

MYCOTIC OTITIS EXTERNA
(Otomycosis)

Otitis externa in which mycotic organisms have invaded the skin of the ear canal causing the formation of dry, scaly accumulations of epithelium, cerumen and dirt. Removal of the scaly deposits often causes bleeding. The condition may extend to and involve the tympanum. Mycotic infections are common in ears with bacterial infection and purulent otitis externa. This type of otitis is commonest in heavy-eared breeds and those dogs that spend much time in the water or swamps. Culture of the organism on Sabouraud's medium is necessary for positive diagnosis.

Treatment is based first on elimination of moisture from the ear canal. Adequate ventilation is mandatory and can best be accomplished in pendant-eared dogs by taping the ears over the top of the head. The ear canal should be thoroughly cleaned of all superficial scaly deposits with a wire loop or cotton swabs saturated with alcoholic phenylmercuric nitrate solution (1:1,500). Fungicidal ointments (℞ 369, 470, 480) or thymol preparations (℞ 479) should be applied until the scaliness has disappeared.

PARASITIC OTITIS EXTERNA
(Otodectic mange, Ear mange, Otoacariasis)

Otitis externa caused by the ear mite *Otodectes cynotis*. The dog, cat, fox, rabbit and ferret are affected. The mites live on the surface of the skin of the ear and ear canal, and feed by piercing the skin and sucking lymph, with resultant irritation, inflammation, exudation and crust formation.

Clinical Findings and Diagnosis: Ear mites cause the animals to shake their heads and to scratch or rub the affected ears. There is a waxy, dark-brown, sometimes flaky exudate in the ear canal. With an otoscope the small, white or flesh colored mites will be found on the dark exudate. Mites can also be observed by examining the exudate with a hand lens or under a low-power microscope.

Treatment: Instillation of a bland oil, such as mineral oil, or a cerumenolytic agent (℞ 467) into the ear canal, followed by gentle massage aids in the cleaning process and kills many of the mites. The use of a wire loop will avoid packing the heavy exudate against the tympanic membrane in the cleaning process. After cleaning, an acaricide such as rotenone (℞ 466) or dimethyl phthalate (℞ 478) or a protective-type solution in an oil base (℞ 473) should be applied and the treatment repeated every third day for 4 applications. This extended treatment will prevent reinfestation by destroying newly hatched parasites. In severe cases, the entire body of the animal should be treated weekly with a parasiticidal powder or dip to kill those mites not in the ear canal. If chronic inflammatory changes are present, a protective ointment (℞ 474) or antibiotic-corticosteroid preparation (℞ 408, 465, 469, 480) should be used until the inflammation subsides. Antibiotic ointments are useful for concurrent bacterial infections.

TUMORS OF THE EXTERNAL EAR

Any tumor of the skin or cartilage may be encountered in the external ear. Adenomas of ceruminous glands are probably the most frequent tumors in the ear canal of dogs and cats. Tumor-like polyps of hypertrophied tissue are common in the ear canal of dogs and cats with long-standing irritation or infection. Malignant tumors are uncommon.

Treatment: Surgical removal is the only satisfactory method of treatment. Lateral resection of the conchal cartilage is often necessary for removal. Concurrent otitis should be treated.

HEMATOMA OF THE EAR

A soft, fluctuating swelling containing blood, usually on the inner surface of the pinna, but occasionally on the outer surface. It occurs commonly in dogs, cats and pigs, and is a particular problem of dogs with pendant ears. It is rare in other species. The hematoma may be small or involve the entire pinna. The cause is trauma, either due to bite wounds or to violent shaking of the head caused by otitis externa. Dicoumarol poisoning may predispose swine to hematoma formation.

Treatment: Small hematomas may be treated by aspirating the blood with a syringe and a fine hypodermic needle and firmly bandaging the ear to the top of the head or to a roll of bandage for 7 to 10 days. Large hematomas require surgical evacuation of the blood clot. The loose skin is then apposed to the cartilage with many sutures placed through all layers of the ear, and the ear is firmly bandaged. Any coexisting otitis must be treated or the hematoma may recur or be produced in the other ear. Wounds in the pinna should be treated at the time of surgery. The animal may require sedation postoperatively to prevent head shaking or scratching of the ear. The bandage and most of the sutures should remain in place for 10 to 14 days.

DERMATITIS OF THE PINNA

Dogs with erect ears are subject to a specific dermatitis of the tip of the pinna resulting from fly bites especially if they are confined outside and can't escape from flies. Dry crusts form from oozing serum and blood following the bites. The use of fly or mosquito repellents or the application of pastes made from flea powders may prevent continued bites and permit healing. Affected dogs should be housed in fly protected areas and ointment (℞ 472) applied to the lesion.

OTITIS MEDIA AND INTERNA

An inflammation of the tympanic cavity arising from infection extending from the external ear canal or from the eustachian tube. Hematogenous infection is possible but rare. Otitis media due to extension of infection from the external ear canal, or due to penetration of the ear drum by a foreign object, occurs in all species, but is common in the dog, cat and rabbit. Extension of infection from the eustachian tube is seen in the dog, cat and pig. Otitis media can quickly lead to otitis interna, and can result in loss of equilibrium and deafness in the affected ear.

Clinical Findings: The signs of otitis media and otitis externa are similar. Head shaking, rotation of the head to the affected side, a painful ear, the presence of a discharge in the ear canal, and inflammatory changes in the ear canal are usually present. If otitis interna is superimposed, head rotation to the affected side will be pronounced. The animal will circle and fall to the affected side and often will be unable to rise. Nystagmus and incoordination may be present, and in severe cases the disease can terminate with death of the animal due to meningitis or abscess formation in the cerebellum.

Diagnosis: Otitis media should be suspected in cases of severe purulent otitis externa, or whenever penetrating plant awns are found in the ear canal. The diagnosis can be confirmed by finding the tympanic membrane ruptured.

Otitis interna should be strongly suspected if the previously mentioned signs are present. Extension of infection from the eustachian tube will cause a discolored and raised or bulging tympanic membrane. In otitis media and interna of long duration, the presence of fluid in the tympanic cavity, or sclerotic changes in the bone of the tympanic bulla may be detected radiologically.

Treatment: Because of the possibility of damage to hearing and the vestibular apparatus, systemic antibiotic therapy should be instituted as soon as the diagnosis is made. Chloramphenicol (℞ 17), ampicillin (℞ 7, 8) or tetracyclines (℞ 77) should be used until the results of bacterial sensitivity tests are known. If the ear drum is ruptured, the tympanic cavity should be carefully cleaned using an otoscope, long alligator forceps, flushes of detergent solutions and rinses of saline. Aqueous solutions containing neomycin and polymyxin B should be placed in the ear canal and the tympanic cavity, in addition to the systemic therapy. The ear drum will heal in time.

In the case of otitis media and interna with a clean, normal external ear, but an abnormal tympanum, incising the tympanum may be advantageous to permit culture of the fluid, relief from pressure and thus the pain, and removal of the inflammatory exudate which could cause a permanent hearing deficiency. Systemic therapy using the antibiotic selected by sensitivity testing should be continued for at least 10 days, and possibly for up to 6 weeks or longer in cases of otitis interna. Any associated otitis externa should be carefully treated. In chronic otitis media with sclerosis and osteomyelitis of the tympanic bulla, a bulla osteotomy may be necessary.

Prognosis: Otitis media with an intact tympanum responds well to systemic antibiotic therapy, but when chronic otitis and a ruptured tympanum are present, the chances of successful treatment are reduced. Otitis interna carries a guarded prognosis. Some neurologic signs (such as the head tilt) may persist for the remainder of the animal's life, or the signs may abate after many months. Animals recovering from otitis interna should be given adequate time to adapt to the neurologic deficiencies inflicted by the disease.

DEAFNESS

Deafness in animals can be acquired or congenital. Acquired deafness occurs because of bilateral occlusion of the external ear canals as in chronic otitis externa or because of destruction of the middle ear as in acute or chronic otitis media. Other causes of acquired deafness are trauma to the petrous temporal bone, loud noises, canine distemper, drugs (hygromycin, streptomycin, kanamycin, neomycin, salicylates), neoplasms of the ear or brain, and old age. Obviously unilateral deafness or partial loss of hearing is possible in some of the above instances.

Congenital deafness can occur in any species or breed. A syndrome in cats causing white fur, blue eyes and deafness results from an autosomal gene that is fully dominant with complete expression in the production of white fur, with incomplete expression for deafness and with incomplete dominance in the production of the blue iris. Deafness is due to the total or partial agenesis of the organ of Corti, spiral ganglion and cochlear nuclei. White coat color also is associated with congenital deafness in other animals. In the dog, the breeds commonly affected at the present time include the Dalmatian, bull terrier, Scotch terrier, border collie and fox terrier. This list changes with time due to breed popularity and the elimination of the defect as it becomes a problem. Cocker spaniels were known, for example, to have a hereditary deafness but it is no longer common in that breed.

Diagnosis: Diagnosis of deafness is difficult in the young or in animals kept in groups; it is only when the animal is observed as an individual at an age when responses to stimuli can be predicted that deafness becomes obvious. The main sign is failure of response to auditory stimulus. An example of this is failure of noise that excites other dogs to awaken a sleeping dog. Less obvious signs are unusual behavior such as excessive barking, a voice change, confusion when given vocal commands and lack of movement of the pinnae. Electrophysiologic methods of conducting auditory testing have been used on cats, but the technique is not in general use. In the case of acquired deafness, otoscopic examination of the external ear, radiographic examination of the tympanic bullae and a neurologic examination may determine the cause. In congenital deafness, these procedures will reveal normal structure and function (apart from absence of hearing). A careful history and shrewd observation of the animal are necessary in the diagnosis of deafness.

Treatment: Successful removal of an occlusion of the external ear canal will eliminate deafness from this cause. Deafness due to bacterial infections of the middle and internal ear may respond to early antibiotic treatment. Relief from deafness due to loud noise, trauma, or viral infections is dependent on time. Hereditary deafness may be eliminated from a species by test breeding to determine the nature of the inheritance so that the responsible carriers can be eliminated from the breeding program.

INFECTIOUS DISEASES

POX DISEASES

Acute viral diseases of man, animals and birds, excluding dogs and cats. Typically, widespread lesions of skin and mucosae occur that progress from macules through papules (pimples), vesicles and pustules before encrusting and healing. In some animal poxvirus infections, however, vesiculation is not clinically evident, but microvesicles can be seen on histologic examination and in some, proliferative lesions are characteristic. In the lesions of most poxvirus infections multiple intracytoplasmic inclusions can be found, which represent sites of virus replication in infected cells.

Poxvirus diseases affect man (smallpox or variola major and the milder alastrim or variola minor); animals (cow pox, swine pox, sheep pox, etc.) and birds (*see* FOWL POX, p. 1097). Infection with poxviruses is acquired either by inhalation, ingestion or through the skin (e.g. smallpox, sheep pox, lumpy skin disease). In certain instances the virus is transmitted mechanically by biting arthropods (e.g. fowl pox, swine pox). Infection may be followed by generalized lesions (e.g. smallpox, sheep pox) or remain localized (e.g. cow pox). Immunization against some poxvirus infections is practiced using strains of virus of reduced virulence, the classical example being the control of smallpox in man by strains of live vaccinia virus. The origin of this virus, which is maintained in the laboratory for immunizing man, is obscure.

The poxviruses can be classified according to their physicochemical and biological properties. The viruses of smallpox, alastrim, cow pox, monkey pox, etc. are immunologically closely related to vaccinia virus, but differ in this respect from the other poxviruses. The avian poxviruses, the myxoma viruses and some of the other poxviruses (e.g. swine pox) are species specific. The viruses of orf, (q.v., p. 247) milkers' nodes (q.v., p. 243) and bovine papular stomatitis (q.v., p. 101), grouped under the genus *Parapoxvirus*, differ morphologically from the other poxviruses.

COW POX

A mild, eruptive disease of milk cows with lesions occurring on the udder and teats. Once considered to be common, it is now extremely rare.

Etiology: The virus of cow pox is closely related antigenically to vaccinia and smallpox viruses. Indeed, cow-pox virus and vaccinia are only distinguishable, if at all, by sophisticated laboratory techniques. Some outbreaks in cows are due to infection with vaccinia from recently vaccinated humans.

Clinical Findings: The disease spreads by contact during milking. After an incubation period of 3 to 7 days, during which cows may be mildly febrile, papules appear on teats and udder. Vesicles may not be evident or may rupture readily, leaving raw ulcerated areas that scab over. Lesions heal within a month. Most cows in a milking herd may become affected and lesions accompanied by fever can occur on the hands, arms or face of milkers, if they have not been vaccinated.

Diagnosis: Cow pox or vaccinia infection may be confused with bovine herpes mammillitis (q.v., p. 848). Because of the similarity in the appearance of the lesions, laboratory confirmation is required.

Pseudo-cow pox (*see* below) is a much milder disease.

Control: Measures to prevent spread within a herd must be based on segregation and hygiene.

PSEUDO-COW POX

(Milkers' nodes, Paravaccinia)

A common, mild infection of the udder and teats of cows, caused by a poxvirus, which is widespread throughout the world.

Etiology: The virus of pseudo-cow pox is related to that of contagious ecthyma (q.v., p. 247) and bovine papular stomatitis (q.v., p. 101). These viruses are grouped under the genus *Parapoxvirus* because they have similar characteristics and are somewhat different morphologically from vaccinia virus. They have a limited host range and have not been propagated in fertile eggs. They will grow in some cell cultures though relatively poorly.

Clinical Findings: Lesions begin as small red papules on teats or udder. These may be followed rapidly by scabbing or small vesicles or pustules may develop before the formation of scabs. Scabs may be prolific but can be removed without causing pain. Granulation occurs beneath the scabs, resulting in a raised lesion that heals from the center leaving a characteristic horseshoe or circular ring of small scabs. This stage is reached in about 7 to 12 days. The granuloma, which can remain for several months, gives the affected teats a rough feel and appearance, and further scabs may form. The infection spreads slowly throughout milking herds and a variable percentage of cows show lesions at any time.

Man may become infected with painless but itchy, purplish red nodules that are generally present on the fingers or hands. These lesions cause little disturbance and disappear after several weeks.

Diagnosis: The scabbed lesions may be confused with warts or mild traumatic injuries to teats and udder. Scabs examined with the electron microscope will frequently show the characteristic virus particles.

Control: Control of infection within the herd is difficult but depends essentially on taking hygienic measures to destroy the virus and prevent transmission. Little immunity appears to develop.

SWINE POX

An acute often mild infectious disease characterized by skin eruptions, which affects only swine. The disease is present in the U.S.A., particularly in the midwest, and has been reported from all continents, though the incidence is generally low.

Etiology: Two different viruses have been identified: In some outbreaks vaccinia virus is involved, in others swine pox virus is the cause. The disease described here is that caused by the latter.

Swine pox virus is distinct from other poxviruses and does not protect against infection with vaccinia virus. It will grow on pig cell cultures, but not embryonated eggs. It is relatively heat stable and survives for about 10 days at 37°C.

Clinical Findings: The disease is most frequently seen in young pigs, 3 to 6 weeks old, but all ages may be affected to varying extents. Following an incubation period of about 7 days, small red areas may be seen on the skin, which develop into papules. These are most frequent on the face, ears, inside the legs and on the abdomen. Within a few days pustules develop or sometimes small vesicles may be seen. The centers of the pustules become dry and scabbed, and are surrounded by a raised inflamed zone so that the lesions appear umbilicated. Later dark scabs (1 to 2 cm in diameter) form which give affected piglets a spotted appearance. These eventually drop or are rubbed off without leaving a scar. Successive crops of lesions can occur so that all are not at the same stage. The early stage of the disease may be accompanied by mild fever, inappetence and dullness. Few pigs die of uncomplicated swine pox.

Virus is abundant in the lesions and is transferred from pig to pig by the biting louse (*Haematopinus suis*). The disease may also be transmitted, possibly between farms, by other insects acting as mechanical carriers.

Control: Recovered pigs are immune. There is no specific treatment. Eradication of lice is important.

SHEEP POX AND GOAT POX

Serious, often fatal, diseases characterized by widespread skin eruption. Both diseases have the same geographic distribution and are confined to parts of Southeastern Europe, Africa and Asia.

Etiology: The poxviruses of sheep and goat pox (*Capripoxvirus*) are now considered to be related antigenically and in their physicochemical characters. They are also related to the virus of lumpy skin disease (q.v., p. 246). Reports on the natural susceptibility of sheep to goat poxvirus and *vice versa* are conflicting; at least some strains seem capable of infecting both species.

Clinical Findings: The incubation period in sheep pox is 4 to 8 days, and goat pox 5 to 14 days. The diseases of sheep and goats present a similar clinical picture, but the disease in goats is generally less severe. Fever and a variable degree of systemic disturbance occur. Eyelids become swollen and mucopurulent discharge crusts the nostrils. Widespread skin lesions develop that are most readily seen on the muzzle, ears and areas free from wool or long hair. Palpation will detect lesions where these cannot be readily viewed. Lesions start as erythematous areas on the skin, which progress rapidly to raised, circular plaques with congested borders caused by local inflammation, edema and epithelial hyperplasia. Though microvesicles are present histologically, vesicles and pustules are not evident clinically. Virus is abundant in the skin lesions at this time. As lesions start to regress necrosis of the dermis occurs resulting in the formation of dark hard scabs sharply separated from the surrounding skin. Regeneration of the epithelium beneath the scabs takes several weeks. When scabs are removed a star-shaped scar free from hair or wool remains. In severe cases lesions can occur in the lungs. In some sheep and in certain breeds the disease may be mild or the infection inapparent.

It has been suggested that transmission may be airborne, or occur by direct contact with lesions, or mechanically by biting insects.

Diagnosis: The disease in either species must be differentiated from the milder infection, orf (q.v., p. 247), which mainly causes crusty, proliferative lesions around the mouth.

Immunity: Infection results in solid and enduring immunity. Live attenuated virus vaccines give more enduring immunity than do inactivated virus vaccines. Live attenuated lumpy skin disease virus can also be used as a vaccine against sheep and goat pox.

LUMPY SKIN DISEASE

An infectious, eruptive, occasionally fatal disease of cattle characterized by the appearance of nodules on the skin and other parts of the body. Secondary infection often aggravates the condition. It occurs in southern and eastern Africa and in recent years has been extending northwest through the continent.

Etiology and Epidemiology: The causal virus is related to that of sheep pox. The prototype strain is known as the Neethling poxvirus. Lumpy skin disease appears epidemically or sporadically. Frequently new foci of infection appear in areas far removed from the initial outbreak. Its incidence is highest in wet summer weather, but it may also occur in winter. It is most prevalent along water courses and on low ground. Since quarantine restrictions designed to limit the spread of the infection have failed, biting insects have been suspected as vectors but outbreaks have occurred under conditions where insects practically could be excluded. Because the disease can be transmitted by means of infected saliva, contact infection must be accepted as a method of spread. Sheep are suspected of being possible carriers in Kenya.

Artificial infection can be produced by the inoculation of cutaneous nodule suspensions or blood taken during the early febrile stage, or by feed or water contaminated with saliva from infected animals.

Clinical Findings: A subcut. injection of infected material produces first a painful swelling and then fever, lacrimation, a nasal discharge and hypersalivation, followed by the characteristic eruptions on the skin and other parts of the body in about 50% of susceptible cattle. The incubation period varies from 4 to 14 days.

The nodules are well circumscribed, round, slightly raised, firm and painful and involve the entire cutis and the mucosa of the gastrointestinal, respiratory and genital tracts. Nodules may occur on the muzzle and within the nasal and buccal mucous membranes. The skin nodules contain a firm, creamy gray or yellow mass of tissue. The regional lymph nodes are swollen and edema develops in the udder, brisket and legs. Secondary infection sometimes occurs, causing extensive suppuration and sloughing. As a result, the animal may become extremely emaciated and may have to be destroyed.

The nodules either regress in time or necrosis of the skin results in hard, raised areas ("sit-fasts") clearly separated from the surrounding skin. These slough off to leave an ulcer, which on healing leaves a scar.

The morbidity varies from 5 to 50% and the mortality from 1 to 75%. The greatest loss is sustained from the decrease in milk yield, the loss in condition and the rejection or reduced value of the hide.

Diagnosis: The disease may be confused with **pseudo-lumpy skin disease** caused by a herpesvirus (bovid herpesvirus 2). These diseases can be very similar clinically, though in some parts of the world, the herpesvirus lesions seem confined to the teats and udder of cows and the disease is called herpes mammillitis (q.v., p. 848).

Pseudo-lumpy skin disease is said to be a milder disease than true lumpy skin, but differentiation depends essentially on isolation and identification of the virus. Histologic and ultrastructural examination of nodules may be helpful. Pox-like intracytoplasmic inclusion bodies or eosinophilic intranuclear herpesvirus inclusions may be seen in the nodules, depending on the cause.

Dermatophilus congolensis is also a cause of skin nodules in cattle (*see* DERMATOPHILOSIS, p. 929).

Prophylaxis and Treatment: Quarantine restrictions are useless. Prophylactic vaccination by means of attenuated virus offers the most promising method of control. Goat pox and sheep pox virus passed in tissue culture have also been used.

Good nursing and administration of sulfonamides and antibiotics to control secondary infection are recommended.

CONTAGIOUS ECTHYMA

(Contagious pustular dermatitis, Sore-mouth, Orf)

An infectious dermatitis of sheep and goats, affecting primarily the lips of young animals. Encountered in all parts of the world, it occurs most commonly in late summer, fall and winter on pasture and winter in the feedlots. The condition may occur in very young lambs in early spring and occasionally in mature sheep that do not have immunity from natural exposure. Man is occasionally affected and there are reports of the disease in dogs after eating infected carcasses.

Etiology: The causal poxvirus (genus *Parapoxvirus*) is related to those of pseudo-cow pox (q.v., p. 243) and bovine papular somatitis (q.v., p. 101). Infection occurs by contact. The virus is highly resistant to desiccation, having been recovered from dried crusts after 12 years. It also is resistant to glycerol and to ether.

Clinical Findings: The primary lesion develops on the skin of the lips, with frequent extension to the mucosa of the mouth. Occasionally, lesions are found on the feet, usually in the interdigital region and around the coronet. Ewes nursing infected lambs may develop lesions on the udder. In very young lambs, the initial lesion may develop on the gum below the incisor teeth. The lesions develop as papules and progress through vesicular and pustular stages before encrusting. Coalescence of numerous discrete lesions often leads to the formation of large scabs, and the proliferation of dermal tissue produces a verrucose mass under them. Where the lesion extends to the oral mucosa, secondary necrobacillosis frequently develops.

The course of the disease is from 1 to 4 weeks, within which time the scabs drop off and the tissues heal without scarring. During the active stages of the infection, the more seriously affected lambs fail to eat normally and lose condition. Extensive lesions on the feet lead to lameness. Mastitis may result in ewes with lesions on the udder.

Diagnosis: The lesion is characteristic. The disease must be differentiated from ulcerative dermatosis (q.v., p. 249), the virus of which produces a different kind of reaction leading to tissue destruction and the formation of crateriform ulcers. Ecthyma usually affects younger animals than does ulcerative dermatosis, although this criterion can only be used presumptively. A positive differentiation may be obtained by the inoculation of susceptible and ecthyma-immunized sheep.

Immunity and Vaccination: Sheep recovered from a natural attack are highly resistant to reinfection. Despite a multiplicity of immunogenic virus strains, with an occasional exception the presently employed commercial single-strain vaccines have produced satisfactory immunity in all parts of the U.S.A. Sheep immunized against contagious ecthyma are susceptible to the virus of ulcerative dermatosis.

Vaccines should be used cautiously to avoid contaminating uninfected premises and vaccinated animals should be segregated from unprotected stock until the scabs have fallen. A small amount of the vaccine is brushed over light scarifications of the skin, usually on the inside of the thigh. Lambs should be vaccinated at about 1 month of age. For best results, a second vaccination about 2 or 3 months later is suggested. Nonimmunized lambs going into infected feed lots should be vaccinated.

Treatment: Antibacterials may help to combat secondary infection. Where indicated to repel screwworm attack, appropriate repellents and larvicides should be applied to the lesions. The virus is transmissible to man and the lesions, usually confined to the hands and face, are more proliferative in man and occasionally are very distressing. Veterinarians and sheep handlers should exercise reasonable protective precautions. Diagnosis in man is established by transmitting the virus to sheep. A complement-fixation test may be of value in the diagnosis.

ULCERATIVE DERMATOSIS OF SHEEP

(Lip and leg ulceration, Venereal balanoposthitis and vulvitis)

An infectious, ulcerative viral disease of sheep manifesting itself in 2 somewhat distinct forms, one characterized by the formation of ulcers around the mouth and nose or on the legs (lip and leg ulceration) and the other as a venereally transmitted ulceration of the prepuce and penis or the vulva (balanoposthitis and vulvitis).

Clinical Findings: The lesion, regardless of anatomic location, is an ulcer with a raw, easily bleeding crater varying in depth and extent, containing an odorless creamy pus and covered from the beginning with a scab. Face lesions occur on the upper lip, between the border of the lip and the nasal orifice, and on the chin. The ulcerative process may, in very severe cases, perforate the lip. Foot lesions occur anywhere between the coronet and the carpus or tarsus.

Posthitis lesions partially or completely surround the preputial orifice and may become so severe as to produce phimosis. In rare cases, the ulcerative process may extend to the glans penis so that the animal becomes unfit for natural breeding. In the female venereal form, the edema, ulceration and scabbing of the lips of the vulva have less serious consequences.

There are no noticeable early systemic reactions. Very often, the disease remains unrecognized until the lesions have reached such an advanced stage that signs of lameness or disturbed urination become apparent.

Diagnosis: This depends entirely upon recognition of the characteristic ulcerative lesion. Differentiation between this lesion and that of orf (q.v., p. 247), which is essentially proliferative in character, is fundamental. The question of the similarity of the agents of ulcerative dermatosis and orf is not clearly defined, but inoculation of sheep previously immunized against orf will help in arriving at a diagnosis. It is also difficult and, in some instances, virtually impossible, without resorting to sheep inoculation, to differentiate between bacterial balanoposthitis (q.v., p. 857) and ulcerative dermatosis.

Prophylaxis and Treatment: Infected animals should be isolated and those with genital lesions should not be bred. The time taken to recover varies from 2 to 8 weeks and is not greatly influenced by treatment. Treatment, therefore, is usually not attempted unless (1) the animals are to be bred in a short time, (2) lip lesions interfere with eating, (3) foot lesions make the animals so lame that they are losing flesh, or (4) secondary bacterial infections become serious.

Treatment, when given, consists of removing the scabs and all necrotic tissue from the ulcers and applying any one of the following preparations: silver nitrate (styptic pencil), 30% copper sulfate solution, 4% formaldehyde solution, 5% cresol (sheep dip) or sulfaurea powder. Foot and lower leg lesions can be treated conveniently with copper sulfate or formaldehyde solutions in foot bath troughs.

PAPILLOMATOSIS

(Warts)

Warts of the skin or oral mucosa are self-limiting benign tumors occurring at multiple sites, chiefly in the young, of many species. They have not been clearly shown to occur in cats. They may be cauliflower-like, as usually seen in cattle, or small, scattered horny elevations. Isolated, individual small pedunculated growths that are not true warts can also develop on the skin. These do not change in size and generally do not create a problem.

Etiology and Transmission: Wart viruses are host-specific under natural conditions. The virus appears to infect the basal cells of the epithelium causing some cells to degenerate, while others are stimulated to excessive growth and wart formation. New virus particles form in the degenerating cells and may completely replace the nuclear material when the cell reaches the surface; thus, there is much infective virus at the surface of the wart. The virus is quite resistant and may contaminate fences, stanchions or other objects. Skin wounds from such objects frequently lead to infection of susceptible animals. Tattoo instruments or hypodermic needles will transmit the infection in cattle.

Clinical Findings: Cattle: Warts commonly occur on the head, neck and shoulders, and occasionally on the back and abdomen. The extent and duration on an animal depends upon the area affected and dosage of virus, as well as the degree of susceptibility. They may last for a year or longer. Papillomatosis becomes a herd problem when the infection occurs in a large group of young susceptible cattle. Immunity to re-exposure usually develops 3 to 4 weeks after initial infection with the virus, although warts may not be seen until about 2 months after infection. They have been known to recur, probably from loss of immunity.

The bovine wart contains a fibromatous element. This is particularly prominent in the venereal form of the disease in young cattle. **Fibropapillomas** may be a serious problem on the penis of young bulls and can cause dystocia when affecting the vaginal mucosa of heifers.

There is a form of persistent **cutaneous papillomatosis** in herds of older cattle in which the warts are small and occur in succession. Although a papilloma-like virus can be seen in such warts, it has not been experimentally transmitted to test animals. Similar persistent warty growths can occur on the teats and udder of dairy cows. Wart virus has been found in tumors of the urinary bladder of cattle, possibly as a secondary infection of the tumor, which probably developed from a carcinogen in bracken fern eaten by the animal. Wart-like lesions in the mouth, esophagus, rumen and reticulum are the result of proliferative (papular) stomatitis virus infection (q.v., p. 101) and not bovine papilloma virus.

Horses: Warts are common when young horses are kept together. The small, scattered warts usually appear on the nose and lips, presumably at the sites of abrasions when colts nuzzle each other. They cause no inconvenience and regress in a few months. The fibrosarcoma-like skin tumors produced in the horse by inoculation with bovine papilloma virus and equine sarcoid, which contains bovine papilloma virus genome, have no relation to equine cutaneous papillomatosis.

Dogs: Oral papillomatosis is often seen in young dogs and is caused by a virus that does not produce warts on the skin. The oral warts may be quite extensive at times. Oral papillomatosis has also been observed in coyotes, but its relation to the disease in dogs is unknown.

Rabbits: Both cutaneous and oral warts occur in rabbits. Rabbits immune to one kind are susceptible to the other. The cutaneous papillomas are found as keratinized horny growths in cottontail rabbits in some sections of Midwestern U.S.A. These contain a virus (Shope papilloma virus) that will produce skin papillomas of the domestic rabbit. The skin lesions do not contain infective virus but some become malignant carcinomas.

Oral papillomatosis may occur in colonies of domestic rabbits and can be transmitted to wild rabbits. The small, white, nodular or cauliflower-like warts are multiple. They are caused by a virus different from that of cutaneous papillomatosis.

Goats: Warts have been described in goats affecting various skin areas, and some of those on the teats and udder become carcinomas.

Monkeys: A transmissible cutaneous papillomatosis has been reported in monkeys, but the species specificity was not established.

Deer: A cutaneous fibromatosis occurs in white-tailed deer and is caused by a papilloma-like virus found only in the epithelium covering the tumors. Deer are not susceptible to the bovine papilloma virus.

Diagnosis: Warts can be readily recognized. Whether they can be regarded as infectious in an individual animal depends upon such circumstances as age of the animal and lesion, previous contacts, and presence of warts on other animals of the herd.

Treatment and Control: Infectious papillomatosis is a self-limiting disease, although the duration of warts on individual animals varies considerably. A variety of chemicals have been advocated for treatment without agreement on their value. Surgical removal is recommended if the warts are sufficiently objectionable. Surgical intervention in the early growing stage of a wart may lead to recurrence and stimulation of growth; therefore, warts should be removed when near their maximum size or when regressing. Affected animals may be isolated from susceptible animals, although with the long incubation period, many will have been exposed to the infection before a problem is recognized.

Vaccines of wart tissues containing formalin-killed virus have been used for treatment with limited success. Since wart viruses are mostly species specific, there is no merit in using a vaccine of wart tissue derived from one species on another species of animal, except possibly to prevent equine sarcoid.

When the disease exists as a herd problem it can be controlled by prophylactic vaccination using a suspension of ground wart tissue in which the virus has been killed with formalin. Autogenous vaccines appear to be more efficacious than the commercially available vaccines. It may be necessary to begin vaccination as early as 4 to 6 weeks of age in calves with about 0.4 ml vaccine intradermally at 2 sites, and repeating the dose in 4 to 6 weeks and at a year of age. Immunity to infection with the virus will develop in a few weeks, but this immunity is not related to the unknown mechanism involved in regression of the wart. Since exposure to the virus may have occurred prior to vaccination, as with a contaminated tattoo instrument, the vaccine-induced immunity may develop too late to prevent development of warts. A program of prophylactic vaccination must be in effect for about 3 to 6 months before its preventive value will be noted. It should be continued for at least a year after disappearance of the last wart since infective wart virus may still contaminate the premises. Stalls, stanchions and other inert materials can be disinfected with formaldehyde fumigation, but this must be done with high humidity and temperature to be effective.

BLUETONGUE

A noncontagious, insect-transmitted viral disease of sheep, cattle, goats and wild ruminants. The disease occurs widely on the African continent and to a lesser extent in North America, Asia and Europe. Recently, the virus was isolated from insects (*Culicoides* spp.) in Australia, and serologic evidence of its presence was also found in cattle and feral water buffalo; however, there is currently no clinical evidence that bluetongue disease exists in ruminants on that continent.

Etiology and Transmission: Bluetongue (BT) virus, an orbivirus, is a member of the family Reoviridae; 20 antigenic serotypes have been identified in the world, 4 in the U.S.A. Under natural conditions, the virus is biologically transmitted by biting insects of the genus *Culicoides*. Cattle are an important reservoir for sheep and other susceptible ruminants while some wild ruminant species may also be reservoirs.

Clinical Findings: The usual incubation period in sheep is 5 to 10 days. In chronologic sequence of appearance, clinical signs include: dyspnea with panting; hyperemia of the muzzle, lips and ears; pyrexia (up to 107.5°F [42°C]); depression; inflammation, ulcers, erosions, and necrosis of the mucosa of the mouth, especially the dental pad. Disease signs that may appear, depending on the severity, include a swollen and cyanotic tongue; lameness due to coronitis; torticollis; vomiting, pneumonia, conjunctivitis and occasionally alopecia. Bluetongue in sheep in the U.S.A. is much milder than in Africa with mortalities ranging from 0 to 30%. Cattle are commonly inapparently infected but some may develop clinical signs similar to those observed in infected sheep (*see also* "MYCOTIC" STOMATITIS, p. 99). If cattle become infected during gestation they may abort or give birth to offspring that are immunologically tolerant to the virus. Congenitally infected calves may have minimal to severe abnormalities (arthrogryposis, hydranencephalus, etc.) and dysfunctions (ataxia) at birth and subsequent reexposure of tolerant animals to BT virus may result in severe clinical disease and death. Also, the virus has been shown to be present in the semen of infected bulls. In white-tailed deer and pronghorn antelope the virus often causes a peracute fatal hemorrhagic disease.

Diagnosis: Clinical diagnosis can be confirmed by direct isolation of the virus in chicken embryos inoculated intravascularly, certain cell cultures, or susceptible sheep. The virus can also be grown (less readily) in suckling mice and hamsters inoculated intracerebrally. Viruses isolated can then be identified by fluorescent antibody or serum neutralization tests. An indirect presumptive diagnosis can be made by testing for antibody rise to the virus in paired serums from recovered animals. Serologic tests include complement fixation, agar-gel diffusion, and serum neutralization.

Bluetongue viremia is primarily associated with red blood cells and the virus can coexist in infected animals with high concentrations of its specific neutralizing antibody. Therefore, washed red blood cells are often necessary for isolation of the virus.

Bluetongue disease is often misdiagnosed, depending on the animal species involved, as photosensitization, "mycotic" stomatitis, bovine viral diarrhea, infectious bovine rhinotracheitis, the mucosal disease form of bovine viral diarrhea, malignant catarrhal fever, vesicular stomatitis, epizootic hemorrhagic disease of deer, contagious ecthyma, grub in the head, as well as foot-and-mouth disease.

Prevention and Control: A monovalent (serotype 10), modified live virus vaccine of cell culture origin is available only for use in sheep in the U.S.A. Modified live virus vaccines with all 4 serotypes found in the U.S.A. and killed virus vaccines are being developed. The live vaccine should not be used in nonendemic areas during the vector season as the insect vector can become infected with the vaccine virus. Passage of the vaccine virus through the insect is known to increase its pathogenicity for sheep. Pregnant ewes should not be vaccinated in early gestation as this frequently results in hydranencephalus and other deformities in lambs. Passive immunity in lambs lasts about 6 months and vaccination during this time may interfere with development of active immunity. In an outbreak, the decision whether to vaccinate will depend on the existing circumstances. Measures to reduce bites on susceptible ruminants by reducing biting insect populations in the area should help to minimize the extent of the disease.

FOOT-AND-MOUTH DISEASE

(Aphthous fever, Aftosa, Epizootic aphthae)

An acute, highly communicable disease chiefly confined to cloven-footed animals. Cattle, swine, sheep, goats, buffalo (including the African buffalo), bison, yak, camel, dromedary, deer, reindeer, moose, elk, North American deer, llama, chamois, alpaca, vicuna, giraffe, elephant, most antelope spp., mole, vole, rat, water rat, coypu and hedgehog are generally considered the natural domestic and wild hosts. Some wild animals develop only minimal clinical signs but, nevertheless, serve as important reservoirs of infection. The dog, fox, cat, rabbit, mouse, muskrat, squirrel, rat, chicken and other fowl, turtle, snail, monkey and snake can be infected artificially but are not believed to have important roles in the spread of the disease, though all might become mechanical carriers. Man, despite his frequent and sometimes intensive exposure, becomes infected only occasionally, when ill-defined predisposing factors are encountered.

Etiology and Epidemiology: The causal agent is a rhinovirus. Types O, A, C, Southern African Territories types SAT 1, SAT 2, SAT 3, and type Asia 1 are all immunologically distinct and afford no effective cross-protection. In addition, numerous subtypes exist, which are important epidemically because a continuous "antigenic drift" occurs among strains. The disease is endemic in certain parts of Europe, Africa, Asia and South America. A disease-free control zone has been established in Central America. As the result of the strictest sanitary measures, the disease has not become established in North America, Australia or New Zealand. Great Britain experiences rare but sometimes serious outbreaks.

The virus is inactivated rapidly by low or high pH, sunlight and high temperature, and also by certain atmospheric contaminants. However, it may remain viable for 5 to 10 weeks in "protected" locations during cool weather, and especially in the presence of tissues or other organic detritus. It is present in the fluid and tissues of the vesicles, as well as in the blood during the febrile stages; at times it is demonstrable in the saliva, milk, feces and urine of living animals or in the meat, bone marrow and lymph nodes of dead animals. Exposed or recovered cattle may carry the virus, principally as an inapparent pharyngeal infection, but such carriers have not been proved to transmit the disease to susceptible animals.

The disease spreads as a result of contact with infected animals, fomites or vehicles; the use of infected semen has been suggested as a possible cause of outbreaks. Flocks of birds may be mechanical vectors, as may rodents, flies and other arthropods. There is good evidence that FMD has been spread by the primary movement of milk from farms to dairies and to consumers. The virus is excreted in the milk during the prodromal phase and pasteurization may not be fully effective. FMD virus is also excreted in exhalations and may survive as an aerosol for several hours. At night or in the absence of bright sunlight and certain atmospheric pollutants, virus can be carried by air streams for at least 40 miles. Relative humidity above 70%, winds, and the presence of dense animal populations downwind tend to enhance aerial spread.

Pigs tend to excrete more virus than cattle or sheep, but the severity of clinical manifestations varies with the strain of virus and the susceptibility of the animal population in the locality. Morbidity in some herds and flocks may approach 100%. Young healthy animals on a high nutritional plane appear to be the most susceptible. The disease may be difficult to detect in sheep kept under extensive husbandry systems. Mortality rarely exceeds 6% in any species but occasionally it may exceed 50%, as a result of an apparent predilection of certain strains for muscular tissues, and for the myocardium in particular. However, great economic losses usually occur as the result of impaired general productivity and of the disruption of normal commerce caused by quarantines, embargoes and interference with normal agricultural practices. Clean-up operations and slaughter policies are also a source of serious expense.

Clinical Findings: The usual incubation period is 2 to 5 days, but extremes of 1 to 18 days or longer have been reported. Onset may be abrupt. The acute disease is characterized by high fever, which in mild cases may be absent or unnoticed. This is followed by eruption of various sized vesicles in the mouth and on the feet. The mouth lesions are small and blanched at first, later becoming large convex vesicles filled with a straw-colored fluid. Vesicles may appear on the mucous membranes at the border or on the dorsal surface of the tongue, on the buccal surfaces of the cheeks, on the gums and inner surfaces of the lips, on the palate, on the margins of the dental pad, or along the margin of the angles of the mandible. Anorexia may be complete. There may be severe salivation, and the animal may open and close its mouth with a characteristic smacking sound. Lameness is common. The feet may become swollen, hot and painful about the coronary bands and interdigital spaces. Eruptions similar to those found in the mouth appear on one or more feet. Vesicles may also occur in the rumen, on the udder, teats, conjunctivae, nasal passages, perineum and other thin-skinned areas. The vesicles usually rupture within 24 hours, leaving a raw, eroded area that heals rapidly in uncomplicated cases.

Secondary bacterial invasion of the ruptured vesicles, particularly those of the feet, may occur. Other complications are abortion, mastitis, pneumonia and septicemia.

Diagnosis: The main signs are fever, salivation and lameness. The appearance of vesicles in the oral cavity and nostrils, and on feet and teats, permits only a clinical diagnosis of one of several viral vesicular diseases.

In cattle, the diagnosis of FMD is complicated by the fact that the lesions are indistinguishable from those of vesicular stomatitis (q.v., p. 259). In swine, the lesions are similar to those of vesicular stomatitis, vesicular exanthema (q.v., p. 261) and swine vesicular disease (SVD, q.v., p. 258). A differential diagnosis is usually made on the results of comparative complement-fixation tests, often after a preliminary passage of virus in cultures of bovine thyroid or porcine kidney cells. Identification of the virus is usually made by the complement fixation test. However, virus neutralization, agar-gel diffusion precipitation, and fluorescent antibody tests may be used also. The type involved is differentiated by complement fixation (CF) or by virus neutralization tests. Subtypes of FMS virus are identified by cross complement-fixation tests employing a series of reference strains.

Partial differentiation of FMD, vesicular stomatitis, SVD and vesicular exanthema has been made by inoculation of a number of species of animals with the infectious material, with subsequent development of the typical disease in only those species known to be susceptible to the particular virus. Usually cattle, swine and horses are inoculated by scarification of the epithelium of the tongue. When cattle and swine develop typical vesicles preceded by a rise in temperature, a diagnosis of FMD is made. A diagnosis of vesicular stomatitis is made when typical vesicular disease is reproduced in all 3 species. The viruses of SVD and vesicular exanthema affect only swine among the domestic animals. Animal inoculation may be abortive because of nonviability of virus in the sample or predilection of the strain for one host species. Because of the importance of an accurate diagnosis, tests should be made only by authorized personnel properly trained to deal with the vesicular diseases. CF tests must be regarded as more accurate than animal inoculation.

In many countries, including the U.S.A., all suspected cases must be reported immediately to the regulatory officials.

Control: Where the disease is controlled effectively by legislation, the following measures are supervised strictly by government inspectors: rapid laboratory diagnosis and subtyping; immediate quarantine of infected premises, including control of movement of persons and vehicles until at least 14 days after eradication; inspection of adjacent farms; slaughter and disposal of all infected and susceptible in-contact animals; thorough cleansing and disinfecting of premises; after a waiting period of 6 weeks, restocking with a small number of susceptible "indicator" livestock.

For practical disinfection, a 2% solution of commercial lye (sodium hydroxide) is used, though a 4% or stronger solution of sodium carbonate and soft soap is less corrosive and is usually adequate. Hypochlorite solutions and trisodium phosphate have been used by some workers. Citric acid and some iodophores are efficacious. Strong acids are even more rapidly effective, but are used only on surfaces that are resistant to corrosion. None of these chemicals may penetrate adequately through straw and manure (which must be burnt). Phenolic disinfectants are generally ineffective. Pasteurization of milk by HTST methods may fail to kill all the viral particles.

Prophylaxis: In countries where the disease is endemic, drastic measures of eradication are not always economically feasible. Control is based on a modified system of vaccination and quarantine, using vaccines specific for the type and subtype of virus involved. Subtype matching of field and vaccine strains is usually very important, especially with SAT strains.

Chemically inactivated vaccines prepared from FMD virus propagated in cattle, in pig kidney or baby hamster kidney cell culture systems, and suspended in an adjuvant, have been used with considerable success in some countries. However, the immunity is not long-lived, and wanes after 4 to 6 months, necessitating revaccination. Vaccines containing one or more immunotypes of the virus are produced in several countries. Vaccination of swine with aluminum hydroxide-adjuvant vaccines is often less successful than vaccination of cattle and sheep, though recently oil-adjuvant vaccines have been used with excellent results. Vaccines prepared with attenuated virus have been used on a limited scale in restricted areas, but all tend to suffer from the general disadvantages of live vaccines. All vaccines are best deployed to produce a peripheral "cordon sanitaire" some miles deep surrounding active outbreaks, or to give "blanket" coverage to whole areas of a country. If the latter system is used, annual revaccination is essential. Vaccines should never be used in close proximity to infected premises as some vaccinated animals may excrete virus after exposure to FMD. Protection afforded by polyvalent or type-specific sera is short-lived (about 2 weeks), and their use has been discontinued.

Virucidal drugs have been tested on an experimental scale, but treatment of clinical infection is contraindicated at present, and a slaughter policy should be mandatory.

SWINE VESICULAR DISEASE (SVD)

Typically a transient disease of pigs in which vesicular lesions appear in the mouth and on the coronet of the feet. The lesions are similar to those in foot-and-mouth disease (FMD, q.v., p. 254) but generally heal more rapidly, especially in mild cases. Nervous signs have been described but are rarely observed in the field. The disease is of minor economic importance in itself and assumes importance only because of the difficulty of differentiating it clinically from other vesicular diseases.

Diagnosis: Effective differentiation can be achieved only in the laboratory and depends mainly upon serologic methods some of which are relatively quick, and to a lesser degree on the susceptibility of different tissue cultures and range of pH susceptibility of the virus. The electron microscope can be used to differentiate the virus from those of vesicular stomatitis or vesicular exanthema. Inapparent infections occur and can only be detected by serologic investigation. SVD virus is indistinguishable from the widely distributed human Coxsackie virus, and differs only in host pathogenicity.

Distribution: The disease was first identified in Italy in 1966 and has subsequently been seen in Hong Kong, Japan and a number of countries in Western Europe. Very energetic steps have been successful in eradicating the disease from some countries, e.g. Britain, Switzerland and Germany.

Control and Prevention: Spread from country to country appears to take place when pork or pork products from infected pigs reach garbage-fed swine in the recipient country and initiate outbreaks. Countries free of the disease can therefore protect themselves by banning the import of pork products from countries where the disease occurs. In countries free of SVD, any suspected outbreak should be reported immediately to the proper authorities.

If the disease does appear, important control measures are the efficient sterilization of all garbage fed to swine and control of the movement of swine. The disease can spread readily from pig to pig by both direct and indirect contact. Infected pigs excrete large amounts of virus and this leads to severe contamination. Unlike FMD, the disease does not spread long distances by aerosol but it remains infective for very much longer periods than FMD in buildings and trucks; disinfection of premises, trucks and equipment must be thorough. The most effective disinfectants are strong alkalis or acids, though hypochlorites can be used in the absence of other organic material.

VESICULAR STOMATITIS

The disease caused by the vesicular stomatitis viruses, like foot-and-mouth disease, is characterized by a febrile response accompanied by vesicles on the mucous membranes of the mouth, epithelium of the tongue, soles of the feet, coronary band, and occasionally in other areas of the body. Cattle, horses and swine are naturally susceptible. However, the agents have a wide host range, which includes deer, bobcats, raccoons and monkeys and experimentally many rodents and cold-blooded animals. Human infections have been recognized in endemic areas and in laboratory workers. The disease has been confirmed only in North and South America.

The rod-shaped virus belongs to the rhabdovirus group, which parasitize not only mammals but fish, insects and plants, a diversity of hosts unknown for any other group of viruses.

Etiology and Epidemiology: In a herd, 50 to 75% of the animals show clinical evidence of the disease; nearly all will develop antibodies. It is not as contagious as foot-and-mouth disease. The virus, found in abundance in the clear vesicular fluid and the vesicular coverings, is most infective at the time the vesicles rupture or shortly thereafter. Five or 6 days later, however, the lesions may be innocuous, indicating that the virus is short-lived. There are 2 serologically distinct viruses, the New Jersey and Indiana viruses, and there are 3 subtypes of the Indiana virus. There is no cross-immunity between the 2 viruses nor between the viruses of vesicular stomatitis, foot-and-mouth disease, vesicular exanthema and swine vesicular disease.

Vesicular stomatitis usually occurs epidemically in temperate regions and as an endemic disease in warmer regions. It occurs during the warm season of the year and can spread very rapidly, affecting thousands of animals within a few weeks. An insect is believed to be the vector. The reservoir for the virus is not known in all cases but phlebotomine sandflies have been shown to fill both roles for Indiana virus.

Clinical Findings: The incubation period is 2 to 5 days. Frequently, excessive salivation is the first sign. Examination of the mouth may reveal blanched, raised vesicles. The lesions vary in size; some are no larger than a pea, while others may involve a portion or the entire surface of the tongue. In the horse, the lesions are principally confined to the upper surface of the tongue, but may involve the inner surface of the lips, angles of the mouth and the gums. In cattle, the lesions may occur also on the hard palate, lips and gums, sometimes extending to the muzzle and around the nostrils. Secondary lesions involving the feet of horses and cattle are not exceptional. In natural infections in swine, foot lesions are frequent and lameness is often the first sign observed. Immediately before or simultaneously with the appearance of the vesicles, there may be a rise in temperature. Ordinarily, there are no complications and the disease is usually self-limiting with recovery in about 2 weeks. In dairy herds, the loss of milk production may be serious and, in some instances, mastitis is a sequela. Recovered and vaccinated animals are immune to naturally acquired infection for over a year.

Diagnosis: Vesicular stomatitis, while economically important, is of particular significance because of its similarity to foot-and-mouth disease, vesicular exanthema and swine vesicular disease. Therefore, outbreaks must be accurately identified. When vesicular stomatitis affects horses under natural conditions, there is no serious diagnostic problem because horses are not susceptible to foot-and-mouth disease. The diagnosis is made upon the distribution and character of the lesions and the disease may be differentiated from horse pox by the absence of papules and pustules. When the disease occurs in cattle or swine, a diagnosis is made by recovering the virus from the vesicular coverings or fluid in embryonating chicken eggs or in cell cultures and identifying the agent by the complement fixation or virus neutralization tests. Antibodies in serums of recovered animals can also be detected by the same tests. Diagnosis of the disease by animal inoculation tests can be made as described under foot-and-mouth disease (q.v., p. 254).

Suspected cases should be immediately brought to the attention of state or federal authorities.

Prophylaxis and Treatment: There is no specific treatment for vesicular stomatitis. Secondary infection of the abraded tissue and other sequelae should be treated symptomatically. Vaccines are available in a few countries of the American tropics.

VESICULAR EXANTHEMA

(San Miguel sea lion virus disease)

First observed in swine in 1932 as an acute highly infectious viral disease characterized by fever, formation of blisters on the snout, on the mucous membranes of the mouth, on the sole of the feet, between the toes, and on the coronary band. In swine, the clinical disease is indistinguishable from foot-and-mouth disease, q.v., p. 254, vesicular stomatitis, q.v., p. 259, and swine vesicular disease, q.v., p. 258. Originally confined to California, the disease became widespread in the U.S.A. during the 1950s, but a vigorous campaign to eradicate the disease was successful. In 1959, the country was declared free of vesicular exanthema (VE) and has remained so to date. The disease has never been reported as a natural infection of swine in any other part of the world. Since 1972, a virus indistinguishable from vesicular exanthema virus (VEV), designated as San Miguel sea lion virus (SMSLV), was isolated from a number of marine sources including aborted sea lion pups, nursing elephant seal pups, from vesicular lesions on flippers of these animals, and seal meat produced in Alaska for mink feed, and finny fishes collected from tidal pools. SMSLV is capable of producing the disease in swine.

A large number of immunologic distinct types of the virus, a calicivirus, have been demonstrated: at least 13 types of VEV from swine populations and at least 8 of SMSLV from marine sources. African green monkeys are susceptible, and serum antibodies have been demonstrated in researchers working with the virus.

Presumptive diagnosis in swine is based upon fever and the presence of typical vesicles, which break within 24 to 48 hours to form erosions. A diagnosis can be confirmed using complement fixation or neutralization tests. Suspected cases of vesicular exanthema should immediately be brought to the attention of regulatory authorities.

RINDERPEST

(Cattle plague)

An acute viral disease of cloven-hoofed animals, particularly cattle and buffalo, characterized by fever, erosive stomatitis and gastroenteritis.

Etiology and Epidemiology: The causal agent is an RNA virus antigenically related to the viruses of canine distemper, human measles and pest of small ruminants (q.v., p. 263). Although all strains of the virus are immunologically identical, they vary markedly in virulence and infectivity. The virus is heat-labile but it will remain viable for weeks in the cold and for months in frozen animal products.

The disease is endemic in parts of Asia and equatorial Africa. Morbidity and mortality may exceed 90% except in endemic areas where the indigenous cattle and buffalo possess a high degree of innate resistance. All domestic and most wild ruminants are susceptible, including sheep and goats. Native swine of Southeast Asia and wild pigs of Africa suffer severely but European breeds of swine show only a mild transient fever.

Spread requires close direct or indirect contact between infected and susceptible animals. The virus is present in all tissues and fluids of infected animals and can be isolated from the blood and nasal secretions 1 or 2 days before the onset of fever. It is excreted in the expired air, nasal and oral secretions and feces. Entry is usually through the mucosa of the upper respiratory tract.

Clinical Findings: A prodromal fever follows an incubation period that varies from 3 to 15 days. Within 1 or 2 days of the onset of fever, nasal and lacrimal discharges appear together with anorexia, thirst and depression. The fever reaches its peak 2 to 3 days later when oral lesions emerge. The nasal discharges become mucopurulent, and the breath is fetid. Diarrhea appears as the fever declines and is followed by dehydration, abdominal pain, labored painful respiration and death. The convalescence of surviving animals is long. Recovery confers a permanent immunity and calves of immune dams are protected passively for several months.

Lesions: Gross changes are most apparent in the digestive tract. In the mucosa of the lips, tongue and buccal cavity, small necrotic foci lose their debris to become superficial erosions which may coalesce. Congestion and hemorrhage of the mucosal surfaces of the abomasum and intestine are prominent; involvement of the crests of the mucous membrane folds results in streaks of inflammation and hemorrhage. The virus also has an affinity for lymphoid tissues, consequently severe necrotic erosion of Peyer's patches is often evident.

Diagnosis: Experienced veterinarians, in countries where the disease is endemic, make presumptive diagnoses of rinderpest from clinical signs and necropsy findings. In countries free of rinderpest, a presumptive diagnosis must be confirmed by isolation and serologic identification of the virus or by detection of specific antigens or antibodies. The current prevalence of the viral diarrhea-mucosal disease complex (q.v., p. 266), which produces similar changes, enhances the need for confirmatory diagnosis. *See also* PEST OF SMALL RUMINANTS, below. The specimens required are blood in anticoagulant, lymph node, tonsil and spleen.

Jembrana disease, initially confused with rinderpest when first encountered in Indonesia, is now believed to be a rickettsiosis.

Control: Small areas of infection, in otherwise rinderpest-free countries, are customarily eliminated by strict quarantine and slaughter. When the disease is widespread, control can be achieved through vaccination. The Plowright tissue culture vaccine has a potential for rinderpest eradication. Strains attenuated by passage through goats or tissue cultures are used as live-virus vaccines. One inoculation confers an immunity of several years' duration. It is only through the persistent, large scale use of rinderpest vaccine that cattle raising is profitable in much of Africa, the Middle East and Asia.

PEST OF SMALL RUMINANTS

(Peste des petits ruminants, Pseudorinderpest of goats and sheep, Stomatitis-pneumoenteritis complex of sheep and goats, Kata)

An acute or subacute viral disease of goats and sheep characterized by fever, necrotic stomatitis, gastroenteritis and pneumonia.

Etiology: The infectious agent of pest of small ruminants (PSR) is a member of the morbillivirus group of the family Paramyxoviridae, is closely related to rinderpest (q.v., p. 262), canine distemper and measles viruses, and grows in various cell cultures. PSR virus is heat labile but maintains viability for several weeks in the cold and for several months in frozen animal tissues. It is inactivated at pH 3 and by ether or chloroform.

Epidemiology: The disease has been reported in West Africa. Sheep are less susceptible than goats, and cattle are only subclinically infected. Surviving animals develop a dual immunity, to PSR and to rinderpest.

Clinical Findings: The acute form is characterized by a sudden rise of temperature to 104 to 107.5°F (40 to 42°C). Affected animals appear ill and restless, and have a dull coat, dry muzzle and depressed appetite. The mucous membranes are congested. Early, a serous nasal discharge is observed; later it becomes mucopurulent and causes a fetid odor to the breath. Diarrhea develops during the later stages of the disease, and the animals become emaciated. The animal dies 5 to 7 days after onset of fever. In the subacute form the animal dies in 14 to 21 days or occasionally survives. The disease is more severe in young animals and morbidity and mortality are higher. Secondary latent infections are activated and may complicate the clinical picture of the disease.

Lesions: Lesions are similar to those of rinderpest, mainly erosive stomatitis, abomasal congestion and enteritis. Bronchopneumonia is a constant finding.

Diagnosis: A presumptive diagnosis can be made on clinical, pathological, and epidemiological findings; but because of the similarity of PSR to other diseases (e.g. rinderpest), virus isolation and identification is essential for laboratory confirmation. Detection of virus-neutralizing antibodies at a rising titer in surviving animals is also diagnostic.

Control: Cell-cultured rinderpest vaccines are used to protect goats and sheep against PSR. Sanitary measures should be applied in case of outbreak.

MALIGNANT CATARRHAL FEVER

(MCF, Malignant head catarrh, Snotsiekte, Catarrhal fever, Gangrenous coryza)

An infectious, usually fatal disease of cattle caused by a virus and characterized by a catarrhal, mucopurulent inflammation of the upper respiratory and alimentary epithelia, keratoconjunctivitis, encephalitis, rapid dehydration and enlargement of the lymph nodes. It is reported in most countries where cattle are raised.

Etiology and Epidemiology: The causative viruses occur as several strains with differing antigenic characteristics, cultivability and host susceptibility. In Africa, MCF virus is a herpes-type virus which is closely associated with the WBC and with lymph node tissue. It remains active outside the body only for a short time. The causal virus of North American MCF appears to be different and has not been fully characterized. The incubation period of both agents varies from 2 weeks to 5 months or longer, but most often is 3 to 9 weeks. Sheep and latently infected cattle may serve as clinically normal carriers. Most commonly the disease is sporadic in occurrence with only individual animals being affected. Rarely it occurs in outbreak form with high morbidity and mortality. This is always in association with comingling of cattle and lambing ewes, which act as carriers of the infection.

Clinical Findings: The course of the disease varies from the peracute condition of 1 to 2 days to an extreme of 4 weeks (usual range, 4 to 14 days). In chronic cases, cattle become severely emaciated and anorectic. Signs most commonly observed are clear, copious nasal discharge and lacrimation, followed by a mucopurulent, dark, nasal discharge with encrustation of the nostrils. The earliest signs may consist of temperature elevation and congestion of the oral mucosa.

Five syndromes have been described: peracute, intestinal, head and eye, benign and chronic. The head-and-eye form, the commonest, is characterized by a profuse mucopurulent nasal discharge, focal necrosis of nasal mucosa, and severe keratoconjunctivitis with purulent ocular discharge. There are erosions on the buccal mucosa and the muzzle is covered with tenacious scabs. There is fever, depression, toxemia and severe dyspnea. Other signs that may be noted are partial cloudiness to complete opacity of the cornea, external swelling of superficial lymph nodes of the head and neck, and scabby lesions of the coronets, dewclaws and teats.

Most sporadic cases are of the head-and-eye form. During outbreaks of disease, nervous or intestinal forms may predominate and may occur together. The intestinal form is accompanied by severe diarrhea, with much tenesmus, and the oral mucosa may become eroded or ulcerated. The nervous form is signaled by excitability, hyperesthesia and muscular tremors. Occasionally, these may progress to epileptiform convulsions or an aggressiveness suggestive of rabies.

Lesions: Three changes characterize the histopathology of MCF: (1) lymphocytic vasculitis with a tendency to affect muscular arteries, (2) lymphoid necrosis and depletion, and (3) reticuloendothelial hyperplasia. Lymphopenia of circulating blood reflects the extensive destruction of lymphocytes. Neutrophilia may occur in late stages when tissue necrosis is extensive. These changes occur in virtually all organs but may be most severe in the alimentary tract, eye, meninges, pituitary, kidney and skin. They are the basis for foci of necrosis and ulceration that occur on organ surfaces. The retropharyngeal and anterior cervical lymph nodes are usually edematous and hemorrhagic.

Treatment and Control: Treatment is of little value, although some animals survive, and administration of antibiotics or sulfonamides for control of secondary bacterial infection, and supportive therapy (fluids) may be worthwhile in valuable individuals. Affected animals should be isolated, and the separation of sheep and cattle may be helpful. The incidence usually is not high enough to justify herd disposal or the development of a vaccine. The prognosis is grave, with death usually occurring within 10 days. In recovering animals, the convalescence is very slow; others may linger on for weeks and even then may relapse. Blindness occasionally persists.

BOVINE VIRAL DIARRHEA

(BVD, Mucosal-disease complex)

An infectious disease of cattle caused by a virus (family Togaviridae, genus *Pestivirus*), characterized by erosions and hemorrhages of the alimentary tract and manifested clinically by diarrhea and dehydration. In addition to classic diarrheal disease, BVD virus is associated with congenital anomalies of the brain (cerebellar ataxia), a debilitating syndrome of young calves with arthritis (weak calf syndrome), and a chronic ulcerative disease of the alimentary tract of older cattle (mucosal disease).

Incidence and Occurrence: Classic enteric BVD occurs worldwide. Primarily a disease of yearlings, and up to 2- and 3-year olds, it can occur in calves and is occasionally observed in adult cows. Although calves may receive passive antibodies in colostrum, these wane in a few months and the calves may then become infected from older cattle. Morbidity is high on the basis of serologic evidence but low from a clinical viewpoint: many cattle have subclinical viral diarrhea which leaves them with detectable antibodies and future protection from the disease. Likewise, the mortality is low when based on serologic evidence but high in those animals showing obvious clinical signs, particularly severe diarrhea.

Transmission: The transmission of BVD under natural conditions is by direct contact with clinically sick or carrier animals, or by indirect contact (contaminated feed). The incubation period is from 1 to 3 weeks under natural conditions and 7 days experimentally.

Clinical Findings: Calves with BVD are dull, depressed and anorectic. There is complete rumen stasis and sometimes mild bloat. Early temperatures vary from 104 to 106°F (40 to 41°C), but these usually return to normal or below in 1 or 2 days and before the animal starts to scour. The diphasic temperature elevation has not been observed in field cases. Heart and respiratory rates are generally increased. Profuse watery diarrhea is usual and the feces may contain mucus, blood and have a foul odor. Tenesmus may be present but defecation is usually effortless. Severe diarrhea causes rapid dehydration. Oral lesions are present in about 75% of clinical cases when the animals start to scour. Typically there is diffuse reddening of the oral mucosa, then mottling of the mucosa with pinpoint lesions which generally enlarge to 1 to 2 cm as shallow epithelial erosions. Sites of erosions include the hard palate, soft palate, dorsum and sides of the tongue, gums and commissures of the mouth. In early cases, the cheek papillae are hyperemic and their tips will slough, leaving blunt, shortened papillae as the disease progresses. The tongue is usually difficult to grasp and pull from the mouth because of the greasy, necrotic cells on its surface. Additional signs occur sporadically in individual animals. These include hyperemic, encrusted external nares, erosions of the coronary band and interdigital cleft, corneal opacity and abortions. Laminitis and respiratory signs have been reported but their direct association with BVD is unconfirmed. Leukopenia with relative lymphocytosis is common early in the disease. Leukocytosis may occur with secondary bacterial infection. The course of the disease varies from 2 to 3 days up to 3 weeks. Cattle with acute BVD can die in 48 hours. Most frequently, affected cattle will be anorectic, exhibiting oral lesions and mild diarrhea for 2 to 4 days, then gradually recover and come back on feed. But if diarrhea is profuse, the prognosis is always grave. Also, failure to make an early diagnosis means the animal will have no salvage value because of dehydration and emaciation. The occasional animal that survives the acute disease is usually so badly debilitated as to be an economic liability and will eventually die from secondary necrobacillosis or mycotic infections.

BVD virus can cause abortion in pregnant cows and cerebellar hypoplasia of calves when they are infected *in utero* before 165 days of gestation.

Lesions: Foci of degenerate epithelial cells containing degenerate virus comprise the basic lesions. These develop with edema and vasculitis immediately below epithelial surfaces. This results in erosions of the esophagus, forestomachs, abomasum and intestine. Epithelial necrosis occurs but is more prominent in mucosal disease where ulceration is marked especially in the oronasal areas. Catarrhal enteritis may be severe in more chronic forms of the disease.

Necrosis of lymphoid tissues occurs, particularly in those associated with the intestine. In the chronic types of mucosal disease, hemorrhage results in dark-red necrotic foci in the ileum representing affected Peyer's patches. Virus is present in vascular and lymphoid tissues and may occur in brain, kidney, eye and other viscera. Animals with mucosal disease die with a febrile systemic infection and circulatory collapse.

Control: Cattle with BVD cannot be effectively treated. A modified live-virus vaccine is available which induces significant antibody titers and offers an immunity that can be useful, but its duration is as yet unestablished. The best program would be to vaccinate calves at 6 to 10 months of age. The economic justification for vaccination is not well defined. The incidence of the fatal disease is so low in most herds, and the naturally occurring protective antibody is so prevalent in most cattle populations, that widespread vaccination does not seem warranted. Routine use has also been discouraged by reports that the vaccine can precipitate the clinical disease in certain circumstances, which unhappily have not been accurately defined.

BORDER DISEASE

("Hairy shaker" disease)

Border disease (Britain) or "hairy shaker" disease (New Zealand) is a congenital disorder of lambs which occurs in many countries, including Western U.S.A. It is caused by infection of the fetus with a virus closely related to, or identical with certain strains of bovine viral diarrhea virus.

Affected flocks will probably first be recognized at lambing time by the presence of a number of undersized lambs with excessively hairy and sometimes excessively pigmented fleeces. Some of these exhibit involuntary muscular tremors of variable severity that may be confined to the head and neck or affect the whole body. The tremors are reduced at rest and exacerbated with movement. These hairy lambs have a poor survival rate and many die before weaning. However, in the few that survive, the nervous signs will gradually disappear within 3 or 4 months. In affected flocks there is an associated infertility problem with up to 8 times the normally expected number of ewes failing to give birth to lambs. Abortions occur at all stages of pregnancy, some of the aborted fetuses being mummified and many of those occurring late in pregnancy having obviously hairy fleeces. There are no characteristic placental lesions but the aborted fetuses are almost always undersized.

Incidence: Up to half of the hairy lambs seen alive may show nervous signs, but usually the proportion is much less than this. The number of lambs affected may be quite small in the first season in which the flock becomes infected, but the incidence may subsequently increase in the following 2 or 3 seasons to as high as 50% of the lamb crop and then decline to a very low incidence.

Diagnosis: The clinical picture in a flock will usually allow a diagnosis. Some normally smooth-coated breeds of sheep have genetically controlled hairiness of the fleece but confusion should not arise because such lambs will not have any associated nervous signs. Histologic evidence of hypomyelinogenesis provides confirmation. The disease agent is present in the tissues of affected lambs and fetuses and experimentally may be transmitted to ewes in the first 2 months of pregnancy parenterally or by the oral or conjunctival routes.

Control: Introduction of sheep from infected flocks should be avoided. Ewes which have given birth to affected lambs acquire a strong immunity to subsequent infection with the same strain of virus. Susceptible ewes in their last third of pregnancy may be exposed to infection without any apparent ill-effects on their progeny though surviving lambs may remain persistently infected and capable of disseminating the disease in subsequent seasons.

The natural mode of transmission is unknown and the possibility of spread by the venereal route has not been excluded. There are currently no methods available for the artificial stimulation of immunity.

INFECTIOUS BOVINE RHINOTRACHEITIS (IBR), INFECTIOUS PUSTULAR VULVOVAGINITIS (IPV) AND ASSOCIATED SYNDROMES

IBR is an acute contagious viral infection characterized by inflammation of the upper respiratory tract. Bronchopneumonia may result when complicated by bacterial infection. The virus may invade the placenta and fetus via the maternal blood stream, causing abortion or stillbirth usually in the last third of gestation although abortion at any time is possible. It also causes encephalitis in 2- to 3-month-old calves and produces severe oral and gastric necrosis in newborn calves. The enteric form of IBR causes high mortality in affected calves under 3 weeks of age and chronic ulcerative gastroenteritis in feedlot cattle.

The virus also causes infectious pustular vulvovaginitis (IPV), an acute contagious disease of cattle characterized in the female by inflammation, focal necrosis and pustule formation on the mucosa of the vulva and vagina, and occasionally in the male by similar lesions on the skin of the penis and prepuce. Vesicle formation does not occur. Venereal transmission is usual although the infection may be transmitted by equipment brought into contact with the genitalia. With the possible exception of South America, the virus is found worldwide.

Etiology: The virus is present in the nasal and ocular secretions of IBR-infected cattle, in the placental tissues and fluids of those that abort, in the tissues of the aborted fetuses and in the brain of calves affected with encephalitis. When responsible for IPV, the virus is found in the exudate produced in association with vulvovaginitis.

Nuclear inclusions are present in the margins of epithelial lesions early in infection. Only cattle are susceptible to clinical infection with this virus. It is a herpesvirus and produces characteristic necrosis and intranuclear inclusion bodies in cell culture.

Epidemiology: IBR is most prevalent in large concentrations of cattle such as are found in feedlots and large commercial dairy operations, while the genital infection (IPV) is confined mainly to small, reproductively active herds, particularly of dairy cattle.

IBR frequently occurs from one to several weeks after the addition of new animals because clinically normal recovered cattle may shed the virus. Cattle also remain shedders of the virus for variable periods following clinical recovery from IPV. Infection of some animals does not result in disease and can be recognized only by detection of neutralizing antibodies in the serum. Corticosteroids will induce cattle with asymptomatic infection to secrete virus and develop upper respiratory lesions; these drugs should be avoided in affected herds.

Clinical Findings: The incubation period of IBR is generally from 10 to 14 days. Initially, the temperature ranges from 104 to 108°F (40 to 42°C) with a serous nasal discharge which in a few instances contains flecks of blood. The animals are mildly depressed, the respiration rate is accelerated, there is profuse salivation and anorexia is present. Inflammation of the conjunctiva often accompanies the respiratory form of IBR. Corneal opacity is not common unless there is secondary infection with *Moraxella bovis*. The majority of cattle do not show other clinical signs and recover without treatment in 10 to 14 days. In about 10% of cases, more severe clinical signs are noted. The muzzle and external nares become hyperemic and encrusted with a dried exudate. As the disease progresses, the nasal exudate changes from serous to mucopurulent, and an inspiratory dyspnea develops because of the presence of a pseudodiphtheritic membrane in the nasal passages and trachea. When complicated by bronchopneumonia, there is considerable weight loss and recovery is prolonged. The morbidity ranges from 15 to 100%; death losses rarely exceed 5% of the affected animals and are due usually to bronchopneumonia. Cattle that recover have a long-term if not lifetime immunity to the disease.

Calves may be born with the enteric form of IBR or become infected shortly after birth. Some calves will show the respiratory form of the disease as well as an intractable diarrhea. There are oral erosions in most calves, and calves under 3 weeks of age do not respond to therapy.

IPV may exhibit a wide variation in severity. There may be swelling of the vulva with a small amount of sticky exudate on the vulvar hair. Pain is exhibited by reluctance to allow the tail to rest on the vulva and when the animal urinates or the vulva is manipulated in the course of examination. The mucosa is bright red and exhibits varying numbers of small pustules about 2 mm in diameter. These are soft and moist with raised edges and depressed centers. In some cases, the lesions are so numerous that they coalesce to form a plaque. Varying degrees of epithelial necrosis and exudation may be observed in the vagina. Appetite and production are little affected and abortion does not occur as a sequela. While it is probable that fertility is reduced during the acute phase, permanent infertility does not result.

Abortion due to the virus may occur in herds in which there is a recent history of IBR or clinical signs of IBR. Prodromal signs of abortion are not obvious; the abortion is rarely complicated by genital tract infection, and the breeding efficiency of aborting cattle does not appear to be impaired.

Lesions: Petechial to ecchymotic hemorrhages may be found in the mucous membranes of the nasal cavity and the paranasal sinuses of cattle with IBR. The sinuses are often filled with a serous or mucoserofibrinous exudate. As the disease progresses the pharynx becomes covered with a serofibrinous exudate. The pharyngeal lymph nodes may be acutely swollen and hemorrhagic. In the early stages of IBR the trachea exhibits multiple small hyperemic areas or general hyperemia. Later, large quantities of blood are found in or lining the wall of the trachea. The tracheitis may extend into the bronchi and bronchioles and terminate in bronchopneumonia. The pulmonary lymph nodes are extensively swollen.

The erosions found in the oral cavity with enteric IBR are also present in the rumen, abomasum, cecum and colon. Regional lymph nodes are necrotic in severe cases.

Diagnosis: Diagnosis of IBR and IPV is based on the characteristic lesions and signs of illness, the demonstration of a rising serum-antibody titer between acute and convalescent stages, the occurrence of intranuclear inclusion bodies in biopsy material, and the isolation of the virus in tissue culture.

Prophylaxis and Treatment: Two basic types of modified live-virus vaccines are available to prevent the various syndromes caused by the IBR virus. The IM vaccine is widely used in feedlot cattle and the intranasal vaccine in breeding herds. The IM vaccine may cause abortion but can be used in both young and open females. The intranasal vaccine will not cause abortion and is reported to provide faster protection than the IM vaccine. The veterinarian should consult with his client and outline a specific vaccination program for a specific farm. In general, heifers that are vaccinated at 6 to 8 months of age and again just prior to breeding with the IM vaccine will not need to be revaccinated. Cattle that receive the intranasal vaccine may require revaccination each year. Feedlot cattle should be vaccinated as part of a preconditioning program since IBR may occur in unvaccinated cattle. Only healthy cattle should be vaccinated.

There is no specific therapy. All breeding operations should be suspended in the herd infected with IPV until the animals return to normal. Most animals recover without treatment in about 2 weeks. Secondary bacterial infection of either IBR or IPV should be treated with appropriate antibiotics.

BOVINE WINTER DYSENTERY

(Winter scours)

An acute infectious endemic disease of stabled cattle affecting animals of all ages with calves and yearlings being least susceptible. Winter dysentery is characterized by high morbidity, but very low mortality. It leads to dehydration, loss of weight and condition and, in lactating animals, to a sharp drop in milk production.

Etiology: The cause is unknown, but the suddenness of onset and the rapidity of spread from farm to farm, suggest strongly that a virus is involved.

Clinical Findings: The period of incubation is short, varying from 3 to 5 days. The onset is sudden; in many herds, only one animal shows evidence of diarrhea for the first few days, but the infection quickly spreads to the remainder of the herd. Just prior to the onset of diarrhea the body temperature may be moderately elevated. A profuse watery diarrhea with a slightly fetid odor is the main sign. The feces often are dark brown and tend to become darker as intestinal hemorrhage occurs. In some instances, they contain large quantities of mucus and blood. Unless complications occur, the temperature shows little or no change. The appetite is slightly depressed and the pulse and respiration rates are only moderately increased.

Severely affected animals may show evidence of abdominal pain by switching of the tail, kicking at the abdomen, and lying down and getting up at frequent intervals. Coughing is observed in about 30 to 50% of outbreaks.

Lesions: The outstanding necropsy features are dehydration, catarrhal inflammation of the jejunum and ileum, and hemorrhage into the lumen of the gut.

Diagnosis: The seasonal incidence of the disease (mainly from November through April in the north temperate zone), the age and number of animals affected, and the suddenness of the onset, are helpful in arriving at a diagnosis. Bovine viral diarrhea (q.v., p. 266) and coccidiosis (q.v., p. 458) should be considered in the differential diagnosis, along with those toxic agents and nutritional deficiencies that may cause outbreaks of diarrhea in cattle.

Prophylaxis: Owners should watch their animals carefully as they go into barns for the winter season. Newly introduced animals should be kept in isolation for 2 weeks. Any animal suffering from acute dysentery, regardless of cause, should be separated from the main herd until recovered. Veterinarians, inseminators and herdsmen, after handling animals with winter dysentery, should make sure of the cleanliness of their clothing and equipment before working with healthy cattle.

Treatment: Most cattle with winter dysentery do not require treatment since they recover spontaneously. Severely affected animals can be given oral astringents along with fluid and electrolyte therapy.

SCRAPIE

(Tremblante du mouton, Rida)

A relentlessly progressive, fatal neuropathy of sheep and less often of goats, characterized chiefly by intense pruritus, altered gait and debility. Pruritis may be absent, and in these cases trembling is the outstanding clinical sign. The disease is rarely seen in animals less than 2 years of age.

Etiology: Scrapie is usually transmitted from parents to offspring. Lateral transmission may occasionally occur among sheep and goats through ingestion of feed contaminated by fetal membranes voided by affected animals. Experimentally it may be transmitted by inoculation of susceptible animals, by various routes, with suspensions of many tissues, but especially brain, from scrapie-affected animals, with cell-free tissue extracts, or with cell-culture cell-free fluids. Until recently, other features that would permit characterizing the agent as a virus had not been demonstrated, nor had it been identified by electron microscopy; there is now evidence of specific DNA molecules in scrapie infected brain.

The pathogenesis of scrapie may be regulated by a genetically determined susceptibility of the host, or by a genetically determined de-repression of the agent. The scrapie agent is non-antigenic and unusually resistant to ultraviolet and ionizing radiation, heat, hydrolytic enzymes and conventional aldehyde fixatives. Unlike most viruses, scrapie is inactivated by membrane disruptive reagents, including some detergents, phenol and organic lipid solvents.

All goats are susceptible to experimental inoculation of the agent, but susceptibility in sheep is only 5 to 60% depending on genetic constitution. Scrapie has been transmitted to a variety of laboratory animals, including domestic cats. Some subhuman primates have also been found to be susceptible.

Incidence: The disease has been reported in most European countries and has been known in Britain, France and Germany for 200 years. In these countries, it is endemic and waxes and wanes in different breeds over periods of many years. Males and females are equally susceptible. The incidence in affected flocks varies greatly, usually ranging from 4 to 20%. Over long periods, however, it may be less than 4%, while occasionally it may approach 50%. Small outbreaks, usually traceable to the introduction of sheep from endemic areas in Europe, have occurred in Canada, the U.S.A., the Himalayan region of India, and South Africa. Australia and New Zealand are now free of the disease.

Clinical Findings: The onset is insidious. Affected sheep become more excitable, and fine tremors of the head and neck may be observed. The most characteristic feature is intense pruritis, which often begins over the rump, and may extend to other parts. In some cases the pruritus makes it difficult for the animal to feed and rest normally. Nervous signs may be elicited from a quiet but affected sheep through a sudden noise or movement. The wool is dry, separable and brittle, resulting in loss of fleece over large areas. Other areas may be rubbed raw. Sheep will nibble at their limbs in an effort to relieve the itching. Emaciation, weakness and incoordination of the hind-quarters are passive, and inability to rise occurs in the later stages. Occasionally there are epileptiform convulsions. When made to trot, there is often a peculiar high-stepping action of the forelegs, sometimes with galloping movements of the hind legs. Animals live about 6 weeks to 6 months following the onset of signs. Recoveries have been reported, but without an unequivocal means of diagnosis such an interpretation remains subject to question.

Lesions: The only macroscopic abnormalities are abrasion of skin over the rubbed areas, and a small increase in volume of cerebrospinal fluid. The histologic picture is of bilaterally symmetrical spongiform encephalopathy, with hypertrophy of astrocytes and degeneration, including vacuolation, of neurons. These abnormalities vary in intensity and distribution in the different species.

Diagnosis: Scrapie remains as a clinicopathological entity since there has been no detectable immunological response to the agent, which has not been specifically identified. Signs of CNS disturbance, hind-limb compulsive rubbing, with an insidious onset and a protracted course strongly suggest scrapie. For diagnosis, histologic examination should be made of the medulla oblongata in sheep and goats, and of whole brain sagittal sections in small laboratory animals.

Control: Sheep from families in which scrapie has been recognized should not be introduced into other flocks. The eradication program used in the U.S.A. comprises: confirmation of field diagnosis through histopathologic evaluation, quarantine and slaughter of all sheep and goats in the infected flock, identification and slaughter of all exposed animals moved from the flock and their immediate progeny. Similar programs were effective in Australia and New Zealand and are in force in South Africa and Canada. No prophylactic or palliative measures are known.

LOUPING ILL

A viral encephalomyelitis of sheep on the tick-infested rough hill pasture of Great Britain and Ireland. It has also been recognized in cattle, horses, pigs, young grouse and man.

Etiology and Epidemiology: The causal agent is one of the flavivirus group (antigenically related to the tick-borne encephalitis (TBE) complex which included Russian spring-summer encephalitis and Central European tick-borne encephalitis). The disease occurs in spring and autumn, which coincides with periods of maximum activity of all the 3 stages of the tick vector, *Ixodes ricinus*. Of susceptible sheep placed on tick-infested pasture when ticks are active, as many as 60% may die.

On farms where the disease is endemic, the losses are mainly confined to sheep under 2 years old, with an average mortality of 10%; the adults of a closed population are mostly immune as a result of abortive and subclinical infections. When, however, the disease appears for the first time, or after a lapse of several years on a farm, sheep of all ages may be susceptible and losses very high.

Ixodes ricinus also harbors and transmits the infective agent of another distinct disease, **tick-borne** fever. This febrile disease, which may result in abortions, is caused by a Rickettsia-like organism, which can be observed in the cytoplasm of the granular leukocytes. Tick-borne fever is not fatal but since most ticks carry the infection, it aggravates the effects of louping ill.

Clinical Findings: All susceptible animals bitten by infected ticks have a viremia for some days afterwards. During this incubation period, although their temperature is high, they appear relatively normal, but after about 6 to 14 days, the virus in some individuals multiplies in the nervous system and signs of brain and spinal cord damage become obvious. These are muscular incoordination, tremors of the lips, ears and head, circling, staggering and standing apart from the flock with a lowered head. Finally, paralysis occurs and the animal may remain down with occasional convulsions for many hours before dying. In some chronic cases, there may be only paralysis of the hind legs, but young lambs die quickly, and most are found dead in the morning. Although about half of the infected animals show no clinical signs they remain immune for life and can pass on maternal immunity to their lambs in the milk. In some cases, however, if animals experience "stress" during the incubation period, the clinical signs are induced. This is thought to be the cause of a number of cases in lambs transported from sales by truck and which develop the clinical disease when they arrive on tick-free pastures. There is no danger of such animals spreading disease, however, and any ticks that they carry do not survive for long on low ground.

Lesions: There are no macroscopic lesions. Microscopically, there is encephalomyelitis with infiltration of mononuclear cells into the meninges and perivascular spaces, together with diffuse and focal infiltration into the substance of the nerve tissue, and perivascular cuffing. Necrosis and neuronophagia of the motor cells is a constant feature in the ventral horn and brain stem, but destruction of Purkinje cells is variable.

Diagnosis: The disease occurs only on tick-infested farms. Affected animals should be examined for ticks on the head, neck, ears, axillae and inside of the thighs. If the animal has a febrile reaction with no signs of encephalitis, diagnosis of louping ill can be made by examining a serum sample for the presence of specific hemagglutinin-inhibiting (HI) antibodies; the presence of immunoglobulin M (IgM) antibodies is indicative of infection within 28 days and rising titers to IgG is confirmatory. If there is severe encephalitis, the presence of IgM is sufficient presumptive evidence; in animals found dead or sufficiently ill to warrant destruction, the brain can be examined microscopically or used to inoculate mice or tissue culture for the recovery of virus.

Prophylaxis: There is no treatment but a concentrated antigen prepared from BHK tissue cultures infected with louping ill, inactivated with formalin and incorporated in an oil-adjuvant vaccine is now available commercially. Vaccination induces antibodies detectable by HI and neutralization tests and is considered to induce an immunity lasting at least 2 years.

Vaccinated ewes pass on maternal antibodies in the colostrum. The vaccine is best given in the autumn to weaned lambs and sheep about to be bred for the first time the following spring. It may be given in the spring if the ewes are injected 28 days before lambing is due, to ensure that antibodies are transferred in the colostrum.

HOG CHOLERA

(Swine fever)

An acute, highly contagious, viral disease affecting swine of all ages, characterized by sudden onset, high morbidity and mortality, and diverse signs and lesions caused by disparately virulent viral strains. Less virulent strains cause chronic disease with low mortality in mature swine but induce abortions, stillbirths and baby pig losses.

Etiology: The cause, an RNA virus (Togaviridae, *Pestivirus*) related to the bovine viral diarrhea virus, is inactivated readily by sunlight, heat and most disinfectants. Its survival beyond 4 days is unlikely in the pig house environment but it may endure for several months in pickled meat and for several years in frozen carcasses.

Clinical Findings: After an incubation period of 2 to 6 days, the first signs of an acute outbreak are dullness, partial anorexia, transient constipation changing to diarrhea, hyperemia and fever peaking at 106 to 108°F (41 to 42°C) about 4 to 6 days after onset. The skin over the abdomen, ears and snout frequently becomes cyanotic. Variable nervous signs include ataxia, paralysis and convulsions. Morbidity is high; mortality is highest in young pigs. Some deaths may occur suddenly and early but most occur 5 to 15 days after the outbreak begins. Chronic cases may linger for 30 days or more. Recovery often results in stunting.

Congenital infections are common. Infection of sows may result in fetal death, mummification, small litter size, stillbirths, anomalies, weak piglets, or congenital tremor.

Lesions: Viral damage is most evident in the endothelium of blood vessels. Lesions may be obscure in peracute cases, but in acute cases petechial and ecchymotic hemorrhages occur in many organs. Lymph nodes are edematous, congested and hemorrhagic. Strongly suggestive but nonpathognomonic gross lesions are: hemorrhages in the larynx, kidneys and bladder, infarcts in the spleen and kidney, button ulcers near the ileocecal valve and a widened white line at the costochondral junctions. Histologic lesions in blood vessels of the brain are more specific.

Diagnosis: Signs and gross lesions may support a tentative diagnosis but many outbreaks do not fit the usual pattern. Concurrent bacterial infections, e.g. salmonellosis and pasteurellosis, may complicate the changes. Leukopenia (i.e. leukocytes below 10,000/cu mm) in pigs over 5 weeks old and characteristic brain lesions support the diagnosis. The most accurate confirmatory laboratory technique is the fluorescent antibody test on frozen sections of tonsil, or on tissue cultures inoculated with a suspension of tonsil or spleen for virus isolation. Hog cholera must be differentiated from salmonellosis, erysipelas, mulberry heart disease, transmissible gastroenteritis, viral encephalitis (including Teschen disease) and pseudorabies.

Immunity and Vaccination: There is only one main serotype of hog cholera virus although minor variants exist. Recovered animals are immune and immune sows confer protection on their offspring through their colostrum. Short-term passive protection can be provided by injecting hyperimmune anti-hog cholera serum.

Although an inactivated vaccine is available, only the live attenuated vaccine is in general use. Live attenuated vaccines usually are prepared from virus adapted to rabbits (i.e. lapinized) or to tissue cultures, or both. Sows should not be vaccinated near breeding time or in early gestation as the attenuated virus may infect baby pigs *in utero.*

Epidemiology and Control: Hog cholera is seriously endemic in most South American, African, Asian and some European countries. It is absent from Canada and Australia and has been eradicated from Britain and the U.S.A.

The virus is transmitted most readily by pig-to-pig contact and by feeding uncooked pork scraps. The virus can be transmitted between farms by contaminated feed, water or fomites. The maintenance of a closed herd and careful entry restrictions usually exclude it. Less virulent strains cause problems in eradication because the diagnosis of chronic mild disease forms is difficult. For similar reasons, vaccination should cease when an area slaughter program has begun. After slaughter of an infected herd, vacant contaminated premises should be thoroughly cleaned, disinfected and left unused for at least 2 weeks.

AFRICAN SWINE FEVER

A highly contagious, usually fatal, viral disease of pigs with signs and lesions resembling those of hog cholera. African swine fever (ASF) was confined to Africa until 1957 when it suddenly appeared in Portugal. It spread to Spain in 1960, thence to France in 1964 and Italy in 1967. The disease was eradicated from France and Italy. ASF was in Cuba during part of 1971. In 1978, ASF was diagnosed in Sardinia, Malta, Brazil, The Dominican Republic and Haiti.

Etiology and Epidemiology: ASF virus remains unclassified, not fitting into recognized viral groups. It is in all fluids, tissues and excretions of acutely infected swine and is periodically found in discharges from carriers. It is exceptionally hardy, retaining infectivity after 18 months at room temperature, after 1 hour at 56°C, or in commercially processed hams after 6 months. Blood smears remained infectious after 24 hours exposure to 1% sodium hydroxide but not to 2%. It is relatively resistant to trypsin and acids but is ether sensitive. It has been passed in rabbits, embryonating eggs and tissue cultures. The attenuated viral strains so evolved have not provided protective immunity nor have killed-virus vaccines.

Only swine are naturally susceptible to ASF. In Africa, outbreaks of ASF in domestic swine often follow contact (probably via ticks) with wart hogs, bush pigs or forest hogs, all of which can be inapparent carriers. *Ornithodoros* and certain argasid ticks can act as vectors of ASF virus for up to 12 months. ASF virus also can survive in a complete tick cycle by transovarian passage from infected female ticks to their offspring. ASF also is readily transmitted to swine by direct and indirect contact. In Portugal and Brazil, the initial outbreaks appear to have been caused by feeding swine pork scraps in garbage from international aircraft.

Clinical Findings: The first sign of ASF is fever; temperatures of 105 to 108°F (40.5 to 42°C) occur from 5 to 15 days after natural infection. There is an early leukopenia. After about 4 days of fever or about 24 to 48 hours before death, animals usually stop eating and become listless, incoordinated and cyanotic. The pulse and respiration are accelerated and about one-third cough and have dyspnea. Vomiting, diarrhea and eye discharges are sometimes observed. Death often occurs within 4 to 7 days after the onset of fever. With ASF acquired from wild animals, mortality in domestic swine frequently approaches 100%. However, in Portugal and Spain, natural passage through domestic swine has somewhat modified the severity of ASF and resulted in a relatively high percentage of survivors. The survivors are usually carriers for life, although the virus is not continually present in the excretions.

Lesions: Generalized viral damage to the walls of small blood vessels results in varying degrees of edema, congestion and hemorrhage, with some thrombosis. A frequently severe cyanosis of hairless areas is sharply demarcated and edematous. Cutaneous ecchymoses occur on the skin of the legs and abdomen. Pleural, pericardial and peritoneal fluids are excessive. Petechiae occur in the mucous membrane of the larynx, urinary bladder, in the renal cortex and visceral surfaces of organs. Edema is often prominent in the mesenteric structures of the colon and adjacent to the gallbladder.

Diagnosis: Any suspect hog cholera-like disease should be reported immediately to state and federal authorities. The lesions of hog cholera and ASF are too similar to be certain of a differential diagnosis by gross pathology; however, there are minor differences that may be somewhat helpful. The "button ulcers" of hog cholera rarely occur in acute ASF. Severe edema of the lungs and walls of the gallbladder and excessive pericardial, pleural and peritoneal fluids are common in ASF and rare in hog cholera. For laboratory diagnosis samples of the blood and spleen should be taken preferably 2 to 3 days after onset of fever.

The suspect virus may be replicated in swine bone marrow or buffy coat (leukocyte) cultures. Swine red blood cells will adsorb to the leukocytes that are infected with fully virulent ASF virus and later the virus causes cytolysis of the leukocytes. These reactions do not occur with hog cholera virus, nor with attenuated strains of ASF from most chronic cases. Fluorescent antibody tests readily differentiate the 2 viruses. The identification of attenuated ASF virus from chronically infected animals is more readily accomplished through immunoelectroosmophoresis, reverse radial immunodiffusion, or indirect immunofluorescence tests to identify the serum antibody. Swine immunized with hog cholera virus will become infected if challenged with ASF virus as the suspect agent.

Control: The spread of ASF to Europe and Brazil and the absence of a vaccine intensify the international hazard. Cooperative international efforts to prohibit the movement of infected animals, products or vectors help, but veterinarians everywhere must be alert to the recognition of ASF and have access to a competent diagnostic service. A diagnosis must be followed by strict quarantine and slaughter.

RABIES

An acute encephalomyelitis caused by a virus. It is a natural disease of dogs, cats, bats and wild carnivores. However, all warm-blooded animals are susceptible. The disease is worldwide except for some countries that have eradicated or remained free of rabies due to their natural protection as islands and by enforcing rigorous quarantine regulations. It is endemic and at times epidemic throughout the Western Hemisphere in bats, dogs, foxes and skunks.

Mode of Transmission: The virus may be recovered from the CNS and salivary glands, as well as most tissues of infected animals. In nature, it is transmitted from animal to animal by means of a bite introducing the virus-bearing saliva. Rarely, rabies may be transmitted by viral contamination of fresh, already existing wounds. Virus may be present in the saliva and be transmitted by an infected animal several days prior to the onset of clinical signs.

Incubation Period: The incubation period is variable, but generally is within 15 to 50 days. In rare cases, it may be much longer, even several months.

Pathogenesis: Infection takes place by the deposition of infected saliva in or near a nerve. The virus is carried to the CNS via the nerve trunks. Experimentally, it has been shown to reach the spinal cord within 24 hours and can be demonstrated in the cord tissue within 4 to 5 days. The virus may remain at the site of inoculation for half the incubation period, which justifies the infiltration of hyperimmune serum in the region of the bite. The virus travels upward in the cord and finally reaches the brain after a variable time. The virus usually travels centrifugally from the CNS and reaches the salivary glands via their nerve supply. Hematologic spread can occur but is rare. Although the disease is usually considered fatal once signs appear, recovery has occurred both in animals and man.

Clinical Findings: Rabid animals of all species exhibit signs that are typical of rabies, with minor variations peculiar to carnivora, ruminants, bats, and man. The clinical course of the disease, particularly in dogs, can be divided into 3 phases: the prodromal, the excitative and the paralytic. The term "furious rabies" refers to animals in which the excitative phase is predominant, and "dumb or paralytic rabies" to dogs in which the excitative phase is extremely short or absent and the disease progresses quickly to the paralytic phase. In any animal, the first sign is a change in behavior, which may be indistinguishable from a digestive disorder, injury, foreign body in the mouth, poisoning or an early infectious disease. Temperature change is not significant and inability to retain saliva may or may not be noted. Animals usually stop eating and drinking and may seek solitude. There is frequently irritation or stimulation to the urogenital tract as evidenced by frequent urination, erection in the male and sexual desire. After the prodromal period of 1 to 3 days, animals either show signs of paralysis or become vicious. Carnivora, swine and, occasionally, horses and mules bite other animals or people at the slightest provocation. Cattle will butt any moving object. The disease progresses rapidly after the onset of paralysis.

Paralytic Form: This is characterized by early paralysis of the throat and masseter muscles, usually with profuse salivation and inability to swallow. Dropping of the lower jaw is common in dogs. Owners frequently examine the mouth of dogs and cattle, searching for a foreign body, or administer medication with the bare hands. These animals are not vicious and rarely attempt or are able to bite. The paralysis progresses rapidly to all parts of the body with coma and death in a few hours.

Furious Form: Furious rabies represents the classical "mad-dog syndrome" in which the animal becomes irrational and viciously aggressive. The facial expression is one of alertness and anxiety, with pupils dilated; noise invites attack. Such animals lose all caution and fear of natural enemies. There is no evidence of paralysis during the excitatory stage. Dogs rarely live beyond 10 days after the onset of signs. Dogs with this form of rabies frequently roam streets and highways, biting other animals, people and any moving object. They commonly swallow foreign objects, feces, straw, sticks and stones. Rabid dogs will chew the wire and frame of their cages, breaking their teeth, and will follow a hand moved in front of the cage, attempting to bite. Young pups apparently seek human companionship and are overly playful, but bite even when petted, usually becoming vicious in a few hours. As the disease progresses, muscular incoordination and convulsive seizures become common. Death is the result of progressive paralysis.

Rabid domestic cats and bobcats attack suddenly, biting and scratching viciously. Foxes frequently invade yards or even houses, attacking dogs and people. Rabid foxes and skunks are responsible for most pasture cattle losses, and have attacked dairy cattle in barns.

Rabies in cattle follows the same general pattern, and those with the furious form are dangerous, attacking and pursuing other animals and man. Lactation ceases abruptly in dairy cattle. Instead of the usual placid expression, there is one of alertness. The eyes and ears follow sounds and movement. A most typical clinical sign in cattle is bellowing of a character that can hardly be mistaken once encountered. This may continue intermittently until approaching death.

Horses and mules show extreme agitation evidenced by rolling as with indigestion. As with other species, they may bite or strike viciously and, because of size and strength, become unmanageable in a few hours. Such animals frequently suffer self-inflicted wounds.

The vampire bat is confined at present to South America, Trinidad, Central America and Mexico. These animals fight among themselves but rarely attack other animals except to feed. Their sole food is fresh blood. Although preferring cattle, they may feed on any animal, including man, by biting and lapping blood from the bite wound. Cattle losses are severe in infected areas. Rabies contracted from vampire bats is almost exclusively of the paralytic form and is commonly referred to as "derriengue."

In North America there are immense numbers of insectivorous bats, both as solitary individuals and in large colonies, which may become infected and transmit rabies. Rabid bats have been found widely distributed throughout the continent. Several human deaths due to rabies have been attributed to infections from bats.

Differential Diagnosis: Clinical diagnosis is usually possible but may be difficult; in the prodromal stage, rabies may easily be confused with other diseases. Inability to swallow saliva in all species of animals is suggestive of an obstruction in the throat, a foreign body lodged between the teeth, or ingestion of irritating substances. Furthermore, many animals will fight when injured, when provoked, or for possession of food or a mate. Normal cats, particularly males, at times make sudden unprovoked attacks on other animals or man. All of these behavior patterns may be present in rabies, but can also be unrelated.

If there is human exposure to an animal suspected of having rabies, an evaluation of the circumstances should be made, e.g. the species of animal, was it provoked, is rabies present in the area? Dogs or cats may be killed immediately but must be submitted to a laboratory for examination. If the animal is not killed it must be confined for a period of 10 days. Should suspicious signs appear, the animal should be killed in a manner that will not damage the head. Rapid laboratory evaluation is essential.

Wildlife acting in an abnormal manner should be considered rabid until proved otherwise. The same is true of bats that may be observed flying in the daytime, resting on the ground, attacking people or animals, or fighting. Insectivorous bats, though small, can inflict a wound with their teeth and should never be caught or handled with bare hands.

The fluorescent-antibody staining technique combines the speed of histologic techniques with the greater sensitivity of biologic examination. The test is based on direct visual observation of a specific antigen-antibody reaction. When properly used, it can establish a highly specific diagnosis within a few hours, and it has become the test of choice in most laboratories. Although utilized by many laboratories as a back-up procedure, results of the mouse inoculation test rarely disagree with the fluorescent antibody test.

Control Methods: Rabies control programs work best on a country-wide basis and should include the following: (1) mass vaccination of dogs and cats—this is the single most effective measure, (2) elimination of stray dogs—strays should be collected and held by a local pound or humane shelter for several days and, if unclaimed, killed humanely. Attempts to lower the number of the wildlife vectors by trapping or other means are of questionable value. It is recognized that when the population drops so does the incidence of rabies; however, attempts to cause this by trapping are difficult and expensive and the results are more psychological than real.

Immunoprophylaxis: Vaccines derived from a variety of tissue culture or chicken embryo origins are available, both live and inactivated. Some require annual revaccination, others protect adequately for 3 years. All must be given IM. The National Association of Public Health Veterinarians, Inc., P.O. Box 13528, Baltimore, Maryland, issue an annually revised compendium of animal rabies vaccines available in the U.S.A., including recommendations for their use. Those responsible for or connected with any control or regulatory program should obtain and read the current compendium.

Management of Dogs and Cats Bitten by Rabid Animals: Unvaccinated dogs, cats and other pets bitten by a known rabid animal should be killed immediately. If the owner is unwilling to do this the animal should be placed in strict isolation for a minimum of 4 months. If the exposed animal is a dog and has been vaccinated within 3 years with a vaccine providing 3-year immunity, it should receive a booster within 7 days of the exposure. Dogs and cats vaccinated with a one-year vaccine, must have been vaccinated within the previous year to be considered safe when given a booster.

Human Immunization: It is strongly recommended that all veterinary practitioners receive pre-exposure immunization. Following the immunization regimen, serum should be tested to determine if protective antibodies have been obtained.

PSEUDORABIES

(Aujeszky's disease, Mad itch, Infectious bulbar paralysis)

An acute viral infection of the CNS of nearly all subhuman mammals, although primarily associated with swine. Swine are significantly more resistant than other susceptible species and some develop latent infections from which they may release virus while remaining asymptomatic. The disease in the other species is almost invariably fatal and often marked by pruritus.

Etiology: The causal agent, *Herpesvirus suis*, is a double-stranded, enveloped DNA virus. The virus (PrV) replicates readily in many cell cultures lines.

Epidemiology: The presence of the disease in an area is dependent upon the presence of swine or virus-laden swine tissues used for food; other species play only a minor role in the spread of the disease. Once the course of infection has developed enough for viral release it is usually only a matter of hours before the victim is immobilized and moribund, minimizing viral spread. The most notable exceptions have been lateral infections among sheep; even so, the source of infection has been swine. While some birds have been shown to be susceptible, no records of natural infections are to be found. However, mechanical transfer of virus-contaminated materials by birds seems possible.

The most important means of spread is by direct contact between infected and susceptible swine. The highest concentration and most lengthy persistence of virus available for infection is in the fluids of the oronasalpharynges of infected swine. Viremia is of low order and intermittent, consequently the viral spill from blood into urine and into feces is also not great. Transmission by contact with contaminated excreta or venereal contact seems possible but unlikely. Some recovered swine will shed significant amounts of virus under poorly understood conditions for an indeterminate period. New foci of infection are often initiated by such swine.

Clinical Findings: Fatality is much higher in baby pigs than in weanlings. The infection usually has been initiated 48 hours prior to the onset of the first signs of sneezing and coughing, followed quickly by pyrexia, anorexia and dullness and then by neurologic involvement manifested by trembling, excited ambulations, incoordination, tonoclonic spasms, convulsions, coma and death. Weanlings follow a similar pattern but fewer die. If they live beyond the sixth day of illness, recovery often occurs. Shoats and mature animals have a much higher rate of recovery. Pregnant swine may abort embryos and macerated fetuses depending on the stage of pregnancy at infection. Less common signs are pruritus, and in protracted cases, blindness.

The disease in cattle and sheep most often follows a short clinical course of 36 to 48 hours. There is a brief excitement phase in which cattle occasionally are aggressive; there is trembling and apparent anxiety as respirations and salivation increase, accompanied by much licking of the nares. As the neurologic involvement deepens, pruritus may develop with savage efforts to relieve the itching, culminating in incoordination, recumbency, convulsion, exhaustion, coma and death.

The disease in dogs and cats follows a course similar to that in ruminants with certain exceptions. Dogs have not been found to be aggressive; the length of the syndrome is more variable. In cats the excitement phase is preceded by a period of sluggishness. At the onset of salivation, mewing becomes persistent and the cat resists being caught. Pruritus may or may not be present in dogs or cats.

Lesions: The most constant gross lesion is congestion of the vessels of the meninges covering the brain. Less frequently there is necrotic tonsillitis and diffuse necrotic foci in the liver, spleen and lungs, which are FA positive for PrV. Even less often, vesicles in the skin of the nares and mucosa of the buccal cavity are present. Microscopic lesions of the CNS are those of encephalomyelitis, meningitis and ganglioneuritis. In the tonsils, liver, spleen and lungs there are necrotic foci of parenchymal cells. Occasionally eosinophilic intranuclear inclusions may be found in glial cells or neurons.

Diagnosis: Diagnosis may be made on the syndrome and history. Sudden onset with respiratory signs changing in 24 to 48 hours to deep neurologic involvement in a significant number of groups of young pigs with attendant dullness, pyrexia, and anorexia strongly suggests the disease even before any mortality has occurred. Abortions require FA procedures to identify viral antigens in tissues of aborted embryos or fetuses, especially if abortions are not accompanied by convincing signs of the disease in others of a group.

Laboratory procedures to support diagnosis also include virus isolation in cell culture with tonsillar tissue being of prime value, and subcut. inoculation of rabbits with suspect tissue suspensions. Tests for virus neutralization by serum from recovered animals serves to identify those that have been infected. Other tests for this purpose that may be used are immunodiffusion and rocket electrophoresis.

A skin test based on delayed hypersensitivity will identify a high percentage of recovered animals and therefore may be used in the field as a screening test for herds whose immune status is unknown. It may be conducted on the farm, and results are available in 24 hours.

Control: An attenuated vaccine has been found to be effective in reducing mortality on farms where losses had frequently occurred. A killed vaccine is also available. Neither vaccine prevents infection by field virus, which is shed by the challenged vaccinates for a variable period. Antiserum is useful in an outbreak to save baby pigs but is not commercially available.

Management is important in maintaining a susceptible herd of swine. The following procedures are basic to the objective: (1) Add only serologically negative swine to the herd. (2) Avoid traffic from infected premises and eliminate public access to swine quarters. (3) Avoid accessibility of the herd to wild animals. (4) Provide separate equipment to service each group of animals.

No therapeutic drugs are useful. Animals not yet affected should be removed from the group promptly, isolated and observed frequently for further action.

Public Health: Recorded human infections are subject to skepticism because of serious omissions and an absence of such records for 40 years. Nevertheless, respect is due the virus since several species of subhuman primates have been found to be susceptible.

SPORADIC BOVINE ENCEPHALOMYELITIS (SBE)

(Buss disease)

SBE has been observed in the U.S.A., Japan, Australia, Czechoslovakia, Hungary and South Africa, suggesting a worldwide distribution. It has not been reported in the U.S.A. for some time.

Etiology: SBE is caused by a strain of *Chlamydia psittaci.* While all chlamydial strains contain an identical group-specific antigen, cell walls of SBE strains contain an antigen that is similar to that found in ovine polyarthritis strains but not in those causing abortions or pneumonia. SBE organisms are found in the brain and spinal cord, in serous exudates, blood, lymph nodes and internal organs indicating a systemic infection. They are excreted in the feces and urine.

Clinical Findings: The incubation period varies from 6 to 31 days. Inactivity and depression mark the clinical onset of SBE. The affected cattle become anorectic and develop fever, which persists until death or recovery. Excessive salivation, dyspnea and mild diarrhea are additional clinical signs in the early stage. Recovery may follow this stage, but most often affected cattle develop nervous signs and have difficulty in walking. They develop a stiff gait, stagger, circle and fall over small obstacles. The limbs become weaker and signs of paralysis develop. During the terminal stage, the cattle can hardly rise and may exhibit opisthotonos. The course of the clinical disease lasts from 10 to 14 days, but in some instances affected cattle may not die for a month. Cattle of all ages may be affected, but the disease is seen more often in younger cattle. The disease occurs sporadically with a low morbidity, but the mortality of the stricken cattle is over 50%.

Lesions: Nonpurulent, aseptic meningoencephalomyelitis occurs. Macroscopic lesions in the CNS are due to hyperemia and edema. After an acute course, few pathologic changes will be found although the peritoneal and pleural cavities may contain increased amounts of fluid. Cattle with chronic disease have serofibrinous exudates in the body cavities. Fibrinous pericarditis, pleuritis and lobar pneumonia may then also be found. Microscopically, all parts of the brain may have vasculitis with perivascular cuffing and parenchymal foci of inflammation composed predominantly of mononuclear cells.

Diagnosis: A definite diagnosis can only be made by isolating and identifying the causative agent from the brain or by histologic examination of the CNS. When typical clinical signs have been observed, a diagnosis of SBE can often be reasonably well substantiated by the serofibrinous peritonitis.

Demonstration by complement fixation of increasing group-specific chlamydial antibody titers in paired serum samples of affected cattle may confirm the clinical diagnosis. Subclinical intestinal infections of cattle with chlamydiae are common, and these strains also stimulate development of group-specific antibodies.

Treatment and Control: No specific means of prevention and control are known. The causative chlamydial agents are sensitive to tetracyclines or tylosin. High doses of these antibiotics (25 to 50 mg/kg/day of oxytetracycline) are given as early as possible in the course of the disease for at least 4 to 5 days. The fever should drop significantly 24 hours after initiation of treatment.

EQUINE ENCEPHALOMYELITIS

(Equine encephalitis)

The equine encephalitides constitute a group of diseases of Equidae characterized by similar clinical nervous disturbances and generally high mortality. The causal arboviruses infect a variety of other vertebrate hosts including man. These diseases are serious although sporadic public health problems. **Borna disease,** a meningoencephalomyelitis of horses, is not of arbovirus etiology and is not known to be pathogenic for man.

Etiology and Epidemiology: Horses may be infected by either alpha (Group A) or flavi (Group B) arboviruses. Alpha viruses include eastern equine encephalomyelitis (EEE), western equine encephalomyelitis (WEE) and Venezuelan equine encephalomyelitis (VEE), while Japanese B encephalitis (JE) is the most notable equine pathogen in the flavivirus group. EEE occurs principally in Eastern Canada and the East Coastal and Gulf States of the U.S.A., but has been identified in the Southwestern States, Mexico, South and Central America and some Caribbean islands. WEE occurs principally in Western Canada, Western and Central U.S.A. and Mexico. Both EEE and WEE have been found to cause clinical disease in horses in the states of Florida, Louisiana and Texas. The Venezuelan virus is widely distributed in South and Central America, Mexico and, in 1971, in Texas caused an outbreak in horses and human beings.

The Japanese B virus is widely distributed in the Far East causing encephalitis of man and horses, although mortality in horses is low (less than 5%). The virus causes abortion in swine but provides no other signs in this species. JE virus has a cycle involving arthropod vectors, birds and mammals. It has not been identified in the Western Hemisphere.

An unrelated and as yet unclassified virus causes Borna disease in Europe, where it has occurred for years usually during the spring and early summer. Clinically, the disease resembles the North American encephalitides. The incubation period is 4 weeks or longer, the course 1 to 3 weeks, the mortality usually high and characteristic inclusions (Joest's bodies) develop in ganglion cells of the brain.

The 3 American viruses, eastern, western and Venezuelan, are maintained in nature by an arthropod-bird or -rodent reservoir from which infection is transmitted to mammalian hosts by biting insects, principally mosquitoes of the genera *Aedes, Anopheles, Culex* and *Culiseta.* Mosquitoes act as biologic vectors, i.e. the viruses multiply in the body and persist in the salivary gland. Transmission by arthropods other than mosquitoes is probably unimportant. Wild birds serve as a principal reservoir for eastern and western encephalomyelitis virus. Forest rodents are the most probable reservoirs of Venezuelan virus. Reservoir hosts tend to develop viremia with blood titers adequate to infect mosquitoes, thereby actively contributing to the cycle of virus survival. The horse may be regarded as a dead-end host with the western virus. Horses infected with eastern virus may develop a viremia adequate for infecting mosquitoes, but do not contribute significantly to transmission or persistence of the virus in nature. The Venezuelan virus produces a viremia adequate for infecting mosquitoes, and unlike the other 2 viruses, may also spread between horses and to man by contact or aerosol.

These diseases are more frequent in pastured than in stabled horses and are concentrated in areas having the appropriate combination of reservoir hosts and mosquitoes.

Clinical Findings: Signs include fever, impaired vision, irregular gait, wandering, reduced reflexes, circling, incoordination, yawning, grinding of teeth, drowsiness, pendulous lower lip, inability to swallow, inability to rise when down, paralysis and death. Those with mild cases may slowly recover in a few weeks but mortality in horses is about 20 to 50% from the western type of virus, over 90% from the eastern type, and up to 75% from the Venezuelan type.

Lesions: No characteristic gross lesions are observed. Microscopically, hemorrhage, degeneration of nerve cells in the cerebral cortex, thalamus, hypothalamus and other parts of the CNS can usually be demonstrated. Perivascular cuffing with polymorphonuclear and mononuclear cells may be present. Inclusion bodies are present only in Borna disease.

Diagnosis: A presumptive diagnosis may be based on clinical signs, history and seasonal occurrence and is aided by knowledge of endemic areas or known epidemic activity of a virus type. Demonstration of typical histopathologic lesions of a viral encephalitis strengthens the diagnosis. Further support and improved specificity result from positive virus neutralization or hemagglutination inhibition tests on acute-phase and convalescent serums. Because of the high mortality and rapid death of horses affected with eastern equine virus, it is difficult to obtain paired serums in this disease. However, horses with eastern virus encephalitis often have developed antibody 2 or 3 days after signs appear. Specific diagnosis is dependent on recovery of the virus from brain tissue and subsequent serotyping.

In the differential diagnosis, botulism, rabies, tetanus, listeriosis, fungal toxicosis, chemical poisoning, and plant poisoning must be considered.

Prophylaxis and Treatment: No specific antiviral agents are available. Supportive treatment and good nursing will aid in the recovery of mild cases. Since the encephalitides are primarily spread by mosquitoes, control measures should be directed against these arthropods. Removing horses from pasture and stabling them is advisable when epidemic outbreaks occur.

Highly effective vaccines are available in combinations of EEE, WEE and VEE; and EEE and WEE and for VEE alone. The combination vaccines are chemically inactivated and available in forms suitable for either intradermal or IM injection. The combination vaccines may also be obtained with inclusion of tetanus toxoid. Since monovalent VEE vaccine is a modified live virus preparation of tissue culture origin it should not be used in pregnant mares or very young foals. Annual spring vaccination for EEE, WEE and VEE is recommended in endemic areas and for horses that may be moved into endemic areas during the summer or early fall.

TESCHEN DISEASE

(Porcine poliomyelitis, Talfan disease)

A viral disease of pigs, analogous to human poliomyelitis, and characterized mainly by spinal paralysis.

Etiology and Epidemiology: The causal enterovirus is resistant to wide variations in pH, to many enzyme actions, and to most bacterial disinfectants. It is inactivated rapidly by formalin and by temperatures over 60°C, but may survive several days at room temperatures and long periods in the frozen state. There is only one main antigenic type.

The Teschen virus infects only the pig, in which it causes a subclinical infection of the alimentary tract, particularly the intestine. Occasionally, it gains access to the CNS causing overt disease. The virus is excreted in the feces for 1 to 3 months, after which a local intestinal immunity develops. In herds in which the virus is endemic, infection of the alimentary tract occurs early in life while the CNS is protected by circulating colostral antibodies. These are superseded by antibodies actively stimulated by the infection itself.

A puzzling epidemiologic feature is that although both virulent and avirulent strains of the virus occur in most areas of the world, including North America, serious outbreaks of the disease have been recorded only in mid-Europe and Madagascar. In other countries the disease is sporadic and mild or unrecognized.

Clinical Findings: In severe outbreaks morbidity and mortality may be high, affecting all age groups. The main sign is an ascending paresis progressing to a flaccid paralysis. Pigs so affected may continue to eat if they can get to food. A few pigs may show other nervous signs. In the milder outbreaks, which occur in most Western countries, the disease appears as a mild posterior paresis affecting small numbers of pigs, usually about 8 to 12 weeks of age.

Lesions: There are no gross lesions. Histologic lesions are confined mainly to the gray matter of the posterior brain and spinal cord. The lesions are typical of viral infections, and include neuronal degeneration, glial cell proliferation, and vascular congestion and cuffing.

Diagnosis: A presumptive diagnosis can be made from the clinical picture and absence of gross lesions. The nature and distribution of the histologic lesions provide supportive evidence, but are not specific to Teschen disease. Further evidence may be obtained by demonstrating a rise of neutralizing or complement-fixing antibodies in paired serum samples from early and late stages of the disease. However, a definitive diagnosis can only be made by demonstrating the presence of the virus in the CNS in early cases. This is usually done by isolating the virus in porcine kidney cell cultures.

The disease must be differentiated from Aujeszky's disease, edema disease, hog cholera, encephalitic forms of vomiting and wasting disease, rabies, arsenic poisoning, and various less common forms of poisoning.

Treatment and Control: There is no treatment. Vaccines are used in mid-Europe but not elsewhere.

PORCINE STREPTOCOCCAL ARTHRITIS AND MENINGITIS

Two recently described, similar syndromes occurring in pigs, but affecting different age groups are caused by 2 antigenically distinct streptococci, both belonging to Lancefield Group D. *Streptococcus suis* type 1 (De Moor's group 5) causes polyarthritis and sometimes meningitis in pigs between 1 and 6 weeks of age. *Streptococcus suis* type 2 (De Moor's group R) causes mainly meningitis and sometimes arthritis at any age up to 6 months, most commonly in pigs weighing 40 to 200 lb (18 to 90 kg). The type 1 disease is of minor economic importance; the type 2 disease may cause an annual herd mortality as high as 2 to 4%.

Etiology: Both agents form aerobic β-hemolytic colonies typical of streptococci on horse blood agar. In smears prepared from lesions they appear as diplococci or short chains. They are differentiated from each other and from other streptococci by slide agglutination tests and precipitation tests using antisera prepared against their respective capsular polysaccharides.

Epidemiology: The disease caused in piglets by type 1 probably occurs throughout the world, but epidemics in feeder pigs caused by type 2 have been recorded only in Europe. Both spread from herd to herd mainly through the movement of carrier pigs. The streptococci are thought to be carried in the nasopharynx. Outbreaks sometimes occur in closed herds. Once the disease appears in a herd, it becomes endemic, clinical cases occurring sporadically in individuals or in small groups of pigs from time to time.

Cases of human meningitis caused by type 2 have been reported, mainly in slaughterhouse personnel, the infection gaining entry through cuts and wounds.

Clinical Findings: Most pigs within a herd probably become infected, but usually few exhibit clinical signs. Minor damage to joints, for example by rough handling, may predispose to arthritis caused by type 1. Stresses of forced movement, mixing or overcrowding seem to predispose to clinical flare-ups of the meningitis caused by type 2.

The incidence of clinical cases caused by type 1 is usually low but that caused by type 2 varies widely from herd to herd, sometimes affecting 10 to 20% of the growing pigs. Most respond to treatment if administered early enough, but will remain unthrifty or die if treatment is delayed by even a few hours. In large feeder pig units the only sign noted may be sudden death.

Both organisms are thought to gain entry to the body via tonsils and adenoids, and initially cause a septicemia which may last several days, and which, in the absence of other lesions, may have a surprisingly small effect on the general appearance of the pig. Both organisms have a predilection for joints and meninges.

Affected joints become painful, swollen and warm and contain an excess of joint fluid. The pigs become lame and sometimes appear paralyzed.

Meningitis caused by type 2 is sudden in onset, acute and severe. Affected pigs become uncoordinated and soon are unable to stand. They lie on their sides continuously paddling. The eyes tend to protrude, marked nystagmus occurs and the mucous membranes of the eyelids are bloodshot. Death usually occurs within 24 to 48 hours. The incubation period may be as short as 24 hours or up to several weeks.

Lesions: Carcass lymph nodes may be enlarged and congested, and there may be fine strands of fibrin in the peritoneal cavity. Affected joints are grossly obvious when incised. Histologic examination may be necessary to confirm the meningitis.

Diagnosis: This is based on clinical signs, gross and histologic lesions, the demonstration of streptococci in smears and cultures of brain and joints, and the accurate typing of the causal agent.

Treatment and Control: Prompt treatment with penicillin or other suitable antibiotic is usually effective for controlling type 1 but may not be so for type 2 infections. Attempts have been made to eradicate type 2 from badly affected herds by massive blanket therapy, both by injection and feed medication, with some success in small herds. To date bacterins have proved ineffective. Where the disease is troublesome in feeder pig units buying pigs from a variety of sources, it is advisable to exclude those with endemic type 2 infection.

TRANSMISSIBLE GASTROENTERITIS (TGE)

A rapidly spreading viral disease of swine, characterized by profuse diarrhea and vomiting. The disease results in severe dehydration and high mortality in pigs infected during the first week or 2 of life. In older swine, morbidity may be high but mortality is low. Most outbreaks occur in winter and early spring.

Etiology: The causal coronavirus can be grown in porcine kidney cell cultures. It proliferates in the epithelial cells of the small intestines and may be found transiently in other organs without causing obvious changes. It does not affect common laboratory animals but may infect dogs and foxes subclinically and may be excreted in their feces for up to 2 weeks. It may also be excreted by experimentally inoculated starlings for short periods. The virus is readily transmitted through feces and fomites; airborne infection may occur in confined spaces. Pigs may shed virus up to 8 weeks after infection. The virus is very labile to sunlight and heat but may remain infective for years when frozen.

Clinical Findings and Diagnosis: The incubation period in newborn pigs is 14 to 30 hours; it may be as long as 4 days in older pigs or with mild strains of virus. The most pronounced sign, scouring, is often preceded by vomiting. Vomiting is less frequent after the first day of illness. In baby pigs, the diarrhea is at first watery and light green or yellow. It may contain curds of undigested milk and often drips from the anus without expulsive efforts. Dehydration is rapid and thirst is evident; even the youngest pigs drink water copiously and they continue to suck the sow as long as they have sufficient strength. As dehydration progresses, the feces tend to become thicker. Diarrhea continues in surviving piglets for 5 to 9 days. Most fatalities occur 2 to 6 days after the onset. Mortality in pigs infected on the first day of life approaches 100%; it is much lower in pigs 3 or more days old at infection and deaths are unusual in pigs over 4 weeks of age. In weaned and older swine projectile expulsion of brownish or yellowish watery feces may continue for 1 to 5 days. Vomiting is rare in shoats and older animals, except in sows infected near parturition. Sows infected late in pregnancy sometimes have elevated temperatures, but depressed body temperatures are commonly found in other pigs.

A different clinical picture, described as **endemic TGE**, has been seen in large herds in which continuous farrowing is practiced. Most sows in such herds are immune and their pigs are protected by lactogenic immunity until late in lactation or weaning. As the pigs lose this protection they develop relatively mild disease which may not be recognized as TGE. Losses are relatively low but such herds may be an important means of carrying the virus over summers. Virus may also persist for long periods in herds to which susceptible feeder pigs are added frequently. Transient diarrhea occurs in each freshly introduced batch of pigs.

Lesions: The primary lesion is loss of intestinal epithelial cells resulting in extreme shortening of the intestinal villi. This may be seen best 1 or 2 days after infection and before regeneration starts by placing bits of jejunum under water and comparing them with a hand lens or dissecting microscope with duodenal mucosa taken from near the pylorus. Chyle, easily seen in the mesenteric lymphatics of normal and most pigs with enteric colibacillosis, is absent in pigs with TGE. In early stages of the disease, the stomach is usually filled with coagulated milk and the intestine is distended with clear or brightly colored fluid and gas containing bits of milk curd. In later stages the pig is dehydrated, distension of the intestine is less pronounced, but the stomach remains filled. The stomach wall in the fundic region is often severely congested in the terminal stages of the disease. Inflammatory changes are rare early in the disease but may later occur in any part of the intestine.

Diagnosis: Diagnosis of TGE is strongly suggested by the appearance of rapidly spreading diarrheal disease affecting all ages of pigs and fatal only in piglets. The clinical appearance in endemically infected herds, however, may not be obviously different from diarrheas caused by rotavirus or bacteria. A specific diagnosis of TGE requires laboratory procedures, such as the fluorescent antibody technique applied to frozen sections of the jejunum, preferably of pigs killed at the onset of disease, or cell cultures inoculated with intestinal materials.

Porcine Epidemic Diarrhea: Two diseases of pigs, both of unknown cause, have been reported under this heading. The "type I" disease, occurring only in older animals is still of unknown cause. Attempts to isolate an infectious agent from pigs suffering from the "type II" disease, which resembles TGE and occurs in both younger and older pigs, have so far been unsuccessful, but recently virus-like particles demonstrable by electron microscopy have been reported. These resembled coronaviruses but the affected pigs did not have increasing antibody titers against TGE or hemagglutinating encephalomyelitis virus. Until the disease(s) is better understood, little can be said other than that it should be considered in the differential diagnosis of TGE.

Prophylaxis and Treatment (of TGE): During an endemic, persons, animals or public conveyances of any kind from infected, or possibly infected, areas should not be allowed on TGE-free farms. If new stock must be introduced, they should be isolated from the herd for a month or until farrowing is completed.

When an outbreak occurs, it is advisable to separate sows near term as widely as possible in small groups or individual houses even when they apparently have been exposed. This practice may not be entirely effective, depending upon the efficiency of personnel, but it usually delays spread. Each day of age gained by baby pigs before infection occurs decreases losses. New sows about to farrow should not be added to an infected herd for 2 or 3 months after an outbreak.

Sows recovered from natural infection transmit a type of immunity to their pigs. This protection is unrelated to colostral circulating antibodies; it depends upon the presence of antibody (mainly IgA) in milk and is effective only as long as such milk is in the gastrointestinal tract of the piglets. Largely because of this mechanism of lactogenic immunity, difficulty has occurred in the development of vaccines. A modified live virus vaccine for IM use is licensed in the U.S.A. IM injected TGE virus, whether attenuated or virulent, stimulates good titers of antibody in serum and colostrum but within days of parturition the titers in milk become too low to prevent disease.

Planned infection of sows early in pregnancy with virulent virus stimulates effective immunity but should be used only where it is inevitable that sows will be exposed on farrowing and where there is no danger of spreading the disease to neighboring droves. This is best carried out by grinding or chopping intestinal tract material from infected pigs from the same drove and mixing it with the sow feed after withholding feed for one day. Sows thus immunized should be isolated from infected pigs at farrowing to reduce the exposure of their pigs to virus.

There is no specific treatment. Some practitioners have observed benefit from orally or parenterally administered antibiotics or sulfonamides in animals more than 4 or 5 days old at onset. Dehydration may be combatted by supplying fresh water or hypotonic saline solution to the piglets. In some instances it has appeared useful to wean pigs old enough to eat dry feed. Careful attention to providing a warm, draft-free, dry environment may increase the survival rate.

VOMITING-AND-WASTING DISEASE

(Ontario encephalitis, Viral encephalomyelitis of piglets)

A viral disease of young pigs characterized by vomiting, constipation, anorexia, and either chronic emaciation or acute encephalomyelitis.

Etiology and Epidemiology: The causal coronavirus, the **hemagglutinating encephalomyelitis virus**, grows in pig kidney cell cultures and affects only pigs. Infection appears to be widespread in North America and Western Europe, but is usually subclinical. In herds in which it is endemic a herd immunity exists, and although occasionally individual piglets may develop clinical signs these are rarely diagnosed. However, if the virus enters a susceptible herd during the farrowing period, several litters may be affected simultaneously, and the morbidity and mortality in these may be high.

Clinical Findings: The virus infects all age groups but usually only piglets of 5 to about 21 days of age show clinical signs. Initial signs are anorexia, depression, constipation and a variable amount of vomiting. Intestinal stasis occurs and the abdomen may become bloated with gas. Some piglets suffer pharyngeal paralysis and are unable to drink. After 1 to 3 days the disease progresses in 1 of 2 ways. In some outbreaks pronounced signs of CNS derangement develop and the affected piglets soon die. In other outbreaks, central nervous signs are minimal but the anorexia and constipation persist and the piglets slowly waste away, dying over periods of 1 to 6 weeks.

Lesions: There are no distinctive gross lesions. Histologically, nonspecific lesions typical of viral encephalitides may be found in the brain stem, cervical cord and paravertebral ganglia. These are constant findings in the encephalitic syndrome and may sometimes be found in the wasting syndrome.

Diagnosis: In large outbreaks a fairly firm diagnosis can be made from the clinical and postmortem findings. Diagnosis can be confirmed by demonstrating a rise of neutralizing antibodies. Isolation of the virus from affected piglets is difficult and unreliable. The disease must be differentiated from bacterial meningitis, hypoglycemia, agalactia, hog cholera, Teschen disease and pseudorabies.

Treatment and Control: There is no treatment, and control is difficult. Herdsmen must be encouraged not to sell out and repopulate in the face of an outbreak since the worst loss is usually over by the time diagnosis is made. Usually, a herd immunity develops rapidly and no further overt clinical cases will be seen. Sanitation and isolation are the only protection for a susceptible herd.

SWINE DYSENTERY

(Bloody scours, Vibrionic dysentery, Hemorrhagic dysentery, Black scours, Mucohemorrhagic diarrhea)

A common, important mucohemorrhagic diarrheal and exudative disease, which occurs in most swine-producing countries.

Etiology: A spirochete, *Treponema hyodysenteriae*, is the only agent involved in the transmission of swine dysentery, but other anaerobic bacteria that are normally present in the colon of pigs are necessary in addition to *T. hyodysenteriae* to produce the disease in gnotobiotic pigs.

Epidemiology: The disease is transmitted by ingestion of fecal material from affected or clinically normal swine carrying *T. hyodysenteriae*. New outbreaks in herds from which the disease was previously absent usually follow the introduction of new stock. Once the disease has entered a herd, it usually spreads slowly at first, requiring close contact between pigs or the movement of relatively large amounts of infective feces. It may take several weeks or months to build up to a high morbidity. It remains permanently endemic and is difficult to eradicate.

Any age of pig is susceptible but the incidence is highest between 15 and 75 kg. The incubation period is usually 7 to 14 days, but it may be considerably longer. In field cases the death losses in weanling pigs may be as high as 30% and the morbidity over 90% but in most cases the mortality is low and the morbidity about 25 to 50%.

Clinical Findings: The first evidence of the disease in most herds is the appearance of yellow-to-gray, soft feces combined with a slight reduction in appetite. As the disease progresses the feces may become watery, contain blood, mucus and a whitish mucofibrinous exudate, with staining of the perineal region; this leads to dehydration, weakness, emaciation, rough coat, incoordination and increased thirst. The body temperature may rise in some animals, however this is not consistent.

The course of swine dysentery is variable. Remissions and recurrences are common. Some surviving animals may be stunted or unthrifty, but most that are treated properly return rapidly to normal.

Lesions: These are confined to the large intestine, cecum and rectum. In a few cases the terminal ileum may be affected. Changes noted in the early cases are hyperemia and edema of the walls and mesentery of the colon. The mesenteric lymph nodes may also be swollen. The mucosa is swollen and covered by mucus. Later, thick mucofibrinous pseudomembranes containing blood may be covered with a thin, dense fibrinous exudate that may be mistaken for marked necrosis, but necrosis is superficial. Lesions may involve all or part of the large intestine and have a tendency to become somewhat diffuse in the latter stages of the disease.

Diagnosis: A provisional diagnosis can be made on the combined evidence of the history and epidemiology, clinical signs, gross and microscopic lesions, response to treatment and the demonstration of large numbers of treponemes in colonic mucosal scrapings or feces, particularly mucus. In fixed smears they appear as gram-negative sinuous organisms and in fresh wet mounts examined under phase-contrast or darkfield microscopy as motile serpentine organisms. Diagnosis can be confirmed by fluorescent antibody tests (FAT) using specific absorbed labeled antiserum and by anaerobic culture, preferably from colonic scrapings.

Nonpathogenic commensal treponemes, morphologically similar to *T. hyodysenteriae*, are common in the large colon and may lead to mistaken diagnoses. In other types of diarrhea (e.g. chronic scours after weaning) they may be present in large numbers. Furthermore, they cross-react with *T. hyodysenteriae* in FATs if unabsorbed antiserum is used. In culture they tend to be less hemolytic than *T. hyodysenteriae*.

Swine dysentery may also be mistaken for salmonellosis, severe acute trichuriasis, gastric ulcers, chronic scours after weaning, intestinal adenomatosis, colonic torsion, and other conditions that can cause blood in the feces.

Prophylaxis: The disease is not readily transmitted from herd to herd on boots, farm equipment, or trucks provided sensible hygienic precautions are taken. Although flies, rats and dogs have been shown to carry the infection for short periods experimentally, they do not appear to be important as vectors in the field, nor do cats, mice, birds or the wind. The main method of spread from herd to herd is via pigs, usually as subclinical carriers.

Consequently, herds that are free from swine dysentery can be kept free for long periods, provided replacement breeding stock is introduced only from sources that are also known to be free. Furthermore, farms that are severely affected with swine dysentery can be depopulated, cleaned and disinfected and repopulated from a clean source with reasonable chances of success. This should be carried out in warm dry weather since the infective agent survives longer in winter. It also survives for limited periods in lagoons and slurry pits, providing a source of reinfection.

Where repopulation is impractical, the disease must be controlled by strict attention to hygiene, husbandry, prevention of stress and overcrowding and the judicious use of drugs. The disease may be hard to control on high-density diets, and frequent changes of ration tend to exacerbate it. The morbidity and severity of the disease is related to the amount of fresh infective feces ingested. A cleanup of the pens and reduction of crowded conditions sometimes leads to dramatic improvements.

The disease is usually hardest to control in large feeder-pig operations where weaners are purchased from a wide variety of breeder herds. New arrivals should be quarantined in groups and two 3- to 6-day periods of water medication and pen cleaning carried out before they enter the main units. Where the supplying herds are few in number it may be advisable to medicate before shipping as well as on arrival.

Several chemotherapeutic agents are useful as feed additives to aid in suppressing swine dysentery; they include carbadox (0.0055%), lincomycin (℞ 45), virginiamycin (℞ 84), arsanilic acid or sodium arsanilate (℞ 674), tylosin (℞ 82), and furazolidone (℞ 119). Trials in the U.S.A. and elsewhere with nitroimidazoles such as ronidazole, 0.006 to 0.012% (60 to 120 ppm) in feed or drinking water, have shown useful activity. All these compounds must be used in conjunction with good husbandry and hygienic practices. They are most effective in keeping the disease subclinical, after the overt clinical signs have been controlled by water medication.

Treatment: Gentamicin, lincomycin (℞ 45), nitroimidazoles, tylosin (℞ 82), and arsenic compounds (℞ 674), appear to be most efficacious; because of the loss of appetite and increased thirst, acute infections are best treated with water medications or injectables. However, nitroimidazoles are not registered for use in the U.S.A. and gentamicin has not been registered for use in swine in the U.S.A. Water medication must be thorough and pens cleaned for good effect.

SALMONELLOSIS

A disease of all animals caused by many species of salmonellae and characterized clinically by 1 or more of 3 major syndromes:

septicemia, and acute and chronic enteritis. The clinically normal carrier animal is a serious problem in all host species. The disease occurs worldwide and the incidence is increasing with the intensification of livestock production. Young calves, piglets, lambs and foals are all susceptible and usually develop the septicemic form. Adult cattle, sheep and horses commonly develop acute enteritis and chronic enteritis may occur in growing pigs and occasionally in cattle (*see also* DIARRHEA OF NEWBORN ANIMALS, p. 172 and DIARRHEA IN WEANED AND ADULT HORSES, p. 167).

Etiology and Epidemiology: The species that most commonly cause disease in mammals include: *Salmonella typhimurium* and *S. dublin* (cattle); *S. choleraesuis* and *S. typhimurium* (swine); *S. typhimurium* (horses). The source of infection includes the feces of infected animals that can contaminate feed and water, milk, fresh and processed meats from abattoirs, plant and animal products used as fertilizers or feedstuffs, pasture and rangeland and many inert materials. The organisms may survive for months in wet, warm areas such as in feeder pig barns or in water dugouts. Rodents and wild birds are also sources of infection. The prevalence of infection varies between species and countries and is much higher than the incidence of clinical disease, which is commonly precipitated by stressful situations such as sudden deprivation of feed, transportation, drought, crowding, recent parturition and the administration of some drugs. The disease is common in hospitalized horses that have been subjected to prolonged surgical procedures.

The usual portal of infection is oral, and following infection the organism multiplies in the intestine causing an enteritis. Invasion may follow and result in septicemia with subsequent localization in brain and meninges, pregnant uterus, distal aspects of the extremities and tips of the ears and tail, which can result respectively in meningoencephalitis, abortion, osteitis and dry gangrene of the feet, tail and ears. The organism frequently also localizes in the gallbladder and mesenteric lymph nodes and survivors intermittently shed the organism into the intestine and thus out in the feces.

Clinical Findings: Septicemia: This is the usual syndrome in newborn calves, lambs, foals and piglets, and outbreaks may occur in pigs up to 6 months of age. Illness is acute; depression is marked, fever (105 to 107°F [40.5 to 41.5°C]) is usual and death occurs in 24 to 48 hours. In pigs, a dark red-to-purple discoloration of the skin is common, especially of the ears and ventral abdomen. Nervous signs may occur in calves and pigs. The case fatality rate may reach 100%.

Acute enteritis: This is the common form in adults and it may also occur in calves of 3 to 6 weeks. Initially there is a fever (105 to 107°F [40.5 to 41.5°C]) followed by severe, watery diarrhea, sometimes dysentery and often tenesmus. In a herd outbreak, several hours may lapse before the onset of diarrhea, and the fever may disappear with the onset of diarrhea. The feces vary considerably: they may have a putrid smell and contain mucus, fibrinous casts and even shreds of mucous membrane; in some cases large blood clots are passed. Rectal examination causes severe discomfort, tenesmus and commonly dysentery. Abdominal pain is common and severe in the horse. Affected horses are severely dehydrated and may die within 24 hours after the onset of diarrhea; the case fatality rate may reach 100%. A marked leukopenia and neutropenia are characteristic of the acute disease in the horse.

Subacute enteritis: This may occur in adult horses and sheep on farms where the disease is endemic. The signs include mild fever (103 to 104°F [39 to 40°C]), soft feces, inappetence and some dehydration. There may be a high incidence of abortion in cows and ewes, some deaths in ewes after abortion and a high mortality rate due to enteritis in the lambs under a few weeks of age. In cattle the first sign may be fever and abortion followed several days later by diarrhea.

Chronic enteritis: This is a common form in pigs and adult cattle. There is persistent diarrhea, severe emaciation, intermittent fever and poor response to treatment. The feces are scant and may be normal or contain mucus, casts, or blood. In growing pigs, rectal stricture may be a sequela if the terminal part of the rectum is involved. Affected pigs are anorexic, lose weight and their abdomen becomes grossly distended. The lesion is obvious on digital palpation and necropsy.

Dogs and cats rarely develop septicemia from salmonellae, although outbreaks in puppies and kittens have been reported. Dogs and cats may act, however, as asymptomatic carriers and many of the types important in other domestic mammals and man have been isolated from them.

A number of *Salmonella* spp. appear in foxes, especially in young kits and produce a peracute enteritis. Mink and other fur-bearing carnivores also may be affected. Several rodents such as guinea pigs, hamsters, rats, mice and rabbits are susceptible (*see* pp. 1155 et seq.). Rodents commonly act as a source of infection on farms where the disease is endemic. Pet turtles are a common source of infection in man.

Diagnosis: This is dependent on the clinical signs and on the laboratory examination of feces, tissues from affected animals, feed (including all mineral supplements used), water supplies, and feces from wild rodents and birds which may inhabit the premises. The clinical syndromes are usually characteristic but must be differentiated from several similar diseases: **In cattle:** enteric colibacillosis; coccidiosis; the alimentary tract form of IBR; bovine viral diarrhea; hemorrhagic enteritis due to *Clostridium perfringens*, types B and C; arsenic poisoning, secondary copper deficiency (molybdenosis), winter dysentery, paratuberculosis, ostertagiasis and dietetic diarrhea. **In swine:** enteric colibacillosis of newborn pigs and weanlings, swine dysentery, hemorrhagic enteritis due to *Campylobacter sputorum* var. *mucosalis* and the common septicemias of growing swine, which include erysipelas, hog cholera, pasteurellosis and hemophilosis. **In sheep:** enteric colibacillosis, septicemia due to *Hemophilus* sp., or pasteurellae and coccidiosis. **In horses:** septicemia due to *E. coli*, *Actinobacillus equuli* and streptococci and colitis-X disease.

The lesions are those of a septicemia or a necrotizing fibrinous enteritis. Special cultural techniques are usually necessary to recover the organism. Serum agglutination tests are useful as an indicator of herd infection. Because of the intermittent shedding of the organisms from infected animals it is usually necessary to conduct repeated fecal examinations before the organism is recovered or the animal can be identified as negative.

Treatment: Broad-spectrum antibiotics (℞ 17, 116) are used parenterally to treat the septicemia, and nitrofurans (℞ 122) may be given orally for enteric infection. Ampicillin (℞ 7, 8) may also be useful for the treatment of septicemic salmonellosis in all species. Treatment should be continued daily for up to 6 days. Oral medication should be given in drinking water, since affected animals are thirsty due to dehydration and their appetite is generally poor. Fluid therapy to correct acid-base imbalance and dehydration is necessary. Calves, adult cattle and horses need large quantities of fluids (℞ 579). Horses affected with acute enteric salmonellosis are severely acidotic and hyponatremic and may need to be treated initially with 5% sodium bicarbonate given IV at the rate of 6 to 9 qt/1,000 lb (5 to 8 L/400 kg) body wt. This is followed by balanced electrolytes containing potassium to correct the hypokalemia that may follow the correction of the acidosis. Septicemic salmonellosis in swine usually responds favorably if treated early. However, the enteric form is difficult to treat effectively in all species. Although clinical cure may be achieved, bacteriologic cure is difficult, particularly in adult animals, because the organisms become established in the biliary system and are intermittently shed into the intestinal lumen, which causes chronic relapsing enteritis and contamination of the environment.

Control and Prevention: Since *Salmonella* spp. survive for long periods in the environment, and recovered animals act as reservoirs of infection, the ideal of scrupulous sanitation and elimination of carriers is impractical; however, the rate of infection can be reduced. In swine herds, the general layout and design of pens should be directed towards minimizing transmission. If calves must be purchased from a variety of sources, they should be kept in isolation for at least 3 weeks after the date of arrival. Infected animals should be identified with the use of serial fecal examinations and raised in isolation. Newborn animals should be reared in isolation away from older infected animals. A periodic thorough cleanup, disinfection and interval of vacancy of animal pens is indicated.

Vaccines have given inconsistent results. A killed autogenous vaccine made from the isolate on the affected farm is given to the dam in late pregnancy, and the young are vaccinated several weeks after birth. A vaccine composed of live avirulent strains of *Salmonella* has been used recently in calves and pigs, and the immunity is reported to be superior to that produced by bacterin.

Major changes in rations should be avoided. Animals to be transported should be handled carefully and rested at intervals. Horses to be hospitalized for surgery should be checked for salmonellae and carefully monitored following prolonged surgery for evidence of enteritis; postoperative antibiotic therapy should not be given unless indicated. Medication of the feed and water supplies of susceptible, exposed animals has been attempted with some success, e.g. for cattle furazolidone in the feed or water, to provide 8 mg/lb of body wt daily for 7 days; for pigs, 0.41 gm/gal. of drinking water for 7 days.

PARATUBERCULOSIS

(Johne's disease)

A chronic infectious disease of ruminants characterized by progressive muscle wasting and diarrhea that is at first intermittent then becomes persistent. The principal lesion is in the intestinal wall and is manifested there by the characteristic thickening in cattle. With few exceptions the disease is fatal.

Although it is a disease of the intestinal tract, the bacillus *Mycobacterium johnei* (Johne's bacillus) has also been isolated from mesenteric lymph nodes, udder, and reproductive tracts of both sexes. Johne's disease is nearly always brought into a clean herd by the introduction of an infected animal which may itself be only a subclinical carrier of the infection. Infection usually occurs by ingestion of infected feces. The organism can survive in fecal material and contaminated soil for more than a year.

Clinical Findings: Calves are more susceptible than older cattle but because of the long incubation period most cases are seen in 2- to 6-year-old animals. However, a few cattle less than 2 years of age will show signs, especially if nutrition or management is suboptimal. A persistent or recurrent diarrhea is the chief sign. Temperature and appetite usually remain normal. The animal gradually loses weight and the hair-coat color may fade.

Lesions: The lower part of the small intestine, the ileocecal valve and the adjacent cecum may be found to be much thickened, and the mucosa thrown up in folds.

The disease in **sheep and goats** is similar but scouring is less marked than in the disease in cattle and thickening of the intestines is less obvious. **Pigs** can be infected, at least experimentally, and thus are potential shedders.

Diagnosis: Intradermal and IV Johnin allergic tests, and complement fixation and immunofluorescence tests are of value in detecting infected herds, but they are insufficiently reliable for individual diagnosis. Detecting early (subclinical) cases is most difficult. Ziehl-Neelsen staining of a fecal sample from an animal with an advanced clinical case will reveal the acid-fast organisms in about one-third of samples. Negative findings do not rule out the disease. Repeated sampling of the feces or biopsy of the ileo-cecal lymph nodes are indicated. Culturing of feces is the method of choice for detecting subclinical shedders, but positive results are unavailable for 6 to 8 weeks, and negative results mean little. Contamination of the cultures with other microorganisms is sometimes a problem. At necropsy the organism may be found in the intestinal lining or the adjacent lymph nodes, either histologically or by culture.

Prophylaxis and Treatment: No satisfactory treatment is known. In some countries, regulatory agencies provide assistance in handling Johne's disease. However the lack of reliable diagnostic methods for preclinical cases is a major problem.

Intrauterine infection occurs and therefore calves from dams which have or develop the disease should not be reared. The prevalence of clinical disease can be reduced if young calves are separated—immediately at birth—from older cows and anything contaminated with their feces. Calfhood vaccination is of value in preventing clinical disease and reducing fecal excretion. However, such vaccination may interfere with the interpretation of subsequent tuberculin tests and bovine vaccination is not authorized in many countries. Even where vaccination is practiced, it should be used in conjunction with sanitary precautions to minimize exposure.

CANINE HEMORRHAGIC GASTROENTERITIS SYNDROME

An acute onset of intestinal hemorrhage in mature dogs characterized by collapse, bloody diarrhea, a rapid course and death of untreated animals.

Etiology: The cause is unknown, but the administration of endotoxin to dogs causes similar findings. Hemorrhagic gastroenteritis has also been associated with clostridial infection.

Clinical Findings: Vomiting and dysentery, the latter often of a jam-like consistency and with a characteristic odor, are the common signs. The rectal temperature is normal or subnormal, the abdomen is painful upon palpation, but dehydration as judged by skin turgor is not common. CNS signs and petechial hemorrhage may be found but are uncommon.

Laboratory Findings: Barium meals may pass slowly, if at all; the abdomen of such dogs may be found to have ileus of the small intestine. An elevated packed cell volume (PCV), red cell count and hemoglobin concentration are characteristic of the disease. The white blood cell count may be low, normal or elevated. In most cases the platelet count is low or low normal. A PCV greater than 70 is a sign of serious illness.

Diagnosis: The diagnosis is on the basis of the clinical findings and the elevated PCV.

Treatment: For mild cases, food and water are withheld for 12 to 24 hours and atropine (℞ 511) and an antidiarrheic preparation (℞ 495) with an antibiotic (℞ 9, 25) are given. For severe cases in which signs of shock are present or the PCV is greater than 60, lactated Ringer's solution (℞ 588) or a similar polyionic solution are given IV rapidly through a large gauge needle until the PCV is normal. The rate of fluid infusion should then be slowed to a rate that will maintain hydration. Sodium bicarbonate (1 to 3 mEq/kg) can be added to the fluids given to severely affected dogs to combat the acidosis that occurs. The infusion of fluid will result usually in a rapid recovery even in seemingly hopeless cases. Corticosteroids (℞ 140) may also be valuable in severe cases. Treatment and observation should continue for 24 hours.

CANINE PARVOVIRAL ENTERITIS

A gastroenteritis of acute onset and varying morbidity and mortality, caused by a parvovirus, that became a notable problem during the summer of 1978. Although dogs of all ages have been affected, puppies appear to be more susceptible.

Clinical Findings: Peracute deaths have been described but more frequently the disease has been characterized by dehydration, inactivity, diarrhea that is liquid and bloody or sometimes liquid and brown, and vomiting. The anterior abdomen is painful when palpated. The body temperature is normal or subnormal in older dogs and as high as 106°F (41°C) in pups. After 2 or 3 days of illness in one outbreak, some dogs developed a cough and some developed corneal edema. The white blood cell count may be low, normal or elevated, depending presumably upon the stage of the disease. The blood urea nitrogen, SGPT and alkaline phosphatase concentrations in the blood were normal in one kennel outbreak involving young dogs.

Lesions: The important findings are those of a hemorrhagic enteritis that involves the entire intestinal tract. At histologic examination, the entire epithelial layer including the crypt cells of the villi are found to be involved. The crypt cells are necrotic. The lymphoid tissue is often necrotic or depleted. The lesions are similar to those of feline panleukopenia, q.v., p. 330.

Diagnosis: At present, the diagnosis is made by the typical histopathologic findings of loss of intestinal mucosal epithelium. The virus can be isolated from feces. A diagnosis based on clinical signs may become possible when more experience is gained with the disease but the findings of vomiting, anterior abdominal pain, cough, "blue eye" and diarrhea make an outbreak in a kennel difficult to distinguish from infectious canine hepatitis (q.v., p. 335) or canine distemper (q.v., p. 332).

Treatment: Prompt, intensive care including fluid therapy (℞ 588), atropine (℞ 511) and antibiotics (℞ 10, 25) has been associated with 100% recovery. Treatment may have to continue for 72 hours. Indwelling catheters should be placed in the jugular veins of severely ill pups for long-term fluid therapy. Isolation of puppies from boarding dogs and isolation of dogs that have travelled to shows is advisable.

CANINE CORONAVIRAL GASTROENTERITIS

A highly contagious enteric disease marked chiefly by vomiting and diarrhea. The disorder was found in show dogs in the U.S.A. in 1978 and in military dogs in Germany a few years earlier. The cause is a coronavirus.

Clinical Findings: The signs are similar to those of parvoviral infection, (*see* above) in that anorexia, diarrhea, vomiting and mental depression, often of sudden onset, are described. The feces are liquid or loose and may contain blood and mucus and often have a particularly fetid odor. Dehydration may be severe and pups may die suddenly. Fever occurs in some cases. The white blood cell count is not low in dogs with this disease. Experimental infections caused only mild disease; the incubation period was 24 to 36 hours.

Lesions: Lesions in experimental infections were not severe, consisting of dilated loops of intestine filled with watery green-yellow material. Naturally occurring cases had severe lesions with frank hemorrhage in the intestinal mucosa and enlarged congested mesenteric lymph nodes. The microscopic lesions were atrophy and fusion of intestinal villi and deepening of crypts, increase in cullularity of the lamina propria, flattening of epithelial cells and discharge of goblet cells.

Diagnosis: A history of a contagious gastroenteritis in a kennel should suggest viral enteritis as a possibility. Finding typical coronavirus particles in fresh feces with an electron microscope confirms the diagnosis. Histopathologic examination of fresh small intestine also will provide important evidence to support a diagnosis of coronaviral infection.

Treatment: There is no specific treatment but supportive fluid therapy and antibiotic treatment as described for canine hemorrhagic gastroenteritis (q.v., p. 304) or canine parvoviral enteritis should be used.

PNEUMONIA (LG. AN.)

In cattle, sheep and swine of all ages, pneumonia is a common pulmonary lesion that frequently becomes clinically significant; it also occurs in horses. Pneumonia is often a major economic problem when groups of young animals, for example calves or pigs, are kept close together either indoors or in yards. Outdoors, grazing animals may develop pneumonia due to parasitic invasion of their lungs; this is an important problem in young cattle and sheep in several areas of the world. For details see BOVINE RESPIRATORY DISEASES, p. 911, and THE EQUINE RESPIRATORY DISEASE COMPLEX, below, and consult the index for the specific pneumonias of each species.

THE EQUINE RESPIRATORY DISEASE COMPLEX

Of the 10 or more viruses associated with acute equine respiratory disease, only those causing arteritis, influenza and equine herpesvirus 1 infection (rhinopneumonitis) produce clinical syndromes and epidemiologic patterns sufficiently distinctive to suggest an etiologic diagnosis. If available, serologic or virologic confirmation should be sought.

The following viruses have been incriminated as causes of acute equine respiratory diseases but their significance is obscure: equine herpesvirus 2 and -3; equine paramyxoviruses (parainfluenza 1, 2, 3); equine rhinoviruses 1 and -2; reoviruses; and equine adenoviruses.

Infection with any of these viruses may be complicated by proliferation of bacteria or mycoplasmas.

EQUINE VIRAL RHINOPNEUMONITIS (EVR)

Etiology and Epidemiology: Equine herpesvirus 1 (EHV-1), the virus of equine viral rhinopneumonitis, produces acute respiratory catarrh upon primary infection, resulting in annual outbreaks among foals in areas with dense horse populations and sporadic episodes elsewhere. The age, seasonal and geographic distributions vary and are probably determined by immune status and aggregation of horses. In individuals, the outcome of exposure is determined by immune status, pregnancy status and possibly age. Mares may abort several weeks to several months after clinical disease or asymptomatic infection. The reservoir is the horse; a latent carrier state may exist. Transmission occurs by direct or indirect contact with virus-laden nasal discharge, aborted fetuses or placentas.

Clinical Findings: After an incubation period of 2 to 10 days, fully susceptible horses may develop any of the following signs: fever (102 to 107°F [39 to 41.5°C]) persisting 1 to 7 days and accompanied by leukopenia (neutropenia and lymphopenia), congestion and serous discharge from nasal mucosa and conjunctiva, malaise, pharyngitis, cough, inappetence, sometime edematous mandibular lymph nodes, and sometimes constipation followed by diarrhea. Frequently bacterial infections with mucopurulent nasal exudate and coughing follow. The infection is mild or inapparent in horses preconditioned immunologically.

In certain outbreaks mild-to-severe CNS signs may occur, which usually include incoordination and ataxia and, in more pronounced cases, paresis of the hind quarters. Myeloencephalitis with recovery of the virus has been reported and it has been suggested that neuritis of the cauda equina may be a sequela of EHV-1 infection.

Pregnant mares may abort fresh (minimally autolyzed) fetuses 3 weeks to 4 months after asymptomatic infection. Abortion is most common in the 8th to 11th months of gestation (sometimes occurring earlier). It is usually sudden, without premonitory signs, and followed by prompt placental expulsion and unimpaired subsequent breeding performance.

Diagnosis: Abortion due to EHV-1 can be tentatively diagnosed when pulmonary edema and, in some cases, grossly evident fetal hepatic necrosis are present in spontaneously aborted, minimally decomposed fetuses with petechiation throughout. Finding intranuclear inclusions in hepatic cells and bronchiolar or alveolar epithelium confirms the diagnosis as does virus isolation. Immunofluorescent techniques may more quickly confirm the diagnosis. Serology on aborting mares is diagnostically unproductive.

Immunoprophylaxis: Immunity following natural infection appears to be a combination of both humoral antibodies and cellular immune factors. Immunity to reinfection of the respiratory tract may persist for less than 3 months but multiple infections lead to a degree of resistance that prevents the appearance of clinical signs of respiratory disease. Immunity to infection leading to abortion is related to the degree of resistance of the upper respiratory tract to productive viral infection. Diminution of such resistance leads to development of a cell-associated viremia, which may lead to infection of the fetus.

Intranasally administered modified live vaccine is used on farms where infection has been a problem. Caution is advised in vaccination or introduction of recently vaccinated animals onto farms free of the disease because of the hazard of vaccine-virus-induced abortion. Parenterally administered live viral vaccines are licensed in some countries but excluded in others. With all live vaccines caution is indicated in breeding areas. Parenterally administered killed viral vaccine is given to pregnant mares during the fifth, seventh and ninth months of pregnancy as an aid in the prevention of abortion. The vaccine is also recommended for use in young horses as an initial 2-injection immunization series and a yearly booster as an aid in prevention of EHV-1 respiratory disease. Other vaccines are available in some countries.

Infection by Other Herpesviruses: Equine herpesvirus 2 (EHV-2) is found ubiquitously on the respiratory mucosa, conjunctivae and in the leukocytes of horses with a variety of diseases of diverse etiology as well as in clinically normal horses of all ages. Its role in the pathogenesis of any disease of the horse remains obscure. Equine herpesvirus 3 (EHV-3) is the cause of equine coital exanthema (q.v., p. 392), a benign progenital exanthematous disease.

Sanitary Management: On small farms with horses in close contact, little is accomplished by attempted isolation after abortions begin. Isolation and strict sanitary precautions are useful in the event of an abortion by a newly introduced mare, especially on large farms with separated groups of mares or in areas where abortion storms are rare or unknown. Efficient quarantine measures should be imposed on unknown mares arriving on a stud farm.

Treatment: Medication is seldom indicated. Confinement with careful observations during the febrile period and several days thereafter is necessary so that serious secondary infections may be handled promptly. There are no treatments for fetal infection. Some prenatally infected newborn foals may survive with diligent care and antibiotics (℞ 27, 50, 66, 76) until 48 to 72 hours after the temperature has returned to normal and the pulmonary congestion and edema are resolved. (*See also* p. 313.)

EQUINE VIRAL ARTERITIS
(Epidemic cellulitis, "Pinkeye")

An acute contagious viral disease characterized by fever, catarrh, edema and abortion.

Etiology and Epidemiology: Presently unclassified, the arteritis virus is distinct from other equine viruses. Spread is by contact with respiratory secretions. The disease is not commonly diagnosed. It occurs in sporadic outbreaks, which are usually attributable to movements of horses. Mortality is low. Clinical signs are most severe in very young or very old horses and those in poor physical condition. Abortion storms occur in which up to 80% of pregnant mares may abort. The disease may occur in epidemic form among horses at race meetings. The virus apparently varies greatly in virulence between outbreaks.

Clinical Findings: After an incubation period of 1 to 8 days, fever and leukopenia may be accompanied by lacrimation, conjunctivitis, nasal congestion and discharge, slight icterus, weakness, depression, anorexia and weight loss. Less consistent findings are: CNS disturbance, photophobia, colic, diarrhea, icterus, and edema of the eyelids, conjunctiva, legs, ventral body wall and sometimes the sheath, scrotum and mammae. Abortion occurs during the febrile period or shortly thereafter. The commonest form of clinically evident viral arteritis is a mild, febrile disease with apparent myalgia, dependent edema of the limbs, scrotal edema, mild conjunctivitis and palpebral edema. The severity of signs of diseases may vary greatly in individuals.

Lesions: In addition to lesions observable in the animals, the occasional fatal case may have pulmonary emphysema, pulmonary and mediastinal edema, excess fluids in the pleural and peritoneal cavities, enteritis, edema of the intestinal submucosa, and splenic hemorrhage and infarcts. Most gross lesions are attributable to vascular lesions consisting of histopathologically evident thrombus formation, endothelial swelling, and a characteristic degeneration and necrosis of the media of arteries and venules, particularly smaller ones.

Diagnosis: Clinical diagnosis usually requires a composite of signs and lesions in several horses. Differential diagnosis includes equine viral rhinopneumonitis (EVR), equine influenza, and sometimes African horse sickness, equine infectious anemia and purpura hemorrhagica.

The occurrence of abortion during or just following illness is a valuable diagnostic feature because abortion rarely accompanies influenza and the mare is usually healthy at the time of EVR abortion. Fetuses aborted due to EVR (q.v., p. 308) usually have characteristic lesions, while those aborted due to arteritis have neither specific lesions nor inclusion bodies.

Since few laboratories work with this virus, it is advisable to get instructions from the laboratory prior to collecting specimens for serologic or virologic diagnosis.

Prophylaxis and Treatment: There is no specific treatment; antibacterial drugs and symptomatic therapy are indicated, and good nursing and absolute rest with very gradual return to activity are essential. Since experimentally developed vaccines are not commercially available, prevention is contingent on good hygiene and isolation.

EQUINE INFLUENZA

An acute, highly contagious febrile respiratory disease.

Etiology and Epidemiology: Presently, 2 immunologically distinct influenza viruses are endemic among horses throughout the world. Myxovirus A-equi-1 has probably been present for decades. Myxovirus A-equi-2 was first recognized in 1963 as a cause of widespread epidemics, which subsided leaving the virus established endemically. The endemic state is maintained throughout the year by sporadic clinical cases, and by mild or inapparent infection of susceptible horses which constantly join the population by birth, immigration or waning immunity. It is not known if a carrier state exists. Consequences of exposure are largely determined by previous immunologic conditioning, and in susceptible animals vary from mild inapparent infection to a severe disease that is rarely fatal except in very young, very old or otherwise debilitated patients. Epidemics are propagated by contact with respiratory secretions and result when one or more actively infected horses join an aggregation of susceptible horses assembled for show, sales, training or racing.

Clinical Findings: The incubation period is usually 1 to 3 days with a range of 18 hours, to 5 and rarely 7 days. The onset is abrupt, with temperature up to 107.5°F (42°C), usually lasting less than 3 days unless bacterial infection follows. Coughing is observed early and may persist for several weeks. Nasal discharge is scant. Expiratory dyspnea, anorexia, weakness and stiffness are sometimes present. Mildly affected horses recover spontaneously within 2 to 3 weeks, but those severely affected may convalesce for 6 months. Recovery from the incapacitating signs and cough are hastened by completely restricting strenuous activities.

Complications such as bacterial infections, chronic bronchitis, asthmatic conditions and pulmonary emphysema are best prevented by restricting exercise, controlling dust, providing superior ventilation and practicing good stable hygiene.

Lesions: Usually no lesions are observed in live patients. At necropsy, interstitial pneumonia, bronchitis, peribronchitis and perivasculitis may be seen.

Diagnosis: In individual cases, laboratory assistance may be needed to differentiate influenza from equine viral rhinopneumonitis, equine viral arteritis and miscellaneous equine respiratory viral infections (q.v., p. 307). Equine influenza is usually diagnosed on observation of fast-spreading disease with rapid onset, high fever, weakness and cough; virologic or serologic study require instructions from a consenting laboratory.

Prophylaxis: Where available, bivalent inactivated vaccines should be administered annually. Probability of exposure can be reduced by isolation of new additions to stables and by minimizing contact with other horses.

Treatment: Horses without complications require only rest and nursing but antibiotics (℞ 27, 50, 66, 76) are indicated when fever persists beyond 3 to 4 days or when purulent nasal discharges or pulmonary involvement are evident. Restricted exercise is mandatory (*see* **Clinical Findings, above**).

COMPLICATIONS OF EQUINE VIRAL RESPIRATORY DISEASES

Bacterial infections may appear during or following viral infections and produce a mucopurulent nasal exudate, persistent fever, lymphadenitis, persistent cough, leukocytosis, laryngitis, bronchitis or pneumonia.

Upper respiratory inflammation may extend into the sinuses, eustachian tubes or guttural pouches. Toxicosis or pleuritis may accompany pneumonia. These complications are more frequent and more severe at collection points and racing and training grounds than on farms. *Streptococcus zooepidemicus*, a common secondary invader, is isolated frequently from the upper respiratory tract and sometimes from lungs or pleural exudate. *Actinobacillus equuli*, *Bordetella bronchiseptica*, *Pasteurella* spp. and *Escherichia coli* are isolated less frequently. *Pseudomonas aeruginosa* may be involved in persistent coughing and other upper respiratory complications. Isolation of *Str. equi* indicates primary or secondary strangles (*see* below). Mycoplasmas of unknown significance are sometimes isolated.

PROPHYLAXIS AND TREATMENT OF RESPIRATORY DISEASES AND THEIR COMPLICATIONS

Prophylaxis: Vaccines of variable effectiveness are available for equine influenza, viral rhinopneumonitis and strangles. General recommendations are impossible in view of the various views of different national regulatory agencies and the rapid development of new vaccines. The cost and hazards of each vaccination must be weighed against the probability of exposure and potential losses in economic and sentimental value. The strength of arguments supporting vaccination increase with the probability of exposure.

Treatment: Most acute equine respiratory disease is clinically diagnosed tentatively as rhinopneumonitis, arteritis, influenza, or influenza-like conditions lacking distinctive signs and possibly due to numerous viruses (q.v., p. 307). Rarely is a definite laboratory diagnosis available when therapy is instituted.

Regardless of etiology, restricted exercise, careful observation and confinement in comfortable, draft-free quarters with palatable feed and fresh water are fundamental. Confinement should begin at onset of fever and continue at least 10 to 14 days or longer, if complications appear. Failure to restrict exercise contributes to severity and duration of illness and development of serious sequelae.

Antipyretics and corticosteroids may obscure signs and mask the need for antibacterial therapy, which should be instituted when fever persists beyond 3 to 5 days or when mucopurulent nasal or pharyngeal exudate appears. Penicillin (℞ 66) and streptomycin (℞ 73), or both, are common initial choices, with supplementation with sulfonamides (℞ 96, 102, 105) and the addition of broad-spectrum antibiotics (℞ 27, 39, 50, 76) to the regimen in unresponsive cases.

Persistent coughs unresponsive to antibiotic therapy require rest and may respond to therapy with iodides (℞ 595, 601, 605) or nitrofuran (℞ 121) or pharyngeal applications of corticosteroid-antibacterial combinations.

STRANGLES

A contagious suppurative regional lymphadenitis of Equidae only, characterized by the occurrence of abscesses in lymph nodes draining the upper respiratory and buccal mucosae.

Etiology and Epidemiology: The causal agent, *Streptococcus equi*, is a β hemolytic, antigenically equine streptococcus (Lancefield Group C). In its endemic form, strangles is a disease of the young but animals of any age without previous infection or in which immunity has lapsed may contract it. The source of infection is the diseased animal or an environment contaminated by pus from strangles abscesses. *Str. equi* is capable of surviving in infectious form for months on fomites or in barns. Whether the asymptomatic carrier stage exists is unknown. Concomitant or predisposing viral infections are not requisite but apparently contribute to the rapid spread of strangles.

Clinical Findings: The incubation period for experimental strangles is 3 to 6 days. Usually the first sign noticed is refusal to consume feed and water. A temperature as high as 106°F (41°C) and catarrhal inflammation of the upper respiratory mucosa and lymphadenitis of the lymphoid nodules of the pharynx develop in the first day or two. Mucopurulent nasal discharge appears when these multiple small abscesses drain. Affected animals are reluctant to swallow and may stand with the neck extended. The infection spreads to the dependent intermandibular and parapharyngeal lymph nodes, which become abscessed. The parapharyngeal nodes are those most commonly involved and the infection may extend from this site to the anterior cervical nodes. The disease is usually contained at the parapharyngeal level and when the abscesses mature and drain, fever lyses and in most cases rapid healing occurs. The course of the disease is approximately 2 weeks for individuals but the course of an outbreak in a herd may extend over several months. If prophylactic measures are not adopted, the disease recurs with the addition of new horses to the herd and with the advent of each crop of foals.

Morbidity in the epidemic form is usually high and mortality low (less than 2%). Death when it occurs is frequently the result of infection of the CNS or formation of abscesses in viscera. Nonsuppurative myocarditis may result; electrocardiography has detected abnormalities in about half of the horses affected. These persist for a few days to as long as several months. Purpura hemorrhagica (q.v., p. 48) may occur as a sequela or even during the course of the more chronic forms of the disease. Empyema of the guttural pouches may occur. However, most horses appear to recover without sequelae.

A more chronic form known as **bastard strangles** may occur. This disease affects individuals only and is not epidemic. It is characterized by abscess formation in many areas of the body over a period of weeks or months and by rapidly progressing cachexia and intermittent fever. This form of disease is likely conditioned by failure of some patients to muster a serviceable immune response and to confine disease to the lymph nodes of the upper respiratory tract. Treatment of horses with penicillin at an inopportune moment in the course of events that lead to the primary immune response may contribute to the development of "bastard strangles" because of the modification of streptococcal cell wall antigens by the antibiotic.

Diagnosis: When strangles occurs in epidemic form, its clinical features are difficult to mistake. High fever and the formation of abscesses in the lymph nodes of the head and pharyngeal region are almost pathognomonic. Infection of the upper respiratory mucosa and lymph nodes by *Streptococcus zooepidemicus* secondary to viral disease may mimic strangles but the fever and the characteristic rapid development of abscesses serve to differentiate the disease clinically. Definitive diagnosis depends on identification of *Str. equi*, preferably from pus obtained upon surgical drainage of mature abscesses. Strangles abscesses that drain naturally are rapidly invaded by *Str. zooepidemicus* and may confuse bacteriologic diagnosis. Identification of *Str. equi* from one horse (whether or not typical signs of strangles are seen) is reliable warning of the imminence of this disease in the herd.

Prophylaxis: Horses with mucopurulent nasal discharges or other suggestive signs should be isolated and cultures made before such animals are added to herds free of strangles. If *Str. equi* is identified from these, they should be kept in strict isolation until they are free of the infection.

A killed bacterin may be administered as a 6 ml total dose IM, in three 2-ml injections given 2 to 4 weeks apart. Vaccinated horses may experience a transient fever, and a local reaction at the site of the injection, the severity of which varies considerably. Abscess formation at the site of the injection usually is caused by immunization of animals in the incubative stage, or those recently recovered from the disease. A severe local reaction following the first or second injection contraindicates continuing the series. Vaccination failure due to antigenic differences in *Str. equi* strains has not been observed.

Treatment: *Str. equi* is very sensitive to penicillin, and resistance to this antibiotic is rare. Sulfamerazine and sulfamethazine are also effective. Early, prompt and continued treatment (℞ 62, 96, 102) may prevent abscess formation. Once begun, treatment must be continued until the temperature has remained normal for several days. After phlegmon or abscess formation occurs, systemic treatment may only prolong the course of the disease.

Complete rest and nursing should be provided. Abscesses may be hot-packed, and when mature should be surgically drained. Severe dyspnea usually indicates compression of the pharynx or larynx from a retropharyngeal abscess and a tracheotomy may become necessary.

PASTEURELLOSIS OF SHEEP

Pasteurellosis of sheep is caused almost invariably by *Pasteurella haemolytica*. There are 2 distinct syndromes: biotype A strains cause **pneumonia** in flocks and sporadically in individuals; biotype T strains cause a **peracute septicemia.** The factors that predispose sheep to the different forms of the disease are poorly understood. One or more of environmental stress situations, immune deficits or prior viral infection (e.g. parainfluenza 3 virus) are usually involved.

P. haemolytica is present in the nasopharynx, tonsillar tissues, lungs and small intestines of healthy sheep. Disease should not be attributed to pasteurellae unless they are recovered in large numbers, appropriate lesions are found and other causes eliminated.

Enzootic pneumonia is the term given to flock outbreaks of pneumonia caused by biotype A. It occurs in sheep under all conditions of management. In lambs under about 2 months of age the disease is more often septicemic than pneumonic. An outbreak usually starts suddenly with sheep dying or acutely ill with obvious respiratory disease. Other sheep in the flock show signs of mild respiratory involvement—coughing and mild oculo-nasal discharge. Mortality rarely exceeds 10%. Physical stresses have been suggested as precipitating factors. Concurrent parainfluenza 3 virus infection has also been incriminated as a predisposing cause. At necropsy of sheep with the acute disease there is fibrinous pericardial effusion and a clear pleural exudate with fibrin clots. The lungs are enlarged, edematous and bright purplish red, sometimes without distinct areas of consolidation. In sheep that have survived longer, the lesions are more sharply demarcated and a darker red, and there are adhesions between the pleurae. Diagnosis depends on the recovery of large numbers of *P. haemolytica* biotype A from the lesions described. Biotype T strains are rarely isolated under these circumstances.

The administration of oxytetracycline at a dose of 1 to 3 mg/lb (2 to 7 mg/kg) daily is the therapy of choice. Vaccines against *P. haemolytica* are available but the value of those currently available is not fully established.

The **septicemic form of the disease** (other than in lambs) is caused by biotype T strains. The epidemiology is poorly understood. The disease often manifests itself a few days after sheep, especially those about 6 months old, have been moved to better nutrition. Deaths often occur in those in best condition and continue for a few days, total mortality being as high as 20%. Affected sheep are usually found dead. Those seen alive are dull, unwilling to move, have dyspnea, a frothy discharge from the mouth and, unless in the terminal stages, an elevated temperature. At necropsy, there is evidence of a septicemia. Hemorrhagic exudative inflammation of the abomasal mucosa and blood splashing on the visceral peritoneum, in the neck and beneath the parietal pleural are prominent features. The kidneys may show cortical softening as in pulpy kidney disease. Pure cultures of *P. haemolytica* biotype T are recovered from the organs and heart blood. Acute toxicoses, metabolic disorders and septicemias caused by organisms other than pasteurellae should be considered under differential diagnosis. Antibiotic therapy cannot often be applied and the value of vaccination is in doubt. Gradual introduction to food of increased nutritive value should be practiced.

P. haemolytica also causes mastitis, meningitis and arthritis.

PASTEURELLOSIS OF SWINE

The commonest syndrome, an important complication of mycoplasma pneumonia, q.v., p. 319, is usually caused by *Pasteurella multocida*. It is a **bronchopneumonia**, sometimes with pericarditis and pleuritis. Primary **sporadic fibrinous pneumonia** due to pasteurellae with no epidemiological connection with mycoplasma pneumonia occurs generally in pigs over one year old. In both primary and secondary forms there is a tendency to develop chronic thoracic lesions and polyarthritis. Diagnosis is based on necropsy findings and the recovery of pasteurellae from the lesions.

Septicemic pasteurellosis and meningitis occasionally occur in piglets. *P. haemolytica* has been recovered from aborted fetuses. Septicemia also occurs in adult pigs. There are no distinctive lesions and the pathogenesis is obscure.

Control of the secondary, pneumonic form of the disease is based on the prevention or control of mycoplasma pneumonia. Early and vigorous antibiotic therapy for all forms of the disease is indicated to prevent chronic sequelae. An increasing resistance to penicillin, streptomycin and tetracycline has been noted among the pasteurellae.

SWINE INFLUENZA
(Hog flu, Pig flu)

An acute, highly contagious respiratory disease caused primarily by a Type-A influenza virus.

Etiology: Although the virus is the primary cause, outbreaks are frequently complicated by *Haemophilus influenza suis* (*see also* GLASSER'S DISEASE, p. 353) and sometimes by other bacteria. Stress is an important predisposing factor. The virus is unlikely to survive outside living cells for more than 14 days except in very cold conditions. It is readily inactivated by disinfectants.

Epidemiology: The disease is most common in the Midwestern U.S.A. during the fall and winter. It occurs occasionally in other states, and some other countries (e.g. Germany, Czechoslovakia and Kenya). In the U.S.A., outbreaks occur frequently in autumn on different farms within an area. It is thought that the virus is widely seeded before the outbreaks begin. Outbreaks are provoked by the onset of cold inclement weather, or other stress factors. The disease then spreads rapidly within a herd mainly by airborne infection.

One mechanism of survival between epidemics involves the swine lungworm as a vector. Lungworm eggs containing the virus are passed in the feces of infected pigs and ingested by earthworms, and the infected earthworms are eaten by pigs. The lungworm larvae then migrate to the lungs. The pigs remain clinically normal and noninfective until the disease is precipitated by stress.

The virus may also survive between outbreaks in a subclinical form in carrier pigs. It has been isolated from the lungs of recovered pigs 3 months after infection.

Clinical Findings: A typical outbreak is characterized by sudden onset and rapid spread through the entire herd, often within 1 to 3 days. The main signs are depression, fever, anorexia, coughing, dyspnea, muscular weakness, prostration, and a mucous discharge from the eyes and nose.

The mortality is generally about 1 to 4%. The course of the disease usually varies from 3 to 7 days, with recovery of the herd almost as sudden as the onset. However, some pigs may become chronically affected. In herds that are in good condition, the principal economic loss is from stunting and delay in reaching market weight.

Lesions: The lesions are usually confined to the chest cavity. The pneumonic areas are clearly demarcated, collapsed, and purplish red. They may be distributed throughout the lungs but tend to be more extensive and confluent ventrally. Nonpneumonic areas are pale and emphysematous. The respiratory airways contain a copious mucopurulent exudate and the bronchial and mediastinal lymph nodes are edematous, but rarely congested. There may be severe pulmonary edema or a serous or serofibrinous pleuritis. Histologically, the lesions are primarily those of an exudative bronchiolitis.

Diagnosis: In typical outbreaks, a fairly firm presumptive diagnosis can be made on clinical and pathologic findings alone but, in atypical outbreaks, it may be necessary to confirm the diagnosis by laboratory tests. Embryonated hens' eggs can be used to isolate the virus from nasal swabs or affected lung tissue in the early acute stage of the disease, or a retrospective diagnosis can be made by taking serum samples during the acute and convalescent stages and demonstrating a rise in specific antibodies using the hemagglutination-inhibition test.

Control: Prevention of swine influenza is not practical except in conditions where pigs can be reared free from lungworms. Experimentally, vaccines may confer some protection but it is doubtful whether they are justified economically. There is no specific treatment, but antibiotics, good husbandry and freedom from stress help to reduce losses.

MYCOPLASMAL PNEUMONIA OF SWINE

(Enzootic pneumonia, EP, Virus pneumonia of pigs, VPP)

A chronic, clinically mild, infectious respiratory disease of pigs, characterized mainly by its ability to become permanently endemic in a herd and to produce a persistent, dry cough, sporadic "flare ups" of overt respiratory distress, and a high incidence of lung lesions in slaughter pigs.

Etiology: The terms "virus pneumonia" and "enzootic pneumonia" are frequently used to describe a characteristic disease syndrome now known to be caused primarily by *Mycoplasma hyopneumoniae* (*suipneumoniae*). It is a fastidious pleomorphic organism, smaller than most bacteria, and difficult to see clearly under ordinary light microscopes. It can be cultured in specially prepared media, but its isolation from field cases is difficult. It is rapidly inactivated in the environment and by disinfectants, but it may survive longer periods in cold weather. It appears to be host-specific. Field investigations suggest that different strains of *M. hyopneumoniae* vary in pathogenicity.

In addition, mycoplasmal pneumonia is frequently complicated by other mycoplasms, bacteria and viruses, which also affect the severity of the disease. There is some evidence that certain strains of *Mycoplasma hyorhinis* and perhaps some viruses may themselves act as primary agents to produce a syndrome resembling mycoplasmal pneumonia.

Epidemiology: Mycoplasmal pneumonia occurs worldwide. In most countries where modern pig farming methods are practiced, the lungs of between 30 and 80% of the swine slaughtered show pneumonic lesions of the type associated with mycoplasmal infection. Pigs of all ages are susceptible but within a herd pigs become infected in the first few weeks of life either by their dam, or other young pigs after mixing. The incidence of lung lesions is highest in pigs between 2 and 4 months of age. Immunity develops slowly, the lung lesions regress, and adult pigs may recover completely.

Economic Importance: Clinical outbreaks of mycoplasmal pneumonia may impair growth rate and feed conversion. The effect is enhanced where large number of pigs are closely confined in poorly ventilated buildings under poor husbandry conditions. The effects of the disease are uneven and unpredictable, placing limits on the efficiency and flexibility of large production units. However, in good modern units with good disease control mycoplasmal pneumonia remains largely subclinical and of little economic importance.

Clinical Findings: In herds in which the disease is endemic, the morbidity is high but clinical signs may be minimal and mortality is low. Coughing is the commonest sign and is most obvious when pigs are roused. The disease tends to flare up sporadically in individual pigs or groups of pigs into a clinically severe pneumonia. A common predisposing factor is a change of weather, usually to hot, humid conditions, but other stresses, such as transient viral infections, may also cause flare-ups. The disease is usually more severe when it first enters a herd, and pigs in all age groups may be affected.

Lesions: The lesions in the lungs are gray or purple, and commonest in the apical and cardiac lobes. Old lesions become clearly outlined. The associated lymph nodes may be enlarged. Histologically, inflammatory cells are present in the bronchioles, there is perivascular and peribronchiolar cuffing, and extensive lymphoid hyperplasia.

Diagnosis: A diagnosis based on clinical, pathologic and epidemiologic findings is adequate for most practical purposes. When necessary, *M. hyopneumoniae* can be demonstrated in touch preparations of the cut surface of the affected lung, identified by the fluorescent antibody technique, and sometimes isolated and identified in culture. Certain serologic tests, principally the complement fixation test, are used sometimes on a herd basis.

Mycoplasmal pneumonia should be differentiated from swine influenza (q.v., p. 317), pasteurellosis (q.v., p. 317), *Bordetella* pneumonia, severe ascariasis, lungworm and other pneumonias.

Control: When the disease first enters a herd, mass treatment with macrolide antibiotics such as tylosin or one of the tetracyclines helps to control the severity of signs. When the disease flares up in herds in which it is endemic, treatment of individual pigs with antibiotics usually results in a remission of the overt signs, presumably by controlling secondary bacteria.

Inactivated mycoplasmal cultures have been developed as vaccines but so far their merit cannot be judged.

The economic effects of the disease can be reduced, sometimes eliminated, by improvements in housing and husbandry, paying particular attention to ventilation and overcrowding.

In large intensive units, it may be advisable, where possible, to start with foundation stock from breeding herds that are mycoplasma-pneumonia-free and to adopt precautions against direct and indirect contact with other herds. The problem is that many herds that are set up in this way do not remain free of mycoplasmas for long periods, particularly in pig-dense areas.

In the U.S.A. and parts of Europe most of the mycoplasma-pneumonia-free supply herds were established originally by the specific pathogen-free (SPF) swine repopulation technique. Other methods of eradicating the disease have proved less reliable. However, in Britain conventional purebred breeding herds have been found in which enzootic pneumonia could not be detected and these have been used to supply pneumonia-free stock. The biggest difficulties with mycoplasmal-pneumonia-free herd programs are the breakdown rate and the difficulty of ensuring that the causal agents of the disease are indeed absent from all the herds enrolled.

CONTAGIOUS BOVINE PLEUROPNEUMONIA

A highly contagious pneumonia generally accompanied by pleurisy. It is present in Africa, parts of India and China, and minor outbreaks occur in the Middle East. The U.S.A. has been free of the disease since 1892, Britain since 1898 and Australia since 1973.

Etiology: The causal organism is *Mycoplasma mycoides* subsp. *mycoides*. (*See also* CONTAGIOUS CAPRINE PLEUROPNEUMONIA, p. 323.) Susceptible cattle become infected by inhaling droplets coughed out by affected cattle. Urine droplets are a possible additional source. The incubation period of the disease varies from 2 to 17 weeks following contact, with most cases occurring within 5 to 8 weeks. In some localities susceptible herds may show 100% morbidity with high mortality, but lower rates of infection are commoner. Some infected animals may, however, show few outward signs of the disease, but the lung lesion often becomes necrotic and is then surrounded by a fibrous capsule. Within this sequestrum the organism may remain viable for up to 10 months. Such animals are carriers and may be infective, but whether in this state or when breakdown of the sequestrum occurs, is not clear. As carriers may not be detectable clinically or serologically they constitute a serious problem in control programs. There are no other natural hosts.

Clinical Findings: The signs, which are typical of pneumonia and pleurisy, are high temperature (up to 107°F [41.5°C]), anorexia, thirst, and painful, difficult breathing. The animal often stands by itself in the shade in hot climates, its head lowered and extended, its back slightly arched and the elbows turned out. Respiration is rapid, shallow and abdominal and, if the animal is forced to move quickly, the breathing becomes more distressed and a soft, moist cough may result. In acute cases the disease progresses rapidly, animals lose condition and breathing becomes very labored, with a grunt at expiration. The animal becomes recumbent, with death ensuing in a few hours. Less acutely affected cattle exhibit signs of varying intensity for 3 to 4 weeks. Often in these cases, the lesion gradually resolves and the animal makes an apparent recovery.

Lesions: The thoracic cavity may contain up to 10 L of clear yellow or turbid fluid mixed with fibrin flakes, and the organs in the thorax are often covered by thick deposits of fibrin. Varying areas of one or both lungs may be involved, the affected portion being enlarged and having the consistency of liver. On section, the typical marbled appearance of pleuropneumonia is evident—due to the thickening of the interlobular septa and subpleural tissue enclosing gray, yellow or red hepatized portions of the alveolar lung tissue. In chronic or carrier cases, the lesion is sequestered in a thick, fibrous tissue capsule and is necrotic; it retains its structure both at gross and microscopic examination.

Diagnosis: Diagnosis is made on clinical and postmortem examination. Confirmation is obtained from the complement fixation test on serum, the precipitin test on lesions (to detect specific antigen) and bacteriologic and histologic examination of lesions. Subclinical disease is detected by use of the complement fixation test. As soon as an outbreak is suspected, slaughter and detailed postmortem examination of a suspect animal are advisable.

Control: In developed countries, where cattle movement can readily be restricted, the disease can be eradicated by quarantine, blood testing and immunization with live vaccine. Where cattle cannot be confined the spread of infection can be limited by vaccination. Tracing of the source of infected cattle detected at abattoirs, blood testing and imposition of strict rules for cattle movement can also contribute to the control of the disease in such areas. The disease is "notifiable" in many countries, where it is by law eradicated by slaughter of all infected and exposed animals..

Treatment is not recommended because necrotic lesions may already be established and these will continue to harbor live organisms.

CONTAGIOUS CAPRINE PLEUROPNEUMONIA

A contagious pneumonia with pleurisy, which occurs in goats in many parts of the Middle East, Africa and Asia, less commonly in Mediterranean countries, Mexico and the U.S.A.

Etiology: Until recently *Mycoplasma mycoides* subsp. *capri* has been regarded as the sole responsible organism but *Mycoplasma mycoides* subsp. *mycoides* (the large colony type recently described) is now commonly isolated. (*See* CONTAGIOUS BOVINE PLEUROPNEUMONIA, p. 321.) In addition, a different mycoplasma known only as F38 has been responsible for a number of outbreaks of contagious caprine pleuropneumonia in Kenya. The disease appears to be transmitted by infective aerosols. The incubation period is from 2 to 28 days, and on sickening the animal rapidly deteriorates and may die within 7 days. Morbidity can be from 60 to 100% and mortality may approach 100%. The greater incidence in winter may be due to housing of animals where optimal conditions for transmission occur.

Clinical Findings: Loss of condition, weakness and a staring coat are constant features. Copious nasal discharge, loss of appetite, a cough and signs of respiratory involvement may be present and abortion may occur.

Lesions: The thorax contains excess straw-colored fluid and the consolidated lung is usually covered with soft spongy fibrin. The pneumonia area is sometimes confined to one lung and the characteristic features are distension of interlobular septa with fluid and the variation in color of the lobules according to the stage of consolidation. Lesions seldom if ever become necrotic and sequestered; they may slowly resolve. Histologically both bronchopneumonia and lobar pneumonia are seen. Pericarditis often occurs.

Diagnosis: The clinical signs, epidemiology and postmortem appearance are used to establish a diagnosis. The causative organism should be isolated and identified but isolation may be difficult in some cases. The filamentous forms of the mycoplasma can often be detected on dark ground microscopic examination of the pleural fluid from acute cases. There are no serological tests in general use, but complement fixation tests may be useful.

Control: Quarantine of affected flocks is desirable. Vaccines, both killed and live, have been used but their efficacy has not yet been established. Treatment with tylosin daily at 4.5 mg/lb (10 mg/kg), IM for 3 days has been effective.

FELINE RESPIRATORY DISEASES

The feline respiratory disease complex comprises several syndromes characterized by sneezing, rhinitis, conjunctivitis, salivation, lacrimation and oral ulcerations. The important diseases are **feline rhinotracheitis** (FVR), and **feline calicivirus infection** (FCI), with **chlamydial** (FPN) and **mycoplasmal infections** being of lesser importance.

Etiology: Probably 40 to 45% of feline upper respiratory infections are a result of infections with FVR virus, a herpesvirus. Feline caliciviruses may account for another 40 to 45% of naturally occurring upper respiratory infections in cats. Dual infections also occur frequently with the feline herpesvirus and calicivirus. Other agents such as *Chlamydia psittaci* (pneumonitis), mycoplasma (PPLO), and reovirus are believed to account for most of the remaining 10 to 20% of the feline respiratory infections. The importance of the reovirus as a feline pathogen is unknown.

Natural transmission of these agents occurs by aerosol droplets and fomites, and the viruses may be carried from an infected to a susceptible cat by a handler. The agents persist in an infected cat for up to 11 months and may be shed continuously (caliciviruses) or intermittently (herpesvirus) by an apparently recovered cat. Stress may precipitate a secondary attack.

The incubation period is generally short (2 to 6 days) with FVR and 5 to 10 days in the case of pneumonitis and as long as 19 days with reovirus.

Clinical Findings: The onset of **FVR** is marked by fever, frequent sneezing, conjunctivitis, rhinitis and often by salivation. Excitement or movement may induce sneezing. The fever may reach 105°F (40.5°C), subside and tend to fluctuate from normal to 103°F (39°C). Initially, a serous nasal and ocular discharge occurs, which soon becomes mucopurulent and copious. By this time depression and anorexia are evident. Ulcers may appear on the dorsal surface of the tongue and ulcerative keratitis occurs in some patients with cases of FVR. FVR tends to be most severe in young kittens. Signs in adults may be limited to sneezing and a slight serous conjunctivitis and rhinitis. Signs may persist for 5 to 10 days in milder cases, and up to 3 to 6 weeks in severe cases. Mortality is generally low and prognosis is usually good except in young kittens and aged cats. The owner should be cautioned that the illness is often prolonged and a marked weight loss may occur, and occasionally the disease is complicated by bacterial infections. Abortions and generalized infections have been associated with the respiratory form of FVR infection.

There are many strains of **feline caliciviruses** that cause a variety of clinical illnesses, from mild to severe infections. Some caliciviruses induce a mild disease that is associated with fever, anorexia, salivation and ulcers, which may occur on the tongue, hard palate, or on the nostrils 2 to 3 days after infection. The ulcers usually heal rapidly and the infected cat is eating 2 to 3 days after the onset of illness. Others may cause a severe infection resulting in a fatal pulmonary edema and interstitial pneumonia. If the disease is not fatal, the course tends to be only 7 to 10 days. Serous rhinitis, conjunctivitis and an acute febrile response are common signs in feline calicivirus infections. The feline calicivirus appears to have a predilection for the epithelium of the oral cavity and the deep tissues of the lung.

Chlamydia psittaci (**feline pneumonitis**) infections are primarily characterized by a conjunctivitis. In acute infection the conjunctivitis is later accompanied by fever, serous lacrimation and an ocular discharge that becomes purulent. The animal tends to improve but may relapse.

Mycoplasma (PPLO) may infect the eyes and respiratory passages of the cat; characteristically they produce a severe chemosis (edema) of the conjunctiva and a less severe rhinitis.

Lesions: Lesions are generally confined to the oral cavity, respiratory tract and conjunctiva. In FVR the conjunctiva and nasal mucous membranes are reddened, swollen and covered with a serous to purulent exudate. In severe cases focal necrosis of the mucosa of the nasal passages and turbinates may occur. The larynx and trachea may be mildly inflamed. The lungs may be congested and show small areas of consolidation; however, the pulmonary lesions are not usually remarkable in FVR. Ulcerative glossitis and ulcerative stomatitis may occur. The characteristic histopathologic lesion of rhinotracheitis is the acidophilic intranuclear inclusion body in the epithelial cells of the tongue, nasal membranes, tonsils, epiglottis, trachea and nictitating membrane. Inclusion bodies are transitory. Inclusions do not occur in calicivirus infections.

The characteristic lesions of the caliciviruses are the ulcerations of the oral mucosa. Lesions on the tongue or hard palate appear as vesicles, which subsequently rupture and ulcerate. Ulcerations occasionally occur on the epithelial covering of the median septum between the nostrils. The more virulent caliciviruses produce a cytolytic effect on the epithelial cells lining the bronchioles and alveoli. This results in an acute pulmonary edema and subsequent interstitial pneumonia with an accumulation of a seropurulent exudate in the alveoli and bronchioles. Conjunctivitis and rhinitis are common in feline calicivirus infections.

In the case of pneumonitis, Giemsa-stained sections will demonstrate elementary bodies in the cytoplasm of mononuclear cells of the conjunctiva and the alveolar and bronchial exudate. Mycoplasma occur as extracellular coccoid bodies.

Diagnosis: A presumptive diagnosis is based on the typical signs of sneezing, fever, conjunctivitis, rhinitis, lacrimation, salivation and oral ulcers. Cytologic examination of Giemsa-stained conjunctival scrapings is of diagnostic value for the feline pneumonitis agent and mycoplasma. A definitive diagnosis is based upon isolation and identification of the agent from the nasal and ocular secretions.

Prophylaxis: Modified live-virus FVR vaccines are available. Some of these vaccines are combined with an avirulent, broadly antigenic calicivirus to produce a feline rhinotracheitis-calicivirus vaccine, of which there are 2 types. The **first** type is for parenteral administration; 2 doses are recommended, the first when the kitten is 9 weeks of age or older and the second 3 weeks later. If a kitten is vaccinated before 9 weeks of age, it is recommended that it be revaccinated every 3 to 4 weeks until it is at least 12 weeks old. Annual revaccination is recommended unless the kitten is kept isolated or is in a nonendemic environment in which case booster doses every 6 months are recommended. The **second** type of feline rhinotracheitis-calicivirus vaccine is administered intranasally (IN). After reconstitution of the lyophilized vaccine, one drop is placed in each eye and the remaining vaccine is dropped into the nasal passages. Healthy kittens, 12 weeks of age or older, receive one vaccination. If under 12 weeks of age at the time of vaccination, a second dose is administered at 12 weeks of age or older. Transient sneezing may be observed 4 to 7 days after vaccination. Annual revaccination is recommended.

Almost immediate protection against rhinotracheitis is afforded by the intranasal vaccine. It is said to be protective against calicivirus exposure 72 hours after vaccination. The parenteral vaccines do not afford protection to a fully susceptible cat until several days after the second dose of vaccine. The disadvantage to the IN vaccine is the reaction (sneezing) that occurs after vaccination. The owner should be warned that this reaction is likely to occur.

A feline rhinotracheitis-calicivirus modified live-virus vaccine combined with an inactivated tissue-culture-origin panleukopenia vaccine is available. It is administered in the same manner as the parenteral feline rhinotracheitis-calicivirus vaccines. A feline rhinotracheitis-panleukopenia vaccine is also available.

A modified live feline rhinotracheitis-calicipneumonitis vaccine is also available. It may be given by the IM or subcut. route. As for other parenteral rhinotracheitis-calicivirus vaccines, 2 doses (3-week interval) are recommended, as is annual revaccination.

A modified live vaccine of egg origin is available for the prevention of pneumonitis. The vaccine is administered IM. It is indicated in catteries or on premises where a definite diagnosis of *Chlamydia psittaci* infection has been made. Kittens are vaccinated at weaning time and yearly thereafter. A combination FVR-calicivirus and pneumonitis vaccine is also available for parenteral administration.

The avoidance of exposure to sick cats, overcrowding and stress provides excellent protection against the upper respiratory diseases.

Treatment: Treatment is largely symptomatic and supportive but the broad-spectrum antibiotics (e.g., ℞ 1, 3, 13, 16, 40, 50, 56, 79) are useful against secondary invaders as well as directly against *Ch. psittaci*. Nasal and ocular discharges should be removed frequently for the comfort of the patient. Nose drops containing a vasoconstrictor and antibiotics (℞ 468, 475) and a bland ophthalmic ointment containing antibiotics (℞ 48, 389, 391) may be helpful. If dyspnea is severe, the animal may be placed in an oxygen tent. Supportive fluids (℞ 584, 589, 592) may be indicated to correct dehydration and force-feeding may be necessary to prevent the severe weight loss. Antihistamines (℞ 555) may be beneficial early in the course of the disease.

FELINE INFECTIOUS PERITONITIS AND PLEURITIS

A contagious viral infection of domestic cats and larger Felidae occurring in all ages, but more commonly in 6-month to 2-year-old cats.

Etiology and Epidemiology: The causal coronavirus is related antigenically to porcine transmissible gastroenteritis virus and canine coronavirus, but the viruses do not appear to be cross-protective. The mode of natural transmission has yet to be established, but the disease has been transferred by inoculation of susceptible cats with urine, blood, ascitic fluid, or suspensions of various tissues from affected cats.

Clinical Findings: The acute infection usually is asymptomatic but transient conjunctivitis or signs of low-grade upper respiratory infection may occur in some cats. The classic chronic disease, which develops weeks to months or years after infection in seropositive cats, is characterized by anorexia, depression, ascites, leukocytosis and pyrexia. More severely affected cats are moribund with a subnormal temperature. Some cats are anemic and exhibit vomiting or diarrhea.

Lesions: In the effusive, or "wet" form of the disease serosal surfaces of the abdominal and pleural cavities may be dull and granular and may be covered with fibrinous exudate. Pale yellow to dark amber fluid that may be clear or slightly cloudy and syrupy, with a high specific gravity (1.018 to 1.047), may be present in the peritoneal and pleural cavities. Few cells occur in the proteinaceous exudate but there may be whitish fibrin flakes. Variant forms of the disease include granulomatous peritonitis and pleuritis, meningoencephalitis, pneumonia, uveitis and nephritis.

Diagnosis: Presumptive diagnosis is based on the history of a persistent antibiotic-resistant fever, chronic debilitation and the presence of fluid exudates in body cavities. Moderate to severe anemia, relative neutrophilia and mild lymphopenia occur commonly. A shift in the protein A/G ratio, caused by hypergammaglobulinemia, is found in most cases. Homogenous "ground glass" fluid density may obscure detail in thoracic or abdominal radiographs. Infected cats develop moderate to high antiviral antibody titers. Immunofluorescent microscopy can be used for serologic confirmation of infection.

Control: Methods of prevention are not known. Treatment is ineffective.

FELINE INFECTIOUS ANEMIA

An acute or chronic anemia of domestic cats in many parts of the world caused by a rickettsial agent which multiplies within the vascular system.

Etiology: The causative agent, *Haemobartonella felis*, is a small, coccoid, rodlike, or ringlike organism, the dimensions of which vary from a diameter of 0.2 to 1.0 μ for the coccoid forms and up to 3.0 μ in length for the rod forms. The organisms are usually found in varying numbers on the surface of erythrocytes, but are occasionally seen free in the plasma. They appear as dark red-violet bodies in thin blood smears stained with Giemsa stain. The number of red cells affected varies with the severity of infection and with the stage in the life cycle of the parasite. The disease can be transmitted experimentally by parenteral or oral transfer of small amounts of infected whole blood into susceptible cats.

In experimentally induced cases the incubation period varies from 1 to 5 weeks, and recovery does not induce immunity to reinfection.

Methods of natural transmission have not been established; however, there appears to be a higher incidence among 1 to 3 year old cats, particularly males. A significant portion of the cat population may carry the infection in a latent form, which becomes exacerbated in the presence of various debilitating diseases or stresses. Infected cats may form antibodies to their own erythrocytes, resulting in autoimmune hemolytic anemia.

Clinical Findings: Any anemic cat may justly be suspected of having feline infectious anemia. In acute cases, there is usually a fever of 103 to 106°F (39 to 41°C). Jaundice, anorexia, depression, weakness and splenomegaly are common signs. In chronic or slowly developing cases there may be normal or subnormal temperature, weakness, depression and emaciation, but there is less likely to be jaundice and splenomegaly. Dyspnea in both instances varies with the degree of anemia. Gross necropsy findings are not distinctive. The spleen and mesenteric lymph nodes may be enlarged and a bone marrow hyperplasia may be present.

Diagnosis: Laboratory confirmation depends upon identification of the parasite in the peripheral blood or bone marrow. A series of smears over a period of several days may be required for an accurate diagnosis, because the erythrocytic bodies show up only periodically. Certain artifacts may be mistaken for blood parasites and must be carefully eliminated. The organisms are readily demonstrated in the affected cells when stained with acridine orange and examined by ultraviolet microscopy.

Blood cell changes typical of a regenerative anemia are present in positive smears. These include diffuse basophilic granules in the larger cells, nucleated erythrocytes, anisocytosis, Howell-Jolly bodies and an increased number of reticulocytes. Red cell counts may fall as low as 1 million per cubic millimeter. Hemoglobin values of 7 gm or less per 100 ml of blood are seen. Mean corpuscular volumes (average cell size) increase. There is a moderate increase in WBC counts with monocytosis in the acute forms of the disease, normal counts in the chronic forms and leukopenia in the moribund cases of the disease.

Prophylaxis and Treatment: Blood transfusion is the most effective treatment, particularly in acutely anemic animals. From 30 to 80 ml of whole blood should be given and repeated as required, perhaps every second or third day. Oxytetracycline (℞ 56) or tetracycline hydrochloride (℞ 76) should be given in full doses. To prevent relapses, drug treatments should be continued over a period of 10 to 20 days. Thiacetarsamide sodium (Caparsolate), an arsenical compound, given IV is reported to be effective; dosage is 0.5 ml/10 lb (0.1 ml/kg) on day 1, and repeated on day 3. Toxic reactions may occur, and transfusion should precede dosing if the hematocrit is less than 20%. The successful use of oxyphenarsine hydrochloride has been reported, as has the administration of prednisolone, to decrease the rate of hemolysis and reverse the depression associated with severe anemia.

In view of limited knowledge about the transmission of this disease, little can be recommended with reference to prophylaxis. Extreme care, however, should be exercised in selecting blood donor cats for general transfusions. Such donors should be checked for evidence of the carrier state by trial transfusion into susceptible experimental kittens.

FELINE PANLEUKOPENIA

(Feline infectious enteritis, Feline distemper, Feline agranulocytosis, Feline ataxia)

A highly contagious disease of cats, characterized by sudden onset, fever, anorexia, depression, dehydration, marked leukopenia and high mortality.

Etiology and Epidemiology: The disease is caused by a small DNA virus that attacks all members of the cat family (Felidae) and the raccoon, coati mundi, and kinkajou in the raccoon family (Procyonidae). Panleukopenia virus or the antigenically identical **mink enteritis virus** causes gastrointestinal disease in mink. All secretions and excretions of affected animals contain virus and the infection spreads through direct contact or by means of material contaminated with virus.

Clinical Findings: The incubation period varies from 4 to 10 days. With the onset of fever, animals stop eating, vomit and become depressed and weak. Diarrhea may occur 2 to 4 days after the initial temperature rise. Extreme dehydration occurs rapidly although affected cats seem to desire water. Shortly before the temperature becomes elevated, there is a decrease in leukocytes; later the leukopenia increases markedly to the point that sometimes few leukocytes can be found. The granulocytes are chiefly affected so that a differential cell count will show the few remaining cells to be of the lymphoid series. If the cat recovers, a compensatory leukocytosis may occur. The course of the disease seldom exceeds 5 to 7 days. Mortality is high, especially in young cats, and losses from 60 to 90% are reported. Infection of kittens *in utero* or within a few days after birth results in the destruction of the external granular layer of the cerebellum (cerebellar hypoplasia), which is manifest clinically by incoordination noted when the kitten begins to walk (**feline cerebellar ataxia**).

Lesions: These correlate closely with signs of illness. There is marked dehydration and emaciation except in very acute cases where gross changes may be negligible. The first changes are found in lymph nodes and consist of hyperplasia, edema and necrosis. Later, the red marrow of the long bones may become semifluid and appear fatty. Reddening may be seen in the terminal portion of the ileum and sometimes extends to involve most of the small intestine. Microscopically, the epithelium of the villi of affected portions of the intestine shows degeneration and the intestinal wall may be edematous. The liver, kidneys and spleen may appear slightly swollen. Degeneration of liver cells and tubular epithelium of the kidney is seen. Intranuclear inclusion bodies are found in the cells of the intestinal epithelium and lymph nodes; however, these can be found only early in the disease and may not be found in cats surviving 3 to 4 days. When recovery occurs, a marked myelogenous cellular response is seen.

Prophylaxis and Treatment: Recovered cats are immune. Feline tissue culture origin attenuated (modified live) virus or inactivated vaccines are recommended. Combinations of modified live feline rhinotracheitis virus and calicivirus inactivated panleukopenia vaccines are also available. The attenuated vaccine should not be given to pregnant cats or kittens less than 4 weeks of age because of the possibility of inducing feline cerebellar ataxia in the kittens. Annual revaccination is recommended.

Feline homologous antiserum offers good temporary protection for 7 to 10 days but it may interfere with subsequent use of vaccine if given within 2 to 3 weeks. Antiserum may be indicated, at a rate of 2 to 4 ml/kg of body wt subcut., for use in susceptible cats that have been exposed to panleukopenia or in colostrum-deprived kittens immediately after birth.

Since antibodies, passively transmitted to the kittens by an immune dam, may interfere with the establishment of active immunity, it is recommended that kittens be vaccinated after weaning at 8 to 10 weeks of age. If tissue-culture-origin inactivated vaccines must be used, a second dose is recommended 2 weeks after the first. To assure that maternally transmitted antibodies are no longer at a possibly interfering level, a third dose at 16 weeks of age is recommended. If tissue-culture-origin attenuated virus vaccines are used, the second dose should be given when the kitten is 14 to 16 weeks of age. If the kitten is 12 weeks old or older when first vaccinated with attenuated virus vaccine a second dose is unnecessary.

Tissue culture origin attenuated or inactivated vaccines will confer protection against virulent panleukopenia virus exposure 72 hours or possibly slightly less after vaccination.

Treatment should be aimed at combating dehydration, providing nutrients and electrolytes, and preventing secondary infection. During the first few days, treatment should be parenteral since most patients with panleukopenia will vomit oral medication. Whole-blood transfusions are valuable: Ten to 20 ml of blood per kg of body wt should be administered daily or every other day during the acute phase of the disease. Dehydration should be counteracted with fluids given IV or subcut. at a minimal rate of 20 mg/kg of body wt per day. A balanced electrolyte solution, Ringer's or lactated Ringer's (℞ 588, 589), is preferred for this treatment. Broad-spectrum antibiotics, e.g. tetracycline (℞ 79), oxytetracycline (℞ 50, 56), chloramphenicol (℞ 16), amoxicillin (℞ 1), ampicillin (℞ 3), cephaloridine (℞ 13) or gentamicin (℞ 40), may be of value in combating secondary infections. Given at the rate of 4 ml/kg of body wt per day in the very early stages of the disease antiserum may be of some value.

CANINE DISTEMPER

A highly contagious viral disease of dogs characterized by a diphasic temperature elevation, leukopenia, gastrointestinal and respiratory catarrh, and frequently pneumonic and neurologic complications.

Etiology and Epidemiology: Canine distemper is caused by a specific paramyxovirus closely related to the viruses of measles and rinderpest. The virus is universal and unless isolated, most dogs are exposed as puppies. Transmission occurs by the aerosol droplet route and by contaminated objects. The incubation period is 6 to 9 days but the premonitory signs are subtle, so sickness may be unobserved until 2 to 3 weeks after exposure. *In utero* transmission has been observed. The disease occurs in the Canidae (e.g. dogs, foxes, wolves), the Mustelidae (e.g. ferret, mink, skunk), most Procyonidae (e.g. raccoon, coati mundi), and some Viveridae (binturong).

Clinical Findings: Canine distemper begins with an elevated temperature lasting 1 to 3 days. The fever then subsides for several days before a second elevation, which lasts a week or more. A leukopenia, especially lymphopenia, accompanies the initial fever and the white blood cell count may remain low, fluctuate, or a neutrophilia may ensue and remain throughout the course of the disease. Mucopurulent material accumulates in the medial canthus of the eyes, the conjunctivae are reddened, photophobia is evidenced by squinting, and a mucopurulent nasal discharge is often present. The dog is usually depressed and anorectic and often develops diarrhea. Hyperkeratosis of the footpads ("hardpad" disease) and the epithelium of the nasal plane may be observed in some cases. Neurologic signs frequently are observed in patients that exhibit this hyperkeratosis. A dog may seemingly recover from the above signs, with the exception of the hyperkeratosis, and then develop nervous complications manifest as: (1) localized twitching of a muscle or group of muscles (chorea, flexor spasm, hyperkinesia) such as in the leg or facial muscles, (2) paresis or paralysis often beginning in the rear quarters manifest as ataxia followed by ascending paresis and paralysis; (3) convulsive seizures characterized by chewing movements of the jaw with salivation (petit mal, chewing gum fits) which become more frequent and severe, and the patient may then fall on its side and paddle its legs, running in place, often with involuntary urination and defecation (grand mal seizure, epileptiform convulsion). A single patient may exhibit 1, 2 or all 3 of these nervous manifestations in the course of the disease. The consequences of infection vary from a mild, inapparent infection to severe disease manifested by most of the above signs. The course of the disease may be as short as 10 days, but more often is prolonged for several weeks or months, in exceptional cases, with intervening periods of abatement followed by a relapse. Sometimes when recovery seems imminent, permanent neurologic residua, as noted above, appear. **Old-dog encephalitis** (ODE), a condition marked by encephalitic signs of ataxia, compulsive movements such as head pressing or continual pacing, and an incoordinated high-stepping gait, may occur in the adult dog without a previous history of respiratory, digestive or other signs indicating distemper. Convulsions and neuromuscular twitching (chorea) do not seem to occur with ODE. Although distemper virus antigen has been found in the brain of dogs with ODE by fluorescent antibody staining, it seems not to be infectious and complete virus has not been isolated. ODE is definitely associated with canine distemper virus but the pathophysiology of the disease is currently unknown (*but see* p. 12).

Lesions: The virus of canine distemper produces cytoplasmic and intranuclear inclusion bodies in respiratory, urinary and digestive epithelium, and an interstitial giant-cell pneumonia. Other lesions depend upon the severity of the attack and the extent of secondary bacterial infection. These may include inflammation of the mucous membranes of the gastrointestinal tract, enteritis, bronchopneumonia and a pustular dermatitis of the lower abdomen. (Occasional hyperkeratosis of the footpads and nose occurs.) Lesions found in the brain of dogs with neurologic complications include neuronal degeneration, gliosis, demyelination, perivascular cuffing, nonsuppurative leptomeningitis and intranuclear inclusion bodies predominately within glial cells.

Diagnosis: Distemper should be considered in any febrile condition in puppies. While the typical clinical case is not difficult to diagnose, sometimes the characteristic signs fail to appear until late in the disease. The clinical picture may be modified by superimposed toxoplasmosis, coccidiosis, ascariasis, infectious canine hepatitis, and numerous viral and bacterial infections. Distemper is sometimes confused with leptospirosis, infectious canine hepatitis, or lead poisoning. A febrile catarrhal illness with neurologic sequelae justifies a diagnosis of distemper. Clinical diagnosis is best confirmed at necropsy by histopathologic lesions or by immunofluorescent assay of viral antigen in tissues. In living patients, conjunctival, tracheal, vaginal or other epithelium, or the buffy coat of the blood, can be examined with these procedures. These samples are usually negative when circulating antibody is present in the diseased dog. The diagnosis can then be made by demonstration of virus-specific IgM.

Prophylaxis: Successful immunization of pups with modified canine distemper live-virus vaccines depends upon the absence of interfering maternal antibody. The age at which pups can be immunized can be predicted from a nomograph if the serum antibody titer of the mother is known; this service is available in many diagnostic laboratories. If it is not available, many alternative procedures may be used. One is to vaccinate the pup with modified live-virus vaccine when it is first seen after weaning (usually about 8 to 9 weeks of age), and to repeat the vaccination at 3 to 4 months of age to immunize those dogs that the first dose left unprotected due to interference by maternal antibody. Administration of doses of vaccine at 2-week intervals more nearly approaches the ideal. Anticanine distemper serum (10 to 30 ml subcut.) has been used to passively protect dogs; however, because it may block active immunization, the use of antiserum for short-term protection is discouraged. Active immunization with modified live-virus vaccines is more efficacious. A modified live-virus measles vaccine and a combination of modified live measles and modified live canine-distemper vaccine are available. These vaccines must be administered IM. The measles or combination vaccine should be administered to pups 6 to 7 weeks old. The pup so vaccinated should receive a modified live-virus distemper, or distemper-hepatitis, or distemper-hepatitis-leptospirosis vaccine at 14 to 16 weeks of age. Many varieties of attenuated distemper vaccine are available and should be used according to manufacturer's directions. Modified live-virus vaccines are generally recommended and annual revaccination is suggested.

Treatment: At the first suspicion of distemper, some clinicians administer repeated large doses of anticanine distemper serum (10 to 30 ml), others immediately give modified live-virus vaccine. Both these procedures are of questionable value once clinical signs have developed. Other treatments are directed at limiting secondary bacterial invasion, supporting the fluid balance and the overall well-being of the patient, and controlling nervous manifestations. These include antibiotics, electrolyte solutions, protein hydrolysates, dietary supplements, antipyretics, nasal preparations, analgesics and anticonvulsants (*see* PRESCRIPTION section, p. 1525 et seq.). No one treatment is specific or uniformly successful. Good nursing care with attention to the comfort of the patient is essential, but despite all effort some individuals will fail to make a satisfactory recovery.

Treatment for chorea is usually unavailing, but it may be treated as are other neurologic manifestations of distemper, with antispasmodics and sedatives.

INFECTIOUS CANINE HEPATITIS (ICH)

A contagious disease of dogs with signs varying from a slight fever and congestion of the mucous membranes to severe depression, marked leukopenia and prolonged bleeding time.

Etiology and Epidemiology: The causal adenovirus (canine adenovirus 1, CAV-1) produces characteristic intranuclear inclusion bodies in hepatic and endothelial cells. Dogs of all ages are susceptible. Exposure usually occurs by ingestion of virus. Airborne transmission is not considered a problem except in the rare respiratory form of the disease. Direct transmission can occur during the acute illness, when the virus is present in all secretions and excretions. The virus then localizes in the kidney and is eliminated in urine for months afterwards. Virus-containing urine from recovered dogs can spread the disease. Indirect infection may also occur through fomites. The incubation period is 5 to 9 days. The disease occurs worldwide, antibodies being detectable in almost 80% of adult dogs. Most infections are asymptomatic.

Clinical Findings: The disease varies from a slight fever to a fatal illness. The first sign is an elevation of temperature above 104°F (40°C), lasting from 1 to 6 days. Usually, a "saddle type" temperature curve is seen, with an initial elevation for a day, then a drop to near normal for a day, followed by a secondary rise. Tachycardia out of proportion to the fever may be observed.

On the day after the initial temperature rise, leukopenia develops, and persists throughout the febrile period. The degree of leukopenia varies, and seems to be correlated with the severity of the illness. If the fever is of short duration, leukopenia may be the only sign, but if the fever lasts more than a day, acute illness develops.

Signs are apathy, anorexia, thirst, conjunctivitis, serous discharge from the eyes and nose, and occasionally signs of abdominal pain. Intense hyperemia or petechiae of the oral mucous membranes may be seen, as well as enlarged tonsils. Vomiting may also be observed. There may be subcut. edema of the head, neck and trunk.

There is direct correlation between the severity of illness and the clotting time. Controlling hemorrhage may be difficult. Interference with blood clotting is manifested by hemorrhage around deciduous teeth and appearance of spontaneous hematomas, and may be demonstrated by nicking the edge of the lip or an ear. However, disseminated intravascular coagulation is commonly seen, which may be significant in the pathogenesis of the disease. Respiratory signs are not usually seen in dogs with ICH; however, the ICH adenovirus has been recovered from dogs with signs of infectious tracheobronchitis and the respiratory signs reproduced in susceptible dogs exposed to the nebulized isolate (*see* INFECTIOUS TRACHEO-

BRONCHITIS, p. 904). Foxes may show convulsions intermittently during the course of illness, and terminal paralysis involving one or more of the limbs or the entire body. Nervous involvement is unusual in the dog; however, the severely infected dog may evidence a terminal convulsion and brain stem hemorrhages are commonly observed.

Upon recovery, dogs eat well but regain weight slowly. Seven to 10 days after the disappearance of acute signs, about 25% of the recovered dogs develop "hepatitis blue eye," a transient unilateral or bilateral corneal opacity that disappears spontaneously. In mild cases of ICH, the transient corneal opacity may be the only sign of disease observed.

Chronic hepatitis may develop in dogs having low levels of passive antibody when exposed. Simultaneous infection with the viruses of ICH and distemper is sometimes seen (*see* CANINE DISTEMPER, p. 332).

Lesions: Endothelial damage results in intraocular hemorrhages, bleeding in the mouth, "paint brush" hemorrhages on the gastric serosa, and hemorrhagic lymph nodes. Hepatic cell necrosis produces varying color changes in the liver, which may be normal in size or swollen. The gall bladder wall may be edematous and thickened; edema or petechial hemorrhages of the thymus may be found.

Diagnosis: Usually, the abrupt onset and prolonged bleeding time suggest ICH. Clinical evidence is not always sufficient to differentiate infectious hepatitis from distemper. The diagnosis is confirmed if characteristic intranuclear inclusion bodies are found in the liver.

Prophylaxis: Attenuated live-virus (modified live-virus) vaccines are available. These vaccines are often combined with distemper vaccine or with distemper and leptospira vaccines or with distemper, parainfluenza and leptospira vaccines. Immunization against ICH is recommended at the time of, and following the schedule recommended for, canine distemper immunization. Attenuated ICH vaccines have been known to produce transient unilateral or bilateral opacities of the cornea and to be shed in urine. Recently, a CAV-2 attenuated live-virus vaccine became available that protects dogs against CAV-1 and CAV-2 infection. This vaccine does not produce corneal opacities or uveitis and the virus is not shed in urine. Improved safety for dogs is the primary advantage of this product. It is available in the same combinations as CAV-1 (ICH) vaccine, i.e. with leptospira bacterin or parainfluenza vaccine or both. Annual revaccination against ICH is recommended.

A passive protection (which interferes with active immunization) is transferred by immune bitches to puppies. As in distemper, 82% of puppies became immune to ICH when vaccinated at 9 weeks of age.

For temporary protection, distemper, hepatitis and leptospira antiserum is available. An inoculation of antiserum, 0.5 to 1.0 ml/kg of body wt, will protect a dog against virulent virus. It should be repeated every 10 days. The use of antiserum may interfere with attempts to stimulate active immunity by vaccination for 10 to 21 days after the antiserum injection.

Treatment: Daily blood transfusions are helpful in seriously ill dogs. In addition, 5% dextrose in isotonic salt solution plus 5% protein hydrolysate in an amount of 250 to 500 ml daily should be given, preferably IV. In patients with prolonged clotting time, subcut. administration of fluids may be dangerous. A broad-spectrum antibiotic, e.g. tetracycline (℞ 79), oxytetracycline (℞ 49, 50), chloramphenicol (℞ 16), amoxicillin (℞ 1), ampicillin (℞ 3), cephaloridine (℞ 13), or gentamicin (℞ 40) should be administered. Since the use of the tetracyclines during tooth development (late prenatal, neonatal, and early postnatal periods) may cause discoloration of the teeth, tetracyclines should not be used in puppies before the eruption of their permanent teeth. Although the transient corneal opacity that may be seen in the course of ICH or be associated with vaccination with attenuated ICH vaccines usually requires no treatment, atropine ophthalmic ointment (℞ 387) may be used to alleviate the painful ciliary spasm that may be associated with this condition. The patient should be protected against bright light when the problem occurs. Corticosteroids are generally considered to be contraindicated in the treatment of the corneal opacity associated with ICH. It is advisable to vaccinate against canine distemper or to give antidistemper, hepatitis and leptospira serum (℞ 127) to prevent simultaneous infection with distemper.

CANINE HERPESVIRUS INFECTION

A fatal viral infection of infant puppies. The virus may also be associated with a vesicular vaginitis in the adult female.

Clinical Findings: Fatal cases of canine herpesvirus infection usually occur in puppies 1 to 3 weeks old although occasional fatal cases may occur in puppies up to 1 month of age, rarely in those as old as 4 months. Typically the onset of disease is sudden and death occurs in young puppies after an illness of 24 hours or less.

Older dogs exposed to or experimentally inoculated with canine herpesvirus may develop a mild rhinitis or a vesicular vaginitis. Some investigators have linked canine herpesvirus with abortions, stillbirths and infertility. There is currently no evidence of association of the canine herpesvirus with infectious tracheobronchitis (q.v., p. 904).

Transmission of canine herpesvirus is usually by contact between susceptible puppies and the infected oral or vaginal secretions of their dam.

Lesions: The characteristic lesions in natural and experimental infections consist of disseminated focal necrosis and hemorrhages. The most pronounced lesions are seen in the lungs, cortical portion of the kidneys, adrenal glands, liver and in the intestinal tract. All lymph nodes are enlarged and hyperemic and the spleen is swollen. Lesions may also occur in the CNS. The basic histologic lesion is that of necrosis with hemorrhage occurring in the adjacent parenchyma. Most often an inflammatory reaction is absent. Single, small basophilic intranuclear inclusion bodies are commonest in areas of necrosis in the lung, liver and kidneys. Occasionally, they occur as faintly acidophilic bodies located within the nuclear space.

Diagnosis: This condition may be confused with infectious canine hepatitis, but it is not accompanied by the thickened, edematous gallbladder often associated with the latter (q.v., p. 335). The focal areas of necrosis and hemorrhage, especially those that occur in the kidneys, distinguish it from hepatitis and toxoplasmosis. Canine herpesvirus causes serious disease only in very young puppies. The rapid death and characteristic lesions distinguish this infection from canine distemper. The virus can be isolated from tissues by cell culture techniques.

Prophylaxis and Treatment: There is no available vaccine. Infected bitches develop antibodies and litters subsequent to the first infected litter receive maternally transmitted antibodies in the colostrum. Puppies that receive maternal antibodies may be infected with canine herpesvirus but no disease results.

Removal of puppies from affected bitches by cesarean section and rearing them in isolation has been successful in preventing deaths under experimental conditions. However, infections have been noted even in cesarean-derived puppies.

Deaths may be reduced when infected puppies are reared in incubators at elevated temperatures (95°F [35°C], 50% relative humidity). Puppies so reared must be given adequate fluids and supportive therapy. Anticanine distemper serum may be of some benefit early in the course of the disease as this serum may contain some antiherpes antibodies. Treatment is generally unsuccessful.

CANINE RICKETTSIAL DISEASES

CANINE EHRLICHIOSIS

A septicemia of Canidae caused by cytoplasmic rickettsiae in the circulating leukocytes. The disease occurs world-wide.

Etiology: The cause, *Ehrlichia canis*, appears as colonies of coccoid bodies in the leukocytes' cytoplasm. The brown dog tick, *Rhipicephalus sanguineus*, is the natural vector. The disease is transmitted through the egg, and all stages of the tick are infective. The blood of diseased or recovered dogs is infective by inoculation.

Clinical Findings: After an incubation period of 1 to 3 weeks, signs are fever, serous nasal and ocular discharges, anorexia, depression, weight loss, anemia, thrombocytopenia, leukopenia and an increased sedimentation rate. Signs may be mild and transitory or may persist for several weeks with marked variation in severity and duration.

More severe signs are recurrent fever, mucopurulent nasal and ocular discharges, vomiting, fetid breath, emaciation, lymphadenopathy, splenic enlargement, erosions of the buccal mucosa and skin, edema of the legs and scrotum, ascites, hydrothorax and gastroenteritis. Less common signs are erythematopustular eruption of the axillae and groin, hyperesthesia, convulsions, hysteria and paralysis.

E. canis infection complicated by concurrent pathogenic *Babesia*, *Haemobartonella* or *Hepatozoon* is common and more severe, causing high mortality.

Especially in German shepherd dogs, marrow hypoplasia may be signaled by sudden epistaxis as long as 60 to 120 days after early signs of infection have disappeared. Other signs, singly or in combination, are anemia, melena, hemorrhages in the eyes, petechiae and ecchymoses on the abdomen and in the mucosa of the penis, buccal cavity and conjunctiva. Earlier signs may recur. Hematologically there is severe pancytopenia. Secondary bacterial infections are common. Usually, death occurs within a few hours to several days after hemorrhaging begins; survivors may show bleeding episodes intermittently. *E. canis* persists in the blood of recovered dogs, perhaps for life.

Lesions: Grossly, there are ulcerations in the alimentary canal, pulmonary edema, mottling of liver and kidneys, splenic enlargement, lymphadenopathy, hemorrhages throughout the subcut. tissue and major organs. Histologically, many organs show perivascular plasma cell infiltration; in dogs dead from hemorrhages, severe bone marrow hypoplasia is evident.

Diagnosis: Clinical diagnosis is confirmed by Giemsa-stained blood films revealing clusters of *E. canis* in the cytoplasm of mononuclear cells and neutrophils. Infected cells are demonstrable also in impression smears from the lungs. Additionally confirmatory are the demonstration of *E. canis* serum antibody and an indirect fluorescent antibody test.

Babesiasis (q.v., p. 426) may mask, or occur with, ehrlichiosis. Both diseases cause similar signs after transmission by the same tick.

Treatment: Tick control should be enforced. To clear the infection intensive broad-spectrum antibiotic therapy is required (e.g. ℞ 78). Concurrent infections should be treated. Supportive therapy, e.g. blood transfusions and good nursing, are important.

Prophylaxis: Tick control is imperative. In endemic areas, tetracycline given orally at 3 mg/lb (6.6 mg/kg) body wt as single daily doses is preventive. Without intensive therapy, recovered dogs remain chronically rickettsemic and should not be used as blood donors.

SALMON POISONING DISEASE (SPD)

An acute infectious disease (not a toxicosis) of Canidae in which the infective agent is transmitted through the various stages of a fluke with a snail-fish-dog life cycle.

Etiology: SPD is caused by infection with *Neorickettsia helminthoeca*. The disease is sometimes complicated (salmon poisoning complex) by a second agent, the Elokomin fluke fever agent which is capable of causing disease (q.v., p. 341) in its own right. The transmitting vector is a small fluke, *Nanophyetus salmincola*. The dog becomes infected by ingesting trout or salmon that contain rickettsia-infected, encysted metacercariae of the fluke. These may occur throughout the fish, but are especially numerous in the kidney. In the dog's intestine, the larval flukes are released, embed in the duodenal mucosa, and introduce one or both of the causal agents. Fluke infection alone produces little or no clinical disease.

The infection is apparently maintained by the elimination of infected fluke ova in the feces of the host. From these, ova develop larval stages which may successively infect the snail and the fish and culminate in the metacercarial stage in the fish. A second dog, eating such fish, completes the parasite cycle and at the same time becomes infected with the rickettsia. There is some belief but no solid evidence that dog-to-dog transmission occurs both by aerosol and per rectum by dirty thermometers.

Age, sex and breed appear to be of no importance. The disease may appear at any time, but is more frequent when fish are most accessible. Infected fish are found in the Pacific Ocean from San Francisco to the 59th parallel (off the coast of Alaska). SPD in dogs is most frequently reported from northern California to Puget Sound. It is more prevalent west of the Cascade Mountains but is also seen inland along the rivers of fish migration. Mortality in untreated natural infections ranges from 50 to 90%.

Clinical Findings: Signs usually appear suddenly 5 to 9 days after eating infected fish and usually persist for 7 to 10 days. During the first or second day of signs, the body temperature reaches 104 to 106°F (40 to 41°C) and persists or falls slightly during the next few days and is accompanied by great depression and anorexia. After a febrile peak the temperature drops to below normal before death ensues. At first, there may be diarrhea or the feces may be scanty, frothy and yellowish, but usually soon become bloody. Sometimes almost pure blood is passed. Vomiting occurs at this time. Dehydration and extreme weight loss are conspicuous in the later stages. Thirst is marked but drinking leads promptly to vomiting. Nasal or conjunctival exudate may be observed.

The diagnosis is supported if fluke ova are found in the feces. The ova are oval, yellowish brown, rough-surfaced, about 50 to 75 μ in size and possess an indistinct operculum. During the first day or two, ova may be too scanty to be found readily in direct smears. All lymph nodes are usually enlarged.

Lesions: SPD appears to affect chiefly the lymphoid tissue and intestine. Alimentary tract lymph follices, lymph nodes, tonsils, thymus and, to some extent, the spleen show enlargement with microscopic necrosis, some hemorrhage and hyperplasia. A variable but often severe hemorrhagic enteritis is seen throughout the intestine. This seems to arise from damaged lymph follicles. Microscopic necrotic foci also appear apart from follicles. Flukes embedded in the duodenum account for little tissue damage.

Prophylaxis and Treatment: No vaccine or other prophylactic is currently available. Immunity in recovered cases is strong and persistent. Various sulfonamides given orally or parenterally have been successful in treatment. Dosage at therapeutic blood levels should be maintained at least 3 days. Experimentally, good results have been obtained with chlortetracycline, chloramphenicol and oxytetracycline. The best results follow administration of large divided doses. If the animal is dehydrated, IV fluid therapy is essential to avoid nephrotoxic effects. General supportive treatment, aimed at correcting and maintaining fluid and electrolyte balance, providing nutritional requirements and controlling diarrhea, often is essential unless there is a prompt favorable response. Treatment in the late stages may not be beneficial.

ELOKOMIN FLUKE FEVER

A fluke-transmitted disease resembling rickettsial infections, of the canine family, bears, raccoons and ferrets. It is seen alone or as a complicating agent in the salmon poisoning complex. It utilizes *Nanophyetus salmincola* in the same manner as described for SPD (*see above*). The Elokomin fluke fever agent (as yet unnamed) resembles *Neorickettsia helminthoeca* but is differentiated from it by animal cross-protection, serum neutralization and its wider host range. This agent produces a mortality of less than 10%.

Clinical Findings: The incubation period is longer than seen in SPD, 9 to 14 days on primary isolation. The temperature curve is of the plateau type with persistence of fever for 4 to 7 days. The bloody diarrhea is absent as is the severe dehydration. Generalized somatic lymph node enlargement is striking. Although the mortality is low, many dogs will exhibit severe persistent weight loss. Fluke eggs are seen on fecal examination. The lesions of uncomplicated Elokomin fluke fever resemble those seen in the salmon poisoning complex, in which it plays a part, except that the severe intestinal lesions are lacking. Treatment and prophylaxis are as for salmon poisoning disease (*see above*).

EQUINE EHRLICHIOSIS

An infectious noncontagious sporadic disease of northern California horses characterized by fever, depression, ataxia, leg edema, thrombocytopenia, leukopenia, mild anemia and low mortality.

Etiology: The cause, *Ehrlichia equi*, shows characteristics similar to those of the etiologic agents of tick-borne fever and bovine petechial fever. *E. equi* is present in cytoplasmic vacuoles of neutrophils and eosinophils during the acute disease states. Giemsa or Wright-Leishman stained blood films reveal one or more loose aggregates (morulae or inclusion bodies, 1.5 to 5.0 μm in diam.) of blue-gray to dark blue coccoid, coccobacillary or pleomorphic organisms within single cytoplasmic vacuoles. The vector, reservoir and mode of transmission of *E. equi* are unknown.

Clinical Findings: Generally the disease is mild to moderately severe; occasionally it may fulminate. After an incubation period of 1 to 9 days, body temperature rises abruptly to 106°F (41°C) or more and persists 1 to 12 days (average 6) during which mild anemia, leukopenia and thrombocytopenia occur and morulae appear in the cytoplasm of circulating granulocytic leukocytes, in up to 50% of the neutrophils. Signs include anorexia, ataxia, depression and icterus. Subcut. edema, usually only of the legs, develops consistently in adult horses; in some the ventral abdomen and prepuce become edematous and the testes of mature males may swell, then atrophy.

Lesions: Grossly, petechiae and edema occur in the subcutis and beneath the superficial fascia of the legs and testes. Inflammation of small arteries and veins, fascia, subcutis, ovaries and testes is common.

Diagnosis: Demonstration of the characteristic morulae is diagnostic. An indirect fluorescent antibody test has been described. In northern California, ehrlichiosis must be distinguished from equine infectious anemia, piroplasmosis, viral arteritis and leptospirosis.

Treatment: Oxytetracycline (℞ 50) is specific against *E. equi*. Tetracycline IV, 10 mg/kg body wt for 8 consecutive days, has cleared *E. equi* infection. Solid sterile immunity follows recovery from the clinical disease.

EQUINE INFECTIOUS ANEMIA

(Swamp fever)

An acute or chronic viral disease of Equidae, characterized by intermittent fever, depression, progressive weakness, loss of weight, edema and progressive or transitory anemia. The disease tends to become an inapparent infection but occasionally results in death. It is found wherever there are horses.

Etiology: In acute cases, the virus is in all tissues and discharges. It persists in blood leukocytes of all infected horses for life. The virus is quite stable in the presence of serum but is readily inactivated by common disinfectants that contain detergent.

Transmission is by transfer of blood cells from an infected horse. Insertion and withdrawal of a hypodermic needle may provide adequate contamination for transmission. Ordinarily, the disease is detected only sporadically, but it may spread in epidemic form from obviously ill horses when bloodsucking flies are abundant or if contaminated surgical instruments are used.

Clinical Findings: The incubation period usually ranges from 1 to 3 weeks but may be as long as 3 months. Horses experiencing active disease will have a decreased packed cell volume and a decreased platelet count but an increased number of monocytes. In horses infected for several months, blood may contain leukocytes with stainable iron and have an elevated gammaglobulin level.

Lesions: In acute cases, hemorrhages are occasionally found on the serous surfaces and mucous membranes. The spleen is enlarged and the splenic lymph nodes are swollen. In subacute and chronic cases, necropsy reveals emaciation, pale mucous membranes, subcut. edema, especially along the ventral abdominal walls and limbs, splenomegaly and enlarged abdominal lymph nodes. The yellow marrow of the long bones may be replaced by red marrow. Intravascular clotting with emboli is frequently observed in advanced terminal cases.

Microscopically, there is reticuloendothelial cell proliferation in many organs and periportal and perisinusoidal collections of round cells in the liver with accumulations of hemosiderin in the Kupffer's cells. Perivascular lymphoid infiltrations may occur in the other organs also. Proliferative glomerulitis is present in some horses and there is glomerular deposition of immunoglobulins (IgG) and complement (C3).

Diagnosis: The clinical diagnosis of EIA should be confirmed by the immunodiffusion or "Coggin's" test. This serological test is simple and highly accurate. It has replaced the older procedure of injecting blood into a susceptible horse to produce clinical disease. Foals nursing infected dams will be temporarily positive in this EIA test and tests in recently infected horses may be negative for a week or so until antibody forms.

EIA should be suspected when a horse is presented with a history of weight loss, accompanied by periodic fever. In addition, several horses in a group may develop similar signs following the introduction of new animals into a herd or death of a horse on pasture.

Treatment and Control: No specific treatment or vaccine is available. General supportive therapy may help in an individual case, but an infected horse, especially one exhibiting clinical signs, should be considered a likely source of infection for other horses. Whenever a diagnosis is established, the infected horse should be promptly isolated from other horses and maintained in isolation, if it is not to be killed. The horse fly is an important vector, thus stabling during the fly season helps to prevent spread of the infection.

Control of stable flies and mosquitoes might also be desirable by repeated spraying or by screening. Equipment that may cause skin abrasions or absorb secretions or excretions should be avoided or disinfected between horses. Hypodermic needles and the like should be sterilized between horses. Foals born to infected mares frequently become infected *in utero* or postnatally, especially if the mares show clinical illness. Thus, all foals out of infected dams must be isolated from other horses until freedom of infection can be established by the disappearance of the maternal antibody.

AFRICAN HORSE SICKNESS

An insect-borne disease of Equidae in which the mortality rate is high. Since the early 1700s the disease has increased to become a major endemic plague throughout Southern and Equatorial Africa.

Etiology: African horse sickness is caused by a double stranded RNA virus of the family Reoviridae, genus *Orbivirus*, with 9 immunologically distinct serotypes. Natural transmission occurs seasonally via insect vectors and not by contact. Gnats (*Culicoides* spp.) are the principal vectors but the disease has also been transmitted experimentally by mosquitoes. The disease disappears between insect seasons, and recovered animals have not been found to be carriers of the virus. Dogs have been infected by eating infected horse meat, but the role of dogs in the spread of the disease is not significant. Cattle and sheep are refractory.

Clinical Findings: The incubation period is less than 10 days. The disease may take either an acute pulmonary or a more chronic cardiac form although at necropsy the lesions generally indicate some degree of mixing of the forms. Infection of partially immune horses results in a mild, transient fever.

Horses with the pulmonary form rarely recover. They develop a high (over 105°F [40.5°C]) temperature but continue to eat and appear quite normal until the last 24 to 36 hours when pulmonary edema causes increasingly difficult respiration. Terminally there is severe, labored respiration with coughing as the bronchi and upper respiratory passages fill with fluid. The horse dies of anoxia.

Horses with the cardiac form are also febrile. The animals continue to eat, but they soon develop localized areas of edema subcut. on the head and neck. The occurrence of edema in the supraorbital and frontal region is characteristic. It may also involve the lips, intramandibular and cervical areas. Stocking or dependent edemas, which appear terminally, are secondary to cardiac insufficiency. Conjunctivitis, often hemorrhagic and edematous, is common as are petechiae on the ventral surface of the tongue.

Lesions: The dominant gross lesions in the pulmonary form are intestinal and alveolar edema, with effusion of fluid filling the bronchi terminally. In the cardiac form, in addition to the changes apparent in the live animal, there is hydropericardium, edema and hemorrhage of the coronary fat, myocarditis with varying degrees of hemorrhage, and necrosis that is often more striking histologically than grossly. Hemorrhagic gastritis is common. Lymphoid tissue is grossly swollen and histologically reactive. There may be hepatic congestion.

Diagnosis: The clinical and pathologic changes are usually adequate for a diagnosis in endemic areas. Virus isolation from equine blood at the height of fever may be accomplished in day-old mice or tissue culture and identified by neutralization with known sera. A rise in antibody titer is also diagnostic of recent infection.

Immunity and Control: All 9 viral serotypes can be grown in tissue culture and used to produce a satisfactory attenuated vaccine. Vaccine containing all of the serotypes present in the region of use should be administered annually.

Control is also facilitated by the destruction of insect vectors. Countries free of African horse sickness must prevent the entry of either infected equine animals or vectors. Horses from infected countries should be quarantined for 30 days in insect-free isolation and tested for virus. Because of the multiplicity of strains, antibody is not an index of either the current presence or absence of virus, and should not be a factor in judging safety for importation.

CORYNEBACTERIUM PSEUDOTUBERCULOSIS INFECTION

(Caseous lymphadenitis, Pseudotuberculosis, Lymphangitis)

Caseous lymphadenitis occurs throughout the world wherever **sheep** are raised. It is common in North and South America, New Zealand, Australia, and many European countries. It occurs also in goats and deer. It has been observed more frequently in range flocks than in small bands of sheep raised on individual farms. It is a chronic disease, in which clinical signs and lesions may not be observed until several months after infection. The superficial, particularly the precrural and prescapular, lymph nodes usually are the primary sites of the lesions. Later, the visceral lymph nodes may be involved, particularly the mediastinal, bronchial and sublumbar. In generalized cases, the lesions may be distributed throughout the lungs, liver, kidneys and spleen, and the corresponding lymph nodes. The disease is seldom fatal; the rate of frequency is determined largely from meat-inspection records.

The affected lymph nodes become enlarged by abscesses containing a cheesy, greenish, odorless pus. In lesions of long standing, this pus becomes a rather dry, firm mass, usually arranged in concentric "onion ring" layers within a thick fibrous capsule. The capillaries surrounding the abscesses are filled with masses of organisms and leukocytes.

Some affected animals in the early stages of an extensive involvement of the lymph nodes are found in excellent condition at the time of slaughter, but if allowed to live, gradual emaciation develops, followed by general weakness and death.

Sheep of 3 to 6 years of age contain the highest percentage of infected animals. Twenty percent of all animals found infected on postmortem inspection are condemned. *C. pseudotuberculosis* is believed to enter the body largely through skin abrasions, principally at the time of shearing. Animals may become infected through the unhealed navel, and docking and castration wounds.

Ulcerative lymphangitis in horses resembles the cutaneous form of glanders. It is characterized by nodules, ulcers and inflammation of the lymph vessels, especially in the region of the fetlock, but occasionally extending up the leg. The nodules may enlarge to 2 to 3 cm in diameter. They are tough and rather insensitive at first, but later become soft and painful, and finally rupture, exuding a greenish white pus. The onset is slow and usually manifests itself by pain. The marked involvement of the lymph nodes, so characteristic of the disease in sheep, is absent in the horse. Infection by inhalation of contaminated dust may also occur, the primary lesions then developing in the lungs.

Chronic single or multiple abscesses, known as **false distemper,** is another manifestation in horses. The disease is characterized by abscess formation, most frequently in the pectoral region, but in some animals extending to involve the mammary gland. These abscesses may reach a size of 5 to 20 cm; there is extensive peripheral edema. The abscesses may be a manifestation of systemic infection and develop slowly over several weeks. Systemic disturbance seems confined to leukocytosis and neutrophilia. Abscesses most often rupture externally, discharge viscid, creamy pus and heal spontaneously. Generalized involvement occurs occasionally, in the form of abdominal abscesses, often perirenal. External abscesses may be found concomitantly. Vague clinical signs, such as depression, anorexia and loss of weight are recorded. Pathogenesis and transmission are unknown. Distribution corresponds to that of sheep raising areas of the world.

In **cattle,** there have been a few reports of this infection. It has been found in a case of bronchopneumonia in a cow and also in calves and in the so-called "skin lesions or tuberculosis" of cattle in Utah, California and Idaho. In areas where skin lesions are commonly found, *C. pseudotuberculosis* has been frequently isolated from the lesions taken by biopsy or at postmortem examination of lesion-free tuberculin-reactor animals.

Diagnosis: Serologic tests alone are not diagnostic. Diagnosis of caseous lymphadenitis in sheep can be made by careful palpation of external lymph nodes or by the appearance of the characteristic lesions at necropsy. The organism can be easily isolated from the lesions of all infected animals. In ulcerative lymphangitis and in all other forms of lymphangitis in horses (q.v., p. 49), a positive diagnosis must be established in order to rule out the possibility of glanders (q.v., p. 409).

Prophylaxis and Treatment: Prevention of the disease in **sheep** is directed toward reducing the opportunities for infection of wounds sustained during shearing and around feed bunks and watering troughs. Where the disease is prevalent, the younger sheep should be shorn first. The older animals should be sorted by palpating the superficial lymph nodes and all suspected animals shorn last. Shears and other equipment should be thoroughly disinfected whenever an abscess is accidentally incised. As the animals are shorn, they should immediately be turned onto pasture or open range. This reduces the exposure of sheep with shearing wounds to infected animals with ruptured or incised abscesses and to the dust of contaminated yards or holding paddocks. Vaccines have been unsuccessful. The infection can be reduced if young sheep are carefully examined for skin lacerations immediately after shearing. All wounds must be cleaned, treated, and the skin sutured if necessary. Penicillin-streptomycin topical ointment or other appropriate antibacterial therapy (℞ 66) should be begun at once and continued until wounds are healed.

The great majority of cases of ovine caseous lymphadenitis go untreated because the disease is usually diagnosed for the first time in animals of good condition at the time of slaughter. When the lesions are so extensive that general signs are apparent, the patient is usually beyond successful treatment. Encapsulated abscesses rarely regress in response to therapy; surgical intervention may be advisable in valuable animals.

In horses, the disease seems to be less prevalent where the animals are kept under conditions of good husbandry and stable management. In the lymphangitis form without abscesses, administration of oxytetracycline, 2 mg/lb (4.4 mg/kg) of body wt IV, daily for 5 days or longer is useful. Bandaging and continued local antibiotic treatment of infected areas should be repeated as indicated.

When chronic abscesses are present, antibacterial therapy prolongs the disease by delaying their maturation. This may be hastened by use of ointments or heat. Irrigation of the drained abscess cavity with suitable antiseptics and systemic administration of oxytetracycline may hasten healing. Prognosis is poor if internal abscesses develop.

ERYSIPELOTHRIX INFECTION

Erysipelothrix rhusiopathiae (*insidiosa*) is a cosmopolitan bacterium capable of living for long periods in water, soil, pasture, decaying organic matter, slime on the bodies of fish, and in carcasses, even after smoking, pickling or salting. It is capable of invading the tissues of animals, birds and man with production of some fairly distinct and other less well-defined diseases. The former include swine erysipelas in its various forms; nonsuppurative arthritis in lambs and, less frequently, in calves; post-dipping lameness in sheep; acute septicemia in turkeys, ducks and occasionally geese and other birds (q.v., p. 1058); and erysipeloid in man.

In acute disease, *E. rhusiopathiae* usually occurs as a slender, gram-positive, nonmotile, nonsporulating rod, about 1- to 2-μ long. In chronic lesions and old cultures it often appears as a mixture of rods and filaments up to 20 μ in length. It is resistant to certain commonly used antiseptics, such as formaldehyde, phenol, hydrogen peroxide and alcohol, but is readily destroyed by caustic soda and hypochlorites. It is very sensitive to penicillin, less so to the tetracyclines and streptomycin and insensitive to most sulfonamides.

SWINE ERYSIPELAS

An infectious disease, manifested in a variety of forms, affecting mainly growing swine. It is fairly common in many swine-raising areas of the world. Although acute septicemic swine erysipelas causes death, probably the greatest economic loss comes from the mild, chronic nonfatal forms of the disase.

Etiology: *Erysipelothrix rhusiopathiae,* the causal agent, can be isolated readily on blood agar plates from the tissues of acutely sick pigs and also from the tonsils of many apparently normal ones. On farms where the organism is endemic, pigs are exposed naturally to *E. rhusiopathiae* while they are young and have maternal antibodies, and thus develop a degree of active immunity without visible disease. The organism is excreted from infected animals and survives for short periods in most soils (may be longer in cold weather, and if soil is moist and low in organic matter). Recovered animals and those chronically infected may be carriers of the organism for months. *E. rhusiopathiae* can cause an allergic response in the joints of sensitized pigs that results in chronic sterile lesions similar to those observed in rheumatoid arthritis in man.

Clinical Findings: The disease occurs in several forms; acute septicemia, a skin form, chronic arthritis and vegetative endocarditis. These may occur together, in sequence, or separately.

Swine with acute septicemia may die suddenly without previous manifestation of illness. This occurs most frequently in suckling pigs (rarely before 3 weeks), or in 100- to 200-lb (45- to 90-kg) pigs. Most acutely infected animals have high temperatures of 104 to 108°F (40 to 42°C), walk stiffly on their toes, lie on their sternums or lie about separately rather than piling in groups. They squeal readily when handled or when submitted to any type of body pressure, and shift weight from foot to foot when standing. Skin discoloration may vary from erythema and purplish discoloration of the ears, snout and abdomen, to urticaria (diamond-skin lesions) over all areas of the body, particularly the lateral and dorsal parts. The lesions may occur as variably sized pink or light purple areas that become raised and firm to the touch within 2 to 3 days of illness. Later they may disappear or progress to a more chronic type of lesion, such as diamond-skin disease or even necrosis and separation of large areas of skin. The tips of the ears and tail may become necrotic and drop off in long-standing untreated cases.

Clinical cases are usually sporadic, affecting individual pigs or small groups. Sometimes larger outbreaks may occur. Mortality may vary from 0 to 100%, and death may occur up to 6 days after the first signs of illness. Untreated animals may develop chronic arthritis or vegetative valvular endocarditis; these conditions may also occur in pigs that have shown no previous signs of septicemia, particularly in vaccinated herds. Valvular endocarditis is commonest in mature or nearly mature pigs and is manifested by fatigue, heavy respiration, cyanosis or sudden death, which usually results from embolisms. Chronic arthritis produces intermittent mild lameness, but the affected joints are frequently difficult to detect clinically. Mortality in chronic cases is low.

Lesions: In the acute infection the lesions are similar to those of many other septicemias. Lymph nodes are usually enlarged and congested, the spleen swollen, pulpy and purplish and the lungs edematous and congested. Petechial hemorrhages in sparse numbers may be found in the kidneys. The skin changes have already been described.

In cases of valvular endocarditis, metastatic embolism and infarctions may occur, particularly in the kidneys, brain or heart. In cases of arthritis, which may involve one or more legs, the joint enlargement is firm due to a thickening of the joint capsule and the capsular ligaments. Granulation tissue forms in the articular cavity. There may be erosion of the articular cartilage, with periostitis and osteitis. Ankylosis may occur.

Diagnosis: The diagnosis of acute erysipelas may be difficult in swine showing only high temperature, poor appetite and listlessness. Since *E. rhusiopathiae* is so sensitive to penicillin, the marked improvement within 24 hours following its use provides support for the diagnosis. If typical diamond-skin lesions develop, these are diagnostic. Chronic forms of arthritis and endocarditis are difficult to diagnose specifically since other agents can cause similar syndromes. At necropsy, demonstration of *E. rhusiopathiae* in stained smears or cultures confirms the diagnosis.

Prophylaxis and Treatment: Either killed bacterins or live-culture immunizing strains of low virulence for swine and man are used. The formalin-killed, aluminum hydroxide-absorbed bacterin does not infect other species of animals or man, and it confers an immunity that in most instances will protect the pig from acute forms of the disease until it reaches market age. An oral vaccine of low virulence is also used. Breeding stock should be revaccinated at least once each year.

Vaccination raises the level of immunity, but does not provide complete protection. Acute cases may still occur following stress, and little protection is provided against the arthritic or cardiac forms of the disease. Some antigenic variation occurs between bacterial strains so that a vaccine may not be equally effective against all wild strains.

If cases of acute erysipelas suddenly occur in an unvaccinated herd, antiserum may be administered to in-contact pigs. Penicillin is the drug of choice in affected pigs. Penicillin treatment is sometimes combined with antiserum to provide a longer action.

NONSUPPURATIVE POLYARTHRITIS IN LAMBS

An acute arthritis of one or more of the diarthrodial joints, usually of the limbs, following entry of *E. rhusiopathiae* through wounds or the unhealed navel. Calves also are sometimes affected.

Etiology: The infective agent, which apparently is widely distributed in alkaline soils and pastures, gains entry to the body usually through wounds of young lambs, particularly at docking and castration. After a transient septicemia, the organism becomes localized in one or more joints, without leaving evidence of specific infection of the wound through which it entered. Poor condition of the lambs at the time of the operation and adverse weather afterwards appear to predispose to a high infection rate.

Clinical Findings: The characteristic lesion is an acute nonsuppurative arthritis manifested by heat, pain and only slight swelling of the joint tissues. The joints most commonly involved are the hock, stifle, elbow and knee. Complete recovery usually occurs in 2 to 3 weeks, but because affected lambs are reluctant to move, growth is often seriously depressed. In about 10 to 15% of cases, the infection persists with the production of chronic arthritis and permanent enlargement of the joint. The mortality is usually low, a few animals dying from acute septicemia or from complications arising from the enforced decubitus.

In outbreaks following docking and castration, the incubation period is remarkably constant, the first cases appearing 9 to 19 days after the operation, and practically all subsequent cases developing within 5 days. The incidence may reach 50% but in most outbreaks it does not exceed 10%.

Diagnosis: In outbreaks following docking and castration, a presumptive diagnosis can be made from the history and clinical signs. In sporadic cases, recourse may be had to isolation and identification of the organism from affected joints. The disease must be distinguished from polyarthritis due to other bacteria (e.g. streptococcal joint ill), white muscle disease and other causes of lameness.

Prophylaxis and Treatment: The adoption of strict antiseptic techniques and the maintenance of hygienic conditions for docking and castration are highly desirable, but cannot be relied upon to prevent the disease. The so-called "bloodless" methods of carrying out both operations may reduce the chances of wound contamination, but outbreaks are known to follow all of the methods commonly used. Vaccination should be considered where the disease is a recurring problem.

Penicillin, administered as early as possible in the course of the disease, is the best form of therapy.

POST-DIPPING LAMENESS IN SHEEP

A laminitis arising from an extension of a focal cutaneous infection, caused by the penetration of *E. rhusiopathiae* through small skin abrasions in the region of the hoof. The condition, which normally occurs in outbreaks, has been described in most of the large sheep-raising countries.

Etiology: With time and repeated use, dipping solutions or suspensions of insecticidal agents, which exert little or no bacteriostatic activity, become heavily charged with numerous species of bacteria. *E. rhusiopathiae* is a common contaminant and its presence in the vat, sometimes in enormous numbers, leads to the infection of any or all skin wounds made during the dipping operation. Small skin abrasions in the region of the hoof and fetlock joint, made by scraping the legs against the sides of the vat, are particularly common. Erysipeloid lesions extending from these leg wounds to the laminae of the hoof cause the acute post-dipping lameness.

Clinical Findings: Two to 4 days after dipping, a variable number—up to 90%—of the flock are lame in one or more legs. At this stage, the affected leg appears normal except that the hoof and pastern are hot and painful on pressure. Later there is a variable degree of depilation, sometimes extending as far as the carpus or tarsus.

In many outbreaks, most sheep recover spontaneously in 2 to 4 weeks with nothing more serious than a slight loss of body weight. In others, however, the mortality may rise to 5% and, in young sheep particularly, a higher proportion may develop signs of acute and, later, chronic arthritis.

Prophylaxis and Treatment: The addition of copper sulfate to the dipping wash at the rate of 3 to 5 lb/1,000 gal. (1.5 to 2 kg/3,785 L) is an effective means of control. Other agents with bacteriostatic activity against *E. rhusiopathiae* are also used. Where therapy is indicated, penicillin is the antibiotic of choice.

ERYSIPELOTHRIX INFECTION IN MAN

The most common type of *Erysipelothrix* infection in man, the result of wound infection with *E. rhusiopathiae*, is known as erysipeloid. This sometimes occurs in veterinarians whose hands become infected while carrying out necropsies on swine or turkeys. These infections apparently lead to immunity since reinfection rarely occurs.

After an incubation period of 1 to 5 days, the skin at the point of inoculation becomes swollen, painful and red. If untreated, the process may extend to involve the entire hand. It is accompanied by an itching, burning or prickly sensation. There may be fever as well as swelling and tenderness of nearby joints and the regional lymph nodes. Suppuration is absent. Most cases follow a mild course to recovery within 2 to 4 weeks. Antiserum in doses of 5 to 20 ml usually brings about quick relief and recovery. Large doses of penicillin are indicated in treating the infection.

Two other forms of infection occur in man. One is the diffuse or generalized form consisting either of a slow spread of erysipeloid over most of the body or eruption in areas remote from the site of entry. This is usually accompanied by fever and joint pains. A septicemic form of variable symptomatology and duration has also been observed. There may be joint pains and endocarditis. The skin eruption which accompanies this is of value in suggesting the diagnosis. Blood culture is positive.

GLÄSSER'S DISEASE

A fibrinous polyserositis of swine. The classic syndrome is caused by encapsulated strains of *Haemophilus suis* or *H. parasuis* (*influenzae suis*). Stress factors, such as weaning or transport, predispose to the disease. Similar syndromes may be caused by *Mycoplasma* spp., notably *M. hyorhinis*. (*M. hyosynoviae* commonly causes arthritis, but not polyserositis.)

The disease is usually mild with a low morbidity, but it may be severe with a high morbidity when the organism first enters a susceptible herd. After an incubation period of 1 to 5 days, septicemia occurs with fever (106 to 107°F [41 to 41.5°C]), anorexia and depression. Some pigs become lame with warm swollen joints. Occasionally, mild CNS signs may be observed. In severe outbreaks, which are not common, respiratory dyspnea and coughing may be noted. Some pigs may die early in the disease, but in others the fever may subside after several days. They may remain lame and debilitated for variable periods but most eventually recover.

The classic lesion is a pronounced serofibrinous or fibrinopurulent exudate, associated with pleuritis, pericarditis, peritonitis, polyarthritis and meningoencephalitis, which is usually subclinical. The diagnosis "Glässer's disease" is based on the typical signs and lesions but the precise cause may be difficult to determine. Neither

Haemophilus nor *Mycoplasma* are easily demonstrated in smears but they may be isolated in cultures.

Haemophilus infections usually respond well to penicillin and streptomycin (℞ 66), and to sodium sulfathiazole (℞ 110). *Mycoplasma* infections may respond to tylosin, lincomycin or erythromycin, but fixed doses have not been established.

STREPTOCOCCAL LYMPHADENITIS OF SWINE

(Jowl or cervical abscesses, SLS)

A benign infectious and contagious disease characterized by the development of one or more heavily encapsulated abscesses in the soft tissues of the ventral or lateral or both aspects of the neck. Pork industry losses are large because of product devaluation.

Etiology and Epidemiology: In herds where it is endemic, streptococcal lymphadenitis occurs in each new generation of pigs and in healthy adult swine introduced for breeding purposes. The causal *Streptococcus* first colonizes in the palatine tonsils, from which large numbers reach the regional lymph nodes via the lymphatics. Recovered swine continue to carry the *Streptococcus* in their palatine tonsils. It has been shown experimentally that carrier pigs may infect contact pigs for at least 21 months after initial infection. The agent has been isolated from deep nasal swabs of sows on premises where the disease was endemic.

Clinical Findings: Experimentally, initial high fever for 5 or more days, depression, reduced feed intake, and constipation occur. These signs may be overlooked in field cases, and the principal observation is cervical abscessation, the developing abscesses becoming visible about 21 days after the initial infection. As a rule, affected swine appear thrifty and make satisfactory weight gains.

Pathogenesis: Scattered miliary abscesses develop in the swollen, affected lymph nodes within 7 days after infection. By about 21 days, abscesses measuring 5 to 8 cm in diameter are common and these destroy the internal structure of affected nodes. Incidence commonly exceeds 50% in a given lot of market hogs and may approach 100%. Developing abscesses reach the skin, rupture, and drain in 7 to 10 weeks. No tendency for deep-seated abscesses to drain into the pharynx has been reported. The drained lesions heal by granulation leaving a dense fibrous subcut. tract which is absorbed after several weeks.

Diagnosis: A tentative diagnosis, made on finding abscesses in several pigs, may be confirmed by identifying the agent. Swine that have only deep-seated abscesses may escape detection until they reach the packing plant.

Prophylaxis and Treatment: The introduction of carrier swine must be avoided. Agglutinin titers are detectable for some weeks after recovery and may permit reliable detection of carriers. A modified live vaccine is available for prophylactic use in 10-week old pigs. The *Streptococcus* is quite sensitive to a broad range of antibiotics, including penicillin and the tetracyclines, and has shown little tendency to develop resistant strains. Once pigs have visible lesions, antibiotic therapy is of doubtful economic value. If diagnosis can be established early, antibiotics mixed in feed (℞ 29, 60) will prevent the development of additional abscesses. Continuous feeding of low levels of antibiotics (25 to 50 gm/ton [0.0025 to 0.0055%] of feed) can be used as a prophylactic measure.

TRANSMISSIBLE SEROSITIS

(Chlamydial polyarthritis)

An infectious disease affecting sheep, calves and swine. Dogs are susceptible experimentally. Chlamydial polyarthritis of sheep was first described in Wisconsin, and has since been recognized in Western U.S.A., Australia and New Zealand. The disease was identified in calves from the U.S.A., Australia and Austria, and in pigs from Austria, Bulgaria and the U.S.A. Strains of the causal agent, *Chlamydia psittaci*, isolated from affected joints of sheep and calves are identical, but strain-specific antigens in their cell walls distinguish them from *Chlamydia* causing abortions or pneumonia in sheep and cattle. The agent can be isolated most consistently from synovia of affected joints. It is excreted in feces, urine and conjunctival exudates.

Clinical Findings: Chlamydial polyarthritis is observed in lambs on range, from farms and in feedlots. Morbidity may range from 5 to 75%. Rectal temperatures of affected lambs vary from 102 to 107°F (39 to 41.5°C). Varying degress of stiffness, lameness, anorexia and conjunctivitis may occur. Affected sheep are depressed, reluctant to move and often hesitate to stand and bear weight on one or more limbs, but they may "warm out" of stiffness and lameness following forced exercise. The highest incidence of the disease among sheep on range occurs between late summer and December.

The disease affects calves from 4 to 30 days of age, which are readily detected because they do not want to move and seek to rest.

They may have fever, are moderately alert, and usually nurse if carried to the dam and supported while they are sucking. They usually have diarrhea, which can be severe, and assume a hunched position while standing. The joints and tendons of the limbs are usually swollen, and palpation causes pain. Navel involvement and nervous signs are not observed.

Chlamydial polyarthritis may be recognized in slaughter pigs as well as in young piglets. The affected piglets become febrile and anorectic, and may develop nasal catarrh, difficulties in breathing and conjunctivitis. This condition has not been clearly differentiated from other infections leading to polyserositis and arthritis in pigs.

Lesions: The most striking tissue changes in chlamydial polyarthritis of lambs and calves are in the joints. Enlargement of the joints of polyarthritic lambs is not often noticed, but in long-standing, advanced cases, slight enlargement of the stifle, hock and elbow may be detected. In affected calves, periarticular subcut. edema and fluid-filled, fluctuating synovial sacs contribute to enlargement of the joints. Most affected joints of lambs or calves contain excessive, grayish yellow turbid synovial fluid. Fibrin flakes and plaques in the recesses of the affected joints may adhere firmly to the synovial membranes. Joint capsules are thickened. Articular cartilage is smooth, and erosions or evidence of marginal compensatory changes are not present. Tendon sheaths of severely affected lambs and calves are distended and contain creamy, grayish yellow exudate. Surrounding muscles are hyperemic and edematous, with petechiae in their associated fascial planes.

Diagnosis: The history of the disease and careful examination of the pathologic changes in the joints and other organs can be valuable diagnostically. Cytologic investigations of synovial fluids or tissues may reveal chlamydial elementary bodies or inclusions in affected cells. Isolation and identification of the causative agent from affected joints confirms the diagnosis. Bacteriologic cultures of affected joints are usually negative, but *Escherichia coli* or streptococci may occasionally be isolated. If the joints of young calves are arthritic and navel lesions are absent, chlamydial polyarthritis should be considered.

Clinical and pathologic features distinguish chlamydial polyarthritis from other conditions that cause stiffness and lameness in lambs. Lambs with mineral deficiency or osteomalacia usually do not have fever. The abnormal osteogenesis in these 2 conditions and the distinct muscle lesions of white-muscle disease are virtually pathognomonic. In arthritis caused by *Erysipelothrix rhusiopathiae* there are deposits on and pitting of articular surfaces, periarticular fibrosis and osteophyte formation. Laminitis due to blue-tongue virus infection can be differentiated clinically and etiologically.

Detailed microbiologic investigations are required to differentiate chlamydial arthritis in animals from mycoplasmal arthritis.

Control and Treatment: If begun early, therapy with long-acting penicillin or tetracyclines or tylosin appear to be beneficial. More advanced lesions do not respond satisfactorily. Daily feeding of 150 to 200 mg of chlortetracycline to affected lambs in feedlots reduces the incidence of chlamydial polyarthritis. One has to keep in mind that intestinal chlamydial infection is probably the first event in the pathogenesis of this disease.

LISTERIOSIS

(Listerellosis, Circling disease)

A sporadic, specific, bacterial infection most commonly manifested by encephalitis or meningoencephalitis in adult ruminants, by septicemia with focal hepatic necrosis in young ruminants and monogastric animals, and by septicemia with myocardial degeneration or focal hepatic necrosis in fowls (*see* AVIAN LISTERIOSIS, p. 1060). The various manifestations of infection occur in all susceptible species. Abortion and perinatal infection may occur in all susceptible mammals, but abortion with encephalitis has not been observed.

Etiology and Epidemiology: Listeriosis is caused by ***Listeria monocytogenes***, a small, motile, gram-positive, nonspore-forming, extremely resistant, diphtheroid rod. Although it grows well on most of the commonly employed bacterial media, it is sometimes difficult to isolate from infected tissues and body fluids.

Listeriosis in its various forms is ubiquitous. The organism has been isolated from at least 42 domestic and wild mammals, 22 species of birds, as well as fish, crustaceans, insects, sewage, water, feedstuffs and earth. The natural reservoirs of the parasite have not been determined. Listeriosis of cattle and sheep is most prevalent in cold weather and seldom occurs during the summer or in areas of warm climate. Outbreaks often occur 2 to 4 days after a sudden drop in temperature. Reported exceptions are listeriosis in sheep and goats in Central Asia during the extremely hot, dry summer months.

The encephalitic form is only one manifestation of listeriosis, and it seems possible that each form may have a unique pathogenesis. There is evidence, for example, that infection through the eye or upper respiratory tract leads to encephalitis via the trigeminal or facial nerves, or both, and experimental oral or IV exposure of pregnant sheep or goats consistently leads to abortion without signs of CNS involvement. However, other evidence supports possible hematogenous entry into the brain. Ectoparasites may play a role in transmission. Removal or change of silage in the ration often stops spread of listeriosis in feedlot animals; feeding the same silage months later may produce new cases. Listeriosis in ruminants has occurred 10 to 14 days following feeding of apparently contaminated silage. Corn silage has been much more commonly implicated in outbreaks in sheep than in cattle. The alkaline pH of spoiled silage appears to enhance the multiplication of *L. monocytogenes.* A nonbacterial listeriosis-enhancing agent (LEA) has been demonstrated in the blood of infected sheep and in the lymph nodes and blood of cattle with the viral diarrhea-mucosal disease complex. Intranasal exposure of sheep with a combination of LEA and *L. monocytogenes* results in listeric encephalitis. Many animals are nonclinical carriers.

Clinical Findings: The most readily recognized form of listeriosis in ruminants is encephalitis. It may affect animals of all ages and both sexes and may appear as an epidemic in feedlot cattle or sheep. The course in sheep and goats is rapid and death may occur 4 to 48 hours after the appearance of signs; occasionally, the animal may survive for several days. In cattle, the disease is less acute and signs may last 4 to 14 days. Spontaneous recovery is uncommon but may occur. Survivors may exhibit manifestations of permanent CNS injury. Lesions are often localized in the brain stem and the signs indicate dysfunction of the third to seventh cranial nerves.

At the onset of the disease, the infected animal becomes solitary. It crowds into a corner or leans against stationary objects as if unable to stand. When walking, it often moves in a circle. Circling is not a constant sign, but when present it is always in one direction. Marked elevation of temperature, anorexia, conjunctivitis and blindness may be present. Marked depression, incoordination and paralysis of the muscles of the jaw, eye and ear as well as stringy salivation and nasal discharge are conspicuous signs. There may be intermittent twitching of the facial muscles, strabismus and drooping of one or both ears, but frank convulsions are rare. The muscles of the head, neck and forelegs usually are more tense than in the posterior part of the body. Terminally, involuntary and aimless running movements are common. Many cows display only a paralysis of the facial and throat muscles, which makes eating and drinking impossible.

The disease may occur on the same premises in successive years. The number of animals involved in an outbreak usually is small but may reach 30% in a flock of sheep or goats and 10% in a herd of cattle. Mortality is high.

L. monocytogenes has been associated with abortion and perinatal death in many animals in addition to sheep, goats and cows, and may be more common than is generally suspected. Abortion usually occurs in late gestation. Focal necrosis of the fetal liver may be masked by autolytic changes. However, *L. monocytogenes* can often be recovered from the placenta and various fetal organs. In some instances, the bacterium can be isolated from the genital tract of the dam and may be shed in the milk for periods varying from days to months. Usually the dam shows no signs of illness or residual damage from listeric abortion. However, fatal septicemia secondary to metritis has occurred. Encephalitic signs and abortion do not usually occur simultaneously on the same premises.

Lesions: In the encephalitic form there are usually no gross lesions. At times, however, the meninges appear slightly inflamed with a few very small gray foci, and the amount of cerebrospinal fluid may be increased. The brain may appear slightly congested and, occasionally, sheep brains may be so hyperemic that the entire brain is bright red.

The septicemic form is commonest in the monogastric mammals. The principal lesions is focal hepatic necrosis. It has been observed in swine, dogs, cats, domestic and wild rabbits, and many other small mammals. These animals may play an important part in the transmission of the disease. This form also has been found in young lambs and calves before the rumen is functional. In young calves, death occurs before 3 weeks of age and often is preceded by dysentery. At necropsy, in addition to focal hepatic necrosis, there is frequently a marked hemorrhagic gastritis and enteritis involving only the small intestine. Though rare, septicemia has been reported in all the domestic ruminants and deer.

Diagnosis: At present, there is no satisfactory antemortem diagnostic test. Listeriosis can be confirmed only by isolation and identification of the specific etiologic agent. Specimens of choice are the brain from animals with CNS involvement and the aborted placenta and fetus. If primary isolation attempts fail, ground tissue should be held at 4°C for several weeks and recultured. Occasionally, *L. monocytogenes* has been isolated from the spinal fluid, nasal discharge, urine, feces and milk of clinically ill ruminants. For isolation from these sources, the use of embryonated hens' eggs or IP inoculation of mice may be preferable to nonliving media. Serologic tests may be of value in some instances but, in general, have proved to be unsatisfactory because many healthy animals show high titers against the bacterium.

In sheep it may be difficult to distinguish between listeriosis and pregnancy toxemia but in pregnancy toxemia, facial and ear paralysis are less likely and ketonuria is a common finding. In cattle the localizing signs of listeriosis, if present, help to differentiate it from thromboembolic encephalitis, polioencephalomalacia and lead poisoning. Rabies must always be considered in the differential diagnosis of listeriosis in both cattle and sheep and sometimes can be ruled out only by laboratory examination. Other causes of brain abscesses, while rare, may be clinically indistinguishable from listeriosis.

Prophylaxis and Treatment: A satisfactory therapeutic agent has not been found, particularly for sheep and goats. Any of the tetracycline antibiotics (e.g. ℞ 27) in high doses appear to be the medication of choice, but may be followed by fatal relapse despite additional therapy. It is difficult to maintain therapeutic levels in the brain with these antibiotics. Supportive therapy including fluids and electrolytes is required for those animals having difficulty eating and drinking.

Results with autogenous bacterins have been inconclusive. In an outbreak, affected animals should be segregated. If silage was being fed, use of the particular ensilage should be discontinued on a trial basis. Spoiled silage should be routinely avoided. Corn that is ensiled before it is too mature is likely to have a more acid pH, which discourages the multiplication of *L. monocytogenes.*

Public Health Importance: Despite the apparently low invasiveness of *L. monocytogenes,* all suspected material should be handled with caution. Aborted fetuses and necropsy of septicemic animals present the greatest hazard. Owners and veterinarians have developed fatal meningitis, septicemia and papular exanthema on the arms after handling aborted material. In encephalitis of animals, the bacterium is usually confined to the brain and presents little danger unless the brain is removed. Pregnant animals, including the human, should be protected from this infection because of danger to the fetus.

L. monocytogenes has been isolated from the milk of cows following abortion and from some cases of mastitis. Such infected milk is a hazard because the organism may survive certain forms of pasteurization and thus expose humans who drink raw or ineffectively pasteurized milk. The concept that animals serve as a reservoir for infection of man may be questioned since the organism has been isolated from the feces of a significant number of apparently normal people as well as animals. Low-grade infections in man may be commoner than is generally suspected and, in pregnant women, may lead to death of the fetus. Perinatal infections account for almost 75% of all the cases of listeriosis reported in man during the past few years. Meningitis or meningoencephalitis accounts for most of the remainder. Other manifestations of listeric infection are conjunctivitis, endocarditis and urethritis.

TUBERCULOSIS

An infectious disease caused by certain pathogenic acid-fast organisms of the genus *Mycobacterium.* Although commonly defined as a chronic, debilitating disease, tuberculosis occasionally can assume an acute, rapidly progressive course. The disease affects practically all species of vertebrate animals, and before control measures were adopted, was one of the major diseases of man and domestic animals. The signs and lesions are generally similar in the various species.

Etiology: Although the disease in all species is known as tuberculosis, the causative agent in all of them is not identical; 3 main types of tubercle bacilli are recognized: human, bovine and avian. Since tubercle bacilli do not multiply except in infected animals, the principal reservoirs of these types in nature are the animal species for which they are named. The 3 types differ not only in distribution, but also in cultural characteristics and pathogenicity. The 2 mammalian types are much more closely related to each other than to the avian type.

All 3 types may produce infection in host species other than their own. The human type is most specific; it rarely produces progressive disease in the lower animals other than primates and, occasionally, dogs and parrots. The avian type is the only one of consequence in birds, but is also pathogenic for swine, cattle and sheep, though natural infection in the latter is rare. The bovine type is the most cosmopolitan and is capable of causing progressive disease in almost all warm-blooded vertebrates.

Pathogenesis: The disease commences with the formation of a primary focus, which in man and cattle is in the lung in about 90% of cases; the primary lesion in poultry is nearly always in the intestinal tract. (*See* AVIAN TUBERCULOSIS, p. 1078.) Lymphatic drainage from the primary focus in mammals leads to the formation of caseous lesions in the corresponding lymph node and this lesion, together with the primary focus, is known as the "primary complex." This primary complex seldom heals in animals, but may progress slowly or rapidly.

Wherever the organisms localize, their activity stimulates the formation of tumor-like masses called tubercles. Because of the continued growth of the organisms these tubercles enlarge often until they become of great size. Sometimes, large masses of new tissue develop on the serous membranes of the body cavities. As the granulomas grow, necrosis of their central portions occurs. Finally, these are reduced to cheesy masses which have a tendency to undergo calcification. In mammals, tubercles may become enclosed in dense fibrous tissue and the disease become arrested. When the bacilli escape from the primary foci they travel via the lymph and blood streams, lodge in other organs and tissues to establish other tubercles. When the blood stream is invaded by numerous tubercle bacilli from a local lesion, many tubercles develop in the major organs. The acute form of generalization, known as miliary tuberculosis, is often rapidly fatal. If small numbers of bacilli enter the circulation from the primary complex, one or more isolated lesions are formed in other organs. These generalized lesions may become encapsulated and remain small for long periods, usually causing no detectable signs.

Clinical Findings: The signs exhibited depend upon the extent and location of the lesions. Small lesions, located in deep lymph nodes, may occasion no clinical signs, but enlarged superficial lymph nodes provide a useful diagnostic sign. If the disease is progressive, the general signs are weakness, anorexia, emaciation and low-grade fluctuating fever. In mammals, the organs of the thoracic cavity usually are involved. When the lungs are extensively diseased, there is commonly an intermittent, hacking cough. The principal sign of tuberculosis commonly is the chronic wasting or emaciation that occurs despite good feeding and care.

Diagnosis: Clinical diagnosis is usually possible only after tuberculosis has reached an advanced stage. Most individuals have become shedders of bacilli by this time and are a menace to other animals. Radiology is used only in monkeys and the small domestic animals. The most certain and practical method of reaching a specific diagnosis in large domestic animals is to apply the tuberculin test. This test depends upon the fact that animals infected with tuberculosis are allergic to the proteins contained in tuberculin and give characteristic delayed hypersensitivity reactions when exposed to them. If tuberculin is deposited in the deep layers of the skin (intradermally). a local reaction characterized by inflammation and swelling is induced in infected animals, whereas normal animals fail to give such reactions.

Animals suffering from infection with either human- or bovine-type tubercle bacilli react about equally well to tuberculin made from either type of organism. When testing for avian-type tuberculosis, whether in birds or mammals, the avian-type organism must be used, as such animals react less strongly to tuberculin made from the mammalian types.

The dose used in the intradermal tuberculin test is 0.1 ml of a suitable tuberculin in mammals and 0.5 ml in chickens. In the U.S.A. the larger mammals are usually injected in one of the folds at the base of the tail, swine in the skin behind the ear, and chickens in the skin of the wattle. The injection sites are examined by observation and palpation for the characteristic swellings 48 hours after injection for swine and chickens, and in 72 hours for cattle.

Nearly all countries are now using a strain of *Mycobacterium bovis* for the preparation of their mammalian tuberculin. Heat concentrated synthetic-medium tuberculin (OT) is still used in some countries, but a majority (including the U.S.A.) are now using a purified protein derivative (PPD) tuberculin at a protein concentration of 1 mg/ml (3 mg/ml in Australia). PPD tuberculins are preferable because they are easier to standardize, more stable and more specific. PPD tuberculins are particularly important in the comparative-cervical (c-c) tuberculin test used to differentiate responses caused by mammalian tuberculosis from heterospecific reactions. In cattle, the c-c test is performed by injecting avian and bovine PPD tuberculins into separate sites in the skin of the neck. The difference in the size of the 2 resultant responses usually indicates whether tuberculin sensitivity is caused by infection with human or bovine type bacilli rather than by the avian type, the Johne's bacillus, or a transient sensitization from other mycobacteria in the environment. These organisms are responsible for many of the false positive tuberculin reactions which are a major problem both in areas where tuberculosis has been nearly eliminated and in those areas where infection with *M. bovis* was relatively low. The incidence of reactors with no gross lesions can be greatly reduced by the use of the c-c test applied by experienced personnel; however, the c-c test is contraindicated in known *M. bovis* populations.

Control: Mammalian tubercle bacilli grow only *in vivo*. The main reservoirs are man and cattle. The prevalence of the disease in such reservoirs determines the disease incidence in other species.

There are 4 principal approaches to the control of tuberculosis: (a) test and slaughter, (b) test and segregation, (c) immunization and (d) chemotherapy. Until the discovery of the antituberculosis drug isonicotinic acid hydrazide (INH) there was no practical therapeutic agent available for the treatment of bovine tuberculosis. Reports from South Africa indicate that it is economically feasible to treat cattle with isoniazid. The disadvantages are so great, however (up to 25% refractory cases, emergence of drug resistant strains, elimination of INH in the milk, and the danger of relapse when the drug is withdrawn) that the treatment of bovine tuberculosis is not allowed in the U.S.A. or in many other countries.

The test-and-slaughter method consists of the application of the tuberculin test and the slaughter of reacting animals. This method has been widely used in the U.S.A., Canada, New Zealand and Australia. In most European countries, where test-and-slaughter would have been impracticable, varying forms of test-and-segregation have been used, with test-and-slaughter only in the final stages.

While BCG (Bacillus of Calmette and Guerin) vaccine is the most successful immunizing agent in humans and reduces the severity of the initial disease in cattle, it does not completely prevent infection and vaccinated cattle react to the tuberculin test. Countries that attempted to use vaccination as the basis of a control program have ultimately abandoned the procedure in favor of the test-and-slaughter method.

TUBERCULOSIS IN CATTLE

This disease used to be very prevalent, particularly in dairy cattle but control programs have greatly reduced the incidence in many countries. A number of countries have virtually eradicated bovine tuberculosis from cattle. A few infected herds continue to be discovered in parts of the U.S.A., which launched the first major eradication program in 1917. The source of infection is usually other infected cattle although in some European countries pulmonary or genitourinary tuberculosis of man caused by bacilli of the bovine type is the source of infection in up to 60% of reinfected herds.

Tuberculous animals with open lung lesions throw infected droplets into the air by coughing. Such animals also swallow sputum and thus contaminate pasture and cowsheds via the feces. Adult animals are infected by the inhalation of airborne dust particles as well as contaminated feed and water facilities. Young calves may be infected by drinking unpasteurized infected milk.

Early lesions are usually found in the chest and sometimes in the lymph nodes of the head or intestines. In advanced stages of the disease, lesions may be found in many organs and tissues that are seldom affected primarily; thus, infection of the udder, uterus, lymph nodes, kidneys and the meninges occurs with varying frequency. The skeletal muscles are very seldom affected, even in advanced cases. Tuberculosis of the udder is of special significance because of contamination of milk with infective organisms.

TUBERCULOSIS IN SWINE

Swine are subject to infection with all 3 types of tubercle bacilli. Infection is most often contracted by the ingestion of infected materials; hence the primary lesions are in the intestinal tract and associated lymph nodes, particularly the submaxillary. With bovine-type bacilli, generalization is often severe and rapid, but infection with the avian or human type is usually limited to the lymph nodes of the head and to the intestinal tract and associated lymph nodes.

Lesions caused by the avian and human types tend to be fleshy and firm and are not strongly invasive, whereas the bovine bacillus usually causes a rapidly progressive disease with caseation and liquefaction of the lesions. Differentiation has to be confirmed by isolating the organism and typing it. Lesions resembling those of tuberculosis are also produced in pigs by certain of the opportunist mycobacteria.

TUBERCULOSIS IN SHEEP

The disease is rare in sheep, but when it occurs the bovine type causes a condition similar to that in cattle. The avian bacillus may also cause severe progressive lesions.

TUBERCULOSIS IN DOGS

Dogs may be infected by the human or bovine type. Up to 10% of dogs necropsied in some cities, when spittoons were commonly used, were found to be tuberculous. The infection now is much less common in most countries, but dogs may still be infected from a human source and may in turn infect man, especially children. The short-nosed breeds appear to be more susceptible and males are more commonly affected than females.

Tuberculous lesions in the dog usually resemble neoplasms, especially the sarcomas. Often the tubercles are grayish white and are circumscribed. The large liver lesions are yellowish with depressed centers and crenated hemorrhagic edges. Some of these lesions have soft almost purulent centers; others appear as ragged bloody cavities or may take the form of small, multiple gray nodules scattered throughout the liver substance.

Lung lesions usually consist of grayish red bronchopneumonic areas; some break down to form cavities. These may open into the pleural cavity or communicate with a bronchus. Early spreading lesions vary from areas of acute congestion to hepatization. The pulmonary and pleural lesions are invariably exudative in type and there may be a large quantity of straw-colored liquid in the chest. Such lesions may cause collapse of the lower portions of the lung.

False negative tuberculin tests are common in the dog; radiographs and a history of exposure are helpful aids to diagnosis. Because of the public health significance, affected dogs should be destroyed as should all dogs on premises being depopulated of cattle because of bovine tuberculosis.

TUBERCULOSIS IN CATS

The cat, unlike the dog, is resistant to infection with human tubercle bacilli. It is considerably more susceptible than the dog to experimental bovine-type infection, and most natural infections arise from the ingestion of infected milk, primary lesions being found in the intestinal tract. However, primary respiratory infection does occur and infected wounds sometimes give rise to tuberculous sinuses. At one time, up to 12% of cats necropsied in parts of Europe were found to be tuberculous but, with the elimination of tubercle bacilli from the milk supply, the disease has become rare.

In general, lesions in cats resemble those in dogs. Few isolated primary foci have been recorded and it appears that infection is followed by rapid generalization. Lesions and discharges are usually rich in bacilli.

The tuberculin test is considered unreliable in the cat and radiographic diagnosis is often difficult. Isolation of the bacilli provides evidence of infection, but negative culture results are of questionable value. Because of the public health significance, affected animals should be destroyed as should all cats on premises being depopulated of cattle because of bovine tuberculosis.

BRUCELLOSIS

A specific contagious disease primarily affecting cattle, swine, sheep, goats and dogs, caused by bacteria of the *Brucella* group and characterized by abortion in the female, to a lesser extent, orchitis and infection of the accessory sex glands in the male and infertility in both sexes. The disease is prevalent in most of the world. Brucellosis occasionally affects horses where it frequently is associated with fistulous withers and poll evil. The human disease, also called undulant or Malta fever, is a serious public health problem.

BRUCELLOSIS IN CATTLE
(Contagious abortion, Bang's disease)

Etiology: The disease in cattle is caused almost exclusively by *Brucella abortus*, but occasionally *Br. suis* or *Br. melitensis* are isolated. Bovine brucellosis is now less prevalent in the U.S.A. than formerly because of vaccination and eradication programs; a few states are virtually free of the disease.

Epidemiology: The appearance of the infection in a nonvaccinated herd that has been free of brucellosis is characterized by rapid spread and many abortions. In the herd in which the disease is endemic, the typical infected animal aborts only once after exposure, and subsequent gestations and lactions appear to be normal. Following exposure, most cattle develop a bacteremia and a positive blood serum agglutination reaction; the remainder either resist or recover rapidly from infection. The positive blood reaction usually precedes abortion, but in some animals it may be delayed. The organism is shed in the milk and in uterine discharges and the cow may suffer from temporary sterility. The bacteria are found in the uterus during pregnancy, during the period of uterine involution and, infrequently, for a prolonged time in the nongravid uterus. Many infected cows shed brucellae from the uterus at subsequent normal parturitions following an abortion. Secondary infection contributes to the infertility and, by prolonging the period of involution, also may prolong the presence of *Br. abortus* in the uterus and its discharges. The organism is shed in the milk for a variable length of time, some animals shedding it for life. The extremes of susceptibility are seen in the naturally immune cow that never becomes infected and the very susceptible animal that suffers repeated abortions.

Natural transmission of the disease is through ingestion of the organisms that are present in large numbers in the aborted fetus, membranes and uterine discharge. Cattle may ingest feed or water that is contaminated with brucellae and occasionally lick the contaminated genitals of other animals or recently aborted fetuses. Venereal transmission by infected bulls to susceptible cattle by natural service may occur but is rare. Cows may be infected by means of artificial insemination when the *Brucella*-contaminated semen is deposited in the uterus but not when it is deposited in the mid-cervix. Brucellae may enter the body through mucous surfaces, the conjunctivae, injuries and even through the intact skin.

Mechanical vectors, such as dogs, other animals and man can act as a means of spreading infection. Under certain circumstances, the organism will live for weeks outside the body. Brucellae have been recovered from the fetus, and from manure that has remained in a cool environment for more than 2 months. Exposure to direct sunlight kills the organism in a matter of a few hours.

Clinical Findings: Abortion of the fetus is the most obvious manifestation of the disease. Establishment of the carrier state in a large proportion of animals may lead to a 20% reduction in the milk yield of infected cows, the production of dead calves at term and an increased frequency of retained placenta. In uncomplicated abortions, there usually is no impairment of the general health.

In the bull, the seminal vesicles, the ampullae, the testicles and the epididymides may be infected which results in the organism being shed in the semen. Agglutinins may be demonstrated in the seminal plasma of such bulls. Abscesses of the testicles may occur. The organism has been isolated from arthritic joints.

Diagnosis: Diagnosis must be based on bacteriologic or serologic examination. *Br. abortus* can be recovered from the placenta, but more conveniently in pure culture from the stomach and lungs of the aborted fetus. The organisms may be isolated from the genital tract after abortion or normal calving for periods of up to 10 weeks in 50% of infected animals. Most cows cease shedding from the genital tract when uterine involution is complete. The reservoirs of permanent infection are the reticuloendothelial system and the udder, and it frequently is possible to isolate *Br. abortus* from the milk.

Blood serum agglutination tests are the standard methods of diagnosing bovine brucellosis. These tests may also be used to detect antibodies in milk, whey and semen plasma. Vaginal mucus tests for

Brucella agglutinins also may be of some diagnostic value. Agglutination at serum dilutions of 1:100 or above for nonvaccinated animals, 1:200 for calves vaccinated between 3 and 9 months of age, or positive brucellosis card-test results, are considered positive for brucellosis.

The latter test differs from the conventional agglutination tests in that it utilizes an acidified, buffered antigen and only a single test dilution. The advantages are selective detection of antibodies most likely to be associated with *Brucella* infection and the ability to conduct the test within a few minutes after blood collection.

Screening diagnostic procedures: (1) Milk ring test—In the official control and eradication of brucellosis on an area basis, the milk ring test has proved to be a highly efficient and accurate diagnostic procedure for locating infected dairy herds. Milk samples are collected from each herd at the milk-processing plant or creamery, or at the farm where the milk is collected in large tanks. The brucellosis status of dairy herds in any area can be determined and the disease eradicated by applying the milk ring test at 3- to 4-month intervals with necessary follow-up blood tests of the positive herds and slaughter of reactors. The cost of such a program is approximately one-tenth of that required to blood-test the cattle of all herds in the same area, whereas the efficiency of the 2 methods in locating infected herds is comparable.

(2) **Market cattle testing**—Nondairy herds in an area also may be screened for brucellosis by testing the marketed cattle. This program is based upon blood testing of nonproductive or surplus adult cattle destined for slaughter through intermediate and terminal markets or at abattoirs. Reactors are traced to the herd of origin, and the remaining cattle in these herds are tested. The unit cost for detecting a reactor by this method is only a fraction of that incurred by area blood testing of the cattle in all herds.

Brucellosis-free areas can be achieved and maintained, both effectively and economically, by a system which combines utilization of both the milk ring test on all dairy herds and the market cattle testing program on all nondairy herds.

Supplementary tests may be employed in herds from which brucellosis has not been eradicated despite the continued conscientious application of standard eradication procedures. Utilization of a battery of these tests improves the possibility of detecting the infected animal or animals that have resided in these herds as undetected reservoirs of infection. Supplementary tests currently used include complement fixation, rivanol precipitation, and mercaptoethanol agglutination tests. These tests are designed to detect primarily the IgG antibodies that are associated specifically with *Brucella* infection. Another supplementary diagnostic procedure is testing of quarter milk samples with milk or whey agglutination tests. The latter procedure is often an excellent method for detecting chronic infection in the udder of cows that may have equivocal blood serum reactions.

Control: No practical effective treatment is known, and efforts are directed at control and prevention. Eventual eradication of the disease depends upon testing and elimination of reactors. Many individual herds have been freed of the disease by this method. The infected herd is tested at regular intervals until 2 or 3 successive negative tests are obtained. When reactors are found, they are removed and the premises thoroughly cleaned and disinfected.

Clean herds must be protected from reinfection. The greatest danger is from replacement animals. Where possible, new additions should be vaccinated calves or nonpregnant heifers. If pregnant or fresh cows must be used, they should originate from brucellosis-free herds and be negative to serologic tests. It is advisable to segregate such replacements from the herd for at least 30 days and retest them before permitting them to associate with the main herd.

Vaccination with *Br. abortus* Strain 19 (5 ml subcut.) is widely used in calves and is effective in increasing resistance to infection. Resistance is not complete and will break to some extent, depending upon the severity of exposure. Experimental evidence indicates that the immunity following calfhood vaccination does not decline with the passage of time. A small proportion of these animals become persistent positive or suspicious reactors to the agglutination test, with attendant confusion in diagnosis.

Another vaccine, *Br. abortus* 45/20 bacterin in adjuvant, has gained widespread acceptance in some countries. Most studies indicate that 45/20 vaccine, when used as recommended, may induce immunity comparable with that of Strain 19. Current recommendations require 2 initial injections at specific intervals and annual booster injections thereafter. The principal advantage of this vaccine is that agglutination test reactors seldom occur after vaccination, since 45/20 is a nonsmooth strain of *Br. abortus*. However, it does interfere with diagnosis when the complement fixation test is used. Disadvantages of 45/20 bacterin are the necessity of giving numerous injections at specific intervals and the attendant economic cost, and occasional objectionable local reactions at the site of injection.

Vaccination as the sole means of control has been effective; the degree of reduction of reactors is directly related to the degree that calfhood vaccination is practiced. However, when it is desired to go beyond control to eradication, test and slaughter are necessary, and continued vaccination poses the problem of interpretation of "positive" test reactions.

BRUCELLOSIS IN GOATS

A disease with signs similar to those of brucellosis in cattle occurs in goats. Caprine brucellosis in man (Malta fever) was the first *Brucella* infection to be recognized and described. The disease in goats is prevalent in most countries where goats and sheep are a significant part of the animal industry, and was fairly common in the Southwestern U.S.A. until recent years. At the present time, it occurs rarely in this country.

The causal agent usually is *Brucella melitensis*, but occasionally *Br. abortus* is found. Infection occurs primarily through the ingestion of the organism, but conjunctival, vaginal and subcut. inoculation will produce the disease. Abortion occurs about the fourth month of pregnancy. Rarely, arthritis and orchitis occur, and keratitis and chronic bronchitis may be caused by infection with *Br. melitensis*. The diagnosis is made by bacteriologic examination of the milk or of the aborted fetus, or by the serum agglutination test. In the interpretation of this test, if any animal in the herd shows a titer of 1:100, all goats reacting at 1:50 or 1:25 should also be considered infected. The disease is controlled by the slaughter of reacting animals.

Two *Br. melitensis* vaccines have shown promise of preventing caprine brucellosis in controlled experiments and field trials. One is a killed vaccine suspended in an adjuvant and the other is an attenuated vaccine (Rev. 1 *Br. melitensis* vaccine). Vaccination for the control of caprine brucellosis should be considered only in countries where the incidence of the disease is high.

BRUCELLOSIS IN SWINE

The clinical manifestations of the disease in swine vary considerably, but they are similar in many respects to those of brucellosis in cattle and goats. The disease often is self-limiting within the individual animal to a greater degree than in cattle. Despite this self-limitation, the disease has remained in some herds for years. Brucellosis due to *Brucella suis* also occurs in other domestic animals and man. Epidemics of human brucellosis occur among packing-house workers and the usual source is infected swine.

Etiology: The disease in swine is caused almost exclusively by biotypes of *Br. suis*, but *Br. abortus* is also occasionally found. The disease is spread mainly by direct animal-to-animal contact, usually through the ingestion of infected material. Infected boars may transmit the disease during service, and the organism can be recovered from the semen.

Swine raised for breeding purposes constitute the important source of infection. Although of infrequent occurrence, natural transmission from infected weanling pigs has been reported. Some suckling pigs may become infected by contact with infected sows, but the majority reach weaning age without becoming infected. The effects of brucellosis usually are more severe in breeding swine than in young pigs, but both age groups are susceptible.

Clinical Findings: Following exposure to *Br. suis*, swine develop a bacteremia in which the organism may persist in the blood stream for periods varying up to 90 days. During and following the bacteremic stage, it may become localized in a wide variety of tissues. Signs depend considerably on the site or sites of localization. Common manifestations are abortion, temporary or permanent sterility, orchitis, lameness, posterior paralysis, spondylitis and, occasionally, metritis and abscess formation in the extremities or other areas of the body.

There is much variation in the incidence of abortion, from as high as 50 to 80% of the females in some herds, to no observed abortions in others. Abortions also may occur early in gestation and be unobserved. Usually, sows or gilts that abort early come in heat a short time afterward and are rebred.

Sterility in sows, gilts and boars is common and may be the only manifestation of brucellosis. In swine herds where sterility is a problem, it is logical to test for brucellosis before attempting treatment. In sows, the sterility may be permanent, but is more frequently of a temporary nature. Orchitis, usually unilateral, may occur. Fertility appears to be lowered, but complete sterility may or may not ensue.

Diagnosis: The principal means of diagnosis of swine brucellosis is the brucellosis card test. Various other serum-agglutination tests or complement fixation tests may also be used. It is generally accepted that the tests are effective in determining the presence or absence of brucellosis in the herd, but have limitations in detecting brucellosis in individual animals. Thus, entire herds or units of herds, rather than individual animals, must be considered in any control program.

Prophylaxis and Control: In almost any sizable herd of swine, low-titered reactions occur in the absence of infection. These same low-titered reactions occur in herds where infection is present and a few infected swine may have no detectable agglutinin titer. The brucellosis card test is usually more accurate than conventional agglutination tests since low-titer agglutinins due to causes other than *Brucella* seldom react with it. Supplementary tests designed for cattle can also be used for swine. Caution should be used in the purchase of individual swine that exhibit a low-titered agglutination response, unless the status of the entire herd of origin is known. Swine should be held in isolation upon their return from fairs or shows before entering the main herd. All replacements should be purchased from herds known to be free of brucellosis, or failing this, should be tested, kept in isolation for 3 months and retested before being added to the herd.

Vaccination is unreliable. Control is based on test, segregation and slaughter of infected breeding stock. The following plans can be used to eliminate brucellosis from a herd:

1. Sales of entire herd for slaughter: This plan is usually the quickest, surest and most economical. Replacement of the infected breeding herd should be from herds free from infection and may be made after the premises and equipment are cleaned and disinfected. The replacement herd should be placed on clean ground (free of swine for at least 60 days).

2. Test, segregation and delayed slaughter of infected herds: This plan is recommended for use in purebred herds only where it is desired to retain valuable bloodlines. The procedures to be followed are: (a) Separate and isolate (on clean ground) the weanling pigs at 6 weeks of age or younger. Market the remainder of the herd as soon as practicable. (b) Test the pigs saved about 30 days before breeding and save only gilts that are negative. Breed only to known negative boars. (c) Re-test the gilts after farrowing. If infection is disclosed, repeat plan 2 or abandon in favor of plan 1.

3. Slaughter of reactors only: This is not generally recommended except in herds where only a very few reactors are found, no clinical signs of brucellosis have been noted, and there is doubt that the reactor titers were caused by *Brucella* infection. In this plan, retest the herd at 30-day intervals, removing reactors until the entire herd is negative.

Swine breeders in the U.S.A. should be encouraged to validate their herds. Details of procedures for validating herds and areas are available from State Veterinarians in each state.

No practical recommendations can be made for treating infected swine.

BRUCELLOSIS IN DOGS

While dogs occasionally become infected with *Br. abortus*, *Br. suis*, or *Br. melitensis*, these are sporadic occurrences, usually in dogs closely associated with infected herds of domestic livestock. Transmission of *Brucella* spp. from dogs to man and other animals is known. Dogs have been considered to be relatively resistant to *Brucella* infection and in most cases the disease appears to be self-limiting. However, in 1966 it became apparent that endemics of abortion among kenneled dogs were caused by a newly described organism, *Brucella canis*. The dog appears to be the definitive host of this organism; infection in man has been reported. In some breeding kennels the disease has caused reduction of the number of pups weaned to one-fourth that of levels before infection. The disease is rapidly disseminated among dogs closely kenneled, especially at the time of breeding or when abortions occur. Transmission is congenital or venereal or by ingestion of infective materials. All ages and both sexes appear to be equally susceptible.

The main clinical feature is abortion without premonitory signs during the last trimester of pregnancy. Stillbirths and conception failures are also predominant features of the disease. Prolonged vaginal discharge usually follows abortion and repeated abortions during successive pregnancies are common. Infected dogs also develop generalized lymphadenitis and, in males, epididymitis, periorchitis and prostatitis frequently occur. Bacteremia is a constant finding and it persists for an average of about 18 months after exposure. Pyrexia is not characteristic.

Diagnosis is based on isolation of the causative agent or serologic tests. The organism can usually be readily isolated from vaginal exudate, aborted pups, blood, urine, milk, or semen of infected dogs. The most commonly used serologic test has been the agglutination test. The antigen for use must be prepared from *Br. canis* or *Br. ovis* as these organisms show little cross-reaction with other *Brucella* spp. Nonspecific agglutination reactions sometimes occur with serums from dogs proved not to have been infected.

Attempts at immunization or treatment have not been uniformly successful. The most successful control measures have been based on elimination or isolation of infected dogs identified by positive cultural or serologic results. Management factors are also important as the incidence of infection has been observed to be much lower in kennels where dogs were caged individually.

BRUCELLOSIS IN HORSES

Horses can be infected with *Brucella* spp., especially *Br. abortus* or *Br. suis*. Suppurative bursitis, most commonly recognized as "fistula of the withers" or "poll evil" (q.v., p. 571) is the most frequent ailment associated with brucellosis in horses. Occasionally, abortion in mares caused by *Br. abortus* or *Br. suis* has been reported. It appears, however, that the commonest manifestation of equine brucellosis is localization of the organism in tissues such as muscles, tendons and joints. In some recent surveys positive results to serum agglutination tests were obtained in as high as 44% of 421 horses sampled. However, most were positive only at low dilutions, and there is little evidence to indicate the significance of the titers. Until the relationship between infection and agglutinin titers is established no specific recommendation for treatment or control of brucellosis in horses can be made.

EPIDIDYMITIS OF RAMS

(*Brucella ovis* infection)

A specific bacterial disease of sheep, characterized in the ram by epididymitis, orchitis and impaired fertility; in the ewe by placentitis and abortion; and in the lamb by perinatal mortality. The disease has been reported in New Zealand, Australia, the U.S.A., South Africa, Kenya, France, Romania, Czechoslovakia, the U.S.S.R. and South America. It is almost certainly present elsewhere. Epididymitis in rams may also be the result of other infections.

Etiology: The causal agent, *Br. ovis* is not known to cause natural infection in other species. Rams as young as 8 weeks have been infected experimentally by various nonvenereal routes. The disease can be transmitted among rams by direct contact but ram-to-ram transmission is increased during the mating season when clean rams acquire infection by serving ewes previously served by infected rams. Active infection in ewes is unusual but has developed after mating with naturally infected rams. Contaminated pastures do not appear important in spreading the disease. Active infection is frequently persistent in rams, a high percentage being capable of shedding the causative agent in semen over periods in excess of 4 years.

Clinical Findings: The principal clinical manifestations are lesions of the epididymis, tunica and testis of the ram and placentitis in the ewe, with abortion and perinatal death of lambs. In recently infected rams, the lesions may develop rapidly, the first abnormality detectable being a marked deterioration in semen quality associated with the presence of inflammatory cells and organisms in the semen. An acute systemic reaction is rarely observed in the field. Following regression of the acute phase—which may be so mild as to go unobserved—lesions may be palpated in the epididymis and scrotal tunics. Epididymal enlargement may be unilateral or bilateral, the tail of the epididymis being involved more frequently than the head or body. The most prominent lesion in the epididymis is the development of spermatoceles of variable size containing partially inspissated spermatic fluid. The tunics frequently become thickened and fibrous, and extensive adhesions develop between the visceral and parietal layers. The testes may show fibrous atrophy. In most cases, these lesions are permanent; in a few, palpable lesions are transient, while in others, organisms may be excreted in defective semen over long periods without clinically detectable lesions.

Lesions in the fetal membranes of infected ewes vary from a superficial purulent exudate on an intact chorion to a marked edema of the allantochorionic mesenchyme, usually with necrosis of the uterine surface of the allantochorion and fetal cotyledons.

Diagnosis: Since not all infected rams show palpable abnormalities of the scrotal contents (nor are all cases of epididymitis due to this specific infection), the remaining rams must be further examined following palpation. Rams shedding organisms, but without lesions, must be identified by cultural examination of semen samples. Repeated examinations may be necessary to identify those rams that shed the organism only intermittently. Microscopic examination of stained semen smears may also be helpful. Fluorescent antibody staining is a highly specific diagnostic aid. Serologic tests used for eradication and accreditation have included complement fixation, hemagglutination inhibition, indirect agglutination and gel diffusion. Allergic tests have also been utilized more particularly in Romania, the U.S.S.R. and South America.

Control and Treatment: The incidence and spread of the disease may be reduced by the regular examination of rams prior to the breeding season and the culling of those with obvious genital abnormalities. Since the incidence of infection in rams rises sharply with age, there are advantages in isolating the younger, clean rams from older, possibly infected rams and keeping the ram flock young.

Immunization of rams has been practiced extensively in New Zealand using two doses of killed *Br. ovis* cells in adjuvant. Immunization of weaner rams with Elberg's Rev. 1 live vaccine has been recommended in South Africa. It is an attenuated *Br. melitensis* vaccine. Since infection in ewes apparently originates almost exclusively from the use of infected rams, lamb losses through infection of ewes may be controlled economically by restricting vaccination to rams.

Chlortetracycline and streptomycin used together have been shown to effect bacteriologic cures. Except in specially valuable rams, such treatment is uneconomic, and even if the infection is eliminated, there is no certainty of a return to unimpaired fertility.

EPIDEMIC BOVINE ABORTION (EBA)

(Chlamydial abortion of cattle)

An infectious disease of cattle manifested primarily by abortion, which has been reported in Western U.S.A. and Europe. It is part of a syndrome known as "foothill abortion" that has appeared in California in cows pastured on foothill terrain.

Etiology and Transmission: One abortifacient agent isolated to date from fetuses aborted from cows pastured in California foothills is a strain of *Chlamydia psittaci* that is similar, if not identical, to the one causing ovine chlamydial abortion, known also as endemic abortion of ewes (EAE, q.v., p. 377). Other incidental isolations of chlamydial agents from ticks and rodents in areas where cattle have aborted suggest the existence of a vector-reservoir cycle of these organisms in nature, with cattle being an incidental host. However, tick-transmitted chlamydial abortion has never been demonstrated experimentally. Recently, *Ornithodoros coriaceus* ticks collected in the field and found free of chlamydiae have been demonstrated to transmit an abortifacient agent by exposure to pregnant cattle. It appears that EBA is a disease complex likely caused by a number of tick-transmitted agents. Chlamydial infection leading to abortion may occasionally be an additional etiologic factor. Further study is needed to clarify the true etiology of EBA.

In epidemic areas, only heifers in their initial pregnancy and cattle introduced from areas free of the disease are affected. The abortion rate varies from 25 to 75% in such animals. In susceptible herds, cattle of all ages are affected.

Clinical Findings: Naturally infected cattle show few if any signs of infection other than abortion, which occurs usually between the fifth and seventh months of gestation. Occasionally, calves are born alive but invariably die within several days. Temporary retention of the placenta sometimes occurs but the cow's reproductive capacity is not affected. Pregnant cows infected experimentally with the chlamydial agent develop a transient hyperthermia shortly after inoculation.

Lesions: The subcut. tissues of aborted fetuses may be edematous and the abdomen distended by excessive amounts of peritoneal fluid; erythema may be present over the skin of the flank and abdomen. Petechial hemorrhages may be scattered throughout the subcut. tissues, over the ventral surface of the tongue, the mucosa of the trachea and the oral cavity, and in the conjunctiva. The liver lesions are the most characteristic of the disease: the liver may be enlarged, granular and friable, and from pale red to reddish orange. About 50% of the fetuses exhibit one or more of the gross lesions associated with the disease; the remainder show no gross changes.

Placentitis and severe necrosis of cotyledons occur in acute cases. The inflammatory exudates in cotyledons are highly infectious and contain large numbers of chlamydiae-infected nonnuclear cells.

Histopathologic lesions consist of focal or diffuse granulomatous changes which may involve most of the fetal organs, but are found most frequently in the liver.

Diagnosis: Tentative diagnosis can be made clinically when typical lesions are present. In their absence diagnosis is based on herd history, circumstances of the outbreak, and histopathologic findings. Isolation of the chlamydial agent from fetal tissues is generally unsuccessful (probably because it fails to survive the long interval between infection and abortion and not all fetuses become infected), but chlamydiae are readily isolated from infected, necrotic cotyledons. Serologic evidence obtained by complement fixation testing is of little diagnostic value since a high percentage of cattle are seropositive for chlamydial antibodies stimulated by the presence of an avirulent chlamydial agent normally inhabiting the gut. Other than isolation and identification of abortifacient chlamydiae from placental or fetal tissues, the only diagnostic test of value is the demonstration of chlamydial antibodies in the serum of the aborted fetus. However, seroconversions occur only in infected, immunocompetent fetuses.

Prophylaxis and Treatment: Field observations indicate that an immunity develops in response to chlamydial infection but it persists only in cattle maintained in areas where the disease is indigenous. This suggests that constant re-exposure to the agent, or agents, is required to maintain the immunity at a protective level. It appears that immunity is cell mediated. An inactivated vaccine prepared from the bovine chlamydial abortion agent and administered intradermally protects against challenge infection. Field trials of the vaccine have given indifferent results because data interpretation was hindered by low rates of naturally occurring chlamydial abortion in test and control animals as compared with those due to other causes. Prophylactic therapy with tetracycline compounds at the level of 2 gm per cow daily throughout pregnancy has been shown to be effective under experimental conditions. However, field application of this measure using antibiotic-incorporated protein-molasses blocks or alfalfa pellets is limited because of material and labor costs and difficulty in maintaining serum antibiotic concentrations at a constant level.

ENDEMIC ABORTION OF EWES (EAE)

(Chlamydial abortion of ewes)

An infectious disease of sheep manifested by abortion and to a lesser extent by stillbirth or premature lambing. The disease has been reported in Scotland, Germany, Hungary, Romania, Bulgaria, South Africa and the U.S.A.

Etiology and Transmission: The causative agent is a strain of *Chlamydia psittaci* that is similar to, if not identical with, the one that causes bovine abortion (q.v., p. 375). Strains recovered from aborted fetuses of either sheep or cattle can be used to reproduce abortion in either species. The organisms from ovine tissues can be propagated in the yolk sac of chicken embryos, in mice by nasal instillation and in guinea pigs by IP inoculation. The natural mode of transmission of the agent appears to be by ingestion although the disease can be produced experimentally by parenteral inoculation. There is no evidence of venereal or arthropod-mediated transmission.

The epidemiology of the disease is not completely understood. It is believed that lambs in aborting flocks become infected during birth or shortly thereafter through ingestion of infectious materials. Open ewes may also become infected at this time. In either case, the infection remains latent until conception occurs. The agent then invades the placenta and fetus, and abortion ensues. Infected ewes may deliver normal lambs at term; occasionally only one lamb of a set of twins will be infected. Ewes that become infected during late gestation may not abort (or deliver prematurely) until the subsequent gestation.

Clinical Findings: Abortion, stillbirth or premature lambing, occurring usually during the second gestation and frequently accompanied by placental retention, are characteristic of the disease. Placental retention occurs more frequently when the ewe aborts than when delivery is premature, and persists from 2 to 10 days. Ewes may carry dead fetuses *in utero,* which sometimes mummify before being expelled. Such ewes lose condition rapidly and some may die shortly after aborting. Apart from these cases, the disease has little effect on the ewe.

Lesions: Placentitis with necrosis of the cotyledons and edema and thickening of the intercotyledonary spaces are the principal lesions. Fetal membranes of the EAE-infected ewes resemble closely those of cattle aborting from brucellosis. The subcut. and muscle tissues of aborted fetuses are edematous and hemorrhagic, and blood-tinged fluids are present in the serous cavities.

Diagnosis: Laboratory assistance is essential in differentiating chlamydial abortion from ovine abortion due to other causes. Placentitis, and the demonstration of intracellular elementary bodies in impression smears from the surface of the cotyledons, provide a tentative diagnosis. Isolation and identification of causative chlamydiae constitute a conclusive diagnosis. Since many ewes normally harbor chlamydial agents in their intestines (and contamination of the placenta with these agents may occur during abortion), isolation of chlamydiae from internal fetal tissues is of more diagnostic value than when isolated from the placenta. Because chlamydia-positive sera are common among flocks naturally infected with intestinal chlamydiae, serologic findings are of no diagnostic value. Campylobacteriosis (q.v., p. 387) causes a very similar syndrome.

Control: Moderate control of chlamydial abortion by vaccination has been reported from Scotland, but this measure had limited success in the U.S.A. Tetracycline compounds are effective in controlling the abortion, but the cost and problem of administering the antibiotic is a major disadvantage. Since the infection is transmitted predominantly at lambing time, precautionary measures such as segregation of aborting animals, and the careful disposal of infected placentas and fetuses are probably the most effective available means of limiting spread of the disease.

Treatment: Tetracycline therapy is recommended for the treatment of infected newborn lambs and ewes that have carried dead fetuses for some time prior to abortion. However, effective doses have not yet been established. Secondary bacterial infection resulting from placental retention lends itself to antibiotic treatment.

LEPTOSPIROSIS

A contagious disease of animals and man due to infection with *Leptospira* spp. These are very slender, helical organisms having a characteristic hook in one or both ends. In dogs, cattle, pigs, sheep, goats and horses, infections are usually asymptomatic, but they may result in a wide variety of disease conditions including fever, icterus, hemoglobinuria, abortion and death. Following acute infection, leptospires frequently localize in the kidneys and are shed in the urine, sometimes in enormous numbers for months or years. They survive well in surface waters, and leptospirosis is essentially a water-borne disease.

The common mode of natural infection is from contact with urine or by intake of urine-contaminated feed or water. Artificial infections are readily established by the conjunctival or vaginal routes and through skin abrasions. If shedder animals are introduced into a herd that has been free of the disease, leptospirosis is rapidly disseminated and abortions may occur among animals in the middle or last third of gestation. Clinical signs may be severe, mild or absent. Recovery is associated with high levels of circulating antibodies and the disappearance of leptospires from the animal except those localized in the kidneys. Leptospiral abortions are not characterized by retention of the fetal membranes or impaired fertility and subsequent pregnancies are usually normal. Most outbreaks of the disease are therefore self-limiting, but the control of some may require rodent depopulation or fencing the herd from surface waters in addition to immunization and chemotherapy.

Diagnostic Procedures: Serologic methods: Of the more than 100 antigentically distinct leptospires, only 6 or 7 cause disease in domestic animals. There is remarkably little cross-immunity, and dual and even treble infections have been reported. Antibodies first appear in the serum of infected animals by the sixth or seventh day, and titers rise rapidly to a very high level. The titer then declines to a more or less constant level that may persist for years. A single positive serologic result indicates either vaccination, passive immunity from the milk of the dam, or past infection. Serological confirmation of a clinical diagnosis of leptospirosis requires the demonstration of a rising titer in consecutive serum samples, the first taken as early in the disease as possible and the second after an interval of 7 to 10 days. Vaccination with bacterins stimulates only low levels of agglutinins. The carrier or shedder state cannot be diagnosed serologically. The serologic methods commonly used include the "plate" agglutination, microscopic agglutination, and complement fixation tests.

Primary isolations are made by inoculating 1 ml of blood, collected during the acute state of infection, into laboratory animals or suitable media. A series of 4 or 5 inoculations should be made to ensure isolation. Similarly, urine may be examined for leptospires 2 weeks or longer after acute infection. Negative results do not rule out infection, however.

Histopathologic examination: A clinical diagnosis of leptospirosis can be confirmed by the demonstration of the organisms in sections of kidney and liver stained by the silver-impregnation method of Levaditi or the Warthin-Starry technique. Leptospires do not stain with the common aniline dyes.

Microscopic examination: Fresh material in the form of tissue scrapings from liver or kidney substance or the centrifuged deposit from freshly collected urine may be examined by means of the dark-field microscope. In some cases, the characteristic motile organisms are readily seen, but the method is hazardous and requires interpretation by an expert. A fluorescent antibody technique is being studied.

LEPTOSPIROSIS IN DOGS

(Canine typhus, Stuttgart disease, Infectious jaundice)

Leptospirosis in dogs is usually due to infection with *L. canicola* or *L. icterohaemorrhagiae*. *L. pomona* infections have been reported, but are usually inapparent.

Etiology: Infections with *L. canicola* are much more prevalent than those with *L. icterohaemorrhagiae* and frequently produce epidemics of the so-called hemorrhagic type of leptospirosis. The icteric type of leptospirosis is usually due to *L. icterohaemorrhagiae;* rats are a reservoir of infection.

Clinical Findings: Dogs of all ages may be affected. The incidence is much greater in males. The incubation period is 5 to 15 days. In severe cases, the disease may have a sudden onset, characterized by slight weakness, refusal to eat, vomiting, a temperature of 103 to 105°F (39.5 to 40.5°C) and often a mild conjunctivitis. At this stage, clinical diagnosis is difficult. Within 2 days, there is a sharp drop in temperature, depression is more pronounced, breathing is labored and thirst is marked. Icterus may appear as the first manifestation of the illness and vary in intensity from lemon to deep orange. Muscular stiffness and soreness, particularly of the hind legs, as evinced by unwillingness to rise from a sitting position, and pain are usually detected on palpation of the anterior dorsal abdomen or lumbar area. The oral mucous membranes may at first show irregular hemorrhagic patches resembling abrasions or burns, which later become dry and necrotic and slough in sections. A slimy salivary secretion around the gums is at times tinged with blood. Swallowing is difficult. In some cases, the tongue may show necrotic patches or the entire tip may slough. Animals with more advanced disease show profound depression and muscular tremors, with the temperature dropping gradually to subnormal, reaching as low as 97°F (36°C). Bloody vomitus and feces may be seen, indicating severe hemorrhagic gastroenteritis. Frequent urination with albumin, pus cells and casts in the urine indicate acute nephritis. The eyes become sunken and the vessels of the conjunctiva are injected. The pulse becomes thready and, in severe cases, uremia develops. Mortality seldom exceeds 10%. In fatal cases, death occurs usually 5 to 10 days after onset. Chronic, progressive nephritis frequently follows acute *L. canicola* infections. In such cases, death may not occur until long after the initial illness has subsided.

The leukocyte count may rise to 35,000; the BUN may also be elevated. Other laboratory findings are variable, depending on the severity and stage of the disease.

Lesions: Hemorrhagic gastroenteritis is often the predominant lesion. The tissues may be uniformly bile-stained. The liver is engorged and the lymph nodes are often hemorrhagic. The myocardium may be diffusely hemorrhagic. The organs may have a uremic odor. The kidneys are enlarged in the acute phase and may have gray foci or mottling at their cortico-medullary junction as in acute interstitial nephritis. Oral ulcers and tongue sloughs may be present in the uremic animal. Chronic cases have varying degrees of interstitial nephritis.

Diagnosis: Diagnosis is made on the basis of clinical and necropsy findings, histopathologic demonstration of leptospires in the kidneys or liver, demonstration of leptospiruria, and serologic tests.

Prophylaxis: To reduce the chances of exposure, owners are well-advised to keep their dogs leashed. During epidemics of leptospirosis, confinement to the owner's premises may be recommended. Bivalent bacterins are available, but apparently must be administered every 6 to 8 months to maintain a significant antibody level.

Chemoprophylaxis (℞ 73) may be recommended for dogs at high risk (show or stud dogs). If leptospirosis is diagnosed in a kennel dog, treatment of all dogs in the kennel should be considered (℞ 73).

Treatment: Penicillin and streptomycin (℞ 66) are recommended for acute infections; dihydrostreptomycin (℞ 73) is recommended in heavy doses for termination of the carrier-shedder state.

Dehydration and acidosis can be treated by giving 0.17M lactate solution, alone or in combination with saline-dextrose solution, and high doses of soluble B-vitamins. If the patient is in the anuric phase of the disease, excessive fluid volume must not be administered. The animal should be weighed daily and the fluid volume adjusted so that a 40-lb (18-kg) dog loses approximately 0.2 lb (90 gm) per day. Although expensive and time-consuming, peritoneal dialysis can be lifesaving when used in selected cases with uremia.

LEPTOSPIROSIS IN CATTLE
(Redwater of calves)

Leptospirosis of cattle in the U.S.A. is due to *L. pomona, L. grippotyphosa* and *L. hardjo.*

Clinical Findings: Hemolytic icterus and hemoglobinuria often exist in 50%, or more, of affected young calves. Mortality ranges from 5 to 15%. The acute clinical syndrome occurs in only 2 to 4% of adults, and deaths are rare. Total morbidity may exceed 75% in older stock and usually approaches 100% in calves.

In calves, the classical case presents fever, prostration, inappetence, dyspnea, icterus, hemoglobinuria and anemia. Body temperature rises suddenly to 105 or 106°F (40.5 to 41°C). Hemoglobinuria rarely lasts longer than 48 to 72 hours. As it subsides, the icterus rapidly clears and is succeeded by anemia. The erythrocytes begin to increase in number on the fourth or fifth day and the count returns to normal 7 to 10 days later. Most affected cattle show leukocytosis. Some degree of albuminuria is commonly present during the febrile peak.

In older cattle, signs of leptospirosis vary greatly and the diagnosis is more difficult. The signs are particularly obscure in dairy herds infected with *L. hardjo;* lowered milk and calf production occur with few clinical signs. A hemolytic crisis is seen only occasionally. In dry cattle, the infection is so mild that it is generally overlooked, but in milking stock, a sharp drop in milk production is noted. The milk is thick, yellow and blood-tinged, although there is no evidence of mammary inflammation. Abortion is common and takes place 2 to 5 weeks following initial infection. It is commonest about the seventh month of pregnancy. An abortion storm in a breeding herd is often the first indication that leptospirosis exists, the mild initial signs having passed unnoticed. Calves reared by cows that have been previously infected acquire through the colostrum a passive immunity which lasts 1 to 2 months. The calves generally have a higher antibody titer than their dams.

Lesions: Anemia and icterus are prominent features in the acute hemolytic form of the disease. The urine is a clear-red or port-wine color. The kidneys show the most significant lesions in the form of reddish brown mottling of the cortex, often sufficiently pronounced to be visible through the intact capsule. The liver may be swollen, with minute areas of focal necrosis. Petechiae in the epicardium and lymph nodes are seen in fulminating cases.

Diagnosis: Serology with paired serum samples, direct culture in media, or animal inoculation techniques are usually necessary to confirm clinical and postmortem findings. The absence of mammary inflammation despite the gross physical changes in the milk is suggestive of leptospirosis. Similarly, elimination of brucellosis, vibriosis and trichomoniasis as possible causes of an abortion outbreak would point to leptospirosis.

Prophylaxis: In the absence of state or federal regulations for the control of leptospirosis, some cattle owners rely on annual vaccinations with commercial bacterins.

Although bacterins confer protection against abortions and death, their efficacy in preventing persistent renal infections has not been proved. Management methods to prevent leptospirosis include: rat control, fencing cattle from potentially contaminated streams and ponds, separation of cattle from swine, selection of replacement stock from herds that have passed serologic tests for leptospirosis, and chemoprophylaxis of replacement stock (℞ 73).

Treatment: No form of treatment will have much effect on the course of the disease once a hemolytic crisis has developed. In the case of valuable animals, the IV transfusion of washed red cells may prove beneficial if the anemia approaches the critical level. Antibiotic therapy—streptomycin (℞ 73), chlortetracycline (℞ 27) or oxytetracycline (℞ 50)—is often successful if it can be given early. Dihydrostreptomycin (℞ 73) is recommended for termination of the carrier or shedder state.

The management of infected herds of cattle merits special consideration. When leptospirosis is diagnosed in pregnant cows during the early epidemic phase, further abortions can be prevented by prompt vaccination of the entire herd and simultaneous treatment of all animals with dihydrostreptomycin (℞ 54). The drug destroys the leptospires in the kidneys and other tissues of exposed and infected animals and provides a measure of protection until active immunity is induced by vaccination. Whether this procedure would be economically advantageous depends on the proportion of seronegative animals in the herd. For example, salvaging 3 or 4 calves offsets the cost of treatment for 100 cows. In dairy herds, the loss of market milk after treatment would have to be considered. Current regulations prevent the sale of milk for 96 hours after treatment with dihydrostreptomycin and animals must be held for 30 days before slaughter for food.

LEPTOSPIROSIS IN SHEEP

Leptospirosis is less prevalent in sheep than cattle, possibly due to less intensive husbandry methods and less frequent association with pigs. In the U.S.A., *L. pomona* is the commonest serotype isolated from sheep. The infection can often be traced to carrier cattle. Clinical features, diagnosis and management of the disease are essentially as already described for mature cattle and calves.

LEPTOSPIROSIS IN SWINE

L. pomona is the organism most commonly encountered in leptospiral infection of swine. Swine act as a reservoir of infection for other animals and man, as apparently healthy individuals can excrete large numbers of organisms in their urine. Swine have been incriminated so often that the disease in man is known in Europe as "swineherd's disease." Swine are also commonly infected with *L. grippotyphosa*. Acute leptospirosis occurs in young pigs due to *L. icterohaemorrhagiae;* this is characterized by fever, icterus, hemorrhages and death. The source of the infection is usually the urine of rats.

Porcine leptospirosis is not a clearly defined entity. In some cases, infection may apparently occur without visible signs, while others show only a febrile reaction lasting 3 to 4 days. More severe clinical signs include poor weight gain, anorexia, intestinal disturbances and occasionally meningitis with rigidity, spasms and circling. *L. pomona* has been isolated from aborted porcine fetuses. Abortions, late in pregnancy, represent the most important single sign of leptospirosis in a herd of swine. They can be terminated by treatment of all sows in the herd (℞ 73). The use of *L. pomona* bacterin in infected or exposed herds is warranted.

LEPTOSPIROSIS IN HORSES

During investigations on the etiology of equine periodic ophthalmia (q.v., p. 226), serologic testing revealed that a high percentage of affected horses carried high titers to *L. pomona* and the organism has been isolated from horses. By artificial exposure to *L. pomona*, periodic ophthalmia has been experimentally produced in horses. Equine leptospirosis is characterized by an elevated body temperature of 103 to 105°F (39.5 to 40.5°C) for 2 to 3 days, depression or dullness, anorexia, icterus and neutrophilia. Periodic ophthalmia or abortion may occur long after the fever has subsided. Other leptospires, e.g. *L. hardjo*, have been isolated from apparently normal horses. The incidence of leptospirosis in horses is not known.

Many cases of leptospirosis undoubtedly occur without being recognized because of the mild transient course, which leaves only the eye lesions as the visible permanent damage. Measures for control and treatment have not been developed.

BOVINE GENITAL CAMPYLOBACTERIOSIS
(Vibriosis)

A venereal disease of cattle caused by *Campylobacter (Vibrio) fetus* subsp. *fetus* and characterized by infertility and early embryonic death. Abortion occurs in a small percentage of infected cows. The distribution is worldwide.

Etiology: *C. fetus* subsp. *fetus* is a gram-negative, curved or spiral shaped rod which is motile by means of a polar flagellum. Exposure to heat, freezing, drying and atmospheric levels of oxygen quickly destroys the organism. There are 2 known biotypes that do not differ in pathogenicity.

Transmission: *C. fetus* is transmitted by coitus under natural conditions. While other possible methods of spread have been suggested, effective control programs can be based on the assumption that the disease is exclusively venereal. The disease may be spread by the use of contaminated semen in artificial insemination and by use of instruments. The infection rate in susceptible females may be almost 100%. Cows develop a resistance to the disease so that in a herd where the condition is endemic, the disease rate drops, but reinfection often occurs.

The disease may spread from one bull to another in an artificial insemination stud when a number of bulls are used on the same teaser. Contact of the penis with the rump or escutcheon of the teaser is believed to be the means of transmission. On occasion bulls may become infected from contaminated bedding.

Clinical Findings: The primary effect is temporary infertility; abortion is of secondary importance. Irregularity of the estrous cycle is a prominent sign. The long cycles are explained on the basis that conception takes place and is interrupted by infection. The embryo is resorbed and a new cycle begins. If the embryo is expelled, it is often so small that the abortion goes unrecognized. The variable degree of endometritis, and the slight vaginitis and cervicitis sometimes produced may also be overlooked.

Under range conditions the first evidence is a high percentage of the herd returning for service after the bulls have been with the herd 60 days or longer. Calving over a long period and an unusual number of open cows in the fall are 2 suggestive signs; great loss of flesh in the breeding bulls, suggesting overwork due to repeated breedings, is another. Conception rates of 40 to 50% or lower occur in newly infected herds. In herds where the disease is endemic, conception rates are usually 65 to 70%, with replacement virgin heifers the most severely affected. Various abortion rates have been reported; most abortions occur about the fifth or sixth month of gestation and are accompanied by placental retention. The placental and fetal lesions are not characteristic enough to be diagnostic.

Diagnosis: The history may include evidence of the introduction of animals from herds where infertility is known to exist. Bovine trichomoniasis (q.v., p. 389) and campylobacteriosis are clinically similar but differ in that pyometra does not occur in the latter disease and trichomonal abortions occur prior to the fifth month of pregnancy. Occasionally, the 2 diseases are found concurrently in a herd. Suspected bovine campylobacteriosis may be confirmed by the following procedures:

1. Isolation of *C. fetus* subsp. *fetus:* The most efficient and specific procedure is the isolation of causative organisms from the herd bulls, which are the principal carriers, or from selected infertile nonpregnant cows detected by pregnancy examination. For cultural examination, preputial fluid is collected by means of a 60-cm plastic pipette equipped with an 85-ml rubber bulb, and cervico-vaginal mucus is aspirated from the anterior vagina with a glass or plastic pipette and a long rubber tube. With bulls, cultural examination can be replaced or augmented by the demonstration of organisms in preputial fluids or in media using fluorescent antibody techniques. *C. fetus* can also be isolated from the stomach contents of aborted fetuses and from associated fetal membranes and fluids. Because of the sensitivity of campylobacters to atmospheric levels of oxygen, samples should be cultured within several hours of collection. Preputial samples can be inoculated into transport medium if longer periods of time must elapse prior to arrival at a laboratory.

2. The vaginal mucus agglutination test: This test is used to make a herd diagnosis and has most application in dairy herds. Samples of cervico-vaginal mucus are collected from cows known to be infertile and examined for the presence of agglutinins against *C. fetus* subsp. *fetus*. Samples from cows in estrus and samples containing blood are not suitable for testing.

3. Fluorescent antibody (FA) stains of sheath-washing from bulls and cervico-vaginal mucus from cows can be used to identify individually infected animals.

Treatment and Control: If there are no gross uterine changes and reinfection is avoided, 75% of cows will recover in a short time, 25% require from 2 to 12 months and a few cows will carry the infection through a normal pregnancy and harbor the infection in the genital tract after parturition. If no reinfection occurs, a herd may be regarded as free of the disease after 2 years. The best method of bringing the disease under control is to use artificial insemination. Semen for this purpose should either be from known uninfected bulls, or be treated with penicillin and streptomycin. *C. fetus* subsp. *fetus* is not transmitted in semen provided it is diluted at least 1:25, and 500 u of penicillin and 0.5 mg of streptomycin are added to each ml of the diluted semen and provided also the treated semen is held at 40°F (4.4°C) for at least 6 hours before being used.

Where natural service must be continued, as in large beef herds, vaccination is effective in controlling the disease. The most important animals to vaccinate are herd bulls and replacement heifers. Vaccination is both curative and preventive in bulls. They should be given 2 subcut. injections initially and annual booster injections thereafter. Vaccination of females is done at least 6 weeks before breeding and may need to be repeated annually. Although spontaneous recovery in the female is the rule, this may be accelerated by the use of intra-uterine infusions of streptomycin (℞ 75) or streptomycin and penicillin (℞ 71).

Two procedures have proven to be effective in treating bulls: in the first, 1 million units of the sodium salt of crystalline penicillin G and 2 gm of streptomycin sulfate in 5 ml of distilled water are emulsified with 20 to 100 ml of peanut oil and infused into the preputial sac where it is retained for 1 hour by bandaging the orifice. Each treatment consists of 3 infusions given on 3 consecutive days. In the second method the bull is given a subcut. injection of an aqueous solution of dihydrostreptomycin sulfate (25 mg/kg) and a preputial infusion of the same solution containing 5 gm, as a single treatment.

OVINE GENITAL CAMPYLOBACTERIOSIS

(Vibriosis)

An infectious disease caused by *Campylobacter (Vibrio) fetus* subsp. *intestinalis* and *C. fetus* subsp. *jejuni* and characterized by abortion. Serious economic loss from this disease occurs in sheep in the Rocky Mountain area of the U.S.A., and in many other parts and other countries.

Etiology and Transmission: Both organisms cause epidemics of abortion in ewes. The route of transmission is oral. Experimental efforts to transmit the disease venereally have not been successful. Carrier sheep shedding organisms in the feces from intestinal and gallbladder infections, or in uterine discharges, aborted fetuses and membranes are probably the major source of infection. Magpies and crows could be secondary reservoirs of infection.

The incubation period of the ovine disease is 10 to 50 days. An outbreak of campylobacteriosis in a flock produces immunity sufficient to prevent the appearance of the disease among exposed ewes for at least 3 years. Repeated outbreaks among susceptible replacement ewes are not uncommon. All ages of ewes not previously exposed or vaccinated are susceptible.

Clinical Findings: Abortion during the last 8 weeks of pregnancy or, in some instances, the delivery of weak lambs at term constitutes the typical syndrome. Fetal death usually occurs 1 to 2 days before abortion. There is usually no indication of the impending abortion but a few ewes may show a prior vaginal discharge. Recovery is prompt and fertility in subsequent breeding seasons is usually good. Occasionally, abortion is complicated by metritis and subsequent death of the ewe. The ewe mortality varies from 0 to 5%. In flocks with previous recent experience with the disease, abortion may be chiefly confined to unvaccinated replacement ewes. Usually, the incidence of abortion does not rise above 10 to 20%. In some outbreaks, however, as many as 70% of the ewes have lost their lambs.

Lesions: In some aborted fetuses, most frequently in those near term, the liver shows typical gray, necrotic foci varying from 1 to 3 cm in diameter. The fetus is usually edematous and the body cavities contain a reddish fluid. The fetal membranes also are edematous and the cotyledons pale and necrotic. There is wide variation in the lesions and it is necessary to have bacteriologic confirmation of the diagnosis.

Diagnosis: A tentative diagnosis can be made by a history of widespread abortion and typical lesions of the fetus and placenta. This may be confirmed by microscopic demonstration of typical *C. fetus* organisms in the stomach contents of aborted lambs or by isolation of *C. fetus* from stomach contents, liver, lung, or placental fluids. Rapid diagnosis, usually accomplished by demonstration of the organism by special staining techniques, is necessary for early treatment and to protect the rest of the ewes in the flock. Cultural methods can then be used for confirmation. Care must be taken to differentiate campylobacteriosis from ovine chlamydial abortion, q.v., p. 377, as this latter disease produces nearly identical clinical findings and can occur concomitantly.

Treatment and Control: Aborting ewes should be isolated and strict hygienic practices adopted; these include removal of aborted fetuses and associated discharges. If possible, unaffected ewes should be moved to a clean area and provided uncontaminated feed and water.

To control an outbreak, ewes should be given bacterin and penicillin and dihydrostreptomycin (℞ 66) at the first treatment followed by the antibiotics only a day later. Abortions usually stop after about a week or 10 days. A bacterin is effective for control if ewes are vaccinated shortly before mating, again in 8 weeks and annually thereafter. In flocks with a history of campylobacteriosis it is recommended that replacement ewes be vaccinated on admission. Feeding chlortetracycline, 80 mg/ewe/day over the last 7 to 8 weeks of pregnancy, will reduce the incidence of abortion, and may be economical in some situations. Usually adequate sanitation is effective and more practical.

BOVINE TRICHOMONIASIS

A contagious, venereal, protozoan disease of cattle characterized by sterility, pyometra and abortion. Distribution is worldwide.

Etiology: The causative pyriform protozoan, *Trichomonas foetus*, is 10 to 15 μ in length by 5 to 10 μ wide. There is considerable pleomorphism, and organisms cultivated in artificial media tend to become spherical. At the anterior end of the organism there are 3 flagella approximately the same length as the parasite. An undulating membrane extends the length of the trichomonad and is bordered by a marginal filament that continues beyond the membrane as a posterior flagellum. A small proportion of organisms are able to survive the freezing procedures used for storing semen. They do not survive drying or high temperatures.

Epidemiology: The organism is found only in the genital tract of the cow and bull. Over 90% of females become infected when bred by a diseased bull. Transmission by artificial breeding can occur, but normal semen dilution methods markedly reduce the chances of spread by this means. It may be assumed that transmission occurs only during coitus and that most bulls remain permanently infected unless properly treated. The infected cow usually recovers spontaneously.

Rarely a cow may remain infected throughout pregnancy and discharge trichomonads from the genital tract following calving. Previously infected cows that undergo 90 days of sexual rest after calving with normal involution of the uterus may be assumed to be free of infection.

Clinical Findings: The most common and important sign is infertility caused by early embryonic mortality and characterized by repeat breeding and irregular estrous cycles. An average of 5 services per conception may be observed in infected herds. If the embryo survives longer than 10 days, the interval between heat periods is extended. If pregnancy continues into the third month, a recognizable abortion may occur. Embryonic or fetal death and the resulting abortion occur prior to the end of the fifth month. Cows that carry their calves beyond this time usually deliver a live calf.

Trichomoniasis is a common cause of postcoital pyometra in cattle and, in infected herds, this complication occurs usually in less than 5% of the animals. It results from the death and maceration of the developing fetus. The corpus luteum and, in some instances, the cervical seal persist so that there is no discharge of pus. More frequently, however, the cervix opens and there is a slight nonodorous uterine discharge. As in all pyometras, estrus does not occur and the condition may persist for many months. Vaginitis, cervicitis and balanitis are rare.

Diagnosis: A tentative diagnosis may be based on the history and clinical signs, but confirmation results upon finding the organism in at least one animal in a herd. The organisms may be found in the placental fluid, in the stomach contents of an aborted fetus, in the uterus for several days after an abortion, and in the exuded pus. In recently infected cows, they can be found in the vagina where they are present in large numbers 12 to 19 days after infection. Subsequently the numbers rise and fall in a regular manner according to the phase of the estrous cycle, being highest 3 to 7 days before each heat period.

In the bull, the organisms are present in the prepuce, frequently in small numbers. While trichomonads may be found in all parts of the sheath and on the penis, they occur in the greatest numbers in the fornix and on the glans penis. Samples should be taken from these areas.

Samples of vaginal mucus are aspirated from the anterior vagina with a glass or plastic pipette and a long rubber tube. Preputial fluid is collected by means of a 60 cm plastic pipette equipped with an 85-ml rubber bulb. Diagnosis is simplified and efficiency improved by culturing samples for 4 to 7 days at 37°C prior to microscopic examination using 100× power.

A larger volume of fluid may be examined if no cover slip is used. The organisms may not be numerous and careful systematic examination is often necessary. Identification can be made at low power and is based on the size and shape of the organisms as well as the characteristic, aimless, jerky motion. Only living organisms are used for diagnostic purposes.

Diagnosis in the bull may be made by breeding several virgin heifers and examining the vaginal fluid 12 to 19 days after service. By careful attention to detail, diagnosis should be more than 90% accurate in the bull.

Treatment and Control: Control measures are based on the assumption that transmission occurs only during coitus. Animals with pyometra or other genital abnormalities should be treated or eliminated from the herd. The remainder of the cows will recover if artificial breeding is used for at least 2 years. If artificial insemination is not possible, the herd can be divided into exposed and unexposed groups. Service in the unexposed group is resumed, using uninfected bulls. In the exposed group, recognizable uterine disease is treated and the entire group is allowed 90 days of sexual rest. For breeding, the exposed herd should be divided into as many groups as possible, with one bull for each group. Bulls and cows should be re-examined for reinfection in any group. Control can also be gained in very large herds by eliminating all bulls over 4 years of age and using only young bulls for mating. This method is based upon the relative lack of susceptibility of young bulls to trichomonad infection.

Slaughter, rather than treatment of bulls is recommended. However, successful treatment has been reported by the oral administration of 40% dimetridazole given at 57 mg/lb (125 mg/kg) once daily for 5 days. Diagnostic tests to confirm success of treatment should be commenced after treatment has concluded.

CONTAGIOUS EQUINE METRITIS (CEM)

A highly contagious bacterial venereal disease of horses, first identified in England in 1977. The disease has since been identified in Ireland, where it was probably present in 1976, in Australia, France and in the U.S.A. (Kentucky) in 1978.

Etiology: The causal organism is a micro-aerophilic, gram-negative, pleomorphic rod-shaped bacterium. It is fastidious, cultivated best on horse-blood chocolate-Eugon agar at 37°C in an atmosphere containing 5 to 10% carbon dioxide. The organism is oxidase and catalase-positive, nonmotile, encapsulated and nonsaccharolytic. It is sensitive to a wide range of antibiotics including penicillin, ampicillin, tetracycline, gentamicin and neomycin. Strains of the organism vary in susceptibility to streptomycin.

Clinical Findings and Mode of Spread: When the organism infects the endometrium, acute purulent endometritis results. The infection is accompanied by a purulent, sometimes profuse discharge from the uterus. The infection may be acquired by mares through contamination of the clitoral fossa and sinuses without causing endometritis, in which case mares may become chronic carriers. The disease does not produce clinical signs in stallions but stallions become chronic carriers and transmitters of the disease by contamination of the urethral sinus and sheath. The principal means of spread of disease is by coitus, but lateral spread may occur by human agency.

Diagnosis: Diagnosis depends on the epidemiologic picture, recovery of the organism from the cervix, endometrium, clitoral fossa or clitoral sinuses of mares, or from the sheath, shaft of the penis, urethral sinus or pre-ejaculatory fluid of the stallion. Bacteriologic cultures are best taken on swabs and should be transported to the laboratory without delay in Amies transport medium without antibiotics. Cultures which are delayed in transport should be kept cold. Bacteriologic diagnosis using specimens from the discharge of mares with endometritis is most reliable. Contamination of cultures taken from other sites may cause false negative cultures. Bacteriologic diagnosis of infected stallions is always difficult due to the presence of contaminating organisms. Culture of semen is not a reliable method of diagnosis. Mares that experience endometritis develop complement fixation and agglutinating antibody titers as early as 7 days after infection. Mares that become contaminated (clitoral area) without experiencing endometritis do not become serologically positive. Serologic tests are not applicable for diagnosis of the contaminated stallion.

Treatment: The successful treatment of the contaminated stallion is a relatively straightforward procedure. Chlorhexidine diacetate or digluconate is used to thoroughly cleanse the penis and sheath of the stallion once daily for 5 days. Although the organism exhibits a wide range of antibiotic sensitivity, treatment of mares is less reliable. Many mares appear to recover without treatment but remain clitoral carriers of the organism. Acute endometritis may be resolved in untreated or antibiotic-treated mares in a period of 10 to 14 days, but such mares may remain carriers.

EQUINE COITAL EXANTHEMA

A sporadic, benign, viral disease of horses, primarily venereal in nature.

Etiology and Epidemiology: Equine herpesvirus 3, an antigenically unique herpesvirus, is the cause. The disease affects both sexes and is spread venereally. The virus also appears to spread by means other than coitus; it may occur as a progenital disease of nonbreeding horses.

Clinical Findings: In mares, the disease is usually recognized by the presence of a single or multiple vulvar scabs, the removal of which reveals shallow erosions with ragged edges. Edema is common but there is little evidence of pain. The erosions may coalesce. Erosions may also appear on the skin below the infected vulva. Similar lesions occur on the penis of the stallion. The disease is benign in both sexes: no signs of systemic disease are presented and the lesions heal rapidly unless complicated by infection with secondary bacteria. Clinical disease may appear in carrier animals when their resistance is lowered by stress, including that of parturition.

Diagnosis: The typical appearance of the disease allows ready clinical diagnosis. Virologic diagnosis requires specialized laboratory studies. Serologic tests are of little clinical significance.

Prophylaxis and Treatment: No specific prophylaxis is available. Treatment, consisting of sexual rest, cleansing the local lesions and the use of local antibiotics to control secondary bacterial infection, results in resolution of the disease in 7 to 10 days.

ANTHRAX

(Splenic fever, Charbon, Milzbrand)

An acute, febrile disease of virtually all warm-blooded animals and man caused by *Bacillus anthracis*. In its commonest form, it is essentially a septicemia characterized principally by a rapidly fatal course. It occurs worldwide. Districts where repeated outbreaks occur exist in Southern Europe, parts of Africa, Australia, Asia and North and South America. In the U.S.A., there are recognized areas of infection in South Dakota, Nebraska, Arkansas, Mississippi, Louisiana, Texas and California. Small areas exist in a number of other states.

Etiology: *Bacillus anthracis* is a gram-positive, nonmotile, spore-forming bacterium of relatively large size (4 to 8 μ by 1 to 1.5 μ). The bacilli grow in chain formation, but may occur singly or in pairs. After discharge from an infected animal or an opened carcass they form spores which are resistant to heat, low temperature, chemical disinfectants and prolonged drying. They may persist for long periods in dry products such as feed, animal by-products, stored contaminated objects or in soil.

Outbreaks of anthrax commonly are associated with neutral or alkaline, calcareous soils that have become "incubator areas" for the organisms. In these areas, the spores apparently revert to the vegetative form and multiply when optimal environmental conditions of soil, moisture, temperature and nutrition occur. The organisms then have an increased capability to form more spores as long as environment and biologic competition remain favorable. Cattle, horses, mules, sheep and goats may readily become infected when grazing such areas. Outbreaks originating from soil-borne infection commonly occur after a major climatic change, e.g. a heavy rain after a prolonged drought and always during warm weather. In endemic areas flies and other insects may mechanically transmit the disease from one animal to another. Infection may also be caused by consumption of contaminated natural or artificial feedstuffs, as oil cake and tankage; in some countries bone meal is the commonest source of disease outbreaks. Swine, dogs, cats, mink and wild animals in captivity frequently acquire the disease from consumption of contaminated meat.

Man may develop localized lesions (malignant pustule or malignant carbuncle) from contact with infected blood or tissues, or acquire a fatal pneumonia (woolsorter's disease) from spore inhalation when handling animal by-products. Occasionally, he develops acute meningitis from systemic involvement, or intestinal anthrax from consumption of meat.

Clinical Findings: The peracute form is characterized by its sudden onset and rapidly fatal course. Staggering, difficult breathing, trembling, collapse, a few convulsive movements, and death may occur in cattle, sheep or goats, without any previous evidence of illness.

In acute anthrax of cattle, horses and sheep, there is first a rise in body temperature and a period of excitement followed by depression, stupor, respiratory or cardiac distress, staggering, convulsion and death. The body temperature may reach 107°F (41.5°C), rumination ceases, milk production is materially reduced, and pregnant animals may abort. There may be bloody discharges from the natural body openings. Horses may show fever, chills, severe colic, loss of appetite, extreme depression, muscular weakness, bloody diarrhea and swellings in the region of the neck, sternum, lower abdomen and external genitalia.

The chronic form of anthrax with local lesions confined to the tongue and throat is observed mostly in swine, but occurs occasionally in cattle, horses and dogs.

In swine, some animals in a group may die of acute anthrax without having shown any previous signs of illness. Others may show rapidly progressing swelling about the throat, which, in some cases, causes death by suffocation. Many of the group may develop the disease in a mild chronic form and make a gradual recovery. However, some of these when presented for slaughter as normal animals may show evidence of anthrax infection in the cervical lymph nodes and tonsils.

A cutaneous or localized form of anthrax, characterized by swellings in various parts of the body, occurs in cattle and horses when anthrax organisms lodge in wounds or abrasions of the skin.

The carcass of an animal dead of anthrax should not be subjected to necropsy. *Rigor mortis* is frequently absent or incomplete. There may be dark blood oozing from the nostrils and anus with marked bloating and rapid body decomposition. If the carcass is inadvertently opened, septicemic lesions are observed. The blood is dark, thickened and fails to clot readily. Edematous, red-tinged effusions are present and small hemorrhages are common in the subcutis and are frequently seen in serous and mucous membranes. An enlarged, dark-red or black, soft semifluid spleen is common. The liver, kidneys and lymph nodes are usually congested and enlarged.

Diagnosis: A diagnosis based on clinical signs may be difficult, especially when the disease occurs in a new area. Therefore, a confirmatory laboratory exmaination should be utilized. Blood should be collected aseptically from a peripheral vessel shortly after death and sent to the laboratory on sterile cotton swabs, gauze or suture tape, or as blood smears. The smears should be dried and kept separated during shipment. Tissue specimens obtained at death should be of small size, placed in clean glass containers and sent to the laboratory in sealed, metal mailing tubes surrounded by dry ice and labeled "suspected anthrax." In the case of swine, cervical lymph nodes packed in borax should be sent to the laboratory, as anthrax organisms rarely occur in the blood stream of this species. Usually, ears and splenic tissue are unsatisfactory for making a laboratory diagnosis.

At the laboratory, the methods commonly used in identifying the disease comprise: (1) microscopic examination of blood smears stained with polychrome methylene blue or Giemsa to demonstrate encapsulated bacilli; (2) observance of death of guinea pigs or mice within 48 hours following inoculation of blood or tissue suspension, and organism demonstration from stained smears of the blood and spleen; (3) identification of the organism by its growth and characteristics from culture inoculation of blood or tissue suspension, or both, and (4) the use of bacteriophage identification of anthrax bacilli from nonpathogenic bacilli.

Anthrax must be differentiated from other conditions causing sudden death. In cattle and sheep, the clostridial infections, bloat and lightning stroke may be confused with it. Also, acute leptospirosis, bacillary hemoglobinuria, anaplasmosis, and acute poisonings from bracken fern, sweet clover and lead must be considered in cattle. In horses, acute infectious anemia, purpura, the various colics, lead poisoning, lightning stroke and sunstroke may resemble anthrax. In swine, acute hog cholera and pharyngeal malignant edema, and in dogs, acute systemic infections and pharyngeal swellings from other causes must be considered.

Treatment and Control: Since anthrax is a highly fatal disease, early treatment and rigid control procedures are essential to control it. When an outbreak occurs it is best to use antibiotics for the sick animals and immunize all apparently well animals in the infected herd and surrounding community. In mature cattle and horses, penicillin (℞ 63) gives good responses in the early stages of the disease. Oxytetracycline (℞ 48) given IV daily in divided doses is also useful. Other antibiotics, e.g. chloramphenicol (℞ 16), erythromycin (℞ 39) or sulfonamides (℞ 102, 105, 106, 110) can also be utilized, but they are less effective than penicillin or the tetracyclines. Prophylactic use of penicillin for exposed cattle has been successful.

Anthrax of livestock can be largely controlled by annual prophylactic vaccination of all animals in the endemic area and the initiation of good control procedures. The noncapsulated Sterne-strain vaccine has essentially replaced the previously used Pasteur-attenuated-spore vaccines. It can be used with comparative safety on all species of livestock, and it produces a high degree of immunity.

Specific control procedures, besides therapy and immunization, are necessary to contain the disease and prevent its spread. These procedures are: (1) notification of the appropriate regulatory official of the disease outbreak; (2) rigidly enforced quarantine of the infected premises or area; (3) prompt disposal of dead animals by cremation or deep burial; (4) destruction of manure, bedding or other contaminated material by burning; (5) isolation of sick animals and removal of well animals from the contaminated areas; (6) disinfection of stables, pens, milking barns and equipment used on livestock; (7) use of insect repellents; (8) control of scavengers feeding on animals dead from the disease; (9) general sanitary procedures for persons who contact diseased animals, for their own safety, and to prevent spread of the disease.

CLOSTRIDIAL INFECTIONS

All members of the genus *Clostridium* are relatively large, anaerobic, spore-forming, rod-shaped organisms. The spores are oval, sometimes spherical, and are subterminal or terminal in position. The vegetative forms of the clostridia in the tissue fluids of infected animals occur singly, in pairs, or, rarely, in chains. Differentiation of the various pathogenic and related species is based on cultural characteristics, spore shape and position, and the serologic specificity of the toxin or the somatic antigens. The natural habitats of the organisms are the soil and intestinal tract of animals and man. Pathogenic strains may be acquired by susceptible animals either by wound contamination or by ingestion. The diseases thus produced are a constant threat to successful livestock production in many parts of the world.

The diseases caused by members of the clostridial group can be divided into 2 categories: (1) those in which the organisms actively invade and reproduce in the tissues of the host with the production of toxins that enhance the spread of infection and are responsible for death; (2) those which are characterized by toxemia resulting from the absorption of toxins produced by organisms within the digestive system (the enterotoxemias) or in food or carrion outside the body (botulism). If treatment of the first group is to be attempted, large doses of antibiotic are indicated to establish effective levels in the center of necrotic tissue where clostridia are to be found.

MALIGNANT EDEMA

An acute, generally fatal toxemia of cattle, horses, sheep, goats and swine usually caused by *Clostridium septicum* and often accompanied by other organisms. A similar infection has often been seen in man. The disease occurs worldwide.

Etiology and Routes of Infection: *Cl. septicum* is found in soil and intestinal contents of animals and man throughout the world. Infection ordinarily occurs through contamination of wounds containing devitalized tissue, soil, or some other tissue-debilitant. Wounds caused by accident, castration, docking, insanitary vaccination and parturition may become infected.

Clinical Findings and Diagnosis: General signs, as anorexia, intoxication and higher fever, as well as local signs, develop within a few hours to a few days after predisposing injury. The local lesions are soft swellings that pit on pressure and extend rapidly because of the formation of large quantities of exudate that infiltrate the subcut. and IM connective tissue of the affected areas. The muscle in such areas is dark brown to black. Accumulations of gas are uncommon. Severe edema of the head of rams occurs following infection of wounds inflicted by fighting. Malignant edema associated with lacerations of the vulva at parturition is characterized by marked edema of the vulva, severe toxemia and death in 24 to 48 hours. Similarity to blackleg is marked, and differentiation made on necropsy is unreliable; laboratory confirmation is the only certain procedure. Horses and swine are susceptible to malignant edema, but not to blackleg.

Rapid confirmation of a diagnosis can be made on the basis of fluorescent antibody staining of the *Cl. septicum* cells from a tissue smear. However, *Cl. septicum* is an extremely active postmortem invader from the intestine and demonstration of its presence in a specimen taken from an animal that has been dead for 24 hours or more is not significant.

Prophylaxis and Treatment: Immunization against *Cl. septicum* infection is attained by the use of bacterins as in blackleg. *Cl. septicum* is usually combined with *Cl. chauvoei* (*feseri*) in a blackleg-malignant-edema vaccine (℞ 129). In endemic areas animals should be vaccinated before they are castrated, dehorned or have their tails docked. Calves should be vaccinated at about 2 months of age. Two doses 2 to 3 weeks apart generally give protection. Annual vaccination is indicated in high-risk areas. In these areas, revaccination is suggested following the occurrence of severe trauma.

Treatment with high doses of penicillin (℞ 63) or broad-spectrum antibiotics (℞ 16, 27, 48, 76) is indicated early in the disease. The injection of penicillin directly into the periphery of the lesion may minimize spread of the lesion but the affected tissues will still usually slough.

BLACKLEG

An acute, febrile disease of cattle and sheep caused by *Clostridium chauvoei* (*feseri*) and characterized by emphysematous swelling, usually in the heavy muscles. The disease is worldwide in distribution.

Etiology and Routes of Infection: *Cl. chauvoei* occurs naturally in the intestinal tract of animals. It probably can remain viable in the soil for many years although it does not actively grow there. Outbreaks of blackleg have occurred in cattle on farms in which recent excavations have occurred which suggests that disturbance of soil may activate latent spores. The organisms are probably ingested, pass through the wall of the digestive tract and, after gaining access to the blood stream, are deposited in muscle and other tissues.

In cattle, blackleg infection is usually endogenous, in contrast to malignant edema. Most lesions develop spontaneously without any history of wounds although bruising may precipitate some cases. Commonly, the animals that contract blackleg are of the beef breeds, in excellent health, gaining weight and usually the best animals of their group. Outbreaks occur in which a few new cases are found each day for several days. Most cases occur in cattle from 6 months to 2 years of age but thrifty calves as young as 6 weeks and cattle as old as 10 to 12 years may be affected. The disease usually occurs in the summer and autumn months and is uncommon during the cold winter season. In sheep the disease is not restricted to the young, and most cases follow some form of injury such as shearing cuts, docking, crutching or castration. Endogenous blackleg in sheep is uncommon in the U.S.A.; it is much more common in New Zealand where blackleg is seen more frequently in sheep than in cattle.

Clinical Findings: Onset is usually sudden and a few cattle may be found dead without premonitory signs. There is commonly acute lameness and marked depression. Initially there is a fever but by the time that clinical signs are obvious the temperature may be normal or subnormal. Characteristic edematous and crepitant swellings develop in the hip, shoulder, chest, back, neck or elsewhere. At first, the swelling is small, hot and painful. As the disease rapidly progresses, the swelling enlarges, there is crepitation on palpation, and the skin becomes cold and insensitive as the blood supply to the area diminishes. General signs include prostration and tremors. Death occurs in 12 to 48 hours. In some cattle the lesions are restricted to the myocardium and the diaphragm with no reliable antemortem clinical evidence of the disease.

Diagnosis: The occurrence of a rapidly fatal febrile disease in well-nourished young cattle, particularly of the beef breeds, with crepitant swellings of the heavy muscles suggests a diagnosis of blackleg. The affected muscle is dark red to black, dry and spongy, has a sweetish odor and is infiltrated with small bubbles, but with little edema. The lesions may be in any muscle, even in the tongue or diaphragm. In sheep, since the lesions of the spontaneously occurring type are often small and deep, they may be easily overlooked. Occasionally, the tissue changes caused by *Cl. septicum, Cl. novyi, Cl. sordelli,* and *Cl. perfringens* may resemble those of blackleg, and at times both *Cl. septicum* and *Cl. chauvoei* may be isolated from blackleg lesions. This is particularly the case when the carcass has been examined 24 hours or more after death, giving time for postmortem invasion of the tissues by *Cl. septicum.* Confirmation of a field diagnosis can be made by laboratory examination of tissue specimens. These should be taken as soon after death as possible. The fluorescent antibody test for *Cl. chauvoei* is quickly carried out and is quite reliable.

Control: A bacterin (℞ 129) containing *Cl. chauvoei* and *Cl. septicum* is a safe and reliable immunizing agent for both cattle and sheep. Calves should be vaccinated twice, 2 weeks apart, between 2 and 6 months of age; in high-risk areas revaccination may be necessary at one year and every 5 years thereafter. When outbreaks are encountered, all susceptible cattle should be vaccinated and treated prophylactically with penicillin (℞ 63) to prevent new cases which may develop for up to 10 days until the bacterin has stimulated protection. Treatment of clinical cases may be attempted with the use of penicillin parenterally and multiple injections locally but it is frequently unsuccessful.

BACILLARY HEMOGLOBINURIA

An acute, infectious toxemic disease, primarily of cattle, caused by *Clostridium haemolyticum.* It has been found in sheep and very rarely in dogs. It occurs in the western part of the U.S.A., along the Gulf of Mexico, in Venezuela, Chile, Great Britain, Turkey and probably in other parts of the world.

Etiology: *Cl. haemolyticum* is a soil-borne organism which may be found naturally in the alimentary tract of cattle. It may survive for long periods in contaminated soil or in bones from carcasses of animals that had been infected. Ingested with the feed or water, it ultimately becomes lodged in the liver as latent spores. The incubation period is extremely variable. The onset of the disease is determined by the occurrence of a locus of anaerobiosis in the liver where dormant spores are lying. Such a nidus for spores is most often caused by fluke infection, much less often by high nitrate content of the diet, accidental liver puncture, liver biopsy or any other cause of localized necrosis. When favorable conditions of anaerobiosis occur, the spores germinate, the resulting vegetative cells multiply and release lethal quantities of toxin causing an acute hemolytic anemia.

Clinical Findings: Cattle may be found dead without premonitory signs. There is usually a sudden onset of severe depression, fever, abdominal pain, labored respirations, dysentery and hemoglobinuria. Varying degrees of anemia and jaundice are present. Edema of the brisket may occur. The duration of clinical signs varies from about 12 hours in pregnant cows to about 3 or 4 days in steers, bulls and nonpregnant cows. The mortality in untreated animals is about 95%. Some cattle suffer from subclinical attacks of the disease and thereafter act as immune carriers of the organism.

After death, rigor mortis sets in more rapidly than usual. Dehydration, anemia, and sometimes subcut. edema are present. There is bloody fluid in the visceral and thoracic cavities. The lungs are not grossly affected and the trachea contains bloody froth with hemorrhages in the mucosa. The small intestine, and occasionally the large intestine, are hemorrhagic and their contents often contain free or clotted blood. An anemic infarct in the liver is pathognomonic, being slightly elevated, lighter in color than the surrounding tissue and outlined by a bluish red zone of congestion. The kidneys are dark, friable and usually studded with petechiae. The bladder contains purplish red urine.

Diagnosis: The general clinical picture usually permits a diagnosis. The most striking sign is the typical port-wine-colored urine, which foams freely when voided or on agitation. A low hemoglobin reading or packed cell volume with normal red cells is characteristic. The presence of the typical liver infarct is sufficient for a presumptive diagnosis. The normal size and consistency of the spleen serve to exclude anthrax and anaplasmosis. Bracken fern poisoning and leptospirosis should also be considered. Diagnosis should be confirmed bacteriologically by (1) isolating *Cl. haemolyticum* from the liver infarct where possible, (2) demonstrating *Cl. haemolyticum* in the liver tissue by fluorescent antibody test, or (3) demonstrating the toxin in the fluid in the peritoneal cavity or in a saline extract of the infarct.

Treatment and Prophylaxis: Early treatment with penicillin (℞ 63) or broad-spectrum antibiotics (℞ 16, 27, 48, 76) is essential. Whole-blood and fluid therapy are also helpful.

Cl. haemolyticum bacterin prepared from whole cultures confers immunity for about 6 months. In areas where the disease is seasonal, one preseasonal dose is usually adequate; where the disease occurs throughout the year, semiannual immunization is necessary. Cattle that are in contact with animals from areas where this disease is endemic should be immunized, for healthy animals from such areas may be carriers.

INFECTIOUS NECROTIC HEPATITIS (INH)

(*Clostridium novyi* (*oedematiens*) infection, Black disease)

An acute infectious disease of sheep and rarely of cattle caused by *Cl. novyi* Type B. The organism multiplies in areas of liver necrosis resulting from the migration of liver flukes, and it produces a powerful necrotizing toxin. The disease is worldwide in distribution, wherever sheep and liver flukes coincide.

Etiology and Pathogenesis: *Cl. novyi* Type B is soil borne and frequently present in the intestines of herbivores; it may be present on skin surfaces and a potential source of wound infections. Fecal contamination of pasture by carrier animals is the most important source of the infection. Focal necrosis caused by immature liver flukes migrating through the liver creates the anaerobic conditions necessary for initiation of the infection. There is an increasing number of reports in which the disease is suspected (but yet not confirmed) as the cause of sudden death in cattle and pigs fed on high-level grain diets and in which pre-existing lesions of the liver are not detectable. The lethal and necrotizing toxins damage hepatic parenchyma, and thus aid in enlargement of the infected lesion and the production of a lethal amount of toxin.

Clinical Findings: Death is usually sudden with no well-defined signs. Affected animals tend to lag behind the flock, go down in sternal recumbency and die within a few hours. Most cases occur in the summer and early fall when the liver fluke infection is at its height. The disease is most prevalent in 1-to-4-year old sheep and is limited to animals infected with liver flukes. Differentiation from acute fascioliasis is often difficult, but peracute deaths of animals that show typical lesions on necropsy should arouse suspicion of black disease.

Lesions: The most characteristic lesions are the grayish yellow necrotic foci in the liver that often follow the migratory tracks of the young flukes. Other common findings are the enlarged pericardial sac filled with straw-colored fluid, and excess fluid in the peritoneal and thoracic cavities. There is usually extensive rupture of the capillaries in the subcut. tissue causing the adjacent skin to turn black, hence the common name.

Control: Some reduction in incidence of this disease may be accomplished by reduction of the numbers of snails, usually *Lymnaea* spp., that act as intermediate hosts for the liver flukes or by reducing the fluke infection of the sheep. However, these procedures are not always practical, and active immunization with *Cl. novyi* toxoid is more effective. A long-term immunity is produced by one vaccination. Following this, only new introductions to the flock (lambs, and sheep brought in from other areas) need to be vaccinated. This is best done before the late summer.

BIG HEAD

An acute infectious disease, caused by *Clostridium novyi, Cl. sordelli,* or rarely, *Cl. chauvoei,* characterized by a nongaseous, nonhemorrhagic, edematous swelling of the head, face and neck of young rams. This infection is initiated in young rams by their continually butting one another. The bruised and battered subcut. tissues offer conditions suitable for growth of pathogenic clostridia, and the breaks in the skin offer an opportunity for the organism's entrance. Treatment is with broad-spectrum antibiotics or penicillin.

THE ENTEROTOXEMIAS
(*Clostridium perfringens* infection)

Cl. perfringens is widely distributed in the soil and in the alimentary tract of animals, and is characterized by its ability to produce potent exotoxins, some of which are responsible for specific enterotoxemias. Six types (A, B, C, D, E and F) have been identified on the basis of the toxins produced, but of these, only 3 are of significance.

ENTEROTOXEMIA CAUSED BY *Cl. perfringens* TYPES B & C

Infection with *Cl. perfringens* Types B and C causes severe enteritis, dysentery, toxemia and high mortality in young lambs, calves, pigs and foals. Type C also causes enterotoxemia in adult cattle, sheep and goats. The diseases are listed below, categorized as to cause and host. *See also* DIARRHEA IN WEANED AND ADULT HORSES, p. 167.

Lamb dysentery: *Cl. perfringens* Type B in lambs up to 3 weeks of age.

Calf enterotoxemia: Types B and C in well-fed calves up to one month.

Pig enterotoxemia: Type C in piglets during the first few days of life.

Foal enterotoxemia: Type B in foals in the first week of life.

Struck: Type C in adult sheep.
Goat enterotoxemia: Type C in adult goats.

Clinical Findings: Lamb dysentery is an acute disease of lambs under 3 weeks of age. Many may die before signs are observed, but some newborn animals stop nursing, become listless and remain recumbent. A fetid diarrhea tinged with blood is common, and death usually occurs within a few days.

In calves, there is acute diarrhea, dysentery, abdominal pain, convulsions and opisthotonos. Death may occur in a few hours but less severe cases survive for a few days and recovery over a period of several days is possible. Pigs become acutely ill within a few days of birth and there is diarrhea, dysentery, reddening of the anus and a high fatality rate; most affected piglets die within 12 hours. In foals there is acute dysentery, toxemia and rapid death. Struck in adult sheep is characterized by death without premonitory signs.

Lesions: Hemorrhagic enteritis with ulceration of the mucosa is the major lesion in all species. Smears of intestinal contents can be examined for large numbers of clostridia, and filtrates made for the recovery of the specific type toxins.

Treatment and Control: Treatment is usually ineffective because of severity of the disease, but if available specific hyperimmune serum is indicated and oral administration of antibiotics (℞ 76) may be helpful. The disease is best controlled by vaccination of the pregnant dam during the last third of pregnancy: initially 2 vaccinations a month apart, and once annually thereafter. When outbreaks occur in newborn animals from unvaccinated dams, antiserum should be administered immediately after birth.

TYPE D ENTEROTOXEMIA
(Pulpy-kidney disease, Overeating disease)

An enterotoxemia of sheep, less frequently of goats, and rarely of cattle, caused by *Cl. perfringens* Type D. This is the classic enterotoxemia of sheep. It is worldwide in distribution and may occur in animals at any age. It is commonest in the young, either under 2 weeks of age or in weaned lambs in feedlots on a high-carbohydrate diet or, less often, on lush green pastures. The disease has been suspected in well-nourished beef calves nursing high-producing cows grazing lush pasture. The sudden death syndrome in feedlot cattle has been attributed to *Cl. perfringens* Type D but supportive laboratory evidence is lacking.

Etiology: The causative agent is *Cl. perfringens* Type D. However, predisposing factors are also essential; the commonest of these is the ingestion of excessive amounts of feed or milk in the very young and grain in feedlot lambs. In young lambs, the disease is usually restricted to the single lambs, for seldom does a ewe give enough milk to allow enterotoxemia to develop in twin lambs. In the feedlot, the disease usually occurs in lambs on high-grain diets. As the starch intake increases, it provides a suitable medium for organism multiplication and toxin production. Many sheep carry strains of *Cl. perfringens* Type D as part of the normal microflora of the intestine, and they serve as the source of organisms to infect the newborn. Most such carriers show a demonstrable amount of antitoxin in their sera in the absence of vaccination.

Clinical Findings: Usually, the first indication of enterotoxemia is the occurrence of sudden death in the best conditioned lambs. In some cases, excitement, incoordination and convulsions occur before death. Opisthotonos, circling and pushing the head against fixed objects are common signs of CNS involvement. Hyperglycemia or glycosuria is frequently, but not always, observed. Diarrhea may or may not develop. Occasionally adult sheep are affected; they show weakness, incoordination and convulsions and die in 24 hours. Those acutely affected calves not found dead show mania, convulsions, blindness and death in a few hours. Subacutely affected calves are stuporous for a few days and may recover. In goats there is diarrhea, nervous signs and death in several weeks.

Lesions: Postmortem examination may reveal only a few hyperemic areas on the intestine and a fluid-filled pericardial sac. This is particularly the case in young lambs. In older animals, hemorrhagic areas on the myocardium, and petechial and ecchymotic hemorrhages of the abdominal muscles and serosa of the intestine may be found. Bilateral pulmonary edema and congestion are frequently occurring lesions, but usually not in young lambs. The rumen and abomasum contain an abundance of feed and undigested feed is often found in the ileum. Edema and malacia can be seen microscopically in the basal ganglia and cerebellum of lambs. Rapid postmortem autolysis of the kidneys has given rise to the popular name "pulpy kidney disease" although pulpy kidneys are by no means always found in young lambs, and are seldom found in goats or cattle.

Diagnosis: A presumptive diagnosis of enterotoxemia is based on the sudden, convulsive death of lambs on good feed. Smears of intestinal contents reveal many gram-positive, short, fat bacilli. Confirmation can be made by the demonstration of Type D toxin in the small intestinal fluid. Fluid, not ingesta, should be collected in a sterile vial within a few hours after death, and sent under refrigeration to a laboratory for toxin identification. Chloroform, added at 1 drop for each 10 ml of intestinal fluid, will stabilize any toxin present.

Control: The method of control depends upon the age of the lambs, the frequency with which the disease appears on a particular property, and the details of husbandry. If the disease occurs consistently in young lambs on one property, ewe immunization is probably the most satisfactory method of control. The breeding females should be given 2 injections of Type D toxoid (℞ 130) their first year and one injection, 4 to 6 weeks before lambing, each year thereafter. If the disease occurs only sporadically, it may be best to wait until 1 or 2 cases have occurred and then to passively immunize the single lambs with antitoxin.

Enterotoxemia in feedlot lambs can be controlled by reducing the amount of concentrate in the diet. However, this may not be satisfactory from an economic point of view, in which case immunization of all animals with toxoid when they first enter the feedlot will probably reduce losses to an acceptable level. Two injections 2 weeks apart will protect them through the feeding period. When alum-precipitated toxoids or bacterins are used, the injection should be given at such a site on the animal that the cold abscesses, which commonly develop at the site of injection, can easily be removed during normal dressing and thus do not leave blemishes on the carcass.

TETANUS

A toxemia caused by absorption of a specific neurotoxin from tissue infected by *Clostridium tetani.* Almost all mammals are susceptible to this disease, although cats seem much more resistant than any other domestic or laboratory mammal. Birds are quite resistant, 10,000 to 300,000 times as much toxin being required for a lethal dose on a body weight basis for pigeons and chickens, as is required for horses. Horses are the most sensitive of all species, with the possible exception of man. Although tetanus is worldwide in distribution, there are some areas, such as the northern Rocky Mountain section of the U.S.A., where the organism is rarely found in the soil and where tetanus in man and horses is almost unknown. In general, the occurrence of *Cl. tetani* in the soil and the incidence of tetanus in man and horses is higher in the warmer parts of the different continents.

Etiology: *Cl. tetani* is an anaerobe with terminal, spherical spores, which is found in soil and intestinal tracts of animals and man. In most cases, it is introduced into the tissues through wounds, particularly deep puncture wounds where anaerobic conditions can prevail. Often in lambs, however, and sometimes in other species, it follows docking or castration. Frequently, it is not possible to find the point of entry in a case of tetanus, for the lesion itself may be minor or healed.

Pathogenesis: The spores of *Cl. tetani* are unable to grow in normal tissue, or even in wounds where the tissue remains at the oxidation-reduction potential of the circulating blood, as this is too high for anaerobic growth. Suitable conditions for multiplication are brought about where a small amount of soil, or a foreign object, causes tissue necrosis and allows multiplication of the contaminating spores. The bacteria remain localized in the necrotic tissue at the original site of infection as they cease growing, the bacterial cells undergo autolysis and the potent neurotoxin is released. It is usually absorbed by the motor nerves in the area and passes up the nerve tract to the spinal cord where it causes ascending tetanus. The toxin causes spasmodic, tonic contractions of the voluntary muscles by nerve cell irritation. If more toxin is released at the site of the infection than the surrounding nerves can take up, the excess is carried off by the lymph to the blood stream to the CNS, causing descending tetanus. Even minor stimulation of the affected individual may cause the characteristic muscular spasms.

Clinical Findings: The incubation period varies from one to several weeks, but usually averages 10 to 14 days. First there is localized stiffness, often involving the masseter and muscles of the neck, the hind limbs, and in the region of the infected wound. General stiffness becomes pronounced about a day later, and tonic spasms and hyperesthesia become evident.

The reflexes are increased in intensity and the animal is easily excited into more violent, general spasms by sudden movement or noise. Spasms of head muscles cause difficulty in prehension and mastication of food, hence, the common designation "**lockjaw.**" In the horse, the ears are erect, the tail stiff and extended, the anterior nares dilate and there is prolapse of the third eyelid. Walking, turning and backing are difficult. Spasms of the neck and back muscles cause extension of the head and neck, while stiffness of the leg muscles cause the animal to assume a "sawhorse stance." Sweating is frequently present. General spasms cause disturbance of circulation and respiration, resulting in increased heart action, rapid breathing and congestion of mucous membranes. Sheep, goats and swine often fall to the ground and have opisthotonos when startled. Consciousness is undisturbed throughout the disease.

Usually, the temperature remains slightly above normal during the disease, but it may rise to 108 to 110°F (42 to 43°C) toward the end of a fatal attack. In mild attacks, the pulse and temperature remain nearly normal. Mortality averages about 80%. In the animals that recover, there is a convalescent period of 2 to 6 weeks; protective immunity does not usually develop following recovery.

Prophylaxis and Treatment: Active immunization of valuable animals can be accomplished with tetanus toxoid. If a dangerous wound occurs after immunization, another injection of toxoid to increase the circulating antibody should be given. If the animal has not been previously immunized with tetanus toxoid, it should be treated with 1,500 to 3,000 IU or more of tetanus antitoxin, which will usually give passive protection up to 2 weeks. Toxoid should then be given simultaneously with antitoxin and repeated in 30 days. Yearly booster injections of toxoid are advisable. Mares should be vaccinated during the last 6 weeks of pregnancy and the foals vaccinated at 5 to 8 weeks of age. In high-risk areas foals may be given tetanus antitoxin immediately after birth and every 2 to 3 weeks until they are 3 months old at which time they can be given toxoid. The decision to vaccinate lambs or calves is dependent on the probability of the disease occurring in the area.

All surgical procedures should be conducted with the best possible operative techniques. When large numbers of animals are docked or castrated, instruments should be sterilized before use and thereafter at frequent intervals. After such surgery, animals should be turned out on clean ground, preferably grass pastures. Only the oxidizing disinfectants as iodine or chlorine can be depended upon to kill the spores.

When administered in the early stages of the disease, curariform agents, tranquilizers, barbiturate sedatives, in conjunction with 300,000 IU of tetanus antitoxin every 12 hours, have been effective in the treatment of horses. Good results have been obtained by the injection of 50,000 IU of tetanus antitoxin directly into the subarachnoid space through the cysterna magna in horses affected with tetanus. Such therapy should be supported by drainage and cleaning of wounds and the administration of penicillin (℞ 63) or broad-spectrum antibiotics (℞ 16, 27, 56, 76). Good nursing is invaluable to tide the animal over the acute period of spasms. The patient should be placed in a quiet, darkened box-stall with feeding and watering devices high enough to allow their use without lowering the head. Slings may be useful in cases where standing or rising is difficult.

BOTULISM
(Lamziekte)

A type of food poisoning marked by progressive paralysis, caused by ingestion of the toxin of *Clostridium botulinum*. *See also* BOTULISM (POULTRY), p. 1139.

Etiology: Botulism is an intoxication, not an infection, and always results from ingestion of toxin in food. There are 8 types and subtypes of *Cl. botulinum,* differentiated on the serologic specificity of the toxins, A, B, C-alpha, C-beta, D, E, F and G. Types A, B and E are of most importance in human botulism; C-alpha in wild ducks, pheasants and chickens; C-beta in mink, cattle and horses; D in cattle. Only 2 outbreaks, both in man, are known to have been caused by Type F. Type G, which was isolated from soil in Argentina, is not known to have been involved in any outbreak of botulism either in man or animals. The usual source of the toxin is decaying carcasses or vegetable materials like decaying grass, hay, grain and spoiled silage.

The incidence of botulism in animals is not known with accuracy, but it is relatively low in cattle and horses, probably more frequent in chickens, and very high in wild waterfowl. There are probably from 10,000 to 50,000 birds lost in most years, with losses reaching one million or more during the great outbreaks in the Western U.S.A. The very great majority of birds involved are ducks, although loons, mergansers, geese and gulls are also susceptible. Type C-alpha is involved in duck botulism. The same type is usually responsible for botulism in pheasants. Dogs, cats and swine are comparatively resistant to all types of botulinum toxin when it is administered by mouth.

Most botulism in cattle occurs in South Africa, where a combination of extensive agriculture, phosphorus deficiency in soil and *Cl. botulinum* Type D in animals creates a condition ideal for bovine botulism. The phosphorus-deficient cattle chew any bones with accompanying tags of flesh that they find on the range; if these came from an animal that had been carrying Type D strains of *Cl. botulinum*, it is likely that intoxication will result. A gram or so of dried flesh from such a carcass may contain enough toxin to kill a mature cow. Any animal eating such material also ingests spores of *Cl. botulinum* Type D. These spores germinate in the intestine and, after death of the host, cells invade musculature which in turn becomes toxic and infective for other cattle. Type C strains also cause botulism in cattle in a similar fashion. This type of botulism in cattle is rare in the U.S.A. A few cases have been reported from Texas under the name of **"loin disease,"** and a very few cases have been encountered in Montana. Botulism in sheep has been encountered in Australia, not from phosphorus deficiency as in cattle, but from protein and carbohydrate deficiency. This results in the eating of carcasses of rabbits and other small animals that sheep find on the range.

Botulism in mink usually is caused by Type C-beta strains that have produced toxin in chopped raw meat or fish. Types A and E strains have been involved, but comparatively seldom.

Clinical Findings: The signs of botulism are associated with the paralysis of muscles, and include progressive motor paralysis, disturbed vision, difficulty in chewing and swallowing, and generalized progressive weakness. Death is usually due to respiratory or cardiac paralysis. **"Limberneck"** is not always seen in birds as death may occur without it. The toxin prevents synthesis or release of acetylcholine at motor end plates. Passage of impulses down the motor nerves and contractility of muscles are not greatly hindered; only the passage of impulses from nerves to motor end plates are affected. No characteristic lesions develop, and pathologic changes may be ascribed to the general paralytic action of toxin, particularly in the muscles of the respiratory system, rather than to the specific effect of toxin of any particular organ.

Diagnosis: Diagnosis of botulism can be best made by identification of the specific toxin in the serum, in extracts of liver tissue, in contents of the gastrointestinal tract, or in the food of affected animals. The type of toxin is determined by specific antitoxin neutralization. Isolation of the organism itself is not reliable evidence, for it can be present either in food or in intestinal contents without causing botulism. In any suspected case of botulism, a serum sample should be obtained as quickly as possible. The feeding of suspected material to susceptible animals will provide supportive evidence for the presence of the toxin.

Control: The correction of dietary deficiencies and the dispersal of carcasses should be implemented if possible. The removal of decaying grass or spoiled silage from the diet of animals is also indicated. Immunization of cattle with toxoid with Types C and D has proved successful in South Africa and in Australia. Toxoid is also effective in immunizing mink, and it has been used in pheasants.

Botulinum antitoxin has been used for treatment with varying degrees of success, depending upon the type of toxin involved and the species of host. Treatment of ducks with Type C antitoxin is often successful, as is the treatment of mink. In cattle, however, such treatment is rarely used. Treatment with guanidine hydrochloride, 5 mg/lb (11 mg/kg) body wt, has been reported to overcome some of the paralysis caused by the toxin, but the drug has not as yet been used sufficiently to be certain of its value.

GLANDERS
(Farcy)

A contagious, acute or chronic, usually fatal disease of Equidae, caused by *Pseudomonas mallei* and characterized by serial development of ulcerating nodules which occur most commonly in the upper respiratory tract, lungs and skin. Man, Felidae and other species are susceptible and are usually affected fatally. Glanders is one of the oldest diseases known and once was prevalent throughout the world. It has now been eradicated or effectively controlled in many countries, including the U.S.A.

Etiology: *P. mallei* is present in nasal and skin ulcerative exudate of infected animals and the disease is commonly contracted by ingesting food and water contaminated by the nasal discharge of carrier animals. The organism is susceptible to heat, light and disinfectants and is unlikely to survive in a contaminated area for more than 6 weeks.

Clinical Findings: Following an incubation period of approximately 2 weeks, affected animals usually exhibit septicemia and high fever (up to 106°F [41°C]), and subsequently a thick mucopurulent nasal discharge and respiratory signs. Death occurs within a few days. The chronic disease is common in horses and occurs as a debilitating condition with nodular or ulcerative cutaneous and nasal involvement. Animals may live for years while disseminating the disease. The prognosis is unfavorable. Recovered animals may not develop immunity.

Although nasal, pulmonary and cutaneous forms of glanders are recognized, more than one form may affect an animal simultaneously. In the **nasal** form, nodules develop in the mucosa of the nasal septum and lower parts of the turbinates. The nodules degenerate into deep ulcers with raised irregular borders. With healing of the ulcers, characteristic star-shaped cicatrices remain. In the early stage, the submaxillary lymph nodes are enlarged and edematous, later becoming adherent to the skin or deeper tissues.

In the **pulmonary** form, small tubercle-like nodules, which have caseous or calcified centers, surrounded by inflammatory zones, are found in the lungs. Pulmonary lesions are common. If the disease process is extensive, consolidation of the lung tissue and glanders pneumonia may be present. The nodules tend to break down and may discharge their contents into the bronchioles, resulting in extension of the infection to the upper respiratory tract.

In the **cutaneous** form ("farcy") nodules appear along the course of the lymph vessels, particularly of the extremities. These nodules undergo degeneration, and form ulcers which discharge a highly infectious, sticky pus. The liver and spleen may also show typical nodular lesions.

Diagnosis: The typical nodules, ulcers, scar formation and debilitated condition may provide sufficient evidence for a clinical diagnosis of the disease. Since, however, these signs usually do not develop until the disease is well advanced, specific diagnostic tests should be applied as early as possible. In addition to the mallein test, the procedure of choice, complement fixation is the most accurate of several serologic tests that may be used. Culture of exudate from lesions will indicate the presence of the causative organism.

Prophylaxis and Treatment: There are no immunizing agents. Prophylaxis and control depend upon the early detection and elimination, by destruction, of affected animals, as well as complete quarantine and rigorous disinfection of the area involved. Treatment is given only in endemic areas. Antibiotics are not very effective. Sulfadiazine (℞ 88) given daily for 20 days has been successful.

MELIOIDOSIS

A bacterial infection characterized by suppurating or caseous lesions in lymph nodes and in viscera. Macroscopically the lesions have no characteristic feature; microscopically there is a mixed purulent and granulomatous response. The disease is caused by *Pseudomonas pseudomallei* (*Bacillus whitmori, Loefflerella pseudomallei, Malleomyces pseudomallei*) a somewhat oval, motile, gram-negative bacillus with bipolar staining. The organisms are found in lesions and in discharges, e.g. nasal mucus when the respiratory tract is infected and urine when the kidneys are involved. The organisms are found in water and moist soils in tropical areas and infection would appear to be from the environment rather than from animal to animal transmission.

Infections have been recorded in sheep, goats, pigs, cattle, horses, dogs, a pet bird, a variety of wild animals and man. In the laboratory, hamsters, guinea pigs and rabbits are highly susceptible. Since melioidosis has been recognized frequently in primates imported for research, it is likely that the disease also occurs on occasion in primates sold as pets.

Clinical signs vary with the site of the lesions. In domestic animals it is usually chronic but progressive. In sheep and goats, abscesses in the lungs are common and signs of pneumonia are evident. Nasal discharge occurs if the nasal septum is ulcerated. At times joints are affected and the animal is lame. Signs of encephalitis may be associated with microabscesses in the CNS.

One or more infected abscesses often have been found in clinically normal sheep, goats and pigs. In pigs abscess of the spleen is often seen. Death occurs when the abscesses are extensive or when a vital organ is involved.

Diagnosis is by identification of the organism and should include agglutination with antiserum. Some organisms with many of the bacteriologic features of *P. pseudomallei* do not agglutinate specific antisera and are not pathogenic to guinea pigs. The complement fixation test on serum is a useful diagnostic aid in most species, including man. A hemagglutination test can be used on cattle and pig sera.

There is no effective vaccine. Treatment of clinical cases is generally unsatisfactory in that animals relapse when treatment is discontinued. The organisms are sensitive to kanamycin, novobiocin, tetracycline, trimethoprim-sulfamethoxazole and sulfonamides. Some strains are not sensitive to chloramphenicol.

TULAREMIA

An infection of wild rodents and lagomorphs, especially rabbits, transmitted to domestic animals and man directly or by arthropod vectors, especially ticks and tabanids. The primary domestic animal affected is the sheep in the Western U.S.A., but it may infect any species and has been reported from most continents.

Etiology and Transmission: The causative agent, *Francisella (Pasteurella) tularensis*, a nonspore forming, gram-negative organism, is serologically related to brucellae. It is killed quickly by heat but survives 3 to 4 months in mud, water or carcasses. Transmission in sheep usually follows bites of large numbers of wood ticks, *Dermacentor andersoni*, during the spring months. The disease is reported, but uncommonly, in pigs, foals, and calves. Severe death losses have occurred on fur farms from feeding infected rabbit carcasses. Dogs and cats may be infected by ticks or by ingesting wildlife. Man is infected from handling, skinning, and cleaning infected wildlife or game birds, from eating incompletely cooked infected meat, drinking contaminated waters, inhalation, or arthropod bites. A few cases have occurred following cat bites.

Clinical Findings: Many infections are subclinical. Heavy infestations of infected ticks generally are necessary to create disease in lambs, pigs, or colts. After a 1- to 10-day incubation period, fever (104 to 107°F [40 to 41.5°C]) stiffness, weakness, lassitude, increased respiration, coughing, and diarrhea are common. Wool breaks and weight loss produce economic problems in sheep. Incoordination, prostration and death may follow. The most characteristic lesions found at necropsy are miliary, whitish to yellowish foci (2 to 8 mm) in the lymph nodes, liver, or spleen. Enlarged congested lymph nodes also may be present. Care should be taken in handling tissues and ticks from animals dead of tularemia.

Diagnosis: The occurrence of a heavy tick population in the spring months and appearance of a generalized septicemia may suggest tularemia. Serum agglutination tests are helpful but the reliability varies with different tests and different animal species. Serologic cross-reactions with brucellae also may create confusion. Necrotic foci in the liver, spleen, and lymph nodes are suggestive and provide material for isolation attempts of fluorescent antibody tests. A special culture medium is required. Organisms can sometimes be isolated from ticks taken from dead animals but this does not prove the host animal was infected.

Tularemia should be differentiated from other septicemias and pneumonia. It has been confused with plague (q.v., p. 415) even by experienced researchers.

Treatment and Control: Individual animals respond to treatment with tetracyclines at levels up to 5.7 mg/lb (12.5 mg/kg) of body weight daily. Dihydrostreptomycin is less effective. Control varies with the route of transmission. Tick control and preventing ingestion of contaminated food and water should be the primary considerations.

ROCKY MOUNTAIN SPOTTED FEVER

An acute, infectious, febrile disease of man that varies from a mild to a rapidly fatal infection. It is widely distributed in the Western Hemisphere. Its interest to veterinarians arises in that the etiologic agent, *Rickettsia rickettsii*, is maintained in animals and is transmitted to man solely by certain ticks that feed on animal hosts, including man. It multiplies in the cells of the small peripheral blood vessels resulting in thrombosis and extravasation. The rash starts on the extremities and extends to the body. The disease may be reproduced experimentally in monkeys. Rabbits, guinea pigs, young sheep and dogs are susceptible. Most infections in dogs are subclinical but a mild illness with fever, loss of appetite, and lassitude also occurs.

Epidemiology: The maintenance of the organism in nature depends largely on ticks and the animals upon which they feed—rodents, rabbits and hares. In the U.S.A. 6 species of ticks have been recognized as natural carriers of the organism: *Dermacentor andersoni*, *D. variabilis*, *Amblyomma americanum*, *Haemaphysalis leporispalustris*, *D. parumapertus*. *D. occidentalis* is a potential vector in the Pacific northwest. The infected tick passes the organism through the egg to its offspring, and the ticks, in any stage of the life cycle, may transmit the infection during feeding.

Exposure may be occupational or recreational, or infected ticks may be brought into the household by dogs. Infected starving ticks seem to harbor an attenuated form of the organism. However, after the ticks have been warmed and allowed to feed, the rickettsiae are reactivated and virulent.

Transmission of *R. rickettsii* to man and animals is accomplished in most instances through the bite of a tick. It has also been shown that the crushed tissues and feces of infected ticks may spread the infection to the conjunctiva or abraded skin surfaces.

Diagnosis: Demonstration of the organism in ticks by immunofluorescence is a common procedure; however, isolation from naturally infected animals, including man, is rarely accomplished. Therefore, the Weil-Felix complement-fixation, indirect immunofluorescence, or indirect hemagglutination tests are used.

Control: No vaccines are commercially available for animals or man. Control of tick populations is difficult. Wide-strip spraying with insecticides (℞ 294, 335) and brush control around yards, barns, kennels, corrals, holding pens and along trails will control *D. variabilis* and *A. americanum.* Elimination of the small host mammals has been more effective in *D. andersoni* areas, but is not often practical.

Clothing barriers can be created by having each outer clothing layer overlap the one above it, e.g. trouser legs tucked in socks. Tick repellents also help (*see* TICK PARALYSIS, p. 747). Since ticks seldom attach themselves immediately and must feed for several hours to transmit the organism, removal of clothing twice a day and searching for ticks is effective. Ticks should be removed with extreme care. The tick should be grasped with forceps, gloves or a piece of paper to avoid contamination of the fingers. Care should be exercised to avoid breaking off the mouth parts in the skin. The wound then should be treated with antiseptic.

Q FEVER

A rickettsial infection of man and other animals, usually inapparent, but occasionally causing influenza-like disease in man, sometimes resulting in chronic endocarditis.

Etiology and Epidemiology: The etiologic agent *Coxiella burnetii* has worldwide distribution and reservoirs in ticks, bison, cattle, caribou, sheep, goats, bandicoots and kangaroos. It is resistant to many disinfectants and dessication. In endemic areas, antibody prevalence approaches 80%. The epidemiology of the disease is complex because it involves 2 major patterns of transmission. The first is a disease cycle in wild animals, with transmission by a tick vector or body fluids. The second pattern, independent of the wild animal cycle, occurs in domesticated animals such as cattle, sheep and goats in which the disease is transmitted through milk and placenta, with aerosols of each a major source of infection for man and other animals.

Diagnosis: Rarely diagnosed clinically, infection is confirmed serologically by complement-fixation or agglutination tests or by isolation of the agent from human blood or sputum, milk or placental materials from animals.

Treatment and Control: Man is treated with tetracyclines. Pasteurization of milk and careful disposal of animal placentas reduce infection. An inactivated vaccine has been effective in studies on cattle.

PLAGUE

A disease affecting mainly the lymphatics and lungs caused by *Yersinia (Pasteurella) pestis.* Although plague is a historic scourge of man, wild rodents and rabbits, confirmed cases in cats were first recognized in the 1970's. Three cases of human plague have been associated with the disease in cats. Experimental infection in 5 cats resulted in acute illness within 24 to 48 hours in all. Fever was as high as 106°F (41°C) and 3 of 5 died (days 4, 6 and 20, respectively). Temperature of the 2 survivors returned to normal by day 6. All of 10 dogs infected experimentally showed transient signs of illness with fever as high as 105°F (40.5°C) persisting for as long as 72 hours, but all recovered and were clinically normal by the seventh day after exposure.

Endemic foci of sylvatic plague exist in the Western U.S.A. and several other areas of the world. Fleas are the vectors that are the primary means of spreading *Y. pestis* from these reservoirs although contact with infected rabbit carcasses has been a significant source of infection for man during winter.

In endemic areas, plague should be suspected in cats presenting signs of fever, pneumonia and lymphadenitis. Diagnosis can be confirmed by blood culture or fluorescent antibody test of lymph node aspirate. Since plague in cats often can be rapidly lethal, therapy should be initiated immediately. Streptomycin and tetracycline in combination are effective and, on the basis of evidence from human cases, should be continued for at least 5 days after temperature returns to normal to avoid relapse. Prevention involves eliminating contact with infected wild rodents or rabbits and their fleas.

EPERYTHROZOONOSIS

An uncommon sporadic febrile hemolytic disease of swine, sheep, cattle, cats and other mammals caused by a blood parasite found in the plasma and upon the erythrocytes.

The majority of infections are subclinical and the incidence of overt disease is low. The parasite probably occurs in most countries but the incidence of subclinical infection is not known. Different species of parasite exist in different hosts (e.g. *Eperythrozoon suis*, *E. ovis*), and each appears to be relatively host-specific. Transmission is chiefly by bloodsucking insects, but surgical instruments and hypodermic needles are also incriminated.

In clinical cases there are varying degrees of hemolytic anemia, fever, anorexia, weakness and icterus. Most cases are mild, transient, unimportant, and are usually secondary to other conditions. More severe cases occur in young pigs and cats.

Differentiation should be made from nutritional anemias (q.v., p. 22) and from ictero-anemic conditions due to other infectious agents or toxic substances. Laboratory diagnosis of acute eperythrozoonosis may be made upon demonstration of large numbers of the blood parasite in Giemsa-stained film taken early in the disease. Smears should be made from fresh, noncitrated blood to avoid alterations in parasite morphology.

Tetracycline or oxytetracycline given IM at not less than 3 mg/lb (6.6 mg/kg) of body wt is specific in single doses against *E. suis*. Hematinic drugs, such as sodium cacodylate and iron-dextran are indicated. Chlortetracycline added to the drinking water at the rate of 200 mg/gal. (50 mg/L) is an effective herd treatment. Close confinement in shade to prevent unnecessary exertion is desirable.

ANAPLASMOSIS
(Gallsickness)

A peracute to chronic infectious disease of ruminants characterized chiefly by anemia, icterus and fever.

Etiology and Epidemiology: The exact nature and classification of the causative agent has presented a continuing taxonomic problem even though most authorities now consider it a rickettsia. Anaplasmata (anaplasms or "marginal bodies") are observed in blood smears stained with Wright's or Giemsa stain as small, rounded, basophilic bodies located in the stroma of the erythrocytes near the margins. Anaplasms range in diameter from about 0.3 to 1.0 μ; each is composed of several so-called initial bodies. The initial body is thought by some to be the infective form, capable of invading the erythrocyte and undergoing a type of fission to form the mature body.

Variants of the classic form or related genera occur. *Anaplasma marginale* has been considered the distinct pathogen of the group, causing anaplasmosis. The disease in cattle is endemic in many parts of the world, usually in the tropics and subtropics. It has been reported from most states in the U.S.A., but is most prevalent in the Gulf States, lower plains states, the intermountain west and California. The infection is limited to cattle and related ruminants. Wild ruminants such as deer and antelope may harbor latent *A. marginale* infection, and under some circumstances are important factors in maintaining *Anaplasma* infection. This is particularly true with the black-tailed deer of California located in the coastal range and the western slopes of the Sierra, where they have been shown to be a major reservoir of infection.

In some parts of the world, notably Africa, the relatively nonvirulent *A. centrale* occurs with *A. marginale* and is differentiated from the latter by the more central location of the anaplasm in the erythrocyte. *A. ovis* is normally relatively nonvirulent, but is capable of producing mild anaplasmosis in sheep and goats under certain conditions.

Transmission: Anaplasmosis has been transmitted experimentally in cattle by the bites of numerous species of ticks (*Boophilus, Rhipicephalus, Dermacentor, Hyalomma* and *Ixodes*), by horse flies (*Tabanus*), by stable flies (*Stomoxys*) and by mosquitoes (*Psorophora*). With fly and mosquito vectors, transfer is mechanical in nature and must be immediate to be effective. Ticks, however, ingest infected blood and transfer the infective agent to a susceptible host animal later when feeding is continued on a new host.

Since the infection is easily transmitted by mechanical transfer of infected blood, outbreaks of considerable proportions have been traced to mass operations, such as bleeding, dehorning, castrating, ear-tagging and vaccinating.

Clinical Findings and Course: The severity of the disease varies considerably with age. Calves undergo mild infections, with little or no mortality. In yearling cattle, the disease is more severe, but recovery is the rule. Increasing severity occurs in adult cattle with marked anemia developing and mortality varying between 20 and 50% in older animals. All breeds and types of cattle are susceptible.

The earliest signs include depression, inappetence, indolence and elevation of body temperature, commonly to 104 to 106°F (40 to 41°C). Lactating cows show a rapid fall in milk production. As the disease progresses, marked anemia develops and the animal becomes dehydrated and constipated. Loss of weight is pronounced and dehydration is noticeable in the acute form. In beef cattle, the disease usually is not recognized until the affected animal is extremely anemic and weak. A marked icterus may develop. Not uncommonly, affected animals succumb from hypoxia when moved or handled for treatment. If the animal survives the period of erythrocyte destruction, it usually recovers gradually. Hemoglobinuria does not occur.

The course of the clinical disease may be as short as a day or less in the fatal, peracute form, several days to 2 weeks in the more typical acute and subacute forms. Recovered animals often remain carriers for life but in rare instances spontaneous remission does occur.

Diagnosis: In endemic areas, anaplasmosis should be suspected in mature cattle showing anemia without hemoglobinuria. Icterus often is an important sign. The only incontrovertible evidence of the disease, however, is demonstration of the anaplasms or marginal bodies in the erythrocytes in stained blood smears. Up to 50 or 60% of the red blood cells may be parasitized. In cases where blood cell destruction has been extensive and the course of the disease prolonged, there may be so few anaplasms present in the circulating red cells that positive diagnosis by microscopy is impossible. A complement-fixation test is an effective diagnostic tool and is available in many diagnostic laboratories. A Rapid Card Agglutination (RCA) test using either plasma or serum works well to detect both the acute and carrier infections, unvaccinated herds or those that have not received vaccine for the preceding 4 months.

Necropsy findings are those associated with red blood cell destruction. The blood is thin and watery, and icterus usually is evident. The spleen is enlarged and soft. The liver is turgid and often of a mottled mahogany color. The bile is thick and brownish green, and the gallbladder is distended. If death occurs suddenly without anemia or icterus, there might be confusion with anthrax on the basis of the gross appearance of the spleen.

Prophylaxis: Prevention is a problem because of the difficulty of significantly reducing vector populations. However, the incidence of the disease can be reduced to some extent by killing or repelling vectors on the host with chemical dusts or sprays. For these to be effective, cattle must be dipped, sprayed or dusted at frequent intervals during the vector season. Large biting flies, particularly horse flies, are believed to be the most serious vectors in the Gulf States, while *Dermacentor* ticks appear to be the most important natural vectors in the intermountain west and the West Coast.

Since animals that have recovered remain permanent carriers, they should be conditioned for market and sold for slaughter as soon as possible, if a clean herd is desired. If the potential breeding value of the recovered animal warrants retention, it should be kept reasonably isolated from other cattle during the season of greatest danger of transmission, or treated to destroy the carrier infection (℞ 27).

Spread of the disease by man can be prevented by use of proper precautions during mass procedures, such as dehorning, bleeding, ear-tagging, castration and vaccination. Care should be taken to use individual sterilized needles and properly cleaned and disinfected instruments for each animal.

The inoculation of blood containing *A. centrale*, which gives rise to a mild infection that protects against subsequent infection with the virulent *A. marginale*, is used with considerable success in Africa, Asia, Australia, and parts of South America but is not permitted in the U.S.A.

The use of virulent and attenuated *A. marginale* isolates to induce premunition or a chronic carrier status is widespread throughout the tropical world where anaplasmosis is endemic. The virulent organisms can be administered to susceptible cattle by inoculating blood from a known infected animal or by using infective frozen blood stabilates. Frozen stabilates have the advantage that they can be checked for infectivity, purity of infection and safety prior to use, but have the disadvantage of requiring special handling in the field. Once thawed the stabilate must be used in a matter of minutes.

The use of virulent organisms in adult cattle is hazardous, and treatment at the onset of patent infection with oxytetracycline or chlortetracycline either parenterally (3.2 to 5 mg/lb [7 to 11 mg/kg]) or orally (11 mg/kg for several days) is recommended to moderate the course of infection. The stabilate vaccine has an advantage in that the incubation or prepatent period is usually predetermined so that the time of treatment is known. Virulent *A. marginale* stabilates can usually be given young cattle (up to a year) without treatment.

An *A. marginale* isolate attenuated by serial sheep passage is becoming increasingly popular in Central and South America. Experimental evidence suggests that this organism can be safely used even in adult cattle (except for lactating dairy cattle), where it produces a replicating, subclinical, infection that protects cattle from virulent *A. marginale*. This vaccine is commercially available in many Latin American countries, but is not approved for use in the U.S.A.

A killed vaccine is commercially available and offers some protection. It renders animals serologically positive for about 4 months. Experimental evidence has shown a relationship of vaccination with cases of neonatal isoerythrolysis (q.v., p. 28) in calves born to previously vaccinated cows.

Treatment: The tetracyclines (℞ 27, 60) are effective in acute anaplasmosis, especially if given early in the course of infection, during the period of *Anaplasma* multiplication.

Carrier infection may be eliminated by daily administration of chlortetracycline at 5 mg/lb (11 mg/kg) in the feed for 45 to 60 days, or by IV or IM injections of oxytetracycline at 11 mg/kg daily for 10 to 12 days. Recent success in eliminating infection using parenteral oxytetracycline at 10 mg/lb (22 mg/kg) for 5 days has been reported.

Two new experimental drugs, hetoxal (gloxazone) and Imidocarb, have shown promise but neither are approved for use in the U.S.A. A new experimental oxytetracycline formulation containing 200 mg/ml has now been reported to give sustained blood levels, thus reducing the number of injections required in the treatment of acute anaplasmosis. One injection of this compound at the rate of 9 mg/lb (20 mg/kg) IM is usually sufficient if given early in the course of infection.

Symptomatic and supportive treatment is important. Transfusion of 4 to 12 L of normal bovine blood is often indicated and may be sufficient to start an extremely anemic animal on the road to recovery. The transfusion may be repeated after 48 hours if necessary. Water given in large volumes, by stomach tube, and parenteral administration of dextrose are helpful. Mild laxatives, such as mineral oil, may be administered for the relief of constipation. Saline laxatives are to be avoided because they contribute further to the badly dehydrated state of the animal.

Treatment procedures should be accomplished with as little disturbance to the animal as possible and, in the case of range cattle or animals not used to being handled treatment may be contraindicated, since even mild exertion can produce hypoxia and death. Sick and convalescing animals respond well to careful management and good nutrition on pasture, with access to shade and fresh water. Application of suitable insect repellents adds to the comfort of the animal.

THE TRYPANOSOMIASES

A group of protozoan diseases of both animals and man caused by species of the genus *Trypanosoma*. Members of this genus infecting mammals are divided into 2 sections, principally on grounds of life cycle and pathogenicity. Those in the section Stercoraria normally follow a cycle of development in an insect vector with the forms infective to the mammalian host being transmitted in the vector feces. None cause disease excepting *T. cruzi*. Most members of the section Salivaria follow a cycle of development in tsetse flies (genus *Glossina*) and are transmitted to the mammalian hosts by the bites of the flies during feeding. Exceptions are: first, *T. equiperdum*, which is a venereal infection, and second, *T. evansi* (*equinum*), which is assumed to be transmitted directly (i.e. without a cycle of development) from a parasitemic to a susceptible mammal in the mouth parts of bloodsucking flies when their feeding is interrupted. All salivarian species are considered capable of causing disease, and concurrent infection with 2 or more species can occur.

Many synonyms are extant both for species names of trypanosomes and for the diseases they may cause. However, analysis of trypanosome isoenzyme patterns is now assisting the clarification of nomenclature.

The term "nagana" is now little used but refers to the tsetse-transmitted animal infections (*T. vivax [bovis]*, *T. uniforme*, *T. con-*

golense, *T. simiae*, *T. suis* and *T. brucei*); "sleeping sickness" refers to the tsetse-transmitted human infections (*T. gambiense* and *T. rhodesiense*); "surra" to animal infections with *T. evansi;* "dourine" to the equine infections with *T. equiperdum;* and "Chagas" disease is the infection of man and animals with *T. cruzi*.

The pathogenicity of salivarian trypanosomes in the field may vary with the species of mammal infected, with breeds within a domestic species, with exposure to stress, including intercurrent disease, with the strain of the trypanosome and with the size and frequency of the infective dose or doses. TABLE 1 therefore only describes a commonly accepted pathogenicity of trypanosome species to domestic animals.

TABLE 1. THE COMMONLY ACCEPTED PATHOGENICITY OF SOME MEMBERS OF THE GENUS *Trypanosoma* TO DOMESTIC ANIMALS

Trypanosoma	Dogs	Horses	Pigs	Camels	Cattle	Sheep/Goats
Stercoraria (selected species only):						
T. theileri	R	R	R	R	—	R
T. melophagium	R	R	R	R	R	—
T. cruzi	—	O	—	O	O	—
Salivaria:						
T. vivax	R	**	R	**	**	**
T. uniforme	R	**	R	**	**	O
T. congolense	*	**	*	**	***	**
T. simiae	O	O	***	***	O	O
T. suis	O	O	*	O	O	O
T. brucei	***	***	*	***	*	—
T. gambiense	—	O	—	O	—	—
T. rhodesiense	O	O	O	O	—	—
T. evansi	**	***	—	***	*	*
T. equiperdum	O	**	O	O	O	O

* ** *** degrees of pathogenicity
— subclinical infections
R refractory to infection
O insufficient data

TSETSE-TRANSMITTED ANIMAL TRYPANOSOMIASIS

Distribution: The trypanosomes infecting animals in Africa are related to the distribution of tsetse flies (*Glossina* spp.), which are found between latitudes 14°N and 29°S. A trypanosome indistinguishable from *T. vivax* on grounds of morphology and host susceptibility has been recovered from Mauritius in the Indian Ocean, from 2 islands in the West Indies, from Peru and all countries forming the North and Northeast coastline of South America. Serologic evidence suggests a New World distribution extending from at least 12°N down to the Tropic of Capricorn.

Epidemiology: The natural transmission cycle of tsetse-transmitted trypanosomes involve wild animals, which usually have symptomless infections. The trypanosomes become important when domestic animals become available as alternative hosts.

There are 22 known *Glossina* species, which can be broadly classified into forest, riverine or savanna species according to their preferred habitat. The most important economic situations relate to the transmission of *T. congolense* and *T. vivax* by savanna species whose presence denies the use of thousands of square miles of land to cattle and other livestock. Cattle populations may sometimes persist in relation to low densities of forest or riverine species.

The importance of noncyclical methods of transmission in Africa is probably small as trypanosomiasis ceases to be a problem when tsetse flies are eradicated. However, this raises the question of how *T. vivax* persists in countries where no tsetse flies exist.

Diagnosis: The field veterinarian most often has to rely on the demonstration of trypanosomes using thick and thin blood and lymph node smears and wet blood mounts. Bovine trypanosomiasis is usually seen as a chronic wasting disease associated with a degree of anemia and intermittent fever, and diagnosis is best made on a herd or an area basis. Horses and dogs may, in *T. brucei* infections, show corneal opacity and edema of the limbs and ventral surface of the abdomen. Trypanosomes in all susceptible animals are most easily seen in the initial stage of the infection or in acute cases. *T. simiae* infections in pigs are often acute with death intervening even a few hours after the onset of signs.

Injection of laboratory rodents with blood from suspected animals will reveal most *T. brucei* infections and some *T. congolense* infections, but *T. vivax* will at best only rarely produce a transient parasitemia. *In vitro* techniques are not used in making a diagnosis. Infective *T. brucei* has been grown in fibroblast tissue culture. Recently developed laboratory methods which may assist the field veterinarian are: the use of the hematocrit centrifuge to concentrate trypanosomes in the blood, the anion-exchange column, and an indirect fluorescent antibody test. The antigenic variation of trypanosomes within a species makes difficult the development of species specific serologic methods of diagnosis.

Treatment and Control: It appears that trypanosomiasis can be eliminated, at least from much of Africa, by eradicating the tsetse vectors but this is not always practical. (*But see* SURRA, p. 423.) Drugs are used extensively in the control of trypanosomiasis but their use can only be palliative as reservoir infections in wild animal hosts are not being attacked. A list of drugs commonly used in the treatment of the trypanosomiases in domestic animals is given in TABLE 2 (p. 425). Another drawback to drug prophylaxis is the ease with which trypanosomes become resistant. In order to try to overcome this difficulty some African countries have adopted a procedure whereby a single chemotherapeutic drug is put into common use, reserving diminazene aceturate to control only drug-resistant organisms. Diminazene aceturate was chosen for this role as for many years no field strains of trypanosomes were discovered to be resistant to it. In recent years, however, resistant trypanosome populations have been commonly reported from Nigeria together with isolated cases from other African countries.

Immunization of cattle using vaccines has not yet been successful, at least in part because of the antigenic variation of trypanosomes.

SLEEPING SICKNESS

(Tsetse-transmitted human trypanosomiasis)

T. gambiense and *T. rhodesiense* are morphologically similar to *T. brucei* and are distinguished from this species principally by their ability to infect man if indeed all 3 are not actually one species.

SURRA

(Animal infections with *T. evansi*)

Distribution: It is probable that this trypanosome is derived from *T. brucei* that has become adapted to noncyclical methods of transmission outside the distribution of tsetse flies. Movements of livestock have introduced the trypanosome into new areas and countries. Allegations that *T. equinum* is involved as a second species may be disregarded. The only stated difference is that the kinetoplast does not color with Rumanowsky stains. Such trypanosomes occur spontaneously in isolations of *T. evansi* and can also be induced by trypanocidal drugs. The disease occurs in the Middle East, Asia, the Far East, Central and South America, and in the areas of Africa north of the distribution of tsetse. The distribution of surra in Africa overlaps that of tsetse transmitted trypanosomiasis but delineation is difficult due to the similarities of morphology and animal-host range between *T. evansi* and *T. brucei*.

Epidemiology: All domestic mammals are susceptible to infection but whereas fatal diseases can occur in camels, horses and dogs, the infections of buffaloes, cattle and pigs are usually nonpathogenic and these animals often form reservoirs of infection. The life cycle of the trypanosome has therefore been considered to involve only domestic animals, as, in addition, past reports of infections in wild animals have related to fatal episodes. However, recent demonstration of capybaras being symptomless carriers of *T. evansi* in Columbia and the finding of a natural infection in an ocelot in Brazil have raised the possibility of a natural cycle in wild animals.

The principal method of transmission of surra is assumed to be "direct" by the interrupted feeding of blood-sucking flies. Carnivores can be infected from eating meat derived from parasitemic animals, and the vampire bat is a proven vector in South America under experimental conditions.

Diagnosis: As with tsetse-transmitted trypanosomiasis, the field veterinarian most often has to rely on the demonstration of trypanosomes using thick and thin blood smears, wet blood smears, or lymph node biopsy smears. Clinical diagnosis is not easy as the disease is characterized by a degree of anemia, edema and intermittent fever. Posterior paralysis is said to occur in camels in the Sudan and horses in South America. The disease in dogs is usually more acute with marked edema, opacity of the cornea and rapid emaciation.

Trypanosomes are best demonstrated in early infections and in acute disease. As well as the examination of tissue smears, suspected parasitemic blood may be inoculated into laboratory rodents. No method is known, however, of culturing *T. evansi*. The demonstration of increased serum immunoglobulins by precipitation with mercuric chloride has allowed efficient and simple diagnosis of surra in camels. Unfortunately the technique does not work in cattle with tsetse fly-transmitted trypanosomiasis. The recently developed methods for diagnosing nagana trypanosomes can also be expected to be of use in relation to *T. evansi*.

Control: The control of surra is almost entirely by diagnosis and treatment (TABLE 2). Resistance to suramin is not uncommon, but the organisms remain fully susceptible to quinapyramine sulfate.

DOURINE

(Equine infections with *T. equiperdum*)

Distribution: The disease is recognized on the Mediterranean coast of Africa, the Middle East, Southern Africa and South America. The distribution is probably wider than reported due to the often very chronic nature of the disease.

Diagnosis: The classical signs may develop over periods of weeks or months. Early signs include edematous swelling of the external genitalia with mucopurulent discharge from the urethra in the stallion and from the vagina in the mare followed by gross edema of the genitalia. Later, characteristic plaques 2 to 10 cm in diameter appear in the skin and the animal becomes progressively emaciated. The mortality in untreated cases is 50 to 70%.

Demonstration of trypanosomes from the urethral or vaginal discharges, the plaques on the skin, or peripheral blood is not easy unless the material is centrifuged. Infected animals can be detected with the complement fixation test but only in areas where *T. evansi* or *T. brucei* do not exist, as they have common antigens.

Control: In endemic areas horses may be treated (TABLE 2). Where eradication is required, strict control of breeding and elimination of stray horses has been successful. Alternatively, infected animals may be identified using the complement fixation test and compulsorily destroyed.

TABLE 2. DRUGS COMMONLY USED IN THE TREATMENT OF THE TRYPANOSOMIASES IN DOMESTIC ANIMALS

Drug	Synonyms	Animal	*Trypanosoma*	Main Action
Diminazene aceturate, (℞ 344)	Berenil, Babesin (as the dilactate salt), Ganaseg	Cattle Dogs	*vivax, congolense, brucei,* *evansi, congolense, brucei, evansi*	Curative (with the possible exception of *brucei*)
Quinapyramine sulfate, (℞ 358)	Antrycide sulfate	Cattle Horses Camels Pigs Dogs	*vivax, congolense, brucei, evansi,* *brucei, evansi, equiperdum* *evansi* *simiae* *congolense, brucei*	Curative
Quinapyramine (prophylactic), (℞ 358)	Antrycide prosalt	Cattle Pigs	*vivax, congolense, simiae*	Prophylactic
Homidium bromide, (℞ 345)	Ethidium bromide	Cattle Equids	*vivax, congolense, brucei* *vivax*	Curative
Homidium chloride, (℞ 345)	Novidium chloride Babidium chloride Ethidium chloride	As for the bromide salt		
Prothidium (℞ 354)		Cattle	*vivax, congolense*	Curative and Prophylactic
Metamidium		Cattle	*vivax, congolense*	Not marketed commercially
Isometamidium (℞ 349)	Samorin M & B 4180	Cattle	*vivax, congolense*	Curative and Prophylactic
Suramin (℞ 363)	Moranyl, Naganol, Antrypol, Bayer 205, Naphuride, Germanin	Horses Camels Dogs	*brucei, evansi, equinum* *evansi* *brucei, evansi*	Curative

CHAGAS' DISEASE

(*T. cruzi* infection of man and animals)

The common transmission cycle is between opossums, armadillos, rodents and wild carnivores, and bugs of the family Reduviidae. Distribution is in Central and South America and localized areas of Southern U.S.A. Chagas' disease is of great importance in South America. Domestic animals may become infected and introduce the trypanosome into human dwellings in situations of low standards of living where the bugs will exist. Man then becomes infected by the contamination of wounds or eyes or food with insect feces containing metacyclic trypanosomes. The trypanosome is pathogenic to man, and possibly to young dogs and cats, but other domestic animals act as reservoir hosts.

NONPATHOGENIC TRYPANOSOMES OF DOMESTIC ANIMALS

T. theileri or markedly similar trypanosomes have been detected by culture of peripheral blood on biphasic blood agar from cattle in every continent. Infection with similar trypanosomes has also been detected in domestic and wild buffalo and a variety of other wild ungulates. In the few areas studied, transmission is contaminative following a cycle of development in species of tabanid flies. Although the majority of parasitemias are subpatent, the trypanosomes may be accidentally seen by a veterinarian in a blood smear being examined for pathogenic protozoa, in a hemocytometer chamber, or as a contaminant of primary monolayers derived from bovine tissue. Allegations of pathogenicity have never been proven experimentally.

T. melophagium of the sheep also has a worldwide distribution and is transmitted by the sheep ked. *T. theodori*, reported from goats may be a synonym for the same trypanosome.

BABESIOSIS

(Piroplasmosis, Redwater, Texas fever, Tick fever)

A group of tick-borne diseases of animals caused by species of *Babesia* that develop within the red blood cells of the mammalian host, and within various cells of the tick vectors. Babesiosis is a significant disease problem in domestic and wild animals wherever suitable vectors occur but especially in the tropics. Normally, the parasites are transmitted from affected to susceptible animals by ticks which act as true biologic vectors. In endemic areas, young animals often become infected before they are a year old (they may be protected either by colostral antibodies—for about 2 months—or a temporarily elevated innate resistance). One exposure during this period protects most cattle from subsequent clinical attacks. Losses occur when cattle in the endemic area escape infection in the first year of life, when susceptible cattle are introduced, and when tick vectors become established in previously uninfested areas. The genus *Piroplasma* is no longer used, and has been replaced at least in part by *Babesia*.

Development in the Vertebrate Host: The development in the mammalian host follows a similar pattern in all the large species of *Babesia*, such as *B. bigemina*, *B. caballi*. Within the red blood cell, an anaplasmoid body, consisting mostly of chromatin, is invested with cytoplasm and becomes a signet-ring trophozoite. During this stage the protozoa exhibit rapid ameboid motility, increase in size, and finally form the typical double pear-shaped bodies, 2 to 4 μ in length and 1.5 to 2.0 μ in width, joined at the pointed ends. The daughter parasites escape from the red blood cells with or without lysis, and invade new red blood cells. The so-called small babesiae, such as *B. equi*, *B. bovis* and *B. divergens*, have a similar developmental cycle. In the case of *B. equi*, the number of daughter cells within an erythrocyte is 4, often arranged as a "Maltese cross." This form is diagnostic for *B. equi*.

Transmission, aside from the tick, can be achieved by mechanical means, i.e. contaminated instruments or needles, and rarely by intrauterine transfer.

Clinical Findings: *Babesia* infections may be peracute, acute, chronic or inapparent in nature. The peracute and acute infections are characterized by varying clinical signs and are often referred to as babesiosis in contrast to the term babesiasis, which denotes the chronic, inapparent but persisting form of the disease. Babesiosis is characterized by signs of malaise, inappetence, fever (up to 107°F [42°C]), hemoglobinurea, hemoglobinemia, anemia and hypoxia. Jaundice may occur in protracted cases, but less commonly than in anaplasmosis. CNS involvement may occur and is most often seen with *B. bovis* infections. Incoordination, ataxia, grinding of the teeth and mania followed by coma or death are not uncommon. Deaths occurring from infections with *B. bovis* may be associated with these CNS signs, which are thought to occur as a result of agglutination and packing of the infected erythrocytes in the cerebral capillaries. This sludging effect in capillaries may occur in organs other than the brain, causing a variety of clinical signs. *B. bigemina*, however, is more often associated with severe anemia and hypoxia. Terminally ill cattle also may show CNS involvement in association with *B. bigemina* infections, which are characterized by muscle tremors, incoordination and aggressive behavior. These signs are thought to reflect the severe anemia and hypoxia usually present at this stage.

Young animals have an innate resistance, which in endemic areas is complemented by colostral antibodies. Exposure and infection in such animals often goes unnoticed, but such infections usually result in immunity.

The prepatent period following tick exposure is usually 7 to 20 days depending on the *Babesia* species involved and the level of tick exposure. This average is extremely variable. The inoculation of large volumes of infected blood may result in active replicating parasitemias in as little as 24 hours. The inoculation of small volumes or lightly infected material may produce prolonged prepatent periods.

Diagnosis: A presumptive diagnosis of babesiosis, or acute infection, is often possible on the basis of clinical evidence, a knowledge of the past history of the area, and by the presence of *Boophilus* ticks, or other suitable vectors. A definitive diagnosis is dependent on demonstrating the causative organism in stained blood films. The Romanowsky type stains are usually sufficient for this purpose. Since demonstrable parasitemias may be short lasting, it may be necessary to resort to animal inoculation, using splenectomized calves, which usually show characteristic signs and parasitemias following exposure.

In cases of chronic or inapparent infection, serologic procedures including complement fixation, indirect fluorescent antibody, and indirect hemagglutination tests are useful, if not essential, since a demonstrable parasitemia is rarely observed. These tests will remain positive for an extended period after infection, and in some instances for a short time after the infection has been eliminated. They are useful in identifying carrier animals and serve a useful purpose in incidence surveys.

Treatment: Acute babesiosis responds well to a variety of chemotherapeutic agents if treatment is given soon enough. Animal response to treatment with respect to the disappearance of *Babesia* parasitemias can be quite remarkable.

Compounds such as: 1,3-di-6-quinolyl urea (Babesan) and quinuronium sulfate (℞ 359), are highly effective against *B. bigemina* and to a lesser extent against *B. bovis*. Acriflavins, neutral and acid, reportedly give good results against *B. bigemina* and *B. bovis*. The diamidine derivatives, phenamidine isethionate (℞ 353), dimenazine aceturate (Ganasag) and amicarbalide di-isethionate (Diampron, ℞ 338), are probably the most commonly used compounds in South America, Africa and Australia. Diminazine aceturate is safe and highly effective; the recommended level for the treatment of babesiosis is 3 to 3.5 mg/kg body wt IM. In premunition studies as little as 0.5 mg/kg was found effective in moderating the clinical course of infection and controlling the parasitemias, without eliminating infection. Larger doses will eliminate infection.

Imidocarb dipropionate (℞ 348), one of the most recently introduced compounds for treating babesiosis, is highly effective and safe in the doses recommended (2 mg/kg). In addition to being an effective treatment, it has a chemoprophylactic effect against *Babesia* for up to 6 weeks, probably due in part to the slow elimination of this compound following injection. Occurrence of tissue residues has retarded its widespread usage.

Immunity: There have been reports of killed or noninfective immunogens against babesiosis, but the principal methods now in use to immunize cattle involve the use of premunition, i.e. the intentional induction of infection that progresses to the carrier state. *B. bovis* has been successfully attenuated by passage in splenectomized calves, and this organism plus *B. bigemina* is widely used in Australia and parts of South America in live vaccines. Both *B. bovis* and *B. bigemina* premunition is practiced throughout the world, but if fully virulent organisms are used in older cattle extreme caution is indicated, and treatment should be used as needed.

Vector Control: The eradication of *Boophilus* ticks in the U.S.A. by dipping and spraying programs almost 40 years ago completely eliminated *B. bigemina* and *B. bovis* infections. Where tick eradication is accomplished the cattle babesiae soon disappear. The emergence of resistant ticks and the lack of control of cattle movement are now jeopardizing tick eradication programs, which may well limit the usefulness of this method of *Babesia* control.

Important Species: There are over 70 recognized *Babesia* spp. in domestic and wild animals. The following species are important in domestic animals:

Babesia bigemina—occurs throughout the tropics, subtropics and in some temperate zones of Africa Asia, Australia, North and South America, causing one of the most widespread and important diseases of cattle. It is a large *Babesia*, measuring 4 to 5 μ by 2 to 3 μ. It is primarily transmitted by *Boophilus* but also possibly by *Haemaphysalis punctata* and *Rhipicephalus* spp.

Babesia bovis (*argentina, berbera*)—has a distribution similar to *B. bigemina*, however, the 2 organisms (*B. bovis* and *B. bigemina*) are not always found together. It is a small babesia and usually measures about 2.5 by 1.5 μ. The principal vectors are the *Boophilus* ticks, but also in some parts of the world *Ixodes persulcatus* and *I. ricinus* may be involved.

Babesia divergens—occurs in Northern Europe and possibly in Asia. It is a small babesia measuring less than 2 μ in length, and is usually observed on the periphery of the red blood cell as a double piriform body. The tick vectors are primarily *Ixodes ricinus* and *Haemaphysalis punctata.*

Babesia major—has been reported from Africa and South America, but is mainly of concern in Northern and Central Europe including the U.K. It is slightly smaller than *B. bigemina* (3 to 4 μ) and is transmitted by *Haemaphysalis punctata, Ixodes ricinus* but possibly by the *Boophilus* ticks also.

Babesia motasi—occurs in sheep and goats in Southern Europe and Asia, Northern Africa, Russia and Indochina. It is relatively large, measuring 2.5 to 4 μ in length. It is known to be transmitted by *Rhipicephalus bursa, Dermacentor silvarum* and *Haemaphysalis punctata.*

Babesia ovis—occurs in sheep and goats in most of the tropical world as well as in parts of Southern Europe and Russia. *B. ovis* is smaller than *B. motasi*, ranging from 1 to 2 μ in length. *Rhipicephalus bursa* is the principal vector.

Babesia caballi—occurs in Equidae throughout most of the tropics, and is common in Southern Europe, Asia, Africa, Central and South America; it has been endemic in southeastern Florida since 1962. It is a large babesia, 2.5 to 4 μ in length. The known vectors are *Dermacentor nitens, D. marginatus, D. pictus, D. silvarum, Hyalomma anatolicum, H. dromedarii, H. marginatum, H. volgense, Rhipicephalus bursa* and *R. sanguineus.*

Babesia equi—has even wider distribution in Equidae than does *B. caballi.* It occurs on all continents that extend into the tropical zone. It is a small babesia, develops tetrads and is less than 2 μ in length. The parasites are transmitted mostly from stage to stage by the following ticks: *Dermacentor marginatus, D. pictus, Hyalomma anatolicum, H. dromedarii, H. marginatum, H. uralense, Rhipicephalus bursa, R. evertsi* and *R. sanguineus.* The vector in the U.S.A. is unknown.

Babesia trautmanni—occurs in swine of Europe, Asia, Central and South America and Africa. It is a large babesia, measuring 2.5 to 4 μ in length. It is known to be transmitted by *Rhipicephalus sanguineus* and possibly species of *Hyalomma* and *Dermacentor.*

Babesia perroncitoi—has been reported only in swine in North Africa. It is a small babesia measuring from 1 to 2.8 μ in length. The tick vector is unknown.

Babesia canis—has occurred in dogs on all continents. It will infect most canine animals. It is a large babesia, measuring up to 5 μ in length. The chief vector is *Rhipicephalus sanguineus,* although *Dermacentor marginatus, D. pictus, D. andersoni, Haemaphysalis leachi* and *Hyalomma marginatum* are also known to be vectors.

Babesia gibsoni—occurs primarily in Canidae of India and the Far East, but has been recorded from North America. It is smaller than *B. canis,* and measures 1 to 2.5 μ in length. It is transmitted by *Rhipicephalus sanguineus* and *Haemaphysalis bispinosa.*

Babesia felis—occurs in Felidae of Africa and Asia. It measures less than 3 μ in length and usually divides into 4 daughter cells.

THE THEILERIASES

A group of diseases caused by protozoan parasites of the genus *Theileria*, which invade but do not destroy the red blood cells, giving rise to acute or chronic febrile infections.

Both *Babesia* and *Theileria* are members of the Class Piroplasmasida. *Theileria* appears in the red blood cells during the acute stage of the disease, but multiplication in erythrocytes, while it can occur, is not important. After inoculation into the blood stream of the susceptible animal, the parasites enter lymphoid cells of the spleen, lymph nodes and liver, where asexual multiplication or schizogony takes place. The schizonts in the lymphocytes are called Koch's blue bodies and are of diagnostic value. They are of 2 types, macroschizonts and microschizonts. The particles of the latter break away from the host cell and invade the erythrocytes. The round RBC ring stages are engulfed by the tick and form spindle-shaped microgamonts, which become microgametes. Some of the ring forms develop into round forms considered to be macrogametes. This occurs sometime during the first 5 days in the tick and rounded zygotes have been seen 6 days after tick repletion although no actual union has been demonstrated. The zygotes develop into club-shaped kinetes. This has been shown for both *T. parva* and *T. annulata* with minor differences. Vector ticks enable the infection to be passed on to the next bovine host.

EAST COAST FEVER

(Coastal fever, Theileriasis of cattle, Rhodesian tick fever)

An acute disease of cattle characterized by high fever, swelling of the lymph nodes, emaciation and high mortality, and caused by *Theileria parva*. The disease is a very serious problem in East and Central Africa.

Etiology and Transmission: *Theileria parva* appears in the red blood cells as ovoid, pear-shaped, discoid or rod-shaped bodies varying in size from 0.5 to 3.0 μ. One or more organisms may be found in a red cell. Schizonts or Koch's blue bodies, 3 to 10 μ in diameter, are found within lymphocytes of the spleen, liver and lymph nodes and occasionally are observed free in the blood stream. Transmission is through ticks of the genus *Rhipicephalus*, especially *R. appendiculatus;* however only the nymph and adult stages are infective. An infective nymph, feeding to engorgement, loses its infectivity. There is no transmission through ova.

Clinical Findings and Diagnosis: The onset is characterized by high fever lasting several days, dyspnea, evacuation of dry or liquid hemorrhagic feces, swelling of the external lymph nodes, emaciation and weakness. Up to 90% of the erythrocytes may be parasitized at the peak of fever. Sometimes, there may be a cough, salivation, conjunctivitis and rhinitis. The disease runs an acute course, death usually occurring within 2 weeks. Mortality may reach 90 to 100%. Recovered animals are immune and do not remain carriers as do animals that have recovered from some other theileriases.

Diagnosis is presumptive on the basis of acute, febrile onset with swollen external lymph nodes in cattle in areas known to be endemic for East Coast fever. In the live animal, demonstration of Koch's blue bodies in smears from lymph nodes or spleen is confirmatory. The absence of anemia and icterus aids in differentiating East Coast fever from cattle tick fever. On necropsy, the most characteristic changes are petechial and streaky hemorrhages on the serous membranes and intestinal mucosa, swelling of the lymph nodes, a liver showing friability, brownish discoloration and small grayish white foci, ulceration of the abomasal mucosa, and kidneys showing white nodules and spots. The white foci, nodules or spots on the liver and kidney represent aggregations of lymphocytes. Pulmonary edema is probably the immediate cause of death.

Control: Incidence can be reduced by tick control. The most effective method of eradicating the disease is slaughter of affected and exposed animals and keeping the land free of cattle for 15 months, during which time the infection dies out in the tick population. During this period, nonsusceptible animals such as sheep, goats and horses may be grazed on the land. Infected ticks that engorge on nonsusceptible animals free themselves of the parasite and take no further part in transmission of the disease.

Successful treatment must begin before clinical signs develop, preferably at the time of infection but diagnosis is usually not made until the disease is well advanced. Hitherto, experimental infection was effected by the attachment of ticks, but now it can be brought about by the injection of infective particles derived from infected ticks and cryogenically preserved. This development has led to successful artificial immunization by the "infection and treatment" method using infective stabilates and injections of long-acting oxytetracyclines. In early experiments, doses of n-pyrrolidinomethyl tetracycline (Reverin) proved effective but subsequently immunization, using an oxytetracycline of undisclosed formulation, has been achieved and shows much promise. Chlortetracycline (℞ 27) and oxytetracycline (℞ 48), if given early and repeatedly, will inhibit further development of the schizonts so that no additional red blood cells can be invaded. Pamaquine (℞ 352) causes degeneration of the erythrocytic forms when administered during the incubation period, reducing or destroying the infectivity of the blood for ticks. Experimentally Menoctone, a naphthoquinone, has been successful in treatment of cattle at the time of temperature rise to 39.5°C. It is said to be active against the schizont stages. Also *in vitro* cultures of lymphoid cells infected with *T. parva* were inhibited in growth by folate antagonists. This might result in a new approach to treatment.

OTHER THEILERIASES

Theileria annulata (*dispar*) causes a disease of cattle in North Africa, the Mediterranean coastal area, the Middle East, India, U.S.S.R. and Asia. The disease has been called **tropical piroplasmosis, tropical theileriosis** and **Mediterranean Coast fever.** Transmission is effected by ticks of the genus *Hyalomma.* Signs are generally milder and mortality lower than with East Coast fever. *T. annulata* cultured *in vitro* showed reduced virulence but retained its immunogenicity in field trials and has been used as a vaccine in cattle in Israel, Iran and Russia. Recovery from *T. annulata* infection leaves an immunity which is not sterile but in which the animal is a carrier.

Theileria mutans is a parasite of cattle in Africa. Ordinarily only mildly pathogenic, on occasions it has been implicated in virulent outbreaks of theileriasis as reported at Tzaneen in South Africa (**Tzaneen disease**). Similar mild forms of *Theileria* have been found in Europe, Asia, Australia and the U.S.A. but these are antigenically different; the true *T. mutans* is apparently confined to the African continent. Animals that have been infected with these organisms remain as carriers. *T. mutans* has recently been shown to be transmitted in East Africa by ticks of the genus *Amblyomma. Rhipicephalus* ticks have also been implicated as vectors further south in the continent.

Theileria lawrencei has been described as the causative agent of **corridor disease** of cattle in Southern Africa. The disease occurs in cattle moved to areas occupied by buffalo, which harbor the parasite as a silent infection. The signs and postmortem lesions resemble those of East Coast fever. This parasite is antigenically related to *T. parva* and might be a variant of that species.

Theileriasis of sheep and goats is caused by *T. ovis* and *T. hirci*. *T. ovis* is the more widely distributed of the 2 species occurring in Africa, Europe, the U.S.S.R., Middle East, India and parts of Asia. It is usually nonpathogenic, any mild manifestation that might occur being called benign ovine or caprine theileriosis. *T. hirci* occurs as the cause of malignant ovine or caprine theileriosis in North Africa, Southern and Eastern Europe, the U.S.S.R., India and Asia Minor. The disease is most serious in adult animals with mortalities often exceeding 40%. Signs and lesions are similar to those seen in cattle infected with *T. annulata.*

BOVINE PETECHIAL FEVER

(Ondiri disease)

An infectious disease of cattle characterized by hemorrhage and edema. It has been confirmed only in Kenya at altitudes over 5,000 ft (1,800 m), although it may occur also in neighboring countries of similar topography.

Etiology: *Cytoecetes* (*Ehrlichia*) *ondiri*, the causal agent, can be observed in circulating granulocytes and monocytes during clinical reaction, and in the spleen at necropsy. Initial multiplication of the organism is believed to take place in the spleen, with subsequent spread to other organs. Latent infections occur after recovery in some animals. Immunity lasts for several years.

Epidemiology: The disease is restricted to cattle grazing scrub or forest edge areas, with heavy shade and a thick litter layer giving high relative humidity. It occurs sporadically throughout the year in imported breeds of cattle, of which the Sahiwal may be most susceptible. An arthropod vector is suspected, but extensive attempts to incriminate ticks, biting insects, and mites have failed. Bushbuck (*Tragelaphus scriptus*) are reservoirs of *C. ondiri* in endemic areas, while other species of wild ruminant are susceptible to experimental infection and constitute potential reservoirs.

Clinical Findings: The disease ranges from inapparent to fatal, and is characterized by fever, apathy, and petechiation of mucous membranes. After an incubation period of 4 to 14 days, animals develop a high fever. After a further 2 or 3 days, most animals appear dull and petechiae can be observed on mucous membranes, particularly the lower surface of the tongue and the vaginal mucosa. These hemorrhages enlarge over several days, and then regress. A characteristic marked conjunctival edema and hemorrhage or "poached egg eye" occur in some severe cases. Characteristic hematologic changes are an absence of eosinophils, and a marked fall in lymphocyte counts followed by an equally pronounced drop in neutrophils. The necropsy lesions are widespread hemorrhage and edema, accompanied by lymphoid hyperplasia. No characteristic histologic abnormalities have been described.

Diagnosis: In areas where the disease is endemic, a history of movement to rough grazing, coupled with clinical and postmortem signs, allow a presumptive diagnosis. In other areas, demonstration of the causal organism is necessary, either in Giemsa-stained blood or spleen smears, or by inoculation of tissue suspensions into susceptible cattle or sheep. Blood smears from the recipient animal should be taken and examined daily for 10 days for the presence of *C. ondiri* in the granulocytes and monocytes.

Control and Treatment: In endemic areas, avoidance of rough grazing associated with previous cases is practiced where possible. Dithiosemicarbazone has been used successfully to treat early experimental cases.

HEARTWATER
(Cowdriosis)

A tick-borne septicemic, rickettsial disease of ruminants. It is found in the regions of Africa and Madagascar infested by ticks of the *Amblyomma* species. Occasionally the disease is reported in Europe.

Many ruminants, including antelopes, are susceptible; some such as blesbok and wildebeest develop transient reactions to infection and act as reservoirs. Indigenous breeds of cattle, goats and sheep, appear to be more resistant than imported breeds.

Etiology and Transmission: The causative organism, *Cowdria (Rickettsia) ruminantium,* is transmitted under natural conditions by "bont" ticks, *Amblyomma* sp. This 3-host tick becomes infected either during the larval or nymphal stages and transmits the infection during one of the subsequent stages. The progeny of an infected female tick are not infective.

The rickettsia can be propagated under experimental conditions by serial passage either by inoculation of infective blood or by feeding infected larval and nymphal stages on susceptible animals. Serial passage with blood is possible in ruminants and in ferrets. It is infective for but can not be serially passaged in mice. At room temperature the infected blood loses its potency within a few hours but the organisms may be preserved by freezing.

Clinical Signs and Pathogenesis: The signs are dramatic and pathognomonic in the peracute and acute forms. In peracute cases the animals develop high fever which is rapidly followed by hyperesthesia, lacrimation and convulsions. In the acute form the animals often develop diarrhea and exhibit nervous signs consisting of depression, a stiff gait, high stepping, exaggerated blinking of eyes and chewing movements, and terminating in convulsions and prostration. In chronic cases the signs are less remarkable, and CNS involvement is inconsistent.

The causative organism initially reproduces in the reticuloendothelial cells, particularly in the macrophages, and then invades and multiplies in the vascular endothelium. During the febrile stages the blood is infective to susceptible animals. The development of clinical signs and lesions is associated with injury to the vascular endothelium, which results in the increased vascular permeability and extensive tissue hemorrhages. These conditions precipitate a fall in the arterial pressure and a general circulatory failure. The pathognomonic lesions observed in peracute and acute cases consist of hydrothorax, hydropericardium, edema and congestion of lungs, enlarged spleen; petechial and ecchymotic hemorrhages on the mucosal and serosal surfaces, and there is occasionally hemorrhage into the gastrointestinal tract.

Diagnosis: In the acute forms the diagnosis can be made on the basis of clinical signs. Demonstration of the organism is necessary for definitive diagnosis. This is done with Giemsa stained endothelial scrapings from the aorta or jugular vein or with "squash" smears of cerebral gray matter. A capillary tube flocculation test is also used.

Prophylaxis and Treatment: Control of tick infestation is the most useful prophylactic measure. Infected blood is used as a vaccine in combination with antibiotic treatment at the time of reaction. However, the various rickettsial strains do not cross protect to give complete immunity. Young calves under 3 weeks old, and lambs and kids up to 6 weeks, are fairly resistant and may recover spontaneously from natural and experimental infections. Tetracyclines will usually effect a cure if administered early. Sheep require a higher treatment level (3 to 4 mg/lb [6.5 to 9 mg/kg]) than cattle (2 to 3 mg/lb [4.5 to 6.5 mg/kg]). Tetracyclines in oil (1 to 3 mg/lb [2 to 6.5 mg/kg] body wt) have been useful, as have the sulfonamides.

NAIROBI SHEEP DISEASE

A tick-borne viral disease of sheep and goats characterized by fever and gastroenteritis. Man is susceptible. It occurs only in Kenya, Uganda and Zaire.

Etiology and Transmission: The causal agent is a member of the Bunya-amwera virus group and is closely related to **Ganjam virus,** a tick-borne infection of sheep and goats in India, and to **Dugbe virus,** a tick-borne infection of cattle in West Africa. It is transmitted naturally by all stages of the brown tick, *Rhipicephalus appendiculatus,* in which it can survive for about 2½ years. Other *Rhipicephalus* and *Amblyomma* ticks may also transmit the disease. The virus is shed in the urine and feces, but the disease is not spread by contact. Wild rodents develop asymptomatic viremias and may be reservoirs of infection.

Clinical Findings: A prodromal fever of 1 to 3 days duration follows an incubation period that ranges from 4 to 15 days. Sometimes the fever is diphasic. Illness is manifested by depression, anorexia, mucopurulent blood-stained nasal discharge, and fetid dysentery causing painful straining. Pregnant animals frequently abort. In fatal cases, death follows about 2 days after remission of the fever. The mortality in sheep varies from 30 to 90%. Native sheep are more susceptible than Merinos. Goats generally recover.

Lesions: The main lesions are hyperplasia of lymphoid tissues and hemorrhages of the gastrointestinal and respiratory tracts, gallbladder, spleen and heart. The fetus has dermal hemorrhages. Additional histopathologic findings are glomerulonephritis and myocardial necrosis.

Diagnosis: Confirmation of suggestive signs and lesions requires isolation and serologic identification of the virus. The preferred specimens are blood, mesenteric lymph nodes, liver and cecum.

Prophylaxis and Treatment: Prophylaxis is achieved by control of tick infestation and by vaccination. Attenuated vaccines have been replaced by a more efficient, inactivated, methanol-precipitated vaccine. There is no reliable treatment.

RIFT VALLEY FEVER

A mosquito-borne viral disease of sheep, goats, camels, cattle, buffaloes, antelopes and rodents characterized by a short incubation period, fever, hepatitis and death in young animals, and by abortion in pregnant animals. Man is susceptible. The disease is found in Kenya, Uganda, Rhodesia, South Africa, Mozambique and Egypt. Explosive epidemics occur at intervals of several years, the most recent being in Egypt in 1977.

Etiology and Transmission: The causal agent is an ungrouped arbovirus transmitted by mosquitoes. The East African forest rat may be the main reservoir of infection. Man is usually, and readily, infected through contact with infected animals and their tissues, primarily by aerosols.

Clinical Findings: The incubation period varies from 12 to 96 hours in sheep and cattle and 2 to 6 days in man. Signs manifested are fever, listlessness, anorexia, unsteady gait, mucopurulent nasal discharge, diarrhea and abortion, which often is the only clinical finding in adult animals. The mortality in lambs is very high, but in adults rarely exceeds 30%. In cattle, the death rate is lower. In man, the disease is usually influenza-like but, on occasion, a fatal hemorrhagic fever with neurologic complications may occur. Retinitis and temporary blindness sometimes results.

Lesions: The striking lesions are the bright-yellow necrotic liver, widespread subserosal hemorrhages, enlarged spleen and gastroenteritis. Microscopically there is coagulative necrosis of hepatocytes with the formation of intracytoplasmic hyaline inclusions. Sometimes, eosinophilic intranuclear inclusions are also observed.

Diagnosis: An epidemic in ruminants, characterized by a short incubation period, a high mortality in newborn animals, abortions, necrosis of the liver and contact infection of man, justifies a tentative diagnosis of Rift Valley fever. For a positive diagnosis, isolation in mice or tissue cultures and serologic identification of the virus is necessary. Histologic examination of the affected liver is an aid to diagnosis.

Prophylaxis and Treatment: Removal of stock from low-lying, moist, mosquito-infested regions to higher altitudes, or stabling, is recommended. Attenuated live-virus vaccine protects but must be administered annually. Pregnant animals are immunized with an inactivated vaccine. No specific treatment is available.

WESSELSBRON DISEASE

A mosquito-borne viral disease of sheep and cattle characterized by high mortality in newborn lambs and by abortion in ewes and cows. The virus has also been isolated from dogs with encephalitis. Man is susceptible. Overt disease has been recognized only in Southern Africa but serologic surveys indicate that infection occurs in many species of animals throughout Africa, even in ground-living birds in Ethiopia. The disease resembles Rift Valley fever (q.v., p. 437) in its epidemiology, clinical signs and postmortem findings, but there is no cross-protection. Jaundice is a common sign in affected sheep, whereas this sign is not seen in Rift Valley fever. Both diseases often are present in the same area and are transmitted by the same species of mosquitoes. Vaccination of nonpregnant sheep with a live-attenuated virus is recommended. No specific treatment is available.

CONGO VIRUS DISEASE

A transient disease of African cattle and goats characterized by fever, depression and anorexia. The causal agent, an ungrouped arbovirus, is transmitted by hard ticks (*Hyalomma* spp.) and is similar to, and may be identical with the virus causing Crimean hemorrhagic fever in man. The link between Africa and Eastern Europe and Central Asia is postulated as being the ectoparasites of migratory birds. Virus isolations in suckling mice have been made from ticks, cattle, man and the African hedgehog. Neither vaccine nor treatment is available.

EPHEMERAL FEVER

(Three-day sickness)

An arthropod-transmitted disease of cattle that occurs in Africa, Australia and Asia, and characterized by fever, stiffness and lameness usually followed by spontaneous recovery within a few days. Natural infections also occur in buffalo, hartebeest, waterbuck and wildebeest.

Etiology and Epidemiology: Ephemeral fever virus (EFV) is classified as a rhabdovirus. Isolation of EFV from infected cattle is usually accomplished by intracerebral inoculation of suckling mice with defibrinated blood. Baby hamster kidney (BHK 21) and monkey kidney (Vero) cell lines may be used to grow EFV and to conduct tests.

The disease can be transmitted from infected to susceptible cattle by IV inoculation with as little as 0.005 ml of blood collected during the febrile stage. Although EFV has been recovered from *Culicoides* and mosquito species collected in the field, the vectors responsible for transmission during major epidemics are not known. Transmission by contact does not occur and EFV does not appear to persist in recovered cattle. Most recovered cattle are immune.

The incidence, extent and severity of the disease vary from year to year and epidemics occur periodically. During epidemics the disease appears suddenly in a herd, affecting a number of animals within days or weeks. It is most prevalent in the summer-early autumn period when conditions favor multiplication of biting arthropods. Morbidity may be as high as 50 to 80% but the mortality is usually less than 1%.

Clinical Findings: Common signs are fever, listlessness, inappetence, lacrimation, serous nasal discharge, drooling, dyspnea, atony of fore-stomachs, depression, stiffness and lameness, and decreased milk yield. Affected cattle may become recumbent for 8 hours to more than a week. There is a cessation of lactation in some cows and, following recovery, milk production often fails to return to normal levels until the next lactation. Bulls and other heavy cattle are the most severely affected, but even so, uneventful recovery usually occurs.

Treatment and Control: Treatment is not recommended. Attenuated live-virus vaccines appear to be effective but should only be used in endemic areas. Inactivated-virus vaccines do not protect against challenge with virulent virus, and so cannot be recommended.

AKABANE DISEASE

A newly recognized infective cause of congenital developmental abnormalities in domestic ruminants. The causal agent is Akabane virus, a member of the Simbu group of arboviruses. It has been isolated from several species of mosquitoes and *Culicoides* in Japan, Kenya and Australia. So far the clinical disease has been reported only in Australia, Israel and Japan, affecting calves, lambs and kids.

Clinical Findings and Lesions: The signs seen at birth depend on the species of animal and the stage of pregnancy at which the dam was bitten by infected insect vectors. Calves infected late in pregnancy may be born alive but unable to stand or are incoordinate and on necropsy show a disseminated encephalomyelitis. Those infected earlier are affected with arthrogryposis, and sometimes torticollis, kyphosis, and scoliosis with associated neurogenic muscle atrophy due to loss of spinal motor neurones. (These calves usually cause severe obstetric problems.) Those affected earlier still are usually born alive, walk poorly, and are dejected and blind. These calves have varying degrees of cavitation of cerebral hemispheres; usually extreme hydranencephaly is present. Some calves may be affected with both arthrogryposis and hydranencephaly. Cerebellar cavitation is occasionally seen.

In sheep and goats there may be similar lesions of hydranencephaly, arthrogryposis and spinal cord degeneration. In Australia, micrencephaly is the main lesion encountered.

Abortion with or without CNS developmental abnormalities is also a feature of this disease.

Horses have high prevalence rates of antibodies against Akabane virus but no congenital abnormality has so far been definitely associated with this virus.

Diagnosis: A presumptive diagnosis may be made on the gross CNS lesions, but the disease must be differentiated from other infective and genetic causes of CNS abnormalities. Confirmation of infection may be made by collecting serums from unsuckled affected offspring and their dams, and testing for serum-neutralizing antibodies against Akabane virus.

Transmission and Prophylaxis: The Akabane virus occurs commonly in certain insect species in several parts of the world. In these endemic areas herbivores are bitten and become infected at an early age and develop a solid immunity by the time of breeding. Thus congenital abnormalities are seldom seen in these areas. However, if for any reason, there is spread of the vector and the virus into new areas, then outbreaks of congenital infection may be expected. Similarly, pregnant ruminants from disease-free areas moved to virus-infected areas are at risk.

No vaccine is available and there is no treatment.

ACTINOBACILLOSIS

A disease similar to actinomycosis, but which most often affects soft tissues and lymph nodes. Bony structures may be affected as well. It occurs in cattle, swine, horses, sheep and chickens and rarely in man. Some confusion exists over the taxonomy of the causative agent(s), and several species have been suggested on host preference and biochemical characteristics—*Actinobacillus lignieresii* (cattle and sheep), *A. equuli* and *A. suis* (pigs and horses, especially young animals), *A. seminis* (rams—epididymitis) and *A. salpingitis* (chickens—salpingitis).

In **cattle**, actinobacillosis usually affects the tongue ("wooden tongue") and less frequently other tissue such as skeletal muscle and liver. Small abscesses with a diffuse, extensive connective tissue proliferation are a prominent feature. In **sheep**, actinobacillosis is a purulent disease of the skin, lymph nodes, lungs, and soft tissues of the head and neck. Epididymitis is common in rams. In **swine**, septicemia, suppurative joint lesions, endocarditis, osteomyelitis and pneumonia have all been recorded as have infections of the soft tissue of the head and mammary glands. Septicemia and crippling infections, especially of the joints, occur in **foals** (q.v., p. 455).

Pus from actinobacillosis lesions may contain granules or "rosettes," which are less than 1 mm in diameter, and are smaller than the "sulfur granules" of actinomycosis. Stained smears of the pus will reveal rather short gram-negative bacteria, in contrast to the gram-positive filaments which are demonstrable in actinomycosis.

Circumscribed lesions may be treated by complete excision. The response to iodides is usually dramatic (℞ 596, 601, 605). Systemic or local treatment with antibiotics, e.g. oxytetracycline (℞ 50), streptomycin (℞ 72) and erythromycin (℞ 39), are effective as well.

ACTINOMYCOSIS

A local or systemic chronic suppurative and granulomatous disease of a wide variety of domestic animals (rarely of wild animals). Causative agents include: *Actinomyces bovis; A. viscosus*, first isolated from gingival plaques of hamsters with periodontal disease, but now known to be an important pathogen of dogs and to a lesser extent pigs and goats; and *A. suis*. Where thorough biochemical and serological studies have been carried out, researchers have identified *A. bovis* only from bovine infections. Predominantly human types, such as *A. israelii*, are occasionally recovered from lesions in lower animals, e.g. mandrill, pig.

ACTINOMYCOSIS IN CATTLE

(Lumpy jaw)

Bovine actinomycosis is a chronic disease of the mandible, maxilla, or other bony tissues of the head; seldom does it involve soft tissue. Actinomycosis of the mandible and maxilla is characterized by swelling, abscessation, fistulous tracts, extensive fibrosis, osteitis and granuloma. The teeth loosen and eating is difficult; swelling of the nasal cavity may cause dyspnea and there is gradual emaciation. Incision of the lesion reveals coalescense of abscesses containing a viscid, mucoid, yellow pus and "sulfur granules" 2 to 5 mm in diameter. Fistulous tracts extend through the skin, discharge pus for a period, then indurate leaving indented fibrotic scars in the skin.

Diagnosis: A history of a slow-developing swelling on the maxilla or mandible with fluctuating abscesses or fistulous tracts suggests actinomycosis. For confirmation, pus should be collected in a tube and shaken with saline to dissolve mucus. The contents then are poured into a Petri dish, "sulfur granules" picked out, crushed on a glass slide and stained by Gram's method. Under the oil-immersion objective, *A. bovis* appears as gram-positive filaments, rods, cocci, branching or club-shaped forms. Finding these structures differentiates it from actinobacillosis (q.v., p. 441) and staphylococcosis, which also produce pus containing yellow granules. Further confirmation of the diagnosis can be obtained by bacteriologic and histologic laboratory techniques.

Treatment: Actinomycotic lesions always take a chronic course of many months' duration. Infection of the maxilla or mandible seldom can be arrested, except when diagnosed and vigorously treated at its onset. When the lesions are small and circumscribed, surgery is the treatment of choice. This is followed by packing the wound with gauze tampons soaked in streptomycin solution or tincture of iodine. If the lesion is not circumscribed or if abscessation is advanced, the fistulas and abscesses should be curetted and packed with tampons soaked in tincture of iodine.

Injection of streptomycin around actinomycotic lesions aids persistent cases. The dosage may be 5 gm daily for 3 days or 2 to 6 gm every other day for 5 treatments. Sulfanilamide, sulfapyridine and sulfathiazole have also been used successfully in cattle. One gram per 15 lb (1 gm/7 kg) of body wt daily for 4 to 5 days is recommended. Also, isoniazid (3 to 5 mg/lb [6.6 to 11 mg/kg]) of body wt, orally or IM, for 2 to 3 weeks has been used.

Once rarefying osteitis becomes extensive, treatment prolongs the life of the animal, but complete recovery should not be expected. X-ray therapy at the rate of 500 r every other day for 5 doses will temporarily reduce the size of the maxillary or mandibular lesions. However, irradiation does not destroy the infection and must be repeated.

ACTINOMYCOSIS IN OTHER SPECIES

Swine: *Actinomyces suis* (and *A. bovis?*) causes primary chronic granulomatous and suppurative mastitis in sows. Small abscesses in the udder contain cohesive, viscid, yellow pus surrounded by a wide zone of dense connective tissue. As in cattle, yellow mineralized granules are scattered throughout the pus. Some of the deep-seated abscesses rupture and discharge exudate through fistulas. Large, irregular, granulating skin ulcerations can be seen at the opening of the fistulas. Granulomatous nodules or abscesses also are seen under the skin of the abdomen. Occasionally, *A. suis* causes generalized infection with purulogranulomatous nodules throughout the lungs, spleen, kidneys and other viscera.

The prognosis is poor since one or more mammae are destroyed and the infection does not respond favorably to chemotherapy. It is often necessary to resort to surgical excision of the infected mammary gland to save the life of the sow and make her acceptable for slaughter.

Horses: An anaerobic *A. bovis*-like microbe, synergistic with *Brucella abortus* or *Br. suis*, is an apparent cause of fistulous withers or poll evil (q.v., p. 571). The anaerobe alone causes abscesses with fistulous tracts in the submaxillary, pharyngeal and cervical region. The lymph nodes of the region contain nodules, abscesses and discharging fistulas.

Dogs: *Actinomyces viscosus* causes a chronic granulomatous pleuritis. Frequently, subcut. lesions (abscesses, fistulous tracts) are present as well. The prognosis is poor since the infection usually is noticed too late.

NOCARDIOSIS

Nocardiosis of animals is a chronic infection resulting from soil-borne organisms of the genus *Nocardia*. Etiologic agents are *Nocardia asteroides*, *N. brasiliensis* and *N. caviae*. Cattle appear to be the most frequent animal host. Other animals affected include dogs, horses, cats, sheep, goats and poultry, as well as fish and a wide variety of wild and captive animals. The disease is characterized by generalized purulogranulomatous nodular lesions. Debate still surrounds the taxonomic position of "*N. farcinica*," isolates appearing to be a mixture of mycobacteria and true nocardia.

Clinical Findings: Cattle: Nocardial mastitis has been the predominant infection reported in cattle. Systemic illness—prolonged high temperature, anorexia, loss of condition, increased lacrimation and salivation—may or may not be evident. Affected mammary glands may become enlarged and firm. The whitish, viscid exudate, contains discrete blood clots and small (1 mm diameter) whitish clumps (microcolonies) of bacteria. Small draining sinuses are often formed, while in severe cases the gland may rupture. Metastasis to lungs and supramammary lymph nodes may occur. Bovine farcy, abortion, pulmonary and generalized infections have also been recorded.

Dogs: The signs include fever, soreness, lameness, dyspnea, empyema, enlarged abdomen, lymphadenitis, and fluctuating subcut. or salivary gland abscesses. Granulomatous swellings resembling actinomycotic lesions are seen, frequently on the extremities. Superficial abscesses rupture and discharge pus containing flakes of necrotic tissue. The lungs and bronchial lymph nodes nearly always contain suppurative and granulomatous lesions. Well defined microcolonies are seen in pleural exudates.

Diagnosis: Nocardiosis should be suspected in dogs with unexplained pulmonary disease, with subcut. and salivary gland nodules or abscesses. Chest radiographs have revealed diffuse, noncalcified, soft nodules in several lobes of the lungs.

For diagnostic purposes, pus, sputum, or a biopsy specimen from a lesion is collected, smears are prepared, dried, stained with Gram's stain and examined under oil immersion. The organisms appear as beaded, gram-positive, weakly or irregularly acid-fast, branching filaments 1 μ or less in diameter. *Nocardia* are easily cultured on plain Sabouraud's dextrose agar, which should be incubated at both 25 and 37°C.

Specific diagnosis of mastitis in cattle depends upon culture of clumps in the milk from the affected quarter. Complement-fixing antibodies and precipitins have been demonstrated in the sera of infected cattle. Cutaneous hypersensitivity reactions have proved of diagnostic value.

Prognosis and Treatment: Nocardiosis frequently terminates fatally despite vigorous chemotherapy. Nevertheless, the canine disease has been arrested by daily treatment with oxytetracycline (℞ 50, 56) for up to 3 weeks, with 1 to 2 gm of sulfadiazine (℞ 88) by mouth daily for 6 to 12 weeks and with novobiocin, 25 mg/lb (55 mg/kg) by mouth daily. Cutaneous or subcut. abscesses or nodules should be surgically excised, followed by local application of iodine.

Bovine mastitis caused by *Nocardia* has been successfully treated with udder infusion of 500 mg of novobiocin combined with 25 to 40 ml of 0.2% nitrofurazone, b.i.d. for 3 to 5 days.

SYSTEMIC FUNGUS INFECTIONS

The soil is thought to be the original source of the pathogenic fungi. Fungi exist as saprophytes on specialized substrates such as decaying keratinized animal tissue and dung. An important characteristic of pathogenic fungi is dimorphism—a transient morphologic adaptation to different environmental conditions. While a few mycoses are highly contagious and are passed from animal to animal without resort to a soil-inhabiting phase, most systemic mycoses are noncontagious, each animal becoming infected from the soil reservoir.

Some fungi (primarily pathogens) are able to establish infection in otherwise apparently normal hosts, while others, the so-called opportunists, require some form of host debilitation in order to establish infection. The widespread use of antibacterial agents, both therapeutically and prophylactically in foods, may predispose animals to infection by endogenous yeasts, while the stress of captivity, acidotic metabolic conditions and malnutrition seem important in establishing some opportunistic mycoses. Histoplasmosis, coccidioidomycoses and blastomycoses can be regarded as primary systemic mycoses, while examples of opportunistic systemic mycoses are the phycomycoses, aspergillosis, candidosis and cryptococcosis, although the latter is frequently recorded in seemingly uncompromised individuals. Lesions produced by systemic fungus infections are characterized by granulomatous or pyogranulomatous inflammation with necrosis, nodule formation and sometimes calcification. The close resemblance of mycotic lesions and those seen in tuberculosis, actinomycosis, actinobacillosis, and sometimes malignancies, require differentiation by identification of the causative agent.

A systemic fungal infection is diagnosed by one or more of the following methods: (1) direct microscopic observation of exudates or material from a lesion in 40% potassium hydroxide:Parker black Quink ink (2:1) solution; (2) isolation of the causal agent on antibiotic supplemented (chloramphenicol, 0.05 mg/ml; gentamicin, 0.1 mg/ml) brain-heart infusion, blood or Sabouraud's dextrose agar incubated at both 25 and 37°C; (3) demonstration of characteristic fungal elements using special stains and fluorescent antibody techniques or both on formalin fixed tissue sections; and (4) the demonstration of specific serum precipitins or agglutinins. Skin testing with specific antigens may be of use with some mycoses.

Recent major therapeutic advances are: the demonstration (in a limited range of human trials) that the broad-spectrum imidazole derivative, miconazole, may be effective in the treatment of many systemic mycoses; that oral 5-fluorocytosine may be of use in the treatment of systemic yeast infection, and that a combination of 5-fluorocytosine (flucytosine [68 mg/lb (150 mg/kg)] daily) orally and amphotericin B (20 mg daily) IV is a safe and efficacious alternative to other regimens for human cryptococcosis. The use of such therapy in animals would now seem warranted.

HISTOPLASMOSIS

A disease caused by *Histoplasma capsulatum* and characterized by coughing, dysentery, pulmonary nodules demonstrable by X-rays, emaciation, ulceration of mucous membranes and lymphadenopathy resembling tuberculosis or lymphoma. In the Central U.S.A., histoplasmosis is the most frequent systemic fungus disease encountered in dogs and man. Cats, cattle, horses, sheep, pigs and wild animals also become infected (most, if not all, subclinically), but histoplasmosis is not a serious problem in these species. *H. capsulatum* grows in soil. The disease is not contagious. Infection is acquired by inhalation of the fungus, or rarely by the oral route.

Clinical Findings: Dogs are presented with a chronic intractable cough or diarrhea or both. Enlarged bronchial lymph nodes and pulmonary nodules cause a deep, nonproductive cough. Ulceration of gastrointestinal mucosa is responsible for the diarrhea. Other signs include anorexia, irregular fever, emaciation, vomiting, dermatitis and enlarged visceral lymph nodes. Careful palpation through the abdominal wall frequently reveals enlarged mesenteric lymph nodes. Ulceration of the buccal mucosa and enlarged tonsils sometimes occur. Acute histoplasmosis is nearly always fatal after a course of 2 to 5 weeks. Eight percent of the affected animals slowly develop a cough or diarrhea of 3 months' to 2 years' duration and are classified as having chronic progressive histoplasmosis.

Diagnosis: Histoplasmosis should be suspected in dogs having a therapeutically unresponsive chronic cough or diarrhea. In such cases, the intradermal test should be performed using histoplasmin prepared specifically for dogs. A dose of 0.1 ml is injected intradermally at the lower edge of the flank skin fold. The presence of at least 5 mm of edema or induration at the test site when examined 48 hours later characterizes a positive reaction. Such a reaction indicates present or past infection with *H. capsulatum*. There is some cross-reaction with blastomycosis and coccidioidomycosis, which must be ruled out by signs, lesions or microscopic examination of exudate from a lesion. Rarely, in the terminal stages of acute disseminated histoplasmosis, the animal is anergic and therefore insensitive to histoplasmin.

Chest radiographs reveal enlarged bronchial lymph nodes and nodules in the lung. The pulmonary nodules vary from granulomatous foci, 2 to 5 mm in diameter, to miliary calcifications. Since tubercles in canine tuberculosis do not calcify, the observation of calcified pulmonary lesions on radiographs aids differential diagnosis. In addition, blastomycosis, nocardiosis and coccidioidomycosis must be considered.

Assistance in diagnosis is provided by serology. Five milliliters of clear serum is submitted to a qualified laboratory for complement fixation (CF), latex agglutination, immunodiffusion, and immunofluorescence (FA inhibition) tests. In combination, the last 2 tests can be helpful when sera are anticomplementary. Advantage should also be taken of the opportunity to prove diagnosis by culture, animal inoculation and histologic demonstration of the small organism (1 to 5 μ).

Prognosis and Treatment: Acute disseminated histoplasmosis usually is fatal; however, over half of the animals with the chronic condition will eventually recover with symptomatic therapy. Since *H. capsulatum* is disseminated through the sputum, feces, vomitus and urine, infected dogs should be handled carefully to avoid unnecessary contamination of the premises. Amphotericin B (℞ 364) may be useful but is toxic, and effectiveness depends on the dog's ability to tolerate the drug.

COCCIDIOIDOMYCOSIS

A highly infectious but noncontagious disease of man, cattle, sheep, dogs, wild rodents, cats, horses, pigs, buffaloes and several other mammals, characterized primarily by single or multiple pulmonary and thoracic lymph node granulomas and a tendency to disseminate to other tissues. *Coccidioides immitis*, the causal fungus, is present in the soil of the low-elevation deserts of the Southwestern U.S.A. and similar areas in Mexico, Central and South America. The infection is contracted by inhalation of airborne arthrospores. Few of the total number of animals exposed to spores ever show clinical signs. Of the domestic animals, cattle and dogs are the most important hosts.

Clinical Findings: The onset of coccidioidomycosis in dogs is insidious and the course variable, usually 2 to 5 months, with termination of progressive cases most frequently made at the wish of the owner. Although the dissemination rate in dogs is several times that for man, the majority of infections are subclinical with uneventful recovery. Coughing, dyspnea and other respiratory distress and fever are the most frequent signs. The cough is probably referable to the extensive swelling of bronchial or mediastinal lymph nodes and the granulomas or abscesses in the lungs. Variable appetite, weight loss, listlessness and diarrhea are commonly noted. Pleural, pericardial and peritoneal effusion, as well as cardiac insufficiency, icterus and uremia occur along with granulomas in the pleura, pericardium, heart, liver, spleen or kidney. Lameness and muscular atrophy follow invasion of bones and joints; fluctuating abscesses and ulcers indicate cutaneous dissemination; postural abnormalities or circling point to brain or meningeal infection, and glaucomatous swelling with corneal opacity to involvement of the eye.

Cattle infections are benign and asymptomatic; lesions are limited to lungs and thoracic lymph nodes, and carcass quality is not affected.

Diagnosis: Coccidioidomycosis should be suspected in all cases of intractable illness in animals that have lived in endemic areas. Pulmonary nodules, which rarely calcify, or enlarged lymph nodes may be noticed in chest radiographs of infected dogs. For CF, precipitin, or FA inhibition tests, 5 ml of clear serum, preserved by adding 1 part of 1:1,000 aqueous thimerosal to 9 parts of serum, should be submitted to a qualified laboratory. The coccidioidin sensitivity test will indicate the possibility of exposure. Strict intradermal injection of 0.1 ml of undiluted coccidioidin is made at the lower edge of the flank skin fold. A positive reaction is characterized by a focus of at least 5 mm of edema or induration at the test site 48 hours after injection. Occasionally, a severely infected dog will be anergic, giving negative serologic and coccidioidin tests. Coccidioidin-sensitive animals may cross-react to histoplasmin, but the reaction to the specific antigen is larger. In tissues or smears, the fungus occurs as round, nonbudding, thick-walled bodies, 20 to 200 μ in diameter, known as spherules. Demonstration of endosporulating spherules in exudate or sections of biopsy material is adequate confirmation. The fungus is easily cultured as a cottony white growth on Sabouraud's agar, but cultures are dangerously infective and should be handled only by persons acquainted with the necessary safeguards.

Treatment: Amphotericin B has been used in the dog (℞ 364). Treatment must be accompanied by monitoring the BUN level.

BLASTOMYCOSIS
(North American blastomycosis)

A chronic disease of dogs, horses, cats and man caused by *Blastomyces dermatitidis* and characterized by granulomas, abscesses and ulcers in the lungs, skin and other organs.

Clinical Findings: In dogs, the systemic type of disease is encountered more frequently than the cutaneous form. Depression, fever, anorexia and weight loss are followed by chronic nonproductive dry coughs. Numerous nodules and abscesses are distributed throughout all lobes of the lungs giving them a grayish-white and pink-mottled appearance. Focal or diffuse consolidation of entire lobes may occur. Central necrosis without calcification occurs in the granulomatous nodes. Extension of infection from the lungs results in enlargement and abscessation of the bronchial and mediastinal lymph nodes and pleuritis. Dissemination from the primary pulmonary site results in destructive lesions in bones, peripheral lymph nodes and meninges. Eye lesions, many of which progress to blindness, are evident in about 20% of diseased dogs. Less frequently, blastomycosis is manifested by solitary or multiple skin granulomas which eventually undergo central liquefaction, necrosis and ulceration.

Diagnosis: Blastomycosis should be suspected in dogs with nodules or abscesses in the skin, and respiratory distress. Chest radiographs reveal noncalcified nodules or consolidation of the lungs and enlarged bronchial and mediastinal lymph nodes. For confirmation of the diagnosis, a biopsy of skin nodules should be performed or pus aspirated from abscesses or sputum collected. *B. dermatitidis* appears microscopically as single or budding spherical cells 8 to 16 μ in diameter with a thick refractile wall. In coverglass preparations, the wall gives a "double contoured" appearance. For a complement fixation test, 5 ml of clear serum should be collected.

Prognosis and Treatment: Blastomycosis is usually fatal once infection is disseminated. Cutaneous lesions may persist for months. Surgical excision of cutaneous nodules is indicated since the infection responds poorly to drug therapy. Amphotericin B (℞ 364) is the treatment of choice for canine blastomycosis. Early diagnosis improves the chance of therapeutic success. Caution should be exercised in handling blastomycosis cases, even though contagion has not been established with certainty.

CRYPTOCOCCOSIS

A subacute or chronic disease of dogs, cats, cattle, horses, sheep and goats as well as numerous wild and captive animals and man; caused by the yeast *Cryptococcus neoformans* (*Filobasidiella neoformans, F. bacillispora*).

Clinical Findings: Dogs: Cryptococcosis in dogs usually involves the brain, meninges and paranasal sinuses, resulting in incoordination, circling, rotation of the head, changes in behavior, lameness, hyperesthesia and nasal discharge. Mucopurulent inflammation of the paranasal sinuses, ethmoturbinates and nasal cavity as well as small cystic centers in the brain and meninges are found at necropsy. Subcut. granulomas are seen around the ears, face and feet.

Cats: Cryptococcosis should be suspected in cats, particularly older cats, having chronic nasal and ocular discharge, blindness, incoordination, fever, cough and swelling in the nasal cavity and pharynx. *Cryptococcus* invades the nasal cavity and pharynx causing the formation of expanding masses resembling neoplasms. Posterior extension of the infection from the nasal cavity results in penetration of the cranial cavity and the optic nerves, leading to blindness. Some cats manifest only an intractable chronic respiratory infection; less commonly, the disease is limited to subcut. tumor-like masses. Eventually, most individuals develop signs referable to CNS involvement. Occasionally, cases of generalized infection occur in which the CNS is spared.

Although there is no evidence that this disease is contagious, contact with infected cats should be kept to a minimum.

Cattle: Decreased milk flow, anorexia, severe swelling and firmness of the udder and enlarged lymph nodes are the first signs of infection. After several weeks, the milk becomes viscid, gray-white and mucoid; sometimes the secretion consists of watery serum with flakes. Contaminated udder infusion equipment and drugs are a source of infection. The organism has been isolated from pigeon feces and soil, as well as from milk from apparently healthy cows. A high percentage of cows in a herd may be infected. Rarely, metastatic lesions appear in the lungs following accidental inoculation of the fungus into the udder via the teat canal. Prevention of this type of infection depends on the use of aseptic udder infusion technique and sterile infusion media.

Horses: Respiratory signs and nasal discharge result from nasal granulomas. Granulomatous foci and necrosis occur in the lungs or may be generalized in the viscera. (*See also* EPIZOOTIC LYMPHANGITIS, p. 453.)

Diagnosis: Cryptococcosis should be suspected in dogs or cats with unexplained respiratory and central nervous disease, and in cows with a viscid, gray, mucoid mammary secretion. An indirect FA technique and a tube-agglutination test both for *C. neoformans* antibodies, and a latex agglutination test for cryptococcal antigens have been developed. For maximal diagnostic coverage, all 3 serologic tests should be used concurrently. Exudative secretions, tissue from a lesion or spinal fluid in coverglass preparations should be examined microscopically. Other specimens can be mounted in undiluted Giemsa stain or India ink under a coverglass as an aid to demonstration of the mucoid capsule of the organism. *C. neoformans* in tissues appears as a round, single-budding, thick-walled, yeast-like organism 5 to 20 μ in diameter. The entire organism is surrounded by a refractile gelatinous capsule that stains red with the mucicarmine stain. Biopsy material may be examined histologically or cultured for confirmation of the diagnosis.

Prognosis and Treatment: Pulmonary, cerebral, meningeal, or paranasal cavity involvement is fatal. Amphotericin-B therapy has been evaluated favorably in human infections and in experimental animal cryptococcosis (*see also* p. 445). Its use in the spontaneous disease of animals is probably justified (℞ 364). Spontaneous recoveries occur in accidental cryptococcal bovine mastitis.

CANDIDOSIS

(Candidamycosis, Moniliasis, Candidiasis, "Thrush")

Candidosis is a general term covering diseases caused by mycelial yeasts of the genus *Candida*, especially by *Candida albicans*. Infections are usually restricted to the alimentary canal where the yeasts normally exist as harmless commensals. Dissemination to the skin, placenta, lungs, kidneys and heart may occur. *Candida* species have also been implicated in bovine mastitis. Among animals, candidosis of poultry and other birds is of particular importance (q.v., p. 1116), while infections of piglets and calves seem to be increasing. Other domestic animals found affected include horses, dogs and cats. Cases have also occurred in a variety of captive wild animals. Immature and debilitated animals are most susceptible. Infections are occasionally associated with antibiotic-supplemented diets or prolonged antibacterial therapy.

Lesions occur most frequently in the mouth and esophagus and consist of large single or small multiple, elevated plaques of soft, whitish yellow pseudomembranous exudate on the mucous membranes. When removed, they leave a hyperemic base which bleeds easily.

Since *C. albicans* or related yeasts may be present on mucous membranes as normal commensals or in other specimens as contaminants from the gastrointestinal tract, it is necessary to demonstrate the fungus in lesions associated with a host reaction. Appropriately stained histologic sections are therefore required. Microscopic examination of scrapings from mucosal or cutaneous lesions usually reveal both yeast cells (2 to 4 μ in diameter) and a tangled mass of hyphae. In such cases, the presence of hyphal filaments provides a tentative diagnosis of candidosis. Diagnostically useful immunodiffusion and indirect FA techniques have been developed for the detection of serum antibodies to *C. albicans*. Yeasts of the genus *Candida* grow readily on Sabouraud's dextrose agar.

A satisfactory treatment for avian candidosis (q.v., p. 1116) is not known. Mucosal or cutaneous lesions in other animals can be treated with oral (℞ 368) or topical (℞ 369) nystatin.

THE PHYCOMYCOSES

The phycomycoses are not a uniform group but have in common the presence of broad hyphae that have few septa.

Mucormycosis

An opportunistic fungal infection that usually occurs in the presence of lowered host resistance or in certain metabolic conditions, e.g. acidosis. Causal fungi belong to the genera *Absidia, Mucor, Rhizopus* and *Mortierella*. Infection follows ingestion, or occasionally inhalation of fungal elements from moldy feed. Animal hosts include the cow, pig, horse, mule, goat, sheep, dog and cat as well as many wild and captive animals and birds. The organs chiefly attacked are the gastric and intestinal mucosa and the lymph nodes of the alimentary canal. Dissemination to any organ of the body may occur. Clinical signs observed include diarrhea, convulsions, respiratory distress, abortion and failure to respond to antibiotic therapy.

Cultures may be misleading as the causal fungi are common saprophytes in animal environments, and the chief difficulty lies in deciding whether an isolate is of causal significance or simply a contaminant. Hyphal elements are often associated with blood vessels and may be missed unless the material is thoroughly examined. With histologic techniques the characteristic, coarse, branching, rarely septate hyphae and associated host response can be demonstrated.

Amphotericin B has been used with variable results in treating human mucormycosis.

Entomophthoramycosis

Primarily a disease of the subcut. tissues and nasal mucosa of otherwise healthy animals—horse, mule, man—by *Basidiobolus ranarum* and *Conidiobolus coronatus* (*Entomophthora coronata*). These fungi are ubiquitous and occur in decaying vegetation, soil, and with *Basidiobolus* species, the gastrointestinal tract of reptiles. *Basidobolus* has been found associated with skin lesions and probably gains access to the tissues following minor trauma and insect bites. The mode of infection of *C. coronatus* is probably by inhalation of spores, which then invade the nasal mucosa. Lesions are limited to nasal polyps and granulomas.

Specimens are collected by biopsy or after surgical removal of the lesions. Histologic techniques reveal the characteristic picture of a granuloma in which coarse, irregular, rarely septate hyphae surrounded by a collar of eosinophilic granular material, are readily visible. Nasal polyps in entomophthoramycosis must be distinguished from those of rhinosporidiosis (q.v., p. 454).

Surgical removal of lesions has been found satisfactory.

ASPERGILLOSIS

A primary respiratory and occasionally generalized infection caused by species of *Aspergillus*, especially *Aspergillus fumigatus*.

It is worldwide in distribution and has been recorded in almost all domestic animals and birds as well as many wild species. The disease is characterized by the formation of yellowish caseous nodules or plaques and has been known to affect almost every organ of the body. The most common forms of aspergillosis are respiratory infections in poultry (q.v., p. 1114) and abortion in cattle. Infection of the paranasal tissues of dogs and the equine guttural pouch are probably commoner forms of aspergillosis than the literature would suggest.

Present knowledge on mycotic abortion is limited to the fetus and membranes, for no signs have been noted in the dams prior to abortion. The cotyledons frequently retain much of their maternal caruncle portion, and are greatly thickened, especially at the margins. Central necrosis is also common. The maternal surface of the intercotyledonary areas of the chorion sometimes has a leather-like consistency with discrete-to-confluent thickenings. Skin lesions may be present on the fetus.

Diagnosis is by the demonstration (KOH, histologic) of characteristic regular, septate hyphae in lesions and by isolation of the etiologic *Aspergillus* on Sabouraud's dextrose agar. Diagnostically valuable immunodiffusion precipitin tests are available for respiratory infections in man. Similar tests should be applicable to animals. Aspergillosis in animals must be differentiated from tuberculosis and other granulomatous diseases. As the many causal fungi of mycotic abortion induce similar changes, abortion due to aspergilli should be distinguished by histologic and culture techniques from that caused by phycomycetes and *Candida*.

Amphotericin-B therapy has been evaluated favorably in human infections. Its use in the spontaneous disease of animals is probably justified.

MISCELLANEOUS MYCOTIC INFECTIONS

Epizootic Lymphangitis: A chronic, nodular and suppurative disease of the skin, superficial lymph vessels, lymph nodes and mucous membranes of horses in Europe, Africa and Asia. Infections have also occurred in the mule, donkey and Asian camel. The etiologic agent has been named *Histoplasma farciminosum* (*Cryptococcus farciminosus, Blastomyces farciminosis*) although there is yet no acceptable morphologic and serologic basis for including the organism in the genus *Histoplasma*. Efforts should be made to differentiate the disease from sporotrichosis, glanders, strangles and *Corynebacterium* infection.

Some animals with mild cases recover spontaneously in a month but in most the disease becomes extensive and incurable. Surgical excision of localized nodules or ulcers is the treatment of choice. Emphasis should be placed upon control by slaughter of infected animals, followed by disinfection of the stable and grooming equipment.

Sporotrichosis: A disease of horses, mules, dogs, cats, rats and man caused by *Sporothrix* (*Sporotrichum*) *schenckii* characterized by subcut. and lymphatic nodules which sooner or later ulcerate and discharge pus. Internal organs may be involved, especially in the dog.

Potassium iodide (℞ 601) should be given orally or sodium iodide (℞ 604) IV to the point of producing signs of iodism. The medication is continued for several weeks after apparent recovery to prevent recurrence. Tincture of iodine should be applied to the skin ulcers. If iodine therapy is instituted before dissemination of the infection, the prognosis is favorable.

Rhinosporidiosis: A chronic, nonfatal, granulomatous disease of cattle, horses, mules and man found in warmer countries, especially India. It is characterized by the production of lobulated, soft pink nasal polyps in animals although in man other sites may be infected as well. The etiologic agent, *Rhinosporidium seeberi*, has never been cultured. Rhinosporidiosis must be differentiated from entomophthoramycosis, aspergillosis and cryptococcosis of the nasal cavity; from "nasal granuloma" caused by *Helminthosporium* and from nasal schistosomiasis.

The standard treatment is surgical excision of the infected growths.

Geotrichosis: An opportunistic oral, intestinal, bronchial or pulmonary infection of dogs, man and birds in captivity, caused by *Geotrichum candidum*.

Phaeohyphomycosis: A rather controversial term used to cover all subcut. and systemic diseases in man and lower animals caused by hyphomycetous fungi that develop in the host's tissues in the form of dark-walled (dematiaceous), septate, mycelial elements. Encephalitis and death (up to 30% of a flock) in poultry has been attributed to the thermophilic, pigmented *Dactylaria gallopava*. Other animal examples of phaeohyphomycosis include cutaneous and disseminated infection in fish by a variety of dematiaceous fungi (*Exophiala salmonis*, *E. pisciphilus*, *Scolecobasidium humicola* and *S. tshawytschae*) and a similar range of diseases in captive frogs and toads; the etiologic fungi being *Phialophora* and *Cladosporium*-like species. No method of treatment has been postulated.

Hyphomycosis destruens, a disease of horses characterized by subcut. nodules and cutaneous ulcers, appears to result from infection of a *Pythium* sp. Although a phycomycosis, this disease is an example of oomycosis.

Oomycosis: Aquatic phycomycetes of the class Oomycetes are important and troublesome pathogens of fish, especially aquarium stock. *See* FISH DISEASES, p. 1247 *et seq*.

Eumycotic Mycetomas (Eumycetomas): A supposedly rare fungal disease of dogs, horses, cats and man that induces chronic inflammatory reactions and the development of granulomatous nodular masses on various parts of the body. Available culture findings indicate that only 3 fungi, *Curvularia geniculata, Petriellidium* (*Allescheria*) *boydii* (*Monosporium apiospermium*) and *Helminthosporium spiciferum*, are agents of eumycotic mycetomas in animals. Blackish, or in the case of *A. boydii*, whitish, granules are present in the lesions. Complete surgical excision is the only effective treatment.

INFECTIONS OF YOUNG ANIMALS

(Infective Arthritis, Navel ill, Omphalitis, Omphalophlebitis, Joint ill, Pyemic arthritis, Polyarthritis, Viscosum infection, Sleepy foal disease, Rhinopneumonitis infection)

(*See also* DIARRHEA OF NEWBORN ANIMALS, p. 172.)

These are infectious processes, arising prenatally or soon after birth, caused by a variety of microorganisms. The etiology, pathogenesis and manifestations vary with the species affected, the age when infection is contracted, the species of infecting organisms and the principal site of infection.

Etiology: Foals: Fatal and crippling infections of newborn foals may be caused by *Streptococcus zooepidemicus* (*pyogenes*), *Escherichia coli*, equine herpesvirus 1 (EHV-1, rhinopneumonitis virus), *Actinobacillus equuli* (*Shigella equirulis, Bacterium viscosum equi*), *Salmonella* spp., *Staphylococcus aureus* and *Klebsiella* spp., in approximately that order of incidence. Prenatal infections may be associated with metritis or placentitis. Entry of postnatal infection is by ingestion, inhalation or through the umbilicus. Hypogammaglobulinemia, as a result of deficiency in colostrum or failure of immunoglobulin absorption through the intestinal wall during the first 24 hours after birth, is a predisposing factor.

Calves: Birth-related diseases are less frequent than in foals. The organisms most often involved are *E. coli*, streptococci, corynebacteria, staphylococci, *Fusobacterium necrophorum* (*Sphaerophorus necrophorus*) and pasteurellae. Prenatal infections may occur in herds with a history of uterine infection, but most infections are postnatal, entering through the umbilicus or by ingestion. Prematurely born calves are more likely to be affected than calves carried to term. Incidence is highest in calves separated from their dams at birth and stabled in groups.

Pigs: Pathogenesis is similar to that in calves, with streptococci, staphylococci and diphtheroids being the organisms principally involved; "wolf tooth" wounds may serve as a portal of entry.

Lambs: Contamination of the umbilicus at birth, docking and castration wounds, and unsanitary lambing quarters are the important sources of infection. *Erysipelothrix rhusiopathiae* causes serious mortality, but other organisms cultured from the lesions such as *Fusobacterium necrophorum* (*Sphaerophorus necrophorus*), streptococci and staphylococci are not of great epidemiologic significance. *Corynebacterium pseudotuberculosis* may infect the navel with subsequent abscessation in the liver and other internal organs.

Clinical Findings: Foals: Signs observed depend on localization of infecting organisms. Lethargy, diminishing strength of the suck reflex and inability to get up and stand unaided or hold the suckling position are characteristic of all infections. Convulsions are associated with meningitis and encephalitis; lameness with arthritis and tenosynovitis; increased respiratory rate and colic with pleurisy, pneumonia, diarrhea and peritonitis. An *A. equuli* infection is characterized by extreme sleepiness, nephritis and uremia. EHV-1 infection presents similar clinical signs and must be suspected, even in foals delivered at full term, until a differential diagnosis has been established.

The course of the condition depends on the affected animal's age at onset and nonspecific factors collectively described as resistance. Death may occur within 12 hours or the course may be prolonged into weeks. Recovery depends on the site of infecting organisms and institution of, and response to, therapy.

Calves: The course is usually less acute than in foals with a greater tendency toward development of umbilical abscesses. Signs are those of a septic process, and joint involvement is less frequent than in other species. Umbilical hernias are an occasional complication.

Pigs: Neonatal infections may be manifest as acute septicemia, pneumonia, abscesses of internal organs, encephalitis, or arthritis. Signs are those common to generalized septic infection or pyemia accompanied by such specific localizations as abscessation of the navel, pyo-arthritis or encephalitis followed by retarded growth or stunting.

Lambs: Infection of the navel and castration or docking wounds, with accompanying pyo-arthritis and internal abscesses may reach epidemic proportions. The suppurative type usually appears during the first month. Morbidity is high. Lambs with suppurative infection develop acute lameness and one or more joints become distended with purulent fluid. Nonsuppurative types appear at 1 to 5 months and are accompanied by lameness and stiffness, usually involving all 4 legs, with chronic lameness and retarded development in as many as 20% of a flock. There is little enlargement of joints in the acute stage, but thickening of the capsule may occur in chronic cases.

Lesions: These are typical of septic processes in the umbilical area, joints, liver and other tissues, although lesions associated with

A. equuli are characterized by macroscopic or microscopic abscessation in adrenal and renal cortices. *E. coli* commonly causes pleurisy and peritonitis and the carcass will often have a characteristic odor. Streptococci or staphylococci cause macroscopic abscessation.

Diagnosis: Because of the variety of organisms affecting each species and the frequency of undifferentiated common signs, especially in the very young subject, it is difficult to make an etiologically accurate clinical diagnosis. Specific diagnosis usually must await cultural examination of an accessible abscess or following necropsy. Accordingly, it is desirable to select treatment to cover the infections occurring most frequently or causing the greatest loss. Often, this is dependent on local experience.

Prophylaxis: The prevention of infection depends largely on good management, particularly the provision of a sanitary environment for parturition and upon proper care of the navel immediately after birth. The umbilical cord should not be ligated. The stump may be treated with an antiseptic solution or powder. In foals the cord should be left to rupture naturally when the mare gets to her feet after delivery or by the foal struggling in an attempt to stand for the first time.

Tincture of iodine applied to the umbilical cord is indicated in all species. A small wide-mouth bottle half-filled with tincture of iodine is held against the navel, the newborn and the glass inverted as a unit, held for a moment and then righted. In the fly season, a desiccating healing powder, preferably one with fly-repellent properties, should also be applied. In screwworm areas, the navel of the newborn must be treated promptly with an ointment that kills the larvae and repels the flies. Generally the navel that is properly treated at birth requires little subsequent treatment. The administration of donor colostrum is recommended in cases where the mare leaks milk prior to foaling. If this is not available, an injection of dam's plasma (about 250 ml) may provide a measure of protection; cross-matching foal's cells against donor plasma should always be performed prior to transfusion but this precaution is unnecessary in calves.

Treatment: The treatment of advanced or chronic infections of the newborn is difficult and unrewarding; however, in the early acute stages, or prophylactically, antimicrobial drugs are effective.

In the newborn foal, prophylactic and therapeutic use of antimicrobial compounds should be directed principally at *E. coli* and *A. equuli,* then at *S. zooepidemicus.* Injectable penicillin-streptomycin mixtures (℞ 66) or neomycin (℞ 46) may be effective. The initial dose should contain a minimum of 1 gm of streptomycin and an additional 0.5 gm should be given at 3-hour intervals for at least 4 days; ampicillin (℞ 6) or cloxacillin (℞ 33) are useful in staphylococcal and streptococcal infections. Joint infection should be treated by the intra-articular and IM or IV routes. Umbilical abscesses should be drained and the sac flushed with tincture of iodine.

For prophylactic treatment, neomycin 0.5 gm b.i.d. for 3 days has proved effective. Broad-spectrum antibiotics (℞ 27, 50, 76) and amoxycillin or compounds such as trimethoprim and sulfadiazine may also be used either prophylactically or therapeutically. Salmonellosis, *E. coli* and *Klebsiella* spp. infections may be treated with chloramphenicol (℞ 16), or neomycin (℞ 46) which should be given both orally and parenterally, or nitrofurazone (℞ 122) orally, which should be supplemented by an antibiotic administered parenterally. Chemical cauterization of a patent urachus with silver nitrate sticks or 10% formalin in saline has assisted in stopping urine leakage.

Treatment of calves should follow the same general principles outlined for foals, but economics may dictate only a one-time treatment. Parenteral treatment with broad-spectrum antibiotics or sulfonamide mixture (e.g. ℞ 98) is preferred because of a less definite pattern in the incidence of infecting organisms. Surgical drainage and local treatment is especially important in calves. If a hernia is present care should be taken not to incise it. Because of the long hair surrounding the umbilical area and a heavy umbilical cord, the incidence of screwworm and other fly maggot infestation is greater and should be considered in local treatment of early infections.

Although individual professional attention to lambs and pigs often may not be economically feasible in some herds, great dependence must be put on sanitary management; treatment of the umbilical cord at birth is economically feasible and should be practiced. Injection of repository antibiotics may reduce the risk of immediate neonatal infection.

MAMMALIAN COCCIDIOSIS

Usually an acute infection caused by the invasion and destruction of the intestinal mucosa by *Eimeria* or *Isospora* spp., characterized by diarrhea, intestinal hemorrhage and emaciation. Coccidiosis is a serious disease in cattle, sheep, goats and also in rabbits, in which the liver as well as the intestine may be affected (q.v., p. 1183). It is less often diagnosed but may also result in clinical illness in swine, dogs, cats, and horses. Under modern husbandry conditions (off-floor housing) it is rarely a problem in mink. Intestinal infections also occur in most wild animals but little is known of the etiology.

Etiology: Infection of the host usually results from ingestion of infective oocysts. Oocysts enter the environment when they are discharged in the feces of an infected host. At this time they are unsporulated and therefore not infective. Under favorable conditions of moisture and temperature, oocysts sporulate and become infective; sporulation requires several days to a week or more. Sporulation consists of development of the amorphous protoplasm into small bodies called sporozoites, which lie within secondary cysts or sporocysts within the oocyst. In the genus *Eimeria*, the sporulated oocyst has 4 sporocysts each containing 2 sporozoites, while in some other coccidial genera there are 2 sporocysts each containing 4 sporozoites.

When the sporulated oocyst is ingested by a susceptible animal, the sporozoites escape from the oocyst, invade the intestinal mucosa or epithelial cells in other locations and develop intracellularly into multinucleate schizonts. Each nucleus develops into an infective body called a merozoite; merozoites enter new cells and repeat the process. After a variable number of asexual generations, merozoites may develop into either microgametocytes or macrogametes; each of the former give rise to many microgametes, which fertilize the macrogametes. A resistant wall is formed around the zygotes, which are then called oocysts; these are discharged in the unsporulated state in the feces of infected hosts.

Clinical coccidiosis caused by *Eimeria* or *Isospora* species is more likely to occur under conditions of poor sanitation and overcrowding, or after the stresses of weaning, shipping, sudden changes of feed or severe weather. Coccidiosis predominantly affects young animals, but may occur in older animals that have had little previous exposure to coccidia.

In recent years new knowledge about coccidia has clarified much of the mystery associated with *Toxoplasma*, *Sarcocystis*, *Hammondia* and *Besnoitia*. Each of these genera was originally identified by an encysted asexual stage in the intermediate host but are now known to be coccidians that usually require 2 host species for completion of the life cycle. Eimerian and isosporan species require only one host in which to complete both asexual and sexual cycles.

Pathogenicity: Of the numerous species of *Eimeria* or *Isospora* that may infect a particular host, not all species are pathogenic. Of those species known to be pathogenic, strains often exist that vary in pathogenicity. Concurrent infections with 2 or more species, some of which may not normally be considered pathogenic, also influence the clinical picture. Within a particular species, some stages may be more or less pathogenic than others.

The asexual or the sexual stages of the various species destroy the intestinal epithelium, and frequently the underlying connective tissue of the mucosa. This is usually accompanied by hemorrhage into the lumen of the intestine, catarrhal inflammation and diarrhea. Signs may include discharge of blood or tissue or both, tenesmus and dehydration. Serum protein and electrolyte levels may be appreciably altered but hemoglobin or packed cell volume changes are seen only in severely affected animals.

Besnoitia besnoiti is pathogenic to cattle. In Africa, Israel, Russia and elsewhere *B. besnoiti* is known to cause pyrexia, photophobia, anasarca, diarrhea and swelling of lymph nodes (acute stage). During the chronic stage it is associated with wrinkling of the skin (seborrheic stage), and the hair may fall out. Severe infections cause death. *See* BESNOITIOSIS, p. 464. The pathogenicity of *Hammondia* species is undetermined.

Ingestion of large numbers of oocysts or sporocysts of either *Sarcocystis cruzi* or *S. ovicanis* by cattle or sheep, respectively cause abortions, anemia, fever, loss of appetite and weight, weakness and death. (*See* SARCOCYSTOSIS, p. 465.)

Immunity and Carrier Infection: Most animals acquire *Eimeria* or *Isospora* infections of varying degree while young. Older animals may have sporadic inapparent infections but are usually resistant to clinical disease. Such clinically healthy, mature animals, however, may be sources of infection to young susceptible animals.

Diagnosis: Clinical coccidiosis caused by eimerian species usually is diagnosed by finding appreciable numbers of oocysts of pathogenic species in the feces of the host. Usually, diarrhea precedes the heavy output of oocysts by a day or 2 and may continue after the oocyst discharge has returned to low levels, hence it is not always possible to confirm the clinical diagnosis by finding oocysts in the feces. The numbers of oocysts present in feces are influenced by the number of infective oocysts ingested, stage of the infection, age and condition of the animal, consistency of the fecal sample, and method of examination. Therefore, the results of fecal examinations must be related to clinical signs and ingestinal lesions (macroscopic and microscopic).

A tentative diagnosis of *Toxoplasma, Sarcocystis, Hammondia* or *Besnoitia* in the definitive host is made by examining the fecal material from canids or felids. Differentiation of *Toxoplasma, Hammondia,* and *Besnoitia* must involve subinoculation of mice, rats, or other susceptible hosts and serologic testing. The asexual (cyst) stages of these genera are found in various tissues of the intermediate hosts.

Prophylaxis of clinical coccidiosis is based on controlling the intake of sporulated oocysts or sporocysts by young animals so that the infections become established in immunizing proportions without causing clinical signs of the disease. Good feeding practices, good management and attention to the principles of animal sanitation accomplish this purpose. Young, susceptible animals should be provided with quarters that are clean and dry, and feeding and watering devices should be kept clean and protected from fecal contamination.

Stresses associated with shipping and sudden changes in feed should be minimized; prophylactic treatment as described below may be advisable under conditions conducive to outbreaks of coccidiosis.

Decoquinate (℞ 341) is effective in calves. Continuous low level feeding of sulfaguanidine (℞ 95) or ionophorous antibiotics (℞ 674, 350) during the first month of feedlot confinement has been reported to have prophylactic value in lambs. Amprolium in feed or water (℞ 340) is effective in calves; both amprolium and ionophorous antibiotics have been reported to be effective in lambs and kids.

Treatment: Clinical infections are self-limiting and subside spontaneously within a week or so if continuous reinfection does not occur. Prompt medication may slow or inhibit development of stages resulting from reinfection and thus may result in shortening the course of infection, reducing the discharge of oocysts, alleviating hemorrhage and diarrhea, and lessening the likelihood of secondary infections and mortality. Enteric sulfonamides, such as sulfaguanidine (℞ 94) or the readily absorbed sulfonamides, such as sulfamerazine (℞ 96) or sulfamethazine (℞ 102), may be used. Sulfaquinoxaline (℞ 109) has been reported to give excellent clinical results in beef and dairy calves, sheep, dogs and cats. The soluble sulfonamides may be given orally or parenterally and are thus more effective than enteric sulfonamides. In outbreaks in feedlots or on lush pastures, consideration should be given to prophylactic treatment of healthy exposed animals as a safeguard against additional morbidity.

Amprolium is effective against outbreaks in calves (℞ 340) and has been reported to be effective against experimental and field outbreaks in sheep and goats. Synthetic or natural vitamin K preparations may be used to increase coagulability of the blood in individual animals with severe hemorrhage (℞ 570, 574). If transfusions are given, provision should be made to counteract the anticoagulant added to transfused blood.

Sick animals should be treated individually whenever possible to guarantee therapeutic levels of the drug. Symptomatic treatment for diarrhea may be helpful. Sick and convalescent animals should be provided with clean dry bedding, good shelter, fresh water and appetizing food. It is critical to prevent dehydration.

COCCIDIOSIS OF CATTLE

Eimeria zuernii and *E. bovis* are the species most often associated with clinical cases; *E. ellipsoidalis* and *E. auburnensis* may be mildly or moderately pathogenic. Coccidiosis is commonly a disease of young cattle from 1 or 2 months to 1 year of age. The disease usually is sporadic during the wet seasons of the year, but may occur at any time in severe epidemics in animals confined to feedlots. Particularly severe losses have been reported in feedlot cattle during extremely cold weather.

The pathogenic coccidia of cattle may cause damage to the mucosa of the lower small intestine, cecum and colon. The first-generation schizonts of *E. bovis* appear as white macroscopic bodies in the mucosa of the villi of the small intestine. The incubation period for bovine coccidiosis caused by *E. zuernii*, *E. bovis* or *E. auburnensis* is 15 to 20 days; for *E. ellipsoidalis* it is 8 to 13 days. In light infections the most characteristic sign is watery feces, but little or no blood is apparent, and the animal shows only slight indisposition lasting a few days. Severely affected animals may develop a diarrhea consisting of thin bloody fluid or thin feces containing streaks or clots of blood, shreds of epithelium and mucus. The diarrhea may continue for 3 to 4 days to a week or more; the animal loses its appetite, becomes depressed and dehydrated, loses weight, and the hindquarters and tail become soiled with fecal discharges. Tenesmus is common. Death may occur during the acute period, or later from secondary complications, such as pneumonia. If the animal survives the most severe period, it may recover but may have significant weight loss which is not quickly regained.

Diagnosis, Prophylaxis, Treatment: *See* pp. 460 to 461.

COCCIDIOSIS OF SHEEP AND GOATS

Clinical coccidiosis of sheep and goats is usually caused by *Eimeria ahsata* or *E. ninakohlyakimovae* or both; *E. crandallis*, *E. faurei*, *E. arloingi* and *E. parva* may be mildly or moderately pathogenic. The most serious outbreaks are seen in lambs in feedlots, usually within 2 to 4 weeks after confinement. In farm flocks, coccidiosis is most likely to occur in lambs 1 to 3 months old. Coccidiosis is a sporadic problem of farm-raised goats.

The localization of infection is predominantly the middle and distal thirds of the small intestine, and the large intestine. Small whitish or yellowish white circular lesions are sometimes visible in the mucous membrane, representing groups of developing oocysts of *E. arloingi*. Macroscopic schizonts, similar to those of *E. bovis* in cattle, are just barely visible to the unaided eye in the mucosa of sheep or goats infected with *E. arloingi*, *E. parva* or *E. ninakohlyakimovae*. Lambs with mild coccidial infections show only slight indisposition and inappetence and a transient diarrhea with soiling of the hindquarters. Severe coccidiosis is characterized by copious diarrhea with straining and discharge of dark, liquid, bloody feces, loss of weight and appetite, and dull appearance. Mortality may be 10% or more in severe outbreaks, with pneumonia and other complications developing frequently. The course for animals that recover is from a few to 10 days, following which there is an extended return to normal weight and condition. Schizonts and merozoites of an unknown species of *Eimeria* occur in the mucosa of the abomasum in sheep and goats. The schizonts attain a macroscopic size and are visible as white bodies known as globidia; the effect of these on the host is unknown.

Diagnosis, Prophylaxis, Treatment: *See* pp. 460 to 462.

COCCIDIOSIS OF SWINE

Coccidiosis is less important in pigs than in cattle and sheep. *Eimeria debliecki, E. scabra, E. spinosa* and *Isospora suis* may be pathogenic under certain circumstances. Inflammation may occur in the small or the large intestine. The incubation period is usually 6 to 10 days. Usually, bloody diarrhea is not associated with coccidiosis in swine. Insufficient experimental infections with single species have been induced to enable valid conclusions as to the effects of these on pigs of various ages. Improper sanitation and crowding increase the likelihood that coccidiosis will occur.

Clinical signs are diarrhea, loss of weight, inappetence and general unthriftiness. The disease usually affects pigs 1 to 3 months old, and unless microscopic diagnosis of coccidiosis is made, the signs are likely to be attributed to ascariasis or other factors. The course usually is 7 to 10 days, with many pigs remaining unthrifty.

Diagnosis, Prophylaxis, Treatment: *See* pp. 460 to 462.

COCCIDIOSIS OF DOGS AND CATS

Much knowledge of coccidia in dogs and cats has accrued within the last few years. No *Eimeria* spp. are known to occur in canids or felids. Two species of *Isospora* (*I. felis, I. rivolta*), one species of *Toxoplasma* (*T. gondii*), one species of *Hammondia* (*H. hammondi*), 2 species of *Besnoitia* (*B. besnoiti* and *B. wallacei*) and 4 named species of *Sarcocystis* (*S. hirsuta, S. tenella, S. porcifelis, S. muris*) occur in the intestines (sexual stage) of felids. Four species of *Isospora* (*I. canis, I. ohioensis, I. heydorni, I. burrowsi*), and 6 named species of *Sarcocystis* (*S. cruzi, S. ovicanis, S. miescheriana, S. bertrami, S. hemionilatrantis, S. fayeri*) occur in canids. *Isospora bigemina* (large strain) is now placed with the *Sarcocystis*. The small strain of *I. bigemina* is probably identical to *I. heydorni* and to *H. heydorni*). It is important when possible to differentiate the species because of the etiological implications. Sporocysts of *Sarcocystis* spp. may be infective for herbivores whereas *Isospora* spp. are not. The oocysts of *Besnoitia, Hammondia, Isospora* and *Toxoplasma* are shed unsporulated and generally have a prominent wall. *Sarcocystis* species are shed as fully sporulated oocysts or sporocysts; the oocyst wall is thin and frequently ruptures during passage in fecal material, releasing free sporocysts in the feces.

Isospora canis and *I. ohioensis* are usually nonpathogenic or only moderately pathogenic. However under certain field conditions, severe "coccidial" outbreaks may occur in young puppies. Similarly, *I. felis* may result in illness in kittens. A definite diagnosis can be made with fresh feces for only some of the species. The oocysts of *T. gondii*, *H. hammondi* and *B. wallacei*, for example, are indistinguishable morphologically. The course may vary from a few days to 10 days, but seldom is fatal, unless complicated.

Diagnosis, Prophylaxis, Treatment: *See* pp. 460 to 462. The results of treatment with the usual therapeutic agents are highly variable but sulfamethazine (℞ 102) seems to give consistently favorable results. In the cat, sulfamonomethoxine at 50 to 200 mg/kg body wt, given orally daily for 7 days is said to be a useful prophylactic. In the dog, amprolium, given orally at 300 to 400 mg/kg of body wt daily for 5 days, or spiramycin by the same route at 50 to 100 mg/kg for 6 days, are reportedly effective.

BESNOITIOSIS

A protozoan disease of the skin, subcutis, blood vessels, mucous membranes and other tissues, caused by various *Besnoitia* spp.

Etiology: The causal agent of the cutaneous disease in cattle is *Besnoitia besnoiti* and that of horses and burros *B. bennetti*. *B. jellisoni* and *B. wallacei* have been described from rodents, *B. tarandi* from reindeer, *B. darlingi* from lizards, opossums and snakes and *B. sauriana* from lizards. Viscerotropic strains of *B. besnoiti* have been isolated from African antelope and an unidentified *Besnoitia* sp. has been found in goats. These *Toxoplasma*-like organisms multiply in endothelial, histocytic and other cells, producing characteristic thick-walled cysts filled with bradyzoites.

Transmission: Cyclic transmission with enteric sexual stages in a definitive host, the cat, has been confirmed for *B. besnoiti*, *B. wallacei* and *B. darlingi*. Biting flies may transmit *B. besnoiti* mechanically from chronically infected cattle, and some *Besnoitia* spp. can be transmitted artificially to suitable hosts by inoculation of tissues containing cysts.

Clinical Findings: In cattle the disease commences with fever followed by anasarca. Inappetence, photophobia, rhinitis, swollen lymph glands and signs of orchitis are also seen. Anasarca gives way to sclerodermatitis. The skin becomes hard, thick and wrinkled, and develops cracks allowing secondary bacterial infection and myiasis to develop; movement is painful. There is loss of hair and epidermis causing varying degrees of alopecia. Severely affected animals become very emaciated. Cysts appear in the scleral conjunctiva and nasal mucosa.

Although the mortality is low, convalescence is slow in severe cases. Permanent sterility often occurs in severely affected bulls. Infected cattle often show no clinical signs other than a few cysts in the scleral conjunctiva. Affected animals remain life-long carriers.

In horses, signs are similar to those of cattle.

Prophylaxis and Treatment: In some countries cattle are immunized with a live, tissue-culture-adapted vaccine. Affected animals should be isolated and symptomatic treatment applied.

SARCOCYSTOSIS
(Sarcosporidiosis)

A disease caused by invasion of the endothelium and muscles by the protozoan *Sarcocystis*. As the name implies, *Sarcocystis* form cysts in the muscles of the intermediate host—man, horses, cattle, sheep, swine, birds, rodents, and reptiles—which vary in size from a few micrometers to several centimeters depending upon the host and species.

Etiology: *Sarcocystis* spp. develop in 2-host cycles consisting of an intermediate host (prey) and the final host (predator). Prey-predator life cycles have been demonstrated for cattle-dog (*S. cruzi*), cattle-cat (*S. bovifelis*), sheep-dog (*S. ovicanis*), sheep-cat (*S. tenella*), swine-man (*S. suihominis*), swine-cat (*S. porcifelis*), cattle-man (*S. hominis*) and others. After ingesting musculature containing *Sarcocystis* cysts, the final hosts shed infective sporocysts in their feces. Following ingestion of sporocytes by a suitable intermediate host, sporozoites are liberated and they initiate development of schizonts in vascular endothelia. Merozoites are liberated from the mature schizonts and produce a second generation of endothelial schizont. Merozoites from this second generation subsequently invade the muscle fibers and mature into the typical sarcocysts. Cysts of some species grow so large that they are easily visible with the unaided eye. The presence of such cysts may result in condemnation of the carcass during meat inspection. Other species remain microscopic even though tremendous numbers of cysts may be present in the muscles.

Pathogenicity: Until recently, *Sarcocystis* were considered of doubtful pathogenicity but after artificial infection with *S. cruzi* sporocysts from canine feces, acute disease occurred in calves and abortions, still-births and deaths were produced in pregnant cows.

Similar findings have been made for S. *ovicanis* in lambs and ewes. The clinical signs were similar to those reported from natural outbreaks of sarcocystosis in cattle in Canada, New York and Oregon. Humans may also serve as intermediate hosts and suffer myositis and vasculitis. Humans have also become ill following ingestion of sarcocysts of S. *suihominis* in uncooked pork; clinical signs of nausea, abdominal pain and diarrhea lasted up to 48 hours. They recurred 14 to 18 days later during sporocyst shedding.

Clinical Findings: In most animals, the disease is not evident and the parasite is discovered only at slaughter. In cattle severely affected by S. *cruzi*, the signs include fever, anorexia, cachexia, decreased milk yield, diarrhea, mild spasms, anemia, hyperexcitability, weakness, prostration, and death. Cows in the last trimester of pregnancy may abort. At necropsy, hemorrhages are observed in sheep infected with S. *ovicanis*.

Diagnosis: A presumptive diagnosis of acute sarcocystosis based on clinical findings can be confirmed microscopically by the detection of schizonts in the endothelial cells of the small vessels in the glomerulus of the kidney and in the lung or other soft tissues, but this stage is short-lived and easily missed. In cases of longer duration, young immature cysts were found in striated muscles and nerves. An indirect hemagglutination test revealed circulating antibodies to *Sarcocystis* antigen in very high titers. Antibodies to *Toxoplasma gondii* did not react.

Control: The main factor in the spread of sarcocystosis is the shedding of sporocysts in the feces of carnivores. Because most adult cattle, sheep and swine are infected, dogs and other carnivores should not be allowed to eat dead animals. Supplies of grain and feed should be kept covered; dogs and cats should not be allowed in buildings used to store feed or house animals. Feeding amprolium (100 mg/kg of body wt daily for 30 days) prophylactically has been reported to reduce the damage in cattle inoculated with S. *cruzi*. Vaccines are not available.

TOXOPLASMOSIS

A protozoan infection caused by *Toxoplasma gondii* affecting most species of warm blooded animals including birds and man in most parts of the world.

Etiology: *Toxoplasma gondii* is now considered to be a coccidium which completes its entire life cycle only in the small intestinal epithelium of members of the cat family; asexual and sexual stages develop endogenously and oocysts are shed in the feces. Three forms or stages of *T. gondii* may infect most other vertebrates without completion of the life cycle.

The trophozoite or tachyzoite: This is the actively proliferating form seen in acute disseminated infections and may be present in blood, excretions and secretions and in a wide range of tissues. It is crescent shaped, 4 to 8 μ by 2 to 4 μ and stains well with Giemsa. It survives in the environment or in dead animal tissues for only a few hours.

The cystozoite or bradyzoite: This is the resting form of *Toxoplasma* and is present in both congenital and acquired, chronic or asymptomatic infections. It is found in cysts mainly in brain, skeletal and cardiac musculature. Individual cysts vary in size from 50 to 150 μ in diameter and may have an argyrophilic and Schiff-positive cyst wall. Each cyst encloses many hundreds of closely packed zoites. This form can survive in tissues for several days after death but is readily destroyed by normal cooking and by freezing.

The oocyst: This form is passed in the feces of susceptible cats following ingestion of any of the 3 infective forms (tachyzoites, bradyzoites, oocysts). Following a meal containing *Toxoplasma* cysts, oocysts (10 by 12 μ) appear in the feces after 4 to 5 days and continue to be excreted, often in enormous numbers for 10 to 20 days. These oocysts sporulate in 2 to 4 days and are then infective for a wide range of intermediate hosts. Oocysts are very resistant and may survive for several months under favorable conditions. They are destroyed by dry heat at 70°C, boiling water, strong iodine and strong ammonia solutions.

Clinical Findings: Most infection by *Toxoplasma* is latent or asymptomatic. High prevalence rates of antibodies are seen in sheep and pigs with decreasing rates in dogs and cats and low rates in cattle and horses.

Clinical infection is relatively uncommon in most species, but sporadic cases and occasional endemics are seen particularly in young and stressed animals, and outbreaks of congenital infection have been reported. Generally the clinical infection runs a similar course in most species. In the young the infection is usually acute and generalized, whereas in adults it is often associated with chronic CNS involvement alone. In young animals, particularly puppies, kittens and piglets, signs include fever, anorexia, cough, dyspnea, diarrhea, jaundice and CNS signs. Lesions include pneumonitis, lymphadenitis, hepatitis, myocarditis and encephalomyelitis.

Congenital toxoplasmosis is an important cause of abortions and stillbirths particularly in sheep and sometimes in pigs. In sheep the lesions in the fetal cotyledon consist of multiple white foci of necrosis up to 2 mm in diameter. In the fetus there are extensive areas of leukoencephalomalacia, glial nodules some of which may show central necrosis.

Diagnosis: Demonstration of the characteristic pathology and the presence of *Toxoplasma*-like organisms in tissue sections should be supported by isolation of the organism and serologic testing. Isolation consists of IP injection of suspect material into mice free of natural *Toxoplasma* infection. Some strains of *Toxoplasma* are lethal to mice in 5 to 12 days and Giemsa-stained smears of peritoneal exudate will show many intracellular and free forms of *Toxoplasma* trophozoites. Other strains of *Toxoplasma* are not lethal to mice but will produce a chronic infection with tissue cysts. Mice can be bled after 4 to 6 weeks and their sera examined for *Toxoplasma* antibodies. Also wet squash preparations of brain can be made and examined for *Toxoplasma* cysts.

Several reliable serologic tests are available for the detection of *Toxoplasma* antibodies. *Hammondia* antibody from intermediate hosts reacts with *Toxoplasma* antigen and must be ruled out in serologic tests. The Sabin-Feldman dye test was the first one developed and this may be used in conjunction with the complement fixation test for the diagnosis of recent exposure. The indirect fluorescent antibody and the indirect hemagglutination tests give comparable results to the dye test.

Some of the reported cases of toxoplasmosis diagnosed strictly histologically in all probability are due to other protozoan parasites, e.g. the schizont stage of *Sarcocystis*.

Treatment: For animals other than man, treatment is seldom warranted. Sulfadiazine (73 mg/kg body wt) has been found to act synergistically with pyrimethamine (0.44 mg/kg) in the treatment of acute severe toxoplasmosis in laboratory animals and man. Since these drugs seem to affect only the free organisms it is important that treatment be instituted as early as possible. This therapy may produce a reversible toxic depression of the bone marrow, which may be prevented by B-vitamins and folinic acid.

Transmission and Prophylaxis: A previously unexposed pregnant animal may develop a parasitemia with spread of the infection to the uterine contents; a latent or overt congenital infection may result. In several species of laboratory rodents asymptomatic congenital infection has been transmitted vertically for several generations.

Most *Toxoplasma* infection is probably acquired after birth. In carnivores infection follows ingestion of fresh, infected (and uncooked) meat or carcasses from a wide range of intermediate hosts. In herbivores it is thought that most of the infection occurs from the ingestion of food contaminated by *Toxoplasma* oocysts derived from cat feces. In man infection seems to result both from ingestion of undercooked meat and from accidental ingestion of oocysts.

In any animal species, latent toxoplasmosis may be stimulated to cause an overt generalized infection. This is seen in association with intercurrent infections, e.g. viruses, protozoans, neoplastic diseases, environmental stresses and immunosuppression.

At any one time about 1% of all cats will be shedding *Toxoplasma* oocysts in their feces. Re-shedding of oocysts infrequently follows reinfection by *Toxoplasma* cysts, but may recur if the cats become infected with *Isospora felis*.

The finding of little or no correlation between the prevalence of *Toxoplasma* antibodies in man and contact with pet cats suggests only slight hazard. To minimize oocyst transmission from cats, they should not be fed raw meat nor permitted to kill birds or rodents; litter should be disposed of daily (before sporulation occurs), preferably, by incineration. Pregnant women should avoid contact with cats and their litter. Laboratory personnel working with cats or examining cat feces for worm eggs or *Toxoplasma* oocysts are at particular risk. They should avoid contamination of laboratory benches and instruments and should wear gloves and protective clothing.

A vaccine is not yet available.

FELINE CYTAUXZOONOSIS

An acute, uniformly fatal, protozoan disease of domestic cats, sporadic in heavily wooded areas of Southern U.S.A.

Etiology and Transmission: The clinical and histopathologic features resemble those produced by *Cytauxzoon* spp. in several species of African ungulates. The feline parasite apparently is a new species with an obscure life cycle ending in host cats. Ixodid ticks are suspected as vectors. In stained blood smears erythrocytic forms are round to oval bodies 1 to 2 μ in diameter with a dark red to purple nucleus and pale blue cytoplasm. Numerous merozoites appear within schizonts measuring up to 75 μ in the cytoplasm of reticuloendothelial cells lining the vascular channels in most organs.

Clinical Findings: Anorexia and depression are followed after 3 to 4 days by pyrexia, 104°F (40°C) or higher, and rapidly developing anemia, dehydration and icterus. Body temperature falls to subnormal, dyspnea develops and death follows in the ensuing 3 or 4 days

Lesions: Gross necropsy findings include generalized pallor and icterus, marked enlargement of the spleen and lymph nodes, congestion of mesenteric veins and petechial hemorrhages on the lungs, lymph nodes, epicardium and urinary bladder. Histologically, schizonts appear within reticuloendothelial cells that occlude major venous channels of lung, lymph node and spleen.

Diagnosis: The typical clinical picture in an endemic area is presumptive. Demonstration of erythrocytic parasites in stained blood smears is diagnostic. *Cytauxzoon* spp. must be differentiated from the smaller, denser, more homogenous *Hemobartonella felis*.

Treatment and Control: Irreversible vascular hemodynamic changes and concomitant hemolytic anemia usually are fatal. No chemotherapeutic agent is specific and palliative or supportive treatments only prolong the course. Until the parasite reservoir and mechanism of transmission are clearly identified, general prevention of exposure to ticks or other potential vectors may aid in control.

SULFONAMIDE AND TRIMETHOPRIM THERAPY

Caution: *In all drug therapy it is important to adhere to local laws and regulations governing the use of such products.*

Pharmacology: Mechanism of action: Sulfonamides inhibit bacterial growth by acting as competitive antagonists of PABA, which is essential for the synthesis of folic acid in susceptible bacteria. This action prevents the organism from growing and reproducing and enables the host's defenses to overcome the infection. Sulfonamides are ineffective against organisms that can utilize preformed folic acid.

Spectrum of activity: Sulfonamides as a group possess a rather wide antibacterial spectrum. Susceptible organisms include streptococci, staphylococci, *Pasteurella, Bacillus anthracis, Escherichia coli, Vibrio, Shigella, Haemophilus, Proteus, Actinomyces, Chlamydia,* coccidia and a number of less important infectious agents. Since the spectra of the individual drugs of this group are alike, if an organism exhibits resistance to one sulfonamide, it is likely that it will be resistant to other members of the group.

Absorption: Certain sulfonamides are relatively well absorbed from the gastrointestinal tract, while others are poorly or slowly absorbed. The sulfonamides that are well absorbed include sulfanilamide, sulfathiazole, sulfadiazine, sulfamerazine, sulfamethazine, sulfapyridine, sulfaquinoxaline, sulfacetamide, sulfisoxazole and sulfabromomethazine. The rate of absorption of these compounds varies among different species, but drug levels sufficiently great to treat systemic infections may be obtained in large and small animals by oral administration. The poorly absorbed sulfonamides include sulfaguanidine, succinylsulfathiazole, phthalylsulfathiazole and phthalylsulfacetamide. These compounds are employed for treating infections of the gastrointestinal tract particularly when the lower bowel is involved.

Fate and distribution: After absorption, sulfonamides may occur in the body in 3 main forms: acetylated, protein-bound and in the free form, in varying stages of equilibrium depending upon many factors. The percentage of these different forms varies with the species of animal. For practical purposes, it is perhaps best to consider the acetylated sulfonamide as being therapeutically inactive and the bound form as an inactive reservoir of drug, available for use as it is released from its binding site. In the dog and other smaller animals these compounds are widely distributed in body tissues and fluids. These include eye fluids, peritoneal and pleural fluids, synovial fluids, cerebrospinal fluids, prostatic and bronchial secretions and saliva. Sulfonamides are secreted in the milk following oral or IV administration, but the levels attained in the milk may be insufficient to treat mastitis effectively.

Excretion: Sulfonamides are excreted mainly in the urine where they are found in greater concentration than in the blood. They are also found in the milk, and close attention should be given to the cautions of the manufacturer regarding withdrawal times and periods following treatment during which the milk should not be used for human consumption.

Blood levels: The blood level attained depends on the rate and completeness of absorption, and rates of elimination and destruction of the drug. There is marked variation in blood levels obtained with a particular sulfonamide in different species of animals and also with different compounds within the same species. In general, sulfathiazole, sulfadiazine and sulfapyridine produce relatively low levels when compared with sulfamerazine, sulfamethazine and sulfanilamide. For effective therapeutic action, it is generally recommended that sulfonamide blood levels of 5 mg/100 ml be established and, in severe infections, levels of 10 or 12 mg/100 ml may be desirable. However, there is empirical evidence that, in many cases, such levels are never achieved, yet recovery quickly follows treatment, indicating that in certain disorders the lower concentrations may be quite as effective.

Examples of sulfonamide compounds that produce prolonged blood levels are sulfabromomethazine, sulfadimethoxine and sulfamethoxypyrazine. These are characterized by a high degree of protein-binding and a low percentage of acetylation. In addition long-acting sulfonamide boluses have been prepared for ruminants. The release of drug from these boluses may require days to weeks. The absorption of drug is slow and often erratic, making total reliance on them for therapy unwise.

Toxicology: The toxic effects of the sulfonamides vary with different compounds, species and individual animals. Toxic signs are more likely to occur with prolonged administration of high doses. In animals, the following toxic signs have been observed: anorexia, diarrhea, constipation, emesis, anemia, leukopenia, agranulocytopenia, cyanosis, oliguria, hematuria, crystalluria, skin rash, urticaria, excitement, depression, hyperesthesia, peripheral neuritis and convulsions. In cattle, decreased milk production has been observed following sulfonamide therapy and, in chickens, a reduction in egg production has been reported.

There is little information on the relative toxicity of the different sulfonamides for domestic animals. However, on the basis of experience in man and experimental animals, sulfamerazine, sulfamethazine and sulfadiazine appear to be less toxic than sulfanilamide, sulfathiazole and sulfapyridine. The sulfonamides that are poorly absorbed following oral administration have a very low toxicity when administered orally.

The presence of dehydration enhances the possibility of the sulfonamides crystallizing in the urine with consequent renal damage. Crystalluria may be avoided by ensuring an adequate urine flow through the use of fluid therapy and the use of the more soluble sulfonamides (sulfanilamide, sulfamethazine, sulfisoxazole, sulfacetamide). Another approach in the prevention of renal damage is the use of combined sulfonamides, since it has been shown that in a mixture, the therapeutic activity is equal to the total amount of sulfonamide present, while, on the other hand, each compound possesses its own individual solubility.

Therapeutic Uses: Selection of a sulfonamide: The principal considerations in the selection of a sulfonamide relate to their pharmacologic characteristics rather than any major difference in antibacterial spectrum. Sulfathiazole, for example, is the most potent sulfonamide *in vitro*, but it is excreted so rapidly that it is difficult to maintain effective blood levels. It is also more toxic than either sulfamerazine or sulfamethazine. Sulfisoxazole is highly soluble over a wide pH range and is, therefore, less likely to produce renal damage. For this reason, it is probably the sulfonamide of choice with which to treat urinary tract infections. Solutions of sulfacetamide have a neutral pH and hence are the least irritating for instillation in the conjunctival sac. Sulfadiazine and sulfapyridine attain the highest levels in the cerebrospinal fluid and are probably indicated for the treatment of encephalitis or meningitis caused by sensitive organisms. A mixture of sulfonamides is preferable for the treatment of systemic infections as adequate blood levels can be maintained with little danger of renal toxicity. However, the improved solubility of the newer sulfonamides such as sulfisoxazole, sulfamethoxazole and sulfadiazine have largely eliminated the need for the triple sulfonamide combinations in classes of animals for which they are available.

The poorly absorbed sulfonamides are most frequently employed in treating enteric infections. These compounds do not penetrate the intestinal wall but remain in high concentrations in the lumen. Some investigators are of the opinion that the well-absorbed sulfonamides are of more value in enteric infections since they may act on infections that lie within the wall of the intestine. Phthalylsulfacetamide is poorly absorbed, but it is stated that it penetrates into all strata of the gut tissue and it, therefore, would appear to be a desirable compound for this type of infection.

Local use of sulfonamides: When applied locally, sulfonamides are likely to produce a foreign-body reaction which delays wound healing. For this reason, the use of sulfonamides in clean surgical wounds is not recommended.

Local therapy with sulfonamides appears to be of value in the treatment of certain contaminated wounds of animals. The more soluble compounds, such as sulfanilamide, sulfacetamide, sodium sulfacetamide and homosulfanilamide are less likely to act as foreign bodies. Homosulfanilamide is not inhibited by the high concentrations of PABA found in purulent exudate and necrotic tissue; hence, it is of particular value in the treatment of suppurative lesions; however, it is more likely to delay wound healing than other sulfonamides. A mixture consisting of 9 parts sulfanilamide and 1 part homosulfanilamide is reported to possess desirable characteristics for local wound treatment.

Dosage and Administration: Effective therapy with sulfonamides depends upon the establishment and maintenance of proper blood levels. Sulfonamide dosage is based on the body weight of the animal and is ordinarily expressed in terms of a daily dose. The initial dose is usually equal to a total daily dose and serves to produce a rapid rise in the blood level. Subsequent fractional doses are given at proper intervals to maintain an effective blood concentration.

Sulfonamides are most frequently administered orally as powders, tablets, boluses, capsules, emulsions and soluble sodium salts. In some species, the compounds may be administered in the feed. They can be used to permit chickens salvaged from an epidemic of bacterial disease to reach market weight.

Under certain conditions, IV therapy may be desirable. This is true when it is impractical to use oral administration or when it is deemed necessary to produce effective blood levels quickly. For parenteral administration, solutions of sodium salts are available in concentrations of 5 to 25%. These solutions are highly alkaline and, therefore, they should be given slowly to prevent a "speed shock" reaction and precautions taken to prevent their leakage into perivascular tissues where they may cause marked irritation.

In most conditions that respond to sulfonamide therapy, treatment for a maximum of 6 days is sufficient. In general, if a condition does not show a favorable response within 3 days, it is probable that no response will be obtained. Prolonged therapy should be avoided since it is conducive to toxic reactions. On the other hand, treatment should be continued long enough to avoid the possibility of relapse.

SULFAMERAZINE

Sulfamerazine has limited use in veterinary medicine, principally in mixtures of triple sulfonamides for the treatment of a wide range of bacterial infections in cattle or horses. Respiratory tract infections caused by pasteurellae usually respond well to such combinations. In rabbits, sulfamerazine is of value in the prevention and treatment of hepatic coccidiosis (*Eimeria stiedai*) and in the treatment of intestinal coccidiosis (*E. perforans*). It is effective in reducing the mortality of several poultry diseases including pullorum disease, paratyphoid infections, fowl typhoid and infectious coryza.

Dosage: Sulfamerazine is administered orally to all domestic animals in a daily dose of 60 mg/lb (130 mg/kg) of body wt, divided into 2 fractional doses, given at 12-hour intervals. The sodium salt is given IV in a dose of 30 mg/lb (66 mg/kg) of body wt. For poultry, sulfamerazine may be administered in the feed in a 0.4 to 0.5% concentration or the sodium salt may be mixed with drinking water in a 0.1 to 0.2% concentration.

SULFAMETHAZINE
(Sulfadimidine, Sulfamezathine)

In horses, sulfamethazine is of value in the treatment of pneumonia and upper respiratory infections, such as strangles. It also has been employed with success in fistulous withers, navel ill (joint ill) of foals and against the gram-negative organisms which frequently are involved in enteric and speticemic diseases of foals.

Chronic mastitis of cattle due to streptococci has been treated by udder infusion with a solution of sodium sulfamethazine. Penicillin (100,000 u) often is included in the sulfonamide solution. In acute mastitis complicated by septicemia, sulfamethazine has been employed, either alone or combined with antibiotics, for local and systemic treatment. In calf pneumonia, sulfamethazine or a triple sulfonamide mixture (sulfamethazine, sulfamerazine and sulfathiazole or sulfapyridine) is the sulfonamide of choice. Calf diphtheria, metritis and calf scours respond to sulfamethazine therapy and, in the latter condition, some workers consider it to be more effective than nonabsorbable sulfonamides. Sodium sulfamethazine is also of value in foot rot of cattle. In sheep, sulfamethazine or sulfamerazine appear to be superior to other sulfonamides for treating pneumonia or mastitis due to pasteurellae. Intravenous administration of sulfamethazine should be slow because of the possibility of a severe "speed shock" reaction.

Sulfamethazine has been found useful in the treatment of infectious enteritis, navel ill, pasteurellosis and pneumonia due to *Haemophilus suis* in swine. It also is useful for treating various bacterial infections secondary to canine distemper. In rabbits, it has been used for the treatment of intestinal coccidiosis and in the prevention and treatment of hepatic coccidiosis.

Sulfamethazine is reported to be effective against coccidiosis in chickens and turkeys, although today there are better drugs for this purpose. It may be useful in reducing the mortality rate in pullorum disease, paratyphoid, typhoid, fowl cholera and infectious coryza of chickens.

Dosage: In the horse, cow, sheep, pig and cat, sulfamethazine is employed in an initial dose of 60 to 100 mg/lb (130 to 220 mg/kg) body wt followed by 60 mg/lb (130 mg/kg) body wt, administered in equal fractional doses at 12-hour intervals. Sodium sulfamethazine is given IV in a dose of 60 mg/lb (130 mg/kg) body wt. For poultry, sulfamethazine may be administered in the feed in a concentration of 0.4 to 0.5%, or sodium sulfamethazine may be added to drinking water in a concentration of 0.1 to 0.2%.

SULFADIAZINE

Sulfadiazine is not frequently used for treatment of animal diseases. In general, it appears to be less toxic than sulfanilamide, sulfathiazole, or sulfapyridine. Sulfadiazine is of value in calf pneumonia, but sulfamerazine and sulfamethazine seem more effective. It is useful in treating postdistemper bacterial infections in dogs and in urinary infections of small animals. For these purposes it is often combined with other sulfonamides. In *Salmonella* infections of chickens (e.g. pullorum disease, paratyphoid infections and fowl typhoid), sulfadiazine is reported to reduce the mortality.

Dosage: Sulfadiazine is given orally in daily doses of 60 mg/lb (130 mg/kg) body wt. In the horse, cow, sheep and cat, this amount is divided into 2 doses given at 12-hour intervals, while in the dog and pig, equally divided doses are administered at 8-hour intervals. In poultry, sulfadiazine may be administered in the feed in a concentration of 0.5%.

SULFANILAMIDE

In the horse, sulfanilamide produces fairly persistent blood levels and is effective against the common organisms involved in pneumonia and in upper respiratory infections, such as pharyngitis, bronchitis and strangles. It also has been employed in a limited number of cases of chronic nasal catarrh and sinusitis. It may be of some value in fistulous withers and poll evil. Hemolytic streptococci are frequently involved in infected wounds of horses and local or systemic use of sulfanilamide is reported to be effective in these cases. In sheep, sulfanilamide has been recommended for treatment of joint ill due to streptococci and it is reported to bring about some clinical improvement of infectious enteritis and coccidiosis but newer more effective drugs are available.

Today sulfanilamide is little used in small animals, but is effective in cases of cystitis in dogs due to *Escherichia coli* and streptococci. Bacterial infections secondary to canine distemper may respond to sulfanilamide, but it would appear that other sulfonamides (e.g. sulfamerazine and sulfamethazine) are of more value in these cases.

Dosage: For the horse, cow and pig, sulfanilamide is administered orally in a daily dose of 60 mg/lb (130 mg/kg) body wt. This is divided into 2 fractional doses at 12-hour intervals. For the dog and cat, the daily dose is 90 mg/lb (200 mg/kg) body wt, divided into 2 equal doses at 12-hour intervals.

SULFATHIAZOLE

Sulfathiazole is effective against many common pathogens when tested *in vitro;* however, it is relatively more toxic than sulfamerazine or sulfamethazine and its rapid excretion makes it difficult to maintain effective blood levels. It is used mainly in combination with sulfamethazine and sulfamerazine etc. in triple sulfa combinations. Since the alkaline urine of herbivores tends to insure solubility of sulfathiazole, it is of value in treating urinary tract infections. Sodium sulfathiazole has been employed for foot rot in cattle.

Diseases in swine that have been shown to respond to sulfathiazole therapy are infectious enteritis, pneumonia and pasteurellosis. A 3% sulfathiazole ointment has been employed topically in treating seborrheic conditions of the skin in pigs.

In dogs, sulfathiazole tablets are effective in treating urinary tract infections due to *Staphylococcus aureus, Proteus vulgaris, Escherichia coli* or β-hemolytic streptococci. It is also employed in bacterial infections secondary to canine distemper. In cats, sulfathiazole has sometimes been found useful in treating feline pneumonitis. Topical therapy with sulfathiazole powder has been employed in various skin conditions of this species. Sulfathiazole is reported to reduce the mortality rate in fowl cholera and infectious coryza of chickens. Sulfathiazole other than in combinations is presently available only in the tablet form.

Dosage: In the horse and cat, sulfathiazole is administered in daily doses of 90 mg/lb (200 mg/kg) body wt. For these animals, 3 equal fractional doses are given every 8 hours. The daily dose for the cow, sheep, pig and dog is 120 to 180 mg/lb (265 to 400 mg/kg) body wt and, in these animals, equal fractional doses are administered at 4-to 6-hour intervals.

SULFAPYRIDINE

In cattle, sulfapyridine is of value in vaginitis, calf diphtheria, and pasteurellosis, but sulfamerazine and sulfamethazine are probably superior. It is usually used now only in combination with 2 or 3 other sulfa drugs. Sodium sulfapyridine has been employed IV for foot rot in cattle. Other conditions that respond to sulfapyridine are secondary bacterial infections in canine distemper, pneumonia in dogs and swine, and pneumonitis in cats. In most of these conditions, sulfamerazine and sulfamethazine appear to be safer and more effective.

Dosage: Sulfapyridine is administered in doses of 30 mg/lb (66 mg/kg) body wt b.i.d. In all animals except the pig, this amount is divided into equal fractional doses administered at 12-hour intervals. In the pig, one dose per day is sufficient to maintain adequate blood levels.

SULFAQUINOXALINE

Sulfaquinoxaline is readily absorbed from the gastrointestinal tract and produces persistent blood levels. The drug is excreted partly in the urine and partly through the intestinal tract in the feces.

In the dog and chicken, sulfaquinoxaline may cause hypoprothrombinemia, which can be prevented by the simultaneous administration of vitamin K (℞ 570).

Sulfaquinoxaline is useful for the treatment of coccidiosis of chickens and for the prevention and treatment of this disease in turkeys. Although sulfaquinoxaline is also used as a prophylactic agent against coccidiosis of chickens, other newer and more effective drugs have largely supplanted it. It has been used in combination with amprolium. The combined drugs used at the rate of 0.0006% of each in feed offer protection against all of the common species of coccidia. When used for prevention of cecal or intestinal coccidiosis in chickens, sulfaquinoxaline may be fed either intermittently or continuously.

Sulfaquinoxaline added to mash is useful in controlling mortality from acute fowl cholera (*Pasteurella multocida*). Losses due to fowl typhoid (*Salmonella gallinarum*) in turkeys can often be reduced by giving sulfaquinoxaline in the drinking water.

Dosage: Because of the varied forms in which this drug is prepared, and the several treatment schedules recommended, the directions of the manufacturer should be followed. In mammals, the daily dose is 60 mg/lb (130 mg/kg) body wt orally for infectious diseases, but only 1/10 of this for coccidiosis.

SULFISOXAZOLE

This sulfonamide is relatively soluble and well absorbed after oral administration. In the dog and cow, experimental studies indicate that sulfisoxazole does not produce as prolonged blood levels as sulfamerazine or sulfamethazine. The drug is excreted rapidly in the urine in high concentrations and this, together with its high solubility, recommends it for use in urinary-tract infections. Compared to other sulfonamides, the acute toxicity of sulfisoxazole is relatively low.

In dogs, sulfisoxazole has been used mainly to treat urinary tract infections.

Dosage: A daily dose of 60 to 90 mg of sulfisoxazole per lb (130 to 200 mg/kg) of body wt probably will be needed in most species in order to maintain adequate blood levels. The daily dose should be divided and administered at 6-hour intervals.

SULFABROMOMETHAZINE
("Sulfabrom")

Bromination of the fifth carbon of the pyrimidine nucleus of the sulfamethazine molecule results in a prolongation of the blood levels attained when this compound is given orally or IP. Sulfabromomethazine retains the excellent antibacterial activity of the parent compound and its unique long-acting effects make it particularly attractive as a sulfonamide for use in large animals. Single doses of this compound in cattle result in therapeutic blood levels that persist for 48 hours and longer. The advantages of this property to the practitioner are obvious; unfortunately, prolongation of blood levels does not reliably occur in other species, although the drug is as clinically effective as other sulfonamides. There appears to be little danger of crystalluria occurring, even with repeated doses of sulfabromomethazine.

Dosage: In cattle, sulfabromomethazine is given orally in boluses in doses of 60 to 90 mg/lb (130 to 200 mg/kg) of body wt. The solution may also be given orally as a drench, and solutions of buffered powder may be administered IP at the same dose. These doses may be repeated after 48 hours, if necessary.

SULFACETAMIDE

Compared to other sulfonamides, sulfacetamide possesses a relatively high solubility and readily penetrates the tissues of the eye. These properties recommend it for use in eye infections. It is used topically as a lotion for dermatologic and ophthalmologic infections in small animals.

SULFAGUANIDINE

Sulfaguanidine is employed for treating various intestinal infections in a number of species, but today other sulfonamides, such as succinylsulfathiazole and phthalylsulfathiazole, are considered to be superior for these purposes. It has been replaced by other drugs for the prevention and treatment of coccidiosis in poultry.

Dosage: Sulfaguanidine is given to mammals at an initial dose of 120 mg/lb (265 mg/kg) of body wt, followed by daily maintenance doses of half this. It may be administered to poultry in the feed in a concentration of 1 to 1.5%.

SUCCINYLSULFATHIAZOLE
("Sulfasuxidine")

This sulfonamide is poorly absorbed and is employed for treating infections of the gastrointestinal tract. These include bacillary dysenteries of dogs and cats, calf scours, and necrotic enteritis in swine.

Dosage: Succinylsulfathiazole is administered orally in daily doses of 80 mg/lb (175 mg/kg) body wt b.i.d. This amount may be divided into 2 or more fractional doses.

PHTHALYLSULFATHIAZOLE
("Sulfathalidine")

Phthalylsulfathiazole, being a poorly absorbed sulfonamide, is used for treating intestinal infections only and is of value in calf scours and in infectious enteritis of swine and dogs. It is considered to be less toxic and more effective than sulfaguanidine.

Dosage: The daily dose range for animals is 60 to 135 mg/lb (130 to 300 mg/kg) body wt.

HOMOSULFANILAMIDE HYDROCHLORIDE
("Sulfamylon")

Homosulfanilamide or mafenide acetate differs from other commonly used sulfonamides in being less active against β-hemolytic streptococci and staphylococci. It is less inhibited by the presence of pus and necrotic tissue than other sulfonamides, because it is not antagonized by the high concentrations of PABA found in such lesions.

Homosulfanilamide is primarily employed by local application in the treatment of infected wounds and is especially suitable for infections due to gas-forming bacteria. It is also particularly suitable for treatment of patients with skin burns where it is applied to the burned area in a thick coating twice a day and left uncovered. A powder containing 1 part homosulfanilamide and 9 parts sulfanilamide is reported to be of value in these conditions. For metritis in cattle, introduction of a suspension containing both homosulfanilamide and sulfanilamide powder into the uterus is recommended. Sulfamylon is available as a 5% dental solution and as an 8.5% topical cream.

PHTHALYLSULFACETAMIDE

Phthalylsulfacetamide does not enter the blood stream after oral administration. However, unlike other poorly absorbed sulfonamides which remain largely in the lumen of the gut, it is reported to penetrate all layers of the intestinal wall.

Commercially, phthalylsulfacetamide has been used as an active ingredient in antidiarrheal preparations. Phthalylsulfacetamide is not active until hydrolysed by bacterial enzymes to form sulfacetamide. This compound therefore is activated only in the lower bowel unless extensive craniad movement of bacteria has occurred. It is of particular benefit for the treatment or control of colitis in dogs.

Dosage: The drug is given in a daily oral dose of 40 to 120 mg/lb (88 to 265 mg/kg) body wt. This is divided into 3 fractional doses.

SULFADIMETHOXINE

This sulfonamide is structurally related to sulfadiazine. In cattle it produces prolonged blood levels. The degree of acetylation and protein binding is similar to that of sulfamethazine. Sulfadimethoxine is reported to be effective for a variety of bacterial infections in dogs and cats; these include: tonsillitis, pharyngitis, bronchitis, pneumonia, sinusitis, metritis and dermatitis. Of particular interest is its use in treating salmonellosis in greyhound dogs. This condition does not respond readily to other sulfonamides or antibiotics. Large oral doses 25 mg/lb (55 mg/kg) of body wt, b.i.d. of sulfadimethoxine in conjunction with concentrated globulins have been used with good results in canine coccidiosis. Presumably sulfadimethoxine should be of value in the same diseases in cattle for which other sulfonamides are used. Sulfadimethoxine has been found useful in treatment of cholera and coccidiosis of chickens and turkeys.

Dosage: For cattle an initial dose of 50 mg/lb (110 mg/kg) body wt followed by a daily dose of 25 mg/lb (55 mg/kg) will maintain effective blood levels. Doses employed clinically for dogs and cats have been considerably less than this. An initial dose of 7 to 14 mg/lb (15 to 30 mg/kg) followed by daily doses of 3 to 7 mg/lb (7 to 15 mg/kg) have been used.

OTHER NEWER SULFONAMIDES

Several other new sulfonamides that produce more prolonged blood levels in cattle have been studied; however few have come into widespread use. A number of human and small animal formulations are available for selective therapy. **Sulfaethoxypyridazine** and **sulfamethoxypyridazine** are both rapidly absorbed orally and produce therapeutically effective tissue levels for extended periods of time. **Silver sulfadiazine** is used extensively to prevent *Pseudomonas aeruginosa* infection in topical burns. **Sulfachloropyridazine** is effective against a large number of gram-negative intestinal bacteria such as *Escherichia coli* and *Salmonella* spp. and has been used for treatment of enteritis in pigs and calves. It is rapidly eliminated after parenteral administration, which limits its usefulness.

Salicylazosulfapyridine has been used along with succinylsulfathiazole and phthalylsulfathiazole for the treatment of ulcerative colitis. The bacteria of the lower intestine cleave the salicylazo group leaving sulfapyridine which is active against bacteria; some is absorbed through the gut wall and excreted via the kidneys.

TRIMETHOPRIM

Trimethoprim was developed originally along with pyrimethamine as an antimalarial drug. The mechanism of action was shown to be through interference with folic acid production. Since the sulfonamides, acting through PABA antagonism, also block the same metabolic pathway, the combination of a sulfonamide with trimethoprim produces a supra-additive response. Trimethoprim is presently combined with sulfadiazine (Tribrissen), sulfadoxine (Trivetrin) and sulfamethoxazole (Septra, Bactrim)—(not all are available in all countries).

The combinations are useful for treating both gram-positive and gram-negative infections of the respiratory system, urinary tract, mammary gland and digestive tract. Combination therapy is less likely to allow the formation of bacterial resistance and is effective against a large number of organisms.

Dosage and Preparations: Trimethoprim-sulfonamide combinations are available in injectable and oral table and syrup form. The dosage for cats and dogs (Tribrissen) is 2 to 4 mg/lb (4.5 to 9 mg/kg) trimethoprim and 5 to 10 mg/lb (11 to 22 mg/kg) sulfadiazine, for 2 to 3 days after clinical signs subside. It should not be used for more than 14 consecutive days. The injectable dosage for cattle, sheep and pigs (Trivetrin) is 1.2 mg/lb (2.6 mg/kg) trimethoprim and 6 mg/lb (13 mg/kg) sulfadoxine. In poultry, medication can be achieved by the addition of 64 mg trimethoprim and 320 mg sulfadiazine per gal. (3.8L) of drinking water.

ANTIBIOTIC THERAPY

Caution: *In all drug therapy it is important to adhere to local laws and regulations governing the use of such products.*

Antibiotics are used for the treatment of infections caused by bacteria, fungi, a few large viruses, and protozoa. They may be either **bacteriostatic** or **bactericidal** depending on their mechanism of action and the dosage given. Higher dosages tend to make many of the antibiotics bactericidal. They act primarily through interference with processes essential for the growth, survival or replication of the microbiological cell. Antibiotics are most effective in acute infections when bacteria are in a rapid growth stage and before the organisms have been able to cause extensive physical damage.

Some antibiotics, classified as narrow spectrum antibiotics, are effective against a rather limited number of organisms while others, classified as broad spectrum, are effective against a wide range of gram-positive and gram-negative organisms. Streptomycin, for example, is mainly effective against gram-negative bacteria whereas penicillin G, erythromycin, lincomycin and novobiocin are mainly active against gram-positive bacteria. Under clinical conditions, it is often not possible to establish the exact nature of the causative organisms. Wherever possible the organisms should be cultured and then chemotherapeutic sensitivity should be determined to aid in the selection of an appropriate agent. Direct correlation of *in vitro* sensitivity disc data to the *in vivo* situation cannot be made; however, *in vitro* sensitivity data can be a valuable tool in the selection of the appropriate drug. If an infection fails to give evidence of responding to a particular antibiotic within a reasonable time (approximately 48 hours) or if *in vitro* sensitivity data suggest otherwise, consideration should be given to changing the drug being used.

Development by bacteria of resistance to the effects of antibiotics is a serious problem that occurs more rapidly with some drugs than with others. Administration of drugs indiscriminately, at too low a level or for too long a time can tend to increase the likelihood of drug resistance developing. Drug resistance can also be transferred from some bacteria to bacteria of other types by virtue of resistance factor transfer plasmids, and in addition resistance can develop to several antibiotics by, in some cases, exposure to only one drug.

Antibiotics differ from the sulfonamides and most other antibacterial agents in that only very small amounts are necessary at an infection site to be effective. In addition the sulfonamides tend to be readily inhibited by the presence of organic matter (i.e. pus, blood, tissue debris) at the site of the infection. However, the sulfonamides excel many antibiotics in their ability to diffuse into body fluids and into cavities such as joints, pleural sacs and the subarachnoid space. Most of the commonly used antibiotics are less likely to produce toxic effects than the sulfonamides. Some antibiotics, however, such as the aminoglycosides (streptomycin, neomycin, gentamycin and kanamycin) and colistin can produce serious toxic effects if not handled correctly. Allergic reactions occur to both the sulfonamides and antibiotics (penicillins in particular); however they have rarely caused severe problems in animals.

Antibiotics may be used alone or in combination with other antibiotics or chemotherapeutic agents. Combinations of drugs can give a supra-additive or synergistic response (greater than the sum of the effects of the individual drugs alone), an additive response (equal to the sum of the individual responses) or an infra-additive response or antagonistic (less than the additive effects of the single drugs used alone). Combinations of penicillin and streptomycin give a supra-additive response with some infections and are widely used. Because of the difference in excretion rates between the 2 antibiotics, fixed dose combinations are less satisfactory than separate administration of the 2 antibiotics each to its own required dose schedule. Combinations of a narrow spectrum antibiotic such as penicillin and a broad-spectrum antibiotic such as tetracycline or chloramphenicol can give an infra-additive response. Whenever a specific determination of a pathogen is possible, the proper use of single drug therapy is recommended.

Antibiotics may be applied locally for treating infections of the skin, ear, eye, udder, uterus, intestinal lumen or any accessible area. This allows for a very high concentration of drug to be placed at the site of infection, often much higher than could safely be obtained by systemic therapy. Antibiotics are frequently used for systemic therapy by administering the drug orally or by the conventional parenteral routes, such as IV, IM or subcut. If a local infection is severe or is spread beyond the original site of infection, systemic, as well as local therapy may be required.

A serious hazard of antibiotic usage in animals is that of residues in the food derived therefrom (meat, eggs, dairy products). Antibiotics administered directly into the mammary gland for the treatment of bovine mastitis lead to high concentrations in the milk which, if mixed with milk free of residues, can still lead to a serious problem of contamination. In addition antibiotics may appear in the milk from systemic therapy as well as from drugs administered locally elsewhere in the body (e.g. the uterus). Repository forms of penicillin (e.g. benzathine penicillin) may appear in the milk for 8 to 10 days and should not be used in milking dairy animals. Close attention should be given to the manufacturer's instructions regarding the periods after treatment during which the milk should not be used for human consumption.

Antibiotics may be added to rations to promote growth in animals, to control or prevent diseases caused by many organisms (bacterial, fungal, and protozoal), as an adjunct to individual therapy, or as the sole therapy in poultry, swine and cattle. Antibiotics may also be added to the water supply to treat disease in groups of animals and this may be a preferred method of administration as sick animals frequently will continue to drink when they may not eat. Palatability and solubility may present problems for some of these drugs.

PENICILLINS

The penicillins are a group of antibiotics with similar chemical characteristics, derived from culture of *Penicillium notatum* or *P. chrysogenom*. Several types are commonly produced; they may be divided into the naturally occurring penicillins such as penicillin G and the semi-synthetic penicillins such as cloxacillin and ampicillin, which are produced by the addition of precursor substances to the mold growth medium.

Sodium, potassium, procaine, benethamine and benzathine salts of the penicillins are available. The sodium and potassium salts of penicillin G and the sodium salts of ampicillin are very rapidly absorbed after IM and subcut. administration and can be used, in addition to IV administration, to give rapid high blood levels of drug. Repository forms of penicillin G, such as the procaine, benethamine and benzathine salts, are absorbed from IM or subcut. sites more slowly, and give a lower but more prolonged blood level. The penicillins are widely distributed throughout the body; however, they do not produce high concentrations in the nervous tissue. The acid secretory mechanism of the kidney very effectively removes penicillin from the blood; high concentrations of the penicillins occur in the urine.

Toxicity problems with these compounds are infrequent. The severe allergic reactions encountered in man occur in animals but at a reduced frequency. Acute anaphylactic reactions with dyspnea, salivation, staggering, collapse and in some cases death have been reported following IV or IM administration of penicillin compounds. Local reactions following IM administration and mild reactions of the skin and mucous membranes have been seen in animals receiving penicillin orally or parenterally and should these reactions occur an alternate non-penicillin drug should be chosen for further therapy.

PENICILLIN G

Penicillin G or benzyl penicillin, derived from cultures of *Penicillium notatum* is a naturally occurring penicillin. The sodium, potassium, procaine, benethamine and benzathine salts are commonly available. When it is desirable to obtain high blood levels rapidly, aqueous solutions of sodium or potassium salts are employed. Repository forms, such as procaine penicillin or benzathine penicillin, are used for maintaining blood levels over extended periods. Penicillin G is well absorbed following IM injection, which is the route generally used. Special formulations are available for oral and IV use, however penicillin G is poorly acid stable and a considerable amount of any oral dosage is destroyed in the stomach. Following absorption, penicillin G diffuses to most fluids and tissues and is rapidly eliminated from the body by urinary excretion. Penicillin G crosses into the brain very slowly.

Clinical Indications: Penicillin is mainly effective against gram-positive bacteria. It is effective in the treatment and control of bovine mastitis due to *Streptococcus agalactiae*. When proper sanitary and husbandry measures are enforced, bacteriologic cures can be obtained in 80 to 90% of this type, particularly if treatment is started before extensive changes in udder tissue have occurred. It also is effective against bovine mastitis caused by streptococci other than *Str. agalactiae*. Penicillin is of limited value in staphylococcal mastitis, due to the prevalence of penicillinase-producing strains. Combinations of penicillin and other antibacterial agents are commonly used for the treatment of mastitis. Many types of vehicles have been used for intramammary infusion of penicillin. These include sterile water, oils and ointments. Penicillin G itself does not appear to be irritating to udder tissue.

Penicillin G is of some value in the treatment of infectious cystitis and pyelonephritis of cattle due to *Corynebacterium renale*. In certain cases, alleviation of signs and disappearance of organisms from the urine occurs, but in others, little or no response may be obtained. For best results, penicillin should be employed early in the course of the disease. Most urinary tract infections are caused by gram-negative bacteria or gram-negative, gram-positive mixed infection and therefore do not respond well to penicillin G therapy.

Clinical evidence indicates that penicillin G is of value in a number of bacterial infections in which the exact etiology is unknown. Among these are calf pneumonia and secondary bacterial infections associated with distemper in dogs. Metritis of cattle, often associated with a mixed infection, has been treated successfully by instillation of penicillin suspension directly into the uterus. Penicillin also can be useful in treating anthrax and infections due to *Erysipelothrix* sp.

Penicillin has been employed in the form of ointments or solutions for treatment of localized infections of the skin, eyes and ears. For infected wounds of the skin and in ear infections, penicillin ointments have been used topically with some success. In severe infections of the eye, skin or ears, it is ordinarily desirable to use both systemic and local treatment. Penicillin given orally has shown some merit in the prevention and control of bloat in cattle, however new, more effective anti-frothing agents are now available. As with many agents used in this condition, considerable variation in response occurs.

Added to bull semen in the concentration of 1,000 to 2,000 u/ml, penicillin G is reported to effectively retard bacterial growth for a period up to 8 days. It is also used for this purpose combined with streptomycin (1,000 u of each antibiotic per ml).

Dosage and Administration: The dose varies with the type and severity of infection; in most instances, a dose of 2,000 u/lb (4,400 u/kg) body wt IM is considered to be minimal. In severe infections, this is increased to 5,000 to 10,000 u/lb (11,000 to 22,000 u/kg) body wt, or more. The frequency at which penicillin G is administered varies with the type of preparation. The following is recommended: for aqueous vehicles, every 3 or 4 hours; oil and beeswax, every 12 hours; for repository forms containing procaine penicillin in water or oil every 12 to 24 hours; for benzathine and benethamine penicillin, every 3 days. In severe infections, it may be desirable to use a sodium or potassium salt combined with a procaine salt, since the former gives a prompt high blood level, while the latter maintains a concentration for a prolonged period.

Government regulations now restrict the maximal single dose of penicillin for intramammary infusion in bovine mastitis to 100,000 u. This may be administered in the form of a solution in sterile water, a suspension in oil, or incorporated in an ointment base.

Oral therapy with penicillin G is not widely used for treating infectious diseases of animals. In general, much larger doses are necessary than by the IM route and absorption is variable. Special forms of penicillin (e.g. penicillin V) are available for oral use.

Preparations: Among these are: penicillin powder for aqueous solution, penicillin in oil and beeswax, procaine penicillin in oil, procaine penicillin in aqueous suspension and penicillin tablets for oral use. Ophthalmic ointments containing penicillin appear to be preferable for treating conjunctival infections since they require less frequent application than do solutions. Combinations of penicillin with other antibiotics are commonly available.

Ampicillin, Amoxicillin

Ampicillin is a broad-spectrum antibiotic useful for treating both gram-positive and gram-negative (*E. coli*, *Salmonella* spp., etc.) bacterial infections. It has been used extensively in small animals to treat infections of the gut, the ear and eye and the urinary tract. In large animals ampicillin has been used to treat enteric infections especially in the newborn, to treat urinary tract infections and to treat local infections responsive to the drug. Ampicillin concentrates in high levels in the urine and is therefore particularly suited for urinary tract infections. A slightly modified ampicillin, **hetacillin,** is available for oral or parenteral therapy.

Amoxicillin is chemically very similar to ampicillin, however it is more completely absorbed orally than ampicillin. Amoxicillin therefore gives higher blood concentrations and urine levels than ampicillin does, given at the same dosage. Amoxicillin appears also to have approximately 40% longer half-life than ampicillin.

Oral ampicillin occasionally causes digestive upsets; these are quickly resolved when the treatment is stopped. Hypersensitivity reactions may occur as a result of ampicillin administration and cross sensitivity with the other penicillins can be manifest.

Parenteral therapy with ampicillin as a trihydrate, sodium or potassium salt, has not been as widely used as oral therapy because of cost and the short length of time adequate blood levels are obtained from IM injections. Continuous IV drip therapy can be used in acute conditions requiring ampicillin.

Dosage and Administration: The dosage of ampicillin depends on location and severity of the infection, and size and age of the animal. The oral dosage is 4.5 to 7 mg/lb (10 to 15 mg/kg) q.i.d.; IM dosages of 12 mg/kg require repetition every 2 hours (ampicillin sodium) or every 3 hours (ampicillin trihydrate).

Dosage forms available: Ampicillin is available as an injectable water-soluble powder, as a sodium or potassium salt or as a trihydrate. Tablets, capsules and a suspension are available for oral use.

Amoxicillin is available as a trihydrate in an oral suspension, water soluble powder and as an oral capsule.

Miscellaneous Penicillins

Penicillin V is an acid-stable penicillin particularly suited to oral therapy. Its spectrum of activity is essentially the same as for penicillin G. Its major veterinary use is in small animal therapy. A recommended dosage is 1.5 to 2 mg/lb (3.3 to 6.6 mg/kg) 3 to 4 times daily. It is available as an oral tablet or as the potassium salt in a tablet or oral solution.

Cloxacillin is a penicillinase-resistant penicillin with a spectrum of activity similar to that of penicillin G. The major veterinary use is in dry-cow therapy for mastitis. Intramammary administration of 200 mg offers one of the best hopes for treating chronic staphylococcal mastitis in the dairy cows. Cloxacillin is available as a sodium salt for IM or IV therapy, as an oral capsule and as an intramammary mastitis ointment.

Carbenicillin ("Pyopen," "Geopen") is a semi-synthetic penicillin structurally quite similar to ampicillin. Its major use is to treat gram-negative bacteria resistant to more widely used antibiotics. Its major disadvantages are susceptibility to development of bacterial resistance and cost. Carbenicillin is not penicillinase resistant and not acid stable. A congener of carbenicillin, **carbenicillin indanyl,** is acid stable and administered orally and is rapidly absorbed. Carbenicillin has been found to be synergistic with gentamicin against *Pseudomonas* infections. Carbenicillin is available as a water soluble powder for IM injection. Carbenicillin indanyl sodium is available as an oral 500-mg tablet.

STREPTOMYCIN AND DIHYDROSTREPTOMYCIN

Streptomycin is produced by cultures of *Streptomyces griseus.* Dihydrostreptomycin is formed by chemical alteration of streptomycin. Both streptomycin and dihydrostreptomycin are relatively stable in the dry form or in aqueous solution, and possess similar antibacterial activity.

Streptomycin is adequately absorbed from subcut. or IM sites of injection; absorption from the gastrointestinal tract is minimal. Applied topically, streptomycin has poor powers of penetration. After absorption, it is well distributed in body tissues and fluids, including the pleural fluid. It is mainly excreted in the urine by glomerular filtration.

In large doses over prolonged periods, streptomycin may be toxic, the most significant effect being reversible vestibular disturbances. Occasionally, a permanent loss of hearing may result. For normal short-term therapy using conventional doses, CNS damage or allergic reactions do not constitute a serious problem. Contact dermatitis may develop in persons handling the drug. Dihydrostreptomycin may produce permanent deafness and for this reason its parenteral use should be restricted to those cases in which the infection is not susceptible to other antibacterial therapy. Streptomycin or dihydrostreptomycin can cause fatal hypocalcemia if given IV. If given IM they can also bind and inactivate sufficiently large quantities of calcium to cause staggering, muscle weakness, respiratory paralysis and death. Animals with endotoxemia or severe electrolyte imbalances are more susceptible to this hypocalcemic effect.

Clinical Indications: Streptomycin and dihydrostreptomycin are primarily effective against gram-negative bacteria, although a few gram-positive organisms also are susceptible. Bacteria quite easily acquire a resistance to the antibiotic, especially when exposed to continued low concentrations of the agent. Usage has reduced markedly in the last decade because of bacterial resistance. The major use for these drugs is in combination with other drugs such as penicillin. Another factor mitigating against their use for parenteral administration in food animals is the long withdrawal time (30 days in many jurisdictions).

Both antibiotics are useful in the treatment of bovine mastitis due to gram-negative organisms, particularly *Escherichia coli, Aerobacter aerogenes* or *A. cloacae.* Streptomycin has been used combined with penicillin in the form of a solution, ointment or bougie. These preparations offer the advantage of a wider antibacterial spectrum. Streptomycin is of some value in actinomycosis of cattle due to *Actinomyces bovis*. It has been successfully used in treating calf pneumonia; this should be continued for at least 4 to 5 days. Intrauterine and preputial infusions of streptomycin are reported to be of value in overcoming bovine infertility due to campylobacteriosis. It also has been combined with penicillin and infused in the uterus, for treatment of metritis in cattle.

In the horse, streptomycin has been used for treating cystitis due to *E. coli*.

In dogs, this antibiotic is useful given orally in treating infectious dysentery. Local therapy with streptomycin has been used for treatment of otitis externa.

Streptomycin and dihydrostreptomycin have been widely used orally against enteric infections although resistant bacteria are now a common problem. Streptomycin has been used to treat leptospirosis in cattle, swine and dogs and has been successful in eliminating organisms from urine. By local injection, streptomycin and dihydrostreptomycin are of value in the treatment of infectious sinusitis in turkeys. Chronic respiratory disease of chickens has also been effectively treated with streptomycin given in the water, feed or by inhalation. The drug is also of some value in control of fowl cholera and fowl typhoid.

Streptomycin in concentrations of 250 to 1,000 mcg/ml of bull semen is effective in inhibiting bacterial growth and does not adversely affect spermatozoa for periods up to 20 days. Combinations of penicillin and streptomycin may also be used for this purpose and have the advantage of being effective against gram-positive and gram-negative organisms.

Dosage and Administration: For dogs the recommended maximum daily dose of streptomycin or dihydrostreptomycin is 20 mg/lb (44 mg/kg) body wt by IM or subcut. injection twice a day and for cats 5 mg/lb (11 mg/kg) body wt by IM or subcut. injection b.i.d. In foals, 0.5 gm every 3 to 4 hours are given by IM injection, while in horses, 1 to 2 gm every 3 to 4 hours have been used. Oral medication is indicated for enteric infections and the suggested dose for dogs, calves and swine by this route is 1 gm daily in a single dose or divided into 2 or 3 equal doses. In bovine mastitis due to *E. coli, A. aerogenes,* or *A. cloacae,* the suggested dose is 0.5 gm streptomycin twice daily by intramammary infusion. In acute coliform mastitis, the use of 5 gm by intramammary infusion combined with 5 to 7 gm given IM has been recommended. These doses are repeated twice daily. The usually recommended dose for parenteral administration in poultry is 15 to 50 mg/lb (33 to 110 mg/kg) body wt, a quantity much higher, proportionately, than used in mammals. Streptomycin and dihydrostreptomycin may be toxic to turkeys if they are very ill.

Preparations: Streptomycin is supplied in the form of a powder in sterile vials as streptomycin or dihydrostreptomycin sulfate. For oral medication, streptomycin sulfate is available in solutions for administration in drinking water and dihydrostreptomycin in the form of tablets combined with other agents. Topical ointments containing streptomycin or dihydrostreptomycin alone or in combination with other antibiotics may be obtained, and combinations of dihydrostreptomycin and other antibiotics for subcut. or IM injection are also available. No reliable depot form of this drug has been developed and parenteral doses must be repeated every 6 to 8 hours.

NEOMYCIN

Neomycin is produced by cultures of *Streptomyces fradiae*. Clinically, it is used as neomycin sulfate, a white amorphous powder that is relatively stable in the dry form. Neomycin is soluble in water, but insoluble in organic solvents. Since little or no neomycin is absorbed from the gastrointestinal tract when the antibiotic is given orally, this method of administration is limited to treatment of gastrointestinal infections. When initially introduced, neomycin was not recommended for parenteral use because of its tendency to produce renal damage and toxicity. However, today it is recognized as being reasonably safe when given by injection if proper precautions are taken. These include the restriction of therapy to 5 days or less of recommended dosage. Parenterally administered neomycin can produce a fatal neuromuscular blockade due to chelation of calcium. This is dose related and is exacerbated by the presence of fluid and electrolyte imbalances.

Clinical Indications: Neomycin has a wide range of antibacterial activity and is effective against a number of gram-positive and gram-negative bacteria, including certain strains of *Pseudomonas* and *Proteus* organisms.

Neomycin sulfate is of some value in treating bovine mastitis due to *Pseudomonas* organisms. In reported trials, 29 to 57% of infected quarters were freed of infection. The efficacy of neomycin in the treatment of streptococcal and staphylococcal mastitis is variable. Some reports indicate that it is quite effective, but in other cases, it was found to be inferior to penicillin for these infections. Neomycin preparations are of value for intramammary treatment in some cases of coliform mastitis. It has been used combined with parenteral steroid preparations for treatment of mastitis.

Oral administration of neomycin is used for treatment of bacterial infections of the gastrointestinal tract including salmonella and coliform infections in farm animals and for pre-operative sterilization of the bowel. Indications for systemic administration are not well characterized and neomycin is rarely used parenterally although it has use in the treatment of neonatal septicemias caused by gram-negative organisms in farm animals.

Topical application of neomycin is of value in treating wounds and infections of the skin, ears and eyes. Ointments containing neomycin in combination with other antibiotic substances (e.g. polymyxin, gramicidin) or other agents (e.g. corticoids) are not available.

Dosage and Administration: In bovine mastitis, the recommended dosage for neomycin sulfate is 0.5 gm per infected quarter. This may be administered by intramammary infusion in the form of an aqueous solution, water-in-oil emulsion or as an ointment. For dogs, calves, foals and pigs an oral dose of 5 to 10 mg/lb (11 to 22 mg/kg) of body wt b.i.d. may be used. In young farm animals 3 to 5 mg/lb (6 to 11 mg/kg) b.i.d. may be given by IM injection.

Preparations: Neomycin sulfate is available as a sterile powder for preparing aqueous solutions for topical or oral use. Topical or ophthalmic ointments containing neomycin alone or in combination with other antibiotics are also available. Neomycin is also available for oral therapy in combination with methylscopolamine or scopolamine to treat enteric infections.

KANAMYCIN
("Kantrex")

Kanamycin is an aminoglycoside antibiotic derived from cultures of *Streptomyces kanamyceticus.* It has a wide range of antibacterial activity against gram-positive and gram-negative bacteria, e.g. *Escherichia coli, Salmonella* spp., *Proteus* spp. and *Staphylococcus aureus.* It is poorly absorbed orally and most is eliminated in the feces. It is well absorbed after IM injection and is excreted primarily by the kidneys. It distributes throughout most of the body's extracellular fluid; however very little crosses the blood brain barrier.

The major side effects of kanamycin are the same as those of the other aminoglycoside antibiotics. Nephrotoxicity and ototoxicity occur following high dosages of the drug administered parenterally for a long period of time especially if kidney function is impaired. Kanamycin appears the least toxic of the aminoglycoside group for dogs but as with all members of this group parenteral therapy for periods longer than 5 to 7 days should be approached with caution. In addition, binding of calcium and neuromuscular paralysis can be produced. The dosage for dogs and cats is 5 mg/lb (11 mg/kg) a day, for cattle 10 to 15 mg/lb (22 to 33 mg/kg) b.i.d. The oral dosage for dogs to treat enteritis is 5 to 15 mg/lb (11 to 33 mg/kg) t.i.d. Intramuscular injectable solutions are available as well as tablets, topical ointments and a pediatric syrup.

SPECTINOMYCIN
("Trobicin," "Spectam")

Spectinomycin is derived from a culture of *Streptomyces spectabilis*. It is active against both gram-positive and gram-negative bacteria but it is mainly used for the treatment of gram-positive bacteria, in particular those resistant to penicillin G.

It is used both orally and IM; orally to treat scours in piglets and in feeder pigs (often in combination with neomycin) and as a feed additive it has been shown to improve growth performance of swine. It has some value in treating and controlling *E. coli, Pasteurella multocida* and *Myoplasma* spp. infections.

The dosage for dogs is 10 mg/lb (22 mg/kg) orally b.i.d.; for piglets 50 mg/lb (110 mg/kg) orally; and for chickens 1 to 2 grains per gal. (20 to 35 mg/L) of drinking water.

LINCOMYCIN
(Lincocin)

Lincomycin is derived from cultures of *Streptomyces lincolnensis*. It is active against a large number of gram-positive organisms. Its effectiveness varies with the bacteria being treated, being quite high for *Actinomyces* spp., some strains of streptococci and *Bacillus anthracis*. It is quite effective against clostridial species such as *C. tetani* and *C. perfringens*, and is moderately effective against a number of strains of *Staphylococcus aureus*, *Nocardia* spp. and *Mycoplasma pneumoniae*. It is partially absorbed when administered orally and produces high plasma levels only when administered parenterally. Only a small amount is excreted in the urine. Lincomycin is well distributed throughout the body, however it does not produce high levels in the CSF (40 to 45% of plasma level during meningitis). Oral administration can lead to gastrointestinal disturbances.

A synthetic derivation of lincomycin, clindamycin, has been prepared having the same spectrum of activity as lincomycin.

Lincomycin has been combined with spectinomycin to give it greater effectiveness against *Escherichia coli* in chickens and baby pigs as well as mycoplasmal infections and swine dysentery.

Dosage and Administration: The dosage for the dog and cat is 5 to 10 mg/lb (11 to 22 mg/kg) IM b.i.d. and for swine 5 mg/lb (11 mg/kg) once or twice daily. Lincomycin is available as 0.881% premix for mixing in feed, as an oral solution, an oral syrup, a tablet, a capsule and as a sterile injectable solution for IM or IV administration.

Lincomycin-spectinomycin: This combination is available as feed premix (2.2% lincomycin hydrochloride base equivalent and 2.2% spectinomycin sulfate base equivalent). It is also available as an IM injectable (lincomycin-spectinomycin ration 1:2) and as an oral water soluble powder (lincomycin-spectinomycin ratio 1:2) for water medication.

GENTAMICIN
("Gentocin," "Garamycin")

Gentamicin is an antibiotic of the aminoglycoside family (other important members include kanamycin, streptomycin, neomycin) derived from cultures of *Micromonospora purpurea.* It is active against a large number of gram-negative organisms such as *Escherichia coli, Proteus* spp. and *Pseudomonas aeruginosa* and has been widely used to treat resistant strains of these bacteria. It is quite toxic when used at high dosages for systemic therapy. It causes the binding of free calcium in the extracellular fluids and a marked increase in the excretion of calcium by the kidneys and thus hypocalcemia and tetany or neuromuscular paralysis. In addition it may cause hypotension, nephrotoxicity and ototoxicity. It can decrease the survival rate of animals suffering from severe endotoxemia.

Gentamicin is poorly absorbed from the gastrointestinal tract when given orally. Parenteral therapy requires IM administration, however the blood levels obtained from this route of administration are somewhat inconsistent.

Plasma antibiotic analyses are very helpful in gentamicin therapy. Levels of 10 to 12 mcg/ml tend to result in toxicity in the animal after extended usage, however levels of 5 to 7 mcg/ml appear to be required to obtain maximum therapeutic benefit. Gentamicin distributes well throughout the body; it is excreted largely in the urine. It crosses the placental barrier but does not reach high levels in the nervous tissue. Dogs and cats are given 2 mg/lb (4.4 mg/kg) IM or subcut. twice the first day and once daily thereafter. Gentamicin is available as an ophthalmic ointment, as an ophthalmic solution and as an injectable solution.

VIRGINIAMYCIN
("Stafac")

Virginiamycin is an antibiotic obtained from *Streptomyces virginiae.* It has a limited range of activity but it has been used to treat and control swine dysentery. It is prepared as a feed additive for mixing in the feed at 0.0025% for prevention, 0.005% for control, and 0.01% for treatment of outbreaks of swine dysentery.

TETRACYCLINE
("Achromycin")

This antibiotic is formed by chemical alterations of chlortetracycline. It is well absorbed after oral administration. Intramuscular injections of tetracycline in a propylene glycol vehicle may cause pain and swellings at the injection site. Tetracycline may be given

IV but caution is required to prevent an acute "speed shock" reaction. Following absorption, it is widely distributed in body fluids. Appreciable concentrations of the active form are excreted in urine and feces and, to some extent, in milk. Tetracycline produces a golden-yellow fluorescence of bone, visible under ultraviolet light. The significance of this in bone metabolism is not yet known, but faulty egg-shell formation, enamel hypoplasia of the teeth and inhibition of long-bone growth have been reported. The tetracyclines should be given with care to pregnant animals. It does not appear to delay fracture healing.

Tetracycline has a broad antibacterial spectrum, being effective against gram-positive and gram-negative bacteria and against certain rickettsiae and large viruses.

The toxicity of tetracycline is relatively low. However, following oral administration some dogs and cats may show nausea, vomiting and diarrhea. Oral dosage is not recommended for adult ruminants as the antibiotic is likely to affect the normal bacterial flora of the rumen. *See also* the caution regarding the use of oxytetracycline in the horse, p. 497.

Clinical Indications: Tetracycline is used for a wide variety of infections in large and small animals including: endometritis, pneumonia, tonsillitis, strangles in horses, foot rot in cattle, bacterial infections secondary to canine distemper and feline panleukopenia, bronchitis, pharyngitis, nephritis, calf scours, pyelonephritis, otitis externa and infected wounds.

Dosage: Orally, tetracycline is given to large animals at the rate of 5 to 10 mg/lb (11 to 22 mg/kg) daily in divided doses. The oral dose in small animals is much larger: 25 to 50 mg/lb (55 to 110 mg/kg) daily in divided dose. The dose is much reduced when the drug is given IV or IM, large animals receiving 2 to 5 mg/lb (4.5 to 11 mg/kg) and the small species 5 to 10 mg/lb (11 to 22 mg/kg) in divided doses.

Preparations: Tetracycline is prepared as boluses of 500 mg and capsules of 50, 100 and 250 mg for oral administration. It is also available as a soluble powder of the hydrochloride salt for the preparation of oral solutions, and sterile vials of 100 and 200 mg for making injectable solutions. A phosphate complex of tetracycline, reported to be more completely absorbed from the gastrointestinal tract, is also available.

CHLORTETRACYCLINE
("Aureomycin")

Chlortetracycline is produced from cultures of *Streptomyces aureofaciens*. It is available in the dry state as chlortetracycline hydrochloride, a yellow crystalline powder which is quite stable. It is well absorbed when administered orally and this route may be employed to obtain therapeutic blood levels, except in adult ruminants where it is likely to disturb the normal ruminal microflora. Chlortetracycline seems to be well distributed in the body. It crosses the placenta and attains levels in the fetal blood that are 50% of those observed in the maternal blood. It is excreted mainly in the urine and smaller amounts are eliminated in the feces. Studies in cattle have shown that appreciable amounts are excreted in the milk.

In experimental studies the toxicity of chlortetracycline is low, and there have been few clinical reports on serious toxic reactions in animals. In adult ruminants, high oral doses may produce digestive upset as the result of its effect on the bacterial flora in the rumen. Likewise, dogs and cats may show vomiting, diarrhea and anorexia when the antibiotic is given orally, especially when therapy is prolonged.

Clinical Indications: Chlortetracycline has a broad antibacterial spectrum and is active against many gram-positive and gram-negative bacteria as well as some large viruses and rickettsiae. It has been used to treat streptococcal and staphylococcal mastitis in cattle, but there are other antibiotics of equal or greater effectiveness for this purpose. Chlortetracycline is too irritating to be used for dry cow intramammary therapy. Other infections in cattle have been successfully treated with chlortetracycline; these include metritis, foot rot, shipping fever complex, sinusitis, pneumonia, calf scours, and necrotic laryngitis due to *Corynebacterium pyogenes* infections. Intra-uterine treatment has proved clinically successful in "repeat breeder" cows with subclinical metritis. The antibiotic may be of some value in treating listeriosis of cattle. Chlortetracycline causes a 30- to 60-day disappearance of transmissible anaplasmosis from the blood of carrier animals, and experimental infection can be prevented by feeding the antibiotic. Feeding low levels of chlortetracycline (75 mg/day) reduces the incidence of liver abscesses in feeder cattle.

In dogs, chlortetracycline has been used to treat tonsillitis, pharyngitis, pneumonia, urinary tract infections, coccidiosis and bacterial infections secondary to canine distemper. It may have some beneficial effect against *Leptospira icterohemorrhagiae*. In cats, the antibiotic is used to treat bacterial infections secondary to feline panleukopenia, infectious coryza and pneumonitis.

Several infections of horses—strangles, shipping fever, pneumonia and septicemia in newborn foals—respond to chlortetracycline, but see the caution regarding the use of oxytetracycline in horses, p. 497.

Enteric infections in swine may respond to chlortetracycline therapy; these include necrotic enteritis, salmonellosis and colibacillosis. The use of chlortetracycline at 0.005% in feed produced a marked decrease in the incidence of cervical abscesses in swine.

In poultry, chlortetracycline is of value in the control of infectious synovitis when given in feed at 0.01 to 0.02%. It is also of some benefit in the control of fowl typhoid and bluecomb disease. In pigeons, use of 0.89% of the antibiotic in feed for 30 days is reported to control ornithosis.

Local application of a 3% chlortetracycline ointment has been employed in treating external infections in dogs and cats, including otitis externa, conjunctivitis, blepharitis, keratitis, dermatitis and infected wounds. However, it would appear that 1% ointments and 0.5% buffered solutions are most satisfactory dispensing forms for ocular application by animal owners. Aqueous solutions of chlortetracycline are irritating if applied to wounds.

Dosage and Administration: For oral administration, chlortetracycline hydrochloride is employed in an initial dose of 10 to 25 mg/lb (22 to 55 mg/kg) followed b.i.d. by 5.0 to 12.5 mg/lb (11 to 27.5 mg/kg) body wt.

In the treatment of bovine mastitis, the usual dose by intramammary infusion is 200 to 400 mg every 24 to 48 hours. For this purpose, ointments are ordinarily employed.

Preparations: Chlortetracycline is available as: chlortetracycline hydrochloride capsules, 50 and 250 mg; chlortetracycline hydrochloride tablets, 50 and 250 mg; ophthalmic ointment, 10 mg/gm of base; and topical ointment, 3%. A calcium salt of chlortetracycline is also available for topical and oral administration.

OXYTETRACYCLINE
("Terramycin")

Oxytetracycline is derived from cultures of an actinomycete *Streptomyces rimosus*. In the dry form, crystalline oxytetracycline hydrochloride is quite stable at room temperature, but solutions are unstable and should be administered soon after preparation. A solution of oxytetracycline in propylene glycol is stable and has a good shelf-life.

Oxytetracycline is well absorbed in the gastrointestinal tract and from IM injections. In dogs, oral doses produce peak blood levels within 1 to 2 hours. Single IM injections in dogs result in peak blood levels within 15 to 30 minutes, with significant blood levels persisting for 8 to 12 hours. After absorption, oxytetracycline is well distributed in body tissues and fluids except cerebrospinal fluid. Relatively large amounts of oxytetracycline are excreted in the urine where it is concentrated and, after oral administration, significant amounts appear in the feces.

High levels of oxytetracycline administered orally to adult ruminants may disturb the normal rumen flora. Acute reactions and some deaths have been reported following parenteral administration in cattle. In dogs and cats, oral doses may cause vomiting and diarrhea, especially when therapy is prolonged. Severe tissue irritation occurs after IM injection of oxytetracycline in propylene glycol. Acute, sometimes fatal, enteritis has been reported in horses receiving high dosages of oxytetracycline and normal doses following surgical procedures.

Clinical Indications: In cattle, oxytetracycline is used by intramammary infusion to treat mastitis. Systemically, it has been used to treat a number of diseases including shipping fever, metritis, foot rot, calf scours, acute mastitis and anthrax. It may be used either IV or IM or by including small amounts in feed. In dogs and cats, the antibiotic is usually given orally; occasionally the IV route is employed. Several conditions in small animals show a favorable response to oxytetracycline therapy. These include bacterial infections secondary to canine distemper and feline panleukopenia, pneumonia, enteritis, endometritis and infections of the urinary tract.

Parenteral injections of oxytetracycline are useful in treating anthrax, strangles and pneumonia in horses. For treatment of fistulous withers, a combination of systemic and local therapy has been used. In sheep, diarrhea and enterotoxemia are reported to respond to oxytetracycline in the feed. It also has been used to treat necrotic enteritis, atrophic rhinitis and leptospirosis of swine. In the latter disease, levels of 0.05% in the feed are reported to eradicate shedding of *Leptospira* in urine and to reduce the incidence of abortions. *Eperythrozoon suis* responds to a single IM injection of 3 mg/lb (6.6 mg/kg) of body wt.

For poultry, oxytetracycline administered in feed is of value in the control of infectious synovitis, erysipelas and chronic respiratory disease. Generally, a level of 0.02% in the feed is required. Oxytetracycline in the feed has been used as a prophylactic against diseases of the newborn in several species, including pigs, calves, lambs and poultry.

Topically, oxytetracycline hydrochloride is used in combination with corticosteroids and other antibiotics for the treatment of infections of eyes, ears, skin and wounds.

Dosage and Administration: Oxytetracycline may be administered orally to all species of animals with the exception of adult ruminants, in which it can exert an unfavorable influence on the ruminal microflora. For oral administration, daily doses are recommended, which range from 5 to 10 mg/lb (11 to 22 mg/kg) body wt (livestock), and from 25 to 50 mg/lb (55 to 110 mg/kg) body wt (small animals), given in divided doses every 6 hours. For dogs and cats, the IM dose is 3 to 10 mg/lb (6.6 to 22 mg/kg) body wt daily. In large animals and poultry, the parenteral dosage is 2 to 5 mg/lb (4.4 to 11 mg/kg) body wt daily given IV, IM or subcut. and repeated at 24-hour intervals unless oral therapy is instituted.

Preparations: Oxytetracycline hydrochloride is available as: tablets for oral use in 50 mg and 125 mg; capsules for oral use in 125 mg and 250 mg; boluses for oral use in 250 mg; preconstituted parenteral solutions containing 50 mg/ml; soluble powder for oral use containing 25 gm/lb (55 gm/kg); ophthalmic ointment for topical use containing 5 mg/gm, aerosol spray for topical use containing 300 mg/2 fl oz (5 mg/ml); intramammary preparations containing 30 mg/gm; preparation for topical and intramammary use containing 200 mg/10 ml. **NB:** Some oxytetracycline preparations are irritating and should be used with caution.

ROLITETRACYCLINE
("Reverin")

Rolitetracycline or pyrrolidinomethyl tetracycline is a highly water soluble tetracycline with a spectrum of activity similar to that of oxytetracycline. The major advantage of rolitetracycline (suspension) is that it causes little or no irritation when injected and is very rapidly absorbed from the IM injection site. The distribution and toxic effects of rolitetracycline throughout the body is similar to the other tetracyclines; however because of its very rapid uptake from the IM injection site it tends to be excreted from the body more rapidly. It is available as an IM injectable suspension for large and small animals. The dose is 2 to 5 mg/lb (4.4 to 11 mg/kg) 2 or 3 times daily.

CHLORAMPHENICOL
("Chloromycetin")

Chloramphenicol is produced by *Streptomyces venezuelae* and is also prepared by chemical synthesis. It is a broad-spectrum antibiotic, being effective against gram-positive and gram-negative bacteria and certain rickettsiae and large viruses. It is well absorbed from the gastrointestinal tract and, in dogs, therapeutic blood levels may be obtained by this route. Peak blood levels are obtained in 2 to 4 hours. High levels of the antibiotic are found in the kidney, bile and liver of the dog. Progressively lower concentrations are found in the lung, spleen, heart muscle and brain. The levels found in the fetal blood are nearly as high as in the maternal blood. Although only small amounts of the active compound are excreted in the urine, this may still provide a sufficient concentration for antimicrobial activity in the urinary tract.

Daily doses of 200 mg/lb (440 mg/kg) of body wt have been administered orally to dogs without causing undesirable effects. Other studies in dogs indicate that oral doses of up to 50 mg/lb (110 mg/kg) of body wt given twice daily for periods up to 133 days do not cause significant alterations in hemoglobin levels or red or white blood cell counts. Depression of bone marrow activity has been reported in the cat and dog receiving large doses of chloramphenicol. Very young animals may be more susceptible.

Clinical Indications: In dogs and cats, chloramphenicol is effective in pneumonia, metritis, cystitis, nephritis and bacterial infections secondary to canine distemper and feline panleukopenia. In dogs, infectious enteritis (*Escherichia coli* or *Proteus* organisms) responds to chloramphenicol either alone or in combination with dihydrostreptomycin. Limited studies indicate that it is effective against infectious bronchitis, or so-called "kennel cough," and in salmon poisoning in dogs. In the conditions described above, chloramphenicol was administered orally or IM.

Few reports have appeared on the use of chloramphenicol in large animals. In calves oral administration has been employed in colibacillosis and in limited experimental trials it was found to be of value for treatment of contagious bovine pleuropneumonia due to *Mycoplasma mycoides*. Intravenous use of chloramphenicol has been shown not to produce therapeutic levels in the horse and only under special conditions of very high dosage in the cow. The half-life in the horse is very short, but clinicians continue to report favorable response to therapy in this species.

Local application of chloramphenicol in the form of ophthalmic ointments or ophthalmic solution has been found to be effective in certain ocular infections. These include corneal ulcers and abrasions, keratitis, conjunctivitis and iritis. Ointments may be applied every 3 hours, while solutions require more frequent application (usually every waking hour for the first day and every 2 to 3 hours thereafter). In some cases, oral medication can also increase concentrations of chloramphenicol in the ocular fluids.

Dosage and Administration: In dogs and cats, oral administration appears to be satisfactory using 25 to 75 mg/lb (55 to 165 mg/kg) of body wt given daily in 4 divided doses. Intramuscularly, it has been used for these animals in a dose of 10 to 15 mg/lb (22 to 33 mg/kg) of body wt at 8-hour intervals. For colts and calves, the daily oral dose is 1 to 2 gm, while for lambs 500 mg daily has been employed.

Preparations: Chloramphenicol is supplied in capsules containing 50, 100 or 250 mg. An ophthalmic ointment and powder for preparing solutions as well as a special preparation for IM administration also are available.

BACITRACIN

Bacitracin is obtained from cultures of *Bacillus subtilis*. In the dry state, it is stable except at high temperatures. In solution at room temperature, it is relatively unstable, but, if kept refrigerated no significant loss of potency is noted for approximately 3 weeks. In the form of an anhydrous ointment, it is stable for periods of a year or longer.

Bacitracin is very poorly absorbed after oral administration. Apparently, large amounts of bacitracin are destroyed in the gastrointestinal tract, and only a portion of that given orally can be recovered in the feces. Experimental studies showed that bacitracin was likely to produce renal toxic effects when administered parenterally and, therefore, its use by injection is not recommended. In man, it is used for topical application. Bacitracin is a common feed additive used to prevent enteric disease and to cause increased rates of growth.

Clinical Indications: Bacitracin, like penicillin, is mainly effective against gram-positive organisms. Some organisms that are resistant to penicillin are sensitive to bacitracin and the reverse also is true.

Bacitracin has been employed in a solution by intramammary infusion for treating cases of bovine mastitis due to *Streptococcus agalactiae*. In general, results were as satisfactory as those obtained with penicillin or sulfonamides.

Bacitracin is useful when applied topically in such conditions as infected wounds, otitis externa and conjunctivitis in dogs. Ointments containing 500 u of bacitracin per gram or solutions containing 500 u/ml have been employed. Abscesses may be injected directly with 0.2 to 5.0 ml of the solution. Infectious keratitis in cattle is reported to respond to treatment with an ointment of the above concentrations.

Preparations: Bacitracin is available as tablets as a feed additive and as topical and ophthalmic ointments containing 500 u/gm as ointment base. Ointments containing a combination of bacitracin and other antibiotics also may be obtained.

TYROTHRICIN

Tyrothricin is produced by cultures of *Bacillus brevis*. It is composed of a mixture of several substances, of which **gramicidin** and **tyrocidine** are present in the greatest quantities. Tyrothricin is relatively insoluble in water, but is soluble in alcohol and propylene glycol. Unlike the majority of antibiotics, it is stable under most conditions.

Clinical Indications: Tyrothricin is effective against gram-positive organisms, but its activity against gram-negative bacteria is low.

Little or no absorption of tyrothricin occurs after oral administration and since it is quite toxic when injected parenterally, it is recommended only for topical use.

Tyrothricin is used in the treatment of bovine mastitis due to *Streptococcus agalactiae*, but generally it is irritant to udder tissue. The average dose of 20 mg per quarter is infused, in an aqueous or oily vehicle, into dry cows only—but other more effective products are available for this purpose.

Tyrothricin in the form of a 0.5% ointment or as a solution has been employed in treating infected wounds and for irrigation of osteomyelitic lesions in bone. Wound exudate and tissue debris do not markedly inhibit its antibacterial action. Endometritis of cattle responds to irrigation of the uterus with aqueous or oily solutions containing 2 mg of the drug per milliliter. Repeated treatment may be necessary. For topical therapy, tyrothricin may be combined with other antibiotics or sulfonamides.

Preparations: Tyrothricin is available in aqueous alcoholic solution, emulsion, ointment and cream.

POLYMYXIN

Polymyxin is produced by cultures of *Bacillus polymyxa* (*asterosporus*). Several polymyxins are identified as A, B, C, D and E. **Polymyxin B** has the most desirable therapeutic characteristics and is said to be least toxic. Polymyxin B sulfate is the form ordinarily employed. It is readily soluble in water and solutions remain stable for periods of approximately 2 months if kept under refrigeration.

After oral administration, large amounts of polymyxin appear in the feces and there is little absorption from the gastrointestinal tract. Following IM injection, the antibiotic is rapidly absorbed. In horses severe inflammatory reactions may occur at the site of IM injections. Polymyxin B is prone to cause nephrotoxicity when administered parenterally and must be used at low levels (e.g. 1 mg/lb [2 mg/kg] body wt IM daily).

Polymyxin B is effective against a large number of gram-negative bacteria and its action is accompanied by the development of little bacterial resistance. It is notably effective against many strains of *Pseudomonas aeruginosa*.

Clinical Indications: Initially, polymyxin was recommended for topical use only. However, recent studies report its parenteral use in combination with neomycin. Polymyxin B should be used only in conditions where it is essential; other less toxic alternatives are usually available. The fact that polymyxin B is excreted mainly in the kidney gives this drug usefulness in treating urinary tract infections. For large animals, the recommended dose is 100,000 to 200,000 u/100lb (2,200 to 4,400 u/kg) body wt b.i.d. and for dogs a total dose of 50,000 to 100,000 u. Both polymyxin and neomycin may produce nephrotoxic effects and therefore they should be used parenterally with caution.

Topically, polymyxin, either alone or combined with other antibacterial agents, such as bacitracin and neomycin, is used for treatment of infections of the skin, ear and eye.

Preparations: Polymyxin is available in a sterile parenteral solution containing 100,000 u of polymyxin B sulfate and 100 mg neomycin sulfate per ml. Various types of ointments, tablets and solutions for local use are also available.

ERYTHROMYCIN

("Ilotycin," "Gallimycin")

Erythromycin is produced by cultures of *Streptomyces erythraeus*. It is poorly soluble in water, but readily soluble in alcohol and alcoholic solutions may be further diluted with water. Solutions are stable at room temperature for approximately 24 hours.

Experimental studies on dogs and cats have shown that erythromycin is rapidly absorbed after oral administration and the unmetabolized portion is rapidly excreted in the urine. In dogs, the antibiotic crosses the blood-brain barrier and enters the cerebrospinal fluid in very small amounts. Oral doses of 25 mg/lb (55 mg/kg) body wt have been administered to dogs and cats for periods up to 3 months without producing toxic signs or changes in the formed elements of the blood. A dose of 25 mg erythromycin given IM during the first 24 hours of life is reported to reduce the incidence of, and mortality due to, infectious diarrhea in pigs. Doses of 10 mg/lb (22 mg/kg) daily have been used to treat the condition.

Erythromycin base is readily destroyed by the acid of gastric juice. For this reason, enteric-coated tablets are preferred for oral administration. The consequent delay in absorption may be corrected somewhat by the use of one of its salts such as the propionate.

Like penicillin, erythromycin is primarily active against gram-positive organisms. Bacterial resistance (but not cross resistance to penicillin) is developed relatively quickly. It has a narrow spectrum of activity and is useful against a limited number of conditions (e.g. *Corynebacterium renale, Erysipelothrix rhusiopathiae, Pasteurella multocida*).

Clinical Indications: Erythromycin has been employed in dogs to treat such conditions as secondary bacterial infections of distemper, pneumonia, pharyngitis, urinary tract infections, enteritis, tonsillitis and otitis. In these cases, the antibiotic was administered orally in daily doses of 300 to 600 mg. These amounts are ordinarily divided into 3 to 4 fractional doses.

Preparations: Erythromycin, either as the base or in the form of one of several salts, is available as 100- and 250-mg tablets, as an oral suspension (100 mg of antibiotic in each 5 ml) and as 1% ointment. Combinations of erythromycin and other antibiotics and sulfonamides are also available.

NOVOBIOCIN
("Albamycin," "Cathomycin")

Novobiocin is derived from *Streptomyces spheroides.* It is freely soluble in water, and solutions are stable when refrigerated. The antibiotic is well absorbed when given orally or IM, and peak blood levels are obtained in dogs within 2 to 4 hours. High levels are still present 12 hours later. Following absorption, it is well distributed in most body fluids, but does not readily enter cerebrospinal fluid. Novobiocin is excreted primarily in the feces; only low levels appear in the urine.

Novobiocin is effective chiefly against the same gram-positive bacteria that are sensitive to penicillin, although a few *Proteus* and *Pseudomonas* organisms are sensitive to novobiocin. It is reported to be especially active against staphylococci even if these are resistant to penicillin. Novobiocin has been implicated in skin rash hypersensitivity conditions and in blood dyscrasias and gastrointestinal upsets.

Clinical Indications: Novobiocin has been used for the treatment of a variety of infections in dogs and cats. These include bronchitis, cystitis, metritis, nephritis, pharyngitis, peritonitis, tonsillitis, staphylococcal skin infections, pneumonia and bacterial infections secondary to canine distemper and feline panleukopenia. In cattle, the antibiotic has been used for treatment of pneumonia, metritis and mastitis. In chickens, it is reported to be of value in treating staphylococcal synovitis. It is also of value when a penicillin-resistant pathogen is encountered.

Dosage: In dogs and cats, novobiocin is given orally in a daily dose of 10 to 15 mg/lb (22 to 33 mg/kg) of body wt and IM and IV at the rate of 2 to 7 mg/lb (4.5 to 15 mg/kg) of body wt. For cattle, the IM and IV dose is 1 to 3 mg/lb (2.2 to 6.6 mg/kg) of body wt daily. In all instances, the daily dose is given in 2 equal parts.

Preparations: Novobiocin is available in 250-mg capsules, as an oral syrup (25 mg/ml) and as a sterile powder for parenteral use. Combinations with other antibiotics are also available.

OLEANDOMYCIN

This antibiotic is produced by *Streptomyces antibioticus* and is primarily effective against gram-positive bacteria. For parenteral administration, it is used as the phosphate salt, and for oral use triacetyl oleandomycin gives best results. After IM or oral administration, peak blood levels are observed within 3 hours and maintained for 4 to 6 hours.

Oleandomycin has been used to treat staphylococcal and streptococcal infections such as acne, furunculosis and deep pyodermas in dogs. The phosphate salt may be given in daily IV doses of 250 mg for 7 days, or triacetyl oleandomycin may be used orally in a dose of 250 mg twice daily for 10 to 14 days. In pigs, the antibiotic is reported to increase weight gains and feed efficiency when supplied at 0.002% in the feed.

TYLOSIN

Tylosin is produced by *Streptomycetes fradiae* and is mainly effective against gram-positive organisms, but some gram-negative bacteria, spirochetes, certain vibrios and PPLO (*Mycoplasma*) are also susceptible. It may be given orally or parenterally, usually as the tartrate salt.

In swine dysentery the antibiotic has produced good results and is one of the drugs of choice when given in a dose of 200 mg IM followed by 0.004% to 0.01% in the feed or when supplied initially in drinking water (1 gm/gal [0.25 gm/L]) for 48 hours and then in feed. Tylosin is effective in treating infectious sinusitis due to *Mycoplasma gallisepticum* in turkeys when injected into sinuses in a dose of 1 to 6 mg or when given parenterally or in drinking water. It is also effective in the treatment of calf pneumonia, swine pneumonia and mycoplasma mastitis in cattle.

CEPHALOSPORINS

The cephalosporins are obtained from *Cephalosporium acremontum*. The semi-synthetic derivatives of cephalosporin C are clinically important. They resemble penicillin in their mechanism of action, but are acid stable and penicillinase resistant. Bacteria that are resistant to penicillin G are frequently also resistant to the cephalosporins. The cephalosporins are active against a wide range of gram-positive and gram-negative bacteria. Their major usage is in infections of the urinary tract, and the ear, and of bone and soft tissue, particularly as a second line drug to treat specific susceptible infections. Cephaloridine has been incriminated as a cause of nephrotoxicity.

The cephalosporins may be dived into oral compounds, e.g. cephalexin monohydrate and parenteral compounds, e.g. cephaloridine, cephalothin sodium. Cephalexin (Kelfex) is available as an oral tablet and capsule. Cephalothin sodium (Keflin) and cephaloridine (Loridine) are available as injectable water soluble powders.

NITROFURAN THERAPY

Caution: ***In all drug therapy it is important to adhere to local laws and regulations governing the use of such products.***

The nitrofurans are a group of synthetic antimicrobial compounds, chemically based upon the furan ring to which a 5-nitro group has been added. The nitrofurans are effective against many gram-positive and gram-negative bacteria; certain nitrofurans are also active against protozoa, fungi and some large viruses. They are more bactericidal than bacteriostatic, acting as inhibitors of the carbohydrate metabolism of the bacterial cell. At therapeutic concentrations they do not interfere with phagocytosis; most are less effective in the presence of blood, serum, pus and milk.

Nitrofurans have a low tissue toxicity. Their prolonged use may lead to a few side effects—such as gastrointestinal irritation or depressed weight gain; depressed spermatogenesis has also been reported. Acute toxicity with excitation, convulsions and death occurs when excessive dose levels are used in calves and pigs. Granulocytopenia with death from secondary enteritis, pneumonia and septicemia occurs in calves fed low levels of furazolidone for several weeks. Clinically, only negligible resistance to nitrofurans has been recognized, except in coccidiosis.

In employing the nitrofurans as therapeutic agents, it is important to select the drug most suitable for the infection being treated. The use of nitrofurans has been markedly reduced in a number of jurisdictions due to their potential as carcinogens, e.g. they can no longer be used for intramammary therapy in dairy cows in Canada.

NITROFURAZONE
("Furacin")

Nitrofurazone possesses *in vitro* activity against a wide range of organisms including gram-negative (*Aerobacter aerogenes*, *Brucella* spp., *Escherichia coli*, pasteurellae, salmonellae, vibrios, and some strains of *Proteus* and *Pseudomonas*) and gram-positive pathogens (clostridia, corynebacteria, staphylococci, streptococci and diplococci).

In various dosage forms, nitrofurazone as a topical agent is effective against bacterial infections of surface lesions of the skin, eye, udder and genital tract. It is useful in infectious enteritis in large and small animals and in canine and avian coccidiosis.

The topical preparations of nitrofurazone are applied as a 0.2% ointment directly on the lesion or on gauze, several times daily, or left beneath an occlusive dressing for at least 24 hours. The drug does not penetrate intact skin in therapeutic amounts. Solutions of the same concentration are given (50 to 150 ml) by intra-uterine infusion in genital infections. Nitrofurazone is incorporated with urea in bolus form for the control of postpartum infections.

A suspension containing 2% nitrofurazone and procaine penicillin G is used in treating topical bacterial infections of domestic farm animals as well as dogs and cats.

Nitrofurazone is also available in a 4.59% water soluble powder for use in infectious necrotic enteritis of swine, for the control of outbreaks of cecal and intestinal coccidiosis (due to *Eimeria tenella* and *E. necatrix*) of chickens and in gray diarrhea of mink. The rate of administration in enteritis and coccidiosis is 330 gm (15 gm active nitrofurazone) of the powder in 36 and 50 gal. (135 and 190 L) of drinking water, respectively. For mink, 330 gm (15 gm active nitrofurazone) of the powder is added to every 150 lb (70 kg) of feed. It is given for 1 to 3 weeks. Aqueous solutions of this preparation will deteriorate if allowed to remain in continuous contact with metal for over 7 days.

Nitrofurazone is available in a number of other formulations for topical or oral use in skin, eye or ear infections, and in genital or gastrointestinal infections. In addition, water soluble nitrofurazone can be used to treat enteritis caused by *Salmonella* spp. in chickens, swine and mink.

NITROFURANTOIN
("Furadantin")

Nitrofurantoin is rapidly and nearly completely absorbed from the gastrointestinal tract. The antibacterial spectrum covers most urinary tract pathogens, including many strains of *Proteus* and *Aerobacter*. The drug is useful in the treatment of epidemic tracheobronchitis (kennel cough) in dogs, however its main use is for urinary tract infections in this species. After oral administration, approximately 45% of the dose appears in the urine; it is supposed that its solubility eliminates the danger of crystalluria. Nitrofurantoin is given 3 times a day at the rate of 2 mg/lb (4.4 mg/kg) body wt for 4 to 7 days or longer. It should be given with caution in the presence of renal impairment. It is available as a suspension and as tablets. Common adverse reactions are nausea, vomiting and gastritis.

FURAZOLIDONE
("Furoxone")

Furazolidone is an effective antimicrobial agent for a number of poultry diseases including: coccidiosis, fowl typhoid, pullorum disease, histomoniasis, hexamitiasis, synovitis, and certain susceptible secondary bacterial infections associated with the chronic respiratory disease complex (CRD) and nonspecific enteritis. Furazolidone improves the efficiency of feed utilization in poultry. It is effective in the treatment of bacterial enteritis and infectious hemorrhagic enteritis of swine, and enteritis and *Pasteurella* pneumonia of rabbits as well as gray diarrhea in mink. Furazolidone is available as

11% and 22% premixes. It is also prepared as a 25% dust for aerosol administration in treating CRD and as an oral liquid suspension (100 mg/ml) for treating bacterial enteritis (colibacillosis or white scours) in baby pigs.

Continual treatment in poultry and large animals may give rise to resistant strains of *Salmonella* spp. and coccidia.

METABOLIC DISTURBANCES

KETOSIS IN CATTLE

(Acetonemia)

A metabolic disease of lactating cows occurring within a few days to a few weeks after calving. It is characterized by hypoglycemia, ketonemia, ketonuria, inappetence, either lethargy or high excitability, loss of weight, depressed milk production and occasionally incoordination. In most areas, the incidence is highest in high-producing cows which are being stall-fed.

Etiology: Any factor that causes a reduction in the intake or absorption of dietary carbohydrate precursors can cause primary ketosis. Although theoretically factors that affect the metabolism of absorbed carbohydrates may similarly cause hypoglycemia and primary ketosis, no such factors have been identified. In particular, the claim that a primary cause of ketosis is dysfunction of the adrenal cortex has not been substantiated. Secondary ketosis is commonly caused by a depression of appetite resulting from a primary disease such as metritis, mastitis, traumatic reticulitis or abomasal displacement.

The carbohydrate deficiency hypothesis is based on the observation that, of the various forms of carbohydrate ingested by the ruminant, little is absorbed as glucose. The animal's principal sources of energy are the acetic, propionic and butyric acids arising from microbial fermentation in the rumen; of these 3, propionic acid is generally accepted as the major carbohydrate precursor and the only one having antiketogenic properties. If this is so, the lactating cow receives little or no surplus of carbohydrate beyond that required for the synthesis of the lactose secreted in the milk. An inadequate caloric intake can occur when the food is insufficient or unpalatable or when the balance of ketogenic and antiketogenic substances in the diet is disturbed, e.g. by the feeding of certain silages. The composition of the diet can similarly modify the microbial population of the rumen, and thus influence the relative proportions of the volatile fatty acids produced by fermentation. If the predisposition is to the production of ketogenic VFAs, ketosis is to be expected as a sequela.

In dairy cows a good deal of the etiologic pressure for ketosis derives from the demands for glucose of the cow's metabolic system to provide for lactose production in a profusely lactating mammary gland. If the demand for a direct supply of glucose for tissues cannot be met from the hepatic stores of glycogen, tissues are raided for fat and protein whose metabolism promotes ketogenesis.

Clinical Findings: The signs of ketosis usually appear a few days to a few weeks after calving. They include inappetence, constipation, mucus-covered feces, depression, a staring expression, a very obvious loss of weight, a drop in milk production and a humped back posture suggestive of mild abdominal pain. Most cases are of this wasting, lethargic type but a few show signs of frenzy as though the cow is drunk. Clinical signs include circling, staggering, licking, chewing, bellowing, hyperesthesia, compulsive walking and head pressing. These occur in episodes that last for about an hour and recur at intervals. There is an acetone odor on the breath. Hypoglycemia, ketonuria and ketonemia are always present.

Lesions: There are no specific postmortem lesions.

Diagnosis: While a negative urine or milk test (Rothera's or Acetest) will rule out ketosis, the mere presence of hypoglycemia, ketonemia and ketonuria is not sufficient for a positive diagnosis of ketosis. Any abnormality, such as metritis, pneumonia, traumatic gastritis or mastitis, that causes a cow to go off feed, will produce some degree of secondary or fasting ketosis. Such conditions, of course, may accompany the pure ketotic syndrome. One of the commonest causes of secondary ketosis is left abomasal displacement (q.v., p. 148). In secondary ketosis the positive reaction to Acetest tablets by urine is often neither as rapid nor as severe as in the primary disease. Sometimes, it is advisable to reserve judgment until the response to treatment has been observed. Failure to get a definite and continuing response to glucose or hormone therapy is cause for reconsideration of the signs and possible complications.

Prophylaxis: Animals susceptible to ketosis should be maintained on a relatively high-energy intake before calving, and the level should be increased substantially after parturition. A good guide to optimum feeding is the cow's bodily condition which must be maintained to avoid being overfat or overthin. The protein content of the ration should be moderate only, about 16%, and the concentrate fed to stall-fed cows should aim to about 3 kg/kg of milk produced.

Daily intake of hay to maintain body condition should be of the order of 3 kg hay per 100 kg of body weight. The roughage must be of good quality, palatable, digestible, and nutritious. Wet silage and moldy dusty hay are common precursors to acetonemia in high producing cows. Rations which induce a high production of propionic acid in the rumen may contribute materially to the prevention of ketosis when fed for a few weeks before and after calving. For example, a ration of finely ground and pelleted alfalfa hay plus a steam-heated cereal (flaked corn, barley, etc.), in which the ratio of hay to steamed cereal may be as great as 8:1, effects a high production of propionic acid. For this ration to be effective, the animal must not have access to long hay, straw, shavings or other unground roughage. When large amounts of silage are being fed, its replacement by hay may be advantageous. Addition of sodium propionate (℞ 671) to the feed will reduce the incidence.

Treatment: In thin cows that have been obviously undernourished replacement of carbohydrate is recommended. In fat cows where nutritional imbalance is more likely to be the cause, glucocorticoids are as effective. The IV injection of glucose (℞ 585) is not sufficiently effective, even when repeated daily for 3 to 4 days, to be recommended as a sole form of treatment. However, it is commonly used as an adjunct to either the injection of glucocorticoids (℞ 162, 154) or the oral administration of propylene glycol (℞ 669). An injection of glucose results in a prompt increase in blood sugar that is followed by a decrease within the next several hours to a value usually below normal, but still greater than the pretreatment level;

the blood sugar may not return to normal for several days, even in cows that show a good response.

Following the IM injection of glucocorticoids, blood glucose usually returns to normal within 8 to 10 hours and may rise to a value considerably above normal within 24 hours, especially when the cause is inadequate calorie intake. In such cases a marked improvement in appetite and general behavior usually occurs within 24 hours and a return to normal blood ketone levels by the third to fifth day. Milk production increases rapidly by the second to third day after treatment. Anabolic steroids are currently being used as treatment but no overall recommendation can yet be made.

Sodium propionate (℞ 671), propylene glycol (℞ 669), or lactate mixtures (℞ 610) given orally will bring a recovery in many cases. Compared with other treatments, however, the response is slower and treatment must be extended over a longer period. These substances appear to be of greatest value when used as supportive treatment following the use of glucocorticoids or glucose. Sodium acetate given orally is less effective. Chloral hydrate (℞ 548) sometimes is used in conjunction with other treatments and is especially helpful if hyperexcitability is exhibited. When the appetite has recovered, following any of the above treatments, good feeding is required to restore the animal to full health and production.

Since it is often difficult to distinguish between primary and secondary ketosis, when the patient exhibits signs of other disease conditions, it is advisable to treat both for ketosis and the complicating condition.

PREGNANCY TOXEMIA IN CATTLE

(Fat Cow Ketosis, Fat Cow Syndrome)

A sporadic disease that occurs most commonly in cows that have become fat because of heavy feeding in early pregnancy, but which suffer a severe nutritional stress during the 2 months before calving. Morbidity is low, being highest when pastured cattle run out of natural feed and are not supplemented. When the disease is observable clinically it is usually far advanced and treatment at this stage is unrewarding; the mortality is virtually 100%.

Affected cows are invariably fat, completely anorectic and in the last stages of pregnancy. There is a transitory period of restlessness and incoordination, the pulse is small and fast, and droppings are small and firm. Sternal recumbency follows; there is a greater than normal clear nasal discharge, the skin on the muzzle is dry, cracked, and may peel off; the respiration is rapid and grunting. The cow's condition remains unchanged for 7 to 10 days. Terminally the feces become soft, smelly and orange, but still small in volume; the cow becomes comatose and dies quietly.

Clinical pathologic examination shows marked ketonemia and

ketonuria, hypoglycemia and proteinuria. The hepatic enzyme levels in serum are raised and terminally the blood glucose levels are often raised to high levels. At necropsy there is gross enlargement of the liver which is also obviously fatty. Ostertagiasis is often a significant concurrent disease and the abomasal mucosa may be obviously abnormal.

Treatment is generally ineffective, especially if the cows are already recumbent. Anabolic steroids have the best reputation, and supportive therapy with glucose, fluids and electrolytes IV, and propylene glycol, fluids and electrolytes orally, is recommended.

Prevention is more satisfying but it is the exploitative nature of the pastoral beef cattle enterprise that promotes the occurrence of the disease and largely precludes supplementary feeding.

PREGNANCY TOXEMIA IN EWES

(Pregnancy disease, Lambing paralysis,
Twin-lamb disease, Ketosis)

A disease of preparturient ewes, primarily characterized clinically by impaired nervous function.

Etiology: The primary predisposing cause is undernutrition in late pregnancy, with overfed ewes carrying twins or triplets being more susceptible than ewes in poor condition and those carrying single lambs.

Anything such as storms, transport or other disease conditions that interrupts feed intake may induce the disease. The primary lesion is a hypoglycemic encephalopathy, the result of inability of the ewe to supply sufficient glucose from products of digestion or catabolized tissues to meet the carbohydrate demands of large multiple fetuses and the ewe. The defect appears to be in maintenance of the blood glucose level since utilization of available glucose is unimpaired. As the disease progresses, severe ketosis and acidosis may develop, together with hepatic, renal and possibly endocrine disorders. The blood sugar may rise without alleviating the signs of encephalopathy. At this stage the ewe is refractory to treatment.

Clinical Findings: Early clinical signs may be erratic and difficult to detect. The usual course, lasting 2 to 5 days includes listlessness, inappetence, aimless walking, "propping" against any kind of obstruction, twitching of the muscles of the ears, around the eyes and perhaps of other parts, unusual postures, grinding of the teeth, progressive loss of reflexes, blindness, ataxia and finally sternal decubitus, coma and death.

Laboratory tests usually reveal hypoglycemia early, with normoglycemia or hyperglycemia later, and hyperketonemia. Acidosis and high blood NPN are variable concomitants. Necropsy findings include fatty livers, indistinguishable from those found sometimes in apparently healthy ewes underfed near term. The adrenal glands may be swollen, hyperemic or grayish. The pulmonary changes are associated with recumbency.

Diagnosis: Acute hypocalcemia before lambing offers the main problem in differential diagnosis. In this, the course is shorter (deaths occur within 24 hours), and there is usually a marked, immediate and persistent response to IV calcium therapy.

Prophylaxis: Obesity should be prevented in early pregnancy and adequate good feed supplied during the last 6 weeks of pregnancy. Feed supplementation depends on the condition of the pastures and the weight of the ewes. Where the pastures become poor, heavy feeding may be necessary. If adequate and suitable feed is not available for the whole flock during late pregnancy, early cases can be identified by gentle driving. These can be separated from the flock and given special care and nourishment. Any interruption of feed intake should, if possible, be avoided.

Where the disease is occurring in fat ewes on good pastures, perhaps associated with mild foot conditions, gentle driving for 30 minutes may prevent incipient cases from developing through elevating the blood glucose for a period.

Treatment: Once the advanced signs have developed, no treatment is effective. Mortality of untreated cases is about 80%. With early diagnosis, such as may be made by gentle driving of the flock, particularly where the disease has been induced by relatively sudden fasting, the glucogenic materials, glycerol or propylene glycol, given orally (4 oz [120 ml] b.i.d.) decrease the mortality. Glucose therapy is ineffective because the effect is transient, and insulin is contraindicated. ACTH and glucocorticoids are probably only effective through increasing blood sugar. Cesarean section early in the course of the disease usually leads to recovery and, if near term, the offspring may be saved. Palatable feed and water and protection from extremes of weather should be provided. Twice daily force-feeding with finely ground dried grass given by stomach tube may be a worthwhile practice with specially valuable animals, treatment being continued until the appetite returns.

PARTURIENT PARESIS IN COWS

(Milk fever)

An afebrile disease, occurring most commonly at or soon after parturition, manifested by circulatory collapse, generalized paresis and depression of consciousness.

Etiology: Although the exact cause of this disease is unknown, it is usually associated with the sudden onset of profuse lactation in mature cows. The most obvious and consistent abnormality displayed is an acute hypocalcemia in which the serum calcium level drops from a normal of about 10 mg% to levels of 3 to 7 mg% with an average of 5 mg%. Signs usually appear when the serum calcium falls to 7 mg% or lower. Serum magnesium levels may be elevated or depressed and influence the clinical picture observed, low levels being accompanied by tetany and high levels by a flaccid paralysis and somnolence. The disease may occur in cows of any age but is most common in dairy cows 5 to 9 years old. There seems to be higher incidence in the Jersey breed.

Clinical Findings: Parturient paresis usually occurs within 72 hours after parturition, but occasionally before, during, or even some months thereafter. The disease is sometimes the cause of dystocia arising from inadequate expulsive efforts.

Early in the onset, the cow may exhibit some unsteadiness as she walks. More frequently, the cow is found lying on her sternum with her head displaced to one side, causing a kink in the neck, or turned into the flank. The eyes are dull and staring and the pupils dilated. Anorexia is complete, the muzzle tends to be dry and the extremities are cool. The pulse rate usually is 50 to 85/min, and the temperature normal or subnormal. The digestive tract is atonic with suppressed defecation and a relaxed anus. If treatment is delayed many hours, the dullness gives way to coma, which becomes progressively deeper, leading to death. With approaching coma, the animal assumes lateral recumbency, which predisposes to bloating, regurgitation and aspiration pneumonia. Treatment in the early stages is always more successful and fewer relapses occur. Those cases that occur at or within a few hours of parturition appear to develop more rapidly and be more severe than those that develop at other times. Diseases that may be confused with parturient paresis are: metritis, ketosis, mastitis, grass tetany, acute indigestion, traumatic gastritis, coxofemoral luxations, obturator paralysis, lymphosarcoma, spinal compression and fracture of the pelvis. Some of these diseases and, in addition, aspiration pneumonia and degenerative myopathy, may also occur as complications.

Prophylaxis: The feeding of high-phosphorus, low-calcium diets during late pregnancy helps to prevent parturient paresis, but such rations are difficult to devise in a practical form and, if continued for long periods in heavy-milking cows, may result in dangerous depletion of skeletal mineral reserves. Delayed or incomplete milking after calving, by maintaining pressure within the udder, is of doubtful value in reducing the number of attacks and may aggravate a latent infection into acute clinical mastitis. Massive doses of vitamin

D (20 to 30 million units daily), given in the feed for 5 to 7 days before parturition, will reduce the incidence, but if administration is stopped more than 4 days before calving, the cow is more susceptible. Dosing for periods longer than those recommended should be avoided because of the danger of toxicity. A single IV or subcut. injection of 10 million units of crystalline vitamin D given 8 days before calving is an effective preventive. The dose is repeated if the cow does not calve on the due date. New compounds used in lieu of vitamin D are 25-hydroxycholecalciferol and 1α-hydroxycholecalciferol. After calving, a diet high in calcium is required. It is now a common practice to administer large doses of calcium in gel form by mouth right after calving to ensure a high intake of calcium. Doses of 150 gm of calcium are given one day before, at, and one day after calving.

Treatment: Effort is directed toward returning the serum calcium level to the normal range and must be carried out at the earliest possible opportunity to avoid the occurrence of muscular and nervous damage, and of downer cows q.v., p. 516. This is facilitated by maintaining close surveillance over cows that have calved in the preceding 72 hours. Calcium borogluconate is most commonly used (℞ 607). Preferably it is injected IV but the subcut. and IP routes are also used. Subcut. administration permits slow absorption of the calcium ion and may lessen the danger of cardiac arrest. Strict asepsis and limitation of the volume injected at one site to about 50 ml reduce the chances of local reactions. Animals that relapse or fail to get up after 8 to 12 hours should be re-treated.

In those cases in which there is an accompanying hypomagnesemia, response is better if magnesium (℞ 608) is added to the injectable calcium preparation. In cases complicated by ketosis 250 to 500 ml of 50% dextrose should be given IV. In the absence of blood analysis it is often impossible to decide which element is low, and in the field it is a common practice to treat unresponsive cows with one of a variety of commercial preparations containing not only calcium and magnesium but also glucose and phosphorus.

In the few cases in which there is failure to respond to any other treatment, the udder may be inflated. Each quarter is inflated through a sterile teat tube until firm and, if necessary, the teats are gently tied with gauze to prevent escape of the air. The gauze is removed after 3 to 4 hours and the udder is partially milked out. If necessary, inflation may be repeated 6 to 8 hours later.

PARTURIENT PARESIS IN EWES

A disturbance of metabolism in pregnant and lactating ewes characterized by acute hypocalcemia and the rapid development of hyperexcitability, ataxia, paresis, coma and death.

Etiology: The exact cause is unknown, but the conditions under which field outbreaks take place are fairly well defined. The disease occurs at any time from 6 weeks before to 10 weeks after lambing, principally in highly conditioned older ewes at pasture. The onset is sudden and almost invariably follows—within 24 hours—an abrupt changing of feed, a sudden change in weather or short periods of fasting imposed by circumstances such as shearing, crutching or transportation.

Clinical Findings: Characteristically, the disease occurs in outbreaks. The incidence is usually less than 5%, but, in severe outbreaks, 30% of the flock may be affected at one time. The earliest signs are slight hyperexcitability, muscle tremors and a stilted gait. These are soon followed by dullness, sternal decubitus, often with the hind legs extended backward, mild ruminal tympany and regurgitation of food through the nostrils, staring eyes, shallow respiration, coma and death within 6 to 36 hours.

Diagnosis: This is based on the history and clinical signs. In outbreaks occurring before lambing, pregnancy toxemia offers the main problem in differential diagnosis. A tentative diagnosis of acute hypocalcemia can readily be confirmed by a dramatic and usually lasting response to calcium therapy.

Prophylaxis and Treatment: Treatment consists of IV or subcut. calcium therapy, preferably with some added magnesium (℞ 608). Affected sheep should be handled with care lest sudden deaths occur from heart failure. Prevention is largely a matter of avoiding the predisposing causes.

NEUROMUSCULAR OR SKELETAL PARESIS IN COWS FOLLOWING PARTURIENT PARESIS

(The downer cow)

Cows become recumbent and are unable to rise for many reasons at or about calving time. Sometimes these reasons are obvious, as when there has been severe nerve or skeletal damage, or both, caused by a difficult calving. The reasons may be less obvious, as when a cow first becomes recumbent with an acute coliform mastitis and the observable changes in the milk are still minimal. "Downer cow" is not an acceptable diagnosis since it tends to lump together all cows that remain recumbent for whatever reasons. In most cases, a careful clinical examination, plus clinical pathologic tests when necessary, will allow a specific etiologic diagnosis for the recumbent cow. This is important not only for treating and offering a prognosis but also in providing advice for prevention of future cases. This discussion concerns itself with the specific problem of cows which remain recumbent after treatment for parturient paresis (milk fever, q.v., p. 513).

Clinical Findings: Affected cows are usually drawn to the attention of a veterinarian 12 to 24 hours after treatment for parturient paresis when they are still unable to rise, although they have usually responded well to calcium therapy in all other respects. Vital signs are within normal ranges, they are bright, alert and will eat and ruminate, although their appetite is usually diminished. There are no other clinical abnormalities but when urged to get up they will either not try or make an unsuccessful attempt. In some cases, this unsuccessful attempt is associated with an inability of the animal to extend the fetlocks and flex the hocks. This is an indication of peroneal nerve damage suffered while the cow has been recumbent with parturient paresis. Clinical examination usually will not reveal the severe, ischemic muscle necrosis that can quickly occur in the hind limbs of paretic cows recumbent on concrete floors.

Clinical Pathology: Serum calcium and inorganic phosphorus levels are usually within the lower limits of the normal range after adequate treatment for the initial hypocalcemia. Serum enzymes (SGOT, CPK) are markedly elevated as a result of the ischemic muscle necrosis. Severe muscle damage can occur in as short a time as 6 to 12 hours in a large cow recumbent on concrete and unable to turn herself from side to side.

Treatment: There is little support for many of the treatments that have been suggested. These include the administration of phosphorus, potassium, ACTH, corticosteroids and antihistamines. Additional calcium should not be given to recumbent cows if they do not have other signs of hypocalcemia. The recumbent cow should be moved promptly to an area with adequate bedding and footing (either outside or on a solid manure pack). Most cows will then move from side to side; those that do not should be turned frequently. Adequate nursing and feeding care are essential for good recovery. Most affected cows will try to get up within a week; those that are recumbent for 2 weeks without improvement are unlikely to ever get up. Great care must be taken if "hip-lifters" are used on large cows; they may do more harm than good by adding to the muscle damage. Slings are less likely to cause additional injury although they are more difficult to use.

Prevention: Prevention of parturient paresis (q.v., p. 513) is the first line of defense against cows which remain recumbent after treatment for this condition. Dairymen should be taught to recognize the earliest clinical signs of milk fever so the cows can be treated before they become recumbent. The incidence of "downer cows" is greatly increased if treatment is delayed after the first signs occur. Cows which are candidates for parturient paresis should calve outside, or in a box stall with a dirt floor and straw or a well-bedded manure pack. They should be in one of these areas at least 4 days before and 4 days after calving.

LACTATION TETANY OF MARES

(Transit tetany, Eclampsia)

A condition associated with hypocalcemia and sometimes with alterations in blood magnesium levels, occurring most often in mares about 10 days after foaling or 1 to 2 days after weaning or in nursing mares on lush pasture, but occasionally in nonlactating horses, usually following some stress such as prolonged transport. Uncommon since the passing of the draft horse, it is characterized by incoordination, tetany, sweating, muscle tremors, rapid, violent respiration, and a thumping sound from within the chest, considered by many to be a spasmodic contraction of the diaphragm. While handling may exacerbate signs, affected horses are not hypersensitive to sound, and there is no prolapse of the third eyelid as in tetanus. However stiffness of the gait and a high carriage of the tail are apparent. The body temperature remains close to normal, and the appetite appears unimpaired but during an attack the animal is unable to eat, urinate or defecate. Mildly affected animals may recover spontaneously; severely affected ones go down in about 24 hours, develop tetanic convulsions and usually die within the next day.

Response to IV injections of calcium solutions (℞ 607) given very slowly is generally good. If associated with transport, it may be advisable to incorporate magnesium in the solution (℞ 608). Sedation is often indicated for excitable mares.

TRANSPORT TETANY OF RUMINANTS

(Railroad disease, Railroad sickness, Staggers)

A condition affecting well-fed cows and ewes in the advanced stages of pregnancy, during or immediately after long-continued transportation and stress. It is also reported in lambs being transported to feedlots. The specific cause is unknown, but the condition is believed by some to be a form of acute hypocalcemia brought on by adverse conditions during shipping. Crowded, hot, poorly ventilated railroad cars or trucks with no provision for feed or water seem to be contributing factors.

Clinical Findings: Evidence of the condition is more commonly observed at destination, but may develop while in transit. Early signs of restlessness and uncoordinated movements are followed by a partial paralysis of the hind legs and a staggering gait. Later, in a prone position, the animal assumes an attitude similar to that observed in parturient paresis. A pulse rate of 100 to 120 may be noted, while respiration is rapid and labored. The temperature may be elevated slightly and congestion of the mucous membranes commonly occurs. Extreme thirst may develop, while anorexia is regularly observed with a reduction or complete cessation of peristaltic and rumen activity. Abortion may occur as a complication. Progressive paralysis, gradual loss of consciousness and death result unless suitable treatment is undertaken soon after onset.

Prophylaxis and Treatment: Animals in advanced pregnancy should be given only dry feed for a day or 2 preceding shipment. Loading should be accomplished with a minimum of excitement and overcrowded, poorly ventilated vehicles should be avoided. For transport involving long periods, suitable arrangements should be made to have the animals fed, watered and rested. Promazine hydrochloride or other suitable ataractics given IM one-half hour before loading are effective in alleviating the stress of transportation and may help to prevent the disease. For treatment, IV injections of calcium borogluconate (℞ 607), or calcium borogluconate with magnesium sulfate (℞ 608) given very slowly, preferably with 250 to 500 ml of 50% dextrose solution, followed by stimulants such as amphetamine (℞ 654) are recommended. Sedation is indicated in the presence of hyperexcitability.

PUERPERAL TETANY

(Hypocalcemic tetany, Lactation tetany, Eclampsia)

A disease occurring in bitches, particularly toy breeds nursing a full, active litter, and rarely in queens. It is commonest in the first 3 weeks of post partum but may occur prepartum, during parturition or as late as weaning.

Etiology: The demand for calcium during pregnancy and lactation results in exhaustion of calcium stores and hypocalcemia without accompanying parathyroid disease.

Clinical Findings: The early signs include panting, restlessness, anxiety and whining, drooling and champing of the jaws. Progressively the gait becomes stiff, the animal staggers, collapses and is unable to rise, the head and neck are extended and twitching of local muscle groups or generalized clonic movements occur. Periods of relaxation are short; soon generalized convulsions persist. The pupils are dilated, the mucosae are congested and the temperature is elevated (106.5°F [41.5°C]). The animal is normally conscious. Untreated bitches usually die.

Diagnosis: A history of impending or recent parturition in a nursing bitch or queen coupled with myoclonus or generalized convulsions is diagnostic. Serum calcium levels fall below 7 to 8 mg%.

Treatment: Elevation of the serum calcium following the IV administration of calcium gluconate (℞ 607) causes immediate remission of signs. Administration should be slow to avoid emesis and cardiac conduction disturbances. An additional half dose of a buffered calcium solution can be given by IM injection to avoid recurrence of signs. Following parenteral therapy, oral calcium gluconate and vitamin D (℞ 611) and adequate nutrition are supplied. If needed, sodium pentobarbitol (℞ 551) may be given IV to effect to control the convulsions. Relapses are not uncommon in which case septic postpartum metritis should be investigated. In animals that relapse intermittently, the litter should be removed from the dam for 24 hours or permanently.

Oral or IV corticosteroids (℞ 151) may prevent the occurrence of the disease by decreasing the incorporation of endogenous calcium into bone. Prednisolone should not be given where the possibility of a coexistent metritis exists. To prevent the disease in subsequent pregnancies, close attention must be given to proper nutrition, especially to intake of calcium and vitamin D during the gestation period.

HYPOMAGNESEMIC TETANY IN CATTLE AND SHEEP

(Grass tetany, Grass staggers)

A metabolic disturbance, characterized by hypomagnesemia, occurring most commonly in adult cows and ewes, especially those that are lactating heavily and are grazing on lush grass pastures. It also occurs in cattle of any age or condition, particularly beef cattle that are grazing on wheat or other cereal crops, or that are undernourished and exposed to changeable, cold weather. It is manifested by irritability, tetany and convulsions.

Etiology: Grass tetany may be considered to occur in 2 stages: first, the development of hypomagnesemia and second, a triggering of the clinical conditions. The rate of onset of hypomagnesemia depends upon the degree of deficiency; it is rapid in lactating cows allowed lush pasture after being housed over the winter and slow in undernourished beef cows. The low levels of magnesium and high levels of potassium and nitrogen in grass and wheat pastures combine to limit magnesium absorption. Excitement, act of milking, adverse weather and concurrent low blood levels of calcium are all possible trigger mechanisms.

Serum magnesium levels below 1.5 mg% should be regarded as suspicious and levels below 1.0 mg% as positive for hypomagnesemic tetany. Serum magnesium levels in affected animals may return to almost normal during the convulsive stage. Serum calcium levels are usually moderately depressed (5.0 to 8.0 mg%). The levels of magnesium in the cerebrospinal fluid are low and this is thought to have a causative effect in characteristic convulsive episodes.

Clinical Findings: In the most acute form of the disease, affected cows, which may be grazing in an apparently normal manner, suddenly throw up their heads, bellow, gallop in a blind and frenzied manner, fall and undergo severe paddling convulsions. These convulsive episodes may be repeated at short intervals and death usually occurs within a few hours. In many instances, animals at pasture are found dead without illness having been observed. In less severe cases, the cow is obviously ill at ease, walks with a stiff gait, is hypersensitive to touch and sound, urinates frequently and may progress to the acute, convulsive stage after a period as long as 2 to 3 days. Grass tetany may accompany parturient paresis and the classical signs of the latter disease be obscured by the tetanic convulsions. Similarly, it may accompany ketosis. In all cases of grass tetany, the loudness of the heart sounds and the rapidity of the heart rate are characteristic signs.

The disease in sheep occurs under essentially the same conditions and has the same clinical signs as the disease in cattle.

Prophylaxis: Prevention is largely a combination of increasing the intake of magnesium in danger periods and of management. Daily oral supplements of magnesite or magnesium oxide (2 oz [60 gm] to cattle and 1/3 oz [10 gm] to sheep) can be incorporated in the concentrate feed or in licks containing molasses, but not in mineral blocks. Magnesium alloy "bullets" have been developed for cattle and sheep to give a slow release of magnesium in the rumen. Fertilization with magnesium limestone or magnesium oxide to increase herbage magnesium is successful only with certain soil types. Dusting of herbage with powdered magnesium oxide (110 lb/acre [125 kg/ha]) gives good short-term prevention against grass tetany under suitable weather conditions.

Out-wintered stock should be protected from wind and cold and provided with supplementary food. Potassium fertilization reduces the content and availability to the animal of magnesium in herbage and should be avoided in the spring before the first grazing. Sheep and cattle should have access to hay or dry pasture.

Treatment: Affected animals require treatment urgently. Usually treatment includes administration of magnesium and calcium compounds, and sometimes sedatives if the convulsions and tetany are severe. An IV injection containing both calcium and magnesium is used (℞ 608), but it must be given slowly and the effect on the heart beat watched carefully. A less risky alternative is to give the calcium IV and magnesium sulfate subcut. (℞ 586). Unless the animal is removed from the tetany-producing pasture, and fed hay and concentrate, the blood-magnesium level is likely to fall again to dangerously low levels 24 to 36 houses after therapy. To prevent this, follow-up treatment with magnesium by mouth should be started, giving 2 oz (60 gm) of magnesium oxide daily for at least a week, and then withdrawn gradually.

HYPOMAGNESEMIC TETANY OF CALVES

Tetany in calves, characterized by hypomagnesemia, and commonly hypocalcemia, is clinically identical with grass tetany in adult cattle. Because of its occurrence in 2- to 4-month-old calves on a sole milk diet, or in younger calves on milk replacer or with chronic scours, the disease is considered to be due to inadequate absorption of magnesium from the gut. The inadequacy may be due to a primary deficiency of magnesium in the diet or to rapid passage of the ingesta through the intestines. In the latter case it is necessary to stop the chronic diarrhea. Affected calves require prompt treatment with a 10% solution of magnesium sulfate (100 ml subcut.) followed by the oral administration of 10 to 15 gm magnesium oxide daily. This level of oral dosing with magnesium oxide is also effective prophylactically.

HYPOGLYCEMIA OF PIGLETS

(Baby pig disease, Fading pig disease)

An important primary cause of death in piglets under one week of age, accounting for 15 to 25% of total piglet mortality and a final common pathway to death in other piglet diseases.

Etiology: With only partial gluconeogenic ability, limited energy reserves and essentially no brown fat, the newborn piglet relies on glycogen reserves and, most importantly, frequent nursing. Suckling may be impaired in piglets by severe splayleg, myoclonia, hydrocephalus, weakness from nutritional deficiencies or *in utero* infections. Predisposition to piglet hypoglycemia occurs from any disease of the sow which decreases or inhibits milk production or let down, e.g. MMA (q.v., p. 854), farrowing hysteria or other puerpural disease, agalactia from ergot poisoning or nipple necrosis. Large litter size with an inadequate number of teats precludes proper nursing; malplacement of the farrowing crate's lower rail, impairing access to the udder, can lead to inadequate milk intake and hypoglycemia.

Critical temperature for the newborn piglet is about 73 to 95°F (23 to 35°C). Piglets have effective metabolic response to cold and fully functional peripheral vasoconstriction but their lack of insulating subcut. fat (until 1 to 2 weeks old) allows marked heat loss. In drafty or wet environments, on cold floors or in low ambient temperatures, body temperature maintenance demands rapid glucose utilization depleting glycogen reserves; if then milk intake is impaired, hypoglycemia and death impend.

Clinical Findings: Most piglets within the litter are involved. Initially behavior changes from normally vigorous sucking or play alternating with sleep to solitary lassitude. Individual pigs aimlessly wander with faltering gait, crying weakly. Piglets are gaunt with pale cold clammy skin, hypothermia, poor muscle tone and are unresponsive to external stimuli. As incoordination increases, piglets may stand with legs splayed and use the snout for support. Sternal or lateral recumbency follows, risking crush injury. Terminally, piglets exhibit convulsions with jaw champing, salivation, milk opisthotonos, nystagmus, forelimb, hind limb contraction, coma and death.

Blood glucose levels fall from a normal 90 to 130 mg% to as low as 5 to 15 mg% in affected piglets. Clinical signs usually are manifest when levels fall below 50 mg%. The BUN usually is elevated.

Diagnosis: Hypoglycemia must be differentiated from neonatal bacterial septicemias and from afflictions marked by convulsions, e.g. bacterial meningoencephalitis, viral encephalitides. Generally it can be diagnosed by an examination of the sow and environment for predisposing factors and by piglet response to glucose treatment. Lesions reflect inadequate milk intake with minimal ingesta in the alimentary tract, dehydration, small hard liver and, frequently, a white precipitate in the renal pelvis and ureters.

Treatment and Prophylaxis: Treatment is 15 ml of 5% glucose given IP. Treated pigs should be placed under a heat lamp or in an equivalently warm environment. Response follows within 5 to 10 minutes with shivering and more activity. Severely hypoglycemic and hypothermic piglets may not respond. Sustained energy intake must be provided to avoided relapse.

If oxytocin (℞ 193) administered to the sow to promote milk let down and nursing fails, 30 to 50 ml of 5% dextrose or evaporated milk diluted with one-half volume water can be administered intragastrically to each piglet through a small plastic cannula (avoiding damage to the pharyngeal diverticulae), or IP glucose can be repeated every 4 to 6 hours. Active piglets learn quickly to drink from a dish. Foster suckling of piglets is possible in batch farrowing units; most sows accept piglets quietly introduced during the milk let-down period. Distribution of uneven litters may reduce mortality from starvation and hypoglycemia. Any primary disease of the sow should be treated effectively and any faults within the environment corrected. Newborn piglets should be held in a draft-free creep area heated to give an environmental temperature of 75 to 80°F (24 to 27°C) during the first week of life. Cold-stressed and marginally hypoglycemic piglets are more susceptible to enteric and other neonatal diseases.

Hypoglycemia in calves is uncommon but can occur where calves are kept in cold and wet circumstances and are fed inadequate amounts of milk or poor quality milk replacers. More common in the second and third weeks of life, calves show collapse, hypothermia, bradycardia and pupillary dilatation. Treatment with IV glucose brings dramatic response.

OBESITY

See NUTRITION p. 1263 et seq. for nutritional requirements of various species.

A common nutritional disease caused by excess food intake and inadequate exercise, characterized by excess generalized or localized fat deposition.

Etiology: The incidence of obesity in dogs increases with age and decreased physical activity. It is commoner in spayed females, castrated males and dogs fed home-prepared table food and snacks. Some breeds of dogs tend to be more obese, e.g. dachshunds and beagles. Cats fed a free-choice diet are commonly less obese. Endocrine imbalances, e.g. hypopituitarism, diabetes mellitus, chromophobe adenoma of the pituitary gland, adrenocortical hyperfunction, hypothalamic disorders and hypothyroidism are not significant causes of obesity in most dogs. Obesity reduces the animal's life expectancy and taxes the normal function of all organs.

Clinical Findings: When endocrine dysfunction is suspected, obesity will be one of the evident signs. Frank obesity is obvious to the veterinarian; however, the thickness of the fat layer covering the rib cage is the best assessment. In normal weight animals, the ribs should be barely visible yet palpable. In grossly obese pets, degenerative joint disease, fatigue and dyspnea, cardiac decompensation, enlarged fatty liver, or signs of intestinal dysfunction, e.g. constipation, may be seen. In addition, subcut. fat distribution contributes to episodes of heat intolerance. Obese animals are surgical and anesthetic risks.

Treatment: The caloric intake must be reduced and a regular vigorous exercise program is advised. The owners are advised to decrease the food intake to 60% of that required for maintenance of the dog at its optimal body weight. After changing the regular diet, small meals are fed frequently during the day. Commercial reducing diets are available or the owner can prepare a diet of lean ground beef, cottage cheese and low-calorie vegetables plus minerals and vitamins to be fed in proper amounts. All snacks and table food are eliminated. Most dogs will take 8 to 10 weeks to reduce to their satisfactory weight on a strictly controlled diet and exercise regime. Weight reduction can also be dramatically achieved by nearly complete restriction of food intake. The animal is hospitalized for the duration, fed vitamin-mineral supplements, water and very little else and physically examined daily. Metabolic acidosis and ketosis are not apt to be clinical problems in the dog when fat is mobilized. Unless specific endocrine dysfunction has been diagnosed, hormonal supplementation to reduce weight is contraindicated. Similarly, the administration of appetite depressants or physical stimulants can cause harmful effects.

HIGH-MOUNTAIN DISEASE

(Brisket disease, Pulmonary hypertensive heart disease)

A noninfectious disease of cattle characterized by the clinical signs and lesions of congestive right heart failure. It affects animals residing in high mountain areas of the Western U.S.A. and South America (usually above 2200 m) and has been reported in certain other mountainous areas of the world. The syndrome affects cattle but the possibility exists of it occurring in certain other ruminants (sheep and deer) under extreme stress. A similar disease is of clinical importance in chickens in the Andes Mountains. The incidence in cattle at risk ranges from 0.5 to 5% but is usually less than 2%. Occurrence is dependent upon high altitude, but not exclusively. Newly introduced cattle tend to have a greater incidence than native cattle in some geographic regions. The disease occurs primarily during the fall in North America, with a reduced incidence in winter and still less in spring months. It affects both sexes, all ages and probably most breeds—but not necessarily equally. It is commoner, for instance, in cattle less than one year of age.

Etiology: The disease is related to the chronic hypoxia of a high-altitude environment, which causes pulmonary vasoconstriction and hence pulmonary hypertension. The necessity of some other inciting or causative factor or factors is often indicated circumstantially. Complete absence of the disease on browse-type ranges in certain geographic areas at altitudes as high as 3400 m, with high incidence on nearby nonbrowse-type ranges having similar cattle strains and management procedures, has been documented. Altered chemoreceptor activity and myocardial metabolism have been implicated as possible contributory factors. Marked variation occurs in individual susceptibility (ostensibly inheritable, at least in part). The pathway by which the pulmonary hypertension proceeds to congestive right heart failure varies. In uncomplicated cases it appears related to individual susceptibility and permanent pulmonary vascular damage. Other stresses, such as pneumonia, lungworm infection, subzero weather, chronic pulmonary lesions, or ruptured diaphragm, are often superimposed upon the already partially compromised pulmonary circulation and disguise the etiology.

Clinical Findings: The disease usually develops slowly. Periods of severe cold or other environmental stress appear to precipitate onset of clinical signs. The affected animal is first noted to be depressed and to remain apart from the herd. As the syndrome progresses, subcut. edema may develop in the brisket region and may extend cranially to the intermandibular space and caudally to the ventral abdominal wall. Ascites and marked distension and pulsation of the jugular vein are usually present, and diarrhea may develop. Respiration is labored and the animals may appear cyanotic. They are reluctant to move, may become recumbent and upon forced exertion may collapse and die.

Lesions: Generalized edema is usually present, particularly of the ventral subcutis, skeletal musculature, perirenal tissues, mesentery and alimentary tract wall. Ascites, hydrothorax and hydropericardium are present. The liver lesions, due to chronic passive congestion, vary from an early "nutmeg" appearance to severe lobular fibrosis. The lungs may have varying degrees of atelectasis, interstitial emphysema, edema, and, in some cases, pneumonia. Marked right ventricular hypertrophy and dilatation of the heart are present. Displacement of the cardiac apex to the left gives the heart an enlarged rounded contour. Occasionally, pulmonary arteries contain thrombi. Microscopically, hypertrophy of the media of small muscular arteries and arterioles in the lung is the most consistent finding. This disease must be differentiated from other diseases causing congestive right heart failure in cattle, such as traumatic pericarditis, chronic pneumonia, congenital anomalies and primary myocardial lesions.

Treatment: It is essential that affected animals be moved to a lower altitude with minimal restraint, stress and excitement, where some will recover spontaneously. General supportive therapy, including antibiotics to combat pneumonia, should be administered. Large amounts of effusion can be removed by paracentesis. Digitalis and diuretic (℞ 525, 533, 541, 544) therapy has proven of benefit. Reduction of pulmonary arterial pressure at high altitude can be accomplished by the administration of oxygen and may be of value in the treatment of valuable animals. Since the disease may recur, recovered animals should not be returned to high altitudes. Since an inherited susceptibility is likely, affected cattle should not be retained for breeding.

POSTPARTURIENT HEMOGLOBINURIA

Primarily a disease of high-producing dairy cows that occurs 2 to 4 weeks after parturition. It is characterized by intravascular hemolysis, hemoglobinuria and anemia.

Etiology: The cause is unknown. The disease is rare in beef animals or animals under 3 years of age, and is uncommon more than 4 weeks after parturition. The incidence is generally low but up to 50% of affected animals may die. Diets high in cruciferous plants (such as rape or kale) or beet pulp, and prolonged feeding on phosphorus-deficient diets are said to be predisposing factors. In North America the disease may occur after prolonged stabling. The hemoglobinuria is believed to be associated with hypophosphatemia since serum phosphorus levels are always subnormal (0.8 to 1.4 mg%) in acutely ill cows. In New Zealand copper is thought to be an etiologic factor in the disease; its administration often prevents the disease.

Clinical Findings: Rapid IV hemolysis leads to hemoglobinuria, extreme pallor and a markedly increased cardiac impulse. Dehydration, weakness and a marked drop in milk yield are prominent signs. The temperature may be elevated to 103°F (39.5°C). Some respiratory distress may be seen. Intravascular hemolysis continues for 3 to 5 days and, in cows which recover, the return to normal is slow. Jaundice may occur in the late stages.

Treatment: Transfusion of large quantities of whole blood may be the only effective treatment of severely affected animals. In less severe cases, 2 oz (60 gm) of sodium acid phosphate in 300 ml of distilled water may be administered IV followed by subcut. injections at 12-hour intervals or by daily oral doses of the same amount of phosphate. If injected, sodium acid phosphate should be well distributed in the subcutis to avoid tissue necrosis. Bone meal should be added to the ration.

PORCINE STRESS SYNDROME (PSS)

An acute, shocklike syndrome, often fatal, which may occur following stress including that due to such routine management procedures as handling or moving.

Etiology: PSS results from a heritable defect in ability to maintain homeostasis, so that stress causes excessive stimulation of β-adrenergic receptors, with rapid depletion of ATP, rapid muscle glycogenolysis and excessive production of muscle lactate. Genetic studies indicate recessive inheritance, although penetrance may be incomplete so that some homozygotes are stress-free and some heterozygous carriers are stress-prone. PSS occurs most often in extremely muscular pigs, with the shortest-legged, most compact pigs most likely to be affected. It achieves its greatest incidence in Pietran, Poland China and certain lines of Landrace pigs. Stress-prone pigs tend to be easily frightened and difficult to manage. They may show muscle and tail tremors. PSS and associated behavior appears to be the result of selecting breeding stock from heavily muscled pigs with large, round hams. It is especially frequent in pigs kept in partial or total confinement. Incidents of PSS occur spontaneously but are commonest during periods of activity such as movement to new pens, regrouping, mating and transport. It has been estimated that more than one-third of American pork producers have had pigs with PSS, and it also occurs frequently in Europe and elsewhere. (*See also* ENZOOTISCHE HERZTOD, p. 597.)

Clinical Findings: Impending PSS may be signaled by a rapid tail tremor. Alternating areas of blanching and erythema may be noted in white or light-skinned pigs, followed by cyanosis. Dyspnea is common with open-mouthed breathing and elevated body temperature. Later, muscles become rigid, the pig is reluctant to move, and it may collapse and quickly die. *Rigor mortis* develops within a few minutes. Postmortem examination may reveal pale, soft, edematous muscles (**pale, soft, exudative or PSE pork**), and certain muscles of the ham such as the gluteus medius and biceps femoris may show a two-toned appearance, with pale, edematous areas. In other cases, muscles may be darker than normal (**dark, firm, dry or DFD pork**). A nonlethal variant with acute necrosis of the back muscles has been described in Landrace pigs.

Diagnosis: There are numerous changes in blood constituents with PSS, including an increase in blood lactate with associated acidosis. An efflux of enzymes into body fluids due to an alteration of cell membrane permeability makes it possible to use elevated blood creatine phosphokinase (CPK or CK) levels following stress to help diagnose susceptibility to PSS. The similarity between PSS and the malignant hyperthermia syndrome (MHS) of humans, which results in muscle rigidity during halothane anesthesia, led to the development of the halothane test for susceptibility to PSS. CPK and halothane tests are best administered to 30- to 60-lb (15 to 25 kg) pigs. In some herds, PSS has been found to be associated with blood types in the H-system of red blood cell antigens, and blood typing may be helpful to predict PSS susceptibility. Phosphohexose isomerase (PHI) isoenzyme types have also been found to be associated with PSS in some herds. Genes for PHI and for "H" red cell antigens are known to be closely linked.

Treatment and Control: Pigs showing signs of stress should be allowed to rest, and it may be desirable to tranquilize pigs in advance of possible stress if they are known to be PSS-susceptible. In its early stages, PSS may be treated by IV administration of tranquilizers, fast-acting hydrocortisone, and bicarbonate to help reduce lactate acidosis, but in advanced cases in which the pig is unable to stand, PSS is irreversible. Susceptible pigs should be handled very carefully. They should not be mixed with strange pigs if at all possible, and overheating or overcrowding should be avoided, as should any sudden or drastic changes in management.

Since susceptibility to PSS is simply inherited, appropriate breeding methods can rapidly reduce its incidence. However, associated undesirable reduction in muscularity and growth rate may be evident in herds where genes for PSS are eliminated.

PHOTOSENSITIZATION

A condition in which the presence of a photodynamic agent renders an animal hypersensitive to light. It should be differentiated from sunburn in which the white or lightly pigmented skin of a normal animal becomes inflamed following overexposure to ultraviolet rays. In photosensitization, the active rays are those absorbed by the photosensitizing agent. They often extend into the visual spectrum and usually are quite harmless to the unsensitized animal. In sunburn, the development of lesions is delayed, while in photosensitization, lesions develop very rapidly. The condition is best known in sheep and cattle, but may occur in any animal. It is worldwide in distribution.

Etiology: Photosensitizing substances may be introduced into the body by ingestion or by injection, or become operative through faulty liver function or aberrant pigment metabolism.

Primary photosensitivity: This is caused by the ingestion of photosensitizing agents not normally present in the diet. Long known sources of such compounds are plants of the genus *Hypericum* (St.-John's-wort or Klamath weed) or *Fagopyrum esculentum* (buckwheat). Recently many plants in the families Umbelliferae and Rutaceae have been found to contain photoactive furocoumarins. Only 4 of these plants are currently known to cause photosensitization in livestock or poultry, but it is likely other plants containing furocoumarins are also responsible. In Israel, and in the Southern U.S.A. where it is an introduced but now widespread weed, *Ammi majus* (bishop's-weed) is an important cause of photosensitization when ingested by cattle and it may also cause **photodermatitis** by contact. Sheep flocks grazing in Utah and Nevada ingested spring parsley (*Cymopterus watsonii*) and developed severe painful lesions of udders and teats and, prevented from suckling, 25% of their lambs died of starvation. Seeds of *A. majus* and *A. visnaga,* and plants of *C. watsoni* and *C. longipes* have caused severe photosensitization when ingested by poultry in Israel and the U.S.A. Many other plants have been reported to cause photosensitization, and in the absence of evidence of liver dysfunction it is reasonable to postulate the presence of photosensitizing agents, even though the photoactive principles have not been isolated.

Species of *Trifolium, Medicago* (clovers and alfalfa), *Erodium* and *Brassica* have also been incriminated in serious outbreaks of photosensitization, e.g. "trefoil dermatitis" and "rape scald." Some of these plants are dangerous only at certain stages of growth, e.g. rape and other *Brassica* spp. usually cause trouble only when immature.

Hepatogenous photosensitivity: This constitutes the most important group. In ruminants, liver dysfunction is by far the most frequent cause of photosensitization. The photosensitizing agent is normally absorbed from the alimentary tract and either detoxified by the liver or excreted in the bile. Anything that interferes with these processes results in the agent reaching the peripheral circulation and photosensitization occurs.

Phylloerythrin is one such substance. It is a porphyrin derived from chlorophyll in the alimentary tract of ruminants and some other animals. It has been incriminated as the photosensitizing agent in the following conditions: occlusion of the common bile duct, facial eczema (q.v., p. 532), a syndrome associated with hepatic pigmentation in Corriedale sheep, congenital photosensitivity of Southdown sheep, and poisoning by *Tribulus terrestris* (devil's thorn or puncture vine), *Lippia rehmanni, Lantana camara, Panicum miliaceum* (broomcorn millet), *P. coloratum* (kleingrass), *Narthecium ossifragum* (bog asphodel—believed to cause conditions known as "yellowses" and "alveld" in sheep), *Myoporum laetum* and copper.

Photosensitization has also been reported when liver damage or icterus have been caused by blockage of the common bile duct by hydatid cysts or liver fluke, in leptospiral infections and Rift Valley fever, in lupine mycotoxicosis, in poisoning by *Senecio jacobaea* (tansy ragwort), *Nolina texana* (bunch grass), *Agave lecheguilla* (lechuguilla), *Holocalyx glaziovii*, *Kochia scoparia*, *Tetradymia* (horsebrush or rabbit brush) species, the algae *Microcystis aeruginosa (toxica)*, *M. flos-aquae* and *Anabaena flos-aquae*, phosphorus, aniline, carbon tetrachloride and phenanthridinium. It is likely that phylloerythrin is the photosensitizing agent in at least some of these.

Many of the plants that cause hepatogenous photosensitization are toxic only under certain conditions of growth or climate; e.g. "geeldikkop" in South Africa occurs in sheep that graze *Tribulus terrestris* after it has wilted. Prior to wilting the plant is regarded as good sheep fodder.

Aberrant pigment metabolism: In this type, e.g. congential porphyria (q.v., p. 534), the photosensitizing agents are pigments that are normally absent or present only in minute amounts in the body.

Clinical Findings: The lesions and signs of photosensitivity are the same regardless of its cause. Photosensitized animals show photophobia immediately when they are exposed to sunlight. They seek shade or, if this is not available, turn their backs to the sun. Lesions are confined to white, or lightly pigmented, exposed areas of skin. Erythema develops very rapidly and is followed by edema. If exposure to light is terminated at this stage, recovery occurs promptly. If exposure to light is continued, skin necrosis follows, and the severity of the lesions may be accentuated by trauma from rubbing and by infection. In sheep, the most commonly affected parts are the face and ear, which frequently become thickened and pendulous ("big head"). In cattle, any unpigmented areas may be affected including the tongue, but the teats and udder appear to be especially sensitive.

In St.-John's-wort poisoning, hypersensitivity to contact with cold water has been reported. Affected sheep may develop convulsions and drown in dips or rivers.

Depending on the cause of the particular condition, there may be lesions and signs other than those associated with the photosensitivity. Some of these are described under facial eczema and congenital porphyria.

Prophylaxis and Treatment: Control of photosensitization can be achieved by preventing access to the offending plants. This is true for both primary and hepatogenous photosensitization, but can prove very difficult in practice, especially when plants are toxic only during certain periods depending on climatic factors. Methods which have proved effective are grazing on plants known to be safe or confining stock to small areas and feeding them hay. The former procedure may involve the growing of special crops for grazing during dangerous periods. In facial eczema, (*see* below), fungicides have proved effective in controlling the saprophytic fungi, and management practices designed to reduce litter may prove of value.

In all except primary photosensitivities, the treatment of skin lesions is symptomatic. Attempts should be made to determine the site and cause of primary lesions; however, the stress imposed by photosensitization contributes to the cause of death and symptomatic therapy is helpful.

While photosensitivity remains, animals should be given adequate shade or, preferably, housed and allowed out to graze only during darkness. Corticosteroids, given parenterally, may prove valuable. If the skin becomes infected, sulfanilamide powder in oil may be applied to the areas. In the case of sheep, fly-strike should be prevented.

When photosensitivity has ceased, the skin heals remarkably well, even after extensive necrosis. Yet the prognosis and the eventual usefulness of an animal will be governed by the site and severity of the primary lesions. After most toxic liver injuries, adequate regeneration takes place and normal function is restored.

FACIAL ECZEMA

(Pithomycotoxicosis)

A photosensitization of sheep and cattle arising from liver damage caused by the ingestion of toxic spores of the saprophytic mold *Pithomyces chartarum*, which grows on dead litter in pastures. It is, therefore, a mycotoxic disease and its common name is an unfortunate misnomer.

The disease occurs in New Zealand, Australia, South Africa and probably in North and South America. Warm ground temperatures and high humidity are required for prolific growth of this mold. Outbreaks of the disease are confined to hot periods of summer and early autumn. There may be several toxic periods in one season, separated by intervals when the pastures are safe. By following weather conditions and by estimation of spore numbers on pastures, toxic periods can be predicted and farmers warned.

A highly toxic compound, sporidesmin, has been isolated from cultures of the mold and from spores collected from toxic pastures. When sporidesmin is given orally to sheep or cattle at the rate of 0.5 to 1.0 mg/kg of body wt, it produces typical liver lesions and photosensitization. Rabbits, guinea pigs, rats, mice and chickens are also susceptible to the toxicosis.

Clinical Findings: The primary lesions in sheep and cattle are confined to the liver, gallbladder, bile ducts and the urinary bladder. At an early stage, there is inflammation, edema and necrosis of epithelium. Later, fibroblastic repair results in partial or complete obliteration of bile ducts by scar tissue, and 10 to 14 days after the toxic period, both obstructive jaundice and the secondary lesions of photosensitization occur. Livers become firm and fibrous with increased bile duct proliferation around the portal tracts.

Many photosensitized animals die of liver injury and stress 3 to 4 weeks after the toxic period. Others recover slowly, the skin lesions heal and there is nodular regeneration of the liver, which remains misshapen. Some animals that recover may lose condition or die if exposed to stresses such as pregnancy and lactation.

Animals with milder cases often exhibit no icterus or photosensitization, but they have patchy, pale, fibrosed areas in the liver, particularly in the left lobe. (For treatment *see* p. 531.)

Prevention: The application of benzimidazole fungicides to pastures considerably restricts the buildup of *P. chartarum* spores and so reduces pasture toxicity. Control recommendations specify the spraing of pastures in mid-summer with a suspension of thiabendazole (℞ 372). An area calculated at 1 acre per 15 cows or 100 sheep should be sprayed and animals admitted and maintained on the sprayed areas only when predicted danger periods of fungal activity are current. The fungicide is effective within 4 days after spraying provided that no more than 1 in. (2.5 cm) of rain falls within 24 hours during the 4-day period. After this time heavy rainfall does little to reduce the effectiveness of spraying since the thiabendazole becomes incorporated within the plants. Pastures will then remain safe for about 6 weeks. After this period spraying should be repeated to ensure protection over the whole of the dangerous season.

Experimentally and in field trials, when large daily doses of zinc are given to sheep and cattle over the period of acquisition of sporidesmin, the animals are well protected from the mycotoxin and the liver injury is largely prevented. Optimal protection requires an intake of zinc 20 to 30 times greater than nutritional requirements; this is safe for periods of 10 days but toxic for longer periods or at higher levels. With this low safety factor, accurate methods of dosage need to be established before zinc prophylaxis can become an alternative to spraying pastures with fungicides. Zinc has no therapeutic value once the disease has been established.

Sheep may be selectively bred for natural resistance to the toxic effects of sporidesmin. "Resistant" and "susceptible" Romney sires are bred and selected each year, initially for research but eventually in stud and commercial flocks.

CONGENITAL PHOTOSENSITIZATION IN SOUTHDOWN SHEEP

A heritable defect in the hepatic uptake of certain organic anions leading to photosensitization from the accumulation of excessive quantities of phylloerythrin in the peripheral circulation. It appears to be inherited as a simple recessive. Affected lambs become photosensitive as soon as they commence to graze green plants, and the progressive skin injury usually leads to death within a few weeks because pain and stress interfere with eating. If chlorophyll is excluded from the diet or if affected lambs are not exposed to sunlight, they grow normally, and several generations have been bred by allowing affected sheep to graze only at night and protecting them from the light during the day. Icterus is rarely seen, but bilirubinemia can usually be detected. No histologic lesions can be seen in the liver, but hepatic function tests indicate delays in plasma clearance of bilirubin, sodium cholate and injected test dyes. Elimination of carriers of the heritable factor, therefore, is the only control feasible.

CONGENITAL PORPHYRIA ERYTHROPOIETICA

(Porphyrinuria, Pink tooth)

A rare hereditary disease of cattle, swine, cats and man in which defective hemoglobin metabolism results in the production of excessive quantities of Type I porphyrins in the nuclei of developing normoblasts.

The defect in cattle is inherited as a simple recessive factor and usually confined to herds where inbreeding or close line breeding is practiced. The disease has been recognized in the U.S.A., Canada, Denmark, Jamaica, England, South Africa, Australia and Argentina.

The heterozygous animal appears as a normal individual, but the homozygous recessive animal is affected at birth and shows reddish brown discoloration of the teeth, bones and urine. The urine contains excessive quantities of coproporphyrin I and uroporphyrin I, while the discoloration of teeth and bones is due primarily to uroporphyrin I. Bones, urine and teeth (especially the deciduous teeth) exhibit a marked red fluorescence when irradiated with near-ultraviolet light. Prolonged exposure to sunlight causes typical lesions of photosensitization with superficial necrosis of unpigmented portions of the skin. A hemolytic anemia develops that is characterized by normochromia with macrocytes and microcytes and marked basophilic stippling. Splenomegaly eventually develops and the bones show increased fragility due to a diminished cortex. The animal becomes progressively unthrifty and may die unless protected from the sunlight.

The defect in swine and cats is extremely rare and differs in some respects from that in cattle. Photosensitization is not a feature and the disease is transmitted as an autosomal dominant trait. The disease in swine has been reported only from Denmark and New Zealand; in cats it has been recognized only in the U.S.A.

Diagnosis should be based on the excretion of abnormal uroporphyrins and on the brown discoloration of the teeth which display red-orange fluorescence when irradiated with near-ultraviolet light. Affected animals and their heterozygous sires and dams should be excluded from the breeding program.

MUSCULOSKELETAL SYSTEM

LAMENESS IN HORSES

Lameness may be defined as a departure from the normal stance or gait, occasioned by disease or injury. At least 90% of the cases of lameness are due to pain. The remainder comprise those in which anatomic changes produce what is called "mechanical lameness." Lameness must be differentiated from defective gait caused by faulty conformation and stiffness due to age or fatigue; stiffness usually passes off with exercise. Lameness is not a disease, but a sign of disease, pain, impediment, deformity or weakness.

Terms such as shoulder lameness, hip lameness and hock lameness are often used to describe so-called regional lamenesses. It should be noted, however, that these regional lamenesses do not specifically indicate the structure involved. In shoulder lameness for instance, the term does not indicate whether the causal lesion is in the scapulohumeral joint, tendon of the biceps, the bicipital bursa, or any of the muscles in that region. A horse's action does not denote the precise region involved, although it may give an indication or clue as to the approximate seat of the trouble.

Etiology: The causes of lameness may be classified as (a) predisposing and (b) exciting. Under predisposing causes may be mentioned immaturity or poor condition, faulty conformation, systemic disease, bad shoeing and lack of attention to the feet. Under exciting causes may be listed trauma, either direct or indirect; incoordination of muscle action, as may occur in tired animals; and bacterial infection, especially of tendon sheaths and joints.

Diagnosis: The history may be valuable if it is objective and complete. Lameness may be evident (a) during rest, (b) during progression and (c) on passive movement, manual examination and testing with hoof testers or hammers.

During rest: Pointing of a forelimb may be evident. No significance is attached to the pointing of a hind leg. A horse may "nurse" or favor a leg by holding it off or just in contact with the ground. The attitude or position adopted by the lame leg may give an indication of the cause. In upward fixation (subluxation) of the patella, the affected leg is in most cases rigidly extended backward with the wall of the toe resting on the ground. Abnormal mobility of part of a limb, even while standing, may indicate a ruptured tendon or fractured bone. Adduction or abduction of a leg also may be noted.

During progression: Following the visual examination, the horse should be trotted at once and not walked beforehand, since it may "warm out" of a mild lameness. Most lamenesses are best manifested at the slow trot on hard, even ground. Splint lameness, however, shows up better at a fast trot. It is important that the handler lead the horse with enough slack to permit head movement. A horse lame in the foreleg raises its head when the lame limb bears weight and nods or drops its head when the sound leg is in support. Provided the horse is unshod or shod all around, the sound made by each hoof as it strikes the ground may give an indication as to the lame leg.

If a horse is lame in both front legs and the causes are the same (e.g. navicular disease) or of equal severity, head nod is not apparent. Careful examination will reveal, however, that although the horse seems to be "going even" in front, the gait is "pottery" or stilted and the stride of both legs is shorter than normal. If, however, the lameness in both front legs is of unequal severity, the head nod will be present as in unilateral lameness. In such a case, the less lame leg is very likely to be overlooked unless careful attention is paid to its action. In addition, if the leg with obvious lameness is subjected to nerve blocking in order to desensitize the painful area, the apparent soundness of that leg and the head movement indicate that the other leg also is lame. In suspected hind-limb lameness, attention should be directed to the movements of the croup or quarter. The croup on the affected side generally is raised when the lame leg is in support, the degree of elevation of the croup varying with the seat of lameness. When both hind legs are lame, both legs move stiffly and often the owner believes that the trouble is in the lumbar region. Backing in such cases is accomplished with difficulty.

As the horse is moved toward or away from the examiner, it should be noted whether the legs are carried in a straight line or are adducted, abducted or circumducted while in motion. Attention also should be directed to the body axis to determine whether or not the axis is in the same line as the direction of movement. Trotting the horse along the foot of a hill may give an indication as to the lame limb because of its effect on collateral ligaments.

Trotting the horse in a circle (both clockwise and counterclockwise) may aggravate a lameness scarcely discernible on the straight.

The action of the horse then should be viewed from the side. By this means, variations in the length of stride and diminished flexion of joints are more readily observed.

Some types of lameness in the foot, e.g. fracture of the wing of the os pedis, are best seen when the patient is trotted or turned in a small circle. Finally, a heavy draft horse should be backed in order to ascertain any disability that might hinder the action of backing.

When the lame leg is evident, attention should be concentrated upon it and the following points noted: degree of flexion of the joints, length of stride, adduction or abduction of the limb, placement of the foot, and the height to which the hocks are carried.

Manual examination is carried out to determine the exact site of lameness and should be done in a systematic manner so that every part of the leg will be scrutinized.

Historically, most cases of forelimb lameness involved the foot, while the hock was the most frequently affected region of the hind leg, but in view of the present-day predominance of the light horse, most cases of forelimb lameness are to be found from the fetlock downward. In the thoroughbred in training however, the carpus is frequently involved.

During examination of the lame limb, frequent comparison should be made between it and the unaffected leg. All identifiable structures should be gently but thoroughly palpated, with the foot both on the ground and raised. The presence of heat in a part should be noted.

If the cause of lameness is thought to be in the foot, the shoe should be removed and the hoof thoroughly cleaned and tested for soundness of both wall and sole with a light hammer, and by application of the hoof tester. Excessive wear of the toe or quarter of the shoe may afford a clue as to the cause of the lameness. The foot of the lame leg should always be closely examined, and eliminated as a cause of an apparently more proximal seat of lameness.

Passive movement of a supposedly affected joint is most useful in the forelimb for detecting limitations of flexion in the carpus and fetlock. It should, however, always be interpreted in the light of the normal range of movement of the limb, especially in older horses. This test should also be carried out on the contralateral leg.

With regard to hind-limb lameness, especially when the lameness appears to be in the hip region, a rectal examination should be carried out. Since the stifle and hock joints move at the same time, pain in the stifle may give rise to limitation of hock movement and vice versa. The additional weight of a rider on the horse's back often accentuates lameness.

If, after the above examination procedure has been carried out, a diagnosis has not been made, the horse should be ridden, lunged, or driven for an hour or so, rested for approximately half an hour and re-examined.

Blocking of the nerves to a suspected area is another aid to diagnosis. If, after anesthetizing the nerve supply to the area in question, the horse goes sound, then it may be concluded that the seat of lameness is supplied by the anesthetized nerve. Palmar (volar) nerve blocks offer the best confirmatory evidence of foot lameness. Too much reliance should not be placed on the posterior digital nerve block, either unilateral or bilateral, since anastomotic branches of the nerves concerned may create a false interpretation of the results.

Very often, radiography permits the only reliable method of confirming or denying the physical findings relating to bones and joints and offers a more realistic prognosis than is possible by clinical examination alone.

In the case of muscle lesions, rhythmic muscular contractions brought about by a rhythmically surged faradic current have been used as a means both of diagnosis and treatment. The value of the method varies directly with the ability of the operator.

CURB

A thickening or "bowing" of the plantar tarsal ligament due to strain.

Etiology: Inflammation and thickening may occur after falling, slipping, jumping or pulling. Poor conformation of the hock is a likely predisposing factor in bilateral cases.

Clinical Findings: There is an enlargement over the posterior surface of the fibular tarsal bone, about a hand's breadth below the point of the hock. It is easily seen when observing the animal from the side. A curb that has recently and suddenly formed is characterized by acute inflammation and lameness. The horse stands with the leg at rest and the heel elevated. The chronic case rarely shows lameness.

Treatment: If the condition is due to acute inflammation, cold packs and rest are indicated. Little can be done to overcome the curb that is secondary to poor conformation.

OSSLETS
(Osselets)

An inflammation of the periosteum on the lower anterior epiphyseal surface of the large metacarpal bone and the associated capsule of the fetlock joint. The proximal end of the first phalanx may also be involved. Hence, this condition constitutes a form of arthritis that may progress from the serous to the ankylosing type.

Etiology: The exciting cause is the strain and repeated trauma of hard training in young animals.

Clinical Findings and Diagnosis: The affected horse moves with a short, choppy gait. Palpation and flexion of the fetlock joint produces pain, and examination reveals a soft, warm, sensitive swelling over the front and sometimes the side of the fetlock joint. Radiography in the initial stages may show no evidence of new bone formation in which case the condition is called "green osselets." Later, demineralization of the bone in the area of the distal epiphysis of the large metacarpal bone and the attachment of the fetlock joint capsule to the first phalanx may be seen. This is succeeded by progressive new bone formation or "calcium proliferation" some of which may break off and appear as "joint mice."

Treatment: Rest is very important. The inflammation may be relieved by the application of cold packs over a period of several days. Systemic anti-inflammatory agents such as phenylbutazone may also be employed. Some prefer the intra-articular injection of a corticosteroid; however, this and other forms of anti-inflammatory medication, if used along with continued training or racing lead inevitably to destruction of the joint surfaces.

SORE SHINS
(Bucked shins)

A periostitis of the anterior surface of the large metacarpal or metatarsal bone. The condition is most often seen in the forelegs of young thoroughbreds in training and racing.

Etiology: This condition is generally brought about by concussion. In some cases there is cortical infraction of the cannon bone, constituting either a stress fracture or in others, a "saucer" fracture with associated sequestrum. In milder cases, the condition is associated only with stretching or tearing of the overlying periosteum with consequent subperiosteal hematoma formation and thickening of the superficial face of the cortex.

Clinical Findings and Diagnosis: There is a warm painful swelling on the anterior surface of the large metacarpal or, less frequently, the metatarsal bone. The horse is lame, the stride is short, and the severity of the lameness increases with exercise.

Treatment: The affected horse must be removed from training. The acute inflammation may be relieved by application of cold packs.

Rest is necessary until all soreness and inflammation have disappeared. If the condition is one of cortical infraction, counterirritation and local corticosteroid injections are contraindicated. Local injections of sodium oleate are currently favored as treatment of this condition.

CARPITIS

(Sore knee, Popped knee)

An acute or chronic inflammation of the joint capsule and associated structures of the carpus. Exostoses may be present in old cases. The acute form is common in thoroughbreds in training.

Etiology: The acute form of the disease usually is attributed to concussion from hard training, especially in horses still somewhat "soft." Injury to the front of the knee, especially in hunters and jumpers, is a common cause. Some exostoses may be the result of undetected slab or avulsion fractures of the small carpal bones (*see* below). The inflammation occasionally appears, however, without any obvious signs or history of a causative agent. Poor conformation may play a part.

Clinical Findings and Diagnosis: Lameness usually is evident at once. Swelling is always present in acute cases and may consist of distension of the joint capsule and related synovial structures or be a true soft-tissue swelling. The chronic case may show well-developed exostoses. The diagnosis usually is simple; however, it is necessary to keep in mind the possibility of fracture of the carpal bones. This, as well as the presence of exostoses, can best be determined by radiologic examination.

Treatment: Rest is the best treatment and, when sufficient rest can be given, the prognosis for acute cases is good. Pain may be relieved by aspiration of excess fluid from the joint and the intra-articular injection of a corticosteroid, but adequate rest is still mandatory. This procedure may be repeated after 4 or 5 days if necessary. The presence of degenerative bony changes in the carpus immediately predicates an unfavorable prognosis. Temporary relief may be obtained in some instances by the use of a corticosteroid or phenylbutazone (℞ 150), but knees so affected never are wholly sound again. Anti-inflammatory treatment combined with continued training and racing will accelerate the degenerative process within the knee.

ARTICULAR FRACTURES OF THE CARPAL BONES, PROXIMAL SESAMOIDS AND FIRST PHALANX

Until radiographic examination became common, "popped knees," sesamoiditis and involvement of the proximal end of the first phalanx were often incompletely or incorrectly diagnosed. These productive exostotic lesions frequently begin as fractures of an avulsion, shear, or chip type.

Most fractures of the carpal bones are caused by "shear" stresses; they usually occur towards the end of a race when the possibility of the joint going into maximum overextension is greatest. Most occur in the anterior aspect of the carpal joint especially involving the radial and third carpal bones. Only the latter is commonly affected with the shear fracture and referred to as a slab fracture. Chip fractures of the proximal end of the first phalanx are quite common and must be differentiated from other injuries of the fetlock joint.

Fractures of the proximal sesamoid bones also follow fatigue with coexistent overextension. The lateral proximal sesamoid in the hind leg in the standardbred may be fractured as a result of torque forces induced by shoeing with a trailer-type shoe. The fractures may be apical, of the same leg, basal, multiple, and may involve one or both sesamoids.

Clinical Findings and Diagnosis: Articular fractures often occur towards the end of a race. Chip fractures may produce no signs until the animal is cooling out, when swelling of the fetlock or carpus with accompanying lameness may be noticed. Slab or compression fractures of the carpal bones and severe fractures involving the proximal sesamoids usually result in immediate swelling and severe supporting lameness. In the presence of the initial severe swelling it may be difficult to clinically differentiate between a fracture of the proximal sesamoids and rupture or severe strain of the flexor tendons or the suspensory ligament.

If the fracture is incomplete or if the fragment is small, the animal may be walking relatively soundly in 7 to 10 days following simple anti-inflammatory measures such as rest and cold applications of the point. Intra-articular injection of steroids and administration of phenylbutazone also relieves the inflammatory signs. However, lameness will recur with any strenuous work.

A diagnostic set of radiographs entails the exposure of 6 plates in the case of the carpus, and 4 for the fetlock: anteroposterior, mediolateral, obliques of both the medial and lateral aspects, and mediolateral flexion views are necessary to ensure that the fracture line is not missed. The flexion view may be omitted for the fetlock. A skyline projection may be of value to delineate the extent of a carpal-slab fracture.

Treatment: The combination of intra-articular or systemic anti-inflammatory treatment and continued work usually leads to degenerative changes within the joint. Surgery often is the treatment of choice. The 3 contraindications applying to all surgical interventions into joints are: (1) the chip is very small and does not involve the articular surfaces, (2) there is radiographic evidence of coexistence of degenerative osteoarthropathy, (3) a corticosteroid has been injected into the joint within 8 weeks prior to the date of surgery.

Fractures of the proximal sesamoids may be treated conservatively by allowing stall rest for an extended period (8 to 12 months) to permit fibrous union.

BOG SPAVIN
(Tarsal hydrarthrosis)

A chronic synovitis of the tibiotarsal joint characterized by distension of the joint capsule.

Etiology: Faulty conformation may lead to hock-joint weakness and increased production of synovia, especially in the bilateral case. The unilateral case is more likely to be a sequela to a more acute cause such as a sprain.

Clinical Findings and Diagnosis: The affected horse usually is not lame unless the condition is complicated by bone involvement. Distension of the joint capsule occurs in 3 places. The largest swelling is on the anterior medial surface of the hock, while a smaller swelling occurs on each side of the proximal posterior aspect. Bog spavin, unless complicated by bony changes, rarely interferes with the usefulness of the animal, but does constitute an unsightly blemish. Spontaneous appearance and disappearance may occur in weanlings and yearlings.

Treatment: The excess fluid within the joint capsule may be aspirated and replaced with 5 ml of one of the corticosteroids developed for intra-articular injection (e.g. ℞ 155), and the procedure repeated 3 weeks later if necessary. The condition has a tendency to recur, especially if poor conformation is a contributory cause.

BONE SPAVIN

Spavin is usually described as a periostitis or rarefying osteitis involving the bones of the hock joint, usually the distal 2 rows of tarsal bones on the medial side, and subsequently resulting in exostosis and terminal ankylosis.

Etiology: Among the theories advanced to explain the condition are faulty hock conformation, excessive concussion and mineral imbalance.

Clinical Findings and Diagnosis: The horse tends to drag the toe. The forward flight of the hoof is shortened and hock action is decreased. The heel becomes high. The exostosis often is visible on the lower medial aspect of the hock. When standing, the horse may rest the toe on the ground with the heel slightly raised. The lameness quite often disappears with exercise and returns after the horse has been rested. In so-called occult spavin, there is no visible exostosis and the lameness sometimes is continuous as the bone lesion may be within the articular surface. The spavin test may be a useful aid to diagnosis: the leg is picked up and held with the hock, but not the fetlock, acutely flexed for a few minutes; the lameness will be accentuated for the first few steps immediately after release of the leg. This test, less dependable in older horses, should also be carried out on the other leg. Lameness from a gonitis also is accentuated by the "spavin test."

Treatment: The horse should be rested. Deep point-firing may be performed to hasten ankylosis of the affected bones, but this result is not always achieved. More recently, arthrodesis has been achieved by using a surgical drill and bit. Corrective shoeing consists of raising the heels and rolling the toe. If the exostosis lies under the cunean tendon, tenotomy of this structure may give relief. Wamberg's peripheral neurectomy has also been employed.

SPLINTS

This condition involves primarily the interosseous ligament between the large and small metacarpal (less frequently the metatarsal) bones. This reaction is a periostitis with production of new bone (exostoses) along the involved splint bone.

Etiology: Trauma from concussion or injury, strain from excessive training, especially in the immature horse, faulty conformation, or improper shoeing may contribute to the development of this condition.

Clinical Findings and Diagnosis: Splints most commonly involve the medial rudimentary metacarpal and, occasionally, the small metatarsal bones. Lameness is observed only when splits are forming and seen most frequently in young horses. Lameness is more pronounced after the animal has been worked. In the early stages, there is no visible enlargement, but deep palpation may reveal local painful subperiosteal swelling. In the later stages, a calcified growth appears. Following ossification, lameness disappears, except in occasional cases where the growth encroaches on the suspensory ligament, or carpal articulation.

Radiography is warranted in many cases to differentiate splints from fractured splint bones.

Treatment: Complete rest is indicated. In thoroughbred practice, it is traditional to point-fire a splint, the aim being to accelerate the ossification of the interosseous ligament. However, should radiographic examination disclose a fracture, irritant treatments are contraindicated. Surgical removal of the distal segment is then the treatment of choice. In the case of impingement exostosis against the suspensory ligament, removal of the encroaching exostosis is sometimes carried out. The local use of steroids will delay the consolidation process and is therefore contraindicated.

FRACTURES OF THE SMALL METACARPAL AND METATARSAL (SPLINT) BONES

Fractures of the second and fourth metacarpal and metatarsal (splint) bones are not uncommon. The cause may be from direct trauma as from interference by the contralateral leg, but more often follows prior suspensory desmitis with its resulting fibrous-tissue build-up and encapsulation of the distal, free end of the bone. The usual site of the fracture is through the distal end approximately 2 in. from the tip. Immediately after the fracture occurs, signs of acute inflammation are present at the site. The suspensory ligament usually is involved in the inflammatory process. A supporting lameness is noted; this may recede after several days rest and recur only after working.

Chronic, long-standing fractures cause a supporting lameness at speed, particularly at the trot. Thickening of the suspensory ligament at and above the site results. The fracture usually shows little tendency to heal, with a considerable build-up of callus at the fracture site.

Diagnosis is confirmed by means of an oblique radiograph setting out the bone involved. Surgical removal of the fractured tip and of the callus is the treatment of choice. Such treatment may not beneficially affect the associated suspensory desmitis which should be subjected to the tendon-splitting operation.

TROCHANTERIC BURSITIS
("Whirlbone" lameness)

An inflammation of the tendon of the middle gluteal muscle, of the bursa between this tendon and the trochanter major, or of the cartilage of the trochanter major.

Etiology: This condition is encountered most commonly in standardbreds and, in some cases, is concurrent with a pre-existing spavin.

Clinical Findings and Diagnosis: The weight is placed on the inside of the foot so that the inside wall of the foot is worn more than the outside wall. The stride of the affected leg is shorter and the leg is rotated inward. The horse tends to carry the hindquarters toward the sound side. In long-standing cases, the muscles between the external and internal angles of the ilium are atrophied, giving a flat appearance to the croup. Pressure over the greater trochanter gives evidence of pain.

Treatment: If the inflammation is acute, the animal should be rested and hot packs applied over the affected area. Injection of an intra-articular corticosteroid into the bursa will temporarily relieve the inflammation. In chronic cases, the injection of Lugol's solution (℞ 599) into or around the bursa gives good results.

BICIPITAL BURSITIS

An inflammation of the bursa between the tendon of the biceps and the bicipital groove of the humerus. The usual cause is trauma to the point of the shoulder.

Essentially the condition produces a swinging-leg lameness, the forward phase of flight being shortened. The animal may stumble due to the toe not being lifted sufficiently to clear the ground. In severe cases, a supporting-leg lameness may also be present. Forced extension of the leg usually causes a pain reaction, particularly if the tendon is also involved. Deep digital pressure over the bursa and the tendon of the biceps may elicit a pain response. Radiographs may be of aid if the bursa can be outlined in the more chronic case in which calcification of the bursa is a common sequela.

Rest is indicated, particularly in acute cases. Intrabursal injection of a steroid may be successful. Phenylbutazone and administration of oral steroids (℞ 141) are useful.

ARTHRITIS OF THE SHOULDER JOINT

An inflammation of the structures of the joint itself. These may consist of changes in the joint capsule, or more frequently, bony changes of the articular surfaces of the humerus or scapula, and "joint mice," as seen in osteochondritis dissecans. Occasionally, fractures involving the articular surfaces are present.

Trauma to the point of the shoulder is the usual cause. Bacterial infection of the joint from puncture wounds or of hematogenous origin (pyosepticemia) may be the cause of a purulent arthritis.

A swinging- and supporting-leg lameness is present in severe cases. In milder cases, only the swinging-leg lameness may be noted. The forward phase of flight is shortened. The toe may be worn. The leg often is circumducted to avoid flexion of the joint. Forced extension of the leg pulling the shoulder forward, often causes pain. Radiographs of the shoulder joint, preferably taken with the horse in lateral recumbency, may demonstrate the arthritic changes.

Treatment often is ineffective due to severe arthritic changes. Intra-articular injections of a steroid (℞ 155) may be of some benefit. Systemic steroids (℞ 141) or phenylbutazone (℞ 150) may relieve signs of pain in some animals.

COXITIS

Inflammation of the coxofemoral articulation. Most cases are traumatic in origin, occurring secondarily to tearing the rim of the acetabulum or fractures through the acetabulum. Localization of a systemic infection, particularly pyosepticemia in young animals, is not an uncommon cause.

Both a supporting- and swinging-leg lameness is noted. In severe cases the leg may be carried. In less severe cases the gait is rolling, the affected quarter being elevated as weight is born on the leg. The leg is advanced in a semicircular manner with the forward phase of the stride shortened. The toe may be worn from dragging. The animal often stands with the leg partially flexed, the stifle turned out, and the point of the hock turned inwardly. Atrophy of the heavy muscles of the quarter occurs in cases of long duration. Rectal palpation often reveals an enlargement over the acetabulum, particularly if a fracture through it has occurred. When possible, radiography of the joint may confirm the diagnosis.

The prognosis is poor. Rest is indicated. Intra-articular steroids (℞ 155) may relieve the lameness temporarily in milder cases. Phenylbutazone (℞ 150) is often useful.

GONITIS

An inflammation of the stifle joint. The joint is complex, and the condition may be precipitated by multiple causes: persistent upward fixation of the patella, injuries to the medial or lateral collateral ligaments of the joint, injuries to the cruciate ligaments of the menisci, erosions of the articular cartilage, and bacterial infection of the joint from puncture wounds or of hematogenous origin (pyosepticemia).

The severity of signs is remarkably variable, depending upon the cause and the extent of the pathologic changes. Usually the joint capsule is distended, pouching out between the distal patellar ligaments. Occasionally, the femoropatellar capsule is distended, the enlargement then being noted just below the patella.

A swinging-leg lameness is noted in all cases, the forward phase of flight being shortened. At rest the leg often is turned out from the stifle downward and the fetlock flexed with only the toe touching the ground. In moderately severe cases both a supporting- and swinging-leg lameness is noted. In very severe cases, the leg may be carried in a flexed position. Crepitation may be noted if the menisci, cruciate ligaments, or the collateral ligaments of the joint have been ruptured. Radiographs of the joint may be of considerable value in confirming the diagnosis.

The prognosis is poor if the condition is of long duration or if severe injuries to the articular surface ligaments or the menisci have occurred. Rest is indicated. Intra-articular injections of steroids may be useful. Phenylbutazone (℞ 150) and systemic steroids may relieve the lameness in less severe cases. Those cases due to rupture of ligaments or damage to the menisci rarely respond satisfactorily.

STRINGHALT
(Springhalt)

A myoclonic affection of one or both hind legs manifested by spasmodic overflexion of the joints during progression. The etiology is unknown. Degeneration of the sciatic or peroneal nerve and affections of the spinal cord have been suggested as possible causes. Horses of any breed may be affected.

Clinical Findings: All degrees of flexion are seen, from the mild, spasmodic lifting and grounding of the foot, to the extreme case where the foot is drawn sharply up till it touches the belly and then struck violently on the ground. Mild stringhalt may be intermittent in character and thus may pass unnoticed at the time of examination. The ailment is most obvious when the horse is sharply turned or backed. In some cases, the condition is seen only on the first few steps after moving the horse out of its stall. The signs are often less intense or even absent during warmer weather.

Although it is regarded as a gross unsoundness, stringhalt does not materially hinder the horse's capacity for work, except in severe cases when the constant concussion gives rise to secondary complications. A severe case may also make the horse unsuitable for equestrian sports.

Diagnosis: Diagnosis is based on clinical signs. If in doubt, the animal should be observed as it is backed out of the stall after hard work for a day or two. False stringhalt sometimes appears as a result of some temporary irritation to the lower pastern area.

Treatment: Best results have been obtained by performing a tenectomy of the lateral extensor of the digit using the standard or radical method. In the latter operation, a portion of the muscle is also removed. Prognosis following surgery should be guarded. Improvement may not be evident until 2 to 3 weeks after surgery.

SWEENEY
(Swinney, Shoulder atrophy, Slipped shoulder)

An atrophy of the supraspinatus and infraspinatus muscles of the horse. This atrophy is of 2 types: disuse and neurotrophic.

Disuse atrophy, sometimes involving the triceps also, follows any lesion of the leg or foot that leads to prolonged diminished use of the limb.

Neurotrophic atrophy is due to damage to the suprascapular nerve, which supplies the supraspinatus and infraspinatus muscles.

The resulting syndrome is termed suprascapular paralysis or slipped shoulder. The triceps is not involved in this type of atrophy.

In most cases the condition is due to damage to the nerve through bruising with effusion; occasionally the nerve may be severed as a result of injury.

Clinical Findings and Diagnosis: If there is no evident trauma, pain may be absent and lameness may be difficult to detect until atrophy occurs. If injury is evident, there is usually some difficulty in extending the shoulder.

As atrophy proceeds, there is a noticeable hollowing on each side of the spine of the scapula, especially in the infraspinous area, resulting in prominence of the spine. Since the tendons of insertion of the 2 affected muscles act as lateral collateral ligaments to the humeroscapular joint, atrophy of the muscles leads to a looseness in the shoulder joint. Abduction of the shoulder follows and, in severe cases, is sometimes erroneously diagnosed as a dislocation. The affected limb, when advanced, takes a semicircular course and, as weight is borne by the leg, the shoulder joint moves laterally (shoulder slip). At rest, along with abduction of the shoulder, there is an apparent abduction of the lower part of the limb.

Prognosis: The prognosis of disuse atrophy depends on removal of the primary cause. In neurotrophic atrophy, the prognosis is guarded; a mild case should allow a patient to recover in 6 to 8 weeks, but where damage to the nerve has been severe, recovery may take many months if it occurs at all. If the nerve has been severed, recovery is most unlikely.

Treatment: Treatment for disuse atrophy consists of removing the cause of the failure to use the limb. For neurotrophic atrophy, massage with stimulating liniments or by an electrical vibrator may be of benefit. Rhythmic muscular contractions by faradism have "kept the affected muscles alive" until nerve regeneration has taken place. When improvement begins, pasture exercise for several weeks is beneficial.

FOOT AILMENTS OF HORSES

LAMINITIS
(Founder)

A metabolic problem of multifactorial causation leading to degeneration and breakdown of the union between the horny and sensitive laminae of the hoof. Rotation of the third phalanx, a common sequela to an acute cause, may progress to dropping (flattening), and in advanced cases, perforation of the sole. The formerly held belief that acute laminitis had as one of its clinical expressions an intense inflammation of the laminae with associated congestion of the blood vessels of the hoof has, to some extent, been replaced by the finding that the arterial blood supply through the terminal arch within the hoof is actually decreased, even destroyed, as a result of ischemic necrosis. Laminitis may be acute or chronic and it may involve 1 or all 4 feet. Most commonly both forefeet are affected.

Etiology: The exciting causes are well known and include: drinking of cold water by an overheated animal; ingestion of excessive amounts of grain; concussion during hard, fast road work; hard work by an unconditioned animal; toxemias as sequelae to pneumonia or metritis (so-called "parturient laminitis") and superpurgation. Allergic reactions have been incriminated. Grain founder is the commonest type. Ponies, in particular, have been known to founder when at pasture. The recent increased incidence of laminitis in one foreleg noted when the opposite member has been treated surgically is thought to be due to the prior, excessive use of corticosteroids in some cases.

Clinical Findings: In acute laminitis, onset is sudden. Both general and local signs may appear. General signs include anorexia, a rise in temperature up to 106°F (41°C) with accompanying increase in respiration and pulse rate. In some cases, the pain is so excruciating as to produce clonic spasms and profuse sweating. If the forefeet only are affected, the animal places them forward to relieve them from weight, bringing the hind feet forward under the body for support. If the hind feet are affected, they are placed forward with the forefeet under the body to support the weight. The animal lies down and rises only reluctantly. If standing, the animal resists movement. The first steps are accomplished with intense pain that subsides to a slight extent as the animal "warms up."

Local signs are marked. The affected feet are warm to the touch. The pulse of the digital artery on the affected feet is hard and bounding. Even mild pressure by hoof testers produces great pain. In mild cases, recovery may occur in about 10 days. In severe cases, the prognosis is poor and the condition is likely to terminate in chronic laminitis. Infiltration of serum takes place in the space between the horny and sensitive laminae with the result that the os pedis is displaced so that the anterior portion of this bone points downward. This displacement is assisted by the pull of the deep flexor tendon. The hoof becomes distorted; the anterior wall becomes concave, the hoof longer, the heels higher, and the hoof wall corrugated. It is important not to confuse so-called "grass rings" with the rings produced by chronic laminitis.

Diagnosis: In acute cases, diagnosis is made by consideration of the case history, the posture of the animal, the increased temperature of the hooves, the hard pulse of the digital artery, the expression of pain and anxiety, and the reluctance to move. Mild cases with no visible hoof deformity may be discovered on examination of radiographs of the affected feet, which disclose a lack of parallelism existing between the hoof wall and anterior face of the third phalanx on the lateral projection.

Treatment: Because of the rapidity with which pedal rotation can occur, acute laminitis constitutes a medical emergency. Despite prompt therapy, however, the prognosis should still be guarded because alteration of the hoof architecture can follow subacute and chronic cases. In acute laminitis, especially in cases of excessive grain consumption and provided superpurgation is not the primary cause, a purgative (℞ 501) is recommended. Oral administration of 1 gal. (4L) of mineral oil will act as a laxative and tend to prevent absorption of toxic material from the intestinal tract. Purgation should not be employed in cases following pneumonia or in parturient laminitis of mares. In the latter condition, the uterus usually requires attention. Cold packs or ice packs applied to the affected feet are advocated by some, but others suggest that hot packs used early in the course of the disease might be more beneficial. Antihistamines, though apparently logical, are of doubtful value. Phenylbutazone is the preferred anti-inflammatory agent but meclofenamic acid (Arquel) has also been of value. Digital nerve blocks in the early stages of the disease will permit walking the patient. This procedure has been shown to increase the arterial blood flow through the terminal arch. Nerve blocking and walking, however, are contraindicated once pedal rotation has commenced. Because of its value in hoof keratinization, methionine is useful at doses of 10 gm daily for 7 days followed by 5 gm daily for 21 days.

Treatment of chronic laminitis consists of attempting to restore the normal alignment of the rotated coffin bone by lowering the heels, removing excess toe, and protecting the dropped sole. This may be accomplished by a competent farrier and may require full leather pads or a steel-plate shoe in addition to trimming the hoof. Acrylic compounds may be useful in conjunction with proper trimming to build up the toe and to protect the sole. The hoof should be trimmed and the shoe reset at 6- to 8-week intervals.

THRUSH

A degenerative condition of the horn commencing in the central and collateral sulci and eventually involving the entire frog. The predisposing causes are unhygienic conditions that require the animal to stand in mud, urine- or feces-soaked earth or bedding, failure to clean the hoof at regular intervals and atrophy of the frog as found in contracted hoofs. In all probability, there is more than one causal organism, and among them can be listed *Fusobacterium necrophorum* (*Sphaerophorus necrophorus*).

Thrush may be found in any or all of the feet, but is commoner in the hind feet. A characteristic foul odor always is present. The affected sulcus is moist and contains a black, thick discharge. When probed the sulcus is deeper than normal and sensitive in its depth. The characteristic odor and the black, thick discharge in the sulci of the frog are adequate for diagnosis.

The prognosis is good. Treatment should begin by providing dry, clean standings and cleaning the hoof gently to avoid unnecessary injury to the affected part. Any of the recognized astringent lotions will effect a cure, following removal of the diseased tissue (℞ 640). The use of a bar shoe may help in the regeneration of the frog, after the disease process has been arrested. If the cuneate matrix has been damaged, radical surgery should be employed to remove diseased frog tissue.

CANKER

A chronic hypertrophy of the horn-producing tissues of the foot, involving the frog, the sole and, at times, the wall. It is most often found in the hind feet. Canker is seldom encountered today, being primarily a disease of the heavy draft horse. The cause is unknown.

Clinical Findings: The disease is frequently well advanced before detection, attention being directed to it by the fetid odor. The frog may appear to be intact, but has a ragged, oiled appearance. The horn tissue of the frog loosens easily, revealing the swollen, ill-smelling corium covered with a caseous, whitish exudate. The surface of the corium is not smooth, but shows a characteristic vegetative growth. The disease process may extend to the sole and even to the wall, showing no tendency to heal.

Diagnosis: The offensive odor, the moist appearance, the soft, swollen, sensitive tissue and the loss of the horny frog establishes the diagnosis.

Treatment: The prognosis is not good, compared with thrush in which treatment is highly successful. Treatment must be persistent. All loose horn and affected tissue should be removed. An antiseptic and mild astringent dressing, e.g. 5% picric acid, is applied under pressure and renewed daily at first. Stronger astringents (℞ 640) may be indicated, the dressings being retained by transverse strips of thin metal, springing the ends under the shoe, by means of a metal sole screwed to the shoe, or an adjustable plastic boot. By the latter methods, the horse, if not lame, can be returned to work without the likelihood of the dressings being lost. Maintenance of pressure on the affected part during treatment appears beneficial.

GREASE

(Grease heel, Scratches, Dermatitis verrucosa)

A chronic dermatitis characterized by hypertrophy and exudation on the posterior surface of the fetlock and pastern. The hind legs are more commonly affected. The disease often is associated with poor stable hygiene, but no specific cause is known. Heavy, coarse-legged horses seem most susceptible.

Clinical Findings: Because of the "feather," the disease may progress somewhat before it is noticed. The skin is itchy, sensitive and swollen during the acute stages; later, it becomes thickened and most of the hair is lost. Only the shorter hairs remain and these stand erect. The surface of the skin is soft and the grayish exudate has a fetid odor. The condition tends to become chronic and vegetative granulomatous growths known as "grapes" appear, caused by hypertrophy of the papillae. Lameness may or may not be present. As the condition progresses, there is thickening and hardening of the skin of the affected region, with very rapid hypertrophy of subcut. fibrous tissue. This assumes elephantiasis-like proportions in cases of long duration.

Treatment: The prognosis is guarded, but persistent treatment is usually rewarding. Treatment consists of washing with warm water and castile or green soap, to remove all soft exudate, drying and applying an astringent dressing (℞ 426, 646). If granulomatous lesions appear, they should be cauterized.

CORNS

(Pododermatitis circumscripta)

Bruising of the sole, in the angle between the wall and the bar, usually in the inner quarter and most commonly in the forefeet. Corns may be classified as dry, moist, or suppurating.

Etiology: Predisposition to corns is usually due to faulty foot conformation, such as straight walls that tend to turn in at the quarters, or contracted feet. More direct causes may be excessive trimming of the sole, thus exposing the sensitive tissue to contusion, or neglect of the feet to the extent that they become long and irregular. Shoes allowed to remain on until overgrown by the hoof, or shoes that have been fitted too closely at the quarters, may also cause the condition.

Clinical Findings and Diagnosis: When the foot is raised and the volar surface freed of dirt and loose horn, a discoloration, either red or reddish yellow, is noted at the site of the corn. A supporting leg lameness is an early sign. Tapping with a light hammer over the area or applying pressure with a hoof tester causes great discomfort. If infection has gained entrance, pain is pronounced when pressure is applied, and if not promptly treated, pus may burrow through to the coronet to produce quittor or a suppurating sinus. The clinical signs are adequate for a diagnosis.

Treatment: The prognosis is favorable. In simple uncomplicated dry corns, relief from pressure on the affected area is the first consideration. This may be achieved by shortening the toe if it is excessively long and by applying a bar shoe to promote frog pressure. A three-quarter bar shoe may be of value in relieving pressure.

If the corn is suppurating, it should be drained at once by a surgical opening directly through the sole. Following drainage, the foot should be dressed to permit drainage. Hot foot baths and agents such as Antiphlogistine are helpful. The horse should be kept in a dry, clean, box stall. After infection is controlled in suppurating corns, the cavity should be loosely packed with oakum and a metal or leather sole placed between the shoe and the foot. Systemic antibacterial therapy may be indicated in severe septic cases.

BRUISED SOLE

A term applied to bruises on the palmar aspect of the foot other than those found at the seat of corn. The cause usually is direct injury from stones, irregular ground or other trauma. Bad shoeing, especially in animals with flat feet or dropped sole, also may cause the condition; in this case, the bruised area is usually around the periphery of the sole.

Signs and treatment are very similar to corns, except that in bruised sole, any infection tends to spread more rapidly under the horn of the sole. Persistent bruised sole not responding to treatment should arouse suspicion of pedal osteitis (q.v., p. 561).

PUNCTURE WOUNDS OF THE FOOT

(Suppurative pododermatitis, Gathered nail, "Nail bind")

The results of such wounds vary from a transient indisposition to an incapacity that may necessitate destruction of the horse. In severe cases, an acutely painful foot is the most obvious sign. Abscess formation quite commonly follows within 10 to 14 days of the infliction of the wound.

The foreign body should be removed and the infected area drained. Keeping the foot for several days in a rubber or plastic boot with a generous cotton pad soaked in saturated magnesium sulfate solution is often useful. Tetanus immunization should be carried out in all cases of puncture wounds in the foot. When pain is severe, a palmar nerve block provides temporary relief. Local and systemic antibiotic therapy are valuable.

QUITTOR

A chronic, purulent inflammation of the lateral cartilage of the third phalanx characterized by necrosis of the cartilage, and one or more sinus tracts extending from the diseased cartilage through the skin in the coronary region. Quittor follows injury to the coronet or pastern over the region of the lateral cartilage, by means of which infection is introduced into the deep tissues to form a subcoronary abscess, or it may follow a penetrating wound through the sole.

The first sign is an inflammatory swelling over the region of the lateral cartilage. This is followed by abscessation and sinus formation. During the acute stage, lameness occurs.

The prognosis is guarded. If extensive damage has been done and the tract has invaded the joint capsule, the prognosis is poor. Surgery to remove the diseased portion of the cartilage is the treatment of choice in most instances.

SANDCRACK

(Toe crack, Quarter crack)

Any break in the continuity of the wall of the hoof that begins at the coronet and parallels the horn tubules. Quarter crack is most commonly seen in racing horses.

Etiology: Trauma or hereditary factors are cited as the cause. Excessive drying of the hoof will predispose to the condition. Extensive injury to the coronet may give rise to a condition characterized by build-up and overlapping of the hoof wall at the site of injury. This latter condition is referred to as false quarter.

Clinical Findings and Diagnosis: The presence of a crack in the horn emanating from the coronet is the most obvious sign. Lameness may be present, although the majority of cases show no lameness. If infection is established, a discharge of pus or blood may follow, accompanied by signs of inflammation.

Treatment: Therapy lies almost entirely in the fields of surgery and corrective shoeing, which change the distribution of the weight borne by the hoof. Growth of new horn may be encouraged by the application of a counterirritant (℞ 650) to the coronet over the crack. If the crack has become infected, an antiseptic pack is indicated. Patching techniques using acrylics, fiberglass, etc. may be successful. Complete stripping of the wall caudad to the crack, being careful not to damage the coronet, is often the treatment of choice in an early and severe quarter crack. The hoof is then bandaged tightly with a suitable dressing. The animal is shod with a three-quarter shoe to relieve any pressure over the stripped portion of the wall.

SEEDY TOE

(Hollow wall, Dystrophia ungulae)

A condition affecting the hoof wall in the toe region, characterized by loss of substance and change in character of the horn. It is most often a sequela to mild chronic laminitis.

Lameness is infrequent. The outer surface of the wall appears sound but upon dressing the palmar surface of the hoof, the inner surface of the wall is seen to be mealy. There actually may be a cavity due to loss of horn substance. Tapping on the outside of the wall at the toe elicits a hollow sound over the affected portion. The disease may involve only a small area or nearly the entire width of the wall at the toe.

The prognosis is usually good. The diseased portion should be curetted and packed temporarily with juniper tar and oakum. If the condition is extensive, it may be necessary to remove the outer wall over the affected area.

KERAPHYLLOCELE

(Keratoma)

An inflammatory non-neoplastic growth of horn on the inner surface of the wall, usually at the toe. It is believed to follow a chronic inflammatory process of the laminar matrix caused by "nail bind," mechanical injury to the wall or coronet, or following hoof-grooving.

The disease often is not obvious until the growth is well advanced. Examination of the palmar surface shows that the growth, commonly of a cylindrical shape, has pushed the white line in toward the center of the sole. The prognosis should be guarded, since pressure atrophy of the pedal bone commonly follows severe cases. Surgical removal of the mass is indicated. In mild cases, corrective shoeing may give some temporary relief..

CONTRACTED HEELS

A condition most commonly seen affecting the quarters and heels of the front feet of light horses. It may be caused by improper shoeing that draws in the quarters and does not allow frog pressure, and is favored by excessive rasping of the foot and trimming of the bars. It may follow the use of a hoof-immobilizing shoe as used for fracture of the third phalanx and, in many cases, navicular disease.

The frog is narrow and shrunken. The bars may be almost parallel to each other. The quarters and heels are markedly contracted and drawn in. Lameness is evident when the horse is worked at speed, although it may disappear after exercise. The length of stride is shortened. Excessive heat may be noticed around the heels and quarters and the pulsation in the digital artery may be marked.

The prognosis is guarded as recovery in well-developed cases takes 6 to 12 months. The most important factor in treatment is to restore normal frog pressure. This can be achieved by means of a bar shoe with the addition of shims between the frog and bar to permit direct pressure on the frog. Other types of surgical shoe, e.g. a slipper shoe, may be tried. Thinning the wall of the quarters just below the coronary band with a rasp, or grooving the walls parallel to the coronet, ¾ in. below the hairline, from the heel halfway to the toe, will aid in expanding the heels; second and third grooves should be ½ in. apart, and parallel to the first. A hoof dressing should be applied regularly. As the quarters grow out the operation must be repeated until the heels and quarters are normally expanded.

SIDEBONE

(Ossification of the lateral cartilages)

Ossification of the lateral cartilages of the third phalanx. The disease is commonest in the front feet of heavy horses used at rapid speeds on hard surfaces. It is also frequent in hunters and jumpers, but rare in thoroughbreds.

Etiology: Repeated concussion to the quarters of the feet may be the essential cause. The condition is believed to be promoted by improper shoeing which inhibits normal physiologic movement of the quarters. Some cases arise from direct trauma.

Clinical Findings: Loss of flexibility on digital palpation of either one or both lateral cartilages is indicative of sidebone. Since the rigidity of the cartilages is accompanied by ossification, the cartilages may, in some cases, protrude prominently above the coronet. Lameness may be a sign depending upon the stage of ossification, the amount of concussion sustained by the feet and the character of the terrain. Lameness is most likely when sidebone is associated with a narrow or contracted foot. Mules often have prominent sidebones, yet reveal no lameness. Walking the horse across a slope may exaggerate the soreness. The gait may show a shortened stride.

Diagnosis: Normally sidebone can be diagnosed by palpation or by observation. In some cases when sidebone is suspected but cannot be palpated, radiologic examination may be useful.

Treatment: When lameness is present, corrective shoeing to promote expansion of the quarters and to protect the foot from concussion often is of value. Grooving the hooves, along with a counterirritant (℞ 650) to the coronary region to promote hoof growth, also may promote expansion of the wall.

RINGBONE

(Phalangeal exostosis)

A periostitis or osteoarthritis leading to exostosis involving the first or second phalanx of the horse.

Etiology: The condition may result from faulty conformation, improper shoeing and repeated concussion through working on hard ground. It may follow trauma and infection, especially wire-cut wounds. In light horses, the straining of ligaments and tendinous insertions of muscles in the pastern region are the most frequent causal factors.

Clinical Findings: Lameness due to the inflammation of the periosteum may appear in the early stages before enlargements occur. After these are well developed, lameness may or may not be present, provided the articular surfaces are not affected. However, lameness is constant if such surfaces are involved and, in some cases, the articulation becomes ankylosed.

Diagnosis: A positive diagnosis of ringbone cannot be made prior to the development of enlargements, since it is based on the presence of enlargements on either of the phalanges. Radiography offers the only dependable means of diagnosis in the early stages.

Treatment: Complete rest is the most important requirement. In the early stages with no involvement of the joint, treatment consists of cold and astringent applications. When the acute stage has subsided, but lameness is still present, superficial counterirritation may be used, but only in the early stages before dense bony accumulations have formed. Deep point-firing may be of value as a means of creating ankylosis when the pastern joint is involved. Anti-inflammatory medication may relieve the signs.

NAVICULAR DISEASE
(Podotrochlosis, Podotrochlitis)

The fact that navicular disease has been described as a chronic osteitis of the navicular bone, associated with navicular bursitis and inflammation of the plantar aponeurosis suggests that this is a syndrome rather than a specific disease entity. It is primarily a disease of the forefeet, but on rare occasions it may appear in the hind feet.

Etiology: The cause is unknown. Usually considered a disease of the more mature riding horse, it has been encountered radiographically even in 3-year-olds. The foot in the long-standing case becomes abnormal in conformation, being upright and narrow and having a small frog. Navicular disease is rare in the Shetland pony, donkey and mule. Defective shoeing that inhibits the physiologic action of the frog and the quarters may be contributory. A recent hypothesis suggests the disease consists of arterial thrombosis within the navicular bones.

Clinical Findings: Navicular disease is insidious in onset and rarely appears suddenly. Attention is first directed to the affected foot or feet by the attitude of the animal when at rest. The horse relieves the pressure of the deep flexor tendon on the painful area by "pointing," that is, by advancing the affected foot with the heel off the ground. If both forefeet are affected, they are pointed alternatively. Lameness is manifested early in the course of the disease. The stride is shortened and there is a tendency to stumble. The animal stands more comfortably when shod with the heels high and the toe rolled.

Diagnosis: Clinical diagnosis is not easy until the condition is well advanced. It is arrived at by the history of pointing, followed by the appearance of lameness. Radiography is of assistance in diagnosis and confirmation of clinical suspicions, but mild radiographic signs alone are insufficient grounds for labeling a case as navicular disease, especially in the absence of the typical history and lameness. Posterior digital nerve blocks may be employed. Application of pressure over the navicular bone with a hoof tester assists in locating the sensitive area.

Treatment: The prognosis is poor since the condition is both chronic and degenerative. Rest is indicated. Thinning the quarters with a rasp may offer relief if the foot is contracted. Toes should be shortened to facilitate the "break-over" when the foot is carried forward. A shoe with branches that thicken toward the heel should be used to relieve tension on the deep flexor tendon. Double posterior digital neurectomy may render relief from pain and prolong the usefulness of the animal. Volar and especially median neurectomy should not be done in light horses that work at speed, and no neurectomy should be considered curative. Intrabursal injection of corticosteroid is also more palliative than curative. Systemic nonsteroidal anti-inflammatory agents in the early stages may prolong the working life.

Based on the theory that thrombosis is causative, anticoagulant therapy is being investigated in hopes of maintaining the secondary blood supply, which develops during the first 2 to 3 years of life. The use of warfarin has shown early promise.

PEDAL OSTEITIS

A rarefying osteitis of the pedal bone. Osteoarthritic factors have been cited as causes, although repeated concussion, laminitis, persistent corns and chronic bruised sole also may be incriminated. The signs are those of discomfort referable to the hoof region. There is often tenderness of the sole on percussion and pressure. Before the use of X-rays in diagnosis, the condition often was confused with navicular disease, especially if the inflammatory lesion was in the posterior part of the foot. Rest and shoeing with protection to the sole may give relief in mild cases.

PYRAMIDAL DISEASE

(Extensor-process disease, Buttress foot)

This condition, formerly classified as a type of low ringbone, is usually due to a traumatically induced periostitis and osteitis or avulsion fracture of the extensor process of the third phalanx caused by excessive pull of the tendon inserted on it.

Because of the close association of the extensor process with the distal phalangeal joint, arthritis is very likely to supervene and lameness is seen in most cases. In the early case, heat and pain on pressure may be manifest. An enlargement of the foot just above the coronet is usually present. Systemic anti-inflammatory treatment may be beneficial.

FRACTURE OF THE OS PEDIS

This condition may arise as a result of a penetrating wound of the foot, as a result of concussion—the horse that "pounds" is susceptible to this type of fracture—or as a sequela to neurectomy or to a pathologic process in the bone. A brittle type of foot or "springing sole" predisposes to the condition.

Clinical Findings: The degree of pain manifested is variable, many cases producing moderate lameness that is greatly increased when the horse is turned or made to pivot on the affected leg. Hoof testers usually yield positive results in early cases.

Diagnosis: The signs may suggest the condition, but the only conclusive means of diagnosis is by radiography. More than 2 different views are often required before the fracture line is evident, especially if X-rays are taken immediately after the fracture occurs and if it is of a hairline nature. Radiographic re-assessment 72 hours later, often rebuts a negative diagnosis immediately following the injury.

Prognosis: When puncture wounds are the cause, the prognosis depends on the presence or absence of infection. Fracture following a pathologic process merits an unfavorable outlook. A guarded to favorable prognosis will, however, depend on the fact that the articular surface is not involved and that adequate rest and immobilization of the part are enforced.

Treatment: Insofar as possible, the foot is immobilized by fitting a plain bar shoe with a clip placed well back on each quarter to limit expansion and contraction of the heels. Rest from work for a year is advised, lesser periods not giving as good results. Where infection or sequestration is present, surgery must be performed. Certain fractures lend themselves to repair using the lag-screw principle. A posterior digital neurectomy may be of value if pedal osteitis follows the healing process.

ARTHRITIS AND RELATED DISORDERS (LG. AN.)

(Degenerative joint disease, Polyarthritis)

Inflammation of the tissues associated with a joint. While frequent in all large animals, arthritis is best known in horses because of the importance of interference with locomotion in this species. (*See also* LAMENESS IN HORSES, p. 538.)

Specific Types of Arthritis: Acute serous arthritis usually is due to trauma and involves only one joint. The joint capsule becomes distended with clear, watery fluid, and is evident upon palpation and movement of the joint. The synovial membrane becomes hyperemic and the tissues surrounding the joint edematous and hot.

Purulent arthritis is commonly associated with navel ill of foals, calves and lambs, or follows trauma near or into a joint. It is characterized by distension of the joint with an accumulation of pus or cloudy synovial fluid containing many neutrophils and is extremely painful. The pyogenic organisms enter the joint through wounds or by hematogenous extension. The articular cartilage, subchondral bone and synovial membrane usually sustain permanent damage. The condition may be polyarticular. Early cases appear as **acute serofibrinous arthritis.**

Chronic arthritis (chronic osteoarthritis) is the type of arthritis most commonly seen in the horse. Ringbone and spavin are common examples. Faulty conformation, repeated trauma and undue stress are factors in producing the disease. Most cases lead to periarticular periosteal exostoses, which may become large and extensive. The condition is commonly observed in the stifle joints of older bulls and cows.

Infectious Swine Arthritis is a common term for a group of bacterial and mycoplasmal arthritic infections in younger pigs. In newborn pigs, infectious arthritis is usually due to intrauterine or navel infection with *E. coli*, *Corynebacterium*, *Streptococcus*, or *Staphylococcus*, and treatment is best directed towards reducing the possibility of infection from the environment. Older pigs will sometimes develop arthritis as a sequela to infection with *Haemophilus*, *Erysipelothrix*, or *Mycoplasma*, and although diagnosis in the early stages of the condition is not difficult, the more chronic stages can be confused with articular lesions produced by dietary hypervitaminosis A. The infectious arthritides are discussed under the headings of the specific diseases.

Clinical Findings: Arthritis produces pain and altered function of the joint. If the process is active or recent, the joint capsule is usually distended and the surrounding tissues swollen and hot. Manipulation of the joint causes pain. In long-standing chronic cases, normal movement is greatly reduced and crepitation may be felt when the parts are moved. Careful palpation of the joint for pain and swelling is important and radiographic examination may be necessary for positive diagnosis.

Treatment: Treatment of acute serous arthritis requires absolute rest until the joint has returned to normal. Application of cold water or ice to the part helps to relieve pain. If the joint capsule is distended, aspiration of the fluid with a sterile needle and syringe gives added relief. Provided the joint cavity is sterile, the injection of corticosteroids (℞ 155, 190), usually exerts a prompt anti-inflammatory action and aids in preventing a recurrence of excessive fluid within the joint. Purulent arthritis demands prompt treatment before irreparable damage is done. In these cases, systemic therapy with appropriate antibiotics as determined by sensitivity tests (℞ 63, 73) may be usefully combined with local therapy. Daily aspiration of the joint contents or incision of the joint capsule to provide drainage and replacement with antibiotics (℞ 67, 75) provide a high concentration of the drugs at the site of infection. Phenylbutazone (℞ 150) relieves pain and allows movement so that fibrous restriction of the affected joint is reduced.

Chronic arthritis and periostitis may be treated satisfactorily only if diagnosed early and treated promptly before the lesion becomes extensive or ankylosis occurs. Where early diagnosis is established, radiation therapy may be of value. Other treatments include the use of counterirritants, such as blisters (℞ 647), ultrasonic therapy and point-firing and surgical fusion. After any type of treatment, the patient must be rested for at least 6 months. Treatment usually is unsuccessful in the chronic deforming and adhesive arthritis of old bulls and cows. However, restricted exercise, good feeding, housing and management may prolong the life of the patient, and this may be worthwhile in the case of valuable breeding animals. In bulls that are unable to mount, semen for artificial breeding purposes may be collected with an electro-ejaculator. The intra-articular injection of corticosteroids (℞ 155, 190) may relieve the discomfort.

BURSITIS

Acute or chronic inflammation of a bursa may occur in all species, but is more common and important in the horse.

Etiology and Clinical Findings: The most commonly involved bursae are those that are superficial and located over bony prominences or between tendons. Common locations are the bursae overlying the tuber ischii (car bruise), the olecranon process (capped elbow, shoeboil), the tuber calcis (capped hock), the trochanter major (trochanteric bursitis), the bicipital groove (intertubular bursitis) and the navicular bone (navicular bursitis).

Acute serous bursitis is usually due to severe trauma and is characterized by rapid swelling, local heat and pain. Infection of bursae may be hematogenous or follow penetrating wounds or nonsterile surgical treatment of a serous bursitis. As the bursitis becomes chronic, the local swelling and heat subside, but the area may show evidence of pain on palpation or movement. Atrophy of muscles may occur if the bursitis causes reduced function of a limb.

Treatment: The pain in acute serous bursitis may be relieved by application of cold packs, aspiration of the contents and injection of 2% lidocaine solution. Prednisolone (℞ 155) or its derivatives have proved beneficial when injected into bursae. Phenylbutazone (℞ 150) will give relief from pain. Repeated injections may result in abscess formation. The bursa should not be incised. If the condition becomes chronic, aspiration followed by repeated injection of half-strength tincture of iodine (℞ 648) or Lugol's solution (℞ 599) may cause the swelling gradually to subside. Radiation therapy (q.v., p. 1490) is often beneficial. The application of counterirritants (℞ 647, 649) over the distended area may also help to reduce the swelling. Infected bursae require drainage and systemic treatment with antibiotics. Recovery is slow.

TENOSYNOVITIS

Acute or chronic inflammation of the synovial sheath of a tendon.

Etiology: Synovitis often occurs in conjunction with tendinitis. Most cases arise from excessive strain on the tendons from overwork. Others are caused by bruising of the tissues by bumping against hard objects. Infection of the synovial sheath may come about by penetrating foreign bodies, or by metastasis in certain infectious diseases of horses. Adhesions of the tendon sheath to the tendon will produce a constant effusion of synovial fluid.

Clinical Findings: If primary, the condition usually affects only one synovial sheath. If secondary or metastatic, usually is it seen in several sheaths. Acute synovitis shows the classic signs of acute inflammation together with accumulation of excessive amounts of synovia. If it becomes chronic, pain and heat disappear, but the excess fluid remains. In synovitis due to foreign-body penetration, there is usually exudation of pus and synovial fluid. In horses, chronic synovitis is common in locations such as the synovial sheath of the deep flexor tendon at the hock (thoroughpin) and the sheath of the deep flexor tendon over the distal third of the metacarpus and metatarsus (tendon sheath gall). Thoroughpin should be differentiated from bog spavin (q.v., p. 545) and tendon sheath gall from chronic distension of the capsule of the fetlock joint.

Treatment: In the acute stage, the use of cold packs or cold-water showers, the injection of steroids (℞ 155) into the affected sheath, repeated after 3 or 4 days, and absolute rest are advisable. If infection is present, or if the condition is secondary to another disease, systemic administration of antibiotics (℞ 63, 73) is indicated. For chronic synovitis, application of counterirritants (℞ 647) followed by massage and bandaging results in temporary reduction of the distension. Injection of corticosteroids (℞ 155, 190) into the synovial space may be followed by prompt and more lasting reduction of the swelling; reinjection is dependent on whether the swelling recurs. Because of the associated weakening effect on the tissues, rest for at least 2 weeks is necessary if steroids have been injected.

TENDINITIS
("Bowed tendon")

Acute or chronic inflammation of a tendon. Tendinitis is seen most commonly in horses used at fast work, particularly race horses. The flexor tendons, are more frequently involved than the extensor tendons, and those of the foreleg more commonly than those of the hind. Of these, the superficial flexor is most frequently involved in the common "bowed tendon" of race horses. The primary lesion is a rupture of the tendon fibers with associated hemorrhage and edema. In thoroughbreds, the leading or inside foreleg (which depends on whether they race in a clockwise or counterclockwise direction) is more frequently affected than the other.

Etiology: Tendinitis usually appears during forced exercise. The commonest causes include overexertion without proper training, continuance of training after first signs of tendon soreness have appeared, fatigue and fast work on muddy, rough or hard track surfaces. Improper shoeing, by placing extra strain on the flexor tendons, also predisposes to tendinitis. Poor conformation and training at too early an age also may result in tendon breakdown.

Clinical Findings: During the acute stage the horse is severely lame and stands with the heel elevated to ease the tension on the tendons. The structures involved are hot, painful and swollen. Chronic straining of the flexor tendons and associated ligaments in the cannon region ultimately leads to fibrosis, with thickening, adhesions, and shortening of the tendons. In chronic tendinitis, the patient may go sound while walking or trotting, but the tendon rarely holds up under hard work.

Treatment: Tendinitis is best treated in the early, acute stage. The horse should be given absolute rest by confinement. The swelling and inflammation should be reduced by applying cold packs and the leg may be immobilized in a plaster cast for 6 to 8 weeks, but many clinicians prefer not to use casts. Good results have also been obtained by injecting the inflamed area of the tendon with prednisolone or its derivatives followed by the application of a plaster cast. The injection is made by inserting a 20-gauge needle through the tendon and depositing 0.5 to 1.0 ml of prednisolone as the needle is withdrawn. The injections are spaced at half-inch intervals over the entire area of the swelling. Rapid reduction of inflammation usually follows. If this procedure is used, absolute rest is required for at least 2 weeks as corticosteroids injected into or around tendons may produce collagen necrosis with temporary weakening of the tendon. X-ray therapy, in conjunction with immobilization, may also be used for acute tendinitis.

After removal of the cast, the patient should be given additional rest and the leg supported with bandages for another 4 weeks. Exercise should be mild and gradually increased. Ideally, training should not be resumed until at least a year of rest has been given.

Chronic tendinitis has been treated by deep point-firing directly into the affected tendon, although the results of firing are questionable in many of these cases. A year's rest should be prescribed and is doubtless the chief element in recovery following firing. An alternative is the injection of the tendon at half-inch intervals with a sclerosing agent (℞ 670), after which the horse is rested for 6 to 8 months. For the first 4 weeks after injection, the horse's heels, which are elevated about 1 in. (2.5 cm) with a special shoe, are gradually lowered to normal position and the animal is given light exercise. Surgical treatment, percutaneous and open tendon splitting, volar annular ligament resection, and fascial transplants are widely used, replacing point-firing to a considerable degree.

ARTHRITIS AND RELATED DISORDERS (SM. AN.)

Inflammatory disorders of the joints are common in dogs, but rare in cats. Several distinct types of arthritis are described in human medicine, but their counterparts in animals are not as well defined. Immune mediated arthritides such as canine systemic lupus erythematosis and rheumatoid arthritis are diagnosed with increased frequency in the dog. (*See* DISEASES INVOLVING IMMUNE COMPLEXES, pp. 4, 10.) Traumatic arthritis occurs as a sequela of direct injury to a joint. The exudate is serous or, if bacteria are present, fibrinous or purulent. Septic arthritis may cause erosion of the articular surfaces and extreme pain on movement of the joint. A common cause of arthritis in the dog is that associated with hip dysplasia q.v., p. 574. Osteoarthritis, or degenerative arthritis, is common in dogs and is usually associated with advancing age.

OSTEOARTHRITIS
(Osteoarthrosis)

Osteoarthritis is frequently seen in dogs and is characterized by proliferative and degenerative changes in the affected joint.

Etiology: The cause of osteoarthritis is not completely understood, but the normal aging processes are thought to be contributory. It frequently follows trauma. Three main factors believed to be involved in the pathogenesis are: enzymes, chondrocyte function and nutrition. Degenerative disease of the cartilage is a primary factor. Osteoarthritis of the hip joint may result from luxation, congenital subluxation or an unstable joint. Osteoarthritis of the stifle joint may result from previous ligament injuries, a common one being rupture of the anterior cruciate ligament. Vascular disturbances, metabolic disorders and hormonal imbalances have been suspected. Obesity may be a predisposing factor.

Clinical Findings: Destruction of the articular cartilage occurs in degenerative osteoarthritis. It may be eroded or pitted and may even disappear. Osseous deposition occurs within the joint and as bone proliferation (lipping) at the edges of the joint.

The hip and stifle joints are most frequently affected. Slowly developing lameness is the outstanding sign. Pain of varying degrees is always present. Stiffness on arising is common, but this usually lessens with movement. Crepitus may be present and atrophy of associated muscles may occur.

Diagnosis: The onset is insidious, the course progressive. Although frequently associated with advancing age, osteoarthritis is common in certain of the larger breeds (boxers, collies, Great Danes), which often show premature senility. It may occur in young dogs following trauma or in dogs with congenital abnormalities of the joints. Radiography is the most valuable diagnostic aid. Radiographs of affected joints reveal varying degrees of proliferative and degenerative changes. There may be poor correlation between radiographic findings and the clinical signs. Biopsy of the synovial membrane and analysis of the joint fluid may be useful in determining the etiology and pathologic state of the disease. Other laboratory tests include a complete blood count, protein electrophoresis, and examination for L.E. cells, antinuclear antibodies, and rheumatoid factor.

Treatment: Aspirin (℞ 612) is the drug of choice for relief of pain. Corticosteroids (℞ 154) have proved useful, but should not be used indiscriminately. Phenylbutazone (℞ 150) has also been recommended. Intra-articular injections of certain corticosteroids (℞ 157) may be beneficial in selected cases. Weight reduction should be attempted if obesity is present. Warm, dry quarters should be provided. Other forms of treatment include the use of heat pads or heat lamps, gentle massage of the affected joints and ultrasonic therapy.

In severe osteoarthritis of the hip, excision arthroplasty may be considered. Surgery to repair ruptured ligaments or damaged menisci in the stifle may also be of benefit in retarding the advancement of the arthritis process.

SUPPURATIVE ARTHRITIS
(Septic arthritis)

This condition is usually caused by the introduction of infection into a joint by trauma. The affected joint is swollen, hot and painful, and the body temperature is elevated. Marked lameness is present. Examination may disclose a wound leading into the joint. A discharge composed of pus and synovial fluid may be present. Pus in the joint cavity may have a lytic effect on the articular cartilage, and bone destruction may follow.

Aspiration of the synovial fluid may be attempted and if unsuccessful, surgical drainage of the joint may be necessary. The fluid should be cultured and antibiotic sensitivity tests performed. Appropriate antibiotics should be used locally as well as systemically and administration should continue for several weeks. Intrasynovial injection of antibiotics often aids in shortening the acute inflammatory phase.

BURSITIS

Trauma to the area is the usual cause of bursitis. The commonest site in dogs is over the elbow. Serous bursitis occurs more frequently in the large breeds, particularly Great Danes, Irish wolfhounds and St. Bernards. The weight of these dogs, coupled with the manner in which they customarily lie down, may be contributory. It is seen occasionally in other breeds, such as German shepherd dogs and bloodhounds.

Clinical Findings: A soft to firm swelling occurs at the level of the olecranon process. Palpation reveals very little pain except when the bursa has become infected. The bursal effusion is usually serous. If continued trauma can be eliminated, recovery may occur spontaneously.

The condition usually recurs in the larger breeds and eventually becomes chronic. In chronic bursitis, the endothelial lining of the bursa degenerates and the bursal wall becomes thickened and fibrous. In cases of long standing, the skin over the center of the bursal swelling occasionally becomes eroded and develops into a typical indolent decubital ulcer.

Treatment: The fluid should be aspirated and, if infection is suspected, a cultural examination of the effusion should be made. If infection is present, an antibiotic (℞ 68) should be injected directly into the bursa. In the absence of infection, aspiration of the bursa and injection of corticosteroids (℞ 157, 190) may be beneficial.

In all cases of bursitis, prevention of further trauma to the affected side is essential. Protective, padded bandages may be applied. Mattresses or suitable bedding should be provided.

Surgical removal of the bursal sac may be attempted if it is large, unsightly and chronically affected. Superficial bursae are not essential and may be safely excised. However, deep bursae are important to function and, moreover, may communicate with a joint. Many clinicians prefer to place a Penrose drain through the bursa and to medicate via the tube.

SPONDYLOSIS DEFORMANS
(Spondylitis)

A degenerative condition involving the vertebrae, particularly the lumbar area, characterized by the development of osteophytes at the ends and near the ventral border of the vertebrae. Degenerative arthropathy may occur at the articular processes. The disease usually occurs as a chronic, progressive disease of older dogs. It may occur in all breeds, but is particularly noted in the larger breeds of working or sporting dogs. Ventral protrusion of the nucleus pulposus associated with changes in the annulus fibrosus is one of the known causes of spondylosis.

The majority of dogs with spondylosis deformans reveal no clinical signs. Signs will develop in association with injury or trauma to the ankylosing new bone. Pain becomes evident and affected dogs are reluctant to move with characteristic freedom.

Radiographically the osteophytes have sloping, smooth ventral or lateral surfaces that blend with the cortex of the vertebral body. The disk spaces are of normal width. One or several pairs of vertebral bodies may be involved. Treatment is indicated only in the event of pain. Aspirin alone (℞ 612) or in conjunction with steroids is beneficial. Anabolic steroids and calcium may hasten the repair of fractures involving the osteophytes.

CAPPED ELBOW AND HOCK

Inflammatory swelling of the subcut. bursa located over the olecranon process and tuber calcis, respectively. Trauma from lying on poorly bedded hard floors, kicks, falls, riding the tail gate of trailers, iron shoes projecting beyond the heels and chronic lameness enforcing long periods of recumbency are frequent causes.

Circumscribed edematous swelling occurs over and around the affected bursa. Lameness is rare in either case. The affected bursa may be fluctuating and soft at first, but in a short time, a firm, fibrous capsule forms, especially if there is a recurrence of an old injury. Initial bursal swellings vary in size from hardly noticeable enlargements to those of sizable proportions. Chronic cases may progress to abscessation.

Acute early cases may respond well to cold-water applications, followed in a few days by aseptic aspiration and injection of a corticosteroid (℞ 157, 190). The bursa may also be reduced in size by the application of a counterirritant paint (℞ 647, 649), ultrasonic therapy, or radiation therapy. Older encapsulated bursae are more refractory to treatment. Surgical removal is recommended only for capped elbows, either of the advanced encapsulated type, or those that have abscessed. A shoe-boil roll should be used to prevent recurrence of a capped elbow in those animals in which the condition has been caused by the heel or by the shoe.

FISTULOUS WITHERS—POLL EVIL

Two inflammatory disorders of horses that differ from one another essentially only in their location in the respective supraspinous and supra-atlantal bursae. The following account deals with fistulous withers but, except for anatomic details, the remarks apply in general also to poll evil. In the early stage of the disease a fistula is not present. When the bursal sac ruptures or when it is opened for surgical drainage, and secondary infection with pyogenic bacteria occurs, it usually assumes a true fistulous character. Today it is rarely seen.

Etiology: Evidence suggests that the condition is primarily infectious in origin, and agglutination test titers support the theory. *Brucella abortus* and occasionally *Br. suis* can be isolated from the fluid aspirated from the unopened bursa and outbreaks of brucellosis in cattle have followed contact with horses with open bursitis.

Clinical Findings: The inflammation leads to considerable thickening of the wall of the bursa. The bursal sacs increase in size by distension. Rupture may occur where the sac has little covering support. In older, advanced cases the ligament and the dorsal vertebral spines are affected, and occasionally necrosis is observed in these structures.

The bursitis in the early stage consists of a distension of the supraspinous bursa with a clear, straw-colored, viscid exudate. The swelling may be dorsal, unilateral, or bilateral, depending on the arrangement of the bursal sacs between the tissue layers. It is an exudative process from the beginning, but no true suppuration or secondary infection occurs until the bursa ruptures or is opened.

Prophylaxis: It is reasonable to keep horses separate from *Brucella*-infected cattle, and horses with discharging fistulous withers from cattle.

Treatment: The earlier treatment is instituted, the better the prognosis. The most successful treatment is complete dissection and removal of the infected bursa. The expense of the protracted treatment required in long-standing cases often exceeds the value of the animal. *Brucella* vaccines have not proved helpful. In some cases, iodine therapy appears to be of considerable benefit.

PATELLAR LUXATION

A partial or complete dislocation of the patella, most commonly seen in dogs and horses and occasionally in cattle. Small breeds of dogs are more frequently affected than the larger breeds. Lateral and more commonly dorsal luxations of the patella are also encountered in horses. In ponies it often occurs as a bilateral affliction in the first few months of life. In other breeds of horses, it appears most often as a unilateral condition during the first 2 or 3 years of life. It is often congenital because of malalignment of the limb but may be acquired due to ligamentous strain or muscular weakness.

Dorsal fixation in the horse may be momentary, recurrent or complete. The stifle and hock joints are locked in extension and the fetlock is flexed. If forced to walk, the animal will drag the toe along the ground. The first few times dorsal fixation occurs, the horse usually exhibits signs of varying degrees of pain, particularly in cases of complete fixation. Backing is extremely difficult or impossible. In cattle the gait disturbance is not as well defined as in the horse.

In the dog, intermittent or recurrent luxations are characterized by the animal appearing normal one minute and carrying a hind limb the next. No pain is evidenced and palpation is not resented. Lameness is marked if the leg is used. The luxation is usually medial, the stifle being adducted and the hock rotated outward. The affected limb has a "pigeon toed" appearance. The patella can usually be replaced with little difficulty by applying gentle pressure to the fully extended stifle joint. Persistent luxations cause continuous lameness or abnormal gaits. Rotation of the tibia on the longitudinal axis and bowing of the distal end of the femur and proximal end of the tibia are commonly noticed on radiographs of dogs affected with congenital patellar ectopia; the trochlear groove may be quite shallow. Lateral luxation is infrequent and usually the result of severe trauma. Bilateral luxations are not uncommon in toy breeds and are characterized by difficulty in standing or walking. Patellar luxations may be classified by clinical features: Grade 1.

The patella may be dislocated only if the knee is extended and digital pressure applied. Occasionally traumatic dislocation occurs. Grade 2. While the patella usually lies in its normal position, it may be dislocated on extension and remain so on subsequent flexion. Grade 3. The patella is dislocated most of the time. It may be manually reduced on extension but dislocated again on flexion. Grade 4. The patella is dislocated and cannot be reduced without surgical intervention; the knee cannot be fully extended.

In all cases the treatment is surgical.

RUPTURE OF THE CRUCIATE LIGAMENTS

In dogs, this is a common result of injury to the stifle joint. The cranial (anterior) cruciate ligament is more commonly ruptured than is the caudal (posterior) ligament. Rupture of one or both of these may be accompanied by rupture of the medial collateral ligament, and commonly the medial meniscus is damaged. The lateral meniscus may occasionally be involved. Acute lameness will moderate with time. Chronic lameness and osteoarthritis may result if the stifle instability is not treated.

Joint instability can be demonstrated by the drawer sign (exerting cranial and caudal pressure on the head of the tiba, with the limb held in normal angulation; when the tibia is released it will often slide forward in affected cases). Medial rotation of the tibia must be prevented while attempting to displace the tibial head.

Surgical stabilization of the stifle is indicated. Many methods have been used and they can be grouped into: (1) creation of a prosthetic ligament; (2) suturing the retinaculum of the joint capsule, or adjacent supporting structures or both; (3) a combination of internal and external technique. Partial or total meniscetomy may be indicated. The prognosis is good if osteoarthritis is not severe and joint stability is achieved.

In large animals, the cranial (anterior) cruciate ligament is ruptured more commonly than the caudal (posterior) cruciate ligament. In many cases, the medial collateral ligament of the femorotibial joint is also ruptured or damaged. Bulls are more commonly affected than other large animals. The injury commonly occurs when the bull is hit by another bull on the lateral side of one stifle joint while breeding a cow. Severe mechanical stresses in horses may also rupture these ligaments. Occasionally the same effect results from an avulsion fracture of the intercondylar eminence or spine instead of ligamentous rupture. Severe lameness is evident, often accompanied by sound of crepitation when the animal walks. Distension of the femoropatellar pouch is present between the patellar ligaments.

Motion between the femur and tibia can usually be produced by a quick backward pull on the top of the tibia and then release. Counter pressure should be applied to the hock; sliding motion can be produced in a normal joint. Rupture of the medial collateral ligament is checked by applying pressure from the outside of the stifle joint and pulling outward on the foot. If opening of the joint can be produced on the medial side, one can assume that the medial collateral ligament is ruptured. The injury must be differentiated from fractures of the femur and tibia.

Replacement of the anterior cruciate ligament with a piece of skin has been done successfully in cattle but not in horses. Success in treatment has also been obtained in bulls by immobilization of the affected limb in a modified Thomas splint for a 6-week period. Prognosis is unfavorable because usually there is damage to the medial meniscus in addition to the ligamentous tearing. Arthritic changes are often irreversible.

CANINE HIP DYSPLASIA

A developmental disease of the hip joints that occurs most often in young dogs of the large and giant breeds. The abnormality may vary from slightly poor conformation to malformation permitting complete luxation of the femoral head. The disease is considered to be a polygenic trait with low to moderate heritability. The occurrence of hip dysplasia can be lowered only slightly by selective mating of individual dogs with normal hips, but may be markedly lowered by selection of breeding animals based on family performance and progeny testing. Breeding of dysplastic animals and of normal animals that transmit a high incidence of hip dysplasia to their offspring is to be discouraged. Environment influences manifestation of the defect.

At birth the hip joints appear normal, both physically and radiographically, hence the disease is not congenital. Dysplasia begins to develop some time after birth if the femoral head ceases to maintain normal contact with the acetabulum. At this time, the femoral head and most of the acetabulum are still cartilaginous and the shapes of these 2 parts are easily changed if stresses are altered. Hip joint instability may be caused by inheritance of a shallow acetabulum, an incorrectly angled femoral neck, laxity of joint-supporting soft tissues (muscles, tendons, ligaments and joint capsule), or a combination of these abnormalities. Degenerative joint disease (remodelling change in cartilage and bone) occurs later as a secondary complication of the dysplasia.

Incidence is highest in heavy and rapidly growing pups of large breeds. Up to 50% of some large breeds are affected, but the condition seldom occurs in dogs maturing at less than 25 lb (11 kg). It has not been reported in Greyhounds, which have greater pelvic muscle mass and different pelvic conformation than other breeds. There is no sex difference in occurrence. Hip dysplasia also occurs in other domestic animals but much less commonly.

Clinical Findings: Dogs that develop hip dysplasia may give evidence of pain in the hip joints starting at 5 to 6 months. This is presumably due to erosion of the articular cartilages of the femoral heads and acetabulae and to tearing of the attachments of the ligaments, tendons and capsule of the hip joint. The disease is best diagnosed radiographically and can be detected by 4 to 6 months of age in well-defined cases. Proper positioning for radiographs is extremely important and the ventrodorsal view with the legs extended is standard. In most instances, the lesion is bilateral and consists of a shallow acetabulum with a loosely fitting, flattened femoral head. Signs of osteoarthrosis are often present. Development of hip dysplasia does not occur at the same age in all individuals, and the optimum age for definitive radiographic diagnosis is 24 to 36 months.

Treatment: Pain relieving drugs (℞ 612) or corticosteroids (e.g. ℞ 154) are useful during the period of joint remodelling. Pectineus muscle surgery (pectinotomy, pectinectomy) is frequently beneficial if pain persists after the dog is mature, though its effects may only be temporary. Femoral neck resection also brings relief from pain, and may be performed either initially or after pectineal surgery has been tried. Techniques for total hip replacement have been developed and are being used successfully.

RUPTURE OF THE ACHILLES TENDON

A partial or complete disruption in the continuity of the gastrocnemius and superficial flexor tendons. It may be the result of trauma from automobile accidents, laceration from mowing machinery or wire, extreme stress during a race or hunt, or occasionally, a severe local infection. Lacerations may occur anywhere along the course of the tendon; however, ruptures are usually at the point of insertions on the calcaneus, in connection with an avulsive fracture of the tuber calcis, or at the juncture of the muscle and tendon.

Rupture of the gastrocnemius muscle (q.v., p. 600) produces a gait identical to that of rupture of the Achilles tendon. Careful examination, both radiographic and by palpation, should be carried out to determine the exact nature of the lesion and the possibility of bone involvement.

There is a characteristic alteration of the stance and gait. The animal is no longer able to stand or walk on the toes of the affected limb. The degree of flexion of the hock is increased without concurrent flexion of the stifle. The plantar surface of the metatarsus may touch the ground. On palpation, the tendon is flaccid and sometimes swollen. Pain is not an outstanding sign.

The treatment is surgical, and musculotendinous ruptures require immediate attention. Ruptures with sharp division of the tendon are easier to repair than indistinct lacerations. After surgical repair, the leg should be immobilized in a slightly flexed position for 5 to 6 weeks. Fixation of the tuber calcanei to the tibia with a bone screw has been recommended as a method of immobilization.

DYSTROPHIES ASSOCIATED WITH CALCIUM, PHOSPHORUS AND VITAMIN D

The principal causes of osteodystrophies are deficiencies or imbalances of dietary calcium, phosphorus and vitamin D. Their interrelationships are not easily defined and there may be absolute or relative (i.e. conditioned or secondary) deficiencies of any of the three. Deficiencies must be assessed in relation to availability and growth rate.

An absolute or relative deficiency of calcium causes hyperparathyroidism in all species with the development of osteoporosis (lack of bone) or osteodystrophia fibrosa or both. Calcium deficiency does not cause rickets or osteomalacia in mammals. Absolute deficiency is less common than deficiency conditioned by excess phosphorus.

Phosphorus deficiency causes rickets in growing animals and osteomalacia in adults. There may also be osteoporosis. Phosphorus deficiency occurs mainly in grazing ruminants, being rare in animals consuming grain or meat. Poor appetite and growth rate, pica and abnormalities of gait occur. Decreased milk yield, infertility and, occasionally, anemia (*see* POSTPARTURIENT HEMOGLOBINURIA, p. 527) are seen in cows.

Vitamin D deficiency is the classic cause of rickets (growing animals) and osteomalacia (adults). It usually results from insufficient exposure of animals or their feed to sunshine. It is influenced by deficiencies or imbalances of calcium and phosphorus; high levels of carotene in green feed may also produce signs of vitamin-D deficiency.

Hypervitaminosis D may be iatrogenic or result from accidental dietary supplementation. Hypercalcemia, wasting and metastatic mineralization of tissues (especially kidney, stomach and blood vessels) result. Pseudohyperparathyroidism occurs in some dogs with malignant lymphoma and produces similar signs. The neoplasm probably secretes a parathormone-like substance. Animals grazing plants with vitamin D activity also may show signs of hypervitaminosis D (*see* ENZOOTIC CALCINOSIS, p. 1032).

More than one disease due to deficiencies and imbalances of calcium phosphorus and vitamin D may coincide in an animal or group of animals, and descriptions of such cases as pure deficiencies have confused the interpretation of naturally occurring osteodystrophies. At present, the diagnosis of these osteodystrophies is based on histologic criteria. Bone ash analyses will generally allow separation of the various diseases. Often, phosphorus deficiency is accompanied by hypophosphatemia; vitamin D deficiency by hypocalcemia; calcium deficiency by normocalcemia.

NUTRITIONAL HYPERPARATHYROIDISM
(Osteodystrophia fibrosa)

A condition affecting all species caused by an absolute or conditioned deficiency of calcium. The lesions and signs are related to excess parathyroid hormone secreted in response to declining serum-ionized calcium. In general, growing animals are most severely affected because their requirement for calcium is high, and fast growth rates increase the likelihood of development of disease. This is the most important osteodystrophy of domesticated animals. A large proportion of the osteodystrophies diagnosed as rickets and osteomalacia and osteogenesis imperfecta of kittens and puppies are manifestations of nutritional hyperparathyroidism.

Etiology: Diets consisting solely of grain or grain products (for horses, pigs, cattle and sheep), meat or liver (for dogs and cats) or fruit (for monkeys) cause the condition. The disease also occurs in horses grazing pastures high in oxalates (e.g. *Setaria sphacelata, Cenchrus ciliaris, Panicum maximum*); insoluble calcium oxalate is probably formed in the gut.

Clinical Findings and Diagnosis: The combination of lameness, bone deformities and osteoporosis in young animals should suggest the diagnosis. In kittens and puppies lethargy, obscure lameness, progressing to posterior weakness and hyperextension, and deviation of carpal-metacarpal and tarsal-metatarsal joints may occur within 6 weeks of weaning onto meat diet. Kyphosis, scoliosis, pelvic deformities and fractures, both macroscopic and microscopic, can also occur within this period if no source of calcium is added to the meat. The onset of signs may be delayed, but not prevented, in kittens fed milk. Milk supplies calcium but also phosphorus, and insufficient milk is consumed to balance these minerals.

Radiographs show generalized demineralization. Growth plates are normal unless rickets is superimposed. Bones are soft, may be deformed and often brown due to subperiosteal hemorrhage. Parathyroid hyperplasia is sometimes recognizable grossly; usually microscopic examination is required. Serum calcium is often normal in response to the parathyroid hormone, therefore analyses may be uninformative. Fibrous tissue proliferation in the marrow with irregular trabeculae showing microfractures and osteoclasia are characteristic of the condition. All bones are affected, fast-growing bones most severely. Treated and adult animals may have deformed bones with normal strength and ash. Pelvic deformities in such animals can cause obstipation or dystocia.

In pigs, lameness and bone deformities occur. Fractures of subchondral bone lead to collapse of articular cartilage. In severe cases bones of the head, including the mandibles, are enlarged. Fractures of long bones may occur and some cases of slipped upper femoral epiphyses and femoral neck fractures in sows may be manifestations of nutritional hyperparathyroidism.

The overt effect of nutritional hyperparathyroidism, is well-known in horses as **bran disease, millers' disease and big head.** Many of the obscure lamenesses of horses have been attributed to nutritional hyperparathyroidism and such cases probably constitute a more important effect of the disease. The pathologic changes are similar to those in other species with the provisos that the bones of the head are particularly affected in severe cases and that gross or microscopic fractures of subchondral bone, with consequent degeneration of articular cartilage and tearing of ligaments from periosteal attachments, are a dominant influence on the clinical signs.

Nutritional hyperparathyroidism is rarely reported in cattle and sheep, but is occasionally recognized in feedlot animals. Marrow fibroplasia is not a feature of the condition in these species. Osteoporosis is the dominant lesion.

Treatment: Calcium, given orally, and rest are required. Vitamin D without calcium is contraindicated because it stimulates bone resorption. Phosphorus, along with calcium, as in bonemeal, or milk, is contraindicated because it hinders the establishment of optimum Ca:P ratios. Injectable solutions containing calcium should be reserved for immediate treatment of severe cases in small animals. Parenteral treatment is not an efficient means of supplying calcium in bulk.

A cheap and efficient treatment is calcium carbonate, which contains 40% calcium by weight. Half a gram of calcium carbonate per 100 gm of meat corrects the Ca:P ratio and provides sufficient calcium for kittens and puppies. (Meat may also be deficient in vitamins A and D and in iodine.)

Generalizations regarding requirements for calcium are less meaningful in horses and pigs than in small animals. Factors such as growth rate and activity should be considered. Recommendations for 1.2% calcium and 1% phosphorus in the ration have been made. These levels are nearly twice "normal levels" and will be influenced by the type and therefore the quantity of feed consumed. Zinc at 100 ppm is required with the high calcium.

Horses require a Ca:P ratio of around 1.4:1 and the ratio is apparently quite critical. Calcium should constitute about 0.4 to 0.6% of the ration.

RICKETS

A disease of growing animals characterized by interference with mineralization, and consequently with normal resorption, of growth-plate cartilage and interference with mineralization of bone matrix. Rapidly growing plates in rapidly growing bones are most severely affected.

Etiology: Deficient intake or absorption or both of vitamin D or phosphorus or both are most often causative. In housed animals, vitamin D deficiency is important; pastured animals are more likely to be phosphorus-deficient. Abnormal metabolism of vitamin D as occurs, for example, in uremia or inherited biochemical defects, should be considered in rachitic animals on apparently normal diets, as should improper compounding of the diet. Failure to absorb vitamin D may be caused by steatorrhea.

Clinical Findings and Diagnosis: In severe cases there is lameness associated with enlargement of the ends of fast-growing bones, and deformities of the weight-bearing long bones. Lameness and enlargement of the joints is more commonly due to chronic polyarthritis and, in young, large dogs, to hypertrophic osteodystrophy. Radiographs of rachitic bones show wide growth plates and demineralization. Demineralization in nutritional hyperparathyroidism is accompanied by normal growth plates.

Widening of the growth plate due to failure to resorb cartilage is not pathognomonic of rickets. Any factor which interferes with normal metaphyseal vascularization or sinusoidal invasion of cartilage or both may cause widening of the plate. This point should be considered when interpreting radiographs of single joints. Rachitic animals usually have a Ca:P (mg%) product of less than 30. This is a useful aid to diagnosis if serum is collected before any therapy or dietary change has been instituted. Confirmation of the diagnosis in mild cases requires histologic examination including study of active growth plates and of bone matrix in normal tissue. Since rachitic animals may be hypocalcemic, histologic changes of hyperparathyroidism may be present.

Treatment: Accurate diagnosis is imperative as vitamin D without calcium exacerbates those conditions associated with nutritional hyperparathyroidism. Rickets caused by simple deficiencies of vitamin D or phosphorus should be treated according to standard nutritional recommendations after detailed consideration and, if possible, analysis of the existing diet. Secondary deficiencies require correction of the underlying cause.

OSTEOMALACIA
(Adult rickets)

A failure of mineralization of bone matrix resulting in softening of bone. Osteomalacia occurs in adult animals after bone growth has ceased. Osteomalacia has become a general term applied to soft bones without regard to the reason for the softness. The term is used correctly to describe an osteodystrophy of particular histologic appearance and is not synonymous with soft bones *per se*. According to this usage, osteomalacia is common only in areas of endemic phosphorus deficiency—most of the osteodystrophies diagnosed as osteomalacia are cases of nutritional hyperparathyroidism.

Etiologically the same general comments made for rickets apply to osteomalacia.

Clinical Findings and Diagnosis: There is a herd history of low fertility, poor growth, pica, spontaneous fractures and perhaps anemia. Serum phosphate is low. Radiographs may show a reduction of bone density but even fractured bones sometimes show no evidence of abnormal density and microscopic examination of mineralized bone is required for confirmation of the diagnosis. Affected bones show an increase in the number and width of layers of unmineralized matrix on bone surfaces.

Osteomalacia in cats and dogs is mostly due to chronic renal failure.

Treatment: Phosphorus supplements should be added to the diet. Specific procedures used will depend on economic and management factors and the magnitude of the problem.

DEGENERATIVE ARTHROPATHY OF CATTLE
(Degenerative joint disease, Osteoarthritis)

A nonspecific condition affecting mainly the hip and stifle joints. The condition is characterized by degeneration of articular cartilage and eburnation of subchondral bone, distension and fibrosis with ossification of the joint capsule, excess synovial fluid and osteophytes.

Etiology: Many causes and predisposing factors probably influence the development, age of onset and severity of the condition. Inherited disposition to degenerative arthropathy occurs. Certain conformations, for example straight hocks in beef bulls, are incriminated. Nutritional factors involved in some cases are high-phosphorus, low-calcium rations, which probably influence the strength of subchondral bone. Copper deficiency may also act in a similar way. Theoretically, anything causing irreversible degeneration of articular cartilage can initiate the sequence leading to degenerative joint disease. The role of infection is unclear. Infectious arthritis in calves usually produces severe changes in the hock but degenerative arthropathy rarely involves this joint.

Clinical Findings and Diagnosis: Young bulls fed for show on high-grain diets may become lame as early as 6 to 12 months but most cases are first noticed at 1 to 2 years. Lameness is of gradual onset and usually affects both hip joints. Stifle involvement in young bulls is rare. Signs progress concomitantly with degeneration of cartilage and development of osteophytes. Lameness to the point of incapacitation, with crepitation of degenerate joints, may develop in a few months; however, correlation between pathologic changes and clinical signs is poor. The earliest changes occur in the acetabulum and on the dorsomedial surface of the femoral head.

In cows, the stifle joint is mostly affected and the medial condyle of the femur shows the earliest changes. Onset of signs is later than in bulls, usually occurring in adult animals. Since degenerative arthropathy may result from any of several initiating factors no specific diagnostic tests are available. Diagnosis is based on clinical signs and history.

Treatment: Most animals have irreversible changes in the joints by the time the diagnosis is made. Palliative treatment in valuable breeding animals should be influenced by the knowledge that the condition may be inherited. In general the diet should be carefully inspected, analyzed and if necessary corrected. This is especially important in fast-growing animals. Adequate exercise is indicated and overfattening should be avoided.

RENAL RICKETS

(Renal secondary hyperparathyroidism, Osteodystrophia fibrosa, Rubber jaw)

A metabolic disease characterized by decalcification of bones, particularly of the jaw and head, and caused by increased secretion of parathormone from hypertrophied parathyroid glands. Chronic progressive renal dysfunction is often seen in older dogs and cats (and congenitally in young animals) and prevents the normal excretion of phosphates in urine, hence serum phosphates are elevated with concomitant lowering of serum calcium. The parathyroids respond to low serum calcium with hypertrophy (often mistermed "hyperplasia") thereby increasing their endocrine output. Calcium is drawn from the most actively remodelled bones, primarily the mandible, resulting in local fibrous osteodystrophy ("rubber jaw") as an early sign.

Clinical Findings: Signs of renal insufficiency are present: vomiting, anorexia, polydipsia, polyuria, acidosis, depression, anemia and an ammonia-like breath. The mandible is soft and pliable and the jaws fail to close properly. Swelling and softness of the maxillae may be noted. The teeth are usually loose. Long bones are affected less, but animals may be stiff or lame and with minor trauma, fractures occur. Radiographically, bone density of the skull is decreased, some teeth may be absent, and the compact alveolar bone disappears from the tooth sockets. Abaxial skeletal changes are seen first in the phalanges as thinning of cortical bone. At necropsy, the kidneys are small, firm, have an irregular pitted surface, and are fibrous.

Diagnosis: Signs of skeletal disease associated with renal failure suggest renal rickets. Biochemical evidence includes: hyperphosphatemia, normal or slightly elevated serum calcium, elevated blood creatinine and BUN, nonregenerative anemia, and large volumes of urine with fixed or low specific gravity.

Treatment: There is no satisfactory treatment. Medical management of renal failure (*see* CHRONIC RENAL FAILURE, p. 881) may prolong the animal's life.

HYPERTROPHIC PULMONARY OSTEOARTHROPATHY

(Marie's disease)

A condition in which osseous changes of the limbs are associated with intrathoracic lesions. It has occurred in conjunction with tuberculosis, bronchopneumonia and pulmonary abscesses. More commonly it is associated with primary or metastatic pulmonary neoplasms. It has occurred in association with granulomatous processes in the thoracic cavity and esophageal tumors related to *Spirocerca lupa* infection (q.v., p. 707). The disease is common in the dog but has been reported in horses, cattle, sheep and other animals.

Etiology: The cause is unknown. There is a rapid initial increase in the peripheral blood flow to the lower portion of the limbs, possibly from vagal stimulation. This is followed by connective tissue proliferation in the phalangeal region of the legs, which progresses proximally. The next change is a bony proliferation involving the phalanges and long bones.

Clinical Findings: Affected animals usually are presented with the history that their legs have become progressively thicker during the past few months. The thickening may or may not cause lameness. There is sometimes a history of chronic cough with some dyspnea, especially after mild exercise, together with the obvious leg abnormalities. The appetite and eliminations usually are normal. In advanced cases, there may be a stilted gait or even an inability to stand. There may be pain on movement or palpation of the affected bones and the thickened limbs are warm.

Lesions: The long bones of the limbs (radius, ulna, tibia, fibula, metacarpals, metatarsals and phalanges) are most frequently involved. The affected bones are either partially or completely covered with uneven and irregular periosteal and new-bone deposits on the surface of the cortex. The joint surfaces are not involved, but there may be a swelling of the soft tissue around the joints and a thickening of the joint capsules.

Diagnosis: This is based on physical examination and characteristic radiographic findings. Radiographs reveal extensive proliferation of new bone, almost always bilateral, along the shafts of the long bones. This bilateral distribution of new bone, together with the absence of cortical erosion, helps to distinguish the condition from bone neoplasia. Radiographs of the chest may disclose a lesion in the lung, mediastinum, pleura or thoracic esophagus.

Treatment: There is no specific treatment for the condition, although treatment of the intrathoracic lesion by surgery or chemotherapy may lead to a regression of the bone changes.

OSTEOCHONDROSIS—OSTEOCHONDRITIS DISSECANS

Osteochondrosis is a generalized disturbance in the maturation of cartilage (osteogenesis) and may involve the articular cartilage, the physis or areas of fusion of periarticular ossification centers. It is principally observed during the period of maximum growth rate, e.g. the dog 4 to 7 months and the horse 1 to 2 years of age. The syndrome is most common in medium to large breeds of dogs and more frequent in males. It also occurs in pigs, turkeys and chickens.

With osteochondrosis, the articular cartilage becomes abnormally thickened and small fissures develop in the surface which may penetrate to the subchondral bone. This allows the entry of synovial fluid into the necrotic subchondral bone and the liberation of noxious elements into the joint. This in turn may initiate an inflammatory stage called **osteochondritis dissecans.** The articular cartilage becomes dissected (dissecans) and undermined, resulting in a partially attached "saucer like" plaque. This plaque of cartilage is nourished by synovial fluid and thus may survive for long periods. It is prevented from healing and reattaching to the subchondral bone by joint motion and the presence of synovial fluid. However the cartilage flap may re-attach and heal spontaneously, or be torn loose. The defect will then fill in with fibrocartilage. The dislocated cartilage may fall into the joint space and be reabsorbed or it may attach to the synovial membrane, gain a blood supply, hypertrophy, calcify and form a radiopaque joint mouse.

Fusion defects involving periarticular ossification centers are suspected to be of a similar cause. Examples of united ossifications are: anconeal process, coronoid process, tibial crest, scapular tuberosity, epicondyle of the humerus and olecranon. These defects frequently result in joint instability and osteoarthrosis. Trauma may also result in separation of ossification centers. Physeal plates are physically the weakest area of maturing bone and thus are vulnerable to trauma.

The defect in the metaphyseal growth plate is most commonly seen as a retained cartilage core in the distal ulnar physis in large breeds of dogs. This may result in a premature closure of the distal ulna physis which could lead to valgus deformity of the carpus, anterior bowing of the radius and perhaps subluxation of the elbow.

Etiology: The cause of osteochondrosis, which is characterized by excessive thickening of the cartilaginous growth plates, is unknown. Trauma is a significant factor in the development of focal lesions. The role of mineral imbalance, particularly of calcium, is in question. Experimentally excessive caloric intake (overfeeding) during the growth phase increases the incidence of the disease in susceptible animals and an inherited predisposition is seen in those animals selected for rapid growth.

Clinical Findings: Osteochondrosis is presented as a persistent or intermittent lameness which is usually insidious in onset. Lameness is generally unilateral, however the lesions are frequently bilateral. Occasionally various joints throughout the body may be affected concurrently. The animal may be stiff after resting and lameness is aggravated by exercise. Pain is usually elicited by hyperextension and hyperflexion of the joint. When untreated, the lameness may last for months, or may become permanent because of secondary osteoarthrosis. In chronic cases, severe crepitus may be palpated and muscular atrophy observed. Mild cases are usually self limiting and it is probable that many cases pass unnoticed.

The lesions of osteochondrosis involving the elbow in the dog, osteochondritis dissecans of the medial humeral condyle, ununited coronoid process, and united anconeal process, reflect similar clinical signs and are differentiated radiographically or by exploratory arthrotomy. Osteochondrosis involving the articular facets and vertebrae may result in spinal cord compression and neurological deficits.

Diagnosis: The history, age, species, breed and clinical signs are useful. High quality radiographs taken bilaterally in the appropriate position and with the aid of chemical restraint, are essential. The shoulder lesion is generally observed on a lateral radiograph as a flattened irregularity of the central caudal half of the humeral articular surface.

Ununited anconeal process is visualized from a lateral projection with the elbow in extreme flexion. When diagnosing fusion defects, it is important to know when the growth plates normally fuse. Radiographic projections for differentiating osteochondritis of the medial humeral condyle and ununited coronoid process are a lateral in full flexion, an anteroposterior, and an anteroposterior with a 10 to 20° oblique. In the early stages, these lesions may be difficult or impossible to demonstrate radiographically and may require an exploratory arthrotomy. As the conditions progress, osteophyte production may be seen on the medial epicondyle, the coronoid process, proximal surface of the anconeal process and the cranial head of the radius.

Osteochondritis of the lateral femoral condyle in the dog is observed best from a lateral radiograph in which the condyles are not superimposed. An anteroposterior projection may also be of value. Anteroposterior radiographs of a hock with osteochondritis dissecans may show swelling, and in many cases, a small joint mouse distal to the medial malleolus may be observed.

Treatment: Some animals with osteochondritis heal spontaneously with 4 to 6 weeks of rest and restricted exercise. In early cases, antiarthritic or anti-inflammatory drugs are generally contraindicated as they encourage activity and may retard healing. Surgical intervention of osteochondritis of the shoulder is recommended if the lesion is extensive or if it does not respond to conservative treatment. Joint mice with or without an osteochondritis dissecans lesion should be surgically removed. In chronic advanced osteoarthrosis secondary to osteochondritis, the use of phenylbutazone and other antiarthritic drugs is the only alternative other than fusion of the joint, the application of a prosthetic device or amputation.

It is important to surgically treat lesions involving the stifle and hock as soon as the diagnosis is made. The exception is that removal of an ununited anconeal process is attended with best results when accomplished at 9 months of age. If the lesions are extensive or osteoarthritis is advanced, the prognosis is guarded.

Osteochondritis dissecans in foals may be treated conservatively as in the dog. Surgical correction of shoulder lesions may be considered if the animal is not heavily muscled. Surgical intervention of stifle lesions in the horse is attended with poor results. Lesions involving the hock, when diagnosed and operated on early, provide a more favorable prognosis.

Retained cartilage in most metaphyseal growth plates are asymptomatic and heal spontaneously. The primary exception is cartilage cores in the distal ulnar physis in the dog, which occasionally result in premature closure and asymmetric growth between the radius and ulna. If diagnosed early in the growth phase, stapling the distal radial growth plate and an ulnar osteotomy may correct lateral deviation of the carpus and bowing of the radius. If the animal is mature and the physeal plates are fused, correction of the deviation requires a radial and ulnar osteotomy with stabilization of the radius in the proper attitude.

Compression of the cervical cord and instability of the cervical vertebrae are best treated by stabilization, however with present methods, results are unsatisfactory.

OSTEOMYELITIS

Inflammation of bone, usually caused by pyogenic bacteria but occasionally by fungi.

Etiology: Osteomyelitis may result from contaminated compound fractures, nonsterile orthopedic procedures or penetrating foreign bodies. In the dog and cat, bite wounds may result in penetration to the bone or extension of soft tissue infection to adjacent bone. In the dog, the common sites are the face and legs and in the cat, the sacral and coccygeal regions. Severe dental disease can result in osteomyelitis of the mandible or maxilla. Hematogenous spread, especially of *Staphylococcus aureus* and *Brucella canis* infections, may lead to vertebral osteomyelitis. *Staphylococcus* spp., *Streptococcus* spp. and *Escherichia coli* are commonly involved in osteomyelitis, with *Pseudomonas* spp. and *Proteus* spp. less common. Coccidioidomycosis, blastomycosis and actinomycosis are the commonest of the fungal infections that may involve bone.

Clinical Findings and Diagnosis: Pain, soft-tissue swelling and an elevated body temperature often with depression and anorexia, characterize early osteomyelitis. A leukocytosis with a left shift and an increased sedimentation rate may be noted. The animal may be reluctant to use the limb and if the infection spreads to a joint, the joint may become swollen, painful and result in the limb being carried. As the condition becomes chronic, fluctuant swellings or draining fistulae may develop. Fluid or pus from these areas should be aspirated or a swab taken for bacterial culture and sensitivity testing. Radiographic findings in early osteomyelitis are soft-tissue swelling, periosteal roughening and eventually, new bone production. As the infection progresses, bone resorption becomes evident and sequestra may develop.

Treatment: Effective treatment of acute or early osteomyelitis depends upon identification of the organism and its antibiotic sensitivity, with the use of systemic antibiotics, preferably bactericidal, recommended. Antibiotics of choice include ampicillin, cephaloridine, chloramphenicol, gentamicin and kanamycin (℞ 2, 13, 19, 40, 41). Drainage of the infected site may be necessary.

Successful treatment of chronic osteomyelitis requires long-term therapy, often including surgical intervention. The appropriate antibiotic should be started prior to surgical exploration of the infection site. All sequestra should be removed and fibrous and necrotic tissue debrided. Fistulous tracts should be explored and the bone curetted until bleeding. Internal fixation should not be removed if it is providing rigid support; however, if it is not, it should be removed and replaced with something that will. The surgical wound can be left open to drain and heal by granulation or closed meticulously, eliminating all dead space, providing drainage tubing has been installed. Fenestrated tubing can be implanted to allow flushing of the infected area with large volumes of sterile saline, antibacterials (℞ 126, 603) and enzyme preparations (℞ 593, 594). Tyloxapol (℞ 459) can be flushed into the site to help break up mucoid material and maintain drain patency. During the course of treatment, culture and sensitivity tests should be performed regularly to ascertain the most effective antibiotics. The progress of treatment should be followed both clinically and radiographically. Inadequate antibacterial therapy of acute osteomyelitis may temporarily eliminate overt clinical signs allowing the infection to continue in a suppressed state, thus leading to chronic osteomyelitis. Amputation should be considered as a last resort, after failure of long-term intensive therapy.

ABDOMINAL HERNIA

A protrusion of abdominal contents into the subcutis through a natural or abnormal opening in the body wall. Protrusion through the diaphragm is termed diaphragmatic hernia or rupture (q.v., p. 589). Herniation as a result of a severe blow leading to tearing of the abdominal aponeurosis is frequently called a rupture and not a hernia. The best examples of a nontraumatic hernia are the umbilical and inguinal or scrotal hernias, the latter being merely an extension of an inguinal hernia.

In cattle, the advisability of surgically correcting **umbilical hernia** is moot. While some cases are hereditary, improper care of the newborn in the form of excessive traction of the oversized fetus and cutting the umbilical cord too close to the abdominal wall are other possible causes.

In **scrotal or inguinal hernias** in all species, surgical correction almost invariably involves simultaneous castration. **Perineal hernia** is encountered mainly in mature dogs and differs from the other types of abdominal hernias in that the peritoneal lining of the hernial sac is either absent or thin and degenerate. Although many factors have been cited, the actual cause of perineal hernia is unknown.

Femoral (crural) hernia is rare in domestic animals, especially in the larger species.

Clinical Findings and Diagnosis: Two types of hernia are recognized: reducible and irreducible. The **reducible** type is characterized by a noninflammatory, painless, soft, elastic, compressible swelling. It may vary in size from time to time. The swelling can be made to disappear by manipulation or by placing the patient in a suitable position. The diagnosis of perineal hernia in the dog is made from the presence of a swelling at the side of the anus or vulva, between the tail base and the sciatic tuber. The hernia can usually be reduced more easily if the hind quarters of the animal are elevated.

Irreducible hernias have the same characteristics as reducible ones, except that the contents cannot be returned to the abdominal cavity. This is due either to adhesions between parts of the hernial contents, to narrowing of the ring, or to distension of a loop of intestine. The contents may be incarcerated or strangulated.

Umbilical abscess may be confused with hernia and both are frequently found together, especially in pigs and cattle. Exploratory puncture is sometimes necessary for differentiation. Hematomas may also be confused with hernias. If the area can be reached by rectal palpation, the diagnosis of an inguinal or scrotal hernia can be definitely determined by locating the ring and the contained bowel.

Inguinal hernia in the male pig is common and the process usually extends into the scrotum. Suspending the piglet by the fore legs and simultaneously shaking the animal will cause even a small hernia bulge to become visible. In the female pig, this defect is invariably accompanied by arrested genital development; such animals are sterile and surgery is indicated only when the size of the process is a threat to the growth of the pig to market weight.

Inguinal hernia in the male foal often resolves spontaneously during the first year of life. For this reason, early corrective surgery is not indicated unless the hernia is of such a magnitude that it interferes with the gait of the animal or is strangulated. Strangulated inguinal hernia in stallions is fairly frequent and is characterized by signs of constant and severe abdominal pain. It is readily recognized by rectal palpation. When diagnosed early, the condition often may be relieved by rectal manipulation of the incarcerated intestine with the animal under general anesthesia. If this fails, immediate radical surgery is necessary.

Inguinal hernia is rare in cattle; however, it is sometimes encountered in the male. Surgical correction when carried out to conserve the breeding potential of the bull is not always successful.

Perineal hernia, which may be either unilateral or bilateral, can be surgically corrected. Whether prostatectomy in the mature male dog is indicated at the same time is a matter of debate, although the consensus appears to favor the simultaneous removal of that gland.

Treatment: When treatment is elected, umbilical hernias are usually dealt with surgically, preferably at 3 to 6 months of age. In calves some success has been achieved by applying a binder of broad adhesive bandage (10 cm width) which is removed 3 to 4 weeks later. The client should be advised that the weakness may be heritable.

DIAPHRAGMATIC HERNIA

A break in the continuity of the diaphragm with protrusion of abdominal viscera into the thorax.

Etiology: Trauma is the usual cause. In younger animals it may be congenital and involve the pericardial sac (peritoneopericardial hernia). The defect in the diaphragm may be large or small and may involve any area of the musculotendinous partition. The liver, omentum, intestine and spleen commonly herniate into the thorax. A considerable volume of abdominal viscera may gradually pass through a relatively small tear because of the negative pressure in the thoracic cavity. Adhesions between the abdominal and thoracic viscera are common in long-standing cases. A collection of serous fluid usually is present. In cattle, the diaphragm adjacent to the reticulum may be weakened by penetrating foreign bodies permitting partial herniation of the reticulum.

Clinical Findings: Dyspnea is the main sign. Incarceration of stomach or intestine may cause signs of obstruction, while cardiac compression may cause heart failure (peritoneopericardial hernia). Lung or heart sounds may be inaudible on auscultation of the chest. In traumatic hernia the diaphragmatic line is disrupted, and abdominal viscera may be seen in the thoracic cavity. Radio-contrast materials given orally aid in visualizing viscera penetrating the diaphragm. Fluid may obscure radiographic shadows. The heart shadow is enlarged and globe-shaped with widening of the shadow at the diaphragmatic pericardial junction (peritoneopericardial hernia).

Diagnosis and Treatment: Diagnosis is based on history (trauma), clinical signs and radiographic evidence. Other diseases which cause dyspnea must be considered in the differential diagnosis—pneumothorax, hemothorax, hydrothorax, chylothorax, intrathoracic inflammation and neoplasia. Horses usually have been subjected to extreme exertion or accident preceding diaphragmatic herniation. Auscultation of the chest for intestinal sounds is not a satisfactory examination procedure since these sounds may be auscultated over the chest in normal subjects. Exploratory laparotomy for obscure causes of colic should include examining the diaphragm. Surgical repair is the only treatment. Except in emergencies (*see also* ACCIDENTS, p. 777) strict rest is mandatory before surgery and the traumatized animal must be allowed to recuperate (24 hours or longer). Antibiotics minimize growth of *Clostridia* in an entrapped, hypoxic liver.

MYOPATHIES AND RELATED CONDITIONS IN DOMESTIC ANIMALS

Myopathy refers to diseases appearing primarily in the muscle fibers. There are a number of examples of myopathies among the food-producing domestic animals including some that occur endemically and consequently have been studied intensively. Beyond these, myopathies have been investigated in laboratory animal species and in poultry as models of human disease, and much useful information has resulted.

CONGENITAL MYOPATHIES

Certain problems are congenital in origin, and are exemplified by lesions in the musculature of newborn animals. These include defects in myogenesis as well as degenerative changes that take place prenatally in fully differentiated muscle. Some of these are inherited.

Rigid fixation of the limbs in abnormal positions frequently occurs as a congenital deformity and may cause dystocia or be damaging or lethal to the young themselves. The immobility of the limbs and the axial deformities may result either from primary disease of the muscle or from denervation atrophy due to spinal cord abnormalities. The general name for this syndrome is **arthrogryposis** (*see also* AKABANE DISEASE, p. 440). Examples include genetically determined myopathies causing muscular contractures in newborn lambs of the Welsh mountain and Australian merino sheep, and nonhereditary, nonfamilial arthrogryposis in calves of several breeds that appear to reflect denervation atrophy rather than primary myopathy. An autosomal recessive trait in a Swedish strain of the British large white breed has been reported as responsible for a lethal muscle contracture in swine. Similar patterns of inheritance have been linked to pronounced changes in skeletal musculature accompanied by congenital hydrocephalus in beef calves. In some cases the calves have been born blind. A transient myopathy called "splay leg" (q.v., p. 602), occurs in baby pigs within a few hours of birth.

NUTRITIONAL MYOPATHIES

The commonest and most economically important myopathies of domestic animals are those having their origin in defective nutrition. These characteristically are acute diseases and affect young animals of suckling age. The clinical signs vary widely, depending on the distribution and severity of muscle damage. Frequently they include symmetrical damage to the girdle muscles that result in stiffness or inability to stand. Complications, such as inability to nurse or bronchopneumonia, may lead to prostration and death within a few days to a week or so after onset. Acute cardiac failure is often the precipitating cause of death, especially in calves.

The lesions in heart or skeletal musculature vary from diffuse, light-colored areas to well-defined white streaks or patches, and almost always are bilaterally symmetrical. Most muscles can be involved, but macroscopic lesions are commonest in the heart or in the large muscles of the shoulder girdle, back and thighs; those of the diaphragm and tongue may also be affected. Examples have been described in most of the domestic and laboratory animals, under a variety of names, including paralytic myoglobinuria (azoturia), myositis ("tying or cording up") eosinophilic myositis, polymyositis, muscular dystrophy, white-muscle disease (WMD), nutritional muscular dystrophy (NMD), stiff-lamb disease, white flesh, fish flesh, waxy degeneration and selenium responsive myopathy.

Associated with some of the myopathies, degenerative changes in other tissues often occur, notably liver necrosis, subcut. and pulmonary edema with exudation into the large serous sacs, and steatitis and other changes in the fat tissues. Disease entities of similar etiology exist in which some of these latter changes predominate or constitute, apparently, the sole pathology, as, for example, in exudative diathesis (q.v., p. 1429) and encephalomalacia (q.v., p. 1429) in the chick; steatitis in the cat and mink (q.v., pp. 596 and 1167); multiple necrotic degeneration (heart, liver, muscle and kidney) in the mouse; dietary liver necrosis in the rat and, perhaps, massive liver necrosis in the sheep.

In addition to structural changes in the various myopathies, chemical changes may be detected in the muscle tissue and in the blood and urine. Lowered levels of muscle creatine are generally observed, with increased sodium and decreased potassium. Blood serum from myopathic animals has been shown to contain decreased levels of alkaline phosphatase and glutathione peroxidase, and increased levels of lactic dehydrogenase, serum glutamate oxalacetate transaminase (SGOT), serum creatine phosphokinase and, in some cases, myoglobin. The urine frequently has an increased creatine:creatinine ratio, as a result of increased creatine excretion, and may contain myoglobin.

Many of the myopathies and some of the related conditions listed have been attributed to a deficiency of vitamin E, sometimes induced by the presence of unsaturated fatty acids and other peroxide-forming substances in the diet. More recent evidence has implicated other dietary constituents, particularly selenium, which is now recognized as a required element in animal nutrition. When the selenium content of feeds approaches the critical required level, substances that enhance or interfere with its metabolism become important. Good examples of these are vitamin E and sulfur.

The interrelations between selenium and vitamin E in metabolism remain obscure. Some myopathies and related conditions respond only to selenium, some only to vitamin E, others to either one. While vitamin E cannot satisfy the need for all selenium, it can reduce the amount required to protect against exudative diathesis. The converse is also true. A vitamin E deficiency in chicks apparently leads to the development of encephalomalacia and muscular dystrophy even in the presence of selenium sufficient to protect against exudative diathesis (on a low-methionine, low-cystine diet). Similarly, selenium cannot replace vitamin E to prevent the sterility and myopathy in some experimental animals (rabbits) or encephalomalacia in chicks produced by vitamin E deficient diets. Conversely, a naturally occurring infertility in ewes, sometimes associated with a high incidence of WMD in lambs in the presence of adequate vitamin E responds remarkably to minute supplements of selenium, as does alopecia in rats and primates. The necrotic liver degeneration observed in rats and swine appears to respond to either nutrient.

In general, the disorders covered in this chapter are nutritional, metabolic or congenital derangements. For convenience the myopathies and certain conditions apparently related to them etiologically have been assembled together.

Azoturia and Tying-Up in Horses
(Cording-up, Myositis)

Tying-up or cording-up is thought to be a mild form of azoturia and therefore to have a similar etiology. The former occurs mainly in light horses, the latter in heavier breeds; both are associated with skeletal myopathy.

Etiology: The cause of these entities is unknown, but as some cases of tying-up apparently respond to selenium α-tocopherol therapy it is possible that these substances may be involved. Both conditions are usually but not invariably directly associated with forced exercise after a period of rest during which feed has not been restricted.

Clinical Findings: In both tying-up and azoturia the first signs are profuse sweating and rapid pulse followed by stiffness of gait, particularly of the hindquarters, disinclination to move and, in severe cases, myoglobinuria. In azoturia, the disease quickly progresses to recumbency, often with nervous signs. Elevated serum glutamate oxalacetate transaminase (SGOT) and creatine phosphokinase (CPK) are useful indications of the extent of muscle damage. The prognosis depends on the extent of the muscle damage and is good for those that remain standing. It is also fairly good for those animals that go down because of loss of use of their hindquarters, providing that they remain quiet and contented and the pulse returns to normal within 24 hours. However, survivors sometimes suffer from lameness and prolonged or occasionally permanent muscle atrophy.

The prognosis is bad for nervous, restless, recumbent animals that are not quieted by sedatives or tranquilizers and for those that are forced to continue moving after the signs become apparent. It is also bad if after 24 hours the patient shows progressive inability to roll up on its sternum and retain that position. A weak or irregular pulse is a most unfavorable sign.

Treatment: Good management is important. The patient should be kept as quiet as possible from the time that signs are first recognized, and attempts should be made to keep the animal standing. Close attention should be given to the horse's comfort and precautions taken against the development of decubital ulcers. Nervous, restless individuals, or those showing evidence of pain, should be given sedatives such as chloral hydrate (℞ 548) or tranquilizers (℞ 377, 381, 383). If conditions indicate a period of recumbency, an oily laxative should be given. Quick-acting purgatives, such as arecoline and physostigmine, should not be used.

When signs are slight, there is no previous history of occurrence and serum enzyme levels are not significantly elevated, moderate tranquilization may be sufficient. More severely affected horses should not be moved but should be provided with on-the-spot shelter. They should be rubbed dry and blanketed according to the weather. Selenium-vitamin E appears to give favorable results in many cases and may be given every 4 to 6 months prophylactically.

White Muscle Disease
(WMD, Stiff-lamb disease, Nutritional myopathy, Selenium responsive myopathy)

A myodegeneration most frequent in calves and lambs whose dams have been fed during gestation or longer on feeds, especially legumes, grown in certain areas where selenium is either deficient or unavailable in the soil. It has been recorded in many countries. It has been produced experimentally in several species of animals on low-selenium intake. A similar myopathy occurs naturally in goats, deer, foals and dogs but proof of the etiology is lacking.

Etiology: WMD is associated with low levels of selenium in animal tissues but interfering substances like sulfur, or lack of enhancing substances, like vitamin E, may be involved in precipitating the clinical disease.

Clinical Findings: The congenital type results in sudden death within 2 or 3 days of birth, usually with involvement of the myocardium. The delayed type of WMD is associated with cardiac or skeletal muscle involvement, or both, and may be precipitated by vigorous exercise. Affected animals may move stiffly with an arched back and frequently become recumbent. If the condition is severe enough to prevent nursing, death results from starvation. Sometimes there is profuse diarrhea. In chronic cases there may be relaxation of the shoulder girdle and splaying of the toes. With severe cardiac damage, death may be sudden. In progressive cardiac failure, dyspnea results. In some areas unthriftiness may be the only sign associated with selenium deficiency.

Lesions: Skeletal muscle lesions are invariably bilaterally symmetric and may affect isolated or many muscle groups. Grossly, the affected muscle is paler than normal and may show distinct longitudinal striations or a pronounced chalky whiteness. Cardiac lesions occur as well-defined subendocardial plaques, which are often more pronounced in the right ventricle. With heart involvement, pleural, pericardial and peritoneal effusions, together with pulmonary congestion and edema, are not uncommon.

Diagnosis: In lambs, outbreaks of infectious nonsuppurative arthritis produce a clinical picture similar to that of WMD, and sudden deaths from heart failure might be confused with enterotoxemia. The history and necropsy findings, however, are usually quite characteristic. In mild cases and in very young lambs, laboratory studies such as histopathologic examination, estimation of glutathione peroxidase, SGOT and CPK levels and urinary creatine:creatinine ratios may be necessary.

Prevention: To prevent congenital WMD or WMD occurring

within 4 weeks after birth, ewes are given 5 mg selenium (Se) and cows 15 mg Se, orally or subcut. 4 weeks before expected parturition. For the prevention of delayed WMD lambs are given 0.5 mg Se and calves 5 mg Se at 2 to 4 weeks of age, repeated twice at monthly intervals. A selenium-vitamin E mixture is advocated in some areas.

The addition of selenium to feed for reproducing animals or their young is a useful preventive in areas of known deficiency or unavailability of Se. The recommended supplemental level is for 0.1 ppm of actual Se, calculated on the basis of total dry-matter intake. It is added as sodium selenite, which contains 45.65% actual Se, and because of the minute quantities involved, and the toxicity of excess intake, premixing and thorough subsequent mixing is necessary. In some countries addition of Se to feeds is controlled by law, and appropriate authorities should be consulted.

Treatment: Lambs and calves may be given sodium selenite-vitamin E in aqueous solution, subcut. at the rate of 0.25 mg Se per lb (0.55 mg/kg) of body wt. This may be repeated after 2 weeks, but not to exceed 4 doses. Larger doses are sometimes advocated but caution is advised as they approach the toxic level.

Myopathies in Herbivora Due to Vitamin E Deficiency

Evidence has accumulated indicating the occurrence of myopathies in various herbivores, including rabbits, guinea pigs, calves and lambs, when the diet is low in vitamin E. More commonly these myopathies result from interference with the biologic activity of dietary vitamin E by lipid peroxides formed from unsaturated fats or other similar-acting substances. Routine administration of cod-liver oil to pail-fed calves, for example, has caused a high incidence of this type of myopathy. Experimentally, acceleration of avitaminosis E has been induced by the presence in the diet of organic antagonists, such as tri-*o*-cresyl phosphate, pyridine, *o*-cresyl succinate, carbon tetrachloride and sodium bisulfite, and by ferric chloride.

Clinical Findings: Signs are frequently lacking and sudden death from heart failure following slight exertion is not uncommon. When degeneration of the skeletal musculature occurs, it may result in weakness of stance, an awkward gait and an inability to rise or walk unaided if the large muscles of the limbs are affected. In acute cases following severe exercise there may be myoglobinuria.

Lesions: Pathologic pictures vary considerably, depending on the intensity and duration of the vitamin E deficiency. Creatinuria and myoglobinuria, as general indicators of muscle damage, are usually present. Mild deficiencies cause slight swelling of the muscle fibers and some degree of hyaline degeneration and proliferation of sarcolemmic nuclei. In some severe cases extensive myonecrosis occurs. Changes also occur in the chemical composition of muscle; usually the potassium content falls and the sodium content rises. These changes are not specific for vitamin E deficiency; they also occur in other myopathies, including those caused by a disturbance of selenium metabolism.

Diagnosis: To differentiate vitamin E deficiency from other myopathies, diagnosis should include evaluation of the vitamin E status of the diet in relation to both sources of the vitamin and the presence of factors—especially cod-liver oil and other unsaturated fats—likely to interfere with its metabolism. Presence of natural or synthetic antioxidants in the diet will reduce the influence of such factors.

Treatment: Where simple vitamin E deficiency is apparent, dietary supplementation with α-tocopherol or substances rich in this vitamin should be instituted. Minimum dosages have not been established; however, cures have been reported following daily doses with 5 mg of α-tocopherol to rabbits; 500 mg α-tocopherol, initially, followed by 100 mg on alternate days to lambs; and 600 mg α-tocopherol acetate initially, followed by daily doses of 200 mg, to calves. When the causative diet contains substances antagonistic to vitamin E, these must be removed. Dry concentrates of vitamins A and D may substitute for cod-liver oil, thus removing a potential source of oxidative damage.

Steatitis in Cats or Fur-Bearing Animals
("Yellow fat" disease)

A disease characterized by a marked inflammation of adipose tissue and the deposition of "ceroid" pigment in the interstices of the adipose cells.

Etiology: It is believed that an overabundance of unsaturated fatty acids in the ration, together with a deficiency of vitamin E, results in the deposition of "ceroid" pigment in the adipose tissue. Most naturally occurring and experimentally produced cases have occurred in animals that have had fish, or fish by-products, as all or part of the diet; fish oil may be the primary agent.

Clinical Findings and Diagnosis: Affected cats are frequently plump and well fed, usually young, and may be of either sex. They show loss of agility and general unwillingness to move. Resentment is exhibited on palpation of the back or abdomen. In advanced cases, even a light touch will cause pain. Fever is a constant finding and anorexia may be present.

In mink, kits may be affected with steatitis shortly after weaning, and if untreated, losses may continue to pelting time. Clinical indications appear suddenly; the kits may refuse a night feeding and be dead by morning. Affected animals may refuse their feed and show a peculiar, unsteady hop, which leads to complete impairment of locomotion and coma. At pelting, survivors show yellow fat deposits and hemoglobinuria.

The typical laboratory finding is an elevated leukocyte count, with neutrophilia and sometimes eosinophilia. Biopsy of the subcut. fat shows it to be yellowish brown, with a nodular or granular appearance. Microscopic examination reveals severe inflammatory changes and associated ceroid pigment.

Treatment: Elimination of the offending food from the diet is imperative. The administration of vitamin E, in the form of α-tocopherol, at least 30 mg daily for cats, or 15 mg daily for mink, is necessary. Antibiotics are of doubtful value, in spite of the fever and leukocytosis. Parenteral use of fluids is not advisable unless dehydration exists. Patients should be handled as little as possible.

CARDIAC AND SKELETAL MYOPATHIES AND HEPATOSIS DIETETICA IN SWINE

There are several specific entities of swine in which muscle degeneration may be very extensive, including mulberry heart disease (MHD) and enzootische herztod (EH), and others where the degeneration is frequently less conspicuous, including hepatosis dietetica (HD).

Etiology: MHD and EH are thought to be nutritional in origin; however, EH may be synonymous with the porcine stress syndrome, q.v., p. 528. HD is definitely associated with diets low in selenium and vitamin E.

Clinical Findings: All 3 conditions have certain characteristics in common; losses tend to occur sporadically, affecting rapidly growing pigs between 6 and 16 weeks of age, and death almost invariably occurs suddenly.

Lesions: In MHD the characteristic lesion is a grossly distended pericardial sac containing straw-colored fluid and fibrin flakes, together with extensive hemorrhage throughout the myocardium. Microscopically, in addition to interstitial hemorrhage, there is usually extensive myocardial necrosis together with fibrinoid thrombi in capillaries. If animals survive for a few days, nervous signs are seen, resulting from focal encephalomalacia.

In EH, which has been reported from Europe, there is less pericardial effusion and myocardial hemorrhage than in MHD. Additional lesions are gross pallor of skeletal musculature and degenerative changes in adrenal and thyroid glands.

In HD there is often subcut. edema together with varying amounts of transudate in serous cavities. Fibrin strands adhere to the liver, which has a characteristic mottled appearance caused by irregular foci of parenchymal necrosis and hemorrhage. Focal lesions of myocardial necrosis and, less frequently, skeletal myonecrosis may be apparent.

Prophylaxis and Treatment: For all 3 conditions, MHD, EH and HD, a change of diet is suggested; errors should be corrected and selenium or vitamin E therapy, or both, introduced.

EOSINOPHILIC MYOSITIS IN DOGS

An acute relapsing inflammation of the muscles in dogs. The disease is common in German shepherd dogs and affects most frequently the muscles of mastication. The cause is unknown.

Clinical Findings: The onset is usually abrupt. During an attack, the muscles of mastication swell symmetrically and interfere with drainage from the retrobulbar tissues, producing edema of the conjunctiva, prolapse of the nictitating membrane and exophthalmos. The mouth is held partially open and the animal eats with difficulty. The attacks last from 1 to 3 weeks and are accompanied by a marked eosinophilia. The periods between attacks vary from 3 weeks to 6 months. After each attack, the affected muscles become more atrophied, with each succeeding attack, the severity decreases and the interval between attacks tends to lessen. In late stages of the disease, involvement of the esophagus makes swallowing difficult.

Lesions: During acute attacks the affected muscles are enlarged and doughy in consistency, darkened and hemorrhagic with focal pale areas. The regional nodes are enlarged and firm. During early attacks the lesions are confined to the muscles of mastication; as the attacks continue additional muscles may become involved. The histologic lesion is an acute eosinophilic myositis. Although the eosinophilic infiltration is usually quite diffuse, the actual muscle involvement is patchy. Frequently, necrotic muscle fibers appear to be the focus of the reaction.

Diagnosis: The periodic nature of the disease and its unusual selectivity for site and breed usually makes diagnosis obvious. Eosinophilia is strongly supportive and if any doubt remains, histologic examination of a muscle biopsy can be used to confirm the diagnosis.

Treatment: The disease is progressive and no therapy has yet been able to alter its recurrent nature and course. The use of the corticosteroids (℞ 138, 154), and ACTH (℞ 137), however, has a marked effect in minimizing the discomfort and muscle swelling during an attack.

EOSINOPHILIC MYOSITIS IN CATTLE

A focal myonecrosis associated with large numbers of eosinophilic granulocytes. The cause is unknown in most instances but the presence of degenerate *Sarcocystis* in the center of some of the necrotic lesions suggests that they may be implicated. This condition is seen at slaughter as focal greenish gray discolorations in skeletal and occasionally in cardiac musculature.

MISCELLANEOUS MYOPATHIES

Maxillary Myositis of the Horse: A disease of horses resembling azoturia both clinically and pathologically, except that it is inclined to be more endemic, more chronic in its course and involves more frequently the muscles of mastication and deglutition. Myocarditis is common. The cause is unknown.

Myopathy of Potassium Deficiency: A degeneration of both cardiac and skeletal muscle occurring in rats, rabbits and possibly other species, fed a potassium-deficient ration. Dosing with sodium salts accelerates the process. The lesions present a picture of diffuse degenerative changes, including hyaline degeneration, accompanied by loss of striation and eventual loss of sarcoplasm. Interstitial edema is evident in the early stages. The addition of potassium to the diet arrests the degenerative changes.

Reversible Metastatic Calcification (Nutritional Calcification): A deposition of calcium salts in the soft tissues, especially in the muscles of the limbs, resulting from an excessive intake of milk. (The condition is similar to "milk drinker's syndrome" in man.) It may occur when show calves are kept for an unusually long time on nurse cows. It is seen also in dogs and other experimental animals kept on high-milk diets, especially when there is some additional calcium intake. The considerable inorganic salt deposits in the muscles cause pain and limit movement. A history of high-calcium (milk) intake will have a bearing on the diagnosis. Withdrawal of the offending diets results in spontaneous reabsorption, although this may take some time.

Congenital Myodysplasia in Calves: An inherited myopathy, the result of a recessive factor, marked by the absence of normal skeletal muscle development and associated with hydrocephalus. Grossly, the large skeletal muscles are undeveloped and light in color, having a yellowish tinge. The cranium shows the characteristic enlargement of hydrocephalus. Microscopically, there is a disarrangement of the normal muscle structure resulting in a tangle of undeveloped muscle fibers and connective tissue. Usually the animals are unable to stand and soon die.

Myopathies from Plant Intoxication: Degeneration of skeletal and cardiac muscles results when cattle and some other animals feed on certain plants. *Karwinskia humboldtiana* (*coyotillo*) and *Cassia* spp. have been incriminated, but other species may also cause damage. There is pallor of severely degenerated muscles. Microscopic lesions consist of hyaline necrosis and granular degeneration. Some blood enzymes are elevated and myoglobinuria may occur. Treatment consists of removal of animals from offending range and supplemental feeding.

Rupture of the Gastrocnemius Muscle in Cattle: An acute myopathy of unknown etiology except that it appears to result from undue stress on the muscle. It sometimes is a sequela to parturient paresis. There is no satisfactory treatment.

"Double muscle" (Doppellendigkeit) or Muscle Hyperplasia: A congenital anomaly occasionally occurring in calves and rarely in lambs. The larger muscles are enlarged due to excessive fibers and their outlines show prominently under the skin. The heritable characteristics are not well understood, but evidence suggests that a recessive factor is responsible.

Brown Atrophy of Bovine Muscle (Xanthosis): A brown pigmentation of the skeletal and heart muscles, of unknown etiology, occurring occasionally in debilitated or aged dairy cows. Grossly, the muscles and heart are brown. Microscopically, very minute brown or yellowish granules are visible in these tissues.

Albino Muscle in Cattle: An apparently physiologic anomaly in which all muscles, except the cardiac, diaphragmatic and coccygeal, appear lighter in color than normal. There is no apparent histologic or functional alteration.

Myocardial Lipidosis: A lesion sometimes encountered upon necropsy of animals which have suffered from debilitating diseases, especially those associated with anemia. The myocardium loses its normal tone, and seen through the endocardium, has a freckled appearance. With appropriate staining, minute and more or less regularly spaced globules of lipid can be demonstrated within the myocardial fibers.

Fatty Infiltration of the Muscle: A hyperplasia of adipose tissue within the skeletal musculature. It may arise following myodegeneration, but usually occurs for no adequately explained reason. In its severest form a whole muscle may be replaced by fatty tissue. A mild form is normally observed in fattened animals. It is only diagnosed at slaughter.

Nonspecific Muscular Degeneration in Dogs may be responsive to vitamin E-selenium therapy. Ascorbic acid orally at 4 mg/lb (9 mg/kg) of body wt daily seems to ameliorate idiopathic muscular soreness.

INFECTIOUS CONGENITAL TREMORS (ICT)

(Myoclonia congenita, Shaker pigs, Dancing pigs)

A transmissible infection of the CNS of unborn piglets in which effects are manifested in the newborn with signs continuing for months among those that survive. The disease has occurred sporadically in the U.S.A., apparently at a rather constant level, for more than a century. The description of what presumably is ICT appeared in the German literature in 1854.

Etiology: A virus has been associated with the infection. While it has not been characterized chemically, it is approximately 20 nm in diameter and is of cuboidal symmetry. It has been shown not to be hog cholera virus or pseudorabies virus in fluorescent antibody preparations. Presumptive evidence has indicated that neither swine parvovirus nor swine enteroviruses are involved.

Epidemiology: Significant epidemiologic studies are not available. The incidence is low and occurrence is sporadic. It appears more often in the warmer months of the year in midwestern U.S.A. It is very rare indeed for a sow to have more than one affected litter and in such circumstances the disease is mild and occurs only in 1 or 2 of the pigs. It is common, during a farrowing involving many females, for the pigs of the early farrowings to be most severely affected, with the pigs of the final farrowings being least affected if at all. Lateral spread has not been reported, although silent lateral spread may be a part of transmission.

Clinical Findings: The principal manifestation is tonoclonic spasms of major muscle groups of the neck, trunk, and legs. The muscles of the pelvic limbs are often in tonic spasm, which is apparently painful; piglets so affected place much of their weight on the forelimbs and often rest in a sitting position with the pelvic limbs splayed or abducted as much as 30° from the midline. At rest the tremors are absent. However, with an external stimulus, such as a sudden noise, the pigs arouse and the tremors resume. When the tremors are of sufficient magnitude to preclude suckling, the piglets soon die of starvation. After weaning, affected pigs retain an altered gait; there is a shortened stride with the pelvic limbs a bit more rigid, resulting in a mincing run. At a standstill, the tail may be observed in fine tremor sometimes accompanied by a similar tremor of the flank. Placing a hand on the lumbar area will permit detection of a tremor which is not visible; this lasts at least into maturity. Even when affected swine reach weights of about 150 lb (70 kg) they can be identified by sight in a lot with unaffected swine of the same age. The affected swine are generally smaller and when forced to run, display the peculiar gait.

Diagnosis: The disease is a clinicopathological entity. Diagnosis is made on the basis of history, clinical observations, and findings on gross and microscopic examination for pathological changes. Since microbiological tests are not available, negative microbiological findings support a diagnosis of ICT.

Lesions: Gross and microscopic pathological changes directly related to the infection are vague or nonexistent. Many microscopic changes have been noted, but it is most significant that they are not similar to findings in other common viral infections of the CNS of swine. Changes most accepted are those of mild vasculitis in the brain and major body organs and hypomyelinization in the brain and spinal cord.

Treatment: No vaccines or antiserums are available. Specific treatment has not been developed. However, since death is caused by an inability to suckle, pigs may be saved by helping them to suckle, or by providing them with sustenance artificially until, as the pigs grow older, the intensity of the tremors diminishes. If the piglets survive past the first 5 days, their chances of survival without help are excellent.

SPLAYLEGS IN PIGLETS

(Spraddled legs)

A condition of newborn pigs in which the rear legs are spread apart or extended forward. Appropriately treated pigs usually recover within a few days although few recover if the front legs are also spread. The incidence between litters varies widely but variation in incidence between herds is more marked. The immediate cause of spreading is weakness of the adductor muscles relative to the abductors. Affected pigs are susceptible to overlaying, starvation and chilling because of poor mobility.

Etiology: The incidence can be varied by selective breeding. However, any cause of stretching the adductor muscles increases the incidence. Stretching can result from slippery floors, struggling while legs are caught in cracks in the floor and as the result of damage to nerve pathways from intrauterine viral infections. The general nutrition of the sow (choline and vitamin E levels) may influence the incidence.

Diagnosis: The clinical signs are distinctive. *In utero* infections with hemagglutinating encephalitis virus, enteroviruses, other viruses, and postpartum bacterial meningeal infection should be considered in addition to trauma.

Prophylaxis and Treatment: The herdsman should provide dry, nonslippery floors with no cracks in which the legs can become trapped, especially for the first 2 days. The pigs should be protected from injury by the sow and adequate suckling should be insured. In affected piglets the rear legs should be secured together above the hocks with a loose figure 8 of adhesive tape for 2 to 4 days. Nutritional defects in the sow ration should be corrected.

ADRENOCORTICAL AND RELATED THERAPY

The quantitatively and physiologically important steroid hormones secreted by vertebrate adrenal cortices are (1) the glucocorticoids—cortisol (hydrocortisone), corticosterone and cortisone, (2) the mineralocorticoids—aldosterone and desoxycorticosterone (DOC) and (3) steroids with androgenic activity. In addition to cortisol, cortisone and desoxycorticosterone, a large number of steroids are produced commercially whose biologic activities mimic the effects of the endogenously secreted steroids. (*See also* THE ADRENAL GLANDS, p. 209.)

Pharmacology of the adrenal cortical steroids: 1. The **androgenic steroids** are rarely of clinical importance, and then only when enzymatic deficiencies of the adrenal cortex diminish cortisol secretion. Under these circumstances a secondary increase in pituitary corticotropin secretion stimulates the production of abnormally large quantities of adrenal androgens resulting in the adrenogenital syndrome.

2. The secretion of **mineralocorticoids** permits the body to maintain normal renal secretion or retention of sodium and potassium. Excessive doses stimulate sodium retention by the kidney and excretion of potassium in the urine. With continued administration of the mineralocorticoids, the animal with normal cardiovascular function "escapes" from the sodium-retaining effects, but potassium excretion continues at a high level. Aldosterone is the primary mineralocorticoid secreted by the adrenal cortex, but is expensive to produce. The commercially available mineralocorticoids are the

acetate ester of desoxycorticosterone, DOCA (desoxycorticosterone acetate) and the 9-α-fluoro derivative of cortisol fludrocortisone.

3. **Glucocorticoids** have profound effects on the metabolism of carbohydrate and proteins and also influence lipid metabolism. Pharmacologically their primary effects are characterized by (1) gluconeogenesis, a shift in the amino-acid pool of the skeletal muscle mass and of the stomach and intestine from protein synthesis into the production of carbohydrate, (2) a significant reduction in lymphoid tissue and lymphocyte formation and (3) inhibition or diminution of all aspects of both the acute and chronic phases of inflammation.

The structural and functional integrity of the adrenal cortex is maintained by the secretion of pituitary corticotropin (ACTH). Increasing concentrations of glucocorticoids in plasma tend to suppress the secretion of ACTH by a direct inhibitory action on the pituitary gland as well as by inhibition of the hypothalamic neurohormone (corticotropin-releasing hormone), which stimulates ACTH production. Long-term administration of glucocorticoids thereby depresses the hypothalamopituitary system and leads to functional and in some species morphologic atrophy of the adrenal cortex.

Corticosteroids produce other less tangible effects such as stimulation of appetite, increased activity and a sense of well-being. The last term is borrowed from human medicine, but seems applicable to animals, because of their improvement in behavior and interest in surroundings. Finally, the endogenously produced glucocorticoids, such as cortisol, possess a significant degree of mineralocorticoid activity.

Chemistry and pharmacology of derivatives of cortisol and cortisone: The primary goals in the production of new steroids have been: first, to formulate drugs with more potent anti-inflammatory effects; second, to minimize the sodium-retaining effects of such glucocorticoids; and third, to diminish the undesirable side-effects inherent in the glucocorticoid or anti-inflammatory responses. The first and second goals have been achieved but the third remains elusive. The first major modification was the formation of the Δ-1 steroids by inserting a double bond between carbons 1 and 2 of the steroid A ring to produce prednisolone from cortisol and prednisone from cortisone. For a comparable degree of sodium-retaining effects, the anti-inflammatory responses of the Δ-1 steroids are 3- to 5-fold greater than for the parent compounds. A second modification was halogenation of the endogenous steroid. When a fluorine atom is placed on carbon 9 in the alpha position of cortisol, both glucocorticoid and mineralocorticoid activity, but particularly the latter, are markedly enhanced. This compound, fludrocortisone is used for its anti-inflammatory activity only in topical preparations.

Halogenation in the 9-alpha position of prednisolone and additionally inserting an hydroxyl or methyl group on carbon 16 produces the most marked pharmacologic changes. For example, 16-α-methyl-9-α-fluoroprednisolone, dexamethasone, has anti-inflammatory activity which is 15- to 25-fold greater than that of cortisol and additionally is virtually devoid of mineralocorticoid activity. Other halogenated steroids with this pattern of activity include triamcinolone, betamethasone, fluocinolone and beclomethasone.

The enhanced glucocorticoid and anti-inflammatory activity of these derivatives results from a more avid binding of cytoplasmic receptor protein molecules. Additionally, the 9-α-fluoro compounds undergo a much slower metabolic transformation. The esterification of the hormones with fatty acids, for example, triamcinolone acetonide or betamethasone valerate, alters the distribution of the steroids permitting them a longer sojourn in the body and hence longer lasting biologic effects.

Clinical Application: Although they do not produce primary cures, corticosteroids are used for the treatment of a wide variety of diseases. The hormones usually control signs or check pathologic changes and, in certain instances, gain enough time to permit other drugs to be used to cure the disease. They should be used in the early stages, before irreversible changes have taken place. When steroids are used in the presence of frank or suspected infection, vigorous anti-infective therapy must be included as part of the therapeutic regimen. In view of the breadth of action of these hormones, their clinical application should be restricted to defined routes of administration in the various diseases. Their use should be safeguarded by carefully established diagnoses, since unwanted side effects may complicate indiscriminate use. The 2 principal uses of corticosteroids are: (1) for their anti-inflammatory and anti-allergic actions in a wide range of disorders, (2) for treatment of several metabolic conditions, including stress disease, in which they may possibly act as replacement therapy.

Administration: Because corticosteroids can produce powerful hormonal effects, it is preferable, whenever possible, to use them locally rather than systemically. The routes of administration include: (1) external application for treatment of ear, skin and eye diseases; (2) local injection, such as subconjunctival, intra-articular, periarticular and infiltration of tissue; (3) the oral route and (4) parenteral administration, via the IV or IM route.

External uses: For treatment of ear, skin, or superficial eye lesions, hydrocortisone, prednisolone, betamethasone or dexamethasone, combined with antibiotics, may be used as ointments or lotions. All phases of inflammation, including hyperemia, cellular exudation, swelling and pain, are markedly and often rapidly reduced. The anti-inflammatory action is at the cell level and systemic absorption of corticosteroids has not been reported except where a compound of higher potency has been used. Skin diseases which respond to corticosteroid treatment include dermatitis, alopecia, and certain forms of eczema. Corticosteroids may be combined with antibiotics for the treatment of pustular dermatitis. Miliary eczema in cats, acanthosis nigricans in dogs and nonspecific skin diseases reportedly respond to corticosteroid treatment. However, relapses sometimes occur, particularly if treatment is stopped suddenly. When extensive lesions are present, systemic use of steroids may be required.

Many eye conditions respond to topical use of these substances, e.g. conjunctivitis, keratitis, panophthalmia, periodic ophthalmia and certain postsurgical conditions. The use of corticosteroids for the treatment of superficial corneal ulcers should be initiated only when the lesion no longer stains with fluorescein. Concurrent antibiotic therapy is essential whenever infection is present or impending. The subconjunctival injection of corticosteroids is sometimes used.

Intra- or periarticular use: Several corticosteroids, preferably with antibiotics, are used for cases in which single accessible joints or tendons are affected. Tendon and muscle injuries have been treated with corticosteroids, with variable results. Conditions that have been treated successfully with corticosteroids include arthritis, bursitis, periostitis, synovitis, tendonitis, tenosynovitis and navicular disease in horses. The most spectacular effect of intra-articular injection occurs when it is used in early stages of serous arthritis when changes are not yet irreversible. Corticosteroids and an appropriate antibiotic are also used in suppurative arthritis such as "joint ill" in foals. Where possible, identification of the causal organism from synovial fluid is advised. The parenteral use of an antibiotic is also recommended. Certain forms of stifle lameness in dogs may respond to intra-articular corticosteroid treatment. Periarticular infiltration of shoulder and hip joints in dogs has produced good results. Repeated intra-articular administration may result in decreased synovial fluid and a dry joint. Injections into tendons may result in calcification.

Subconjunctival use: The subconjunctival route of administration is of special value where the deeper structures of the eye are involved. Hydrocortisone, prednisolone, dexamethasone or betamethasone in combination with appropriate antibiotics may be used. The volume of injection is approximately 0.5 ml. More than one injection may be necessary.

Systemic use: Systemic administration has proved valuable in the treatment of bovine ketosis, general arthritic conditions and dermatitis. Clinicians frequently use corticosteroids as supplementary therapy in conditions such as infection, shock, acute mastitis, pneumonia, selected cases of colitis in dogs, eosinophilic myositis, burns, feline enteritis, rodent ulcers (cats), laminitis and following surgery. In most cases, it is essential (a) to use antimicrobial or chemotherapeutic substances or specific sera for treating the primary cause, (b) to discontinue the steroid therapy gradually and (c) to maintain use of the specific antimicrobial therapy for at least 24 hours after the corticosteroid drug administration has been discontinued.

The IV injection of corticosteroids is primarily reserved for emergencies, such as postoperative or traumatic shock, or other severe and acute stress syndromes.

Clinical Evaluation of Steroid Therapy: Most corticosteroids have a wide scope of action and versatility. Because of this versatility and such factors as differences in stages of disease in different animals, it is difficult to devise controlled studies for clinical evaluation of these substances. The glucogenic response can be assessed by changes in the blood sugar and liver glycogen levels. This enables the clinician to determine which preparation has the most powerful gluconeogenic property. However, for other effects the appreciation of these drugs rests largely on individual assessment and experience of clinicians. In general, clinical observation would indicate that steroids are useful in the treatment of:

1. Inflammatory conditions of many types affecting the skin, ears, joints, tendons, muscles and sometimes the eyes. In small animals, 80 to 90% of nonspecific skin conditions appear to improve with steroid treatment. While relapses do occur, the risk of their occurrence may be reduced by gradual withdrawal of the corticoid used.
2. Mastitis: Although some intramammary preparations contain corticosteroids, controlled trials have shown that there is little, if any, advantage in the inclusion of these substances in such formulations. The parenteral use of corticosteroids in certain acute cases of mastitis as adjunctive treatment to appropriate antibiotic therapy can be advantageous.
3. Bovine ketosis: The rationale for using corticosteroids in ketosis is based on their ability to stimulate gluconeogenesis and to promote other nonspecific effects such as stimulating the appetite. On parenteral administration, the steroids produce a rise in blood glucose within a few hours. The acetone content of the urine declines and milk production rises to normal, usually within 48 hours depending on the duration of the disease and the milk yield. Several corticosteroids including betamethasone, dexamethasone, prednisolone, prednisone and trimethyl prednisolone have been used. Blood sugar levels are increased to a varying degree after injection of one of the preparations. Most glucose levels are back to preinjection levels within 38 to 72 hours, except where betamethasone is used as the alcohol suspension, after which increased blood glucose levels

have been maintained for 3 to 4 days. Because of the complex nature of ketosis, however, corticosteroids may not always afford specific treatment. In treating any condition with these substances, the nutritional status of the animal should also be considered and full use should be made of supportive treatment with other agents as indicated.

4. Miscellaneous conditions embracing a wide variety of otherwise unrelated diseases, usually those assumed to be caused or exacerbated by "stress," have been treated with corticosteroids either alone or in combination with other drugs. Clinical impressions of such treatment are generally favorable, but further critical evaluation is required. In infections, corticosteroids should only be used in conjunction with antibiotics or other chemotherapeutic agents. The latter should be continued for a few days after discontinuing corticosteroid administration. Large doses of corticosteroids (0.5 to 1.0 mg dexamethasone per kg of body wt) given IV are of value in the therapy of shock and are also used in conjunction with hypertonic solutions such as 20% mannitol for decompression of the brain and spinal cord. Corticosteroids can also be used to induce parturition in cattle and sheep. *See* ABORTION, p. 832.

Contraindications: In veterinary medicine, corticosteroids are used chiefly to treat acute conditions for a limited period; consequently side effects, although known, are infrequent and easily reversed by withdrawing the drug. However, contraindications do exist. The most important contraindications include: (1) infections, unless full doses of antimicrobial drugs are included; (2) degenerative eye diseases; (3) dendritic ulcers of the cornea; (4) diabetes mellitus; (5) pregnancy toxemia in sheep; (6) chronic diseases in which tissue changes are irreversible; (7) corneal opacity due to infectious canine hepatitis and (8) cardiac and terminal stages of nephritis. It should be recalled that parturition may be induced. Prolonged medication at high dosages may cause a number of serious systemic disturbances, and withdrawal after such medication should be gradual. Adequate warnings and precautions concerning these risks are given in detail in the labelling of the particular steroid, and should be particularly noted.

Dosage: There is no fixed dosage, but usually 1 to 5 mg of cortisone per lb of body wt is recommended for small animals (*see* TABLE for relative potencies). Following remission of the signs of disease the dose is gradually reduced until the drug is either discontinued or a satisfactory maintenance dose is found. This particularly applies to the treatment of chronic skin conditions and to certain forms of lameness. Some dogs and cats have been kept free of signs for long periods on small doses given only once a week.

For the current information on indications, methods of administration, duration of treatment and the precautions to be observed, the reader is advised to follow the recommendations supplied by the manufacturers of the various steroid products available.

RELATIVE BIOLOGIC POTENCIES IN MILLIGRAM EQUIVALENTS OF COMMONLY USED CORTICOSTEROIDS

Corticosteroid	*Potency*	
	Anti-inflammatory	Mineralocorticoid (Na-Retaining)
Hydrocortisone*	1	1
Cortisone	0.8	0.8
Desoxycorticosterone	None	30–50
Fludrocortisone	10	125
Prednisone	4–5	0.8
Prednisolone	4–5	0.8
Methylprednisolone	5–6	0.5
Triamcinolone	4–5	Minimal
Dexamethasone	30	Minimal
Betamethasone	30	Minimal

* Hydrocortisone expressed as unity.

Adrenocorticotropic Hormone (ACTH): This hormone is obtained from the anterior lobe of the pituitary gland. It acts by stimulating the adrenal cortex to produce corticosteroids. Its effects are, therefore, similar to, although slower, than those of cortisone acetate. Its use has been superseded by the corticosteroids. Small doses of ACTH are sometimes used following sudden cessation of corticosteroid therapy to prevent withdrawal signs. It is also used in adrenal stimulation studies for the diagnosis of canine Cushing and Addison's disease.

NEOPLASMS

NEOPLASMS

Persistent, purposeless growths composed of cells that do not respond properly to normal mechanisms controlling cell proliferation. Whether a neoplasm is benign or malignant depends on the extent to which its cells escape growth restraints. Progression of a neoplasm towards more malignant behavior can occur as succeeding generations of cells become increasingly unresponsive to controls.

Neoplasia is generally a multistage process in which one or more events initiate the development of a potentially neoplastic clone of cells and additional events influence whether a recognizable neoplasm will appear. Chemical carcinogens, oncogenic viruses and physical agents such as ultraviolet irradiation are the most important initiators. Their action is influenced by genetic background. Emergence of a neoplasm requires some stimulus for proliferation of the potentially neoplastic cells. Hormonal, immunologic and genetic factors are important modifiers of this stage.

Diagnosis: For each domestic species, patterns and types of common neoplasms are well known. Geographic variations in incidence of certain tumors are also recognized. Clinical and radiographic findings often lead to a tentative diagnosis. Evidence of invasion and destruction of local tissues, and multiple foci are indicators of probable malignancy. Exfoliative cytology of solid masses or effusions is a useful diagnostic adjunct and can sometimes provide a definitive answer.

The most accurate information on the nature and histogenetic origin of a suspect neoplasm is obtained by histologic examination. A pathologist can usually provide a likely prognosis. The entire tumor is submitted for pathologic examination if complete surgical excision is possible. Failing that, punch or wedge biopsies are taken. Care is necessary to ensure that both peripheral and more central portions of masses are represented in biopsy specimens. Diagnosis of hemopoietic and lymphoreticular neoplasms is made by examining blood and either or both bone marrow and lymphoid tissue.

Treatment: Surgery, radiotherapy, chemotherapy, immunotherapy, or combinations of these are the available methods. Neoplasms of skin and adnexae lend themselves to therapy because they are likely to be detected early and are accessible. Many of them do not become malignant, and those that do, tend to metastasize late in the disease process. The majority of tumors arising in deeper tissues, once recognized, cannot be treated successfully with currently established regimens.

Complete surgical removal is the simplest and most effective treatment where feasible and consistent with satisfactory healing and retention of function. An exception to this is that sometimes no action is taken for neoplasms that regress spontaneously such as papillomas in young animals or canine transmissible venereal tumor. Cryosurgery is useful for difficult sites, as in the mouth, rectum, or around blood vessels and nerves. Electrocautery lessens difficulties associated with excessive vascularity or local transference of viable tumor cells or agents.

Radiotherapy is used on radiosensitive neoplasms that are malignant or cannot be completely excised because of their location. Good results are achieved by X-ray irradiation of superficial squamous cell carcinomas, mast-cell tumors and perianal gland tumors. It can also have an effect on other epithelial tumors of the skin and mouth, fibrosarcomas and melanomas. Beta particles from ^{90}Sr are very effective for early squamous cell carcinomas of the eye in cattle and horses. Implantation of γ-ray emitters such as radium and ^{60}Co is occasionally used to combat large inoperable masses. Parenteral ^{131}I is given for thyroid tumors.

Chemotherapy of malignant tumors as practiced in man has had limited usage in animals. With rigorous management it can prolong the life of dogs and cats with generalized neoplasms such as lymphosarcoma for 6 to 12 or more months. A variety of agents is available for cancer chemotherapy. They act by interfering with selective stages in the cell proliferative cycle. Among the more common are: alkylating agents that cross-link DNA strands; antimetabolites that interfere with purine- or pyrimidine-base synthesis; vinca alkaloids that destroy the cell spindle; and steroid hormones that inhibit protein synthesis. Administering a combination of these drugs enables a larger proportion of a neoplastic cell population to be killed and reduces the amount of any one agent needed. The latter is important because anticancer drugs also kill actively proliferating normal host cells. A major problem is the need to monitor closely the bone-marrow function of animals under treatment and to counteract the effects of immunosuppression. Special forms of chemotherapy are hormonal treatments, e.g. an estrogen to reduce perianal gland tumors in dogs, and the topical use of 5-fluorouracil cream for invasive cutaneous neoplasms. *See* CANINE MALIGNANT LYMPHOMA, p. 629.

Immunotherapy appears to be of benefit for warts and for squamous cell carcinoma of the eye in cattle. Its practical value otherwise has not been clearly established.

NEOPLASMS OF SMALL ANIMALS

Most neoplasms in dogs and cats arise in animals more than 5 years old; the probability of a tumor developing increases with age. The pattern of occurrence of neoplasms differs in dogs and cats. They are 5 to 6 times commoner in dogs than cats. Benign tumors outnumber malignant ones in dogs, but the reverse holds true for cats. Most commonly affected sites in dogs are skin and subcutis, and mammary gland. In cats they are skin and subcutis, and lymphoid tissues and bone marrow. Purebred dogs are more frequently affected than mongrels, and the boxer is more prone to neoplasia than other pure breeds. Benign tumors usually grow slowly, appear as round or ovoid masses, are well encapsulated and exert their harmful effect on the host by occupying space or mechanically interfering with other tissues in the body. Malignant tumors are seen in all sizes and shapes, invade and destroy normal tissues and are often disseminated through the blood stream or lymphatics (metastasis). Carcinomas, tumors of epithelial origin, usually spread first by means of the lymphatics and later enter the blood stream and become widely disseminated throughout the body. Sarcomas, tumors derived from mesenchymal tissue, usually spread directly via the blood stream. Variations from these generalities will be pointed out in the following text, which will deal only with the commoner neoplasms found in each organ system. (*See also* DERMOID, p. 221.)

TUMORS OF THE SKIN

Histiocytomas are single or multiple nodules found in the skin of dogs usually under 2 years of age. They most frequently are found on the head, legs and feet. Grossly they are 1 to 2 cm in diameter, domed or button-shaped, and are often ulcerated. The cut surface is pale gray with minute red stippling. Microscopically, histiocytomas are composed of dense accumulations of round cells with ovoid or indented nuclei, abundant cytoplasm, indistinct cytoplasmic borders and many mitotic features. These tumors do not metastasize, but the ulcerated nodules may become infected in which case surgical excision is the treatment of choice. Spontaneous regression commonly occurs if they are not excised.

Mast-cell tumors in the dog are most commonly found as single or multiple nodules on the posterior half of the body, particularly on the scrotum and the limbs. Grossly, they are usually nodules located within the dermis. Frequently the overlying skin is ulcerated. The cut surface is grayish white or tan. Impression smears of the tumor, stained with Wright's stain, will show typical mast cells with metachromatic bluish purple cytoplasmic granules and a round nucleus. Microscopically it is composed of cords and sheets of mast cells with varying numbers of eosinophils scattered throughout the lesion. The tumors infiltrate locally, sometimes with metastasis to the draining lymph node, spleen, liver, kidney, lungs and heart. There is a strong tendency for these tumors to recur locally, making wide excision a necessity in surgical removal. It is reported that the use of corticosteroids will help control mast-cell tumors when they are widespread.

Occasionally in the dog there is widespread systemic invasion of highly anaplastic mast-cell tumors. In the cat, the cutaneous form of mast-cell tumor most often affects the head and neck regions. The commoner form in the cat, however, is a mast-cell leukemia in which there is widespread involvement of bone marrow, blood, spleen and other organs.

Papillomas occur in dogs as single and multiple projecting nodules, most commonly found around the head, feet and mouth (*see* ORAL PAPILLOMATOSIS, p. 115 and PAPILLOMATOSIS, p. 250). They are rare in cats.

Squamous cell carcinomas arise mostly from the skin. Grossly, they have a broad base with an ulcerated surface that extends downward into the underlying tissue. The cut surface is pink or pink-gray. Microscopically, they are composed of large polygonal cells resembling squamous epithelium. The cells form sheets and cords as they infiltrate the dermis and subcutis. Frequently these cells form clusters that contain keratin in their center. These structures are recognized as "epithelial pearls." Squamous cell carcinomas are highly invasive and destructive. They are generally slow to metastasize.

A peculiar form of this tumor, generally considered to result from solar radiation, occurs on the ear tips of white-eared cats. It develops slowly but eventually the entire pinna will be destroyed. Early amputation of the pinna of the ear is required to prevent metastasis.

Basal cell tumors occur as small nodular growths in the skin, usually on the head and neck. This tumor arises from undifferentiated basal cells in the epidermis. Grossly, these spherical nodules may or may not be pedunculated and they frequently ulcerate. The cut surface is firm, gray and lobulated. Microscopically, the basal cell tumor in dogs is composed of undifferentiated basal cells that occur in a ribbon, solid, cystic or medusoid pattern. Basal cell tumors do not often metastasize but recur following incomplete removal. Wide excision is necessary to prevent recurrence. Related to basal cell tumors are **trichoepitheliomas** arising from hair follicles and **pilomatricomas** arising from hair matrix.

Sebaceous gland tumors are the commonest skin neoplasm in dogs; they occur most frequently on the head, especially eyelids and extremities. In appearance and behavior they closely resemble basal cell tumors. The vast majority of sebaceous tumors are benign. They are composed of lobules and nests of cells with variable proportions of sebaceous and undifferentiated basal cells.

Tumors of the perianal gland arise from the modified sebaceous glands normally present around the circumference of the anus, at the base of the tail and in the preputial skin, sacral and lumbar regions. Male dogs are more commonly affected than females and the tumor usually occurs in the older age groups. Grossly, the tumors appear as smooth, spherical masses in the subcutis; often they ulcerate and bleed. The cut surface is tan and has a definite capsule and a firm, rubbery lobulated surface. Microscopically, polyhedral eosinophilic cells densely clustered in an expanding mass are observed. The tumor is usually benign and grows slowly. A rare malignant form of this tumor is a nonprojecting mass most easily detected by rectal palpation. Adenocarcinomas of the perianal gland metastasize readily to the iliac and sublumbar lymph nodes, which may obstruct the colon as it enters the pelvic canal. Partial control of the benign form of the tumor can be achieved by the use of stilbestrol. Hormone treatment is particularly useful in controlling the bleeding that accompanies ulceration of these tumors. Definitive treatment requires surgical excision of the tumor.

Melanomas are tumors found mostly in the skin and oral cavity of the dog. They are rare in cats. Grossly, they appear as solitary, small, raised nodules that may or may not be ulcerated. The cut surface is often visibly black. Microscopically, melanomas are composed of immature elongate cells that usually contain melanin granules in their cytoplasm. The cells form whorls, sheets and small packets. Melanomas of the skin are usually benign whereas those of the oral cavity and digits are malignant. Early wide excision of the primary nodule is essential.

Smooth, firm, ovoid **cysts** are commonly found in the skin and subcutis of dogs. Sometimes a small communication exists between the lumen of the cyst and the skin surface through which drainage of the cyst contents occurs. Grossly, the cysts contain either pale-yellow, curdy exudate or dry, crumbly, brown material. Microscopic differentiation has to be made between epidermal inclusion cysts, intracutaneous cornifying epithelioma, or cystic tumors of the basal cell, trichoepithelioma or pilomatricoma type. Since cells are continually shed into the cyst lumen, expression of the cyst contents only provides temporary relief. Frequently, the wall of the cyst is ruptured while trying to express its contents, allowing the contents to escape. This produces an intense inflammatory reaction resulting in persistent purulent drainage from the area. Consequently, regardless of the type of cyst, surgical excision of the entire cyst is the treatment of choice.

TUMORS OF LYMPHOID AND HEMOPOIETIC TISSUES

Lymphosarcomas (malignant lymphomas), malignant tumors arising from lymphoid tissues, are the commonest specific tumor in cats. They are the fourth most frequent category of tumor in dogs, behind tumors of the skin, mammary gland and digestive system. Lymphosarcomas are classified according to both anatomic pattern of tumor distribution and cell type. In dogs, multicentric involvement of lymph nodes and to a lesser extent liver, spleen and other organs, is the predominant anatomic pattern. Next most common is the alimentary form where lesions are principally in the gastrointestinal tract and associated nodes. Thymic, dermal or leukemic (bone marrow, blood, spleen and liver) involvement is much less frequent. Lymphosarcoma in the cat occurs at an earlier age than other malignant tumors, presumably because of the causative role of the virus of feline leukemia, q.v., p. 631. The alimentary tract and related lymph nodes are the most commonly affected sites in cats, followed by the thymus. The multicentric, leukemic or solitary organ pattern of involvement is less often found. Grossly, affected nodes are enlarged and on cut section are usually homogeneous, soft and pinkish gray to cream-colored. Necrosis, hemorrhage, or both can be present in large or rapidly expanding masses. Other organs have either soft, pale nodular masses or diffuse, pale enlargement. Histologically, the tumors consist of lymphoid cells with one or other of the various stages of differentiation predominating. Prolymphocytic, lymphoblastic and histiocytic types of cells are the usual ones.

Myeloproliferative disorders, which are persistent, irreversible proliferations of one or more of the cellular elements of bone marrow, are important in cats. The feline leukemia virus also seems to play a role in the causation of these diseases. Clinically, cats usually are presented because of a severe, unresponsive anemia resulting from replacement of normal bone marrow by immature cells. Where evidence of maturation is detected, it is usually towards the erythrocytic series (erythremic myelosis) or a mixture of erythrocytic and granulocytic cells (erythroleukemia). The abnormal cells are present in blood and cause hepatosplenomegaly by their accumulation in these organs. Lymph nodes are usually mildly affected and other organs marginally so. The nature of the myeloproliferative disorder can be established by careful examination of blood and bone marrow. These disorders are infrequent in dogs, the best recognized being granulocytic (myelogenous) leukemia. Neoplastic and often immature granulocytic cells replace normal bone marrow, invade the blood and cause hepatosplenomegaly. Lymph nodes and other organs are less affected. Hematologic examination of blood and bone marrow is necessary for diagnosis and to differentiate granulocytic leukemia from the leukemoid response produced by conditions such as pyometra.

TUMORS OF THE VASCULAR SYSTEM

Hemangiomas usually are seen as a single mass in the cutis or subcutis, often on the limbs or in the spleen. Grossly, the tumor in the skin is a spongy, encapsulated mass that has a dark-red cut surface that oozes blood. In the spleen this tumor is circumscribed, dark red-black and when cut, oozes red-black fluid. Microscopically, the tumor is composed of a spongy mass of thin-walled vascular spaces lined with low-lying flat endothelium. Hemangiomas are slow-growing tumors. They do not metastasize, and surgical excision is curative. **Hemangiosarcoma,** the malignant counterpart of the hemangioma, may also occur in the skin but is usually found in the spleen, liver, or in the right atrium of dogs. Grossly, in the spleen this tumor may reach a size of 15 to 20 cm in diameter and contains large areas of clotted blood due to infarction. Microscopically (excluding areas of infarction and necrosis), the tumor is composed of large immature endothelial cells which form ill-defined vascular channels. This tumor grows rapidly and metastasizes early. If splenectomy can be performed before metastasis has occurred, it may be curative. Thorough examination of the abdominal viscera and a chest radiograph should be taken in conjunction with splenectomy.

TUMORS OF THE RESPIRATORY TRACT

Adenocarcinomas of the nasal cavity arise from nasal epithelium in both dogs and cats. These tumors are destructive and invasive. Radiographically they are seen as a dense mass filling the nasal cavity on the affected site. Grossly, the tumors appears as a reddened, rough, ulcerated, bleeding mass occupying the nasal cavity frequently causing purulent discharge from the nares. Microscopically it is composed of cords or nests of columnar epithelium, some of which may form mucus-secreting glands or exhibit squamous cell metaplasia. The tumor grows primarily by local invasion and is destructive to the normal structures of the nasal cavity. There is no satisfactory treatment. **Fibrosarcomas** and **osteosarcomas** also form similar destructive masses in the nasal and paranasal regions.

Primary tumors of the lung are uncommon and are found usually in animals over 8 years old. They arise from the epithelium of bronchi (**bronchogenic carcinoma**) or from cells lining bronchioles and alveoli (**bronchiolo-alveolar tumors**). Bronchogenic carcinomas tend to occur in more hilar regions. Most are adenocarcinomas, a few are squamous cell carcinomas, and in the dog anaplastic varieties occur. Grossly they are generally large, grayish, irregular masses, often with smaller scattered nodules formed by spread through airways and lymphatics. The bronchogenic carcinoma is usually widespread before diagnosis is made; consequently, there is no effective treatment. Bronchiolo-alveolar tumors are found mostly in the dog, often as solitary peripheral nodules. The neoplastic cells line alveolar walls. They usually spread slowly by local extension so these tumors are amenable to treatment by lobectomy. Occasionally, bronchiolo-alveolar tumors follow a highly malignant, locally invasive course.

TUMORS OF THE GASTROINTESTINAL TRACT

(*See also* TUMORS OF MUSCLE, p. 619.)

Adenocarcinomas are infrequent tumors that might occur anywhere in the digestive tract from the stomach to the rectum. They arise from the mucosa and infiltrate the muscularis. Grossly, they are invariably recognized by a large mucosal ulcer that has a raised, thickened, umbilicate margin. The cut surface of the unulcerated portion of the tumor, which has a firm gray appearance, can be seen occupying the zone between the serosa and the mucosa. Adenocarcinomas that involve the large and small intestine grow in an annular fashion and produce constriction of the gut, with subsequent partial obstruction. Microscopically, the tumor is composed of irregular, poorly formed glands with extensive fibrous stroma surrounding them. These tumors are locally invasive and metastasize to the draining lymph node. Occasionally, the tumor may become implanted on the peritoneal surface of the abdominal cavity and will appear as numerous tiny nodules. Early resection of the tumor can be curative.

Adenocarcinoma of pancreatic acinar cells occurs infrequently and may arise in any portion of the pancreas. Grossly, it is usually seen as a small, firm, white nodule in the parenchyma of the gland. Microscopically, it tends to be composed of large cuboidal or columnar cells arranged in irregular acinar formation. This tumor metastasizes very early, first to the liver, then to other organs, frequently as numerous small, gray nodules throughout the abdominal cavity on the mesentery, omentum and peritoneum. The widespread metastases are often conspicuous and the primary nodule in the pancreas may be overlooked.

Tumors of the islet cells of the pancreas are usually functional. Due to their insulin production, clinical signs of hypoglycemia (ataxia, weakness, convulsions, fainting) aid in their diagnosis. Grossly, the tumor appears as single or multiple, firm yellow to red nodules in the pancreas. Microscopically, groups of islet cells form a slowly expanding mass within the gland. Carcinomas of islet cells are more common than adenomas in dogs. The carcinoma of islet cells metastasizes via the lymphatics to the regional lymph nodes, liver and peritoneal surfaces.

TUMORS OF CONNECTIVE TISSUE

Fibromas may occur anywhere but are most commonly found in the skin and subcutis and the wall of the vagina. Grossly, they are usually circumscribed, firm spherical nodules with a rubbery, pearl-gray surface. Microscopically, fibromas are composed of broad bundles of mature fibroblasts, which produce appreciable amounts of collagen. Surgical removal is the treatment of choice.

Fibrosarcomas most commonly arise in the skin and subcutis in both cats and dogs, also the oral and nasal cavities in dogs on the limbs and around the head. Grossly, they are irregularly shaped, poorly encapsulated, lobulated, white fleshy masses. The cut surface is usually gray and may have blotchy zones of red and yellow, representing hemorrhage and necrosis, respectively. Microscopically, the tumor is composed of plump or spindle-shaped cells arranged in irregular whorls with little evidence of collagen production. These tumors expand rapidly by infiltrative growth. They are late to metastasize, but when metastasis occurs, it is widespread. Early complete surgical excision is the only means of treatment. This is often difficult due to the infiltrative nature of the tumor.

Lipomas are common in old dogs and occur as single or multiple nodules in the subcutis of the back, sternum and abdomen. Grossly, they are usually well-defined spherical or lobulated masses, which look like normal fat on the cut surface. Microscopically, the tumor cells are indistinguishable from normal fat cells. These tumors grow slowly and need only be removed when they mechanically interfere with normal structures. **Liposarcomas** are very rare in dogs and cats. These tumors are poorly defined masses that grow by infiltration rather than by metastasis. Their biologic behavior is similar to that of a fibrosarcoma.

Hemangiopericytomas occur only in the skin and subcutis of dogs. They are most often found on the extremities and in the subcutis of the trunk. Grossly, they are poorly encapsulated, often infiltrating between the fascial planes and muscle bundles of the limbs. The tumor is mottled gray and has a firm consistency. The microscopic pattern is variable but is usually a collection of elongate cells arranged in short interlacing bundles or in a whorled pattern around small vascular spaces or collagen bundles. Hemangiopericytomas spread primarily by infiltration and have a strong tendency to recur following surgical removal. Because of this tendency to recur, it is recommended that, when the tumor occurs on a limb, amputation rather than local excision be performed. Hemangiopericytomas are similar in many respects to the much less common **neurofibroma.**

TUMORS OF MUSCLE

Leiomyomas are benign and arise from smooth muscle cells. They are most frequently found in the gastrointestinal tract, uterus and vagina. These tumors usually form a single, large, spherical mass that has a smooth, translucent gray-pink surface. Microscopically, the tumor mass is composed of spindle-shaped cells with elongate blunt-ended nuclei arranged in irregular broad fasciculi. Leiomyomas grow slowly by expansion and exhibit little tendency to infiltrate locally. The much less common malignant form of the tumor, **leiomyosarcoma,** appears in the same locations as the benign counterpart, but metastasizes readily to the regional lymph nodes. Complete surgical excision is usually curative.

Rhabdomyomas are very rare in dogs and cats. They arise from striated muscle and should all be considered potentially malignant. Histologically, the cells are similar to those of a pleomorphic fibrosarcoma except that cross-striations can be visualized in the cytoplasm of some cells, thereby identifying the cells as arising from striated muscle.

TUMORS OF CARTILAGE AND BONE

Tumors containing cartilage are most often found as part of a mixed mammary tumor in dogs. **Osteochondromas** are benign, cartilage-capped tumors arising from the surface mainly of the scapulae, ribs, vertebrae and pelvis. Multiple lesions (osteochondromatosis) are more common in cats. Malignant transformation of multiple lesions sometimes occurs. Grossly, **chondromas** appear as single masses of varying size. The cut surface is translucent blue-gray and frequently contains red-brown areas of necrosis. Microscopically, the cells in the benign tumor closely resemble mature hyaline cartilage, with peripheral collections of immature chondrocytes. Chondromas and the malignant counterpart, **chondrosarcomas**, grow primarily by expansion. Tumors arising from cartilage should be considered potentially malignant regardless of their histologic appearance. Consequently, radical excision is the treatment of choice.

Osteosarcomas are common in dogs, particularly the giant breeds, and affect the long bones more often than the axial skeleton. There are breed differences in distribution pattern, however. On the limbs, this neoplasm is usually located in the metaphysis of long bones. These tumors are firm and may contain spicules of mature bone or cartilage. They destroy normal bone and stimulate periosteal proliferation by their presence, thus producing the characteristic radiographic "sunburst" effect. Microscopically, the tumor cells are quite pleomorphic in appearance and may produce mature bone spicules, immature bone spicules, cartilage and fibrous connective tissue. Osteosarcomas are very invasive locally and they metastasize readily, particularly to the lungs. Early amputation is necessary when the tumor is located on a limb. This tumor always carries a poor prognosis.

TUMORS OF THE LIVER

Hepatomas occur infrequently in dogs and are even less common in cats. Grossly, these tumors are large multilobular spherical masses that are separated from normal liver tissue by a thin, distinct capsule. They are soft and usually protrude above the surface of the liver. The cut surface is usually yellow-gray and often has irregular zones of dark-red hemorrhage. Microscopically, the tumor cells appear very similar to normal liver cells, but they form solid sheets of cells without the orderly cord arrangement of normal liver; central veins, portal triads and bile ducts are absent. The tumors grow by local expansion. Secondary metastases may occur within the liver, causing numerous, smaller, ill-defined spherical masses. Extrahepatic metastases are rare. Surgical removal of a single liver lobe, when feasible, may be curative.

Bile duct carcinomas arise from the epithelial cells lining the bile duct and usually form a single large mass frequently with secondary intrahepatic and extrahepatic metastases. Grossly, they usually form a spherical, nonlobulated, poorly encapsulated mass. The cut surface is gray-white and firm. Microscopically, the tumor cells form incomplete and poorly defined bile ducts, which may contain mucin. Besides being locally infiltrative, they metastasize readily to the regional lymph nodes and abdominal viscera. There is no effective treatment.

TUMORS OF THE KIDNEY

Adenocarcinomas of the kidney are usually seen as a unilateral mass arising from the renal tubular epithelium. Grossly, the mass is spherical, white and yellow with deep-red striae visible on the cut surface. It is usually well demarcated from normal kidney parenchyma although a visible capsule may not be present. Microscopically, the tumor cells form incomplete tubules amidst varying amounts of fibrous connective tissue. Adenocarcinomas metastasize early and often there will be a tumor in the opposite kidney by the time the diagnosis is made. The primary lesion grows by expansion in the affected kidney and may metastasize to the regional lymph nodes. Early diagnosis of the tumor in a single kidney and the removal of that kidney may be curative.

Embryonal nephroma arises from the metanephros and is composed of multipotent, undifferentiated, vestigial renal tissue. It is unilateral, rare in dogs and cats, and is detected in young animals usually under a year of age. Grossly, the tumor is large, encapsulated and may fill most of the abdomen. The cut surface is divided into many lobules by connective tissue stroma and is soft, fleshy and white-gray. Fluid-filled cysts of varying size may be visible on the cut surface. A small zone resembling kidney tissue can usually be found compressed along one border of the tumor. Microscopically, the tumor cells may form tubules, incomplete glomeruli, connective tissues, cartilage and bone, illustrating the primitive tissue from which this tumor arises. Surgical removal in the absence of metastases is curative even when the tumor has reached immense size.

Transitional cell carcinomas arise from the transitional epithelium in the urinary tract. They are found in the renal pelvis, ureter, bladder or urethra of dogs and are extremely rare in cats. Grossly, they appear as pedunculated or sessile masses, which are ulcerated and friable on the luminal surface. The cut surface is gray to yellow, firm and often blotched with red. Microscopically, the tumor cells may form acini or they may undergo patchy areas of squamous metaplasia. Transitional cell carcinomas metastasize early to the regional lymph nodes and are locally invasive. Surgical removal is generally impossible.

TUMORS OF THE TESTICLE

Sertoli cell tumors arise in the seminiferous tubules of dogs and are often found in retained testicles, but may be present in one or both scrotal testicles. The opposite unaffected testicle is invariably atrophic. Over 25% of Sertoli cell tumors produce signs of feminization in the dog (atrophy of the uninvolved testicle, bilaterally symmetrical alopecia, nipple enlargement, prostatic enlargement, attraction for other males). Grossly, the tumor appears as a lobulated, grayish yellow, greasy mass within the contours of the testicle and may enlarge the overall size of the testicle. The cut surface is coarsely lobulated and contains soft red areas. Microscopically, the tumor is composed of numerous tubules filled with Sertoli cells separated by thick collagenous septa. It grows primarily by expansion and seldom metastasizes. Castration is curative.

Seminomas are usually seen as a solitary nodule arising from the spermatogenic epithelium of the seminiferous tubules. Like Sertoli cell tumors they are more frequent in retained testicles. Grossly, they are small, firm, whitish gray spherical nodules within the parenchyma. Microscopically, the tumor cells form solid masses of large, round, germinal epithelial cells with prominent nucleoli. The tumor cells can be seen to have broken out of tubules and invaded the interstitium of the testicle. Although seminomas are potentially malignant, they grow primarily by expansion within the gland. Metastasis is uncommon in dogs. Castration is curative.

Interstitial cell tumors are common in aging dogs. They often appear as solitary nodules under 1 cm in diameter; bilateral involvement is common and sometimes they occur together with other testicular tumors. They exert no known hormonal effect on the dog and rarely distort the size or shape of testis. Grossly, the tumor appears as a light-brown, spherical mass with zones of deep reddish-brown hemorrhage scattered throughout the cut surface. Microscopically, the tumor cells form sheets which are interrupted by zones of hemorrhage. The tumors grow slowly by expansion and are the least likely testicular tumors to metastasize. Castration is curative.

Adenocarcinomas of the prostate gland are seen in the dog as focal or diffuse tumors arising from prostatic epithelium. The gland may or may not be enlarged. Differentiation clinically from prostatic hyperplasia is often difficult. The tumor may block one or both ureters, causing secondary hydronephrosis. By rectal palpation the prostate gland containing an adenocarcinoma might be felt to be adherent to the floor of the pelvis due to fibrous adhesions developed between the neoplastic gland and the normal intrapelvic tissue. Grossly, an affected gland may be larger or smaller than normal and it is usually somewhat asymmetric. The cut surface of the tumor is gray, firm and often distinct from the normal glandular tissue. Adhesions to the pelvic wall and the neck of the bladder are common. Microscopically, the tumor cells may form solid cords or ill-defined acini. Inflammatory cyst formation and fibrosis often accompany the tumor. The tumors metastasize early and widely. Invasion of the neck of the bladder is common. There is no known effective treatment, since complete surgical removal of the neoplastic tissue is generally impossible. (*See also* PROSTATIC NEOPLASMS, p. 879.)

TUMORS OF THE OVARY AND UTERUS

Granulosa cell tumors arise from the ovarian follicles. They have the potential to secrete estrogen or androgen. Clinical signs when present are usually attributable to hyperestrinism. Grossly, the tumor is usually seen as a large unilateral multilobulated grayish yellow mass. The cut surface frequently contains numerous follicle-like structures. The tumors grow by expansion and metastasis sometimes occurs. If the tumor ruptures, implantation of tumor cells may occur on the peritoneum, forming numerous small botryoid masses. Ovariohysterectomy is curative in the absence of metastasis.

Dysgerminomas are rare ovarian tumors in dogs and cats. They have a smooth, glistening surface and the cut surface is grayish pink. Microscopically, they have the histologic features of a seminoma. There is no known hormonal effect on the host. Dysgerminomas should be considered potentially malignant. Ovariohysterectomy is curative.

Adenocarcinoma of the uterus is a rare tumor in dogs and cats which arises from the glandular epithelium of the uterine mucosa. It is usually found close to the cervix, hence both intact and spayed female dogs may have this tumor. It usually occurs in dogs over 10 years of age. Clinically, a persistent sanguinous discharge from the vagina in an old female is suggestive of adenocarcinoma of the uterus. Grossly, the tumor is broad-based and penetrates through the mucosa into the muscular layers of the uterus. The luminal surface is frequently ulcerated and the tumor can grow in annular fashion around the organ. The cut surface is pink-tan and firm. Microscopically, the tumor cells form irregular ill-defined acini amidst abundant fibrous stroma. These tumors are locally invasive but eventually metastasize. Early surgical removal of the uterus or uterine stump including the cervix may be curative.

MAMMARY TUMORS

Mammary tumors are among the most frequent tumors in dogs, representing 25% of neoplasms in female dogs. They occur most frequently in intact bitches and are extremely rare in male dogs. Ovariectomy of bitches before first estrus dramatically reduces the risk of mammary neoplasia, ovariectomy after one estrus period reduces it to a lesser degree, and those neutered after maturity (2½ years) have the same risk as intact bitches. The caudal 2 mammary glands are more often involved than the anterior 3 glands. Grossly, mammary tumors appear as single or multiple nodules in one or more glands, ranging in size from 1 to 25 cm. The cut surface is usually lobulated, gray-tan and firm, often with small and large fluid-filled cysts. Mixed mammary tumors, those which contain both neoplastic epithelial tissue as well as neoplastic mesenchymal tissue, are usually benign and often have grossly recognizable bone or cartilage present on the cut surface. Microscopically, mammary tumors may be divided simply into 4 categories: (a) *Adenomas*—rare benign growths of glandular epithelium. (b) *Adenocarcinomas*—frequently fast-growing tumors composed of glandular epithelium, which often metastasizes to the lungs. (c) *Benign mixed mammary tumor*—the most frequent tumor, which contains neoplastic epithelial and mesenchymal tissue. These tumors grow slowly, may reach considerable size and may undergo malignant transformation after a certain time. (d) *Malignant mixed mammary tumor*—grossly resembles its benign counterpart and has a tendency to rapidly increase in size. Histologically, either the epithelial or mesenchymal component may have the characteristics of malignant growth, as seen by invasion of lymphatic and blood vessels, anaplasia and metastasis. Most often the epithelial components metastasize.

From a practical standpoint mammary tumors should be regarded as potentially malignant regardless of the size or the number of mammary glands involved. Treatment requires mastectomy, ovariohysterectomy and removal of the appropriate (draining) lymph nodes. The caudal 3 glands on each side have a common lymphatic system and drain into the inguinal lymph node. The anterior 2 glands also have a common lymphatic system and drain into the axillary lymph node. Since the malignant mammary tumors metastasize readily to the lungs, radiography should always be performed prior to surgical removal of affected glands in order to rule out previous metastasis.

TUMORS OF THE ADRENAL GLANDS

Adenomas of the adrenal cortex are frequently seen in old dogs. They have no known hormonal effect. Grossly, they appear as discrete small-to-large tan-yellow nodules within the cortex that may encroach upon the medulla or may project irregularly from the surface of the gland. Microscopically the tumor cells are large polygonal cells with foamy cytoplasm that form solid nodules. These benign tumors grow slowly by expansion and are usually recognized only at necropsy. Therapy is not considered necessary. Occasionally the tumors are functional and clinical signs of cortisol excess (Cushing's-like disease) are produced.

Carcinoma of the adrenal cortex is rare in dogs. Histologically, it may be confused with tumor of the adrenal medulla, **pheochromocytoma.**

TUMORS OF THE PITUITARY GLAND

Pituitary gland tumors may be **adenomas** or **adenocarcinomas.** They are uncommon and can be responsible for producing canine Cushing's-like disease and diabetes insipidus. Grossly, the pituitary gland is enlarged asymmetrically and may expand dorsally via the infundibulum into the hypothalamus. The cut surface of the tumor is gray, firm and frequently contains irregular zones of hemorrhage. Microscopically, the tumor cells may be recognized as chromophobe cells or, much less frequently, pituitary acidophils and basophils. Tumors of the pituitary gland grow by dorsal expansion and invasion of the hypothalamus since the gland normally lies in a closely confined osseous crater at the base of the skull.

TUMORS OF THE THYROID GLAND

Tumors of the thyroid gland are most frequently **carcinomas** in dogs but **adenomas** in cats. At the time of diagnosis approximately 25% of these tumors are present in both glands. Grossly, adenomas are small, well demarcated, pale tan nodules. Some are predominantly cystic. Carcinomas are larger, multilobular, invade adjacent structures, and often have areas of necrosis and hemorrhage. Microscopically, the tumor cells are cuboidal epithelial cells which may form ill-defined acini or grow in broad, solid sheets. Invasion of blood vessels by the tumor cells is common and subsequent thrombosis and infarction may contribute to the gross cystic appearance. Thyroid carcinomas metastasize to the opposite gland directly via the lymphatic communication at the hilus of the 2 glands. Metastasis also occurs to the lungs, cervical lymph nodes and viscera. Bilateral thyroidectomy is advisable regardless of the gross absence of nodules in the opposite gland. Care should be taken to leave the anterior parathyroid glands in place. Daily administration of thyroid hormone is essential for the remainder of the dog's life following surgery.

AORTIC BODY TUMORS

Aortic body tumors arise from the chemoreceptor cells in the aortic body and are usually found in the sinus transversus pericardii, the space between the aorta and the pulmonary artery at the base of the heart (**heart-base tumor**). There is no known hormonal function of these tumors. Brachycephalic breeds such as boxers and Boston terriers have a higher incidence of this tumor than other dogs. Grossly, the tumor is a firm, fleshy, nodular, spherical mass that infrequently obstructs the pulmonary artery or the aorta, although it is closely applied to each of these major vessels. The cut surface is lobulated, pink and firm. Microscopically, the tumor is composed of small, cuboidal to polyhedral cells with pale eosinophilic or vacuolated cytoplasm. Usually, these tumors do not directly invade the atria, aorta or pulmonary artery, but may be seen in small blood vessels or lymphatics. Aortic body tumors grow principally by expansion. Metastasis is uncommon. There is no known effective treatment.

Carotid body tumors have a similar appearance and biologic activity, but are located at the junction of the carotid arteries near the angle of the mandible. They are more often malignant than aortic body tumors.

TUMORS OF THE CENTRAL NERVOUS SYSTEM

Astrocytomas arise from the glial astrocytes and are most often found in the cerebrum. Compression of the third or fourth ventricle, or sylvian aqueduct may produce secondary hydrocephalus. Grossly, this tumor appears as an ill-defined mass within the nervous tissue that may be firm or soft and gelatinous. The cut surface is gray to pink and may contain small zones of hemorrhage and necrosis. Formalin fixation of the brain frequently more clearly differentiates the neoplastic tissue from normal brain. Microscopically, the tumor appears in various patterns ranging from sheets of fibrous stellate cells to large nests of undifferentiated fusiform, polygonal or rounded cells. These tumors grow by local infiltration and rarely metastasize. There is no known treatment.

Oligodendrogliomas are also derived from glial cells and are seen most commonly in the cerebral hemispheres. Grossly they are well demarcated, pink to gray and soft. Microscopically, the tumor is composed of cells closely arranged with scant cytoplasm and uniform, dark, round or oval nuclei. This tumor grows by local expansion. There is no known treatment.

Meningiomas are commoner in cats than dogs. The tumor arises from the leptomeninges and usually encroaches upon the brain. Grossly it is seen as a well-lobulated, spherical, firm, white mass that compresses adjacent areas of normal brain tissue. They are often multiple in cats. Microscopically, the tumor cells are usually spindle-shaped and arranged in well-defined whorls. Meningiomas grow by expansion, causing compression atrophy of the underlying brain. Invasion of the CNS by these tumors is rare. There is no known treatment. However, if this tumor were diagnosed early enough, it could be surgically removed, since it rarely invades nervous tissues. The signs produced are caused by compression atrophy of the adjacent nervous tissue.

NEOPLASMS OF LARGE ANIMALS

Cattle: Over 100 types of neoplasia have been recorded in cattle. While there has been extensive reporting on the occurrence of neoplasia in cattle as accomplished by governmental meat-inspection services, a detailed discussion of them will not be undertaken. The commonest tumor of cattle is the viral papilloma (q.v., p. 250); however, since this is benign most cases are not reported. Of the malignant tumors, the commonest is squamous cell carcinoma of the eye and orbit (q.v., p. 628). Lymphoid tumors (q.v., p. 633) are probably the second commonest malignancy of cattle. Studies of bovine malignant lymphoma indicate rates as high as 40 per 100,000 cattle in the U.S.A. and even higher rates in some European countries.

At a lower level of incidence are tumors of the genital tract. Multiple schwannomas affecting particularly the brachial plexus, intercostal and cardiac nerves, are found occasionally at slaughter.

Horses: The commonest tumor in horses is the cutaneous "**sarcoid,**" which usually appears on the skin of legs, ventral trunk and head. Sarcoids and papillomas (warts) in young horses are probably virus-induced; however, sarcoids do not ordinarily regress spontaneously within a reasonable amount of time and must be removed surgically. Recurrences at the surgical site are frequent. **Squamous cell carcinomas** of the eye and tumors of the genital tract are next in frequency, but are much less common than tumors of the skin. The genital tract tumors include **ovarian tumors** in mares and **squamous cell carcinoma** of the penis in stallions or geldings.

In old gray horses, **melanomas** are the commonest tumors, and these can metastasize widely from the usual primary perineal site, giving rise to signs of colic and general loss of condition. Squamous cell carcinomas of the penis, mostly the glands, are cauliflower-like or smooth tumors, slow to metastasize, and sometimes respond well to surgical removal although they tend to recur. Squamous cell carcinomas of the vulva of mares occur at a slightly lower incidence.

Tumors found in the mouth, nasal cavity and throat regions are **squamous cell carcinomas, fibrosarcomas** and **carcinomas** from the nasal sinuses and salivary glands. Signs of swallowing difficulty may be present but often the tumor is discovered as a visible and palpable mass in the ventral neck region. Older horses show a moderately high incidence of **cholesteatomas** of the brain, and are rather prone to **thyroid** and **pituitary adenomas,** the latter often associated with a long hair coat.

Visceral tumors are rare in the horse. **Hemangiosarcomas** of the liver and spleen are the commonest neoplasms of these organs, although **hepatic carcinomas** and **lymphoid tumors** do occur. **Lipomas** of the peritoneal cavity and skin are moderately prevalent. Any of these visceral tumors can give rise to signs of colic and chronic inanition. Gastric **squamous cell carcinomas** in older horses may be accompanied by a persistent anemia as well as emaciation.

In the mare, **granulosa cell tumors** and **teratomas** occur in the ovary. The former are commoner and are often associated with abnormal sexual behavior and infertility. In the stallion, **seminoma** is the commonest (but still infrequent) testicular tumor. **Mammary carcinoma** has been reported in the mare.

Sheep: Lymphoid tumors are the most commonly encountered neoplasm of sheep. **Hepatic tumors** are less often seen and, in some areas of the world, **squamous tumors of the skin** are quite frequently encountered. **Tumors of the skeleton** (mostly cartilaginous) are commoner in sheep than in other large animals, while a moderately high incidence of **ovarian tumors** parallels the situation in cattle. Neoplasms of the nasal passages and sinuses are not infrequent. **Renal tumors, pulmonary adenomatosis** and **carcinoma of the eye** may be encountered with moderate frequency. A high regional incidence of **intestinal carcinoma** is found in New Zealand and Australian sheep. Very few other tumors have been recognized in sheep.

Pigs: The incidence of tumors in pigs is low, probably in large measure because of the short life of pigs in commercial herds. Those neoplasms most often encountered necessarily occur in young animals and are believed to have a congenital or hereditary basis. The most important are **malignant lymphoma, embryonal nephroma, congenital rhabdomyomas** of the heart and **melanocytic tumors** (q.v., p. 625) in certain breeds. In some swine herds there is strong evidence for the influence of hereditary factors or vertical transmission of a possible causative virus in determining the distribution of cases of malignant lymphoma.

OCULAR CARCINOMA IN CATTLE

(Cancer eye)

A term used clinically to designate any apparently malignant neoplastic growth involving the eye and orbital region. This is almost invariably a squamous cell carcinoma originating on the bulbar or palpebral conjunctiva, eyelids, membrana nictitans, or lacrimal lake.

Incidence and Etiology: Ocular carcinoma is the commonest neoplasm of cattle. Significant economic loss results from condemnation or reduction in salvage value of carcasses and from a shortened productive life-span. The disease seldom occurs before 4 years of age and has a peak incidence at 8 years of age. A hereditary basis has been demonstrated that is apparently related more to ocular and circumocular pigmentation than to the neoplastic process itself: pigment in the lid epithelium and limbus has a significant inhibitory effect on tumor development and both forms of pigmentation are heritable. High levels of sunlight and nutrition appear to have an important influence on enhancing the disease. Involvement of the IBR virus has been suggested but not proved.

Clinical Findings and Diagnosis: On the bulbar conjunctiva, evolution of the neoplasm proceeds from a hyperplastic plaque, sometimes with an intervening papillomatous stage, to a carcinoma. On the lids, the sequence may proceed from keratosis or focal ulceration to carcinoma. Some carcinomas appear to develop *de novo* and not from benign precursor lesions. The most frequent tumor sites are the lateral and medial aspects of the corneoscleral junction (limbus). Metastasis to parotid lymph nodes occurs late and in about 5% of the cases.

Treatment: A recently developed hand-held high-frequency electronic device, using an ordinary 12-volt battery as a power source, offers promise as a field treatment. The electrodes of the device are placed on the tumor and the tumor tissue heated to 50°C for 30 seconds. Tumors with diameters greater than 2 cm may require surgical removal of the tumor surface before thermal treatment. Cryotherapy utilizing a double freeze-thaw cycle and freezing to −25°C has resulted in a 95% cure rates for tumors less than 5 cm in size with well-defined margins. Liquid nitrogen spray units were most successful. Cryotherapy is rapid, economical, requires minimal pre- or postoperative medication and may be repeated.

As ocular squamous cell carcinomas may have a genetic basis, culling of affected animals should be considered.

Immunotherapy, primarily in the form of IM injection of an extract of tumor tissue or injection of the lesion with BCG cell-wall vaccine, has also been used with variable but dramatic success. However, these methods are still experimental and injection of BCG into the lesion is not permitted in the U.S.A. Radiation therapy is successful in treating squamous cell carcinoma but the requirements for specialized equipment facilities and cost make it impractical for routine field cases.

CANINE MALIGNANT LYMPHOMA

(Lymphocytoma, Lymphosarcoma, Lymphocytic leukemia)

A progressive, fatal disease of dogs characterized by proliferation of the lymphoid series of cells usually originating in solid lymphoid organs (lymphosarcoma) or bone marrow (lymphocytic leukemia) with variable signs depending on which organs are involved.

Incidence: Malignant lymphoma is the commonest hemopoietic neoplasm of dogs, with an incidence in the general population reported as high as 24:100,000 dogs. All breeds are affected although the incidence in boxers is significantly higher than for any other purebred dog. No sex prevalence has been found.

Clinical Findings: The commonest early clinical sign is a painless, bilateral, superficial lymphadenopathy, often first noticed in lymph nodes about the throat and neck. Subsequently, there is a gradual development of nonspecific signs including anorexia, weight loss, anemia and inactivity as neoplastic cells progressively infiltrate visceral organs. In the alimentary form, signs are associated with gastrointestinal obstruction; diarrhea may be present in 80% of affected dogs. Hypercalcemia, due to development of pseudohyperparathyroidism, may be seen in 10% of dogs with malignant lymphoma. If untreated, affected dogs usually die within 1 to 2 months of diagnosis.

Lesions: Commonly all superficial and various internal lymph nodes are enlarged to 3 to 10 times their normal size (multicentric form). Affected nodes are freely movable, firm, gray-tan, bulge on cut surface, and have no cortical-medullary demarcation. There is frequently hepatosplenomegaly with either diffuse enlargement or multiple, variable sized, pale nodules disseminated in the parenchyma. Other less commonly involved organs include the alimentary tract, kidney, heart, tonsils, pancreas and bone marrow.

In the alimentary form of the disease, the second most commonly encountered anatomic form, any part of the gastrointestinal tract or mesenteric lymph nodes may be affected but superficial lymph nodes and spleen are rarely involved.

True lymphocytic leukemia is a rare form and must be differentiated from lymphosarcoma because it requires different treatment. This disease is characterized by a normal to elevated white blood cell count with a predominance of lymphoid cells in peripheral blood and bone marrow. There is frequently a diffuse splenomegaly. Although neoplastic lymphocytes may also be encountered in the blood and bone marrow in lymphosarcoma, they then represent a leukemia secondary to spill-over from neoplastic infiltrates in solid lymphoid organs. Most lymphosarcomas have a normal hematologic profile, except for a normocytic, normochromic anemia. In the later stages an absolute neutrophila may develop (granulocytic leukemoid reaction).

Other less commonly encountered types of lymphosarcoma include an anterior mediastinal form with primary involvement of the thymus and an extranodal form which includes skin or a single organ (e.g. kidney) involvement.

Different cytologic forms (stem cell, lymphoblastic, histiocytic, prolymphocytic, lymphocytic) and histologic patterns (diffuse and nodular) have been described in canine malignant lymphoma. There is no consistent correlation between anatomic form, cytologic form, or histologic pattern.

Diagnosis: Microscopic examination of lymphoid tissue is required for positive diagnosis since lymphadenopathies may be due to causes other than lymphoid neoplasia. Examination of peripheral blood or bone marrow is usually not helpful except in terminal stages of the disease or in the rare cases of true lymphatic leukemia. A viral etiology for canine malignant lymphoma has not been established and serological tests comparable to those used in the diagnosis of feline or bovine leukemia are not available.

Treatment: Although there is no known cure, the disease can be temporarily controlled by the judicious use of combination chemotherapy. Average survival times (in dogs other than those in advanced stages) of 8 months after diagnosis may be expected. Numerous treatment regimens have been been designed but a useful one for cases of multicentric lymphosarcoma utilizes a repeating 4 week cycle: week 1—vincristine (0.025 to 0.05 mg/kg daily, IV); week 2—cyclophosphamide (10 mg/kg daily, IV); week 3—vincristine as per week 1; week 4—cytosine arabinoside (30 to 50 mg/kg, subcut.). The alimentary form does not respond well to chemotherapy and, if the lesion is localized, surgical resection should be attempted.

True lymphocytic leukemia may be cytologically classified as either well differentiated or poorly differentiated. The latter form is more refractory to chemotherapy and has a poor prognosis. However, prolonged remissions of the well differentiated form may be achieved with chlorambucil at 0.2 mg/kg, orally for 7 days, followed by a reduced dosage of 0.1 mg/kg daily, until it no longer controls the disease or signs of toxicity appear.

Periodic clinical and laboratory examinations are imperative during the course of all chemotherapeutic regimens, as the drugs are cytotoxic. Adverse reactions include bone marrow suppression and increased susceptibility to infection. Anabolic steroids and prophylactic use of antibiotics may be used to prevent these occurrences. Transfusions may be necessary.

FELINE LYMPHOSARCOMA AND LEUKEMIA

(Feline Visceral Lymphoma and Leukemia, Lymphosarcoma)

Lymphosarcoma is the most frequently diagnosed feline neoplastic disease. Thymic, multicentric and alimentary forms are recognized: the thymic form is common in young cats, while involvement of the abdominal organs typically occurs in older animals. Lymphoid and myeloid leukemia occur with lesser frequency.

Etiology and Epidemiology: Feline leukemia virus can be demonstrated in cats with lymphosarcoma: in 90% of thymic, 70% of multicentric and 35% of alimentary cases. It is present in the mouth of infected cats and transmission occurs by cat-to-cat contact and also congenitally. There is no evidence that infected cats pose a threat to human health. Cats may experience subclinical infection and develop immunity to disease. Alternatively, they may become persistently infected. These cats have a marked predisposition to the occurrence of neoplasia or one of the nonmalignant diseases associated with feline leukemia virus infection (q.v., p. 633). The incidence of disease is greatest in cats living in households where other cats have had lymphosarcoma previously.

Clinical Findings: Frequently the affected cat undergoes a chronic wasting disease marked by anemia, lethargy and anorexia. Thymic lymphosarcoma may cause dyspnea, dysphagia and coughing. Radiographs may indicate the presence of a mediastinal mass, or the thoracic architecture may be obscured by pleural effusion. In the latter case, the presence of large numbers of immature lymphocytes in stained smears of aspirated pleural fluids will differentiate lymphosarcoma from other causes of hydrothorax. The signs of the abdominal form often are those of intestinal obstruction. One or more mesenteric lymph nodes frequently are enlarged. The wall of the stomach or intestine may be thickened diffusely, or it may contain a discrete tumor. Uremia can result from extensive renal involvement. Hepatic involvement can cause anemia and jaundice. Enlargement of involved viscera may be evident in radiographs of the abdomen. In the multicentric form, the superficial lymph nodes are grossly enlarged. Cats with lymphosarcoma usually do not develop leukemia. Primary involvement of hemopoietic tissue usually causes a nonregenerative anemia. The reticulocyte count is low, and the packed red cell volume may decrease 8 to 15%. Nucleated erythrocytes may be present in stained smears of peripheral blood. When immature lymphocytes are observed in these smears, a bone marrow biopsy should be performed. In lymphoid leukemia, more than 40% of the nucleated cells in marrow aspirates will be lymphocytes.

Lesions: Thymic lymphosarcoma originates in the precardiac mediastinum. The anterior ventral thorax may be filled with white, lobulated tumorous tissue embedding the heart and displacing the lungs dorsally and posteriorly. The abdominal organs affected by lymphosarcoma are, in decreasing order of frequency, intestine (ileum), kidneys, liver, mesenteric lymph nodes, and spleen. In the multicentric form most of the lymph nodes and the spleen are involved.

Diagnosis: Lymphosarcoma may be diagnosed by the detection of tumors in affected organs. The nature of these masses should be confirmed by biopsy and cytologic examination. Hematologic changes in cats with lymphosarcoma are seldom pronounced but hematology may be useful in the diagnosis of lymphoid and myeloid leukemia. The strong association between persistent infection with feline leukemia virus and lymphosarcoma makes laboratory testing for the detection of feline leukemia virus group-specific antigen in blood a useful diagnostic procedure.

Control: Methods for the prevention of lymphosarcoma and leukemia have not yet been developed. Chemotherapy programs have been developed with the goal of extending the affected cat's life. Long-term remission occurs in some cases, but survival of 3 to 6 months is commoner. These cats must be considered as potential sources of infection for other susceptible cats in close and continuous contact with them. Feline leukemia virus may be eradicated from closed households of cats by the removal of cats that test positive for the virus in the blood, combined with a program of quarantine and disinfection.

FELINE LEUKEMIA VIRUS-ASSOCIATED DISEASES

In addition to causing neoplasia (*See* FELINE LYMPHOSARCOMA AND LEUKEMIA, p. 631), feline leukemia virus also causes nonmalignant disease conditions. The better characterized of these illnesses include nonregenerative anemia and immunosuppression. The latter condition predisposes the leukemia virus-infected cat to many infectious diseases including feline infectious peritonitis, q.v., p. 327, and feline infectious anemia, q.v., p. 328. Other diseases that have been associated with leukemia virus infection include enteritis, glomerulonephritis and fetal absorption or abortion. The presence of feline leukemia virus in affected animals is best demonstrated by testing for viral group-specific antigen in the blood.

BOVINE LEUKOSIS

(Bovine leukemia, Lymphosarcoma, Malignant lymphoma)

Bovine leukosis is an inclusive term and is preferred because persistent lymphocytosis (leukemia) is not always present and lymphosarcoma refers specifically to the tumor. Bovine leukosis virus (BLV) is one etiologic factor in the adult form of lymphosarcoma. Bovine leukosis occurs, with or without leukemia, in 4 forms:

The **adult multicentric form, lymphosarcoma,** the commonest malignant neoplasm affecting cattle aged 3 years and older, involves scattered lymph nodes in the pelvic region, heart, uterus and glandular stomach. Lymphocytosis with immature lymphoblasts and slight lymph node enlargement may exist for months when, often at parturition, enlarged lymph or hemal nodes suddenly appear. Other signs relate to specific area or organ involvement. Loss of weight and milk production and, usually, death follow. At necropsy the lymphosarcoma, showing hemorrhage and necrosis, usually is confined by a greatly enlarged lymph node capsule wherein normal lymphatic tissue has been partially or completely replaced. Focal or diffuse tumor growth may occur in visceral organs, retrobulbar tissue, spinal meninges, heart (especially right atrium) or extended from affected lymph nodes and thymus.

The **juvenile form**, relatively uncommon, occurs from before birth to 1 year of age and involves nearly all lymph nodes, liver, spleen, kidneys and bone marrow.

The **thymic form**, not common, which occurs in cattle ½ to 2 years old, involves the thymus and some scattered lymph nodes. Lesions may extend from the larynx to the thorax.

The **skin form**, rare, occurs in 2-to-3-year-old cattle. Lesions may regress and regression may be followed later by the adult form. Localized lesion of edematous, congested tumor growth, a few millimeters to several centimeters in diameter, are scattered in the corium; anemia may occur.

BLV infection is identifiable only in the adult form of bovine lymphosarcoma. In some areas more than half the dairy herds harbor BLV infection, with a lesser incidence in beef cattle herds. BLV appears to spread from dam to daughter *in utero* and by colostrum, milk, insects or contact. Infection can develop in older cows previously serologically negative, indicating horizontal transmission. Artificial insemination from infected bulls does not transmit the infection.

Sheep develop all 4 clinical forms of leukosis observed in cattle. Chimpanzees can develop persistent antibody levels after experimental BLV infection but BLV has not been isolated from them nor have they developed lymphosarcoma. The potential hazard of BLV to man has been investigated by serologic studies of veterinarians in dairy cattle practice, people with various forms of leukemia and cancer, and farm families drinking raw milk from BLV-infected dairy cattle. Despite anecdotal reports suggesting possible association of human and bovine leukemia, these and other extensive studies based on geographic distribution indicate BLV is not oncogenic for man.

Serologic diagnosis of BLV infection in adult lymphosarcoma by immunodiffusion test detects antibody against the glycoprotein-70 BLV envelope antigen. Similar testing utilizing viral nucleoprotein is a less sensitive detector.

B-lymphocytes are the principal cells in both bovine and ovine lymphosarcoma; increased thymidine uptake by bovine cells is an index of transformation to neoplasia. Lymphocytosis classifications by "lymphocyte keys" are unreliable indices of BLV infection because false positive results ensue from chronic infections, mastitis, parasitism, etc., and false negative results occur in cattle when BLV infection does not cause lymphocytosis.

BLV infection persists for years with 10% of infected cows developing clinical signs. Usually when 30% of a herd is serologically BLV-positive clinical disease occurs, although no lymphosarcoma may develop even with a 75% infection rate. The juvenile, thymic and skin forms of leukosis produce no serologic evidence.

Anticancer drug therapy is impractical in bovine lymphosarcoma.

If only a few cows are infected they should be removed from the herd. Any infected cows retained should be segregated and not allowed to nurse replacement calves.

HEREDITARY MELANOMA OF SWINE

(Cutaneous melanoma, Cutaneous melanoepithelioma, "Blood warts")

A benign, heritable, cutaneous tumor of swine. Melanomas, often highly malignant in other species, are clinically benign in swine. Many affected swine survive for several years without apparent signs of metastasis.

Incidence and Etiology: Slaughterhouse surveys on swine of all breeds indicate an incidence of not more than 1:200,000. Tumors occur exclusively in pigmented swine, most frequently of the duroc breed and, occasionally, in Hampshires, Hampshire-duroc crosses and Hormel miniature swine. In affected herds, melanomas can occur in 60% of all litters farrowed but litter incidence usually is 10%.

Litter incidence increases after inbreeding for several generations. Recorded matings in affected duroc herds indicate transmission via a non-sex-linked recessive gene of incomplete penetrance. Unaffected littermates of melanomatous pigs are suspected carriers. Attempts to transplant tumors have been unsuccessful.

Clinical Findings: On newborn piglets, melanomas vary from darkly pigmented pinpoint spots to lesions 2 cm in diameter. Tumors vary in growth rate but reach maximum size usually when swine are 6 to 8 months old. Tumor regression, through unknown mechanisms, may follow castration or partial tumor removal surgically, or it may be spontaneous. The tumors, usually less than 6 per animal, occur more frequently over the dorsal region around the base of the ears, midback, loin, tailhead and flanks, less frequently on the abdomen and legs. Early metastasis is evidenced by regional lymph node enlargement. Affected swine show few clinical signs despite the extensive lymphatic involvement but posterior paralysis and secondary gastric ulceration have occurred in advanced cases. Metastasis may progress beyond the lymphatic system to the liver, lungs and kidneys.

Lesions: Adult swine show circular or oval, circumscribed, blue-black to black, hairless lesions with glistening surfaces up to 5 cm in diameter raised to 3 cm above the skin. Large tumors may ulcerate, bleed or ooze a black, pigmented discharge; secondary infection is common. Macrophages, after invading the neoplasm, distribute melanin pigment to the dermis, subcut. fat and local lymphatics and neoplastic melanocytes move via the lymphatics to other organs.

At necropsy the gray-black lesions are readily recognizable by their color in the lymphatic system and nodes. Metastasis may have progressed beyond the lymphatic system to the liver, lungs, kidneys and proceeded to the bone marrow, adrenals, heart and meninges.

Control of swine melanomas depends on eliminating affected and carrier animals from breeding. Breeding records should identify the carrier bloodlines. Replacement swine should be acquired only from melanoma-free herds.

NERVOUS SYSTEM

CLINICAL EXAMINATION OF THE NERVOUS SYSTEM

To diagnose and locate a lesion of the nervous system, a complete and methodic neurologic examination must be performed. An understanding of neuroanatomy, neurophysiologic concepts and neuropathologic processes is a requisite to the final interpretation of the nervous dysfunction. In conjunction with clinical assessment and diagnostic aids, the problem may be defined as diffuse or localized. Although an exact diagnosis may not be made clinically, the clinician can often define the disease as teratologic, inflammatory, metabolic or toxic, degenerative, neoplastic or traumatic.

A neurologic examination typically consists of obtaining the history and assessing the mental state, gait and posture, cranial nerve reflexes, spinal reflexes, sensory perception, postural and attitudinal reactions. Important aids in diagnosis are cerebrospinal fluid, plain and contrast radiography.

History Taking: Many neurologic diseases have a breed incidence and familial relationship. Environmental conditions often indicate a toxic or infectious cause. Information regarding age of onset, vaccination status and duration of illness is important.

Physical Examination: This will aid in establishing the role of musculoskeletal, liver, renal, pancreatic, cardiac and endocrine disorders that may mimic or contribute to nervous dysfunction.

Gait and Posture: Exercise will exacerbate motor tract and proprioceptive deficiencies. It assists in distinguishing tetraparesis, paraparesis, hemiparesis and monoparesis. A head tilt with ataxia and perhaps circling may signify a vestibular disturbance. A base-wide stance, hypermetric gait and head tremor are pathognomonic for cerebellar disease. Paraplegic or tetraplegic animals should be assisted to their feet if possible and observed for any perceptible movement or support in the limbs.

Demeanor: Assessment of the mental state of the patient helps to identify cerebrocortical disease and occasionally thalamic and midbrain dysfunction. Clinical manifestations include varying degrees of depression, excitation, seizures, circling activity, head pressing, and loss of consciousness.

CRANIAL NERVE EXAMINATION

This consists of simple testing of all 12 cranial nerves. Deficiencies may occur spontaneously with no other involvement of the nervous system. In conjunction with signs related to brain function, cranial nerve palsies can help to localize a lesion within the brainstem.

I. Olfactory: *Tests:* (1) Observation by owner. (2) Observe reaction to chemicals such as cloves, benzene, xylol (avoid substances which will irritate the trigeminal nerve, such as camphor or phenol).

Diseases: Head trauma, toxic damage, neoplasms.

II. Optic: The optic nerves extending from the retina to the optic chiasma also carry the afferent fibers of the pupillary light reflex center of the midbrain. A lesion of the optic nerves causes varying degrees of blindness and pupillary light reflex abnormalities. Lesions of the optic tract, optic radiation, or occipital cortex lesions usually produce a contralateral blindness with normal pupillary light reflex, i.e. a lesion of the left cerebral hemisphere will cause a right-sided blindness with normal pupil reactions. Unilateral optic nerve lesions will cause blindness on the same side with pupillary light reflex deficiency.

(1) Visual Tests: Perform the *menace test* by making a threatening gesture towards each eye, taking care to avoid excessive air current or touching the hair. *Obstacle testing* may be necessary when visual acuity is in doubt. It is useful to blindfold one eye at a time to detect asymmetrical blindness. *(2) Pupillary light reflex:* A bright focal light is directed into each pupil towards the temporal retina and the pupil observed for immediate constriction. The opposite pupil should constrict consensually. *(3) Ophthalmoscopic examination* detects local eye diseases. Choroid retinitis or papilledema may be associated with central or peripheral nervous diseases.

Diseases: Optic neuritis (distemper, toxoplasmosis, reticulosis), neoplasms, vitamin A deficiency.

III. Oculomotor: This nerve carries efferent parasympathetic fibers from the pupillary light reflex center to the ciliary ganglion whose fibers innervate the constrictor muscle of the pupil. Also it is the motor nerve to the levator palpebrae muscle, dorsal, medial and ventral rectus muscles, and the ventral oblique muscle of the eye.

Tests: 1. Perform the light reflex test as for the optic nerve. 2. Observe for ptosis of the upper eyelid and ventrolateral strabismus.

Diseases: Trauma, retrobulbar or midbrain inflammation, listeriosis, hydrocephalus.

IV. Trochlear: This is the motor nerve to the dorsal oblique muscle of the eye.

Test: Observe for dorsomedial strabismus.

Disease: Polioencephalomalacia of ruminants.

V. Trigeminal: This comprises 3 main sections. The mandibular is the motor nerve to the muscles of mastication, the floor of the oral cavity and ventral arcade, and to the skin of the ventrolateral head. The ophthalmic and maxillary nerves are sensory to the skin of the dorsolateral head, mucous membrane of the roof of the oral cavity and the dorsal arcade, mucous membrane of the nasal cavity; and sensory to the eyeball, including the cornea (pain).

Tests: (1) Observe for a "dropped jaw" with weak tone and masticatory movements. Neurogenic atrophy of the masseter and temporal muscles will develop quickly. (2) Stimulate the medial and lateral canthi of the eyes to elicit the *palpebral reflex* (closure of the eyelids). An avoidance reaction to stimulation of the cornea and oral and nasal mucosae assesses the sensory function of the fifth nerve.

Diseases: Inflammatory, traumatic and neoplastic lesions of the medulla, idiopathic dropped jaw syndrome of dogs.

VI. Abducens: This is the motor nerve to the lateral rectus and retractor bulbi muscles of the eye.

Tests: (1) Observe for medial strabismus. (2) Elicit the corneal reflex (V) with the eyelids held open and observe for retraction of the eyeball and prolapse of the third eyelid.

Diseases: See Trigeminal Nerve (V).

VII. Facial: This is the motor nerve to the muscles of facial expression (ear, eyelids, nose and mouth).

Tests: (1) Elicit the palpebral, menace and corneal reflex for orbicularis oculi motor function. (2) Examine the nose for deviation (with unilateral lesions), for drooling of saliva and accumulation of food in the vestibule due to paralysis of the buccinator muscle, and for pendulous lower lip.

Diseases: (1) Peripheral lesions occur with inner ear diseases and trauma to superficial nerve branches. Idiopathic neuritis also occurs in dogs. (2) Diseases involving the medulla at the level of the facial nucleus.

VIII. Vestibulocochlear: There are 2 main divisions of this nerve; the first, the *cochlear nerve,* functions to provide the sense of hearing.

Test: Total deafness is easily detected by creating loud noises near the sleeping animal.

Diseases: Congenital and drug induced deafness, otitis interna.

The second branch of the vestibulocochlear (VII), the *vestibular nerve* allows maintenance of normal posture, muscle tone, and equilibrium.

Tests: (1) Observe for head tilt, ataxia and tendency to fall, roll, or circle with unilateral or asymmetrical lesions. (2) Check for the presence of abnormal nystagmus with the head in normal position (resting nystagmus) and with the head held in a deviated position (positional nystagmus).

Diseases: (1) Trauma or inflammation of the inner ear. (2) Distemper, listeriosis (medullary lesions).

IX. Glossopharyngeal; X. Vagus: These provide sensory and motor control of the pharynx, larynx, and of the visceral systems and the heart (vagus).

Tests: (1) Check for the absence of a *gag reflex* in association with dysphagia. (2) Observe for abnormal vocalization and inspiratory dyspnea. (3) Abnormal heart rate and gastrointestinal activity may occur with increased or decreased vagal activity.

Diseases: Laryngeal hemiplegia in horses, rabies, tumors and inflammatory lesions of the caudal medulla, guttural pouch infections.

XI. Spinal Accessory: This nerve is generally not tested in a neurologic examination, as malfunctions are difficult to detect clinically. In large animals, atrophy of the sternocephalicus muscle may be noted.

XII. Hypoglossyl: This is the motor nerve to the tongue and geniohyoid muscles.

Test: Observe for muscular control of the tongue. Muscle atrophy will occur with chronic conditions. The tongue is deviated with unilateral lesions.

Diseases: Trauma, caudal medullary lesions as in listeriosis, rabies.

SPINAL REFLEXES

In conjunction with the gait examination, evaluation of spinal reflexes will assist in localizing of focal spinal lesions. Additional tests are required to determine the causes of the problem. The qualitative assessment can distinguish between upper and lower motor neuron disease which will influence the prognosis.

Flexor Reflex: *Functions:* (1) In the forelimbs, the integrity of the spinal segments of the brachial plexus, which supply the muscles of flexion, is assessed. Areflexia or hyporeflexia of the forelegs in association with tetraparesis or tetraplegia, would indicate a cord lesion involving primarily the lower cervical segments (C6 to T1 inclusive). (2) Flexion of the *pelvic limbs* depends upon sciatic nerve function (flexion of the tarsus and stifle), derived primarily from cord segments L6 to S1 and upon segments L1 to L7 for hip flexion.

Test: In small animals, compress the toes of each limb, in turn, with a pair of forceps. In large animals, pain may be applied with forceps on the skin of the distal limb. Observe if all joints of the limb are flexed fully in response to the stimulus. Areflexia associated with a spinal lesion indicates lower motor neuron damage that may be irreversible. It is important to note that the spinal cord segments L3 to S3 overlie vertebrae L3 to L6 and the spinal cord terminates at L6 to L7 in the dog and in the sacral region in horse, ox, pig and cat. A compressive sacral lesion will affect the cauda equina in all species.

Patellar Reflex: *Function:* This stretch reflex assesses the femoral nerve and the L4 to L6 cord segments, chiefly; the cranial part of the biceps femoris muscle attaches to the patella and contributes to this reflex.

Test: Lightly tap the patellar tendon with a percussion instrument, which will elicit extension of the stifle. This test should be performed with the animal in lateral recumbency.

Perineal Reflex: *Function:* This tests the integrity of the pudendal nerve and the S1 to S3 cord segments which control the bladder, rectum and anus.

Test: Touch the anus and observe for constriction of the sphincter and depression of the tail.

Cutaneus Trunci Reflex: Pin pricks applied to the skin of the thorax and abdomen result in contraction of the cutaneus trunci muscle. This reflex arc uses the cutaneous branches of the lumbar and thoracic spinal nerves as afferent pathways and the caudal pectoral nerve of the brachial plexus as the efferent pathway. The reflex is used to localize cord lesions between the site of afferent stimulation and brachial plexus levels. A similar reflex can be elicited in the cervical region; the afferent limb of the arc is the cervical nerves and the efferent limb is the facial nerve which supplies the cervical cutaneous muscles.

Release Phenomena: When the upper motor neuron pathways that influence spinal reflex activity are interrupted, exaggerated reflex activity may be noted. This means that the lesion must be cranial to the affected spinal segments. *(1) Crossed extensor reflex:* When performing the flexor reflex in a limb, observe if the opposite limb automatically extends. *(2) Passive manipulation:* Observe for increased extensor tone while pushing the limbs into a flexed position. Clasp-knife extensor rigidity is the usual type found in domestic animals.

Conscious Sensory Perception: During the examination of the spinal reflexes, sufficient stimulus should be applied to cause vocalization or head movement of the patient.

Attitudinal and Postural Reactions

These tests require complete integrity of the brain, spinal cord and peripheral nervous system. They also assist in detecting subtle deficiencies of the system.

Tonic Neck and Eye: With the animal standing, elevate the nose and observe that the eyes coordinately adjust to the center of the palpebral fissure (dog and cat). Simultaneously, the forelimbs should extend with no tendency to knuckle or collapse.

Proprioceptive Positioning: Displace each digit by turning it onto its dorsum or by abducting or adducting the limb widely. The animal should immediately replace the leg to a normal position. Conscious proprioception is often the first modality to be affected with subtle lesions of the nervous system.

Placing: Small animals may be carried toward a table top; upon seeing the table, the animal will normally anticipate placing its forepaws upon the surface. If blindfolded, the animal will place the forepaws on the table only upon contacting the limbs with the edge of the table. In large animals, the tactile placing reflexes can be examined by blindfolding the animal and walking it over level ground without obstacles. Normal placing of the limbs indicates that the proprioceptive reflex pathways are intact. A common sign of loss of proprioceptive sense is crossing of the limbs in an animal with an otherwise normal standing attitude.

Extensor Postural Thrust: This can be tested in small animals. Hold the animal upright by its thorax and lower the back legs to the ground. The limbs will extend to support weight.

Hopping: This can be tested in small animals only. While holding the other 3 limbs off the ground, force the animal to move or hop on the fourth limb. Motor and proprioceptive weakness, cerebellar incoordination and cerebrocortical deficiency may be detected with this procedure. The test examines the proprioceptive pathways, which in large animals can be examined as described under Placing (above).

Righting: Observe if the animal can right itself from lateral recumbency. A small animal suspended upside down by the hips will attempt to hold its head up when the trunk is rotated from side to side.

Cerebrospinal Fluid

Examination of the pressure and composition of cerebrospinal fluid may assist determination of the etiology of CNS disorders.

Examination can be carried out by puncture of the cisterna magna in small animals, or the subarachnoid space at the lumbosacral junction in large animals. Elevations of pressure above 170 mm water indicate the presence of space-occupying lesions or a defect in drainage of cerebrospinal fluid into the venous system. Elevation of protein is an indication of encephalitis or meningoencephalitis. Elevation of cellular content suggests infection of the CNS. The presence of neutrophils is indicative of bacterial infections, subarachnoid hemorrhage (erythrocytes are also present) or brain abscess. The presence of increased numbers of lymphocytes is indicative of viral infections or toxoplasmosis. Cultures of cerebrospinal fluid will often demonstrate the causative agent in microbial encephalitis.

INHERITED DISEASES AND CONGENITAL MALFORMATIONS OF THE CNS

Congenital defects of the CNS are common and most can be recognized by structural change, which may involve both the CNS and the skeletal structures, or only the former. Functional defects are rare. Some congenital defects are known to be inherited, others are caused by environmental factors (toxic plants, nutritional deficiencies, viral infections); for many the cause is still unknown. In animals born with a well-developed nervous system (foals, calves, lambs and pigs), inherited neurologic disorders may be recognized at birth. In kittens and puppies, born less well developed, neurologic disorders may not be noticeable until they would normally begin to walk.

CEREBRAL DEFECTS

Anencephaly, nonclosure of the cranial portion of the neural tube and subsequent failure of the cranium to develop, has been described in cattle. Its cause is unknown. The pituitary may be absent and its absence probably is responsible for the prolonged gestation of some calves affected with anencephaly. Associated defects include cleft palate, taillessness, atresia ani and patent fontanelle.

Arhinencephaly, defined as absence of the rhinencephalon, is a rare deformity in cattle characterized by unilateral or bilateral absence of olfactory bulbs, tract or nerves. Prolonged pregnancy may accompany the condition. Breeds involved are Simmental, Guernsey, and Angus. Cause of the deformity is unknown, although it was once assumed to be a dominant lethal mutation.

Exencephaly is a brain entirely exposed or extruding from a large defective skull (acrania). The defect is rare and its cause is unknown.

Agenesis of the corpus callosum, absence of all or part of the corpus callosum, has rarely been described in domestic animals and its cause is unknown.

Hydranencephaly is complete or almost complete absence of the cerebral hemispheres in a cranium of normal conformation. The space is filled with cerebrospinal fluid encased by thin membranous cerebral tissue and meninges.

The congenital syndrome of hydranencephaly, with or without arthrogryposis, occurs sporadically or as epidemics in calves. The chief clinical signs are blindness, incoordination, imbecility and joint problems. Other pathologic changes observed are cerebellar hypoplasia, muscular atrophy, cleft palate, scoliosis and spina bifida. Abortion, stillbirth or premature birth may occur. Several causes have been identified, including hyperthermia and the viruses of ephemeral fever, Japanese encephalitis, bluetongue and Akabane disease (q.v., p. 440).

Hydrocephalus (internal), q.v., p. 668, is common in cattle and other domestic animals. It is defined as excessive accumulation of fluid within the ventricular system. Calves with internal hydrocephalus may be born dead or may die within a few days of birth. In many breeds of cattle, it appears to be inherited as a simple autosomal recessive trait. In Hereford and shorthorn calves it is accompanied by a stenotic aqueduct, cerebellar hypoplasia, myopathy, multiple ocular anomalies, retinal detachment and dysplasia, cataracts, microphthalmia, and persistent pupillary membranes. Hydrocephalus varies considerably; one or both lateral ventricles may be involved, the third ventricle and anterior portion of the aqueduct may be dilated, and the fourth ventricle may be normal. In Hereford calves there may be dorsal kinking and lateral compression of the midbrain with stenosis of the middle part of the mesencephalic aqueduct. Doming of the skull is not consistent in domestic animals. Achondroplastic calves are usually affected with internal hydrocephalus (*see* BOVINE DWARFISM, p. 823).

Meningocele and **meningoencephalocele** are characterized by protrusion of meninges and brain tissue through a cranial cleft (cranioschisis). The herniated portion sometimes forms a large liquid-filled sac. Meningoencephalocele usually occurs in the frontal region (proencephaly), but may be midfrontal, parietal, or occipital. It is not known whether the defect is inherited in most domestic animals, however in piglets it is established as a simple autosomal recessive trait. (Meningoceles occur in the spinal column also, as a type of spina bifida.)

Micrencephaly or microcephaly is rare and has been described as a normal-sized cranial activity only partly filled by brain. In the reported cases, there was a decrease in number of gyri and the corpus callosum and fornix were absent. All animals were stillborn or died soon after birth. Associated defects were micrognathia, multiple ear and eye defects, vesicular cerebral hemisphere and absent septum pellucidum.

Cyclopia and **cebocephalia** are severe defects involving the cranium as well as the facial skeleton. The cause in lambs is ingestion of the range plant *Veratrum californicum* by ewes at day 14 of gestation.

Cranioschisis, a cleft in the cranial skeleton, is usually associated with herniation of the meninges and parts of the brain.

DEFECTS OF CEREBELLUM AND BRAIN STEM

Arnold-Chiari malformation, consisting of herniation of tongue-like processes of cerebellar tissue through the foramen magnum into the anterior cervical spinal canal plus caudal displacement and elongation of the medulla oblongata, pons, and the fourth ventricle, is often associated with spina bifida, hydrocephalus and meningomyelocele. It is rare in domestic animals and of unknown cause.

Cerebellar aplasia, hypoplasia and degeneration: Congenital cerebellar lesions consisting of agenesis, aplasia (absence or imperfect development) and hypoplasia have been described in many species. Their pathogenesis and causes must be re-evaluated in the light of recent findings that prenatal and neonatal infection (kittens with feline panleukopenia virus and calves with BVD virus) may be causative. The main signs consist of ataxia at birth or shortly after, lack of equilibrium, violent muscular movements, coarse tremors and opisthotonos. The pathologic features include atrophy of all or parts of the layers of the cerebellar cortex but particularly, loss of the Purkinje cell layer. Cerebellar hypoplasia in puppies and kittens is often accompanied by hypoplasia of the pons, the inferior olivae and sometimes the optic tracts. Clinical signs consist of tumbling, circling and ataxia; a head tremor is often present.

Another type of cerebellar disorder has been seen in Jersey and other calves in North America. In this condition, the cerebellar white matter is predominantly affected. Lesions also occur in other parts of the brain, the most notable one being a lack of myelin formation. In Britain, a somewhat similar condition of hypomyelinogenesis congenita has been described in newborn paralytic lambs. Throughout the entire nervous system, axis cylinders develop but myelination is deficient. Myoclonia congenita in pigs (q.v., p. 601) may represent a variation of hypomyelinogenesis congenita.

Progressive ataxia is a recently recognized clinical and pathologic entity of unknown etiology in female Charolais cattle. Clinical signs were first noticed in cows 8 to 24 months of age and progressed in 1 to 2 years from slight ataxia involving all 4 limbs to recumbency. Histopathologic lesions consisted of eosinophilic plaques in the white matter of internal capsule, the cerebellar white matter, and the spinal cord. There is myelin breakdown but no phagocytic response.

Cerebellar cortical atrophy has been described in Holstein calves with clinical and morphological features comparable to those of the defect in lambs (**daft lambs**) and dogs. A similar condition has been described in Angus calves as **familial convulsions and ataxia.** The clinical signs usually appeared during the first few hours of life and were characterized by single or multiple, sudden tetaniform seizures of variable intensity, lasting from 3 to 12 hours or longer. Inheritance appeared to be as a dominant mode with incomplete penetrance (20 to 30%). A similar disease was described in Holstein calves in New York and in a Charolais, with clinical and pathologic changes almost identical to those of familial convulsions and ataxia of Angus calves.

Hereditary neuraxial edema and congenital brain edema were first reported in neonatal polled Hereford calves. The calves were unable to rise and lay quietly without struggling. There was incoordination and coarse muscular tonic contraction. Sudden touch or clapping of hands elicited vigorous extension of the legs and neck. Brains were grossly normal. Microscopic examination revealed spongy vacuolar appearance of the central nervous tissue along the long axis of myelinated fibers in white and grey matters.

SPASTIC AND PARALYTIC DISEASES

A group of diseases, some of which are hereditary, with clinical evidence implicating CNS involvement. However, pathogenesis and neuropathologic lesions have not been well defined.

Spastic paresis, which occurs in many breeds of cattle, is characterized by spastic contracture of the muscles and extension of the stifle and tarsal joints of one or both hind legs. It has been referred to as "contraction of the Achilles tendon," "straight hock," and "Elso heel." Spasticity affects the gastrocnemius and superficial flexor muscles and tendons and, in some cases, also the biceps femoris, semitendinosus, semimembranosus, quadriceps, and abductor muscles. It is a progressive disease varying in severity and time of onset, usually noted first in calves from 3 to 6 months of age.

Radiographs of affected hock joints are characterized by increased joint angle, osteoporosis and exostosis involving the distal epiphyseal line of tibia, curvature and exostosis of the dorsal side of the calcaneus, and widening of the epiphyseal line of the calcaneous. There are no CNS lesions. Genetic influence(s) as well as environmental factors interact to express spastic paresis. Affected bulls should not be used for breeding purposes.

Lethal spasm (lethal neonatal spasticity) has been reported in Jersey and Hereford cattle as a simple autosomal recessive trait.

Hereditary **epilepsy** (idiopathic epilepsy) is a convulsive state without discoverable etiologic factors or definite underlying lesions. It has been recorded in Swedish Red cattle as an autosomal recessive, and in Brown Swiss cattle as an autosomal dominant trait. (*See also* below.)

Mannosidosis in Angus and Murray Grey cattle (originally reported as **pseudolipidosis**) is due to deficiency of the enzyme mannosidase and is a simple autosomal recessive trait. Clinically there is ataxia, incoordination, head tremor, aggression and failure to thrive. Most affected calves die within the first 12 months, sometimes shortly after birth. Vacuolation of neurons, macrophages and reticuloendothelial cells of lymph nodes, and exocrine pancreas cells are typical. Affected (homozygous) calves suffer from absolute deficiency of α-mannosidase and heterozygotes have partial deficiency of this enzyme. Therefore, mannosidosis can be controlled by identifying and eliminating heterozygotes on the basis of biochemical testing.

GM_1 gangliosidosis, occurs in inbred Friesian calves in Ireland, and involves a reduction (70 to 80%) in β-galactosidase activity. Clinical signs become evident during the first few weeks of life, and include swaying of the hindquarters, reluctance to move and stiffness of gait. Microscopic lesions are primarily vacuolation of neurons.

Neuronal lipodystrophy, probably hereditary, was described in an 18-month-old inbred Beefmaster bull. This strain of cattle had a history of blindness and intermittent circling for 6 months before coma, periodic clonic convulsions and death.

DISEASES IN WHICH LESIONS HAVE NOT BEEN DEMONSTRATED

A spastic syndrome (remittent or periodic spastic syndrome, crampy neuromuscular spasticity, progressive posterior paralysis, or stretches) is observed in cattle over 6 years of age and is characterized by sudden spastic muscular contractions of one or both hind legs. Early signs occur when the animal arises from a sternal position. The hind legs are stretched and rigid and the muscles of the neck and back exhibit coarse tremors. Initially, attacks may last only a few seconds but progressively they lengthen to last several minutes. At first, the attacks are separated by long intervals which become progressively shorter as the disease advances. The disease is thought to be inherited. No treatment is known to effect a permanent cure; temporary relief may be obtained by the administration of mephenesin (℞ 550).

Epilepsy is a functional disease of the brain characterized by recurrent periodic tonoclonic convulsions, usually of short duration, and apparently similar to epilepsy in man. "Idiopathic" epilepsy (*see also* p. 647) has been described in many species but probably is seen most often in the dog. A high incidence has been noticed in cocker spaniels. The typical history is that of recurrent convulsive seizures with few or no other physical signs. Convulsions may begin in the first year of life, but more frequently begin in the second year. The typical seizure lasts for 1 to 2 minutes and consists of a staring appearance, falling on the side and running movements of the extremities. Evacuation of the bladder and bowel is common during seizures. After the convulsion, the animal may quickly regain its normal state or act dazed and uncoordinated for a few minutes. Convulsions in dogs have also been associated with deficiencies of vitamins A and B, hypocalcemia, intestinal parasitisms, intestinal obstructions and hyperthermia. Convulsions may precede the paralysis of tick paralysis.

Since the cause is unknown, treatment must be aimed at alleviating the clinical signs. The most effective drug in controlling canine epileptic seizures is primidone (℞ 553). Other drugs commonly used are phenobarbital (℞ 552) and diphenylhydantoin (℞ 549). These may be given singly or in combination.

DISORDERS OF THE NERVOUS SYSTEM OF DOGS

A permanent **trembling condition** in the hindquarters and tail occurs in Airedale terriers and is seldom seen until the dogs are at least 6 months old.

Paralysis of the hind limbs of the F_1 of St. Bernard x Great Dane and Great Dane x bloodhound crosses developed when the dogs were 3 months old. Death of motor and preganglion sympathetic neurons in the spinal cord was thought to be inherited.

Heritable cerebellar hypoplasia and degeneration, reported in 12-week-old Airedales, was manifested by signs of ataxia and hypermetria. There was absence and degeneration of Purkinje cells as well as chromatolysis of the neurons of the central cerebellar nuclei.

Hereditary ataxia, a simple autosomal recessive trait, appears in 2- to 4-month old fox terriers. Progression is rapid then slows, but the lengthy general ataxia progresses until the dog is unable to walk. Histologic lesions are bilateral demyelination of the dorsolateral and ventromedial columns of the spinal cord. Ataxia in Jack Russell terriers is similar clinically to that in fox terriers.

A **neutrotropic osteopathy** in 3- to 9-month old pointers, considered to be hereditary, was characterized by toe gnawing, self mutilation, and low sensitivity in distal parts of the limbs. Spinal cord sections revealed demyelination and vacuolar degeneration of the white matter.

Globoid cell leukodystrophy, (Krabbe's disease) reported in Cairn terrier, West Highland white terrier, and miniature poodle, is inherited as a simple autosomal recessive causing deficiency of the galactocerebroside β-galactosidase. Clinically, 2 major syndromes are seen: at 3 to 6 months little pelvic stiffness is seen in some dogs, while in others, a cerebellar disturbance is the main clinical sign. Death occurs 2 to 3 months after the onset of signs of the disease. Total protein content of 80 mg% in the CSF compares with normal

27.5 mg%. Large globoid cells are distributed throughout the white matter of the spinal cord and brain.

Spinal dysraphism in weimaraner dogs is an inherited disorder, although the mode of inheritance is not clear. Major clinical signs are hopping gait, crouching stance, abduction of one limb, and abnormal proprioreception in the hind limbs when the dogs are 4 to 6 weeks old. The disease is not progressive. Spinal cords have duplication, absence, and malformation of the central canal, thinning and absence of central gray matter, and areas of ectopic gray matter in the ventral median sulcus. **Syringomyelia,** or cavitation of the spinal cord may develop in older dogs.

Convulsive seizures appear to be hereditary in certain breeds of dogs: spastic attacks in the Labrador retriever resembled epilepsy (in EEG readings). Tervueren shepherd "fits" probably have an inherited basis. Epilepsy (*see also* pp. 647 and 648) in beagles has a genetic basis. The differences in maximum rates between males (11.9%) and females (2.6%) suggests a genetic hypothesis involving 2 loci, one an autosomal recessive, the other a sex-linked suppressor gene. Epilepsy in German shepherd dogs appears also to be inherited as an autosomal recessive trait. Electroencephalograms may be used to detect at an early age neurological disorders that are likely to manifest as convulsions when the dog is older.

Familial **amaurotic idiocy,** possibly inherited as a simple autosomal recessive, has occurred in the German shorthaired pointer; clinical signs at 6 months of age were nervousness and decreased ability for training. Progressive ataxia and impaired vision developed later. Neurons with soluble and insoluble granules and an increase of CM_2 gangliosides in the cerebral cortex was seen histologically.

Juvenile amaurotic idiocy (AFI) in the English setter, most likely inherited as a recessive, was characterized by reduced vision and dullness, manifest when the dog was 12 to 15 months old. By 18 months, muscle spasms appeared and eventually seizures progressed to severe tonic clonic spasms. Gross pathologic findings were enlarged lymph nodes, and brain atrophy. Histologically, lipid granules were observed in neurons, heart, lungs, liver, and gastrointestinal tract.

Recurrent tetany referred to as Scotch Cramp and usually first seen around 12 months of age, is characterized initially by arching back followed by a stiff-legged gait due to overflexed hind limbs and abducted front limbs. Signs are seen when the dogs are excited or strenuously exercised and regress with rest. It is a simple autosomal recessive and may result from abnormal serotonin metabolism.

Neuronal abiotrophy in the Swedish Lapland, inherited as a simple autosomal recessive, is characterized by a sudden onset of weakness in either thoracic or pelvic limbs when dogs are 5 to 7 weeks old. It progresses to tetraplegia, atrophy of the limbs, and joint flexion. Central peripheral chromatolysis, cell body shrinkage, neurophagia, and axonal and myelin degeneration is seen histologically.

Hallucinatory behavior in the King Charles spaniel is characterized by persistent fly catching in the absence of the stimuli (flying insects).

Note: For spinal cord defects, *see* DISEASES OF THE SPINAL COLUMN AND CORD, below; for hereditary and congenital disorders of the eye and optic nerve, *see* VETERINARY OPHTHALMOLOGY, p. 216.

DISEASES OF THE SPINAL COLUMN AND CORD

It is important to conduct a detailed systematic evaluation of spinal cord dysfunction in the differential diagnoses of paresis, paralysis and paraplegia in animals. Following are some of the commoner pathologic conditions in the various species. (*See also* INHERITED DISEASES AND CONGENITAL MALFORMATIONS OF THE CNS, p. 644.)

DISEASES IN DOGS

Infections which may produce signs of spinal or related involvement include distemper, rabies, Aujeszky's disease, tetanus, botulism, toxoplasmosis, systemic mycoses, meningitis, osteomyelitis and diskospondylitis.

Distemper may occur as an acute or chronic neurologic disease in dogs of all ages. The clinical signs may originate from lesions within the spinal cord, brain stem and cerebellum, or within the CNS in general. It has recently been suggested that the encephalitic signs in old dogs may be the result of a "slow type" of distemper virus characteristic of similar viral manifestations in man.

Rabies and **pseudorabies** in the dog should always be considered as possibilities in appropriate encephalitic disorders. The dog, even though somewhat resistant to **tetanus** toxin, can be affected clinically in deep, penetrating, or massive wounds. **Botulism** is not frequent in dogs but in a recently documented outbreak in hounds, "type C toxin" was isolated from serum and feces. The general flaccid paralysis must be differentiated from tick paralysis and polyradiculoneuritis. The usual antitoxin (A and B) is of little value and treatment is supportive.

Toxoplasmosis in dogs and cats is of prime zoonotic importance. Toxoplasmosis in the nervous system is generally disseminated and is not treatable. (*See* TOXOPLASMOSIS, p. 466.) The clinical signs resemble those of other infections of the CNS. The systemic mycoses affecting the CNS are similarly untreatable.

Meningitis in the dog usually results from an extension or metastasis of another infection. Usual signs are muscular rigidity, fever, hyperexcitability and abnormal spinal fluids. Antibiotics that pass the blood-brain barrier, e.g. chloramphenicol, may be helpful.

Osteomyelitis of the spine generally occurs from wounds and may involve the introduction of foreign bodies. Characteristic bone erosion and proliferation occur with or without clinical signs of meningitis or paralysis. A fistulous tract may be present. Surgical debridement of affected bone, decompression of the cord and antibiotic therapy should be used where indicated.

Diskospondylitis in the dog may be caused by *B. canis* (q.v., p. 370) or a variety of other organisms.

Noninfectious and degenerative diseases showing spinal or spinal-like signs of more prevalent importance are diffuse degenerative myelopathy in the German shepherd dog (German shepherd syndrome), dural ossification, spondylosis, tick paralysis, polyradiculoneuritis (coonhound paralysis) and spinal fibrocartilaginous emboli.

The "**German shepherd syndrome**" is seen in middle to older age (mean 9 years) dogs with no apparent sex predominance. Diffuse demyelination is seen that is usually not associated with compressions such as spondylosis, disks, or dural osseous plaques. The clinical signs of posterior paresis and proprioceptive deficiencies finally result in functional paraplegia over a 1- to 8-month period. Treatment with steroids, phenylbutazone, salicylates and large doses of B-complex vitamins are palliative until neurologic changes have become permanent.

Dural ossification (osseous pachymeningitis) occurs primarily in large breeds after maturity. Bone plaques may cause pressure on the cord and nerve roots which results in pain and gradually increasing paresis. The clinical significance of dural ossification is in question, especially in the German shepherd breed. Spondylosis is characterized by development of ventral bony spurs as seen radiographically, frequently in clinically normal dogs. As ossification completes the "bridging" and progresses dorsolaterally to cause pressure on nerve roots; pain and paresis may result.

Tick paralysis, q.v., p. 747, is usually due to *Dermacentor* infestations. It is characterized by flaccid paralysis, or paresis. It must be differentiated from botulism or coonhound paralysis. Prompt recovery is seen when the ticks are removed.

Many other parasites have been the cause of bizarre signs, when located in CNS tissue. Some of these include *Babesia,* tapeworm and roundworm larvae, heartworms and *Cuterebra* larvae.

Polyradiculoneuritis (coonhound paralysis) is a disorder of ventral spinal roots and nerves which appears pathologically and clinically identical to Guillain-Barre syndrome in man. The disorder has been reported largely in coonhounds 7 to 14 days after a bite or scratch from a raccoon. Signs of weakness, hyporeflexia and flaccid paralysis frequently revert to normalcy after 3 to 6 weeks of supportive nursing care. The cause has been postulated as an autoimmune reaction.

Fibrocartilaginous infarction of the spinal cord may occur, the signs mimicking those of compression or other cord trauma. The ischemic cord infarcts occur when both veins and arteries plug with fibrocartilaginous emboli, suggesting the intervertebral disk as the source. The onset of signs frequently accompanies exercises and is rather acute. The affected dog may exhibit unilateral or bilateral paresis or paralysis in either fore or hind legs. The treatment is supportive (good nursing care, anti-inflammatory agents and antibiotics) and improvement is usually noted within one week, if it is to occur.

The **hereditary** and **congenital** disorders of the spinal column and cord are many (*see also* INHERITED DISEASES AND CONGENITAL MALFORMATIONS OF THE CNS, p. 644) and include metabolic storage diseases (e.g. Krabbe's disease and the various gangliosidoses), cervical spondylopathy (wobblers, instability), occipital dysplasia and cervical vertebral anomalies, spinal dysraphism, syringomyelia, atlantoaxial subluxations, and vertebral malformations such as spina bifida, hemivertebrae and block vertebrae.

The **metabolic CNS storage diseases** are examples of inborn or hereditary errors of metabolism resulting in neurologic signs as the puppy or kitten grows toward adulthood. These signs manifest themselves in bizarre motor deficits as well as mental disturbances, blindness and even convulsions. Examples are gangliosidosis in cats and German shorthaired pointers, and globoid cell leukodystrophy (Krabbe's disease) seen in Cairn and West Highland white terriers. These diseases are progressive, and there is no known treatment.

The **cervical spondylopathy or wobbler syndrome** is a recently recognized disorder seen primarily in larger breeds such as the Great Dane and the Doberman pinscher. The wobbler characteristically suffers spinal cord compression from cervical vertebral instability or from a malformed spinal canal where dimensions of the osseous canal vary greatly from vertebra to vertebra. Any breed can be affected when trauma causes an instability, whereas the true wobbler is hereditary in origin. Hypernutrition with protein and calcium in the growing Great Dane may be involved. The clinical signs are proprioceptive deficits, paresis, and paralysis of the limbs (front, back, or all 4). Often, neck pain is not present. The treatment is surgical or symptomatic.

Occipital dysplasia, which is characterized by an enlarged foramen magnum, is seen in the toy breeds such as the Chihuahua, and is occasionally associated with anomalies of the first 1 to 3 cervical vertebrae (e.g. spina bifida). Such disorders may be asymptomatic, but trauma may cause cerebellar herniation. Occipital dysplasia has been associated with hydrocephalus in the Chihuahua.

Atlantoaxial subluxations have a primary hereditary predilection in some of the toy breeds but can result from trauma. The signs are the result of compression of the spinal cord, and resemble those of disk protrusion. Surgical decompression and stabilization can be effective.

Many **vertebral malformations** such as spina bifida (incomplete closure of the spinal arch), hemivertebra (incomplete fusion of vertebral bodies), and block (incompletely segmented) vertebrae may be entirely subclinical in nature. However, with certain traumas, these abnormal vertebrae may be predestined to cause a cord compression. Surgical correction may be successful.

Neoplasia may be either vertebral or intraspinal. The various spinal bone tumors are manifested clinically by signs of compression of the cord. Meningiomas cause compression of the cord and produce profound pain, paresis, or paralysis. Medullary spinal cord tumors may cause segmental destruction of the cord. Myelography is frequently needed to pinpoint the location.

Compressions of the spinal cord may be due to **spinal fractures, spinal luxations** and **disk protrusions** in addition to many of the aforementioned disorders. Characteristic clinical signs of a spinal cord compression include pain, paresis and incoordination, and paralysis (flaccid or rigid). If the lesion is at the thoracolumbar junction, the knee-jerk reflex is generally exaggerated, while the toe pinch is normal or diminished. The placing reflex is generally absent. If there is no conscious pain response associated with the toe-pinch reflex, the prognosis of recovery is not favorable, regardless of treatment. If extensor rigidity in the front legs is constant and profound, much spinal-cord damage has occurred and the prognosis is unfavorable. Fractures, luxations and disk protrusions should be confirmed by careful radiographic examination. They frequently require surgical decompression. Pain due to mild spinal cord compression may be reduced by salicylates (℞ 612), phenylbutazone (℞ 621) and corticosteroids (℞ 141, 154).

Intervertebral Disk Abnormality

Herniation or calcification of the intervertebral disk with or without protrusion. Disk abnormalities are most commonly found in dogs, but they have also been reported in cats, rabbits and other species. Lesions usually occur in the terminal thoracic and lumbar segments, but frequently affect the cervical region. The most susceptible breeds are the so-called chondrodystrophoid group, e.g. dachshund and Pekingese. The multiple disk changes, often seen in dogs of this group, represent a definite systemic degenerative disease. Clinical neuropathy results from pressure on the spinal cord or nerve roots.

Clinical Findings and Diagnosis: Signs vary with the nature, extent and position of the injury. There may be pain, paresis, flaccid or rigid paraplegia, or evidence of acute progressive ascending paralysis resulting from hemorrhagic myelomalacia or hematomyelia. Pain may be localized over the affected disk or be generalized. An arched back, abdominal tenseness and reluctance to move up and down stairs are signs of thoracolumbar-disk protrusion. Extreme pain on moving the head or neck is characteristic of a cervical disk protrusion. Paresis or weakness may accompany the pain. Thoracolumbar protrusions are usually characterized by hypertonia and hyperreflexia. The paraplegia may be accompanied by urinary and fecal retention or incontinence. Disk protrusions that result in an acute progressive ascending paralysis usually cause respiratory paralysis followed by death within 3 to 7 days.

Positive diagnosis and localization of the lesions are achieved only by careful neurologic and radiologic examination. Contrast myelography may be necessary.

Treatment: The treatment depends largely on the extent of the lesion and the severity of clinical signs produced. Acute progressive ascending myelomalacia does not respond to treatment and is usually fatal. Certain paraplegics will recover with conservative treatment. This treatment consists largely of symptomatic care and good nursing. Complete cage rest, good nutrition and maintenance of urine and fecal elimination are essential. An analgesic (℞ 612) and anti-inflammatory drugs (℞ 621) are indicated if pain is severe. Physiotherapy in the form of hot water baths, whirlpool baths, or ultrasound are helpful.

Surgical treatment is indicated when the location of the herniation can be determined and the spinal cord compression is of relatively few days' duration. Sudden and severe compression may require decompression within a few hours to prevent irreversible damage to the spinal cord. Surgical procedures include disk fenestration, hemilaminectomy, dorsal laminectomy, or a combination of the first 2 of these. Disk fenestration involves lateral or ventral curettage of the affected disk. Hemilaminectomy exposes the cord by removal of one side of the bony arch of the spinal canal. The protruding mass can then be completely removed. Dorsal laminectomy generally allows for decompression but no extensive removal of the offending disk material.

DISEASES IN HORSES

Abnormality of the vertebral column as a result of trauma is the commonest cause of paralysis in the horse. It frequently involves the cervical vertebrae, and results from kicks, accidents during halter breaking, injury while tied to a stationary object, and falls while running. The degree of paralysis is dependent on the location and severity of the accompanying spinal cord lesion.

The terms **equine sensory ataxia,** the **wobbler syndrome, wobbles** or, more recently, **cervical vertebral stenotic myopathy** refer to a syndrome in which there is an abnormality in articulation or formation of the cervical vertebrae causing contusion of the cervical spinal cord. The specific cause is unknown; proposed possibilities include rapid growth rates causing an uneven development of skeletal and muscular structures, nutritional imbalances, congenital and heritable abnormalities. The condition is usually seen initially as a rear-limb ataxia in animals less than 2 years old. A higher incidence is reported in thoroughbred males. The time of onset varies and the course is usually progressive. The signs of pelvic limb ataxia are variable in both type and degree. They include: an asymmetry of stride, an occasional tendency to drag one or both rear legs and to step on or cross one leg over the other when being pushed to the side. When moving the animal in a tight circle, there is a tendency to swing the outside rear limb wide and high during the anterior phase of the stride. Severely affected animals will usually back awkwardly and often collapse. In many cases the forelimbs are also involved but the signs are usually less definite.

Protozoal myelitis, also referred to as **segmental myelitis,** is a focal or diffuse involvement of any area of the spinal cord. It is caused by a protozoan that resembles *Toxoplasma gondii.* It most commonly involves young mature horses, usually affecting only one animal in a group. Many times the animal is initially presented with an obscure lameness. As the condition progresses, one limb is usually more severely affected than the others and the ataxia becomes more severe. Both signs and the rate of progression can be quite variable. There is no effective therapy.

The neurologic form of equine herpesvirus 1 or rhinopneumonitis infection (q.v., p. 308), may occur as the only form of this disease on a farm or it may be associated with either or both the upper respiratory or abortion form of the disease.

Degenerative myeloencephalopathy of horses is often difficult to distinguish from the wobbler syndrome. The onset may occur up to 2 years of age but usually is seen in the first few months of life. The signs are many times equally as severe in the thoracic as they are in the pelvic limbs and usually are more pronounced than in wobbles. There are no gross abnormalities of the spinal cord but histologically there is diffuse degeneration of the neurons of the white matter. The cause is unknown and there is no known effective treatment.

Other proposed causes of spinal disorders in the horse include: equine encephalomyelitis, nutritional deficiencies, primary parasitism or aberrant migration of parasites in nervous tissues, neoplasms of the spinal cord, unidentified substances in certain hybrid pasture grasses, myelitis following rabies vaccination, neuritis of the cauda equina and congenital atlanto-occipital malformation.

DISEASES IN CATTLE

Practically all inflammations or infections involving the spinal cord affect the meninges. True spinal myelitis is rare, except in Aujeszky's disease (q.v., p. 284).

The most frequent pathologic condition is compression causing sudden or progressive paraplegia. Spinal injury and fractures usually are accompanied by sudden motor and sensory paralysis. Tumors and abscesses usually produce progressive motor paralysis. The commonest tumor to be involved is bovine lymphosarcoma (which affects the cord in about 20% of generalized cases) but osteosarcoma, osteochondrosarcoma, angioma and lipoma may occur. Abscesses of the spinal cord are metastatic, usually from umbilical or castration infection, metritis, mastitis or traumatic peritonitis.

Spondylitis is common in mature cattle, especially bulls. Spinal fractures occasionally occur in newborn calves from mineral deficient dams, however, the most frequent occurrence is in 3- to 4-month-old calves that have been on inadequate diets and with little or no exposure to sunshine. Such fractures occur when the calves are turned out to pasture in the spring.

Tubercular spinal spondylitis is now rare. Rabies may cause an ascending paralysis and anesthesia. Temporary paraplegia may occur in the cow in heat after much "riding" by other cows.

DISEASES IN SWINE

The commonest infectious causes of paresis, paralysis, or paraplegia are hog cholera, Teschen disease, brucellosis and pseudorabies. Bacterial toxemias, as seen in edema disease, are also of diagnostic importance. Toxemias due to plant and chemical origin may cause spinal cord damage. Abscesses of the extra dural space usually cause compression of the spinal cord but do not usually invade the dura. Nutritional causes include calcium, phosphorus, vitamin A and various vitamin B deficiencies. Fractures and disk problems have become more numerous in recent years due to the elongation of the bacon-type hog being raised in confinement, and probably to the inadequacy of diets formulated for older types of slower growing pigs.

DISEASES IN SHEEP AND GOATS

Spinal cord irritation and damage in the sheep and goat may be caused by exotoxins of *Clostridium botulinum*, *Cl. perfringens* and *Cl. tetani*. Maternal copper deficiencies of pregnant ewes and does may result in "enzootic ataxia" (q.v., p. 1399). Maternal vitamin A deficiency, congenital syndromes, aberrant migration of *Parelaphostrongylus tenuis*, a meningeal nematode of white tailed deer, and fetal viral infections such as bluetongue may be incriminated. Haloxon, an organophosphate anthelmintic, occasionally causes a delayed spastic paraparesis and ataxia of only the pelvic limbs. The signs usually occur acutely 3 to 4 weeks following worming and persist.

Epidural abscesses (usually metastatic), tumors, ingestion of toxic plants (e.g. *Veratrum californicum*) by pregnant ewes, senile atrophy and focal symmetrical spinal poliomalacia are recorded causes. Spinal cord lesions may follow subacute *Phalaris aquatica* (*tuberosa*) poisoning. Osteodystrophic diseases, vitamin D and mineral deficiencies may cause maldevelopment and fractures of the vertebral column.

FACIAL PARALYSIS

Facial paralysis in the cat and dog is not uncommon and is frequently related to trauma or inflammation of the inner ear and lesions in the medulla of the brain. A transient idiopathic neuritis, similar to Bell's palsy in man, has been observed in the dog. The horse may suffer from facial paralysis as a result of trauma to the superficial branches of the facial nerve as it crosses the mandible. Facial paralysis is occasionally associated with the cauda equina neuritis syndrome in the horse. Trauma to the petrosum of the temporal bone and guttural pouch infections may also damage the nerve. Listeriosis and other inflammatory lesions of the medulla are the common causes in ruminants.

Clinical Findings: Total unilateral facial paralysis is characterized by the absence of a palpebral reflex, immobility of the ear, and flaccidity of the muscles of facial expression with subsequent deviation of the nose toward the normal side. The palpebral fissure is opened widely and in response to the menace test the animal may retract the globe resulting in flicking of the third eyelid instead of blinking.

Depending upon the site and degree of injury to the nerve, total or partial facial paralysis may be demonstrated. For instance, in the horse, damage to the buccal branches may only result in slight deviation of the nose and flaccidity of the lips. Drooling liquids and impaction of food in the buccal area of the mouth on the affected side is common in the horse. The nostril will also fail to dilate actively on inspiration. The site of facial paralysis can frequently be localized to the inner ear by the concomitant vestibular disturbance manifested by a head tilt, nystagmus and incoordination in the acute stages.

Lesions of the brain stem in the vicinity of the facial nucleus may cause bilateral signs. In addition, the presence of limb weakness and other cranial nerve deficits are helpful in differentiating a central disease from peripheral lesions.

Treatment: Traumatic and idiopathic neuritis of the facial nerve often heals spontaneously within a few weeks. Corticosteroids (℞ 143) are useful in controlling acute edema and inflammation (most useful for relief of edema of nervous tissue within 24 hours of injury). Infections must be treated vigorously with the appropriate drug. Protective ophthalmic ointments or surgical closure are necessary to prevent keratitis when the eyelids are paralyzed. With impairment of the prehensile lips of horses, providing wet bulky mashes and deep water containers constitutes important supportive care.

PARALYSIS OF THE FORELIMB

The innervation of the foreleg is commonly damaged by direct trauma, ischemia from restraint or prolonged anesthesia of heavy horses and cattle in lateral recumbency, and occasionally by tumors involving the nerves or rootlets of the brachial plexus. Severe traction on the forelimb resulting in excessive abduction of the shoulder can avulse or severely stretch the entire plexus. The radial nerve is most vulnerable to injury at the level of the first rib and at the humerus where it lies in the musculospiral groove.

Characteristically, any animal with complete brachial plexus paralysis will stand with the elbow dropped and the carpus and metacarpal joint in partial flexion. The limb will be dragged, and weight-bearing causes collapse at the elbow and carpus. Of the 5 major nerves of the plexus (musculocutaneous, axillary, radial, ulnar and median), injury to the radial nerve proximal to the elbow produces the greatest motor disability because the elbow, carpus and digits cannot be extended to bear weight. A lesion of the nerve distal to the elbow will result in knuckling of the digits and carpus only. With severe radial nerve lesions, desensitization occurs over the dorsum of the forearm and digits primarily. Impaired flexion of the digits and carpus occurs with ulnar and median nerve paralysis. Axillary and musculocutaneous nerve damage affects shoulder movement and elbow flexion respectively. Involvement of the first thoracic root often produces signs of Horner's syndrome on the same side as the limb paralysis. Within a week or 2, severe neurogenic muscle atrophy will develop in the denervated muscle groups.

An accurate history and a careful neurologic examination of the foreleg are essential and usually adequate to establish the diagnosis.

Radiographic evidence of fractures may suggest the site of injury. The prognosis is guarded where sensory loss is complete and 2 to 4 months' convalescence may be necessary if nerve regeneration is to occur.

With acute contusion of the nerves, the object is to relieve edema and pressure. Where severance of a nerve(s) is suspected, surgical exploration and repair is indicated. If the foot is continually dragged and prone to laceration, it may be protected with a leather boot. Amputation of the limb in small animals may be necessary in irreversible cases.

OBTURATOR PARALYSIS

A paralysis of adductor muscles of the hind legs resulting from injury of the obturator nerve. This is most frequently associated with dystocia. Occasionally other pelvic nerves are also affected, and the signs are of posterior paralysis or posterior ataxia. The condition is commonest in the cow, but the mare, ewe and bitch may also be affected. Nerve injury occurs when the fetus lies in the pelvic canal for an extended period, or a large fetus is forced through the pelvic canal. There is nearly always some degree of posterior paralysis in cattle when a hip lock exists for more than an hour.

Paralysis or paresis of the muscles of the hind leg result in ataxia or inability to stand. When only the obturator nerve is affected, the animal may lie on its sternum with the hind legs in extreme abduction. Paralyzed animals are bright and alert in contrast to animals with other postparturient diseases such as milk fever, acute mastitis and metritis. The condition should be differentiated from fractures, muscle trauma, tumors and abscesses involving the pelvic nerves and posterior spinal cord.

Treatment consists of good nursing care while the patient is recumbent. Ample dry bedding and easy access to feed and water are essential. Many animals will recover in the recumbent position, but should be turned from one side to the other at least twice daily. Some prefer to raise the animal in a sling each day, but extreme care should be observed in using a hip sling since severe trauma frequently results. Unless recovery occurs in 7 to 10 days, the prognosis is unfavorable. Some animals apparently fail to realize that they have recovered and should be stimulated daily to try to rise. Animals that can stand but are ataxic recover in 1 to 4 days. They should be maintained in an area of good footing so that they do not slip and become discouraged when attempting to rise. Tying the hind feet together with a rope or strap will prevent spreading. If animals are on a slippery surface, tying burlap bags over the feet will provide better traction.

DISEASES OF THE CNS CAUSED BY HELMINTH PARASITES AND INSECT LARVAE

Several helminths, particularly their larval stages, occur in the CNS. Whether actual disease is caused by their presence depends upon several factors, especially location, activity and size. There is also the possibility that helminth larvae entering the CNS may transport and facilitate the multiplication of pathogenic microorganisms. In some instances, lodgement in the CNS may possibly have some biologic significance, such as facilitating, by incapacitation, the capture of the intermediate host, e.g. in coenurosis, but in other instances, migration into the CNS occurs when the parasite enters an unusual host, and it is in such hosts particularly that signs may be encountered. There may be motor weakness, ataxia, staggering, circling, head deviation, paralysis, blindness and drooping of the ear or eyelid. Any nematode whose larval stages have a protracte migratory phase may occasionally reach the CNS.

In contrast to these erratic invaders, there are several parasites for which the CNS is the usual location for some phase of development. This applies particularly to the nematodes, of which several species are neurotropic. A pathologic feature of these nematode infections is that, whereas they have become adapted to their natural hosts, in which they cause little or no damage, when they gain access to other hosts, even closely related ones, they may cause severe damage.

An example of a neurotropic cestode is the larva of *Taenia (Multiceps) multiceps*, which is considered below. This parasite usually occurs in the brain of the sheep. There are no neurotropic trematodes in domestic animals, but the immature forms of *Paragonimus westermanii* sometimes lodge in the brain, where it may be found in the cat, dog, or pig.

CESTODES

Coenurosis

The common names (gid, sturdy, staggers, etc.) describe prominent clinical signs. The disease is found in sheep, cattle, other herbivores and occasionally man. The adult *Taenia (Multiceps) multiceps* occurs in the small intestine of the dog, fox and jackal. Tapeworm segments are voided onto pasture, the eggs are ingested by herbivorous hosts and the oncospheres that are released in the small intestine migrate probably by the blood stream to the CNS where they become coenuri. The cycle is completed when scolices within the *Coenurus* are eaten by the definitive host. Coenurosis is commonest in sheep, less common in cattle.

In infected herbivores, initial invasion can cause acute suppurative meningoencephalitis. In the chronic phase, the mature cyst (which may attain 5 to 6 cm in diameter in 7 months) may cause increased intracranial pressure. Depending on neuroanatomic location, the cyst gives rise to various neurologic signs; these may be general, such as somnolence, inappetence and wasting, or focal, such as turning, circling or other locomotor disturbances.

CYSTICERCOSIS

The definitive host of *Taenia solium* is man; infection occurs from eating pork containing the larval stage (*Cysticercus cellulosae*). Cysticerci may also occur in man when eggs are swallowed and oncospheres reach the muscles. In man, pigs and dogs, cysticerci may occur in the ventricles of the brain often assuming a racemose form. They may cause epileptiform convulsions, various mental signs and disturbance of locomotion.

ECHINOCOCCOSIS

The definitive host of *Echinococcus granulosus* is the dog; infection occurs from eating viscera of sheep and other ruminants containing hydatid cysts; sometimes they occur in the brain producing signs resembling those of tumors. Cerebral infections occur in man, cattle and horses. The definitive host of *E. multilocularis* is the fox; multilocular hydatids have been reported in the human brain, but not in domestic animals. The usual intermediate hosts are rodents. There may be little surrounding reaction in the brain other than a fibrous gliosis, and lymphocytic and eosinophilic infiltration.

NEMATODES

Setaria (Artionema) digitata occurs in the peritoneal cavity of cattle and buffalo; microfilariae reach the blood, are ingested by mosquitoes and thereby transmitted to new hosts, sometimes to abnormal hosts, such as sheep and goats. In such hosts, the infective larvae migrate from the skin and may gain access to the nervous system. In their neural migrations, they cause traumatic focal malacic lesions, with neurologic signs of varied kinds, such as paralysis. A disease, characterized by lumbar paralysis and termed **cerebrospinal nematodiasis** has been ascribed to this nematode. It has been reported in Asian countries, especially Ceylon, India, Japan, Korea and Israel.

Other filarioid nematodes and their larval stages occur in the brain of domestic animals, but are rarely discovered; they include *Parafilaria multipapillosa*, *Dirofilaria immitis* and *Onchocerca* spp.

A few strongyloids, such as *Strongylus* spp. and *Stephanurus dentatus* have been observed to cause lesions in the nervous system of horses and pigs, respectively. *Trichinella spiralis* has been found in the brain, in fatal human cases. Ascarids, particularly those whose larval stages migrate in the tissues of intermediate hosts, e.g.

Baylisascaris columnaris and *Toxocara canis*, frequently gain access to the CNS. *Ancylostoma caninum* has been found in the cervical cord of the dog causing pain, posterior paresis and loss of balance.

Of particular importance, in this regard, are the metastrongyloids or lungworms. Several species in this group undergo a migration through the brain before reaching the lungs or even mature in the CNS, releasing their eggs and larvae via the lungs. The effects of this sojourn in the CNS are not ordinarily manifested in the usual host, but when infective larvae are ingested by other hosts, signs of nervous involvement may occur.

Skrjabingylus spp. are known to cause superficial hemorrhage and meningitis in skunks and weasels. *Aelurostrongylus abstrusus* and *Angiostrongylus vasorum* are lungworms that have been found in the nervous system of cats and dogs, respectively. *Angiostrongylus cantonensis* occurs in the brain of rats and dogs but not in other domestic animals. The metastrongyloid nematodes of ruminant animals are important in northern regions as a cause of neurologi disease. *Parelaphostrongylus tenuis* normally occurs in the white-tailed deer (*Odocoileus virginianus*) in North America without causing disease, but where deer and moose occur in the same location severe effects (**moose sickness**) may occur in the latter, as a result of damage by the worms to the dorsal horn region of the spinal cord. If sheep or goats become infected the worm continues to migrate through nervous tissue causing limping and incoordination followed by almost complete paralysis of the hindlimbs or of the neck, body and all 4 legs.

A similar situation exists in Northern Europe and Asia, where several other species of the genus *Parelaphostrongylus* are found in the CNS of deer and reindeer, in which they may cause neurologic signs, such as paresis and ataxia.

INSECT LARVAE

Larvae of some Diptera find their way into the CNS of animals and cause neurologic signs. Larvae of *Oestrus ovis*, the nasal fly of sheep, normally inhabit the nasal passages and paranasal sinuses. Sometimes the larvae penetrate the ethmoid bone and reach the forebrain, or an associated pyogenic infection of the sinuses spreads to the brain; this results in neurologic manifestations such as head-shaking, a high-stepping gait, incoordination and paralysis.

Larvae of the "warble fly" of cattle, *Hypoderma bovis*, in the course of their migration to the subcut. position, normally reside for several months in the spinal canal, where their presence causes inflammation, and necrosis of epidural fat. Despite such regular intraspinal migration, associated neurologic disorders have seldom been reported. However, transient neurologic signs, varying from a stiff, unsteady gait to severe ataxia and weakness of the limbs, may occur in calves given systemic insecticides, e.g. organophosphates, when large numbers of larvae are present in the spinal canal. Onset is rapid and recovery usually occurs in 48 to 72 hours after the calves receive the insecticide. Supposedly, the syndrome is made manifest by the pronounced irritation of epidural tissues that accompanies rapid killing of many larvae. Cerebral invasion by larvae of *H. bovis* also has been reported in cattle and sometimes occurs in horses. Perhaps the most practical approach to dealing with parasitic infection of the CNS is the use of appropriate and effective prophylactic measures.

Treatment: Attempts have been made to apply various forms of treatment to parasitic infection of the CNS. Surgical removal hardly seems practicable with animals. Successful chemotherapeutic treatment has been reported with diethylcarbamazine for cerebrospinal nematodiasis in India at a dose of 45 mg/lb (100 mg/kg). It should, however, be borne in mind that to kill worms may remove the traumatic effect, but may provoke further damage through toxic or suppurative effects.

MENINGITIS

Inflammation of the meninges is a common sequela to neonatal septicemia of calves, lambs and piglets. It is rare in foals. Fibrinopurulent meningitis may occur in feeder pigs due to *Haemophilus* infection with or without evidence of a generalized polyserositis (*see* GLASSER'S DISEASE, p. 353). Encephalitic listeriosis in sheep, goats and cattle often causes a basilar purulent meningitis. Meningitis of bacterial or mycotic origin occurs sporadically in dogs, cats and horses. Secondary invasion of the meninges is usually associated with pyogenic processes involving the head or adjacent to the vertebral column. In cats, meningeal lesions can occur with primary nasal cryptococcosis and feline infectious peritonitis. Vertebral abscessation and guttural pouch infections may extend to the meninges of horses. Spontaneous meningitis occurs in dogs from which an organism is rarely identified but which often responds to broad-spectrum antibiotics.

In the acute stage, meningitis is classically characterized by high fever, hyperesthesia, pain on movement of the body, and in extreme cases, opisthotonos. If depression, coma or paralysis develops, the infection has advanced to meningoencephalitis or myelitis or both. In the dog, chronic primary meningitis may be manifested by pain only, often in the neck or abdominal region. A cerebrospinal fluid examination is a reliable diagnostic aid for the disease. The neutrophils predominate in numbers varying from several hundred to occasionally a thousand or more per cu mm. The spinal fluid may be opaque from a high cellular and protein content. In chronic bacterial conditions, the percentage of mononuclear cells tends to increase. Mycotic or other granulomatous reactions usually cause a predominance of mononuclear cells in the spinal fluid.

Specific antibiotic therapy is used if a bacterial culture and sensitivity is obtained. However bacterial infections of the meninges may respond to broad-spectrum antibiotics (℞ 7, 8, 20) at dosages 2 to 3 times the usual level and for a prolonged time if necessary. The prognosis is good in dogs with primary meningitis. It is guarded to poor for neonatal and secondary infections. Granulomatous infections are usually untreatable.

Supportive care consists of analgesics, anticonvulsants, fluids, high quality diet and physiotherapy when necessary. Corticosteroids are contraindicated; they may not exacerbate the condition but often mask the response to antibiotic treatment.

HAEMOPHILUS SEPTICEMIA OF CATTLE

(Infectious thromboembolic meningoencephalitis, TEME)

An acute septicemic disease affecting primarily the CNS, characterized by fever, severe depression, weakness, ataxia, blindness, paralysis, coma and death within one hour to several days. It is commonest in feedlot cattle but may occur in pastured animals.

Etiology and Pathogenesis: The causal organism is *Haemophilus*-like (tentative classification, *H. somnus*). It produces a septicemia with diffuse vasculitis and often hemorrhage, thrombosis and infarction in a variety of organs. The severest lesions are usually evident in the brain, but there often is synovitis, serofibrinous polyserositis, retinitis, necrotic laryngitis and pneumonia. Abortion has been attributed to the organism. There is cultural and serologic evidence that the infection rate in healthy cattle is relatively high but the incidence of disease in affected groups of cattle generally is 2 to 5%, although it may be as high as 30%. The fatality rate among diseased animals approaches 100%.

Clinical Findings: Temperatures in the early stages may be as high as 108°F (42°C) but fall to normal or subnormal very rapidly. Other characteristic signs are stiffness, knuckling at the fetlocks, severe depression, ataxia, paralysis and opisthotonos, followed by coma and death within 1 to 48 hours. Most affected animals are blind, and retinal hemorrhages with grayish foci of retinal necrosis may be observed. Other signs such as hypersensitivity, convulsions, excitement, nystagmus and circling occur inconsistently. Occasionally animals are found dead without showing any signs of illness. A marked change in the total and differential leukocyte count is common; a leukopenia and neutropenia occur in severe cases and a neutrophilia in less severe cases. In the CSF, the total cell count is markedly elevated and neutrophils predominate. The organism can be cultured from blood, synovial fluid, CSF and brain.

Lesions: The fundamental lesion of the disease is vasculitis and resulting hemorrhage, thrombosis and infarction. Characteristic gross lesions are evident in the brain (most easily observed on the cut surface) where there are usually multiple focal areas of hemorrhagic necrosis 0.5 to 1.5 cm in diameter. Hemorrhages and less frequently infarcts are evident in the renal cortex, trachea, lung, liver, skeletal muscle, myocardium and serous surfaces. There frequently is mild fibrinous peritonitis, pleuritis, and pericarditis and serofibrinous polysynovitis and necrotic laryngitis.

Diagnosis: Presumptive diagnosis can be made on the basis of clinical signs, examination of cerebrospinal fluid and gross necropsy findings. Confirmation may be obtained by histopathology and culture. The disease must be differentiated from polioencephalomalacia, hypovitaminosis A, lead poisoning and listerial meningoencephalitis.

Treatment and Prophylaxis: Clinically affected animals should be segregated and treated immediately with penicillin and streptomycin IM (℞ 66) or oxytetracycline (℞ 52). Treatment is most effective in the early stages of the disease; after the animal becomes recumbent the prognosis is poor. Animals should be checked at least every 2 hours in feedlots where the disease has been confirmed. Mass medication of the feed or water with a sulfonamide (℞ 99) for 10 to 14 days may be indicated if new cases begin to develop at a rapid rate. However, constant surveillance and immediate treatment of new cases may be more economical. Most outbreaks will run their course in 2 to 3 weeks. A bacterin is available but insufficient information is available on its efficacy.

POLIOENCEPHALOMALACIA

(Cerebrocortical necrosis)

A noninfectious neurologic disease of cattle, sheep, goats, antelope and deer, characterized clinically by amaurosis, anorexia, incoordination and depression of ruminal activity. Animals that do not recover from these early signs either spontaneously or after treatment, progress to a state of recumbency and opisthotonos, and tonic-clonic convulsions. Polioencephalomalacia is the term used in the U.S.A., Canada, Australia and New Zealand while cerebrocortical necrosis is the term used to describe what is apparently the same disease in the U.K., France and Germany.

Etiology: Affected animals are in a state of thiamin depletion. Ruminants normally derive adequate thiamin from symbiotic ruminal activity; the inadequacy is thought to be a result of intraruminal thiamin destruction either by the enzymes of microbes or other dietary sources. Rations rich in readily fermentable carbohydrates appear to result in these intraruminal changes in flora. Cattle fed substantial quantities of molasses without access to forage frequently are affected. Pasture forms occur in North America but particularly in Australia, New Zealand and the U.K. where outbreaks coincide with lush-pasture growth having a high-protein content. Low soil and forage levels of cobalt may potentiate the disease. Structural analogues of thiamin may interfere with thiamin metabolism. Thiamin is a coenzyme in carbohydrate metabolism, and its lack can be expected to cause increases in the blood concentrations of pyruvic, lactic and α-ketoglutaric acids, and a decrease in the activity of the tissue enzyme transketolase, α-ketoglutarate dehydrogenase and pyruvate dehydrogenase. The dependence of neurons and glial cells of the brain on carbohydrate catabolism using these enzymatic pathways accounts for the prominent neurologic signs.

Clinical Findings: The disease occurs more frequently in young cattle on high-energy diets, although it also affects sheep or cattle on pasture. Sudden depression, medial dorsal strabismus, moderate opisthotonos, disturbances of gait and blindness of cortical origin are the usual presenting signs, but a short period of prodromal anorexia may be observed. The rumen usually is contracting, but the action is weak and infrequent. Hyperesthesia, head-pressing, muscular tremors and twitching of ears, eyelids and muzzle may also occur. Elevated cerebrospinal fluid pressures and papilledema (the result of tissue swelling in response to brain necrosis) may be noted 24 to 48 hours after the onset of signs. Unless convulsions follow, temperature, pulse and respiration rates remain within normal limits. Bradycardia and arrhythmias occur occasionally. In untreated recumbent cattle the mortality is close to 100%. The morbidity in feedlot cattle is usually less than 5% but in 3- to 5-month-old calves it may be as high as 50%.

Diagnosis: Clinical diagnosis is based on signs and the exclusion of other etiologic causes by cerebrospinal fluid smears and blood and fecal lead estimations. Blood pyruvate, while often spuriously high due to convulsive activity, may be of assistance in diagnosis. Blood transketolase activity is uniformly depressed. Specific assays for thiaminase in large quantities in feces is considered confirmatory.

Pathologic diagnosis is based on the recognition of cortical and bilateral posterior collicular nuclear necrosis. The use of ultraviolet light at 365 nm in dark conditions will cause autofluorescence of necrotic foci except in mild or very early cases. Characteristic areas of laminar cortical necrosis, symmetrical deeper brain lesions and low thiamin levels in the brain, liver and heart are confirmatory findings.

Included in the differential diagnosis should be lead poisoning, nitrofuran toxicity, hypomagnesemia, vitamin A deficiency, chlorinated hydrocarbon toxicity, infectious thromboembolic meningoencephalitis, brain abscesses and Type-D clostridial enterotoxemia of sheep.

Treatment and Control: Thiamin, alone or in a B-complex preparation, administered IV and IM at a dosage of 1 to 2 mg/lb (2 to 4 mg/kg) by each route ensures rapid activation of enzyme complexes. Continued antagonism and destruction of alimentary derived thiamin may necessitate treatment twice daily for 2 days. Feedlot lambs if treated early respond to the same regimen.

Rapidity of recovery relates directly to the speed of disease recognition and institution of thiamin therapy. Recovery of vision and restoration as an economic unit is often achieved. Since others in the herd are probably also at risk, dietary cereal content should be decreased and additional good quality roughage supplied for a period of 5 days prior to a gradual return to higher energy rations. Supplementary dietary thiamin has questionable prophylactic or therapeutic value. Since carbohydrate metabolism is impaired in the disease, the use of IV dextrose is contraindicated except in the convalescent stages. Animals severely affected for more than 24 hours cannot be expected to respond well to treatment.

HYDROCEPHALUS

The presence of excessive amounts of cerebrospinal fluid (CSF) within the cranial cavity. It may be external, with the fluid accumulating in the subarachnoid space around the brain, or internal with the fluid being contained within the ventricular system. In communicating hydrocephalus the excess fluid is present in both locations.

Etiology and Pathogenesis: Hydrocephalus usually results from: (1) overproduction of fluid by the choroid plexuses, (2) obstruction of fluid flow at some point in the CSF pathway, or (3) inadequate resorption of fluid into the venous system via the arachnoid villi.

In vitamin A deficiency, an increase in CSF fluid pressure and subsequent hydrocephalus may be associated with a decreased absorption of CSF in the arachnoid villi. Other nutritional deficiencies have been cited as possible causes of some forms of congenital hydrocephalus. Other congenital forms are related to mechanical obstruction of the tentorial foramen or cerebral aqueduct, although such obstructions are generally difficult to demonstrate morphologically. Hydrocephalus in small animals occurs most commonly in the small dogs such as the Chihuahua, Boston terrier, Pekingese, beagles and other brachycephalic breeds.

Hereditary forms of congenital hydrocephalus have been reported in Holstein-Friesian and Hereford calves and beagle dogs. These are probably due to a single autosomal recessive gene. Achondrodysplastic calves frequently also have congenital hydrocephalus and the conditions are usually inherited as a simple recessive character. The condition may be acquired, most often by obstruction of the CSF pathways as by a tumor, meningitis or other infectious process involving the cerebral aqueduct or the foramina of the fourth ventricle. In aged horses, cholesteatomas of the choroid plexuses frequently are associated with some degree of internal hydrocephalus.

Clinical Findings: Many cases of congenital hydrocephalus remain subclinical and well-advanced lesions have been observed as incidental findings at necropsies. The most prominent feature of congenital hydrocephalus is an enlarged head. Hydrocephalus may cause open fontanelles and suture lines. The animal may exhibit depression, abnormal reactions to stimuli, incoordination, paralysis, prostration and sometimes convulsions. Loss of vision and papilledema of the optic disk are frequently evident. Occasionally an affected dog will become irritable, resent being handled and whine without apparent cause. Changes in temperament have also been reported in the horse. Pneumoventriculograms have been successful diagnostic aids in dogs.

Vitamin A, multiple B-complex, improved nutrition and diuretics may be beneficial occasionally. Aspiration via cerebrospinal tap is beneficial in the event of overproduction or inadequate resorption. The administration of thiazide diuretics in concert with corticosteroids may be useful. Surgical treatment consisting of various shunting devices has been described. The prognosis, however, is generally unfavorable.

NEONATAL MALADJUSTMENT SYNDROME (NMS)

(Barkers, Wanderers, Dummies, Convulsive foals)

A noninfective condition characterized by gross behavioral disturbances. Affected foals show signs of clonus, generalized convulsions, loss of the sucking reflex and affinity for the mare, apparent blindness, opisthotonos and extensor rigidity of hind and fore limbs, loss of righting reflexes, incessant chewing, sneezing, asymmetrical pupillary apertures, muscular flacidity and coma, wandering or dummy-like behavior. They may be hypoxic and show respiratory distress or acidosis with normal pulmonary function. Signs of cardiac dysfunction as evidenced by a marked jugular pulse, rapid heart-rate and a hard peripheral pulse, may be present in some individuals. Fractured ribs and myocardial damage may be found at necropsy in some cases and histologic changes include pulmonary atelectasis, cerebral hemorrhage, necrosis and edema.

The pathogenesis of NMS is not fully understood. Pressure on the thorax during birth has been suggested as an exciting cause and a relationship to obstetrical procedures, especially cord clamping, has been postulated. Birth asphyxia and hypoglycemia are other possible causes, but more recently attention has focused on cerebral hemorrhage; it has been suggested that this may be related to high intracranial pressure during birth.

The prognosis is poor in most instances.

Treatment: Treatment consists of supportive measures and symptomatic therapy. Anticonvulsant therapy may include phenytoin administered IV or IM at a rate of 2.2 to 4.5 mg/lb (5 to 10 mg/kg) body wt followed by maintenance doses of 0.5 to 2.2 mg/lb (1 to 5 mg/kg) body wt every 2 to 4 hours reducing to 12 hourly intervals according to response. Incoordinated foals require constant supervision to prevent exhaustion from unavailing attempts to stand. Comatose foals should be placed on a rug to avoid pressure necrosis of the skin. In the absence of a suck reflex feeds should be administered by a stomach tube. Mare's milk or reconstituted dried milk should be fed at the rate of 35 ml/lb (80 ml/kg) body wt per day divided into a minimum of 10 equal feeds. Dried milk preparations should be reconstituted to provide 45 cal in 8 to 12 ml water per kg body wt daily. Hypothermia should be countered by raising ambient temperatures and the acidosis dealt with by giving 2.2 to 4.5 ml/lb (5 to 10 ml/kg) of a 5% solution of sodium bicarbonate, IV.

PARASITIC DISEASES

GASTROINTESTINAL PARASITISM (LG. AN.)

The digestive tract is inhabited by many species of parasites. The development of clinical parasitism depends on the number and activity of these parasites, which in turn depend on climatic conditions and management practices, and the resistance, age, plane of nutrition and level of concurrent disease in the host. The economic importance of subclinical parasitism, now well established in ruminants, is determined by the same factors. Animals that show no clinical signs of disease often perform less efficiently, even under feedlot and dairy conditions. Advances in therapy and our understanding of epidemiology make possible control, and even prevention, of most losses from parasites. This goal is accomplished by coordinating management practices, diagnostics and strategic use of anthelmintics as an integral part of comprehensive herd-health programming.

Since the advent of effective broad-spectrum anthelmintics, most worm infections of ruminants are diagnosed and handled as general parasitoses and not as specific infections. Diagnosis, treatment and control of the gastrointestinal helminthiases of ruminants are therefore dealt with collectively following the separate discussions of parasite species rather than under each species (see the table of contents, p. 671).

CATTLE

Haemonchus, Ostertagia AND *Trichostrongylus* INFECTION

The common stomach worms of cattle are *Haemonchus placei* (Barber's pole worm, large stomach worm, wire worm), *Ostertagia ostertagi* (medium or brown stomach worm) and *Trichostrongylus axei* (small stomach worm). In some tropical countries *Mecistocirrus digitatus*, a large worm up to 40-mm long, is present and causes severe anemia. *H. placei* is primarily a parasite of tropical regions whereas *O. ostertagi* and to a lesser extent *T. axei* prefer temperate climates. Adult males of *Haemonchus* are as long as 18 mm and the females are up to 30 mm. *Ostertagia* adults are 6 to 9 mm in length and those of *Trichostrongylus* are smaller about 5 mm.

The preparasitic life cycles of the 3 groups are generally similar. With favorable temperatures larvae hatch from the eggs shortly after they are passed in the feces and are infective from 4 days. In areas with narrow diurnal temperature variations, those months with a mean maximum temperature of 64°F (18°C) and with rainfall over 5 cm are favorable for development of the free-living stages of *H. contortus* but where wide fluctuations occur the mean minimum temperature of 50°F (10°C) is a more accurate criterion. The preparasitic forms of *O. ostertagi* and *T. axei* develop and survive better in cooler conditions but their upper limits for survival are lower. If the temperature is unfavorable or drought conditions exist, embryonated eggs or infective larvae may remain dormant in the feces for weeks until the subsequent emergence of large numbers of infective larvae onto the pasture when conditions become favorable again.

The prepatent period is normally 18 to 25 days. In *O. ostertagi* infections the ingested larvae penetrate the abomasal glands and molt by the 4th day; they remain in the glands for the remainder of the prepatent period growing, and undergo a final molt before emerging to the lumen of the abomasum as young adults.

The presence of larvae in the glands causes hyperplasia of the mucus secreting cells and nodules, which may be discrete or confluent. Severe epithelial cytolysis occurs when the larvae emerge and results in loss of parietal cells with a consequent rise in pH to 6 to 7 and failure to convert pepsinogen to pepsin. A protein-losing gastroenteropathy results and together with anorexia and impaired protein digestion leads to hypoproteinemia and weight loss. Diarrhea is constant. Disease resulting from recent infections is defined as **Type I ostertagiosis** and in this infection the majority of worms present are adults and the condition responds well to anthelmintic treatment. This contrasts with the condition occurring when large numbers of larvae, which have become dormant in the early 4th larval stage, emerge from the glands. This condition, known as **Type II ostertagiosis,** does not respond well to treatment because the majority of worms are in the early larval form and these are resistant to most modern anthelmintics although fenbendazole, oxfendazole and albendazole will remove sufficient numbers to cause a clinical response. The condition of larval inhibition (hypobiosis) is thought to be analogous to diapause in insects and serves to allow *O. ostertagi* to avoid the harmful effects of winter in the northern hemisphere and the hot summer conditions in the south. The factors that cause inhibition are not completely known but cold conditioning of the free-living stages plays a part, while parturition, removal of concurrent infection and the lapse of time may stimulate their emergence.

H. placei also may become dormant over the winter period to resume development in the spring and infect the pastures with eggs at a time suitable for their development. Both the larval and adult stages are pathogenic due to their blood-sucking ability. *T. axei* causes gastritis, with superficial erosion of the mucosa, hyperemia and diarrhea. Protein loss from the damaged mucosa and anorexia causes hypoproteinemia and weight loss. Hypobiosis does not occur to any significant degree with *T. axei*.

Clinical Findings: Young animals are more often affected, but mature animals frequently show signs and succumb to infection. *Ostertagia* and *Trichostrongylus* infections are characterized by profuse watery diarrhea that usually is persistent. In haemonchosis, there may be little or no diarrhea, but possibly intermittent periods of constipation. Anemia of variable degree is a characteristic sign of haemonchosis.

Concurrent with the diarrhea of *O. ostertagi* and *T. axei* infection and the anemia of heavy *Haemonchus* infection, there is often hypoproteinemia and anasarca particularly under the lower jaw (bottle jaw) and sometimes along the ventral abdomen. Very heavy infections can produce death before clinical signs appear. Other variable signs include progressive loss of weight, weakness, rough hair coat and anorexia.

Lesions: In heavy *Haemonchus* infections, there is severe anemia and generalized anasarca. Worms can readily be seen and identified in the abomasum and small petechiae may be seen where the worms have been feeding.

The most characteristic lesion of *Ostertagia* infection is the presence of small, umbilicated nodules 1 to 2 mm in diameter throughout the abomasum. These may be discrete but in heavy infections they tend to collect and give rise to a "cobblestone" or "morocco leather" appearance. Nodules are most marked in the fundic region but may cover the whole abomasal mucosa. The pH rises to 6 to 7 and surplus pepsinogen is reabsorbed and high levels can be found in the plasma. Edema is often marked and in severe cases may extend over the abomasum and into the small intestine and omentum.

In *T. axei* infections the mucosa of the abomasum shows slight-to-medium congestion but superficial erosions, sometimes covered with a fibrinonecrotic exudate, may be seen.

Diagnosis, Treatment and Control: *See* p. 683 et seq.

Cooperia INFECTION

Several species of *Cooperia* occur in the small intestine of cattle; *C. punctata*, *C. oncophora* and *C. pectinata* are the commonest species. The adults vary from 5 to 8 mm in length, are red, coiled and the male has a large bursa. They may be difficult to observe grossly. Their life cycle is essentially the same as other trichostrongylids. These worms apparently do not suck blood. Most of them are found in the first 10 to 20 ft of the small intestine. The prepatent period is 12 to 15 days.

Clinical Findings: The eggs of the *Cooperia* spp. can usually be differentiated from those of the common gastrointestinal nematodes by the fact that the sides are practically parallel, but a larval culture of the feces is necessary to diagnose *Cooperia* infection with certainty in the living animal. In heavy infections with *C. punctata* and *C. pectinata* there is profuse diarrhea, anorexia and emaciation, but no anemia; the upper portion of the small intestine shows marked congestion of the mucosa, with small hemorrhages. The mucosa may show a fine lacelike necrosis superficially. It is usually necessary to make scrapings of the mucosa to demonstrate the worms, which must be differentiated from *Trichostrongylus*, *Strongyloides papillosus* and immature *Nematodirus*.

Diagnosis, Treatment and Control: *See* p. 683 et seq.

Bunostomum INFECTION

The adult male of *Bunostomum phlebotomum* is about 9 mm and the female up to 18 mm in length. Hookworms have well-developed buccal capsules into which the mucosa is drawn, and have cutting plates at the anterior edge of the buccal capsule that are used to abrade the mucosa during feeding. The prepatent period is approximately 2 months. Infection may be by infestion or skin penetration.

Clinical Findings: Penetration of the lower limbs by larvae may result, particularly in stabled cattle, in uneasiness and stamping. The adult worms cause anemia and rapid weight loss. Diarrhea and constipation may alternate. Hypoproteinemic edema may be present but "bottle jaw" is rarely as severe as that seen in haemonchosis. During the patent period, a diagnosis may be made by demonstrating the characteristic eggs in the feces.

On necropsy, the mucosa may appear congested and swollen, with numerous small hemorrhagic points where the worms were attached. The worms are readily seen in the first few feet of the small intestine and the contents are often deeply blood stained. As few as 2,000 worms may cause death in calves. Local lesions, edema and scab formation may result from penetration of larvae into the skin of resistant calves.

Diagnosis, Treatment and Control: *See* p. 683 et seq.

Strongyloides Infection

The intestinal threadworm, ***Strongyloides papillosus***, has an unusual life cycle. Only female worms occur in the parasitic phase of the cycle. These are 3.5 to 6 mm long and are embedded in the mucosa of the upper portion of the small intestine. Small embryonated eggs are passed in the feces, hatch rapidly and may develop directly into infective larvae or into free-living adults. The offspring of these free-living adults may develop into another generation of free-living adults or into infective larvae. The host is infected by penetration of the skin or by ingestion; transmission of infective larvae in colostrum may occur as in other species. The prepatent period is approximately 10 days.

Clinical Findings: Signs are rare, but may include intermittent diarrhea, loss of appetite and weight, and sometimes the presence of blood and mucus in the feces. Large numbers of worms in the intestine produce a catarrhal enteritis with petechial and ecchymotic hemorrhages, especially in the duodenum and jejunum.

Diagnosis, Treatment and Control: *See* p. 683 et seq.

Nematodirus Infection

The adult males of *N. **helvetianus*** are about 12 mm and the females 18 to 25 mm in length. The eggs develop slowly; the infective third stage is reached within the egg in 2 to 4 weeks and may remain within the egg for several months. Eggs may accumulate in pastures and hatch in large numbers after rain to produce heavy infections over a short period. The eggs are highly resistant and those passed by calves of one season may remain alive and infect the calves of the next season. After ingestion of infective larvae the adult stage is reached in approximately 3 weeks. The worms are most numerous 10 to 20 ft (3 to 6 m) from the pylorus.

Clinical Findings: Clinical signs include diarrhea and anorexia. The signs usually develop during the third week of infection before the worms are sexually mature and clinical infections may be seen in dairy calves from 6 weeks onward. During the prepatent period, diagnosis is difficult; during the patent period, diagnosis is easily made on the basis of the characteristic eggs. Relatively small numbers of eggs are produced by this parasite. Resistance to reinfection develops rapidly. Postmortem findings may only include a thickened, edematous mucosa.

Diagnosis, Treatment and Control: *See* p. 683 et seq.

Toxocara INFECTION

The ascarid *Toxocara vitulorum* is a stout, whitish worm (males 20 to 25 cm, females 25 to 30 cm) that occurs in the small intestine of calves under 6 months of age after which they are resistant. Larvae hatching from ingested eggs pass to the tissues and in pregnant cows are mobilized late in pregnancy and pass via the colostrum to the calves. Eggs appear in the feces of calves from 3 weeks of age and are easily recognized by the presence of a thick, pitted shell. In some parts of the world the infection is considered serious, particularly in buffalo calves.

Diagnosis, Treatment and Control: *See* p. 683 et seq.

Oesophagostomum INFECTION

The adults of *Oesophagostomum radiatum* (nodular worm) are 12- to 15-mm long and the head is bent dorsally. The eggs are very similar to those of *H. placei* and often are grouped with them on routine fecal examination. The life cycle is direct. The larvae penetrate the intestinal wall where they remain for 5 to 10 days and then return to the lumen as fourth-stage larvae. The prepatent period in susceptible animals is approximately 6 weeks but in subsequent infections larvae become arrested for some time and many may never return to the lumen.

Clinical Findings: Young animals suffer from the effects of adult worms whereas in older animals the effect of the nodules plays a more important part. Infection causes anorexia, severe and constant diarrhea, which is dark and fetid, loss of weight and death. In older, resistant animals the nodules surrounding the larvae become caseated and calcified thus decreasing the motility of the intestine. Stenosis or intussusception occasionally occurs. Nodules can be palpated *per rectum* and the worms and nodules can readily be seen at necropsy.

Diagnosis, Treatment and Control: *See* p. 683 et seq.

Chabertia Infection

Adults of the large-mouth bowel worm, *Chabertia ovina*, are about 12-mm long and bent ventrally at the anterior end. There is a typical direct life cycle, with the larvae penetrating the mucosa of the small intestine shortly after ingestion and later emerging and passing to the colon. The prepatent period is at least 7 weeks. *C. ovina* larvae and adults may cause small hemorrhages with edema in the colon and the passage of feces coated with mucus. Clinical chabertiasis is seldom if ever seen in cattle.

Diagnosis, Treatment and Control: *See* p. 683 et seq.

Tapeworm Infection

The anoplocephalid tapeworms *Moniezia expansa* and *M. benedeni* are found in young cattle. The tapeworms of this group are characterized by the absence of a rostellum and hooks, and the segments usually are wider than long. The eggs are triangular or rectangular and are ingested by free-living oribatid mites, which live in the soil and grass. After a period of 6 to 16 weeks, infective cysticercoids are present in the mites. Infection occurs by ingestion of the mites; the prepatent period is approximately 5 weeks.

Moniezia is commonly considered nonpathogenic in calves.

Diagnosis, Treatment and Control: *See* p. 683 et seq.

SHEEP AND GOATS

A number of species of nematodes and cestodes are capable of producing parasitic gastritis and enteritis in sheep and goats. The most important of these are *Haemonchus contortus, Ostertagia circumcincta, Trichostrongylus axei*, intestinal species of *Trichostrongylus, Nematodirus* spp., *Bunostomum trigonocephalum* and *Oesophagostomum columbianum. Cooperia curticei, Strongyloides papillosus, Trichuris ovis* and *Chabertia ovina* may also be pathogenic in sheep; these and related species are discussed under helminths of cattle (q.v., p. 676 et seq.).

Haemonchus, Ostertagia and *Trichostrongylus* Infection

The principal stomach worms of sheep and goats are *Haemonchus contortus, Ostertagia circumcincta, O. trifurcata* and *Trichostrongylus axei* and in some tropical regions also *Mecistocirrus digitatus*. Cross-transmission of *Haemonchus* between sheep and cattle can occur, but not as readily as in infections with the homologous species. Sheep are more susceptible to the cattle species than are cattle to the sheep species. For information on the size of these worms and on their life cycles, see the discussion under CATTLE, p. 674.

Haemonchus is commonest in tropical or sub-tropical areas or in those areas with summer rainfall, while *Ostertagia* and *T. axei* are commoner in winter rainfall areas. The latter species also predominate in temperate zones.

Clinical Findings: Ovine haemonchosis may be classified as hyperacute, acute or chronic. In the hyperacute disease, death may occur within a week of heavy infections and without the sheep showing significant signs. The acute disease is characterized by a severe anemia accompanied by generalized edema; anemia is also characteristic of the chronic infection, often of low burdens, accompanied by a progressive loss of weight. Diarrhea is not a sign of haemonchosis; the lesions are those associated with anemia. The abomasum is edematous, and in the chronic phase the pH becomes elevated leading to gastric dysfunction. It should be emphasized that mature sheep may develop heavy, even fatal, infections particularly during lactation.

The lesions, pathogenesis and signs of *Ostertagia* and *T. axei* are similar to those found with corresponding infections of cattle. Even subclinical levels of infection will cause a depressed appetite, impaired digestion and a reduction in the utilization of metabolizable energy. *Ostertagia* is the principal genus involved in the periparturient rise in sheep and causes diarrhea and depressed milk production in the ewe and this output of eggs serves as the main source of contamination for the lambs.

The same type of retarded development (hypobiosis) as recorded in cattle has been seen with both *Ostertagia* and *Haemonchus*.

Diagnosis, Treatment and Control: *See* p. 683 et seq.

INTESTINAL TRICHOSTRONGYLOSIS
(*T. colubriformis, T. vitrinus, T. rugatus*)

The life cycle of intestinal *Trichostrongylus* is direct, the developing larvae burrow superficially in the crypts of the mucosa and develop to egg-laying adults in 18 to 21 days.

Clinical Findings: Anorexia, persistent diarrhea and loss of weight are the main signs. Villous atrophy occurs and results in impaired digestion and malabsorption and protein loss occurs across the damaged mucosa. There are no diagnostic lesions on necropsy and a total worm count should be done to demonstrate the worms and evaluate the condition.

Diagnosis, Treatment and Control: *See* p. 683 et seq.

Bunostomum AND *Gaigeria* INFECTION

Adults of *Bunostomum trigonocephalum* (hookworm) are found in the jejunum. The life cycle is essentially the same as that of the cattle hookworm, as are the clinical findings. As few as 100 may cause clinical signs. *Gaigeria pachyscelis* is found in Africa and Asia and resembles *Bunostomum* in size and form (2 to 3 cm). Larvae of *G. pachyscelis* only enter via the skin. It is a powerful bloodsucker and probably the most pathogenic hookworm.

Diagnosis, Treatment and Control: *See* p. 683 et seq.

Nematodirus INFECTION

The species of *Nematodirus* occurring in the small intestine of sheep are similar in morphology and life cycle to *N. helvetianus*. Clinical *Nematodirus* infections are of considerable importance in Great Britain, New Zealand and Australia where death losses of 20% of the lambs in the affected flocks have been reported. The parasites are endemic in some parts of the Rocky Mountain area in the U.S.A. where they occasionally cause clinical disease in lambs.

In those areas where clinical infections are common, the disease often has a characteristic seasonal pattern. Many of the eggs passed by affected lambs lie dormant through the remainder of the grazing season and the winter, with large numbers of larvae appearing during the early grazing period of the following year. Thus the lambs of one season contaminate the pastures for the next season's lambs and the life cycle can be broken if the same area is not used for lambing each year. Most clinical infections occur in lambs 6 to 12 weeks old. *N. battus* occurs in Great Britain and parts of Europe and appears to be more pathogenic than other species and because of the management techniques used in those areas the disease occurs with great regularity each year. Because the eggs of *Nematodirus* spp. are very resistant and do not hatch except in moist conditions, they accumulate in periods of dry weather and hatch in large numbers after rain, with disease outbreaks occurring 2 to 4 weeks later. *Nematodirus* spp. often occur in low-rainfall regions (e.g. the Karroo in South Africa and inland Australia) where other parasites rarely cause disease.

Clinical Findings: The disease is characterized by sudden onset, "loss of bloom," unthriftiness, profuse diarrhea and marked dehydration, with death occurring as early as 2 to 3 days after the beginning of the outbreak. Nematodirosis is commonly confined to lambs or weaner sheep, but in low-rainfall country where outbreaks are sporadic, older sheep may experience heavy infections. The lesions usually consist of dehydration and a mild catarrhal enteritis, but acute inflammation of the entire small intestinal tract may occur. Counts of at least 10,683 worms, together with characteristic signs and history, are indicative of clinical infections. The affected lambs may pass large numbers of eggs, which can be indentified easily; however, since the onset may precede the maturation of the female worms, this is not a constant finding.

Diagnosis, Treatment and Control: *See* p. 683 et seq.

Oesophagostomum INFECTION

The sheep nodular worm *Oesophagostomum columbianum* is similar morphologically and in its life cycle to the nodular worm of cattle (q.v., p. 678).

Clinical Findings: Diarrhea usually develops during the second week of the infection. The feces may contain excess mucus as well as streaks of blood. As the diarrhea progresses, the animals become emaciated and weak. These signs often subside near the end of the prepatent period, but the continuing presence of numerous adult worms may result in a chronic type of infection in which signs may not develop for several months. The animals become weak, lose weight despite a good appetite and show intermittent periods of diarrhea and constipation.

As resistance develops, nodules form around the larvae and these may become caseated and calcified. Nodule formation is usually more pronounced in sheep than in cattle. Affected sheep walk with a stilted gait and often have a humped back. Stenosis and intussusception may occur in severe cases.

The diagnosis is difficult during the prepatent period, at which time it must be based largely on clinical signs, although the nodules can often be palpated by digital examination per rectum.

Diagnosis, Treatment and Control: *See* p. 683 et seq.

Chabertia INFECTION

The adult worms cause severe damage to the mucosa of the colon with resulting congestion, ulceration and small hemorrhages. Infected sheep are unthrifty; the feces are soft and contain much mucus, and may be streaked with blood. A strong immunity quickly develops and outbreaks are only seen under conditions of severe stress.

Diagnosis, Treatment and Control: *See* p. 683 et seq.

Strongyloides INFECTION

Heavy infections with adult worms cause a disease resembling trichostrongylosis. Infection is usually by skin penetration but can also occur via the milk. Damage to the skin between the claws, produced by skin-penetrating larvae, resembles the early stages of foot rot and may aid the penetration of the causal agents of foot rot. Most infections are transitory and inconsequential.

Diagnosis, Treatment and Control: *See* below.

Trichuris Infection

Heavy infections with whipworms are not common but may occur in very young lambs or in drought conditions where sheep are fed grain on the ground. The eggs are very resistant. Congestion and edema of the cecal mucosa accompanied by diarrhea and unthriftiness is seen.

Diagnosis, Treatment and Control: *See* below.

Tapeworm Infection

The pathogenicity of *Moniezia expansa* in sheep has long been debated. Many earlier observations, which associated this infection with diarrhea, emaciation and loss of weight, did not accurately differentiate between tapeworm infections and infection with certain of the small nematodes (e.g. *Trichostrongylus colubriformis*). It is now recognized that tapeworms are relatively nonpathogenic, but heavy infections may result in mild unthriftiness and digestive disturbances. Diagnosis may be made on the basis of presence of yellowish proglottids in the feces or protruding from the anal opening, or the demonstration of the characteristic eggs on fecal examination. The life cycle involves an oribatid mite which lives in the mat of pastures. The prepatent period in sheep is 6 to 7 weeks. Lambs develop resistance quickly and infections are lost from most sheep by about 4 to 5 months.

Thysanosoma actinioides, the "fringed tapeworm," inhabits the small intestine, as well as the bile and pancreatic ducts. They are commonly found in sheep from Western U.S.A. Their presence has not been associated with clinical disease. *Thysanosoma* is of economic importance because livers are condemned when tapeworms are found in the bile duct during meat inspection. The proglottids are pearl-white and bell-shaped.

Diagnosis, Treatment and Control: *See* below.

DIAGNOSIS OF GASTROINTESTINAL PARASITISM IN RUMINANTS

The clinical signs associated with gastrointestinal parasitisms are shared with many diseases and conditions; however, presumptive diagnosis based on history and signs is often justified and infection can usually be confirmed by demonstrating eggs on fecal examination. In evaluating the clinical importance of fecal examinations, the following points should be remembered: (1) The number of eggs per gram of feces usually is not an accurate indication of the number of adult worms present because of a) negative counts despite the presence of large numbers of immature worms, or b) suppression of egg production by immune reaction or previous anthelmintic treatment, and c) variations in the egg-producing capacity of different worms (significantly lower for *Trichostrongylus*, *Ostertagia* and *Nematodirus* than for *Haemonchus*). (2) Specific identification of eggs is impractical. The ova of *Nematodirus*, *Bunostomum*, *Strongyloides* and *Trichuris* are distinctive but reliable differentiation of the commoner species of ruminant nematode ova is difficult. Fecal cultures will produce distinctive third-stage larvae if antemortem differentiation is important. The advent of safe and effective broad-spectrum anthelmintics has reduced the need for species or generic differentiations of these parasites. In areas where *Ostertagia* spp. predominate, the examination of sera for evidence of elevated plasma pepsinogen levels is a useful aid to diagnosis. Likewise where *Haemonchus* spp. predominate, a packed cell volume estimate on heparinized blood provides a quick guide to the degree of anemia.

In many management situations experience has shown that significant infections can be taken for granted, particularly after favorable temperatures and rainfall conditions in certain seasons. "Diagnostic drenching" is recommended in cases where eggs are few or absent, yet history and signs suggest infections. A clinical response to a safe, broad-spectrum anthelmintic permits a retrospective diagnosis, but the animals should be placed on safe pastures after treatment to avoid reinfection.

Postmortem examinations are the most direct method to identify and quantitate gastrointestinal parasitisms. The demise of one or more animals can provide valuable parasitologic data about the status of the rest of the herd or flock. Routine postmortem examinations are invaluable to diagnosis and are recommended.

On postmortem examination, *Haemonchus*, *Bunostomum*, *Oesophagostomum*, *Trichuris* and *Chabertia* adults (or advanced immature worms) can be seen easily. *Ostertagia*, *Trichostrongylus*, *Cooperia* and *Nematodirus* are difficult to see except by their movement in fluid ingesta. Clinically important infections are easily overlooked with these genera, and the total contents and all washings should be combined and a total worm count done so that the severity of the infection can be evaluated. Samples of digestive contents and scrapings of the mucosa should be examined microscopically (low-power magnification). These smaller nematodes can be stained (5 minutes) with a strong iodine solution. After the background ingesta and tissue are decolorized with 5% sodium thiosulfate, the small nematodes are easily seen. The type and severity of gross lesions may also be of considerable diagnostic value.

Multifactorial causation should be considered in evaluating clinical, laboratory and necropsy findings. Mixed parasite infections are the rule. Shipping fever, nutrition-related digestive disorders, salmonellosis, Johne's disease, viral diarrhea and trace-element deficiencies, fascioliasis, etc., should be considered in making a differential diagnosis.

TREATMENT OF GASTROINTESTINAL PARASITISM IN RUMINANTS

Effective worm control cannot be obtained by drugs alone; however, anthelmintics play an important role. They should be used to reduce contamination and, for this, should be used at times critical for the survival of the free-living stages. Coordination with other methods of control, such as alternate grazing of different host species, integrated rotational grazing of different age groups within the one species (including creep grazing) and alternation of grazing and cropping are other management techniques which when combined with anthelmintic treatment can give economic control.

The "ideal anthelmintic" should be safe, highly effective against adults and immature stages (including hypobiotic larvae) of the important worms, rapidly and completely metabolized, be available in a variety of convenient formulations, economical to use (inexpensive, ineffective drugs are not economic) and be compatible with other commonly used compounds. Several drugs now satisfy all or most of these requirements. Thiabendazole (℞ 265) was the forerunner of the modern anthelmintics, and set a new standard in efficiency and safety. Despite minor weakness against hypobiotic larvae in cattle and 1 or 2 worm species, thiabendazole is still widely used. Following thiabendazole, other benzimidazoles such as cambendazole (℞ 229), fenbendazole (℞ 238, 239), mebendazole (℞ 245, 246), oxfendazole (℞ 247) and albendazole (℞ 222) have been developed, and the last 3 of these compounds are effective against all the major gastrointestinal parasites of ruminants including hypobiotic stages. Levamisole (℞ 244), the pyrantel group (℞ 257) and thiophanate (℞ 266) are also highly effective, safe wide-spectrum anthelmintics.

Apart from drenching or injection, other routes of administration are used in a bid to reduce labor costs. For example, the incorporation of drugs into feed, drinking water, mineral or energy blocks, is particularly useful in feedlot systems or where grazing animals are being given supplementary feeding. Another advantage of these "in-feed" routes is that continuous low-level administration of a drug can be obtained and a reduction in pasture contamination achieved during periods that are optimal for free-living development of the parasite. The disadvantages include erratic consumption of anthelmintic, unacceptable tissue residues and encouragement of drug resistance by continual exposure. Another labor saving route of administration is the "pour-on" dermal treatment developed for some of the organophosphates such as trichlorfon (℞ 337) and now used for levamisole (℞ 244), which is readily absorbed through the skin; this technique is particularly suited to treating range cattle.

Lead arsenate (℞ 243), niclosamide (℞ 248), cambendazole and albendazole, are effective against tapeworms in cattle and sheep; only niclosamide (at 250 mg/kg) has been reported to be effective against *Thysanosoma actinioides*.

Consideration should be given to the following points when treating clinically affected animals: a) providing adequate nutrition, b) movement of stock to safe pastures to minimize reinfection, c) treating all animals in the group as a preventive measure and to reduce further pasture contamination, d) treatment of stock at times when climatic conditions are particularly harmful to the free-living stages and infection pressure is low so that treatment effectively reduces pasture contamination for long periods.

Finally, the development of drug resistance by populations of *Haemonchus contortus* and *Ostertagia* spp. to thiabendazole and some of the other newer anthelmintics has been demonstrated, and while such resistance is currently only a problem at a local level, it should be considered when response to therapy is suboptimal.

GENERAL CONTROL MEASURES FOR GASTROINTESTINAL PARASITISM IN RUMINANTS

The word "control" generally implies the suppression of parasite burdens in the host below that level at which economic loss may occur. To do this effectively requires an intimate knowledge of the epidemiologic and ecologic factors governing pasture larval populations and the role of host resistance to infection.

The goals of control can be summarized as: (1) to prevent heavy exposure in susceptible hosts (recovery from heavy infection is always slow), (2) to reduce overall levels of pasture contamination, (3) to minimize the effects of parasite burdens, and (4) to encourage the development of immunity or resistance.

Strategic use of anthelmintics has a seasonal basis and is designed to reduce worm burdens and thereby the contamination of pastures at periods based on a knowledge of the seasonal changes in infection. Tactical use is based on prompt recognition of conditions likely to favor the development of parasitic disease, e.g. weather, grazing behavior and malnutrition. Strategic and tactical timing of treatment must be based on a knowledge of the regional epidemiology of the various helminthoses.

For example, in Great Britain, where the pattern of disease caused by *Nematodirus* infection in sheep is clearly defined, strategic treatments with 3 doses of anthelmintic at 3-week intervals beginning just before the disease characteristically appears are recommended. Similarly, in Western Europe, pasture levels of *Ostertagia* larvae increase after mid-July; young cattle are dosed before then and moved to a sheep-grazing or grass-conservation area.

In other countries similar controls may be used if the seasonal pattern of the disease is known, but in most regions a tactical use of anthelmintics may be required, e.g. during hot, dry periods.

SHEEP—SPECIAL CONSIDERATIONS

A special strategic treatment is required in most regions to counter the post-parturient relaxation of resistance (parturient rise, etc.) seen in ewes. The precise timing of such treatment will vary between regions and for different species of parasites, but in general, treatment within the month before and again within the month after parturition appears desirable. A treatment 2 weeks before breeding, as part of a "flushing" program, is another strategic application of anthelmintics. Supporting management after a treatment includes movement of sheep from contaminated pastures to cattle pastures, grass conservation areas, root crops or pasture not grazed by sheep for several months. The latter period will vary according to the seasonal pattern of larval mortality in different countries and may be as long as 1 year in some temperate countries.

Sheep are more consistently susceptible to the adverse effects of worms than other livestock. Clinical disease is commoner. Resistance is not strong and frequent treatments may be required, particularly during the first year of life.

CATTLE—SPECIAL CONSIDERATIONS

Worm problems occur most frequently in dairy herds and principally affect segregated groups of calves during the first season at grass. Immunity to the gastrointestinal nematodes is acquired slowly and usually requires 2 grazing seasons before a significant level is attained. In endemic areas cows may continue to harbor low burdens and these may be the cause of suboptimal production. Control of gastrointestinal parasitism in young stock may be achieved by the use of broad-spectrum anthelmintics used in conjunction with pasture management to limit reinfection; the latter includes alternate grazing with other host species, with grass conservation areas or integrated rotational grazing where the susceptible calves are followed by immune adults. Simple pasture rotation of calves is not effective since the bovine fecal mass may protect larvae for several months from adverse environmental factors and rotating calves could therefore be subject to reinfection at a later date.

In beef herds, anthelmintic treatment at weaning is of value particularly if the young weaners are going to feedlots. Further treatment is indicated before feedlot stock are moved to finishing lots. Cattle fattened on grass should receive treatment following weaning and at intervals during the next 12 months. Particular care is needed to avoid type II ostertagiosis and this requires treatment in July with movement to safe paddocks. Treatment with an anthelmintic, effective against hypobiotic larvae, a month before the expected time of outbreaks is also recommended.

SWINE

Hyostrongylus, *Ascarops* AND *Physocephalus* INFECTION

Three types of stomach worms occur in swine; a thin worm, *Hyostrongylus rubidus* (the red stomach worm), and 2 thick stomach worms, *Ascarops strongylina* and *Physocephalus sexalatus*. The thin stomach worm is about 6-mm long and very slender, while the thick stomach worms are 12 mm or more in length and much stouter. The thin stomach worm has a direct life cycle while the thick stomach worms are acquired when swine eat infected coprophagous beetles.

Clinical Findings: These worms are commoner in grazing pigs. When present in large numbers or when the host's condition is reduced by poor nutrition or other factors, they may cause a variable appetite, anemia, diarrhea, or loss of weight. *Hyostrongylus* characteristically is found under a heavy catarrhal or mucous exudate and may produce lesions of the mucosa similar to those of *Ostertagia* in ruminants except that hemorrhages are commoner. Retarded development of larval stages in the mucosa is analogous to that of *Ostertagia*. In sows the retarded worms resume development around parturition. The sow may suffer severe gastritis and in addition contaminate the environment of the young pigs.

Diagnosis and Treatment: Clinical signs other than unthriftiness are not obvious. Fatal hemorrhages have been reported in hyostrongylosis. Fecal examinations may show the distinctive ova of *Physocephalus* and *Ascarops*—small (35 to 40 μ by 20 μ), thick-shelled eggs containing an active larva. *Hyostrongylus* ova resemble those of other strongyle worms, *Oesophagostomum, Necator, Trichostrongylus* and *Globocephalus*, and fecal cultures are required to obtain infective larvae for differential diagnosis.

At necropsy, adult worms, especially *Physocephalus* and *Ascarops* are readily seen. Mucosal scrapings for microscopic examination are essential for detection of immature *Hyostrongylus*.

Thiabendazole (℞ 265), levamisole (℞ 244) and dichlorvos (℞ 234) are effective against *Hyostrongylus*. The newer benzimidazoles are highly effective and will also remove retarded stages. Carbon disulfide (℞ 230), or the complex with piperazine (℞ 250), which releases carbon disulfide in the stomach, are usually recommended against *Physocephalus* and *Ascarops*, but precise data are lacking.

Ascaris INFECTION

The adults of the large roundworm, *Ascaris suum*, are found principally in the small intestine, but they may migrate into the stomach or bile passages. They are 30 cm or more in length and quite thick. A female produces large numbers of eggs (as many as 250,000 per day) that develop to the infective stage in 2 to 3 weeks and are very resistant to chemical agents. When the eggs are ingested, the larvae hatch in the intestine, penetrate the intestinal wall and enter the portal circulation. After a period of growth in the liver, they are carried by the circulation to the lungs, where they pass through the capillaries into the alveolar spaces. About 9 or 10 days after ingestion, the larvae leave the lungs by passing up the bronchial tree and return to the digestive system where they mature in the small intestine. The first eggs are passed 2 to 2½ months after infection.

Clinical Findings: Adult worms may significantly reduce the growth rate of young animals; if they are sufficiently numerous, they may cause mechanical obstruction of the intestine (in which case rupture of the intestine may result), or they may migrate into the bile passages and occlude them, producing icterus. The latter is fairly common, especially in hogs having long periods without feed while in transit to slaughter.

Migration of larvae through the liver causes hemorrhage and fibrosis appearing as "white spots" under the capsule. In heavy infections the larvae can cause pulmonary edema and consolidation, and exacerbate infection of swine influenza and endemic pneumonia. Affected animals show abdominal breathing, commonly referred to as "thumps."

In addition to the respiratory signs, the animals show marked unthriftiness and loss of weight. Permanent stunting may result. The greatest harm comes to pigs up to 4 to 5 months.

Diagnosis: During the patent period, the diagnosis may be made by demonstrating the typical eggs in the feces. However, many young pigs show signs (especially respiratory involvement) during the prepatent period. A presumptive diagnosis can be made at this time on the basis of history and signs, and this can be confirmed by demonstrating immature worms on necropsy. In acute cases in which no worms are found in the intestine, it may be possible to recover larvae from the affected lung tissue.

Treatment: Supportive treatment and therapy for the secondary bacterial invaders may be necessary during the respiratory phase of the infection. Many drugs have been used to remove adult ascarids. Piperazine preparations (℞ 256) have low toxicity and are moderately priced, and for some years this has been the drug of choice. Sodium fluoride and cadmium compounds are inexpensive but are more hazardous to use. Dichlorvos (℞ 234), haloxon (℞ 240), cambendazole (℞ 229), fenbendazole (℞ 238, 239) and pyrantel (℞ 260) are all very effective, have broader spectrums than piperazine and may be administered in the feed. Levamisole (℞ 244) is also effective, has a broad spectrum and can be given in feed or water.

The antibiotic hygromycin (℞ 242) is active against the ascarids when administered as a low-level additive to the feed. Many drugs have been tested for efficacy in destruction of the migratory stages. Pyrantel (℞ 260) shows greatest promise in this regard. The beneficial effects of reduced lung and liver damage deserve close study.

Macracanthorhynchus INFECTION

The adults of *Macracanthorhynchus hirudinaceus* (thorny headed worm) usually are in the small intestine. They may be 30 cm in length and 3 to 9 mm in width, slightly pink and with the outer covering transversely wrinkled. The anterior end bears a spiny retractable proboscis or rostellum by means of which it is firmly attached to the intestinal wall. The eggs are ingested by the grubs of various beetles that serve as intermediate hosts.

The signs are not specific. There is an inflammatory reaction at the site of attachment. This may have a necrotic center surrounded by a zone of inflammation. These lesions can usually be seen through the serosa. The rostellum may perforate the intestinal wall with a resulting peritonitis and death.

Levamisole (℞ 244) is effective. Antemortem diagnosis is difficult, as the ova do not float reliably in salt solutions. Control depends on avoiding the use of contaminated permanent hog lots or pastures.

Strongyloides INFECTION

The life cycle of *Strongyloides ransomi* (intestinal threadworm) is apparently very similar to that of *S. papillosus* of cattle (q.v., p. 697), except that transmission of larval *Strongyloides* occurs through the colostrum, explaining the serious nature of the infection in baby pigs. The adult worms (only females in the parasitic cycle) burrow into the wall of the small intestine. In light and moderate infections the animals usually show no signs. In heavy infections, diarrhea, anemia and emaciation may be observed. Death may result.

Demonstration of the characteristic small, thin-shelled embryonated eggs in the feces or of the adults in scrapings from the intestinal mucosa is diagnostic. *Strongyloides* ova must be differentiated from the larger *Metastrongylus* (swine lungworm) ova, which are also embryonated in fresh feces. At necropsy, immature worms may be recovered from minced tissues placed in a Baermann isolation apparatus.

Thiabendazole (℞ 265) is effective against intestinal infections. Recent studies have shown that mebendazole administered in the feed for several days before and after parturition reduced colostral infections in piglets while it was being fed. Cambendazole is also highly effective against the adult worms.

Oesophagostomum Infection

Oesophagostomum dentatum is the most important of the nodular worms in hogs. The adults are found in the lumen of the large intestine; they are 8 to 12 mm in length, slender and white or gray. The life cycle is direct, with infection resulting from the ingestion of the larvae. These penetrate the mucosa of the large intestine within a few hours after ingestion and return to the lumen in 6 to 20 days. Infective larvae may be carried by flies. Sows have a periparturient rise in worm-egg output and this is an important source of infection for the piglets. The mucosa of the large intestine from the ileocecal valve to the rectum may be covered by a brownish material composed mostly of coagulated serum. The wall is 2 to 3 times its normal thickness. The serosa shows small nodules, a hypersensitive response as a result of previous infections. Heavily infected animals may show anorexia, emaciation and digestive disturbances.

See Hyostrongylus (p. 688) for comment on differential diagnosis when strongyle eggs are found in feces. At necropsy the worms and lesions are readily seen. Scrapings from the mucosa, with microscopic examination, may be required to detect immature worms. Thiabendazole (℞ 265), levamisole (℞ 244), piperazines (℞ 256, 254) dichlorvos (℞ 234), pyrantel tartrate (℞ 260) and the newer benzimidazoles (*see* cattle section, p. 685) are effective.

Trichuris Infection

Trichuris suis is 5- to 8-cm long and consists of a slender anterior portion and a thickened posterior third. Exposure is by ingestion of embryonated ova. Heavy exposure is associated with poor sanitation. Heavy infections with whipworms may cause inflammatory lesions in the cecum and adjacent large intestine accompanied by diarrhea and unthriftiness. The double-operculated eggs are diagnostic. Dichlorvos (℞ 234) and levamisole (℞ 244) are effective.

THE PERIPARTURIENT RELAXATION OF IMMUNITY IN SOWS

During the periparturient period (2 weeks prior to parturition and

6 weeks after) there is a relaxation in immunity of sows and, if infected, a marked increase in their nematode fecal egg count occurs due particularly to *Oesophagostomum* and *Hyostrongylus*. In the second half of pregnancy the number of adult worms present increases and egg output in the period between farrowing and weaning is high. At weaning there is an abrupt drop in fecal egg output and many worms, particularly *Oesophagostomum*, are eliminated. The phenomenon has considerable epidemiologic importance, since the environment of the young is contaminated.

WORM CONTROL

Apart from basic good hygiene in pig houses, control is now based on in-feed anthelmintics. A simple anthelmintic program is as follows: treat sows and gilts 5 to 7 days before farrowing and in mid-lactation; treat weaners prior to entering fattening pens and 8 weeks later; treat fatteners at approximately 50 kg; treat boars at 6-month intervals.

HORSES

Gasterophilus INFECTION

Horse bots are the larvae of bot flies. The adult flies are not parasitic and cannot feed; they die as soon as the nutrients brought over from the larval stage are used, usually in about 2 weeks. The 3 important species in the U.S.A. can be differentiated in any stage of their development. The eggs of *Gasterophilus intestinalis* (the common bot) are glued to the hairs of almost any part of the body, but especially the forelegs and shoulders. The larvae hatch in about 7 days when properly stimulated, usually by the animals' licking. The eggs of *G. haemorrhoidalis* (the nose or lip bot) are attached to the hairs of the lips. The larvae emerge in 2 or 3 days without stimulation and crawl into the mouth. *G. nasalis* (the throat bot) deposits eggs on the hairs of the submaxillary region. They hatch in about a week without stimulation.

The larvae of all 3 species apparently stay for about a month around the molar teeth or embedded in the mucosa of the mouth, after which they pass to the stomach where they attach themselves to the cardiac or pyloric portions and in the case of *G. nasalis* to the mucosa of the first part of the small intestine. After a developmental period of about 8 to 10 months, they pass out in the feces and pupate in the soil for 3 to 5 weeks. The adult emerges after about a month.

Clinical Findings and Diagnosis: Bot infection causes a mild gastritis but large numbers may be present without any clinical signs. The first instars migrating in the mouth can cause stomatitis and, if they enter into pockets alongside the molars, may produce pain on eating. The adult flies are responsible for much annoyance when laying their eggs during the summer months. Specific diagnosis of *Gasterophilus* infection is difficult and can only be made by demonstrating larvae as they pass in the feces at the end of the period of larval development. Infection is often assumed in the fall of the year. History of the individual animals, knowledge of the seasonal cycle of the fly in the particular locality and observation of bot eggs on the animal's hairs are all helpful.

Treatment: Most parasite control programs assume horses are infected in the fall. Dichlorvos (℞ 234) or trichlorfon (℞ 268) have largely replaced carbon disulfide. A single treatment is usually adequate. It should be given approximately a month after the first killing frost has destroyed the flies in the fall. There is no satisfactory method for protecting exposed animals from attack by the adult flies. When applied on a regional basis to all horses, bot control programs markedly reduce fly numbers and larval infections.

Habronema INFECTION

GASTRIC HABRONEMIASIS

The adults of the stomach worms *Habronema muscae, H. microstoma* and *Draschia megastoma* vary in size from 6 to 25 mm. *Draschia* occurs in tumor-like swellings in the stomach wall. The other species are free on the mucosa. The eggs or larvae are ingested by the larvae of house or stable flies, which serve as intermediate hosts. Horses are infected by ingesting the infected flies or the larvae which emerge from flies feeding on the lips.

Clinical Findings: An inflammatory reaction of the mucosa, contributing to gastric irritability, poor digestion and sometimes colic may result from heavy infections with adult worms. *Draschia* produces the most severe lesions, tumor-like enlargements as much as 10 cm in diameter. These may be filled with necrotic tracts and masses of worms. The tumors may rupture and lead to a fatal peritonitis. Larvae of *Habronema* and *Draschia* have been found in the lungs of foals associated with *Corynebacterium equi* abscesses and it is thought that migrating larvae of these species or the large strongyles may allow entry of the bacteria.

Diagnosis and Treatment: Diagnosis is usually established during postmortem examination. Antemortem diagnosis is difficult since the thin-shelled eggs or larvae are easily missed in fecal examinations. Worms and eggs may be found by gastric lavage. An examination of *Musca* or *Stomoxys* taken near stables will often reveal *Habronema* larvae up to 3-mm long, which is a clear indication that horses are likely to be exposed.

Most anthelmintics tested have shown little or no activity against these stomach worms but carbon disulfide (℞ 230) will remove those worms in the lumen.

CUTANEOUS HABRONEMIASIS
(Summer sores, Jack sores, Bursatti)

A skin disease of Equidae caused at least in part by the larvae of the stomach worms. When the larvae emerge from flies feeding on pre-existing wounds, they migrate into and irritate the sore, resulting in the production of a granulomatous reaction. The lesion becomes chronic and healing is protracted. The diagnosis of cutaneous habronemiasis is based on the finding of the granulomatous lesion that is pathognomonic of the condition. Larvae can sometimes be demonstrated in scrapings of the lesions. Many different treatments have been used for summer sores, most of them with poor results. The organophosphate pesticides, ronnel (administered orally) or trichlorfon (given IV), have given encouraging clinical response. Organophosphates applied topically to the abraded surface may kill the larvae. Surgical removal or cauterization of the excessive granulation is usually necessary. The commonly employed screwworm smears containing lindane in pine oil make a good dressing for these lesions. Control of the fly hosts and the regular collection and stacking of manure together with regular anthelmintic therapy will help to prevent *Habronema*.

Trichostrongylus INFECTION

The small stomach worm of horses, *Trichostrongylus axei*, is the same species as found in ruminants. The adults are very small and slender, measuring up to 8 mm in length. The details of the cycle in Equidae have not been carefully studied, but it is known that the larvae penetrate the mucosa.

These worms produce a chronic catarrhal gastritis and may result in rapid loss of condition. The lesions comprise a characteristic thickening of the glandular mucosa with marked congestion and a variable amount of heavy mucous exudate. The lesions may be rather small and circumscribed (in which case they often are irregularly round) or involve most or all the glandular portion of the stomach. Occasionally, the only lesion is a nodular thickening of the mucosa.

Definite diagnosis on the basis of fecal examination is difficult because the eggs are so similar to the strongyle eggs. The feces can be cultured and, in about 5 days, the infective larvae identified.

No drug has been shown to have significant activity against *T. axei* in the horse. This may be due in large part to the protection provided the worms by the heavy mucous exudate. Massive doses of thiabendazole may be worth a trial.

Parascaris Infection

The adults of the equine ascarid *Parascaris equorum* are stout worms up to 30 cm in length, with the 3 lips being very prominent. The life cycle is essentially the same as that of the hog ascarid, the prepatent period being 12 weeks. The infective eggs may persist for years on contaminated soil. Adult animals usually harbor very few worms and the principal source of infection for the young foals is soil contamination with eggs from foals of the previous year.

In heavy infections, the migrating larvae may produce respiratory signs. Foals show unthriftiness, loss of energy, diarrhea and occasionally colic. Intestinal obstruction and perforation have been reported. Diagnosis is based on the demonstration of the eggs in the feces. During the prepatent period, diagnosis is based on clinical history.

On farms where the infection is common, most foals become infected soon after birth. As a result, most of the worms are maturing when the foals are about 2½ to 4 months of age. Treatment should be started when foals are 8 weeks old and repeated at 6- to 8-week intervals until they are yearlings. Piperazine (℞ 256) or piperazine-thiabendazole (℞ 221) are effective against the adult worms and have considerable activity against the immature stages. All of the broad-spectrum equine anthelmintics are effective, therefore, ascarids are readily controlled in a multiple treatment program.

Large-Strongyle Infection

The large strongyles of horses are also known as blood worms, palisade worms, sclerostomes, or red worms. The 3 species and their respective sizes are: *Strongylus vulgaris*, 12 to 25 mm; *S. edentatus*, up to 35 mm; and *S. equinus*, 30 to 50 mm. Under favorable conditions, the larvae develop to the infective stage within 7 days after the eggs are passed. The larvae are resistant to low temperatures. Infection is by ingestion of infective larvae, which exsheath in the intestine and migrate extensively before developing to maturity in the large intestine. The prepatent period is from 5 to 12 months. The larvae of *S. vulgaris* migrate extensively in arteries, being particularly evident in the anterior mesenteric and nearby arteries where they may cause parasitic thrombosis and arteritis. Larvae of the other 2 species may be found in various parts of the body (under the parietal peritoneum, in the liver, pancreas and testicles). These species do not produce lesions in the mesenteric arteries. Mixed infections of these species and small strongyles are the rule.

Clinical Findings: The strongyles are active plug-feeders and blood suckers and the attendant blood loss may lead to anemia. Weakness, emaciation and diarrhea also are commonly observed. The intestinal mucosa is damaged where the worms attack and feed. *S. vulgaris* is especially important because of the damage done to the mesenteric arteries. As a result of the interference with the flow of blood to the intestine and thromboembolism, any one of several conditions may follow. Colic and gangrenous enteritis are the most common and serious. Intestinal stasis, torsion or intussusception and possibly rupture may also occur. Cerebrospinal nematodiasis (q.v., p. 662) can cause a variety of lesions depending on the part of the CNS affected.

Diagnosis and Treatment: Diagnosis generally is based on demonstration of eggs in the feces. Differential diagnosis can be made by identification of infective larvae. Arterial lesions may be palpable per rectum. Serologic diagnosis based on the rise of β-globulin particularly IgG(T) and arteriography of the anterior mesenteric artery have been recommended.

Parasite control programs assume that grazing horses are infected; hence, routine treatments are administered to minimize the level of pasture contamination and reduce the risks associated with migrating *S. vulgaris* larvae.

Phenothiazine (℞ 252) has been the traditional treatment, but because of toxicity, drug resistance and development of drugs with broader spectrums of activity, it is no longer recommended except in combination with other drugs. The long-popular, low-level treatment programs should only be used in conjunction with periodic treatment with other drugs.

Mixing phenothiazine with piperazine salts (℞ 251) in amounts which supply 1.24 gm of phenothiazine and 4.0 gm piperazine base per 100 lb (45 kg) body wt, results in improved efficacy against most large and small strongyles.

There are now a number of benzimidazole anthelmintics that are active against both large and small strongyles and these are efficient nontoxic drugs for strongyle control. Dichlorvos (℞ 234) and pyrantel (℞ 260) in combinations, or alone, are effective against adult worms. Strongyle control, particularly in grazing animals should be on a routine basis. Treatment only removes those forms in the lumen of the bowel and must be repeated at 6- to 8-week intervals to kill larvae emerging from nodules in the bowel wall before they become patent. The frequency necessary for satisfactory control will vary with the value of the animals, their access to pasture, and management practices. Proper programs will reduce contamination, and fecal egg counts can monitor the adequacy of the program. Treatment against migrating worms is difficult. Large doses of thiabendazole (200 mg/lb) will kill migrating *S. vulgaris* in the early stages of development, and colic due to arterial lesions has been successfully treated with this regimen. Fenbendazole has also been shown to be active in high doses against larval stages of large and small strongyles. Many of the new benzimidazoles have given promising results in the treatment of both large and small strongyle larval infections.

Colic may be associated with the use of anthelmintics. Special precautions are necessary when organophosphorus products (trichlorfon and dichlorvos) are used. Concurrent use of other organophosphates and phenothiazine compounds (including tranquilizers) may have untoward effects. Succinylcholine should not be used sooner than 30 days after administration of organophosphates.

SMALL-STRONGYLE INFECTION

Many species in several genera of the small strongyles are found in the cecum and colon. Most of them are appreciably smaller than the large strongyles, but some may be almost as large as *Strongylus vulgaris*. One species, *Triodontophorus tenuicollis*, produces rather severe ulcers in the wall of the colon. Most of the small strongyles do not appear to be blood-suckers. There is apparently no extra-intestinal migration of the larvae in the host, the larval development taking place in nodular enlargements of the wall of the large intestine. Although these are much less important than the large strongyles, they play a part in the development of the common clinical parasitism. See the discussion of the large strongyles (*above*) for the recommended treatments.

Oxyuris INFECTION

The adults of the horse pinworm, *Oxyuris equi*, are found mainly in the large intestine. This species is the largest known pinworm, the female being 7.5 to 15 cm in length. Male worms are smaller and fewer in number. The gravid females pass toward the rectum to lay their eggs on the perineum around the anus; some are passed in the feces, while others crawl out of the anal opening onto the perineum. When the latter occurs, they usually rupture, leaving around the anus a yellowish, crusty mass composed of fragments of worms and eggs. The eggs, which are flattened on one side, become embryonated in a few hours and are infective in 4 to 5 days.

Pruritus is the commonest sign. Rubbing of the tail and anal region, with resulting broken hairs and bare patches around the tail and buttocks, is a characteristic sign and should suggest the presence of pinworms. Samples collected around the perineal region often contain dried female worms or eggs. Application of cellophane tape to the skin of the perineum may be used to recover ova for microscopic examination. The worms also may be found in the feces.

Most of the broad-spectrum drugs recommended for the strongyles are effective against the adult pinworm.

Strongyloides INFECTION

Strongyloides westeri is found in the small intestine. Larvae are passed in the milk from about 4 days onward and diarrhea can be seen in foals from 10 days. Details of the life history of the worm in the horse are not known to differ significantly from that of *Strongyloides* in the pig. Thiabendazole (℞ 265) and cambendazole (℞ 229) are effective.

TAPEWORM INFECTION

Three species of tapeworms of the anoplocephaline group are found in horses: *Anoplocephala magna, A. perfoliata* and *Paranoplocephala mamillana.* They vary in length from 8 to 25 cm (the first one usually being the longest and the last the shortest). *A. magna* and *P. mamillana* usually are in the small intestine, but may also be in the stomach. *A. perfoliata* occurs mostly in the cecum, but may occur in the small intestine. The life cycle is like that of *Moniezia* in ruminants. Diagnosis is made by demonstrating the characteristic eggs in the feces. In light infections no signs of disease are present. In heavy infections, digestive disturbances may occur and anemia has been reported. Ulceration of the mucosa occurs quite commonly in the area of attachment of *A. perfoliata.* Specific treatment is seldom attempted but niclosamide and dichlorophen are recommended.

AMEBIASIS

An acute or chronic enteric disease, common in subhuman primates and sometimes observed in the dog but rare in cattle, swine and cats, and characterized by a persistent diarrhea or dysentery.

Several species of ameba occur in the large intestine of domestic herbivores, but the only known pathogen is *Entamoeba histolytica.* Man is the natural host for this species and usually the source of infection for dogs.

Clinical Findings: *E. histolytica* may live in the lumen of the large intestine as a commensal or invade the intestinal mucosa. In dogs, tissue invasion may result in a mild-to-severe hemorrhagic enteritis, occasionally with irregular macroscopic ulcers. Diarrhea may persist for weeks to months in chronic cases with or without mucus or blood in the feces. Rarely, there may be hepatic abscesses or even septicemia. Patients with acute cases either develop fulminating dysentery, which may be fatal, progress to chronicity or show spontaneous recovery. Amebiasis in subhuman primates tends to resemble the human infection.

Diagnosis: Presumptive diagnosis is based on the demonstration of *E. histolytica* in smears for fresh or specially preserved feces, but its presence may be secondary to other etiologic agents. The pathogenic ameboid form is 20 to 40 μ in diameter and distinguished from nonpathogenic species by the morphology of the nucleus or the presence of ingested red blood cells. The cyst stage is rarely found in dogs.

Treatment of Dogs: Case reports indicate metronidazole (14 to 27 mg/lb [30 to 60 mg/kg] daily orally or twice daily at half the dose for 5 to 10 days) and furazolidone (4.5 mg/lb [10 mg/kg] t.i.d. for 7 days) were effective. Metronidazole is the drug of choice for human amebiasis, but toxic manifestations with rejection are common in dogs.

CANINE HOOKWORM DISEASE

Etiology: *Ancyclostoma caninum* is the principal cause of canine hookworm disease in the U.S.A. *A. tubaeformis* of cats, commonly misidentified as *A. caninum*, has a similar but more sparse distribution. *A. braziliense* of cats and dogs is sparsely distributed from Florida to North Carolina in U.S.A. *Uncinaria stenocephala* is the principal canine hookworm in continental Europe and the British Isles; it is the canine hookworm in Canada and the northern fringe of the U.S.A., where it is primarily a fox parasite. *A. caninum* males are ca. 12-mm, females ca. 15-mm long; the other species are somewhat smaller.

Infection commonly results from ingestion of infective larvae. They mature in the second quarter of the small intestine. A major problem is the infection acquired from colostrum and milk by the pups; prenatal infection is less common. Although oral infections appear to be commoner, comparable infections with either *A. caninum* or *A. braziliense* can result from larval invasion through the skin. Skin penetration is followed by migration through the liver and lungs where they are coughed up and swallowed to reach the small intestine. Such migration also occurs following oral infection with *A. caninum* in a dog with immunity from prior infections. Percutaneous infection is rare with *A. stenocephala;* 95% of the larvae fail to develop, evidently killed in or near the skin.

The elongate (±65 μ) thin-walled hookworm eggs in the early cleavage stages (2 to 8 cells) are first passed in the feces 15 to 20 days after infection; they complete embryonation and hatch in 24 to 72 hours on warm, moist soil.

Clinical Findings: An acute hypochromic microcytic "kennel" anemia in young puppies is the characteristic, and often fatal, clinical manifestation produced by *A. caninum*. Surviving puppies develop immunity. Nevertheless, debilitated and malnourished animals may continue to be unthrifty and suffer from a chronic anemia. Mature, well-nourished dogs may harbor a few worms, i.e. a subclinical infection. These are of primary concern as the direct or indirect source of infection for puppies.

Lesions: The anemia results directly from the blood sucking and the bleeding ulcerations when *A. caninum* shift feeding sites. The amount of blood loss due to a single worm in 24 hours has been estimated at 0.1 to 0.8 ml. There is no interference with erythropoiesis in uncomplicated hookworm disease. The liver and other organs may appear ischemic with some fatty infiltration of the liver. Neither *A. braziliense* nor *U. stenocephala* is an avid blood feeder and anemia does not occur but hypoproteinemia is characteristic. Serum seepage around the worm's attachment in the intestine may reduce blood protein more than 10%.

Dermatitis due to invading larvae may occur with any of the hookworms but has been most frequently reported in the interdigital spaces with *U. stenocephala*. Secondary bacterial infection is reputed to be a serious problem with greyhounds in England.

Prophylaxis: The bitch should be free of hookworms before breeding and not permitted on hookworm contaminated areas before pregnancy. The pups should be whelped and suckled in sanitary quarters. Concrete runways that can be hosed twice a week in warm weather are best. Sunlit clay or sandy runways are good; these can be decontaminated with sodium borate (10 lb/100 sq. ft. [1 kg/2m^2]). Chemical prophylaxis with styrylpyridinium is usually used in combination with diethylcarbamazine (℞ 262) to prevent both hookworm and heartworm infection.

Treatment: Pyrantel pamoate (℞ 259) is currently favored because a single oral dose without starvation or purgation after treatment is highly effective. It has a good margin of safety so that the dose may be repeated if necessary to eliminate those worms that have matured after the first dose when there is continuous exposure to infection. Disophenol (℞ 236) administered as a single subcut. dose acts more slowly but is just as effective. There is a relatively narrow margin of safety against a possible overdose and there is no effective antidote. A second dose should not be administered. Several of the newer drugs such as thenium (℞ 263) and mebendazole (℞ 245) are effective but require multiple doses and some must be given on an empty stomach and followed with a purgative. Dithiazanine iodide (℞ 237) is useful against both *A. caninum* and the microfilariae of heartworm. Bephenium hydroxynaphthoate (℞ 226) is reported to be particularly effective against *U. stenocephala*. When anemia is severe, chemotherapy may have to be supported by transfusion or supplementary iron or both, to be followed by a high-protein diet until the hemoglobin level is normal.

CANINE STRONGYLOIDOSIS

Etiology: The causative organism is a small, slender nematode, a few millimeters long, which, when fully mature, is buried in the mucosa of the anterior half of the small intestine. The worms are almost transparent and at necropsy it is all but impossible to see them with the unaided eye. Some evidence suggests that the species found in dogs is identical with that found in humans (*Strongyloides stercoralis*); it may, however, be a distinct species. Since the disease in man can be quite serious and is resistant to treatment, extreme caution should be exercised in handling infected dogs.

The parasitic worms are all females, an unusual circumstance among nematodes, and the eggs that they deposit in the intestinal mucosa develop parthenogenetically. The eggs embryonate rapidly and hatch before they are evacuated in the feces. Under appropriate conditions of warmth and moisture, extracorporeal development is rapid. The third larval (infective) stage may be achieved in little more than a day. The molted filariform larvae are excellent skin penetrators, but also may infect a host via the oral mucosa. They migrate by way of the circulation and lungs, reaching the intestine usually as fourth-stage organisms which molt and begin their adult life. Progeny may be shed in the feces within 7 to 10 days after infection.

Some of the larvae shed from a patent infection develop into infective larvae; others develop into characteristic free-living male and female worms, which mate and produce progeny that are infective for a new host.

Clinical Findings: Clinical strongyloidosis is a heavy infection that has been building up for some weeks. The disease usually is characterized by a blood-streaked, mucoid diarrhea. Emaciation is prominent and failure to make appropriate growth may be one of the first signs of infection. The appetite usually is good and the animal is normally active in the earlier stages of the disease. In the absence of intercurrent infections, there is little or no elevation of temperature. In advanced stages, the prognosis is grave. Usually, there is shallow, rapid breathing and pyrexia and, at necropsy, evidence of a verminous pneumonia with large areas of consolidation in the lungs. Marked enteritis, with hemorrhage, mucosal exfoliation and much mucus secretion is also seen.

Prophylaxis: Poor sanitation and the association of susceptible dogs and puppies lead to a rapid build-up of the infection in all animals in a kennel or pen. Animals with diarrhea should be promptly isolated from healthy or asymptomatic dogs. Direct sunlight, elevated soil or surface temperatures and desiccation are deleterious to all free larval stages.

Treatment: Dithiazanine iodide (℞ 237) has been a satisfactory anthelmintic for infection in both man and dogs. Thiabendazole will prevent mature *Strongyloide* infections in dogs when fed continuously at levels between 0.01 and 0.05% of the ration. Mebendazole experimentally has been shown to be effective. Diethylcarbamazine (℞ 235) has also been employed successfully.

ASCARIASIS (SM. AN.)

Etiology: The large roundworms (ascaridoid nematodes) of dogs and cats are commonly encountered, especially in puppies and kittens. There are 3 species involved, namely *Toxocara canis, Toxascaris leonina* and *Toxocara cati.* The most important species is *T. canis,* not only because it may readily be transmitted to man, but because heavy infection may occur in very young pups. It has also been recorded in cats. *T. leonina* occurs most often in adult dogs, more rarely in cats. *T. cati* occurs in young cats and only exceptionally in dogs. Distribution varies throughout the world.

These species occur also in wild carnivores and probably gain access to the definitive host by the ingestion of other larvae-infected animals. This mode of infection can also occur in cats with *T. cati* and *T. leonina.* The usual mode of infection with *T. canis* is by prenatal infection of puppies from larvae in the tissues of the bitch. When embryonated infective eggs of *T. canis* are swallowed by adult dogs, the larvae do not reach the intestine after migration, but are distributed in muscles, connective tissue, kidneys and many other tissues. From there they migrate into the developing fetus and eventually reach the intestine within a week or so after birth. At this time, eggs may also be passed by the lactating bitch, as, by licking the feces of her pups, she may swallow some of the larvae which fail to maintain a hold in the intestine of the puppy. Infection with *T. leonina* can be direct by swallowing eggs, as occurs mostly in dogs, the larvae developing in the intestinal wall. It can be indirect, as occurs with cats, by ingestion of rodents, in which larvae may be found encapsulated in the gut wall, mesenteries, diaphragm, abdominal wall and adjacent tissues.

Larvae of ascaridoid nematodes may migrate in the tissues of many animals, including man. Migrating larvae, especially those of *T. canis,* are associated with lesions in liver, kidneys, lungs, brain and eye. The larvae cause mechanical damage and are often associated with granuloma formation and eosinophilia. This is referred to as **visceral larva migrans.**

Clinical Findings: The first indication of infection in young animals is lack of growth and loss of condition. Infected animals have a dull haircoat and are often potbellied. Worms may be vomited and are often voided spontaneously in the feces. In the early stages, pulmonary damage due to migrating larvae may occur; this may be complicated by superimposed bacterial pneumonitis, so that respiratory distress of variable severity may supervene. Cortical kidney lesions (granulomata) containing larvae are frequently observed in dogs.

Diagnosis: Infection in dogs and cats is diagnosed by detection of eggs in feces. It is important to distinguish the spherical, pitted-shelled eggs of *Toxocara* spp. from the oval smooth-shelled eggs of *T. leonina*, owing to the public health importance of the former.

Treatment: Piperazine salts (℞ 256) are highly effective. Hexylresorcinol (℞ 241) is also effective, but should not be used for treating cats. n-Butyl chloride (℞ 228), toluene (℞ 267), or a combination with dichlorophene (Difolin, ℞ 233) and diethylcarbamazine (℞ 235) are widely employed. Dithiazanine (℞ 237) has been reported as effective. Dichlorvos (℞ 234) has proved suitable for removal of ascarids and may be given either by capsule or in older dogs with the daily ration of canned food or meat. Mebendazole (℞ 245) and pyrantel pamoate (℞ 258) are new and effective products. Thiabendazole, fed continuously at levels between 0.01 and 0.05% of the ration, has been reported to prevent the embryonation of eggs of *T. canis* in feces of dogs.

It is important that puppies be treated before eggs appear in the feces, particularly if there are children in the household. It is recommended that the first treatment be given to pups at 2 weeks after birth, also that bitches nursing the puppies be treated at the same time. Repeat treatments are necessary if eggs appear in the feces.

Control: The eggs of *T. canis* tend to adhere to inanimate objects—walls, etc.—and to become mixed in soil and dust. For this reason it is important to prevent accumulation of dog feces near the house. This applies particularly in lactating bitches, whose feces should be collected and burnt throughout the suckling period. As eggs may be adherent to the paws and hair, children should not handle lactating bitches or young puppies until successful treatment has been established.

CANINE TRICHURIASIS

(Whipworm infection)

Etiology: The adults of *Trichuris vulpis* are 40 to 70 mm in length and consist of a long, slender anterior portion and a thickened posterior third. They inhabit the cecum and colon where the worm is firmly attached to the intestinal wall, its anterior end being deeply embedded in the mucosa. Thick-shelled eggs with a bipolar plug are passed in the feces and become infective in 2 to 4 weeks in a warm, moist environment. Although eggs remain viable in a suitable environment for up to 5 years, they are susceptible to desiccation. The life cycle is direct. Following the ingestion of infective eggs, larval development occurs in the jejunum and the adults mature in the large intestine in about 10 weeks, where they may remain for up to 16 months.

Clinical Findings: No signs are seen in light infections, but as the worm burden increases and the inflammatory, and occasionally hemorrhagic, reaction in the large intestine becomes more pronounced, loss of weight and diarrhea become evident. Fresh blood may accompany the feces of heavily infected dogs, and anemia occasionally follows.

Prophylaxis: Besides regular anthelmintic treatment of dogs, advantage should be taken of the susceptibility of the eggs to desiccation. By maintaining cleanliness and eliminating moist areas the infection of dogs can be reduced considerably.

Treatment: There are now at least 4 acceptable treatments. Phthalofyne (℞ 253) has proved quite useful either orally or IV. Dichlorvos (℞ 234) can be administered either by capsule or in feed and glycobiarsol (℞ 672) may be given orally as a tablet or crushed in the feed. Mebendazole (℞ 245) in the feed is effective and the occasional side effects, vomiting or diarrhea, are minimal.

CANINE HEARTWORM INFECTION

(Heartworm Disease Complex)

A clinical or inapparent infection caused by the filarial worm *Dirofilaria immitis*, the adults of which occur primarily in the venous return, right ventricle and pulmonary outflow tracts. Two filarial species have been reported in the U.S.A., *Dirofilaria immitis* and *Dipetalonema reconditum*. Since only *D. immitis* is pathogenic, identification is essential. The cat is an occasional aberrant host for *D. immitis*.

Etiology: Adult females are about 27-cm long and males about 17 cm. The fertilized eggs develop and hatch within the uterus of the female. The precociously active embryos (microfilariae), which are about 315-μ long, are discharged into the blood stream where they remain active for 1 to 3 years, but are incapable of further development until ingested by the intermediate host—various mosquito species. Within the mosquito, development from the microfilaria to the third stage (infective) larva is completed in about 2 weeks. The infective larvae then migrate to the mouth parts and gain entrance into the dog when the mosquito feeds again.

The immature stages develop and grow in the intramuscular fascia or subcut. tissue for approximately 2 months and then begin migration to the right ventricle, arriving 2 to 4 months after infection. An additional 2 to 3 months are required for the worms to reach maturity; thus microfilariae first appear in the peripheral circulation about 6 months after infection. Adults may live and continue to produce microfilariae for several years. The adult worms live in the right ventricle and the adjacent blood vessels from the posterior vena cava, hepatic vein and anterior vena cava to the pulmonary artery.

Geographical Distribution: The disease has a cosmopolitan distribution at sea level in the tropics and subtropics. It is common in coastal China, the Western Pacific Islands and parts of Japan as well as Coastal Mexico, Central America, and the Northern part of South America. In the U.S.A. it occurs frequently in all mosquito-infested areas; until recently it appeared to be endemic mainly in the Southeastern States, with prevalence of disease in mature dogs not kept indoors reaching as high as 50%. It is now nearly as common, where high mosquito densities occur, in the Middle and North Atlantic States and the Midwest extending into Ontario and adjacent areas. It is uncommon on the West Coast but has been reported in northern California and Oregon.

Clinical Findings: Physical examination and a thorough history will usually indicate gradual weight loss, decreased exercise tolerance, cough aggravated by exercise and, in advanced cases, dyspnea, increased temperature, abdominal fluid, cyanotic mucous membranes and periodic collapse. The time and severity of infection along with the individual dog's susceptibility will determine the variation of clinical signs.

In the acute hepatic syndrome (postcaval syndrome), the adult worms obstruct the posterior vena cava causing sudden onset of critical signs, hemoglobinuria, and death within 24 to 72 hours due to hepatic and renal failure.

Lesions: Endarteritis and thromboembolization from alive and dead adult heartworms are the most constant changes in the pulmonary arteries. Periodic episodes of acute inflammation and fibrosis obstruct and mechanically interfere with normal blood flow, resulting in pulmonary hypertension and secondary right heart enlargement (cor pulmonale). Postcaval obstructions exhibit enlarged hepatic venules, thickening of hepatic veins, and centrolobular necrosis. The kidneys show evidence of hemosiderosis of the convoluted tubules with heme casts in the medulla.

Diagnosis: Identification of *D. immitis* microfilariae in blood samples confirms the diagnosis based on history and clinical signs. Heartworm microfilariae are differentiated from microfilariae belonging to *D. reconditum* by size, shape, and movement.

	Dirofilaria immitis	*Dipetalonema reconditum*
Anterior end	Tapered head	Blunt head
Posterior end	Straight	Sometimes hook-shaped
Movement in blood	Side to side movement	Forward movement
Size	315 μ × 6–8 μ	270 μ × 5–6 μ

Microfilariae are usually isolated and identified either in a fresh blood smear, by centrifugation (modified Knott's technique) or by millipore or nucleopore filters.

To complicate diagnosis, some dogs (15 to 20%) do not exhibit circulating microfilariae, thus the term "occult infections." The diagnosis is then based on history, clinical examination and thoracic radiographs. Diagnostic changes occur in the cardiac silhouette and pulmonary arterial segments. Usually the right ventricle and pulmonary arterial segment are enlarged and the lungs exhibit enlarged, tortuous pulmonary arteries which fail to taper peripherally. A dilated postcava, hepatosplenomegaly and ascites are typical in more advanced cases.

Prophylaxis: Because of the serious sequela that may be associated with treatment, prevention is preferable. The accepted prevention is daily administration of diethylcarbamazine (DEC—℞ 235, 262) orally, begun prior to and continued for 2 months after the mosquito season, to kill infective larvae on their migration to the heart. Regions with continuous mosquito populations require year-round daily therapy. The drug should not be given to dogs with microfilariae as a shocklike syndrome, sometimes fatal, may result. Evidence of sterility and impotency among male dogs is either rare or an individual idiosyncrasy and appears not to be a justification for discontinuing such prophylaxis.

Protection of dogs from mosquitoes and biannual treatments for adult worms are alternate methods of prophylaxis. Protection from mosquitoes involves mosquito control and confinement of dogs, which may not be possible.

Treatment: Treatment is primarily directed at destruction of the adult worms but cannot be considered complete unless followed by microfilaricidal therapy and preventive medication to guard against reinfection.

Arsenamide (℞ 225) is the drug of choice for the adult worms. The drug is potentially nephrotoxic and hepatotoxic, requiring pretreatment evaluation of liver function (SGPT) and renal function (both BUN and urinalysis). These tests are indicators of existing problems but do not predict which animals will react to thiacetarsamide. Following treatment, close confinement is required for 3 weeks and limited exercise for the next 3 weeks. Temperature rise and pneumonia may occur within the first 2 weeks as the adults die and fragment into the lungs. Single doses of steroids to reduce inflammation and high levels of antibiotics may give satisfactory results.

Dithiazanine iodide (℞ 237) is the only microfilaricide in general use today. Microfilaricidal treatment should follow treatment designed to kill the adults within 3 to 6 weeks depending on clinical judgment. Levamisole has been reported to be an effective microfilaricide but may also have side effects (CNS). Although both drugs are effective, toxic side effects by either may require using the other to remove microfilariae prior to use of the prophylactic drug (DEC).

SPIROCERCA LUPI IN DOGS

Etiology: Adult *Spirocerca lupi* are bright red worms 30-mm (male) to 80-mm (female) long. They generally are located within nodules in the esophageal wall. Dogs are infected by eating an intermediate host (usually dung bettle) or a transport host (e.g. chicken). The larvae migrate via the wall of the thoracic aorta where they usually remain for about 3 months. Eggs are passed in feces about 5 to 6 months after infection.

Clinical Findings: Most dogs with *S. lupi* infection show no clinical signs. When the esophageal lesion is very large, as it usually is when it has become neoplastic, the dog has difficulty in swallowing and may vomit repeatedly after trying to eat. Such dogs salivate profusely and eventually become emaciated. These clinical signs, especially if accompanied by enlargement of the extremities characteristic of osteoarthropathy, are strongly suggestive of spirocercosis with associated neoplasia, particularly in regions where the parasite is prevalent. Occasionally, a dog will die suddenly as the result of massive hemorrhage into the thoracic cavity following rupture of the aorta damaged by the developing worms.

Lesions: The characteristic lesions are aneurysm of the thoracic aorta, reactive granulomas of variable size around the worms and, often but not always, deformative ossifying spondylitis of the posterior thoracic vertebrae. Esophageal sarcoma, often with metastases, is sometimes associated (apparently causally) with *S. lupi* infection, particularly in hound breeds. Dogs with *Spirocerca*-related sarcoma often develop hypertrophic pulmonary osteoarthropathy (q.v., p. 582).

Diagnosis: A positive diagnosis can be made by demonstration of the characteristic eggs on fecal examination using a flotation method with saturated sodium nitrate or zinc sulfate solution. A gastroscopic examination may occasionally reveal a nodule or an adult worm. Since eggs are sporadically voided in feces and are often missed, a presumptive diagnosis can be made by radiographic examination when it reveals dense masses in the esophagus. Barium will help define the lesion. Spondylitis of the ventral surface of the bodies of posterior thoracic vertebrae is an inconsistent sign of *S. lupi* infection.

Most infections are not diagnosed until necropsy. The granulomas vary greatly in size and location in the esophagus, but are usually so characteristic as to be diagnostic, even if the worms are no longer present. Worms and granulomas may be present in the lung, trachae, mediastinum, wall of stomach, or other abnormal location. Healed aneurysms of the aorta persist for the life of the dog and are diagnostic of previous infection. When sarcomas are associated with the infection, the esophageal lesion is usually larger and often contains cartilage or bone. Metastases of these lesions are frequently present in lung, lymph nodes, heart, liver, or kidney.

Control: Treatment is not practical with information presently available, but in endemic areas dogs should not be fed raw chicken scraps.

Preliminary studies have shown that dithiazanine and disophenol may have some effect on the worms. Surgical removal is usually unsuccessful because of the large areas of the esophagus involved.

STEPHANOFILARIASIS

(Filarial dermatitis of cattle)

Stephanofilaria stilesi is a small filarial parasite responsible for a circumscribed dermatitis along the ventral midline of cattle. The parasite has been reported throughout the U.S.A., but is commoner among cattle in the Western and Southwestern regions. The adult worms are 3- to 6-mm long and are usually found in the dermis, just beneath the epidermal layer. Microfilaria are 50-μ long and are enclosed in a spherical, semirigid vitelline membrane. The intermediate host for *S. stilesi* is the female horn fly, *Haematobia irritans* (q.v., p. 762). Horn flies feeding on the lesion ingest microfilariae that develop to the third stage infective larva in 2 to 3 weeks. The infective larva is introduced into the skin as the horn fly feeds.

Clinical Findings and Diagnosis: The dermatitis develops along the ventral midline, usually between the brisket and navel. With repeated exposure the lesion spreads, often involving skin posterior to the navel. Active lesions are covered with blood or serous exudate, while chronic lesions are smooth, dry and devoid of hair. Hyperkeratosis and parakeratosis occur in the epidermis of the parasitized area.

Deep skin scrapings are macerated in isotonic saline solution and examined microscopically for adults or microfilariae. Microfilariae must be differentiated from *Rhabditis strongyloides* (q.v., p. 928), a small free-living nematode that is occasionally responsible for a moist, superficial dermatitis. The rhabditiform esophagus, so characteristic of that nematode, does not occur in filarial nematodes.

Prophylaxis and Treatment: No treatment is available for stephanofilariasis, but control of horn flies will break the cycle.

ONCHOCERCIASIS

Four species of *Onchocerca* occur in domestic animals in the U.S.A. *O. cervicalis* occurs in the ligamentum nuchae and other sites in horses. In cattle, *O. gutturosa* locates in the ligamentum nuchae, *O. lienalis* in the gastrosplenic ligament and *O. stilesi* in the stifle joint, although there is some debate that these 3 are the same species. Microfilariae are found in the dermis or dermal lymph vessels just below the epidermis. They are most numerous in skin overlying sites occupied by adult females. The microfilariae are slender, 200- to 250-μ long and have a short, sharply pointed tail. The intermediate hosts for *O. cervicalis* are species of *Culicoides*. For *O. gutterosa* and *O. lienalis* and probably for *O. stilesi*, species of *Simulium* are intermediate hosts.

Clinical Findings: The only species that may cause disease is *O. cervicalis*, and there is even doubt about this. The adults are frequently associated with fistulous withers and poll evil (q.v., p. 571), but their contribution to these conditions is probably minor.

The microfilariae are often found in areas of inflammation and as a result, they are often blamed for dermatitis about the face, neck, shoulders and breast. Dermatitis is caused by a multitude of external irritants, allergens and infectious agents (q.v., p. 926), and microfilariae may contribute in some degree.

Microfilariae also accumulate in the eye of horses with equine periodic ophthalmia (q.v., p. 226) but because of their predilection for inflamed areas, microfilariae could easily be in the eye as a result of the disease rather than as the cause. Since the cause has not been clearly defined, however, microfilariae must be considered as possible etiologic agents.

Diagnosis: The most effective method is to excise a piece of skin about 1 or 2 cm in diameter, macerate in isotonic saline solution, and examine microscopically for the characteristic microfilariae. The microfilaria of *O. cervicalis* must be stained with Mayer's hemalum to differentiate it from the microfilaria of *Setaria equina*. The sheath of the latter can be seen at the anterior end. They must also be differentiated from the larva of *Habronema* spp., the etiologic agent of cutaneous habronemiasis (q.v., p. 694). This larva is in the third stage of development and possesses a spiked knob on the caudal extremity.

Treatment: No treatment is available against the adults or microfilariae of *O. cervicalis*. The treatment recommended for dermatitis (q.v., p. 926) is often of value, even when microfilariae are present in the lesions.

ELAEOPHOROSIS

(Filarial dermatosis; Sorehead; "Clear-eyed" blindness)

Elaeophora schneideri is a parasite of mule deer and black-tailed deer inhabiting mountains of the Western and Southwestern U.S.A.; recently it has been found in white-tailed deer in the Southern and Southeastern regions. Adult parasites are 60- to 120-mm long and are usually found in the common carotid or internal maxillary arteries. The microfilariae, about 275-μ long and 15- to 17-μ thick, normally occur in capillaries of skin on the forehead and face. Development in the intermediate hosts, which are horse flies of the genera *Tabanus* and *Hybomitra*, requires about 2 weeks. Infective larvae invade the host as the horse fly feeds, go into the leptomeningeal arteries and develop to immature adults in about 3 weeks. These young adults migrate against the blood flow and establish in the common carotid arteries, where they continue to grow. About 6 months later the parasites reach sexual maturity and begin producing microfilariae. The life span of the adults is 3 to 4 years.

Clinical Findings: Clinical disease has not been reported in mule deer and black-tailed deer; therefore, they are considered to be the normal definitive hosts. When horse flies transmit the infective larva to elk, moose, domestic sheep, domestic goats, sika deer and, possibly, white-tailed deer, development of the larva in the leptomeningeal arteries causes ischemic necrosis of brain tissue, resulting in blindness, brain damage and sudden death. Blindness in these animals is characterized by absence of opacities in the refractive media of the eye, thus the popular name "clear eyed" blindness.

Domestic sheep and goats, especially lambs, kids, and yearlings, may die suddenly 3 to 5 weeks after infection. Death is usually preceded by incoordination and circling, and often by convulsions and opisthotonos. Numerous thrombi occur in the cerebral and leptomeningeal arteries. One or more young adult *E. schneideri* accompany each thrombus. If sheep or goats survive the early infection, 6 to 10 months later they develop a raw, bloody dermatitis on the poll, forehead or face, thus the popular name "sorehead." Lesions occasionally occur on the legs, abdomen and feet. These lesions are an allergic dermatitis in response to the microfilariae lodged in capillaries. Lesions persist, with periods of intermittent and incomplete healing, for about 3 years, followed by spontaneous recovery. Hyperplasia and hyperkeratosis occur in the epidermis of the parasitized area.

Diagnosis: Differential diagnosis involves coenurosis (*Multiceps*), cerebrocortical necrosis (q.v., p. 666) and enterotoxemia (q.v., p. 402). Elaeophorosis should not be considered unless sheep are known to have been in endemic areas of the disease during the summer months. Diagnosis of the disease in lambs, kids, or yearling and calf elk, is usually done at necropsy. Numerous thrombi and parasites will be found in the common carotid, internal maxillary, cerebral and leptomeningeal arteries. Presumptive diagnosis in mature sheep is based upon history, and location and type of lesion. The skin lesion must be differentiated from ulcerative dermatosis (q.v., p. 249). Confirmation is by recovery of microfilariae from the lesion, or postmortem recovery of the adult parasites. A skin biopsy of the lesion is macerated in isotonic saline solution, and allowed to stand for at least 6 hours at room temperature. The skin is strained off and the fluid examined for the typical microfilariae.

Prophylaxis and Treatment: Piperazine salts are effective at 100 mg/lb (220 mg/kg) body wt orally. Complete recovery will occur in 18 to 20 days. No treatment is available for the cerebral form of the disease.

GIANT KIDNEY-WORM INFECTION IN THE DOG AND MINK

Etiology: The giant kidney worm, *Dioctophyma renale*, occasionally occurs in dogs. The females are the largest nematodes known. When adults they range from 75 to 100 cm in length and up to 1 cm or more in diameter. Males are smaller, up to 45 cm in length. When mature, the bright-red adults live in the renal tissues, almost invariably the right kidney. The renal parenchyma is gradually destroyed as the female worm grows and passes eggs in the urine of the host.

The pitted thick-shelled eggs have a bipolar plug and, if ingested by oligochaete annelids, which are parasitic on crayfish, they hatch and infective larvae develop. By ingesting the annelid alone or the parasitized host, or fish that have fed on infected annelid worms, the carnivore becomes infected with *D. renale*. Larvae migrate from the stomach or duodenum of the dog to the peritoneal cavity and occasionally the liver before becoming mature adults in the kidney. Eggs are passed in the urine 4 to 6 months after infection. Reported cases in dogs are relatively few, but the incidence in mink ranges from 2 to 5%.

Clinical Findings and Diagnosis: Signs develop when the parasites approach or reach maturity. The sequence involves a marked loss of weight, as much as one-third to one-half in a few weeks, hematuria, frequent urination, restlessness and evidence of severe abdominal or lumbar pain. The animal may cry, stretch and exhibit a nervous trembling. Anemia may occur secondary to the blood loss. The disease is diagnosed from the signs and the presence of the parasite eggs in the urine. The adult worm may sometimes be detected radiographically.

Prophylaxis and Treatment: Curtailment of the ingestion of raw fish or other aquatic organisms is recommended, especially in areas where the parasite is known to occur in wild animals. Nephrectomy, in the early stages of the infection, leads to rapid recovery.

SWINE KIDNEY-WORM INFECTION

Etiology: The adults of the swine kidney worm, *Stephanurus dentatus*, (25 to 35 mm in length and about 2 mm in diameter) are found in the kidneys, the wall of the ureters and in the perirenal fat. The eggs hatch shortly after being passed in the urine; the larvae reach the infective stage in about 3 to 5 days and are susceptible to cold, desiccation and sunlight. They usually are ingested, but may penetrate the skin through abrasions. They migrate to the liver and, after extensive wandering through the liver tissue and beneath the capsule for 2 to 3 months, most pierce the capsule and enter the abdominal cavity. After some wandering, the larvae settle in the kidney, its adnexa and, occasionally, in other tissues or organs. Patent infections in pigs younger than 5 months of age are required prenatally. The kidney worm is found worldwide and, next to *Ascaris*, is the most important parasite of swine, especially in warm climates.

Clinical Findings: Heavy experimental infections of kidney worms have been shown to affect growth adversely. Pleuritis and peritonitis are quite common. The principal economic loss results from the condemnation of affected organs and tissues on meat inspection. Inasmuch as migrating worms may invade and damage a number of organs and tissues, lesions and signs are variable; most commonly observed are lesions of the liver, kidney and surrounding tissue and lungs. The most severe lesions are in the liver, which shows cirrhosis, scar formation, extensive thrombosis of the portal vessels and a variable amount of necrotic tissue.

Diagnosis: When worms are in the kidney or ureter, or have established communication with them, eggs may be recovered in the urine. Otherwise, a definitive diagnosis is dependent on demonstration of the worms or lesions at necropsy.

Control: Although feeding a concentration of 0.1% thiabendazole in the ration for 14 days has prevented migration of kidney-worm larvae, no satisfactory treatment has yet been developed for the elimination of the adult worm. Experimentally levamisole at 8 mg/kg of body wt was successful in stopping worm-egg production in 4 days and the urine remained free of eggs for 6 weeks following treatment. The parasite is eradicated from a pasture in 12 to 18 months after egg contamination is stopped (longer from shaded feedlots). Only first-litter gilts may be used as breeding stock and these disposed of when their pigs are weaned; this program is effective because the worms may require as long as 10 months to attain significant egg-laying potential. Older boars should also be removed from the infected herd and replaced with young boars from clean herds or the gilts hand-bred. Raising swine on slats cleaned daily will reduce this infection to a low level.

After the kidney worm has been eradicated, the gilts may then be kept in the breeding herd if it is maintained as a closed herd and care is taken to prevent the introduction of infected animals.

TRICHINOSIS

A parasitic disease of primary importance as a public health problem. Human infections are established through the consumption of infected, insufficiently cooked meat, usually pork or bear. Prevalence rates are generally higher in dogs and cats than in swine; natural infections are often reported in wild carnivores. It has also been reported in such animals as rats, beavers, opossums, walruses and whales. Probably all mammals are susceptible.

Etiology and Epidemiology: *Trichinella spiralis* is the causative nematode. Infection occurs by ingestion of muscle tissue containing viable trichinae. The cyst wall is digested in the stomach and the liberated larvae partially penetrate the duodenal and jejunal mucosa. Within about 2 days, the larvae develop into sexually mature adults which mate. The females (3 to 4 mm) penetrate deeper into the mucosa and discharge living larvae beginning by the fourth to seventh day. A single adult female generally produces 500 to 1,000 larvae over a 2- to 6-week period. Following reproduction, the adult trichinae die and usually are digested. The minute larvae (0.1 mm) migrate to the muscle by 2 routes, either following the lymphatic and portal systems to the peripheral circulation or through connective tissue. Those larvae that reach striated muscle penetrate individual muscle fibers and grow to 1 mm in length. As early as 17 days after infection they coil up and are encysted by host reaction; a myositis is produced. They are resistant to digestion and capable of infecting a host if ingested. They may remain viable in the cyst for several years. The diaphragm, tongue, masseter and deltoid muscles are among the most heavily involved muscles. The larvae also may invade organs and tissues other than striated muscle but usually are destroyed by local inflammatory reaction. Heart and nervous system damage may occur.

Infective larvae that may pass through the intestine and be eliminated in the feces before maturation are infective to other animals.

Clinical Findings: Most infections are light and go undiagnosed. In heavy infections that produce serious illness and occasional deaths, 3 clinical phases are evident: The intestinal stage, commencing about 24 hours after ingestion of trichinous meat and continuing through the first week, results in a nonspecific gastroenteritis that may include diarrhea, slight fever, signs of mild abdominal pain, nausea and vomiting. The muscle invasion stage, beginning about a week after infection and usually extending several weeks, is characterized by anorexia, emaciation, muscular pains, dyspnea, edema, low fever and eosinophilia. The invaded muscles are hard, swollen, tense and painful, especially the muscles of respiration, mastication, deglutition and movement. The degree of eosinophilia depends on the host species and may be related to infective dosage. The peak eosinophilia usually occurs 2 to 3 weeks after infection and then declines gradually. Deaths are commonest in this stage. The convalescent stage generally begins 5 to 6 weeks after infection. Signs usually recede, although in severe infections muscular stiffness, neurologic disorders, myocardial weakness, nephritis or pulmonary disorders may be seen as a result of tissue damage.

Diagnosis: Although antemortem diagnoses in animals other than man are rare, swine, dogs and cats with the above signs are prime suspects, especially if there is a history of feeding raw or insufficiently cooked pork. Microscopic examination of a muscle biopsy sample will confirm but not necessarily rule out trichinosis. In animals, biopsy usually is not feasible and examination of muscle tissue normally is not made until necropsy. The fluorescent antibody test and the enzyme labeled antibody test are probably the most reliable of currently available serologic tests for infections in animals.

Prophylaxis: Although infected wild animal carcasses are also important, most domestic animals are infected by eating garbage containing raw or insufficiently cooked pork. The general objectives are to prevent the ingestion by animals or man of viable trichinae present in meat. For swine and other animals this can be accomplished by (1) elimination of feeding of garbage and wildlife carcasses; or (2) cooking all garbage 212°F (100°C) for 30 minutes. Rodent control programs should be carried out as a precautionary measure.

Inspection of meat for viable trichinae at the time of slaughter has proved effective in many countries. Methods of meat inspection and processing in the U.S.A. are currently based on the assumption that all pork may be infected with trichinae; pork products that appear to be "ready to eat" must be processed by adequate heat, freezing or curing to kill trichinae before marketing. Similar pork products lacking the governmental inspection seal or raw pork products should be cooked to at least 170°F (82°C) before eating.

Treatment: Treatment consists mainly of symptomatic and supportive therapy to alleviate pain until the infection has subsided. ACTH and adrenal corticosteroid hormones are commonly used. Infections in man can be treated successfully with thiabendazole, but this is generally less practicable for animals.

LUNGWORM INFECTION

(Verminous bronchitis, "Husk," "Hoose")

An infection of the respiratory tract by any of several parasitic nematodes. Species of veterinary importance include *Dictyocaulus viviparus*, the lungworm of cattle, *D. arnfieldi* in horses and donkeys, *D. filaria*, *Protostrongylus rufescens*, *Muellerius capillaris* in sheep and goats, 3 *Metastrongylus* spp. in pigs, and *Aelurostrongylus abstrusus* in cats.

The cattle lungworm causes economic loss in young animals in Northwest Europe, particularly the British isles; North America, in areas with moderate temperatures and high humidity; and in many other areas of the world. *D. arnfieldi* is becoming commoner in many areas of the world. Donkeys are a common host and may, in some areas, be the reservoir of infection for horses. The sheep lungworms are important pathogens of sheep in Australia, Southeast Europe and North America, causing losses particularly in lambs maintained with ewes. Lungworms are of less importance in swine but outbreaks of the disease occur sporadically. *A. abstrusus* has been reported to occur in up to 20% of free-ranging cats.

Life Cycle and Epidemiology: *D. viviparus, D. arnfieldi* and *D. filaria* have direct life cycles. Eggs laid in the large bronchi are coughed up, swallowed and hatch during passage down the alimentary tract. Larvae are passed in the feces and reach the infective third stage in 5 to 7 days at moderate temperatures (64 to 68°F [18 to 20°C]). Grazing animals ingest the infective larvae that migrate to the lungs via the lymphatic system. The larvae migrate through the alveoli, bronchioles and finally mature in the main bronchi. The prepatent period is 3 to 4 weeks in ruminants and 5 to 6 weeks in Equidae. Viability of infective larvae is enhanced by moderate temperatures and high humidity. Lush pasture, which promotes production of semi-fluid feces, results in larvae being widely spread in the herbage. Some of the infective larvae successfully overwinter in soil and herbage even at low temperatures and can persist in temperate climates for at least one year. The disease is usually observed in young animals during their first season at pasture though occasional outbreaks occur in adult stock not previously exposed to lungworm infection; light infections may persist for many months and these older animals with silent infections are an important source of pasture contamination with larvae.

Transmission and Epidemiology: Eggs of *Metastrongylus* of swine are passed in the feces and are ingested by earthworms in which they develop to the infective stage. *P. rufescens, M. capillaris* and *A. abstrusus* require slugs or snails as intermediate hosts. Ingestion of these intermediate hosts is necessary for infection to occur, but transport hosts may also be involved, particularly with *A. abstrusus.*

Pathogenesis: The pathogenic effect of lungworms depends on their location within the respiratory tract. With *D. viviparus,* during the prepatent phase of infection the main lesion is blockage of small bronchi and bronchioles by an eosinophil exudate produced in response to the migration of developing larvae; this blockage results in obstruction to the passage of air with consequent collapse of the alveoli distal to the block. In the patent phase the irritation caused by the presence of adults in the bronchi produces a bronchitis with much exudation into and blocking of air passages. However, the major pneumonic lesion is caused by a cellular response in which macrophages and giant cells engulf aspirated eggs and newly hatched larvae and consolidation ensues. In some animals a proliferative pneumonia develops due to alveolar epithelialization. Pulmonary edema, emphysema and secondary bacterial infection may occur as complications and bronchiectasis as a sequela. The pathogenic effect of the other lung nematodes has a similar basis but since heavy infections are uncommon, the severity of the lung pathology is usually much less and complications uncommon. (*See also* REINFECTION HUSK IN ADULT CATTLE, p. 917.)

Clinical Findings: The most consistent signs in cattle are tachypnea and coughing. Initially, rapid, shallow breathing is accompanied by a loose husky cough which is exacerbated by exercise. Dyspnea may ensue and heavily infected animals stand with their heads stretched forward, mouths open and drool. The animals become anorectic and rapidly lose condition. Lung sounds are particularly prominent at the level of the bronchial bifurcation. Infected animals are afebrile unless secondary bacterial infection is present.

The signs in sheep and horses infected with *D. filaria* are similar to those in cattle. Pulmonary signs are not usually associated with *M. capillaris* and *P. rufescens* in sheep, though heavy infections are reported to cause unthriftiness. Though pulmonary clinical signs have been described with heavy *Metastrongylus* infections in swine and *D. arnfieldi* in the horse, usually an intermittent husky cough is the only sign. Coughing and dyspnea occur in cats and kittens heavily infected with *A. abstrusus*.

Lesions: In the early prepatent phase of *Dictyocaulus* infections, gross lesions may be absent and the worms may be difficult to see in the bronchioles. By the patent phase plum-colored areas of consolidation are present in the posterodorsal diaphragmatic lung lobes and worms can easily be found by cutting along the bronchi leading to these areas. Interstitial emphysema is a common finding.

The lesions caused by *P. rufescens* in sheep are also found in the dorsal areas of the diaphragmatic lobes. The lesions may be brownish areas of consolidation up to 2 cm in width or smaller, shot-like greenish gray areas of calcification 2 to 3 mm in diameter. Worms may be found in the bronchioles leading to these areas. *M. capillaris* lives in the alveoli and parenchyma and causes the formation of gray nodules under the pleura.

The lesions of *A. abstrusus* are scattered throughout the diaphragmatic lobes of the lung and are yellowish nodules up to 1 cm in diameter. Eggs, larvae and adult worms may be found in the cut surface of a nodule. In horses, lesions are minimal and are usually confined to excess mucus in the bronchi.

Diagnosis: This is made on the evaluation of 4 criteria: clinical signs, epidemiology, the presence of first-stage larvae in the feces and necropsy of animals in the same herd or flock. Larvae will not be found in the feces of pneumonic animals in the prepatent stage of the disease.

First-stage lungworm larvae cannot be recovered using most fecal flotation techniques. The most efficient method for recovering larvae is by a modification of the Baermann technique. A 25-gm fecal sample is wrapped in tissue paper or cheese cloth and suspended or placed in water contained in a tumbler. The water at the bottom of the tumbler is examined for larvae after 4 hours; in heavy infections larvae may be present within 30 minutes. In the early stages of an outbreak, larvae may be few in number or absent.

If an animal is necropsied in the early prepatent phase, worms may not be seen, and microscopic examination by direct smear of the bronchiole mucus may be necessary; in the patent disease the adult lungworms are readily visible in the bronchi, particularly *Dictyocaulus* spp., which are up to 8 cm in length.

Control: Calves should not be pastured with cattle with a recent history of lungworm infection, or placed in pastures recently grazed by infected cattle. Infections usually terminate after approximately 3 months and confer a high level of resistance to subsequent infection. In housed dairy calves the disease is usually the result of such poor husbandry practices as feeding hay from the floor of pens.

Vaccination against the disease is practiced widely in Britain and Northwest Europe. The vaccine is comprised of 2 doses of attenuated (X-irradiated) infective larvae. The vaccine is administered by mouth and the second dose is given from 2 to 5 weeks after the initial dose. The animals are housed during the vaccination procedure and for 2 weeks after the second dose to ensure development of adequate resistance before release to pasture. A similar vaccine is used against *D. filaria* in Southeast Europe.

Those lungworms that require an intermediate host may be controlled by measures designed to eliminate, or to avoid contact with, the intermediate hosts.

Treatment: Several drugs are useful in cattle. Diethylcarbamazine (℞ 235) is highly effective against larval stages (prepatent disease) but not against adults; levamisole (℞ 244) and the newer benzimidazoles, cambendazole (℞ 229), fenbendazole (℞ 238, 239), oxfendazole (℞ 247) and albendazole (℞ 222) are effective against all stages of lungworms and also many of the gastrointestinal helminths, which may cause concurrent infections. All of the latter drugs are effective against lungworms in sheep and pigs, while the newer benzimidazoles are effective against lungworm infections in horses and donkeys. Levamisole and fenbendazole have been used successfully in cats.

Supportive treatment is of value. The animals should be moved to clean pastures or clean well-bedded quarters, and a high level of nutrition maintained.

FLUKE INFECTIONS OF RUMINANTS

Fasciola hepatica, the most important trematode of domestic ruminants, is the commonest cause of liver fluke disease in the U.S.A. and other temperate areas of the world. It is endemic along the

Gulf Coast, the West Coast, the Rocky Mountain Region and other areas. It is present in Eastern Canada, British Columbia and South America. *F. hepatica* is of particular economic importance in the British Isles, Western and Eastern Europe, Australia and New Zealand. *Fasciola gigantica* is economically important in Africa and Asia and has been reported in Hawaii. *Fascioloides magna*, primarily a parasite of North American deer, has been reported to occur in at least 21 states and in Europe. In North America, *Dicrocoelium dendriticum* is confined mainly to New York, New Jersey, Massachusetts and the Atlantic provinces of Canada. It is also found in Europe and Asia.

FASCIOLA HEPATICA
(Common liver fluke)

Etiology: *Fasciola hepatica*, 30-mm long, 12-mm wide and leaf shaped, has a worldwide distribution and a broad host range. Economically important infections occur in cattle and sheep in 3 forms: **chronic,** which is rarely fatal in cattle but often fatal in sheep; **subacute or acute,** primarily in sheep and often fatal; and in conjunction with **"black disease,"** almost exclusive to sheep and usually fatal.

Eggs passed in the feces develop miracidia in about 2 to 4 weeks depending on temperature, and hatch in water. Miracidia infect lymnaeid snails in which development and multiplication occur through the stages of sporocysts, rediae, daughter rediae and cercariae. After about 2 months' development, cercariae emerge from snails and encyst on aquatic vegetation. Encysted cercariae (metacercariae) may remain viable for many months unless exposed to desiccation.

After ingestion by the host, usually with herbage, young flukes are released in the duodenum, penetrate the intestinal wall and enter the peritoneal cavity. The young fluke penetrates the liver capsule and wanders in the parenchyma for several weeks, growing and destroying tissues. It enters a bile duct and matures, beginning to produce eggs about 8 weeks after infection occurred. The prepatent period is usually 2 to 3 months depending on the fluke burden and the adult fluke may live in the bile ducts for years. Prenatal infections have been reported in cattle.

Clinical Findings: Fascioliasis in ruminants ranges in severity from a devastating disease in sheep to an asymptomatic infection in cattle. The course usually is determined by the numbers of metacercariae ingested over a short period. In sheep, acute fascioliasis occurs seasonally and is manifest by a distended, painful abdomen, anemia and sudden death. Deaths can occur within 6 weeks after infection. The acute syndrome must be differentiated from "black disease," infectious necrotic hepatitis (INH, q.v., p. 401). In subacute disease, survival is longer (7 to 10 weeks) even in cases with great damage to livers but deaths occur due to hemorrhages and anemia. Cases of chronic fascioliasis occur in all seasons; signs may include anemia, unthriftiness, submandibular edema and reduced milk secretion, but even heavily infected cattle may not show clinical signs. Heavy chronic infection is fatal in sheep.

Sheep do not appear to develop resistance to infection, and chronic liver damage is cumulative over several years. In cattle, there is evidence of reduced susceptibility following fibrosis of liver tissues and calcification of the bile ducts.

Lesions: Immature, wandering flukes destroy liver tissue and there is hemorrhage. Extensive damage leads to acute fascioliasis in which the liver is enlarged and friable with fibrinous deposits on the capsule. Migratory tracts can be seen and the surface has an uneven appearance. In chronic cases, cirrhosis develops. Mature flukes damage the bile ducts, which become enlarged, even cystic, and have thickened, fibrosed walls. In cattle, cystic ducts are seen and the walls are greatly thickened and often become calcified. Flukes are frequently found in the lungs. Mixed infections with *F. magna* have been reported in cattle.

Tissue destruction by wandering flukes may activate the spores of *Clostridium novyi* (*oedematiens* Type B) and the resulting multiplication of this organism leads to necrotic changes and a fatal toxemia (infectious necrotic hepatitis).

Diagnosis: The eggs, oval, operculated, golden, 130 to 150 μ by 65 to 90 μ, must be distinguished from those of paramphistomes (stomach flukes), which are larger and gray. Eggs of *F. hepatica* cannot be demonstrated in feces during acute fascioliasis. In subacute or chronic disease, the number varies from day to day and repeated fecal examinations, using sedimentation techniques, may be required. At necropsy, the nature of the liver damage is diagnostic. Adult flukes are readily seen in the bile ducts, and immature stages may be squeezed or teased from the cut surface.

Control: Control measures for *F. hepatica* infections are designed to reduce the number of flukes in the host animal and to reduce the snail population in the environment. Routine treatments of livestock in autumn and in late winter are advisable; additional treatments are determined by a knowledge of the local epidemiologic factors. Animals brought into feedlot may require treatment. When drug safety permits, pregnant animals should be treated a few weeks before parturition to ensure that they are not anemic during lactation. Certain products are forbidden in dairy cows.

Older remedies included carbon tetrachloride, hexachlorethane, hexachlorophene, bithionol and Hetol. These compounds had varying degrees of efficacy against adult flukes but treatment was frequently followed by signs of toxicity. More recently a number of compounds have become available such as bromsalans, clioxanide, oxyclozanide, rafoxanide, brotianide, nitroxynil, albendazole and benzenesulfonamides. Some of these compounds (rafoxanide, brotianide and nitroxynil) have increased efficacy against immature and adult flukes.

The selection of a fasciolicide should be based on the disease situation, host animal and local environmental conditions. Contraindications should be observed and use precautions followed. Vaccination of sheep against INH is essential in some countries.

The snail intermediate host may be controlled by drainage of land, by suitable management and by use of molluscicides. The ideal compound would kill snails and their eggs when used in low concentration, and be harmless to mammals and fishes. Routine treatment of an area several times a year may be necessary to achieve adequate control. Copper compounds, sodium pentachlorphenate and Frescon, are the commonly used molluscacides and are very effective if applied correctly.

Suitable management and fencing may be used to exclude grazing animals from snail habitats. Control is complicated by reservoir infections in horses and in wildlife, e.g. deer and rabbits. When sheep and cattle graze together, it is necessary to treat both in a control plan.

FASCIOLA GIGANTICA
(Giant liver fluke)

Fasciola gigantica is similar in shape to *F. hepatica* but is larger (75 mm) with less clearly defined shoulders. It occurs in warmer climates (Asia, Africa) in cattle and buffalo, in which animals it is responsible for chronic fascioliasis, and in sheep, in which the disease is frequently acute and fatal. The life cycle is similar to *F. hepatica* except for species of snail intermediate hosts. The pathology of infection, diagnostic procedures and control measures are similar to those described for *F. hepatica.*

FASCIOLOIDES MAGNA
(Large liver fluke, Giant liver fluke)

Etiology: *Fascioloides magna*, 75-mm long, thick and oval in outline, is distinguished from *Fasciola* spp. by the lack of an anterior projecting cone. It occurs in ruminants, domestic and wild. Deer are probably the normal hosts. The life cycle resembles that of *Fasciola* spp.

Clinical Findings: The life cycle is not completed in cattle. In this host, pathogenicity is low and losses are confined primarily to liver condemnations. In sheep and goats, a few parasites can produce death due to the inability of the host to limit the migration of the flukes in the liver parenchyma.

Lesions: In deer, there is little tissue reaction and the parasites are enclosed in thin fibrous cysts that communicate with bile ducts. In cattle, *F. magna* cause severe tissue reaction resulting in thick-walled encapsulations that do not communicate with bile ducts. In sheep, encapsulations do not develop and the parasites migrate extensively causing tremendous damage. On section, infected livers of cattle, sheep and deer show black tortuous tracts formed by the migrations of young flukes.

Diagnosis: While the eggs of *F. magna* resemble those of *F. hepatica,* this feature is of limited use, as in cattle usually no eggs are passed. Recovery of the parasites at necropsy and differentiation from *F. hepatica* and *F. gigantica* is necessary for definite diagnosis. Where domestic ruminants and deer share the same grazing, the presence of disease due to *F. magna* should be kept in mind. Mixed infections with *F. hepatica* have been reported in cattle.

Control: Little is known of the effects of anthelmintics. Oxyclozanide has been reported effective against *F. magna* in white-tailed deer and rafoxanide has been used successfully against natural infections in cattle. Deer are required for the completion of the life cycle and if they can be excluded from the areas grazed by cattle and sheep, control may be affected. Control of the intermediate host (lymnaeid snails) may be possible once it has been identified in a region and the nature of its habitat examined.

DICROCOELIUM DENDRITICUM

(Lancet fluke, Lesser liver fluke)

Etiology: The lancet fluke is slender and 12 mm long. It has a wide distribution in many countries and will infect a wide range of final hosts including domestic ruminants. Another species, *D. hospes,* is common in Africa. The first intermediate host is a terrestrial snail (*Cionella lubrica* in the U.S.A.) from which cercariae emerge and are aggregated in a mass of sticky mucus (slime-ball). The cercariae are ingested by the second intermediate hosts, which are ants (*Formica fusca* in the U.S.A.), and encyst in their abdominal cavity. One or 2 metacercariae in the subesophageal ganglion of the ant cause abnormal behavior which in turn increases the probability of ingestion by the final host. The young flukes migrate to the liver via the bile duct and begin egg laying, about 10 to 12 weeks after infection.

Clinical Findings and Diagnosis: Clinical signs are not obvious, but in massive infections jaundice may be seen. The eggs are distinctive but are very small (40 μ by 25 μ) and not readily seen upon fecal examination.

Lesions: There does not appear to be any immunity and very heavy infections may accumulate (50,000 flukes in a mature sheep). Cirrhosis occurs and the bile ducts may be thickened and distended. Economic loss is due primarily to condemnation of livers.

Control: The complex life cycle makes an attack on the intermediate hosts difficult unless aggregations of snails and ants can be located and eliminated. Anthelmintics commonly used against *F. hepatica* are not usually effective, but there are reports that Hetolin is very active and that thiabendazole, other benzimidazoles and praziquantel also have efficacy.

EURYTREMA SPP.

(Pancreatic fluke, family Dicrocoeliidae)

Etiology: The fluke is 16-mm long, 6-mm wide and has a thick body. It is a parasite of the pancreatic ducts and occasionally of the bile ducts of sheep, pigs and cattle in Brazil and particularly in Asia. Three species, *E. pancreaticum, E. coelomaticum* and *E. ovis,* are recognized. The first intermediate hosts are terrestrial snails (*Bradybaena* spp.). For the encystment of cercariae second intermediate hosts, grasshoppers (*Conocephalus* spp.) are essential.

Clinical Findings and Diagnosis: There are no obvious clinical signs. *Dicrocoelium*-like eggs can be demonstrated in feces.

Lesions: Light infections cause proliferative inflammation of the pancreatic duct which may become enlarged and occluded. In heavy infections fibrotic, necrotic and degenerative lesions occur. Losses are reported due to condemned pancreas, but the pathogenesis suggests an additional loss of production.

Control: The control of intermediate hosts may not be practical as in the case of *Dicrocoelium*. Treatment with benzimidazoles or praziquantel should be worthy of trial.

PARAMPHISTOMES

(Amphistomes, Stomach flukes, Conical flukes)

Etiology: There are numerous species (*Paramphistomum, Calicophoron, Cotylophoron* spp.) in ruminants in many countries. The adult parasites are pear-shaped, pink or red, up to 15-mm long, attached to the lining of the rumen and reticulum. Immature forms in the duodenum are 1 to 3 mm long. One species, *Gigantocotyle explanatum,* is parasitic in the bile ducts of cattle and buffalo in India.

The life cycle in the snail host resembles that of *Fasciola hepatica,* but the snails commonly infected are planorbids or bulinids. In the ruminant host, the young flukes remain in the small intestine for 3 to 6 weeks before migrating forward to the rumen and reticulum. Eggs are produced 8 to 14 weeks after infection occurs.

Clinical Findings: Adult flukes do not cause overt disease and large numbers may be encountered. The immature worms attach to the duodenal and, at times, the ileal mucosa by means of a large posterior sucker and cause severe enteritis. Affected animals exhibit anorexia, polydipsia, unthriftiness and severe diarrhea. Extensive mortalities may occur especially in young cattle and sheep. Older animals can develop resistance to reinfection but may continue to harbor numerous adult flukes.

Diagnosis: The large, gray, operculated eggs are readily recognized, but in acute paramphistomiasis there may be no eggs in the feces. Examination of the fluid feces in these cases may reveal immature flukes, many of which are passed. Diagnosis is commonly made at necropsy.

Control: The snail hosts may be attacked as described in the control of fascioliasis (q.v., p. 721). The immature flukes in sheep are susceptible to niclosamide, niclofolan and rafoxanide, but resorantel is considered to be the anthelmintic of choice as it is effective against both immature and adult stomach flukes in cattle and sheep.

OPISTHORCHIS FELINEUS

A small, slender fluke 17-mm long, 2-mm wide, parasitic of the bile ducts and pancreatic ducts of cat, dog, fox, pig and man. It is present in North America, Asia and Europe. The miracidium hatches from eggs in the first intermediate host aquatic snail (*Bithynia*) and cercariae develop. They attach to the scales of fish (Cyprinidae), enter the subcutis and become infective.

Clinical Findings and Diagnosis: There are no obvious clinical signs of light infections; ascites, edema and eosinophilia in heavy infections. Operculate eggs 26 by 12 mm containing miracidia can be detected in the feces. Lesions range from slight chronic proliferative inflammation of the bile ducts and pancreatic ducts to fibrosis and biliary cirrhosis with serious necrotic changes in both liver and pancreas.

Control: Control is obtained by prevention of feeding raw fish to dogs. Efficient anthelmintics for both animals and man are niclofolan and particularly praziquantel.

SCHISTOSOMIASIS

(Blood Flukes)

Etiology: Schistosomes are thin elongated flukes, up to 30 mm in length, which live in blood vessels. The female lies in a longitudinal groove of the male. A variety of water snails act as intermediate hosts. Schistosomes pathogenic to domestic animals are widely distributed throughout Africa, the Middle East, Asia and some countries bordering the Mediterranean. In many areas a high percentage of animals are infected and although the majority have low burdens and the infections are asymptomatic, severe outbreaks due to heavy infestation are occasionally reported. Most pathogenic schistosomes are found in the portal and mesenteric blood vessels and the principal clinical signs are associated with passage of the spined eggs through the tissues to the gut lumen. One species, *S. nasale*, is found in the veins of the nasal mucosa, where it causes coryza and dyspnea.

Eggs passed in the feces have to be deposited in water if they are to hatch and release the miracidia. The miracidium then invades a suitable water snail and develops through primary and secondary sporocysts to become cercariae. When fully mature the cercariae leave the snail and swim freely in the water, where they remain viable for several hours. The cercariae invade the final host through the skin and mucous membranes. During penetration the cercariae develop into schistosomula, which are transported via the lymph and blood to their predilection sites. The prepatent period is approximately 6 to 9 weeks.

In southern and central Africa *S. mattheei* is the dominant species, whereas in northern and eastern areas *S. bovis* is more commonly found. The latter parasite also occurs in certain areas of Southern Europe, as well as in the Middle East. In Asia *S. spindale* and *S. japonicum* are widespread. The latter parasite is of particular importance because infected ruminants form a reservoir host for the disease in humans. *S. nasale* occurs in the Indian subcontinent, Malaysia and the Caribbean area.

Clinical Findings: The major clinical signs associated with the intestinal and hepatic forms of schistosomiasis in ruminants develop after the onset of egg excretion and consist of hemorrhagic enteritis, anemia and emaciation. Severely affected animals show rapid deterioration and usually die within a few months of infection, while those less heavily infected develop chronic forms of the disease and may eventually recover. Nasal schistosomiasis is a chronic disease of cattle, horses and occasionally buffaloes. In severe cases there is a copious mucopurulent discharge, snoring and dyspnea but lighter infections are frequently asymptomatic.

Lesions: The intestinal and hepatic forms of schistosomiasis are characterized by the presence of adult flukes in the portal, mesenteric, intestinal submucosal and subserosal veins. The main pathologic effects are, however, associated with the eggs and the granulomas or "pseudotubercles" that form around them, particularly in the liver. Other hepatic changes include medial hypertrophy and hyperplasia of the portal veins, the development of lymphoid nodules and follicles throughout the organ and fibrosis in more chronic cases. Extensive granuloma formation also occurs along the whole alimentary tract but most especially in the small intestine. In severe cases numerous areas of petechiation and diffuse hemorrhage are seen on the mucosa and large quantities of discolored blood may be found in the intestinal lumen. The parasitized blood vessels are frequently dilated and tortuous. Vascular lesions may also be found in the lungs, pancreas and bladder of heavily infected animals.

In nasal schistosomiasis the adult flukes are found in the blood vessels of the nasal mucosa, but again the main pathogenic effects are associated with the eggs. The latter cause abscess formation in the mucosa and they are released into the nasal cavity with the pus following rupture of the abscesses. This eventually leads to extensive fibrosis. In addition large granulomatous growths commonly occur on the nasal mucosa, which occlude the nasal passages and cause dyspnea.

Diagnosis: The clinical history and signs alone are insufficient and it is necessary to identify the eggs in the feces or nasal mucus of affected animals to confirm the condition. Of the terminal spined eggs, S. *bovis* and S. *mattheei* are spindle shaped (150 to 250 μ by 40 to 90 μ), those of S. *spindale* are more elongated and flattened on one side (160 to 400 μ by 70 to 90 μ), while the boomerang-like eggs of S. *nasale* measure 300 to 550 μ by 50 to 80 μ. The oval shaped eggs of S. *japonicum* are relatively small (70 to 100 μ by 50 to 80 μ) with a small lateral spine. In chronic cases of schistosomiasis it may not be possible to find eggs in the feces or nasal mucus and in these cases it is necessary to confirm the diagnosis at postmortem examination by finding adult flukes in the blood vessels.

Control: Control measures for schistosomiasis are rarely practiced on a large scale. The drugs so far developed produce either inconsistent results or have serious side effects. Older remedies include a number of antimonial compounds but great care is required in their use because of their toxicity. More recently a variety of compounds have been shown to have schistosomicidal properties but treatment is generally uneconomic as usually a large number of repeated doses at intervals of 2 to 3 days is required. These newer drugs include stibophen, lucanthone hydrochloride, hycanthone and trichlorfon.

Infection can be reduced by control of the intermediate snail host using molluscacides such as copper sulfate, niclosamide or trifenmorph, or by fencing off infected water bodies and providing clean drinking water. These measures will not only help to reduce the incidence of schistosomiasis but they will also assist in the control of other parasitic trematodes such as *Fasciola gigantica* and *Par-*

amphistomum spp., which similarly have water snails as intermediate hosts and frequently occur in the same localities as schistosomes.

HEPATIC DISTOMATOSIS (SM. AN.)

A slow, inevitably fatal fibrosis of the hepatic duct, due to massive infection with the trematode *Metorchis conjunctus*. The parasite was first recorded in 1934 in dogs in Northern Canada. It has also been reported in South Carolina and the same parasite, or a similar one, has been found occasionally in cats and raccoons in the Northeastern U.S.A. The fluke (*M. conjunctus*) is found in an area extending from the Laurentian Mountains into northern Saskatchewan and in the region south of Hudson Bay. The geographic distribution coincides with that of its 2 intermediate hosts, the snail, *Amnicola limosa porata*, and the suckerfish, *Catostomus commersonii*. Infection of the mammalian host occurs by ingestion of raw fish.

Infected dogs show progressive weakness, ending in complete exhaustion, coma and death. Severe ascites and signs of obstructive jaundice may accompany the infections in cats. The liver is 2 to 3 times normal size. The hepatic duct is distended, thickened and fibrosed, the interlobular connective tissue is hypertrophic. Adult worms may occur in large numbers in the hepatic duct. The diagnosis is made from the presence of the embryonated, operculated eggs in the feces.

All fish fed to dogs in the endemic area should be sterilized by boiling or the equivalent. No specific treatment has been developed.

CESTODES OF DOGS AND CATS IN NORTH AMERICA

Most North American urban dogs and cats eat prepared foods and have restricted access to natural prey. Such dogs may have *Dipylidium caninum*, with its infective stage from the flea, and cats also may have *Dipylidium* sp., although those with access to infected house mice and rats also acquire *Taenia taeniaeformis*. Suburban, rural and hunting dogs have more access to various small mammals and raw meat and offal from domestic and wild ungulates. A number of cestodes can be expected in such dogs (*see* TABLE). On western sheep ranges, and wherever wild ungulates, particularly Cervidae, and wolves are common, dogs may acquire *Echinococcus granulosus*. Sylvatic *E. multilocularis*, previously known only from Arctic North America, now occurs in Midwestern and Western U.S.A. and Canada, but thus far infections in cats or dogs are rare. Humans that

CESTODES OF DOGS AND CATS OF NORTH AMERICA
(In order of their importance)

Name[1]	Definitive Host	Intermediate Host and Organs Invaded[2]	Diagnostic Features of Adult Worm	Remarks
Dipylidium caninum (Double-pored dog tapeworm)	Dog, cat, coyote, wolf, fox and other animals.	Fleas and more rarely lice; free in body cavity.	Strobila 15 to 70 cm in length and up to 3 mm in maximum width. 30 to 150 rostellar hooks of rose-thorn shape in 3 or 4 circles; large hooks 12 to 15 μ, smallest 5 to 6 μ in length. Segments shaped like cucumber seed with pore near middle of each lateral margin.	Probably most common tapeworm of dogs, less common in cats; cosmopolitan. Occasionally infects man, particularly infants.
Taenia taeniaeformis[3]	Cat, dog, lynx, wolf and other animals.	Various rats, mice and other rodents; in large cysts on liver.	Strobila 15 to 60 cm in length, 5 to 6 mm in maximum width. 26 to 52 rostellar hooks in double row; large hooks 380 to 420 μ, small hooks 250 to 270 μ in length. No neck. Sacculate lateral branches of uterus difficult to count.	Common cestode of cats; rare in dogs; cosmopolitan.
Taenia pisiformis	Dog, cat, fox, wolf, coyote, lynx and other animals	Rabbits and hares, rarely squirrels and other rodents; in pelvic cavity or peritoneal cavity attached to viscera.	Strobila 60 cm to 2 m in length, 5 mm in maximum width. Around 34 to 48 rostellar hooks in double row; large hooks 225 to 290 μ, small hooks 132 to 177 μ in length. 5 to 10 lateral branches on each side of gravid uterus.	Particularly common in suburban, farm and hunting dogs, which eat rabbit and rabbit viscera.

Taenia hydatigena	Dog, wolf, coyote, lynx, rarely cat.	Domestic and wild cloven-footed animals, rarely hares and rodents; in liver and abdominal cavity.	Strobila to 5 m in length and 7 mm in maximum width. Around 26 to 44 rostellar hooks in double row; large hooks 170 to 220 μ, small hooks 110 to 160 μ in length. 5 to 10 lateral branches on each side of gravid uterus.	In farm dogs, more rarely hunting dogs; cosmopolitan.
Diphyllobothrium spp.[4]	Man; dog, cat and other fish-eating animals.	Encysted in various organs, or free in body cavity of various fish.	Strobila to 10 m in length and 20 mm in maximum width, but usually smaller. Scolex with 2 grooves (bothria) and no hooks. Genital pores ventral on midline of segment.	Canada; Alaska and various other states of the U.S.A.
Echinococcus granulosus (Hydatid tapeworm)	Dog, wolf, coyote, possibly fox and several other wild carnivores.	Sheep, goats, cattle, swine, horses, deer, moose and some rodents; occasionally man and other animals; commonly in liver and lungs, occasionally in other organs and tissues.	Strobila 2 to 6 mm in length with 3 to 5 segments; 28 to 50, usually 30 to 36, rostellar hooks in double row; large hooks 27 to 40 μ, small hooks 21 to 25 μ in length.	Foci, especially among North American range sheep and dogs associating with them, are known; sylvatic moose-wolf cycle where these animals occur; probably cosmopolitan.
Echinococcus multilocularis (Alveo hydatid tapeworm)	Arctic, red, and gray foxes; coyotes, cat and dog.	Microtine rodents, occasionally in man; in the liver.	Strobila 1.2 to 2.7 mm in length with 2 to 4 segments; along with previous species smallest tapeworm in dogs; 26 to 36 rostellar hooks in double row; large hooks 23 to 29 μ, small hooks 19 to 26 μ.	Alaska and Midwestern U.S.A. and Canada; thus far significant cycle in North American cats and dogs not recognized.

CESTODES OF DOGS AND CATS OF NORTH AMERICA
(In order of their importance)
(*Continued*)

Name[1]	Definitive Host	Intermediate Host and Organs Invaded[2]	Diagnostic Features of Adult Worm	Remarks
Mesocestoides spp.	Many wild canids, felids, mustelids, and other animals including dog and cat.	Complete life history unknown; juvenile tetrathyridia in abdominal cavity and elsewhere of various mammals, birds and reptiles; now known tetrathyridia from body cavity of dogs may enter intestine through intestinal wall.	Strobila 10 cm in length and 2 to 5 mm in width. Scolex with 4 suckers, but no rostellum or hooks. Genital pore ventral in midline of worm. Gravid segments with paruterine organ.	Reported from dog and cat in Midwest and West; in wild animals elsewhere in U.S.A. and Canada.
Taenia multiceps	Dog, wolf, coyote and fox.	Sheep, goats and other domestic or wild ruminants, rarely man; usually in brain and spinal cord.	Strobila 40 to 100 cm in length and 5 mm in maximum width. Scolex with 4 suckers and 22 to 32 hooks in double row; large hooks 150 to 170 μ, small hooks 90 to 130 μ in length. Vagina with reflexed curve near lateral excretory canal. 9 to 26 lateral branches on gravid uterus.	Rare in domestic carnivores in Western North America; more common in wild animals.
Taenia serialis	Coyote, wolf, dog and fox.	Rabbit, hare, squirrel; in subcut. connective tissue, or retroperitoneal, rarely man.	Strobila 20 to 72 cm in length and 3 to 5 mm in width. 26 to 32 hooks in double row; large hooks 110 to 175 μ, small hooks 68 to 120 μ in length. Vagina with reflexed curve near lateral excretory canal. 20 to 25 lateral branches on gravid uterus.	Primarily in wild canids. Considered by some authorities as not distinct from *I. multiceps*.

Taenia crassiceps	Fox, wolf, coyote and dog.	Various rodents and perhaps other animals; subcut. and in body cavities; one record from man.	Strobila 70 to 170 mm in length and 1 to 2 mm in width. Scolex with 30 to 36 hooks in double row; large hooks 126 to 132 μ, small hooks 121 to 140 μ in length. 16 to 21 lateral branches on uterus, sometimes becoming diffuse.	Reported from Canada and Northern U.S.A. including Alaska.
Taenia krabbei	Wolf, coyote, dog and bobcat.	Moose, deer and reindeer; in striated muscle.	Strobila ca. 20 cm in length and 9 mm in maximum width. Scolex small with 26 to 36 hooks in double row; large hooks 146 to 195 μ, small hooks 85 to 141 μ in length. 18 to 24 straight and narrow lateral branches on gravid uterus.	Reported from Canada and Northern U.S.A., including Alaska; considered by some a subspecies of *T. ovis*.
Taenia ovis	Dog, cat (rarely).	Sheep and goat in musculature, but rarely elsewhere.	Strobila 45 to 110 cm in length and 4 to 8.5 mm maximum width. Scolex with 32 to 38 hooks in double row; large hooks 160 to 202 μ in length. 20 to 25 lateral branches on gravid uterus. Vagina crosses ovary on poral side of segment.	Occasionally from farm dogs in Western North America; cosmopolitan.

1 *Taenia polyacantha* recorded rarely from dogs in Alaska is excluded here..

2 In all cases where the life cycle is known, cats and dogs become infected by eating animals, or parts therefrom, which contain the infective metacestode. These intermediate hosts become infected by ingesting tapeworm eggs (except in the case of *Mesocestoides* spp. and *Diphyllobothrium* spp., which have an earlier extra stage), which are passed in the feces of the definitive host.

3 Several other large-hooked *Taenia* spp. occur in the larger wild cats, but most use lagomorphs and ungulates as intermediate hosts, so domestic cats rarely get exposed.

4 Several species of *Diphyllobothrium* have been recorded from North American dogs and cats; they require extensive study before they can be identified with certainty.

CESTODES OF PUBLIC HEALTH IMPORTANCE* **

	Taenia saginata	*Taenia solium*	*Diphyllobothrium* spp.***	*Echinococcus granulosus*	*Echinococcus multilocularis*
Host of adult worm.	Man only.	Man only.	Man; dog, cat and other fish-eating mammals and birds.	Dog, wolf, fox and several other wild carnivores.	Canidae and the domestic cat.
Name or metacestode intermediate.	Cysticercus "beef measles".	Cysticercus "pork measles".	Procercoid in copepod, plerocercoid in fish.	Hydatid cyst.	Multilocular or alveolar "cyst" or hydatid.
Measurements of metacestode.	9 x 5 mm.	6-10 x 5-10 mm.	2 to 25 x 2.5 mm.	Diameter sometimes 150 mm.	Variable, penetrates like neoplastic tissue.
Principal intermediate hosts.	Cattle.	Pig, dog (man may be both definitive and intermediate host).	Copepod first host, then fish.	Sheep, cattle, swine, moose, deer, rarely, dog, cat, man.	Field mice, voles, lemmings, sometimes domestic mammals and man.
Site of metacestode.	Intermuscular connective tissue.	Intermuscular connective tissue. Occasionally, nervous system.	Mesenteric tissues, testes, ovary, muscles.	Commonly in liver and lungs, occasionally in other organs and tissues.	Various organs and tissues.

* *See also* CESTODES OF DOGS AND CATS IN NORTH AMERICA, p. 728.

** Human infections with the metacestodes of *Taenia crassiceps, T. multiceps, T. serialis, Mesocestoides* sp. and other cestodes occur rarely.

*** Since several species of *Diphyllobothrium* infect man in North America, it is no longer advisable to refer to all such infections as due to *D. latum.*

associate with infected dogs may develop metacestodes of *E. granulosus, E. multilocularis, T. multiceps, T. serialis* or *T. crassiceps* in various tissues, or adult *D. caninum* in the gut. The presence of metacestodes in livestock may, furthermore, limit commercial use of such carcasses or offal meats. Generally speaking then, cestodes of dogs and cats are of public health importance.

Adult cestodes in the gut of dogs and cats rarely cause serious disease, and clinical signs if present may depend on the degree of infection, age, condition and breed of host. Signs can vary from unthriftiness, malaise, irritability, capricious appetite and shaggy coat to colic, mild diarrhea, and rarely emaciation and epileptiform fits. Diagnosis is based on finding segments or eggs in the feces. The eggs of *Taenia* spp. and *Echinococcus* spp. cannot be reliably differentiated by microscopic examination.

Treatment and Control: Control of intestinal tapeworms of dogs and cats combines prevention of infection and treatment of infected animals with anthelmintics. Animals that roam freely usually become reinfected with metacestodes available in carrion they find or animals they kill. *D. caninum* is different since it can cycle through fleas that may be associated with confined infected animals.

Arecoline hydrobromide (℞ 224) and arecoline acetarsol (℞ 223) continue to be used against all cestodes in dogs and cats, notwithstanding that they are highly erratic, and frequently produce undesirable side effects. Bunamidine compounds (℞ 200) are effective against mature *Echinococcus* spp. and *Taenia* spp., but they are less effective against immature *Echinococcus* spp., and *Dipylidium* sp.; bunamidine hydrochloride is the more toxic of the two. Niclosamide (℞ 248) and its piperazine salt (℞ 255) are reasonably good against *Taenia* spp. in dogs and cats, but much less effective against *Dipylidium* sp. and *Echinococcus* spp.; vomiting and diarrhea may occur. Dichlorophen (℞ 232) and quinacrine hydrochloride (℞ 356) also are used, although neither is as effective as some of the other drugs listed above.

TICK INFESTATION
(Acariasis)

Ticks are destructive blood-sucking parasites found in most, if not all, countries of the world, but of greater economic significance in tropical and subtropical zones. Infestation generally causes local irritation, resulting in wounds that are susceptible to secondary bacterial infection and screwworm infestation. Heavy tick burdens also result in loss of production of meat, milk, wool and eggs and decreased value of hides. Severe infestation may cause anemia and even death. In some areas and countries, infestation with certain species of ticks requires restriction of movement and export of livestock.

Many ticks transmit serious disease due to protozoa, bacteria, rickettsia and viruses. Various species act not only as vectors but also as reservoirs of a number of diseases in different parts of the world, the most important being babesiosis, anaplasmosis, theileriasis, heartwater, Q fever, Rocky Mountain spotted fever, tularemia, relapsing fever and louping-ill (q.v. INFECTIOUS DISEASES, p. 236 et seq.). Also, tick saliva contains toxins that may cause deleterious effects on the host such as paralysis (q.v. 747) and SWEATING SICKNESS (q.v. 748).

Ticks can survive long periods of starvation depending on environmental conditions. All species suck blood and many, although having a host preference, will feed on a wide range of animals. Ticks are separated taxonomically into 2 families, the Argasidae or "soft ticks" and the Ixodidae or "hard ticks," the latter more important in affecting domestic stock.

The Argasidae usually feed frequently and for relatively short periods of time, lay small batches of eggs following each blood meal and may live for several years. Morphologically, these ticks do not have chitinous plates and sexual dimorphism is slight. The capitulum of the larvae extends anteriorly but, in the nymph and adults, is situated subventrally and generally is not visible dorsally.

The Ixodidae, on the other hand, have chitinous plates and show sexual dimorphism. The scutum of the unengorged female covers a small part of the dorsal surface, whereas in the male the dorsum is almost completely covered by the scutum. The capitulum always extends anteriorly from the body and is visible from above. Females take one large blood meal and die after laying one batch of eggs, while males may feed more than once or not at all and ingest only small quantities of blood at a time.

Life Cycle of Ticks: The whole life cycle, under normal circumstances, usually lasts less than one year, but some 3 host ticks may complete only one life cycle stage a year. There are 3 parasitic stages in the life cycle of argasid and ixodid ticks: the larva, nymph and adult. The larva has 3 pairs of legs compared to 4 pairs in the other stages and may spend the major proportion of its life span away from the host. Once it attaches to a suitable host, it ingests blood or plasma for 3 to 7 days to complete engorgement. From this stage the life cycle differs according to the species.

One-Host Ticks: In these species, e.g. *Boophilus* spp., *Dermacentor albipictus,* the tick remains on the host throughout its entire parasitic life, molting to the nymph and adult on the same host, and leaving the animal only as a replete female.

Two-Host Ticks: In some species, e.g. *Rhipicephalus evertsi,* the larva and nymph both complete this part of the life cycle on the same host, while the adult developing from the nymph attaches to another host.

Three-Host Ticks: In these species the engorged larva drops from the host and molts to the nymph on the ground. The nymph attaches to another animal, not necessarily the same species as the original host, engorges to repletion, again falls to the ground and molts to the adult. This stage attaches to a third host and subsequently, as a fully engorged female, leaves the animal to oviposit. The American dog tick, *Dermacentor variabilis,* is typical of this large group.

In most species of hard ticks, fertilization usually occurs while the female is still attached to the host. The male, once attached to a suitable host, may mate with a number of females. As the larva, nymph and female feed, they increase greatly in size and in some species the replete female may be as much as 300 times the body weight of the unengorged parasite. The male, on the other hand, shows only a small increase in size and weight.

A knowledge of the developmental cycles is essential if we are to apply effectively present methods of control or develop new ones. Since the cattle tick *Boophilus microplus* is an important species infesting cattle and occurs in most of the major cattle-producing countries, its life cycle is outlined below as an example.

The fertilized female tick on repletion falls to the ground and crawls away from light among the surface debris or tussocks of grass. Egg laying may commence in 2 or 3 days and be completed in a week or 10 days during the summer; however, in cooler climates, oviposition may be delayed and extended considerably. The female lays one batch of eggs, *circa* 2,000, and subsequently dies. The eggs are resistant to adverse conditions provided humidity is adequate, but require warmth and humid conditions for hatching. Under laboratory conditions, hatching usually occurs in 14 to 16 days at temperatures around 80°F (28°C) and relative humidity greater than 80%. The adult tick is susceptible to low temperatures and the eggs and larvae to low humidities, consequently the distribution of the parasite is greatly influenced by climatic conditions.

On hatching, the larvae or "seed" ticks climb to the tip of the grass stalks or other vertical objects to await a passing animal. High atmospheric humidity is the most important factor favoring survival of the larvae during this nonparasitic stage; the other limiting factor is the food supply in its unengorged state. Although most die within 90 days, some may survive for about 180 days on pasture, depending on environmental conditions.

Once the larva reaches a suitable host, it attaches to commence the parasitic part of the life cycle (to replete female) on the one host, a period of 19 to 28 days. The nymphs appear by about the 6th day and the adults emerge by the 13th to 15th day. Fertilization takes place soon after the molt and is necessary before the female is able to complete engorgement. The female on repletion falls to the ground and in a few days, under favorable conditions, oviposits to initiate the nonparasitic stage of the cycle.

In general, the life cycle of the Argasidae differs from that of the "hard ticks," most argasids being multi-host ticks. Larvae may require several days and even up to 30 days for engorgement, but nymphs and adults attach for short periods of time, usually less than one hour. Nymphs molt after each meal and some species have a number of nymphal stages before becoming adults. Females feed many times leaving the host after each ingestion to lay small batches of eggs. *Otobius megnini* is an exception in that the larva and nymph remain on the one host and the adult stages do not feed.

Feeding Habits: Ticks may be found attached to most parts of the body, but the most favored sites are the escutcheon, neck, shoulders and head. A number of species attach only or predominantly in the ears of cattle and horses, these being *Otobius megnini,* the spinose ear tick; *Dermacentor (Anocentor) nitens,* the tropical horse tick; *Amblyomma maculatum,* the Gulf Coast tick; and *Rhipicephalus evertsi,* the red-legged tick.

Generally, the immature stages require 4 to 7 days for engorgement, whereas the females remain attached for 7 to 14 days and even longer. The males usually take small blood meals from time to time and may remain on the same host for weeks. In some species, the larvae and nymphs feed on small mammals or birds, and only the adults are found on livestock.

During feeding, salivary secretion is injected into the host and the salivary glands remove excess fluid from the blood meal. Some animals develop a local allergic response to the salivary gland secretion and this local reaction may limit or completely prevent tick infestation. This phenomenon appears to be better developed in the *Bos indicus* group of cattle and, in general, these animals carry substantially lower burdens especially of one-host ticks.

IMPORTANT IXODIDAE

Amblyomma americanum, the lone star tick, is abundant in the Southern U.S.A. from Texas north to Missouri, and eastward to the Atlantic Coast. It also occurs in Mexico, Central and South America. A 3-host tick in which all stages attach to both domestic and wild animals and man, it is active from early spring to late fall. All stages of development are polyhostal. It is capable of transmitting tularemia, Rocky Mountain spotted fever and Q fever to man, and may produce tick paralysis in man and dogs. The scutum of the male has sparse pale markings, while that of the female has a conspicuous silvery white spot near the posterior end. Ticks prefer the more sparsely haired parts of the body and the wounds produced predispose livestock to attack by the screwworm fly, *Cochliomyia hominivorax.*

Amblyomma maculatum, the Gulf Coast tick, is also an important pest of livestock, particularly cattle, in the U.S.A., being found in those states bordering the Gulf of Mexico, north into Arkansas and Oklahoma, and along the Atlantic Coast to South Carolina, Georgia and Florida. This tick also occurs in Central and South America. It is a 3-host tick, the larvae and nymphs generally feeding on birds and small mammals, while the adult stages attack cattle, deer, horses, sheep, pigs and dogs. Livestock are infested principally during the late summer and early fall, but dry summer conditions may delay the seasonal occurrence of this tick. It prefers areas of high rainfall and temperature and is seldom found in large numbers away from the coastal areas. It is dark brown and the scutum of both sexes is ornate, being freely marked with silver lines and spots. Adults tend to attach to the inside of the outer ear, producing an intense inflammation and predispose the ear to attack by the screwworm fly. They also attack the hump region of Brahman cattle and sometimes feed along the top of the neck of all breeds, causing marked irritation where they feed in clusters.

Amblyomma cajennense, the Cayenne tick, is found only in southern Texas in the U.S.A. but is a pest of considerable importance in tropical Central and South America and Mexico. It is a 3-host tick, all stages attacking livestock, deer, dogs, man and a variety of wild animals. It is active throughout the whole year, and is a known vector of Rocky Mountain spotted fever. Adult ticks prefer to attach between the legs and on the abdomen but may be found anywhere.

Amblyomma hebraeum, the bont tick, is found primarily in the Republic of South Africa, Rhodesia and parts of Mozambique and Botswana. It is a 3-host tick and all stages are found on a variety of domestic and wild animals, although adults prefer cattle and antelope. The immature stages also feed on birds, small mammals and reptiles. Adults are most abundant on hosts during the late summer and autumn months and thrive best in a warm, moderately humid climate. Adults prefer bare areas of the body and the long mouth parts produce painful wounds which predispose to bacterial infections and infestation with blowfly larvae. This species is a vector of heartwater in ruminants.

Amblyomma variegatum, the tropical bont tick, is widely distributed in Eastern, Central and Western Africa. It is a 3-host tick; the larvae prefer smaller mammals and birds, but will feed on cattle, sheep, horses, goats, camels and a wide variety of wild mammals, the common hosts for the adult stage. Adults increase in numbers and these remain high during the rainy season but decrease during the dry season when larvae and nymphs are most abundant. Adult ticks prefer the lower parts of the body, under the tail and external genitalia. The scutum is ornate with brightly colored patterns and the legs have white bands. It is a known vector of the virus of

Nairobi sheep disease and transmits the rickettsia causing heartwater in ruminants.

Several other species of *Amblyomma*, namely *A. gemma*, *A. pomposum* and *A. lepidum*, are also economically important ticks on the African continent.

Boophilus is one of the most important genera of ticks affecting domestic stock throughout the world. *B. annulatus*, the North American cattle tick, has been eradicated from the U.S.A. but still exists in the drier parts of Mexico. *B. microplus*, the tropical cattle tick (q.v., p. 735), is widely distributed and has been recorded from Australia, Central and South America, Asia and South Africa. *B. decoloratus*, the blue tick of Africa, and *B. calcaratus*, the cattle tick of North Africa, have been recorded from the African continent. These ticks are predominantly parasites of domestic and wild ungulates, particularly cattle and horses, but may also be found on sheep, goats, pigs and dogs. Ticks are found on most parts of the body and are most prevalent in the warmer months of the year. All are involved in the transmission of babesiosis or tick fever of cattle.

Dermacentor andersoni (*venustus*), the Rocky Mountain wood tick, is found in Western and Northwestern U.S.A. and Canada. It is a 3-host tick with the larvae and nymphs feeding primarily on small mammals while the important hosts for the adult include cattle, horses, sheep, dogs, man and other large mammals. The immature stages are generally found around the head, neck and shoulders of the hosts while adults prefer similar sites, but also the groin and escutcheon. Ticks survive over winter as nymphs or adults. Adults reach maximum numbers during April and May, but may be found from February to July. Nymphs appear early in April and larvae early June. This species has an unusually long life cycle, frequently requiring 2 or 3 years to develop to maturity, especially in colder climates. Ticks are reddish brown. The male scutum is beautifully marked with white or silver while that of the female is almost solidly silver-colored and contrasts markedly with the red-brown of the dorsal surface. This is the most important parasite of Northwestern U.S.A. and is the vector of Rocky Mountain spotted fever, tularemia, Q Fever and Colorado tick fever of man. It is also the chief cause of tick paralysis of man and animals.

Dermacentor variabilis, the American dog tick, is widely distributed over the eastern half of the U.S.A., parts of Western U.S.A., Canada and Mexico. It is a 3-host tick with the immature stages attacking largely small rodents. The common hosts for the adult stage include dogs, cattle, horses, man and most other wild and domesticated mammals. In the Southern U.S.A., all stages may be found on their respective hosts throughout the year, but are generally more abundant in the spring. In more temperate climates, adults are found between April and September being most prevalent in June. In heavy infestations, parasites may be found over all parts of the body, but preferred sites are the neck, axillae, groin, escutcheon and lower body surfaces. The adults are reddish brown, being similar to *D. andersoni*, but have a different geographical distribution. The tick is the most important vector of Rocky Mountain spotted fever in the Eastern U.S.A. and also transmits tularemia. It is an annoying pest of livestock and can also produce paralysis in man and animals.

Dermacentor albipictus, the winter tick (shingle tick), is an important pest of stock in the Northern and Western U.S.A., Canada and northern parts of Mexico. It is a one-host tick, being parasitic on deer, moose, elk, horses and cattle. Heavy burdens inflict severe losses among wild ruminants and range horses and cattle. The ticks prefer the lower parts of the body, especially the dewlap and brisket, but in severe infestations may occur over the entire body causing depression, inappetence, lusterless hair coat, general debilitation and even edema from jaws to flanks. This tick is unusual in that it attacks animals from autumn until early spring. On livestock, the parasitic period ranges from about 28 to 60 days when the replete females drop to the ground and surviving over winter, deposit their eggs the following spring. The eggs hatch in 3 to 6 weeks, but the larvae remain clustered tightly together throughout the summer and do not attach to hosts until the cool weather in the late fall.

Dermacentor nigrolineatus, the brown winter tick, is widely distributed throughout the eastern half of the U.S.A., especially in the Southeast and also in southwestern Texas and New Mexico. It is closely related to *D. albipictus*. The preferred host is the white-tailed deer, but horses and cattle are frequently attacked. It is a one-host tick, occurring on animals only during the fall, winter and early spring.

Dermacentor occidentalis, the Pacific Coast tick, is confined to the Pacific Coast area, from Oregon to Lower California. It is a 3-host tick, the immature stages feeding primarily on a number of small mammals while the common hosts for the adult stage include cattle, horses, deer, sheep, dog and man. Ticks may be found distributed over the body of the host without any obvious site preference. Adults may be found throughout the year, but reach their peak of abundance in April and May during the rainy season. The immature stages are most prevalent in the spring and summer. This tick has been found naturally infected with the virus of Colorado tick fever and the rickettsia of Q fever and is probably implicated in the spread of bovine anaplasmosis.

Dermacentor (Anocentor) nitens, the tropical horse tick, has been found in the U.S.A. only in southern Florida and southern Texas, but is common in Mexico, Central America, the West Indies and the northern parts of South America. A one-host tick, the preferred hosts are domesticated Equidae, but it occurs also on cattle, deer, sheep and goats. The parasitic period on the host varies between 26 and 41 days. All stages may be recovered throughout the year in endemic areas. The preferred site of attachment for all stages is the ear, but ticks may be found on all parts of the body in heavy infestations. This is a serious pest of horses in tropical and subtropical areas and heavy burdens on the ears predispose to attack by the screwworm. It is a vector of *Babesia caballi*, of Equidae.

Dermacentor reticulatus occurs in Asia and southern Europe being parasitic on many domestic and wild mammals. It is a 3-host tick and is involved in the transmission of the protozoa, *Babesia caballi* in the horse and *B. canis* in the dog.

Haemaphysalis leachi leachi, the yellow dog tick, is found primarily on dogs and larger wild carnivores in Africa and Asia. It is a 3-host tick being most abundant during the warmer months of the year. It is the principal vector of *Babesia canis* of dogs in South Africa.

Haemaphysalis longicornis, the New Zealand cattle tick, occurs primarily on cattle in parts of New Zealand, Australia and Japan. Horses, dogs, sheep and various wild mammals may also act as hosts. It is a 3-host tick, being most abundant in the spring and early summer. The male is nonfunctional and the female produces parthenogenetically. Ticks occur on all parts of the body, especially the escutcheon, head and neck regions. It is a vector of *Theileria mutans*, a small blood protozoan of cattle. *H. bispinosa*, a closely related species, occurs in India, Sri Lanka, China and Southeast Asia, and is recorded as a vector of *Babesia gibsoni* of dogs in India.

Haemaphysalis cinnabarina punctata occurs on cattle and other mammals in Europe, Asia, Japan and North Africa. Larvae and nymphs are also found on reptiles, birds and small mammals. This species has been implicated in the transmission of *Babesia bigemina*, *Anaplasma marginale* and *A. centrale* in cattle and *B. motasi* in sheep and goats.

There is much confusion relating to the various species of *Hyalomma*. These are probably the most important parasites of domestic animals in Southern Europe, the Middle East, Northern Africa and from the Southern U.S.S.R. to India. The principal species are *H. excavatum*, *H. marginatum*, *H. detritum*, *H. scupense*, *H. detritum mauritanicum* and *H. dromedarii*. They are usually 2-host ticks though some species may use 3 hosts. *Hyalomma* spp. are vectors of *Babesia caballi*, *B. equi*, *Theileria annulata*, *T. dispar* in horses and cattle.

Ixodes ricinus, the "castor-bean" tick, is common in most of Europe and is found also in North Africa and limited areas of Asia. It is a 3-host tick with the adult stages being recovered from dogs, sheep and cattle and many other mammals. The larvae and nymphs are found largely on birds, small mammals and lizards. This species usually has a long life cycle extending over a period of 3 years. Ticks tend to feed largely in the spring-summer and are found predominantly on the face, ears, axillae and the inguinal region. This species transmits *Babesia divergens*, *B. bovis* and *Anaplasma marginale* in cattle, louping ill, rickettsial tick borne fever of sheep and CTE in man.

Ixodes rubicundus, the paralysis tick of South Africa, is confined to specific mountainous wet areas. It is a 3-host tick, adults being taken from sheep, cattle, goats and a number of a wild animals, especially during the autumn. Predilection sites are the ventral body surfaces and the legs. Immature stages feed chiefly on small mammals and wild Canidae, being most prevalent during the same period as the adults. Paralysis occurs usually during this period of peak activity.

Ixodes holocyclus, the paralysis tick of Australia, is confined largely to scrub country of the northern and eastern coasts. It is a 3-host tick, occurring largely on dogs, domestic stock, man and native fauna, particularly the bandicoot. It is most prevalent during the spring and summer. A single female tick attached for several days can cause paralysis and death.

Ixodes canisuga is often called the British dog tick and has been recovered from the dog, sheep and the horse. It can become a serious pest in dog kennels.

A number of other species of *Ixodes* occur throughout the world and of these *I. scapularis*, *I. cookei* and *I. pacificus* are pests of domestic stock and dogs on the North American continent.

Rhipicephalus appendiculatus, the brown ear tick, is widely distributed in parts of Southern, Central and Eastern Africa. This is primarily a tick of cattle, but is also recorded from other ruminants, horse and dog. It is a 3-host tick and although the immature stages occur on small mammals, they are also found on the larger mammalian host. Adults are most abundant in the spring-summer period while the immature stages occur earlier. The ear is the predilection site although in heavy infestations, ticks may be found on the head, neck, abdomen and genitalia. This species is the most important vector of *Theileria parva*, the cause of East Coast Fever. Other protozoa transmitted by this tick include *T. lawrencei*, *T. mutans* and *Babesia bigemina*, while it is also a known vector of Nairobi sheep disease and Kisenyi sheep disease.

Rhipicephalus evertsi, the red-legged tick, is widely distributed in parts of central and southern Africa. The adult tick is found primarily on cattle, goats, sheep and Equidae and a number of wild mammals. It is a 2-host tick and the immature stages also feed on small mammals. Adults preferably attach to the peri-anal region under the base of the tail, groin and scrotum. This tick is most active in the summer but can occur throughout the whole year. This tick is known to transmit *Babesia bigemina*, *B. equi*, *Theileria parva*, *T. mutans*, *T. ovis*, *Ehrlichia ovina* and *Borrelia theileri*.

Rhipicephalus bursa is widely distributed in southern Europe and Africa and is found primarily on horses, sheep and cattle. It is a vector of a number of protozoan infections, rickettsia and the virus of Nairobi sheep disease. It is a known vector of *Babesia ovis* and *Theileria ovis* of sheep, *B. equi* and *B. caballi* of horses, *B. berbera* (*B. bovis*) and *Anaplasma marginale* of cattle.

Rhipicephalus sanguineus, the brown dog tick, is probably the most widely distributed species of tick in the world and is found throughout the tropical and temperate parts of the world. In North America it is found primarily on dogs and is generally associated with kennels. It is a 3-host tick and adults have also been found on a wide variety of animal hosts besides the dog. It is found throughout the year in tropical areas but in temperate areas it is most abundant between spring and autumn. This tick transmits *Babesia canis* and has been implicated in the transmission of a number of protozoal, viral and rickettsial infections of domestic stock and man.

IMPORTANT ARGASIDAE

Argas persicus, the fowl tick, is widely distributed throughout tropical and the warm-temperature zones of the world. It was a severe pest of poultry in Southwestern U.S.A. and is still a problem in Asia and Africa. It is a complex of closely related but distinct species, occurring predominantly in domestic and wild birds. It is found in greatest abundance during the warmer and drier seasons of the year and attaches primarily beneath the wings and the more sparsely feathered parts of the body. Nymphs and adults attach only briefly, usually at night. Heavy infestations may result in paralysis and death through exsanguination while lower burdens may result in loss of production. This species is the chief vector of the spirochaete, *Borrelia anserina*, and the blood protozoan, *Aegyptianella pullorum*.

Ornithodoros coriaceus, the pajarello tick, is found in California and the west coast of Mexico. This is a multihost tick feeding primarily on cattle and deer, although man and other animals may serve as hosts. The larval stages may remain attached for some 10 to 20 days before repletion, whereas nymphs and adults engorge in 15 to 30 minutes. Adults may survive for 3 to 5 years. It is not known to transmit disease but the bite is reported to be very painful.

Ornithodoros erraticus of northern Africa, Portugal, Spain and the Middle East is primarily of importance in man, but it is possibly a vector of *Babesia* spp. and African swine fever. *Nuttallia danii* has been transmitted experimentally.

Ornithodoros moubata, a species complex of Africa, is an important vector of African relapsing fever in man. This species feeds on man and a variety of wild and domestic animals and in certain parts of southwest Africa is troublesome on sheep.

Ornithodoros savignyi of Africa and Asia and *O. tholozani* of

Central Asia are important reservoirs and vectors of disease producing organisms of man.

Ornithodoros turicata, the relapsing fever tick, and *O. talaje* have been taken occasionally from domestic animals in the southwestern areas of the U.S.A. and Florida. The primary hosts are various species of rodents. Both species also occur in Mexico and the latter also in South America. Although they are not known to be vectors of diseases of livestock, they are important vectors of relapsing fever in man.

Otobius megnini, the spinose ear tick, is a common and important pest in the Southwestern and Western U.S.A., Mexico, Central and South America, Africa and India. It is primarily a parasite of livestock, particularly cattle and horses, although other domestic and wild animals also serve as hosts. The larval and nymphal stages are found in the ears and may remain attached for several months, causing pain, irritation, lopped ears and a foul smelling discharge of wax and tick debris. The nymph is readily identified by the violin-like body and the spines on the integument. The adult is nonparasitic. It is not known to transmit disease but infestation predisposes to screwworm or other maggot attack.

Clinical Findings: Most animals tolerate a few ticks, but become irritated and restless as the numbers increase, and set about to rid themselves of the pests by rubbing, scratching, licking and biting. These efforts, in turn, usually aggravate the situation, leading to the development of irritated or raw areas, which may become secondarily infected.

In large numbers all species will produce anemia. The toxins in the saliva cause irritation at the site of the bite and, in some species at least, systemic effects such as weight loss, inappetence, lethargy or paralysis.

The first evidence of the presence of ticks on small animals usually is the effort of the animal to dislodge them. Ticks in the ear canal cause great distress, often leading to almost hysterical activities of the animal. Head shaking, crying, scratching and inappetence are common signs seen in small animals.

Diagnosis: Frequent sites of tick attachment are the ears, neck, flanks and the interdigital spaces, but ticks can be found over the entire body surface. Ticks, particularly the soft tick, *O. megnini*, frequently are deep in the ear canal and may be located only by the use of an otoscope. Since all 3 stages of ixodid and most argasid ticks may occur on the animal, the size of the tick may vary from that of the tiny larva ("seed tick") to that of the engorged female, generally 0.5 cm or more in length, although some species, *D. andersoni* and *H. dromedarii*, may measure up to 2 cm in length.

Control: Climate and predators afford natural control of ticks. All the ixodid ticks are susceptible to lack of moisture and the geographical distribution of many species is largely controlled by environmental temperature. Predators including birds, rodents and ants, in some areas, play an important role in reducing pasture contamination. Rotation of pastures, especially when combined with chemical treatment, can also reduce infestation of stock. Techniques involving rotation of pastures are especially applicable to the control of one-host ticks where the nonparasitic larval stages are susceptible to the effects of the environment. Various breeds of cattle, especially *Bos indicus* cattle, appear to develop resistance to ticks and through carrying lower tick burdens reduce pasture contamination. The crossing of *Bos indicus* and *Bos taurus* cattle will produce progeny which are generally more tick resistant than the *Bos taurus* parent.

Chemical Control: The most effective method of control is through the appropriate use of chemical pesticides or acaricides. A large number of these are effective against ticks, but in some places various species and strains within a species have become resistant to the recommended levels of some insecticides. The incidence of strains resistant to one or a number of insecticides is increasing but fortunately newer classes of insecticides are effective against these resistant strains. Insecticides may be used as sprays, dips, dusts, aerosols, smears or systemics, but such preparations must be used in such a way to keep residues in food-producing animals to an acceptable level. When only a few ticks are present on an animal, they may be removed manually. Care should be taken to insure that the mouthparts are not broken and left embedded in the host. Most of the irritated areas heal rapidly, with little attention, once the tick is removed properly. Larvae are easily overlooked because of their small size, and treatment of the entire animal best effects their removal.

Ticks on livestock: The control of ticks on livestock is usually a matter of herd or flock treatment, but the same treatment can be applied to individual animals. Ear ticks may be removed from the ear canal manually, but this is usually more difficult and laborious than spraying, dipping or squirt-can treatment.

Although many acaricides are effective in reducing tick populations, a number of them leave undesirable residues in meat or milk. Because no residues of acaricidal agents in milk are tolerated under the requirements of the United States Food and Drug Administration, and only minimal specified residues are permitted in the fat of meat-producing animals, the earlier approval of some materials has been suspended.

In the U.S.A., arsenic (As_2O_3) at 0.175 to 0.19% concentration in solution; pyrethrins plus synergists at 0.1 and 1.0%, respectively, as a wet spray, or 1.0 and 10.0%, respectively, as a mist spray; rotenone, 2 to 4 oz of 5% derris powder per gal. of water; or crotoxyphos at 0.1 to 0.3% in water; have been suggested for tick control on lactating dairy cattle to conform to government restrictions. Current regulations and label directions should always be consulted since these vary from time to time and from country to country.

For control of ticks on beef cattle, horses, sheep, goats and hogs, lindane at 0.025 to 0.03%, dioxathion at 0.15%, toxaphene and/or malathion at 0.5%, ronnel at 0.75%, coumaphos at 0.25 to 0.5% concentrations have been suggested. Toxaphene, lindane, dioxathion and coumaphos are usually recommended as dips. In dipping sheep and goats, the concentration of toxaphene and of coumaphos may be reduced to 0.25 to 0.3%. The 0.5% concentration, for safety, must be restricted to adult cattle, horses and hogs. The recommendations for dairy cattle may also be used for the other species.

Solutions, emulsions or suspensions may be used as dips or sprays. Regardless of the material or method used, it is of prime importance that a uniform dispersion of the acaricide be maintained to avoid erratic dosage and possible poisoning of the animals.

In spraying livestock, freshly mixed dispersions are used and, in a power sprayer, the agitator helps to keep the spray at a uniform concentration. For dips, large quantities of acaricide are used to charge the vat and the dip frequently is re-used over a period of months. It is difficult to stir dipping vats thoroughly and there is the further hazard that the dip may deteriorate on standing, with the result that cattle may be improperly treated. Therefore, although properly dispersed dips are as safe as sprays, there generally is less risk of injuring livestock if spray treatments are employed.

Dips maintained at proper strength are usually more effective than sprays. However, sprays applied thoroughly also give good control. Sprays may be applied at any desired pressure, there being little if any difference in the effectiveness as long as the hair is thoroughly wetted. High-pressure sprays (200 to 400 lb/sq in.) penetrate more uniformly and rapidly and, therefore, are generally preferred.

In addition to dips and sprays, direct application into the ear is often used against ear ticks. Low-pressure sprays of toxaphene at 0.5% concentration may be directed into the ears. Squirt-type oil cans or syringes may be used for the same purpose, with any preparation containing 0.5% of lindane or toxaphene. Ronnel, coumaphos or malathion may be used in the same manner. Repetition of these treatments is usually required, according to the degree of infestation.

In other parts of the world where ticks are of considerable economic significance, a number of newer acaricides have been registered for commercial use particularly against the cattle tick, *Boophilus* spp. Some of the chemicals belonging to these newer classes are: chlordimeform, clenpyrin, chlormethiuron and amitraz. Many of the older acaricides still provide adequate control when used appropriately but, where resistance to the organophosphorus compounds occurs, the use of other classes of chemical is generally recommended. Synthetic pyrethroids are showing promise against resistant strains and will probably be used, mixed with other compounds, in the future.

Ticks on small animals: Dogs may be freed of ticks by treating them with an acaricide. Washes are usually more effective than sprays or dusts as they penetrate the hair better and reach all the ticks. A wash or spray should contain one of: 0.5% of malathion, or 0.05% of lindane or rotenone. Delnav has shown excellent capacity for tick control on dogs and cats when used at concentrations of 0.15 to 0.25%. If a dip is preferred (immersing the dog except for the head), one-half these concentrations should be used. If a dust is preferred, products containing 5% carbaryl, 1% lindane, 4 or 5% malathion, or 3 to 5% rotenone (derris or cube powder) are available. Lindane should not be used on cats. Dichlorvos in collars and as a topical application is also useful.

Pyrethrins (℞ 308), with or without synergizing compounds, are effective tick killers, but have practically no residual activity and in general are comparatively expensive.

Always consult and follow label instructions.

Premises: To avoid reinfestation, houses, barns and kennels may be cleared of ticks, including the brown dog tick, by application of the following: diazinon, dichlorvos, or lindane as 0.5% sprays; malathion as a 2 to 3% spray or 4 to 5% dust; chlordane as a 2 to 3% spray or 5 to 6% dust. These materials should be used on limited areas only, and all possible hiding places should be painted, sprayed, or dusted. Food, water, dishes, or utensils should not be contaminated. Children or pets must not be allowed in treated areas until the acaricide has had time to be effective and the excess chemical has been removed.

Treatment of premises should always be supplemented by treating all animals including the farm dog with a product labeled for such use.

Cautions: The preparations used for tick control may be toxic to man and animals if contacted or ingested in sufficient quantities (*see* TOXICITY OF ORGANIC INSECTICIDES AND ACARICIDES, p. 995) and should be used with due regard for this fact. Manufacturers are careful to recommend their products within specified limitations. In all cases, the recommendation of the manufacturer, as stated on the label, together with precautions on the label, should be followed to the letter. Products must be plainly labeled for animal use. If only plant recommendations appear on the label, then the product must not be used on animals regardless of the circumstances. Home-devised mixtures of various acaricidal agents and additions of detergents to liquid preparations must not be used.

Most acaricides and insecticides are toxic to fish and quantities of these materials should not be allowed to enter streams or ponds.

TICK PARALYSIS

A flaccid, afebrile ascending motor paralysis in domestic and wild animals and man, produced by a neurotoxin generated by some but not all strains of certain species of ticks. Not all infested animals become paralyzed. Pyrexia may precede the clinical syndrome.

Etiology: Although the disease has a worldwide distribution, the species responsible have not been identified in all countries. The incidence largely depends upon the seasonal activity of the transmitting ticks. Important species are: in Australia (*Ixodes holocyclus*), the U.S.A. (*Dermacentor andersoni, D. variabilis*, and possibly *Amblyomma maculatum* and *A. americanum*), Canada (*D. andersoni*), Bulgaria (*Haemaphysalis inermis, H. punctata*), Yugoslavia (*H. punctata, Hyalomma detritum* [*scupense*]), and South Africa (*Rhipicephalus evertsi*). The incidence is highest in spring and summer. In European and Asian U.S.S.R. (*Ornithodoros lahorensis*), Yugoslavia and Crete (*I. ricinus*) and South Africa (*I. rubicundus*), the incidence is highest in autumn and winter. Eleven other ixodid species may be responsible for sporadic cases in animals and man. *Argas persicus* causes paralysis in poultry in South Africa, the U.S.A. and Turkey.

Sheep, dogs and humans appear to be particularly susceptible, one tick frequently being capable of causing complete paralysis. Before the application of effective prophylactic measures in 1958, the annual losses were estimated at several thousand sheep in South Africa. During the last 6 decades more than 400 human cases have been recorded, from Canada (250), U.S.A. (123) and Australia (30), and of these 9% died. Prompt removal of ticks undoubtedly saved many lives. Severe outbreaks with considerable losses of cattle have occurred in Montana and British Columbia. The disease has also been produced experimentally in marmots, guinea pigs, hamsters and other animals.

It is generally accepted that tick paralysis is caused by a neurotoxin produced by the female during feeding because males of some species do not feed on the host; however, adult males of *D. andersoni* (Canada), *Hyalomma truncatum* and *Rhipicephalus simus* (South Africa) have been responsible for tick paralysis in humans.

Clinical Findings: The onset is gradual, paralysis first becoming evident as an incoordination in the hind limbs resulting in an unsteady gait. Reflexes are lost, but sensation may be present. The paralysis ascends over a period of 1 to 2 days from its onset, at the end of which time the victim may be completely immobilized. Further advance results in respiratory failure and death. Immunity is of short duration; reinfestation 14 days after recovery may result in another attack.

Lesions: Generally there is only local irritation at the site of tick bite, with no pathologic changes. However, in South Africa tick paralysis is accompanied by edema of the lungs, hyperemia of the meninges, enlargement of lymph nodes and atrophy of the spleen.

Diagnosis: Tick paralysis in livestock, due to its general appearance, may be mistaken for plant or pesticide poisoning. Full consideration should be given to the fact that the signs do not appear until the tick has been attached and feeding for about 6 days. It also is noteworthy that in livestock, ticks frequently attach themselves in the regions of the head. In humans, any covered portion of the body may provide a site for attachment.

Prophylaxis and Treatment: If possible, tick-infested areas should be avoided during the tick season. Tick-infested animals should be treated with a suitable locally available acaracide. In South Africa experiments have shown that topical application of one of the following compounds protect sheep for a month or more: quinthiaphos (0.03%), chlorfervinphos (0.05%) and camphechlor (0.25%). Prompt treatment or removal of the ticks by hand will check an outbreak. In the U.S.A., if all ticks are removed, signs normally disappear within a few hours with no observable after effects. Tick paralysis in other countries frequently does not disappear after removal of the ticks and, in some cases, paralysis does not develop until after the tick has dropped off on completing its engorgement. In Australia a hyperimmune serum is used to treat humans and dogs affected with paralysis caused by *Ixodes holocyclus*.

Humans frequenting infested areas should wear close-fitting garments of a smooth, tight texture, and tucked-in trousers and shirts. Clothing and the body should be examined daily for ticks. Excellent protection against ticks can be obtained by spraying clothing with insect repellents, such as diethyltoluamide or ethylhexanediol.

SWEATING SICKNESS

An acute, febrile, tick-borne toxicosis characterized mainly by a profuse, moist eczema and hyperemia of the visible mucous membranes. It is essentially a disease of young calves, but adults are not entirely immune. Sheep, pigs, goats and a dog have been infected experimentally. It occurs in East, Central and Southern Africa, and probably in Ceylon and Southern India.

Etiology: The cause is a toxin produced by certain strains of *Hyalomma truncatum* (*transiens*). The toxin develops in the tick, not in the vertebrate host. It is retained by ticks for 20 generations, and possibly more. Attempted experimental transmissions between affected and normal animals by contact or inoculations of blood have been successful.

Graded periods of infestation of a susceptible host by "infected" ticks have different effects on the host. A very short period has no effect; the animal remains susceptible. A period just long enough to produce a reaction may confer an immunity, but if the exposure is prolonged more than 5 days, severe clinical signs and death may result. Recovery confers an immunity, which lasts up to 13 months.

Clinical Findings: After an incubation period of 4 to 11 days, signs appear suddenly and include hyperthermia, anorexia, listlessness, watering of the eyes and nose, hyperemia of the visible mucous membranes, salivation, necrosis of the oral mucosa and hyperesthesia (as in heartwater, q.v., p. 435). Later, the eyelids stick together. The skin feels hot and a moist dermatitis soon develops, starting from the base of the ears, the axilla, groin and perineum, and extending over the entire body. The hair becomes matted and beads of moisture may be seen on it. The skin becomes extremely sensitive and emits a sour odor. Later the hair and epidermis can be readily pulled off, exposing red, raw wounds. The tips of the ears and the tail may slough away. Eventually the skin becomes very hard and cracked, and predisposed to secondary infection or screwworm infestation. The animal is very sensitive to handling, shows pain when moving and seeks shade.

Often the course is rapid, and death may occur within a few days. In less acute cases, the course is more protracted and recovery may occur. The mortality in affected calves varies from 30 to 70% under natural conditions. Morbidity in endemic areas is about 10%. The severity of infection is influenced by the number of ticks as well as the length of time they remain on the host.

Lesions: Emaciation, dehydration, diphtheroid stomatitis, pharyngitis, laryngitis, esophagitis, vaginitis or posthitis, edema and hyperemia of the lungs, congested liver, kidneys and meninges, and atrophy of the spleen are found in addition to the skin lesions described above.

Diagnosis: It is essential to determine the presence of the vector. There is typically a generalized hyperemia with subsequent desquamation of the superficial layers of the mucous membranes of the upper respiratory, alimentary and external genital tracts, and profuse moist dermatitis followed by superficial desquamation of the skin.

Prophylaxis and Treatment: Control of tick infestation is the only effective prophylactic measure. Removal of ticks, symptomatic treatment and good nursing are indicated. Antibiotics (℞ 27, 50, 66) either alone or with costicosteroids, and sulfonamides (℞ 96, 102, 110) are useful in combating secondary infection.

PEDICULOSIS

(Louse infestation, Lousiness)

Various species of biting lice (order Mallophaga) and sucking lice (order Anoplura) infest domestic animals. Sucking lice are known to occur only on mammals. Biting lice are found on both mammals and birds (*see* ECTOPARASITISM of poultry, p. 1116).

Etiology: Cattle are most commonly infested with the cattle biting louse, *Bovicola* (*Damalinia*) *bovis*, and with 3 species of Anoplura, the shortnosed cattle louse, *Haematopinus eurysternus*, the longnosed cattle louse, *Linognathus vituli*, and the little blue cattle louse, *Solenopotes capillatus*. Anoplura less commonly found on cattle include the cattle tail louse, *H. quadripertusus* (Florida and Gulf Coast) and the buffalo louse, *H. tuberculatus* (Old World and tropics).

Horses are commonly infested by 2 species of lice, the horse biting louse, *Bovicola equi*, and the horse sucking louse, *Haematopinus asini*.

Swine are commonly lousy, but only one species is involved, the hog louse, *Haematopinus suis* (Anoplura).

Sheep may become infested with one species of Mallophaga, the sheep biting louse, *Bovicola ovis*, and 4 species of Anoplura, the sheep foot louse, *Linognathus pedalis*, the body louse, *L. ovillus*, the goat sucking louse, *L. stenopsis*, and the African sheep louse, *L. africanus*.

Goats harbor many louse species, the commonest being the goat biting louse, *Bovicola caprae* (Mallophaga), and the goat sucking louse, *Linognathus stenopsis* (Anoplura). Two other Mallophaga, *B. limbata* and *B. crassipes*, are also frequently found.

Dogs and cats may be infested with lice. The parasites involved are *Linognathus setosus* (Anoplura) and *Trichodectes canis* (Mallophaga) on dogs, and *Felicola subrostrata* (Mallophaga) on cats. Other kinds of lice have been found on dogs, e.g. *Heterodoxus spiniger* (Mallophaga).

The Anoplura are bloodsucking lice with mouthparts reduced to stylets which are retracted within the body when not in use. The Mallophaga are provided with obvious ventral chewing mandibles and live on epidermal products as well as blood and exudates when available.

Louse eggs are glued onto hairs or feathers and are pale, translucent and suboval. About 3 or 4 weeks are required to complete one generation, but this varies with species and climatic conditions.

Clinical Findings and Diagnosis: Pediculosis of both types is manifested by pruritus and dermal irritation with resultant scratching, rubbing and biting of infested areas. A generally unthrifty appearance, roughened hair coat and lowered production in farm animals are common. In severe infestations, there may be loss of hair and local scarification. Extreme infestation with sucking lice can cause anemia. In sheep and goats, the rubbing and scratching often results in broken fibers giving the fleece a "pulled" appearance. In dogs, the hair coat becomes rough and dry and, if the lice are numerous, the hair may be matted. Sucking lice cause small wounds which may become infected. The constant crawling and either piercing or biting of the skin causes nervousness in hosts.

To find lice the hair should be parted and an examination, under strong light, made of the skin and proximal portion of the hair coat. The hair of large animals should be parted along the topline, on the neck and dewlap, on and in the ear, on the escutcheon, on the tail base and in the tail switch. The head, legs and feet should not be overlooked, particularly in sheep. On small animals, the ova (nits) attached to the hair are readily seen. Occasionally, where the coat is matted, the lice can be seen when the mass is broken apart. The biting lice are active and can be seen moving through the hair, while the sucking lice usually are found with the sucking mouthparts embedded in the skin.

In dairy herds, the young stock, dry cows and bulls may escape early diagnosis and suffer more severely. Infestations, particularly of the several sucking louse species, may become so severe as to produce signs suggestive of a grave ailment. Young calves may die. Treatment that effectively removes the lice results in prompt improvement.

Pediculosis of livestock in the Northern U.S.A. is most prevalent during the winter. Louse infestations are greatly reduced in severity with the approach of summer.

Transmission usually occurs by host contact. Lice dropped or pulled from the host die in less than a week, but disengaged ova may continue to hatch over a period of 2 to 3 weeks in warm weather. Premises recently vacated by infested stock should, therefore, be disinfected before being used for clean stock.

Treatment: Louse control requires dermal application of insecticides. Zero to very low tolerances for pesticides in milk limits the highly effective insecticides that may be used on dairy cattle and dairy goats to crotoxyphos (℞ 283), crotoxyphos plus dichlorvos (℞ 275) and coumaphos (℞ 277). Additionally, dairy cattle may be treated with crotoxyphos plus dichlorvos (℞ 275), coumaphos (5%, dust) and stirofos (3%, dust). Beef cattle, sheep, goats and swine should be treated with 0.03 to 0.06% coumaphos, 0.015% dioxathion, 0.03% lindane, 0.5% malathion, methoxychlor (℞ 301), 0.5% carbaryl, ronnel (℞ 314), 0.5% toxaphene, crotoxyphos (℞ 283) and crotoxyphos plus dichlorvos (℞ 275). Stirofos (℞ 326) and stirofos plus dichlorvos (℞ 312) may be used as a spray on beef cattle, and 0.5% stirofos may be used as a spray on hogs. Rotenone (℞ 320, 322) should not be used on swine, but is safe for use on other animals where current regulations permit its use.

Spraying or dipping should be thorough, and usually 2 treatments 14 days apart will eradicate lice. Effective spraying requires soaking the hair to the skin: cattle and sheep require a minimum of 1 gal. (4 L), but as much as 3 gal. may be required on large long-haired cattle. At least ½ gal. per head should be applied to swine. Cattle that can be restrained, e.g. dairy cattle in stanchions, can be treated with a low volume mist application of 1% crotoxyphos plus 0.25% dichlorvos. Dipping is more dependable than spraying, but only coumaphos, dioxathion, ronnel, lindane or toxaphene should be used in dips.

Toxaphene should be used at 0.25%, half the spraying strength, for dipping sheep and goats; 0.03% diazinon is an effective spray against lice on sheep. (*See also* Treatment of sheep ked, p. 755.)

Cattle lice can be controlled, but not eradicated, by wintertime use of back-rubber devices or dust bags similar to those used against flies in the summer. Effectiveness depends on frequent use by all cattle in the herd (℞ 280, 283, 288, 297, 314, 336). Only crotoxyphos, dichlorvos, coumaphos (℞ 275, 281, 283), or 3% stirofos may be used on dairy cattle. Cattle louse populations can also be reduced by hand-dusting with 5% malathion, 5% toxaphene or 10% methoxychlor on beef cattle: or 1% rotenone, 3% stirofos, or 1% coumaphos on dairy or beef cattle. A pour-on formulation of 3% fenthion can be used to control lice infestations of beef and nonlactating dairy cattle. Where current regulations permit, chlorpyrifos (℞ 274), which is applied in a low volume to a single spot on the back of an animal, will provide season-long control of lice on beef and nonlactating dairy cattle.

Dogs can be treated with dips, washes, sprays, or dusts containing rotenone (℞ 320, 322), 0.5% methoxychlor, 0.03% diazinon, 5% malathion, or 0.5% coumaphos. On cats, only rotenone and pyrethrum preparations should be used.

Lice on swine can be controlled with dips and sprays of 0.03% lindane, 0.15% dioxathion and 0.5% methoxychlor, and sprays of 0.5% malathion, 0.5% carbaryl, 0.03 to 0.06% coumaphos, 0.5% toxaphene, crotoxyphos plus dichlorvos (℞ 275), crotoxyphos (℞ 283), ronnel (℞ 314), and 0.5% stirofos. Dust formulations of 3% stirofos and 1% coumaphos and a pour-on formulation of fenthion (℞

291) are also effective. Dust formulations of 3% stirofos and 1% coumaphos (℞ 280, 329) and a granule formulation of 5% ronnel (℞ 317) may be used to treat bedding.

The United States Food and Drug Administration (USFDA) and Environmental Protection Agency (EPA) strictly specify tissue residue limits of insecticides and carefully regulate their use in livestock products. Similar regulatory agencies exist in most countries. Regulations elsewhere are not identical to those of the USFDA and EPA, and such regulations, in the U.S.A. and elsewhere, are subject to change. Users of the MANUAL are cautioned to familiarize themselves with pertinent current local laws and requirements. The treatment of meat and dairy animals must be restricted to uses specified on the labels and all label precautions carefully observed. Tissue residue tolerances and minimum drug withdrawal times between treatment and slaughter are given under TOXICITY OF ORGANIC INSECTICIDES AND ACARICIDES, p. 995). Some states have further restrictions on use of pesticides. Note also the cautions given with the prescriptions.

FLEA INFESTATION

Fleas are small, wingless, laterally compressed, bloodsucking external parasites. All adult fleas take blood meals from their hosts and, in feeding, cause intense pruritus and irritation to the hypersensitive host.

Etiology: Several species of fleas infest the dog and cat, 2 of these being the cat flea. *Ctenocephalides felis*, and the less common dog flea, *C. canis*. The flea spends much of its adult life on the body of the host. Eggs are laid either on the ground or on the host from which they fall to the ground. The eggs eventually hatch into larvae, which feed on organic matter in the bedding of the host or in cracks and crevices in floors. When mature, the larva spins a loose cocoon attached to bits of debris and pupates. After about 5 days under optimum conditions, the adult emerges from the cocoon and seeks a host in order to feed and continue its life cycle.

Clinical Findings: Fleas irritate the host by their constant biting and the salivary secretion of toxic and allergenic products. In hypersensitive animals flea bites produce intense pruritus; the animal becomes restless, and bites and scratches. By so doing the animal produces an acute, discrete dermatitis patch ("hotspot") or a chronic nonspecific dermatitis. The former lesions are usually subauricular, interscapular or about the rump or thighs. The chronic nonspecific dermatitis usually is restricted to the lower back and perineum. Secondary infection is a common complication in both syndromes. Self-inflicted trauma often leads to an itch-scratch cycle.

Diagnosis: A careful examination of the animal will reveal the fleas or flea debris in the hair. Fleas often can be found in greatest number around the rump and the tail head.

Treatment: To control fleas, both the animal and its environment must be treated. Many of the insecticides will remove fleas from the host's body, but others will return unless they and the immature forms are killed in the bedding or other places.

To kill fleas on pets, commercial preparations of methylcarbamate, pyrethrum or rotenone powder may be applied. These materials kill quickly and are safe. Powders or sprays containing lindane, malathion, or other organophosphorus compounds (℞ 314) in concentrations recommended by the manufacturer, are also highly effective, but should not be used on cats. "Flea collars" impregnated with organophosphorus compounds are a convenient means of applying these compounds. As with other insecticides, an appreciation of the toxic or allergic potential of the organophosphorus compounds is essential. Pendants containing these compounds also are available but appear to be less effective than the collars. Adequate precautions and instructions should be given to the client.

The use of insecticides should relieve much of the animal's discomfort. Treatment of self-inflicted dermatitis should be directed towards controlling secondary infection and relieving the pruritus. The topical application of bacitracin in combination with neomycin, and polymyxin ointment, with or without hydrocortisone, and the oral or parenteral administration of prednisolone (℞ 153), aspirin, phenobarbital or tranquilizers (℞ 383), achieves these purposes. Care should be taken to clean the dermatitic areas before initiating treatment; 3% hexachlorophene is ideal for the purpose.

Control of breeding places of fleas is easy when the pet has a sleeping box or basket. The old bedding should be discarded and then the box or basket and surrounding area treated with any of the insecticides mentioned below. Animals should not be allowed to reoccupy the area before surfaces are dry. Other areas where the animal spends considerable time should be treated similarly.

If there is a general flea infestation in a home, regular and thorough vacuum cleaning supplemented with 0.5% malathion sprayed along baseboards will control a mild infestation. In truly heavy infestations, it is probably better to call in a professional exterminator as resistance of fleas to insecticides has been reported.

In addition to 0.5% malathion, lindane 0.5% dust, 1% rotenone, and pyrethrum dusts (℞ 323) can be used for flea control in buildings. Chlorinated hydrocarbons cannot be used on cats, but dusts containing rotenone and pyrethrins with synergists give excellent results in feline patients. These powders can be liberally dusted in the hair and also sprinkled around the animal's habitat.

For the hypersensitive patient, a program of hyposensitization with flea antigen (℞ 131) is worth trying. One can expect approximately 25% success. Hyposensitization, when effective, should be repeated yearly before the flea season.

THE SHEEP KED
(Sheep tick)

The sheep ked (*Melophagus ovinus*) is one of the most widely distributed and important external parasites of sheep. It is a true insect, a wingless fly, and not an acarine. The adult is about 7 mm long, of a brown or reddish color and covered with short, bristly hairs. The female gives birth to a single fully developed larva, which is cemented to the wool and pupates within 12 hours. A young ked emerges after about 22 days and may live 100 to 120 days if a female and about 80 days if male. During this time about 10 larvae are produced by each female. The entire life is spent on the host. Keds that fall off the host usually survive less than a week and present little danger of infestation to a flock.

To feed, keds pierce the skin with their mouthparts and suck blood. They usually feed on the neck, breast, shoulder, flanks and rump, but not on the back where dust and other debris collect in the wool. They cause a skin defect in hides called cockle. The lesions create a blemish that affects the grade and value of the sheep skin.

Ked numbers increase during the winter and early spring when they spread rapidly through a flock, particularly when sheep are assembled in close quarters for feeding or shelter.

Clinical Findings: The skin irritation when the keds feed causes sheep to rub and bite, and the fleece becomes thin, ragged and dirty. The excrement of the keds causes permanent discoloration, which is likely to reduce the value of the wool. Infested sheep, particularly lambs and pregnant ewes, may lose vitality and be unthrifty. Keds also transmit *Trypanosoma melophagium*, which is said to be nonpathogenic for sheep.

Control: Shearing removes many pupae and adults. Thus shearing before lambing and the subsequent treatment of the ewes with insecticides to control the remaining keds can greatly reduce the possibility of lambs becoming heavily infested. Sheep are usually treated after shearing and best results are obtained if an insecticide is used whose residue remains at least 3 to 4 weeks. By this means the keds which emerge from the pupae will also be killed. Modern fly dips, giving freedom from blow fly strike for 6 to 20 weeks, will also eradicate the keds.

Dipping: When sheep dipping vats are available, dipping is regarded as the most effective method of treatment. Completely submerging the sheep ensures the destruction of all keds present but in most instances does not kill the pupated larvae, unless a long-acting insecticide is used so that the ked newly emerging from its pupa, is killed by the residue in the fleece of the sheep. Large flocks of range sheep should be treated in a permanently constructed sheep dipping vat. Smaller flocks and farm flocks may be successfully treated in portable galvanized-iron dipping vats or in smaller tanks, tubs or in canvas dipping bags.

Spraying may be as effective as the dipping method, and is more convenient in some areas. Pressures of 100 to 200 lb/sq in. for short wool and 300 to 350 lb/sq in. for long wool are commonly used.

Shower dipping is also sometimes used. In this procedure, the sheep are held in a special pen and showered from above and below until the fleece is saturated. The run-off is returned for recirculation and the concentration of insecticide used is the same as for dipping. The concentration of the insecticide can drop rapidly and become ineffective if the instructions for replenishment are not followed explicitly.

Jetting: This technique involves the forceful application of the insecticide by means of a hand-held multiple-jet comb drawn through the short fleece. Although a little slower, and less effective than dips or sprays, it is thought advantageous for smaller flocks, as it is economical and does not require a permanent installation.

Dusting: Power dusting is a method which fits well into management practices at shearing time. It is rapid and economical, and avoids wetting the animals. Various types of equipment for dusting are available commercially. *See* TABLE, p. 757.

FLIES AND MOSQUITOES

BLACK FLIES AND BUFFALO GNATS

Members of the dipterous family Simuliidae are characterized by a strongly humped thorax, a marked enlargement of the anterior wing veins and the absence of simple eyes. Few species exceed 5 mm in length. Gray, olive and black are their common colors.

The immature stages are aquatic, and most require rapidly flowing water. An exception is the southern buffalo gnat, *Cnephia pecuarum*, which breeds most frequently in relatively slow moving waters of the lower Mississippi Valley. Depending upon the species, eggs of black flies are attached to objects at the water's edge, attached to submerged objects, or scattered over the water surface. Larvae and pupae attach to submerged objects to avoid being washed away by the current. Development from egg to adult may require as little as 3 weeks for some species, while others that overwinter in the larval stage require several months. The adult flies may migrate several miles after emerging.

TABLE OF TREATMENTS FOR LICE AND SHEEP KED IN SHEEP AND NONLACTATING GOATS

Insecticide	Min. Days from Last Application to Slaughter	Formulation, Strength and Method of Treatment	Special Safety Restrictions
Coumaphos	15	WP, 0.06% S or dip	Do not re-treat within 10 days.
Crotoxyphos	0	EC, 0.25% S, 1 gal. (4 L)/animal	Do not use more than once weekly.
Crotoxyphos + Dichlorvos	0	EC, 0.3% + 0.02% S, 1 gal. (4 L)/animal	Do not treat more than once weekly.
Dioxathion	0	EC, 0.15% S or dip	Do not repeat more often than every 2 weeks.
Dioxathion + Dichlorvos	0	EC, 0.15% + 0.005% S or dip	Do not repeat more often than every 2 weeks.
Lindane	30 (S) 60 (dip)	WP, 0.03–0.06% S or dip	Do not treat animals under 3 months of age.
Malathion	0	WP or EC, 0.5% S Wet thoroughly.	Do not treat animals under 1 month of age.
		D, 4 or 5%	
Methoxychlor*	0	WP, 0.5% S or dip WP, 50% as a dust	
Methoxychlor + Malathion	0	D, 5% + 4% Apply after shearing.	
Ronnel	28	EC, 0.25% S	Do not treat more often than once every 2 weeks.
Toxaphene	28	EC, 0.125–0.3% S or 0.125% dip	Do not treat animals under 3 months of age.
Toxaphene + Lindane	30 (S) 60 (dip)	D, 5% + 1% EC, 0.1 + 0.005% S or dip Must wet thoroughly.	Do not treat animals under 3 months of age.
Toxaphene + Malathion	28	EC, 0.25 + 0.025% S or 0.125% + 0.0125% dip	Do not treat animals under 3 months of age.
Toxaphene + Methoxychlor	28	D, 5% + 5% Apply after shearing.	

* For lice only.
D = dust.
EC = emulsifiable concentrate.
S = spray.
WP = wettable powder.

Although the female black fly is a blood feeder, some species are zoophilic, and it may not be readily apparent to man that these tiny gnats are attacking livestock. When animals are under attack, numerous small blood droplets that result from the feeding injury may be apparent on exposed parts of the body such as udders, sheath, ears, etc.

Only 2 of more than 100 species of black flies in North America have caused severe losses of farm animals. The southern buffalo gnat, in outbreak years, has been reported responsible for deaths of thousands of mules and cattle in Louisiana, Arkansas and Mississippi. Attacks by *Simulium arcticum* from the Saskatchewan and Athabaska Rivers in Canada are reported to be severe enough to kill livestock 3 or 4 years out of 10. In 1944 to 1948, more than 1,300 animals were killed.

It is generally believed that the rapid death of animals following attack by large numbers of black flies is due to toxic substances injected by the insects. The serious effects in animals observed in the Saskatchewan black fly outbreaks appeared to be the result of an increase in the permeability of the capillaries with a consequent loss of fluid from the circulatory system into the tissue spaces and body cavities. Tissues are edematous and reveal internal hemorrhages. This is interpreted as due to a direct toxic action without previous sensitization. The possibility of anaphylaxis has not been completely ruled out since animals that suffer 2 fairly closely spaced attacks sometimes fare worse during the second attack.

Certain species of black flies sometimes cause losses to poultry either by direct attack or through the transmission of *Leucocytozoon* disease (q.v., p. 1135).

Control: Since area-wide control of black flies is difficult and expensive livestock men usually resort to repellents for the protection of their animals. Dense smudges may provide some protection. Cold mixed lubricating-oil emulsion has been widely used for years. Temporary relief may be afforded dogs, horses and valuable cattle by frequent sprays of pyrethrum plus synergist and repellent (℞ 309, 310, 311). Horses may be protected with spray, wipe-on or gel of stirofos plus pyrethrins (℞ 331, 332).

If public funds and trained supervisory personnel are available, large-scale control of black flies is possible by treating breeding streams with an approved larvicide. Pesticide treatments involving water surfaces or large land areas are subject to governmental regulation and must be done with due regard for possible deleterious environmental effects and residues in food products.

MOSQUITOES

Mosquitoes of the genera *Aedes* and *Psorophora* sometimes attack livestock in such great numbers that serious production losses, and even deaths, have been reported. Both of these genera lay their eggs on a substrate such as damp soil where they are hatched by subsequent flooding due to irrigation, rainfall, snow melt, etc. Larvae and pupae, known also as "wigglers" and "tumblers," then grow in the relatively still water. After the immatures have completed development, millions of adults may then emerge, all within a short period of time. Some of these mosquitoes have several generations per year, and alternate dry and wet periods due to rainfall or irrigation will bring them out in enormous numbers. The flight habits of adult mosquitoes vary with species, and some *Aedes* are reported to migrate many miles from their aquatic, larval habitat. Usually, these genera overwinter in the egg stage, and the eggs of some species can withstand dry periods of several years. In the rice-growing areas of Arkansas and Louisiana, *Psorophora columbiae* is a severe pest of both animals and man. *Aedes* spp. are pests of livestock, to a greater or lesser degree, all over the U.S.A. and Canada.

Other mosquito genera that are important pests of livestock include *Culex* and *Culiseta*. Unlike the preceding mosquitoes, these deposit their eggs on the surface of standing water, and they usually overwinter in the adult stage. The genus *Culex* is widespread in distribution. *Culex tarsalis*, the important vector of western equine encephalitis, is found in the western, central and southern states of the U.S.A. *Mansonia* spp. are severe on livestock in Florida.

The injury that mosquitoes inflict on livestock mainly consists of severe annoyance and blood losses, and the transmission of several diseases. It also is suspected the toxins injected at the time of biting may cause severe systemic effects. Several diseases, including equine encephalomyelitis, are transmitted by mosquitoes. The microfilariae of the dog heartworm are mosquito-transmitted. In Central and South America, *Dermatobia hominis*, the parent of the notorious and destructive torsalo grub, fastens its eggs to a species of *Psorophora* mosquito which then transmits them to the mammalian host where they hatch as the mosquito feeds. Instances of the apparent transmission of fowl pox by mosquitoes have been reported.

Control: The individual stockman should make every attempt to eliminate or reduce areas on his land that are producing mosquito larvae. Area control of mosquitoes usually involves the cooperation of many individuals and can be carried out successfully only by experienced personnel with proper equipment. In addition to elimination of aquatic breeding sites, area programs generally include extensive use of larvicides or oils. In the case of large outbreaks of adult mosquitoes, particularly when disease transmission is a concern, application of an insecticide active against the adults, e.g. Ultra Low Volume malathion, may be necessary. ***Caution is advised with area programs as many kinds of nontarget organisms, e.g. fish, shrimp, bees, may be exposed to insecticides.***

It is difficult for the individual stockman to protect his animals; residual sprays on the animals do not prevent attack, and currently available repellents will not confer adequate protection during heavy outbreaks. Protection from adult mosquitoes may be provided by ground and, in some cases, by aerial application of an insecticide at the time of maximum infestation (℞ 285, 299, 304). Depending on local conditions, this protection may be short-lived.

Valuable animals should be housed in closed or screened buildings and the mosquitoes inside killed with a fog or aerosol of synergized pyrethrum (℞ 310) or dichlorvos (℞ 285, 286). Temporary relief may be afforded by a spray or wipe-on of materials such as pyrethrum plus repellent, stirofos and pyrethrum or dichlorvos (℞ 285, 309, 310, 311, 330, 331, 332). The insecticidal residual deposits suggested for stable-fly control (p. 762) will aid in mosquito control outside barns.

HORSE FLIES AND DEER FLIES

Horse flies and deer flies belong to the family Tabanidae. They are characterized by 3-jointed antennae with the last segment terminating in a series of rings, the costal vein extending entirely around the wing, large squamae and the almost complete lack of body bristles. Three genera, *Chrysops*, *Hybomitra* and *Tabanus*, contain most of the important pest species in North America. *Tabanus* and *Hybomitra* (horse flies) are generally larger than *Chrysops* (deer flies) and are more serious pests of animals. Various horse flies and deer flies are important pests more or less locally in different parts of the world.

The larvae of horse flies are largely aquatic or semiaquatic. Egg masses of most species so far studied are deposited on vegetation, rocks or debris projecting from the water or near the water's edge. Eggs usually hatch in 5 to 10 days. The young larvae fall into the water, but most of them soon find their way to the mud near shore where the larval period is spent in search of food, which is either organic matter or other forms of animal life. As time for pupation approaches, larvae travel to drier areas a few feet farther from shore where there is less danger of prolonged submergence during the pupal period. Most horse flies studied have a single brood each year, and overwinter in the larval stage.

Female horse flies have bladelike mouthparts that inflict a painful wound and cause a considerable flow of blood, which they then lap up. A few individuals of the larger species can prevent a herd from feeding normally and add to the loss by the overactivity they stimulate. Blood loss becomes a significant factor when dozens of flies feed on an animal for several hours each day during the summer. As many as 200 flies have been seen on single isolated animals. Horse flies take from 0.1 to 0.3 ml of blood at a feeding. Moderate infestations may rob an animal of 100 ml of blood daily over long periods.

Horse flies can transmit the causal agents of anthrax, anaplasmosis, tularemia and equine infectious anemia. They are suspected as transmitters of the virus of equine encephalomyelitis. In the Philippines, they carry the trypanosome of surra between animals, while in Africa, they transmit several typanosomes pathogenic to livestock. In all of the above instances, transmission is purely mechanical, flies never serving as intermediate hosts for the causative agents.

Control: Horse flies are among the most difficult to control of any of the bloodsucking flies. While the majority of the new organic insecticides will kill horse flies even at low dosages, they will not do so fast enough to prevent biting. Repellents are the only present answer and the synergized pyrethrins have given the best results, even though of limited value. Wetting the haircoat heavily (1 to 2 qt/cow) by spraying with an emulsion (℞ 309) is recommended for maximum protection. Protection may last up to 3 days, when treatment must be repeated. Addition of a synthetic repellent may increase effectiveness (℞ 310). Stable flies and horn flies also will be repelled. Allethrin may be substituted for some pyrethrins. Oil-base sprays (℞ 275, 285, 310, 311) afford some protection, but pyrethrin, synergist and repellent concentration must be higher than for less aggressive flies. They are applied from a hand or electric atomizer, using not more than 2 oz (60 ml) per head. Dairy cattle need treatment at each milking. Automatic sprayers are convenient for cows in lactation. Horses may be protected with stirofos, pyrethrins and repellent (℞ 331, 332).

STABLE FLIES

While resembling the house fly in size and general appearance this species, *Stomoxys calcitrans*, has a needle-shaped proboscis that at rest protrudes noticeably in front of the fly's face. The larvae commonly develop in moist, fermenting vegetable matter, and manure contaminated with vegetable matter. Hay or green chop on the ground around outdoor feeding racks is one common habitat for larvae, and refuse from vegetable processing plants is another; others are peanut refuse left in fields to become wet, and bay grasses often washed ashore in windrows along the coastlines of New Jersey and Florida. The cycle from egg to adult can be completed in 3 weeks during the summer, and the females live 4 to 6 weeks.

The "bite" is painful and the wounds bleed freely after the fly has left and are attractive to screwworm flies, house flies and other flies. Both sexes are hematophagous. The decreased production of livestock caused by stable flies is principally due to annoyance and blood loss. Flies also may mechanically transmit anthrax and possibly other livestock diseases. It has been estimated that milk production may decrease as much as 50% during heavy infestations and that weight losses of 10 to 15% may occur.

Control: Since individual stable flies visit their hosts only for short periods, spray applications on the host are not highly effective in reducing populations. Spraying the outside of all livestock quarters on farm premises, as well as fences and other observed resting places, gives some control but is expensive and entirely impractical for range beef herds or even for dairy herds when pastures are well removed from the barnyard. Recommended materials for this purpose are 1% diazinon, 0.25% stirofos plus 1% dichlorvos, 1% ronnel, or 0.5% methoxychlor. Mist or fog applications can be performed in areas such as feedlots, corrals, or holding pens (℞ 285, 299, 304). This operation is also expensive, and results, depending on local conditions, can be variable. Livestock barns should be sprayed with 1% dimethoate, 1% ronnel, 1% stirofos, 1% fenthion, or 1% diazinon to thoroughly control stable flies as well as the ubiquitous house fly.

Synergized pyrethrum, crotoxyphos, stirofos or dichlorvos sprays kill most of the flies that come to feed on animals (℞ 275, 283, 285, 310, 311, 313). Care must be taken to treat well the preferred feeding sites on the legs of animals. Barns should be fogged with synergized pyrethrum (℞ 310) or dichlorvos (℞ 285, 286) to kill stable flies.

Horn Flies

The horn fly, ***Haematobia irritans***, is a small fly (about one half the size of a house fly) that is frequently found in large numbers on the back, the belly, and at times, at the base of the horns of cattle. A blood feeder, its mouthparts are similar in structure to those of the stable fly. The adult spends most of its time on its host, almost exclusively cattle, using the latter both as a resting place and a source of food. Females leave only to deposit eggs on the host's freshly dropped feces.

The horn fly's life-cycle is among the shortest known for flies, and hot, humid weather favors the species. Eggs sometimes hatch in less than 24 hours, larval stages may be completed in as few as 3 days and the pupal period in 6, making a total cycle of 10 days.

Since they occur over the entire U.S.A. and can build up enormous populations in short periods, horn flies can cause great losses in livestock production. As many as 5,000 to 10,000 flies have been reported on a single cow, and the blood loss under these conditions is severe. The flies feed at least 15 times daily and 10,000 flies would extract about a liter of blood a day. Infested animals spend much time fighting the flies and grazing time thereby is reduced. They also crowd together closely for protection and many horn and kick wounds result.

Control: Because of their habit of living almost continuously on the host, horn flies are controlled easily. Methoxychlor (0.5%), crotoxyphos (℞ 275), carbaryl (0.5%), malathion (0.5%), toxaphene (0.5%), coumaphos (0.03 to 0.06%), ronnel (1%), and stirofos (℞ 313, 326) are all highly effective as sprays on beef cattle. Beef cattle may be treated for horn-fly control in pens or chutes by spraying the backs of the cattle with a high-pressure hydraulic sprayer. To control only horn flies, there is no need to completely cover the animals with spray; 1 or 2 qt (1 or 2 L) per head is adequate, not more often than once every 3 weeks. The only sprays permitted on dairy cattle (to avoid residues in milk) are crotoxyphos, dichlorvos (℞ 275, 283, 285), 0.03% coumaphos, and synergized pyrethrum (℞ 309, 310, 311).

Horn flies also may be controlled by using oilers, which are available commercially, or "back rubbers," which are lengths of chain or barbed wire heavily wrapped with feed sacks and suspended loosely between 2 posts about 15 ft (5 m) apart. The sacks are saturated thoroughly with insecticide in number 2 fuel oil or diesel oil. Effective insecticides include 5% methoxychlor, 1% crotoxyphos, 1.5% dioxathion, 2% malathion, 0.1% coumaphos, 0.8% crotoxyphos plus 0.2% dichlorvos, 5% toxaphene, 1% ronnel, 1% stirofos, or 1% stirofos plus 0.25% dichlorvos. Only crotoxyphos, dichlorvos (℞ 275, 283) or 1% coumaphos may be used on lactating dairy cattle.

Daily spraying dairy cattle with an oil-base stock spray (℞ 275, 285, 310, 311) will give excellent horn-fly control. If stock sprays are not used, the dairy farmer may resort to dusts of 0.5% coumaphos, 3% stirofos, methoxychlor (℞ 279, every 3 weeks), or 5% malathion (every 10 to 14 days). Labor can be minimized by using dust bags filled with 3% stirofos or 5% coumaphos in lanes or on pasture. Utmost care must be taken not to allow the dust to contaminate milk or milking utensils, or illegal residues in milk will result.

Dust bags may also be used for horn-fly control on beef cattle, using 3% stirofos, 5% coumaphos, 10% methoxychlor or 5% toxaphene. Horn flies on beef and lactating dairy cattle can be controlled by daily feeding of methoprene (℞ 300) or stirofos (℞ 325). These materials pass through the digestive tract of the cattle and affect the larvae and pupae that develop in the manure of treated cattle. Horn flies on beef cattle can be controlled by feeding ronnel (℞ 318).

Face Flies

The face fly, *Musca autumnalis*, is now common in most of the Northern U.S.A. and Southern Canada. Although the species occurs in Europe and parts of Asia and Africa, it is of no importance there as a pest of livestock. It is morphologically similar to the common house fly, *M. domestica;* members of both species have mouthparts that consist of sponging labellae, both have 4 longitudinal stripes on the thorax. The face fly is slightly larger but this difference is difficult to detect in the field. An entomologist can differentiate them by the closeness and angles of the interior margins of the eyes and by the distinctive coloration of the face and abdomen.

Face flies breed only in fresh feces and therefore their presence and prevalence will depend on how the animals are maintained. Common house flies will breed in almost any type of manure or decaying organic material. Face flies are present if large numbers of flies are found on the face and muzzle of livestock.

Face flies are important primarily as a source of irritation, particularly when they feed around the eyes. Only a few flies are sufficient to cause irritation. When large numbers are present the animals will often bunch up in groups with their heads together. Control is difficult. Since the flies do not follow the host into barns they do not come in contact with residual sprays. Stirofos as a mineral mix or block (℞ 325) will control face flies in manure of beef and dairy cattle. Control of larvae in the field requires the scattering of all feces within 3 to 5 days of deposit.

Several insecticide formulations can be used for control of face fly as well as other flies (℞ 275, 277, 283, 285, 311). At present, the most effective is crotoxyphos or dichlorvos emulsified spray applied to the face of the animal. The addition of a small amount of sugar may increase the attractiveness of the spray. In treating the face, it is necessary to use safe materials at frequent intervals since secretion of tears by the animals will cover or dilute the spray. Dust bags containing a suitable insecticide (e.g. 5% coumaphos or 3% stirophos) have been used with variable results.

BUFFALO FLIES

The buffalo fly, *Haematobia* (*Siphona*) *exigua*, of East, South and Southeast Asia and Oceania is similar in size, appearance, feeding and breeding habits to the horn fly (q.v., p. 762). It is a problem in Australia and New Guinea but not in New Zealand. The bloodsucking flies rarely leave the host except to oviposit or to move to a new host, and are most common on withers, shoulders and flanks.

The eggs, deposited in fresh dung, may hatch in as little as 18 hours. Larvae complete growth in 3 to 5 days and pupation takes a similar time under favorable conditions but the life cycle may be prolonged to several weeks. Populations are highest following the summer rains.

Cattle and buffalo are the preferred hosts but Equidae are also parasitized. Man, sheep, pigs and dogs are attacked when associated with preferred hosts.

The constant irritation and annoyance cause serious damage to cattle, especially those attacked for the first time. Cattle from infested areas are readily recognized by the large raw areas around the eyes on the body that are formed from scratching and rubbing of the animal. Such wounds are attractive to the injurious bush fly found in Australia. Populations up to 1,000 per animal are usually tolerated without much injury, although 2,000 or 3,000 flies per animal is considered a serious infestation. In the Indo-Malayan Archipelago, surra disease and anthrax are considered to be transmitted by this species.

For control measures see control of the horn fly, p. 762.

Head Flies
(Plantation flies)

The head fly, *Hydrotaea irritans*, is a nonbiting muscid found in large numbers in Northern European countries, especially Denmark and Britain, where it is pest of cattle, sheep and other livestock, from early June until late September. Unlike other *Hydrotaea* species, *H. irritans* is univoltine, producing 1 generation each year, with 3 larval instar stages. Eggs deposited in late summer hatch out in the second instar larval stage within a few days. This saprophagous stage lasts a brief spell before developing to the main third stage which is predatory on other insect larvae. Overwintering occurs as late-stage larvae. Adult flies are most active in the vicinity of thickets or woodland in which they shelter between periods of feeding.

In Britain, sheep are mainly affected. Large swarms, attracted by the movement of animals, congregate to feed on the secretions from the eyes and nose, and the cellular debris at the growing horn base. To alleviate the persistent irritation produced by the presence of the flies the sheep scratch and rub their heads which results in the formation of raw wounds or "broken heads," especially on the poll. Flies, attracted by the blood, settle on these self-inflicted lesions and extend the margins by their feeding activity. Sheep of all ages are involved but breeds with horns and without wool on the head are most severely affected.

Head flies also attack man, deer, horses, cattle and rabbits. Although no corresponding "broken head" lesions develop in cattle, the association between the occurrence of summer mastitis (due to *Corynebacterium pyogenes*) and the seasonal activity of head flies is closely linked, especially in Denmark. Head flies may also be involved in the spread of myxomatosis in rabbits.

Control: The development, emergence, and collection of the pest, which occur away from farm areas, precludes the traditional methods of insecticide spraying of generalized breeding sites and resting habitats. Control at the point of contact between the feeding adult insects and the mammalian hosts is also limited in value. With sheep, the retention of organophosphorus compounds or pyrethrin derivatives on the susceptible head areas is of short duration necessitating impractical re-applications in free-ranging animals. From the results of the feeding habits of the fly and its apparent greater contact with cattle it has been postulated that population reductions may be achieved if cattle are sprayed with insecticides; this has still to be proved.

The complete removal of livestock from infested locations during the fly season is the only effective way to prevent damage. The housing of sheep once broken heads have occurred is the only successful method of stopping further fly damage.

SCREWWORMS IN LIVESTOCK

Screwworms were once among the most important pests of livestock in the Southern and Southwestern U.S.A., causing annual losses estimated at more than 200 million dollars. They are obligatory parasites, and under optimal environmental conditions the flies oviposit on almost every wound that occurs—even abrasions as small as tick and fly bites.

It is important to distinguish between screwworms and the secondary maggots, which frequently infest necrotic tissues. Primary screwworm myiasis should be diagnosed promptly so that livestock owners in the community may be alerted to protect their animals.

Biology: Screwworms are the larvae of the blow fly, *Cochliomyia hominivorax*, a member of the family Calliphoridae. The bluish green screwworm fly is similar in appearance to the common blow flies, but differs in that its larval development occurs only in the tissues of living warm-blooded animals.

The screwworm fly deposits 200 to 400 eggs on the edge of a wound in rows that overlap like shingles. After about 12 hours incubation larvae circled with rows of dark spines are visible through the translucent shells and the egg mass has a gray appearance. Upon hatching, the larvae crawl into the wound and burrow into the flesh. The maggots feed on the wound fluids and live tissues and complete their growth in 6 to 8 days. The larvae then drop from the wound and burrow into the soil to pupate. The pupal period varies from 8 days to 2 months depending on temperature. Freezing or sustained soil temperatures below 46°F (8°C) kills the pupae. The adult insects mate when 3 or 4 days old and gravid females are ready to oviposit at 6 days of age. In warm weather, the life cycle may be completed in 21 days.

Full-grown screwworm larvae are about 12 mm long. Since the body is tapered with a pointed anterior end and a blunt posterior end they roughly resemble a screw. A pair of tracheae extend from the posterior spiracles forward into the body cavity. For about one-third of their length, these tracheae are deeply pigmented. They may be seen through the skin of the maggot as a pair of parallel lines and are characteristic of the screwworm. When fully grown or nearly so, the larvae are pinkish.

Clinical Findings: Screwworms feed as a group, burrowing deeply into the flesh. The wound fills with a profuse reddish brown exudate that almost completely covers the larvae and may stain the hair or wool for several inches as it drains.

An aid in recognizing screwworm infestation in range animals is the change in the animal's behavior. Even a small and relatively inconspicuous wound infested with screwworms attracts not only screwworm flies, but house flies and blow flies, which seek the wound primarily to feed on the exudate and are extremely annoying to the infested animal. As the annoyance increases, the infested animal seeks protection by retreating to the densest available shade.

Prognosis: If an infestation continues without treatment for as long as 2 weeks, at a time when ovipositing flies are numerous, the host animal will almost certainly be killed. Wounds treated within 4 days after infestation usually heal within a month.

Bacterial infections often complicate screwworm infestations. In general, cattle are quite resistant to infection and the wounds usually heal promptly with good treatment, but sheep, goats and horses frequently develop secondary infections.

Control: The most important control measures are prevention of wounds when flies are active, the prophylactic treatment of unavoidable wounds, regular and frequent inspection of range animals to detect infestations promptly, and treatment of existing infestations to kill larvae and prevent reinfestation.

Breeding should be controlled so that young are not born during the fly season. The navel of the newborn animal is a preferred site for oviposition and should be treated promptly with a recommended screwworm prophylactic if young are born during the fly season. Castration, dehorning, docking and branding should be carried out in cold weather. If surgery is performed during the fly season, the wound should be coated with a screwworm remedy and the treatment repeated as necessary until the wound has healed.

Flies and ticks should be controlled by the proper use of insecticides. Each animal on pasture should be seen twice weekly. Animals that are not with the herd, but are solitary and in dense shade or other dark places, should be examined closely.

Eradication Program: In 1958, the United States Department of Agriculture (USDA), in cooperation with livestock authorities of the Southeastern States, initiated a program to eradicate screwworms from the Southeast.

Screwworm larvae were reared on artificial media and, 2 days before fly emergence, the pupae were exposed to gamma irradiation at a dosage that caused sexual sterility but no other deleterious effects. Sterile flies were distributed over the entire screwworm-infested region at the average rate of 400 male flies per square mile per week, sufficient to outnumber the native flies. The female mates only once and when mated with a sterile male does not reproduce. There was a decline in the native population each generation until the native males were so outnumbered by sterile males that no fertile matings occurred and the native flies were eliminated. The last case in Florida was found in June 1959 and sterile-fly releases were discontinued in November. The states east of the Mississippi have remained screwworm-free since that time except for brief infestations resulting from import of infested animals from Western States.

In 1962 a more extensive program of eradication was undertaken in the Southwestern U.S.A. In most of the years since 1962, this program has eliminated almost all the losses caused by screwworms in these states. Native populations of flies were eradicated in the winter of 1963-1964 and again in the winter of 1964-1965. Unfortunately the Southwest has been periodically reinfested by fertile female flies from Mexico. There is evidence that the flies are capable of flying over 200 miles, and no natural barrier exists to block their northward movement during favorable seasons. The goal of a joint Mexico-U.S. program started in 1976 is the eradication of screwworms from both countries and the establishment of a permanent barrier in Southern Mexico to protect against reinvasion.

Veterinarians and livestock producers in the U.S.A. and Mexico can greatly assist the eradication effort by promptly reporting all suspected cases of screwworms to regulatory officials. If myiasis is found, larvae should be preserved in 70% ethanol and forwarded for identification.

Treatment: The USDA has developed 2 remedies, either of which can be used for the protection of wounds from screwworm infestation and for treating infestations. EQ 335 is a mixture containing 3% lindane in a gel base. Smear 62 is an older remedy that utilizes benzene as a killing agent and diphenylamine as a protectant against infestation or reinfestation by newly hatched larvae. Ronnel has also been incorporated into a wound dressing similar to EQ 335. All 3 smears are best applied with a 1-in. (2.5-cm) paint brush. Careful application is necessary to be sure that the smear reaches all the many pockets formed by the burrowing maggots in deep wounds. A thin layer should also be applied to the skin surrounding the wound.

Sprays and dusts may also be used for screwworm control. The topical application of a dust containing 5% coumaphos is an economical and effective means of killing the maggots in a wound. In regions where screwworm flies are very active, it is often advisable to spray livestock with either coumaphos or ronnel as a prophylactic measure. If properly applied, these sprays will kill all larvae and protect animals from infestation for 2 weeks or longer.

WOOL MAGGOTS

(Fly strike, Fleece worms)

Several species of blowflies cause myiasis of sheep. Primary flies in the U.S.A. and Canada are the black blowflies, *Phormia regina* and *Protophormia terraenovae*, and the green bottle fly, *Lucilia sericata. Lucilia illustris, Cochliomyia* (*Callitroga*) *macellaria* (secondary screwworm) and some others are usually secondary invaders. *Lucilia cuprina* is the most important primary fly in Australia, *L. sericata* in Great Britain, and *L. sericata* and *Calliphora stygia* in New Zealand.

Eggs are usually laid below the tip of the fleece, and hatch within 24 hours if conditions are moist. Moisture, containing nutriments from serum, feces, etc. is necessary for the survival of the first stage maggot. The second stage larvae can abrade the skin with its mouth hooks, and thus obtain food. Once established, strikes can spread rapidly and attract more blowflies, secondary as well as primary. Bad strikes can be fatal but even mild strikes can cause rapid loss of condition. Strikes should be diagnosed early, and the behavior of a sheep is a good indicator of myiasis. Screwworm, q.v., p. 766, may be suspected if the larvae are associated with wounds.

A common site of strike is the breech where flies are attracted to wool soaked with urine or fecal contamination resulting from scouring. The body of the sheep may also be struck. This is usually associated with heavy soaking rains that cause the development of fleece-rot, often characterized by discoloration by *Pseudomonas* sp., or mycotic dermatitis, q.v., p. 931. The odors and associated moisture attract flies, and stimulate oviposition particularly when the weather is hot and humid.

Other common sites are the heads of horned rams, the wool around the pizzle, the sides where feet with foot-rot come in contact with the fleece, and wounds.

Control: Blow-fly infestation of the breech can be effectively controlled for about 6 to 8 weeks by "tagging," ("crutching") whereby the wool is shorn from the area between the legs and around the tail. Complete shearing will control outbreaks involving other parts of the body. The wool can be removed from around the heads of rams to prevent poll strike and around the pizzle to prevent pizzle strike.

Urine staining of the crutch of Merino ewes can be virtually eliminated by removal of breech wrinkles (the Mules operation in Australia), and fecal contamination can be greatly reduced by docking tails correctly, at the third joint. Causes of scouring should be sought and prevented; the common associated causes are sudden change of food and helminth infection.

Chemoprophylactic measures consist of wetting the wool and skin of susceptible areas with suitable insecticidal and larvicidal preparations such as 2.5% ronnel, 0.03 to 0.06% coumaphos, 0.15% dioxathion, or 0.03% diazinon or other organophosphorus insecticides. These substances may be used as dips or sprays, the aim being complete saturation of the fleece. The most efficient procedure is to force the insecticide into the fleece under a higher pressure ("jetting"); this is usually applied locally—to the breech, along the back, the heads of rams. Protection can be effective for 6 to 8 weeks but in some countries where the primary fly has become resistant to insecticides, e.g. with *L. cuprina* in Australia, protection may only last for 2 to 3 weeks. The application at weekly intervals of agents such as 2.5% ronnel pressurized spray to wounds until healed can be highly beneficial, particularly where screwworm is present.

In small flocks, where individual treatment is carried out, the wool should be completely removed from and around the struck area and the lesions then treated with suitable agents.

Destruction of all carcasses by burning or deep burying (preferably after poisoning of the carcass) has been recommended as a valuable general hygienic measure; however, it may have little effect on the primary "strikes." The main source of primary flies is the struck sheep.

CATTLE GRUBS

(Ox warbles)

Cattle in the Northern Hemisphere are commonly infested by myiasis-causing larvae belonging to the genus *Hypoderma*. The adults are called gadflies, heel flies or bomb flies. Central and South American cattle may be infested by larvae of the genus *Dermatobia*.

Biology: Two species of heel flies (order Diptera, family Oestridae) attack cattle. The smaller species (*Hypoderma lineatum*) develops into the common cattle grub, the other (*H. bovis*) into the northern cattle grub. The adults, hairy flies about the size of honeybees, with a general coloration much like bumblebees, are rapid fliers. Their whitish eggs, about 1-mm long, are fastened to the hairs of the legs and lower portions of the animal's body.

In 2 to 6 days, depending on the temperature, the eggs hatch. The young larvae crawl down the hair to the skin and burrow directly into the tissues. There is a period of several months after the larvae enter the body, during which their movements are not well known. They apparently travel continuously and almost exclusively through connective tissue. They have been found in the connective tissue of the spleen, rumen, intestines, thoracic cavity, muscles, spinal column, heart and esophagus, and rarely, in the CNS. The larvae secrete proteolytic enzymes, which dissolve the tissues, producing readily ingestible food and facilitating their forward movement. The majority of *H. lineatum* congregate for a period of 2 to 4 months in the submucosa of the esophagus, increasing severalfold in size and weight. *H. bovis* migrate along the nerves and congregate for a similar period in the epidural fat of the spinal canal. The larvae, now about 15 mm in length and 1 to 2 mm in diameter, begin their final migration, again through connective tissue. Eventually the larvae arrive in the subdermal tissue of the back, where each secretes an enzyme to make a breathing hole through the skin. Although cysts (called warbles or wolves) are formed around them, the breathing pores remain open. Their presence irritates the cyst walls; the serum exuded into the cysts, and abundant secondary invading organisms furnish food for the larvae. After a 40- to 60-day period of growth in these cysts, during which 2 molts occur, they emerge through the holes, drop to the ground and pupate. By this time, they have grown to a length of 25 mm and a diameter of 8 mm and have changed in color from creamy white to dark brownish gray. The adult heel flies emerge from the pupae in 1 to 3 months, depending on weather conditions. They may mate within an hour after emergence and are ready to spend their brief adult life terrorizing their bovine hosts. The adults do not feed and live an average of a week.

Distribution and Seasonal Activity: In much of the Southern U.S.A. *H. lineatum* is common, but *H. bovis* is absent or rare in native cattle. Elsewhere to the north in North America, both species are pests wherever cattle are raised.

Where both are present, the seasonal events for the 2 species are similar except that those for *H. lineatum* are about 6 to 8 weeks earlier. These events vary considerably from year to year and may be fairly well correlated with local and regional climatic conditions. In Texas, larvae ordinarily make their first appearance in backs of cattle about mid-September; progressing northward, this appearance is gradually later, until in Montana, it is about December 25, and in some of the higher mountain areas, it may be a month or more later. In Texas, the first emergence of the grubs from the back takes place during the last half of November. Where both species are present, grubs may be found in the back for about 5 to 6 months, where only *H. lineatum* is present, for about 4 to 5 months. In Texas, the heel fly season (that time when the flies actively chase cattle) is at its height during January, February and March; in the Northern States, during May, June and July.

Domestic cattle and American bison are the only mammals known to be regularly infested with large numbers of *H. bovis* and *H. lineatum*. Increasing numbers of horses seem to be experiencing light infestation in recent years. On rare occasions, man becomes infested. In these cases, the grub usually is found in the subdermal tissues of the upper extremities. Other species of grubs may be found in the tissues of mammals (*see* CUTEREBRA INFESTATION OF SMALL ANIMALS, p. 775).

Clinical Findings and Diagnosis: Signs of heel-fly attack: During periods of sunshine on warm days, cattle run wildly, often blindly, tails high in the air. Careful observation will sometimes permit detection of a pursuing heel fly. Refuge from the flies is found in shade and in water holes. Not all stampeding of this kind is due to heel fly attacks, however, for this activity occasionally is observed in seasons or regions known to be free of heel flies.

Signs of internal infestation: In otherwise normal cattle, the presence of *H. bovis* and their secretions in the epidural fat of the spinal canal is associated with dissolved connective tissue, fat necrosis and inflammation. Sometimes the inflammation extends to the periosteum and bone, producing a localized area of periostitis and osteomyelitis. Occasionally, the epineurium and perineurium may become involved. In rare, severe cases, paralysis or other nervous disorders may occur. Similarly, the presence of *H. lineatum* in the submucosa of the esophagus may cause inflammation and edema in the surrounding tissues sufficiently severe to hinder swallowing.

Signs of external infestation: The penetration of the skin by the newly hatched larvae produces a hypodermal rash. The points of penetration are painful, inflamed and usually exude a yellowish serum. Grubs in the back may occur from the tailhead to the shoulders and from the topline to a point about one-third the distance down the sides. The cysts or warbles are firm and raised considerably above the normal contour of the skin; in each there is the breathing hole, ranging in size from a very small slit to a round hole, 3 to 4 mm in diameter. Secondary infection may result in large suppurating abscesses. The emergence of the grub, its forced expulsion, or its death within the cyst, usually results in healing of the lesion without complications. Carcasses of cattle infested with cattle grubs show marked evidence of the infestation and may be penalized upon inspection.

The number of warbles in an infested animal may range from 1 to 300 or more; infested herds may have animals with no grubs. Infestations are progressively lighter with age.

Treatment: Some organophosphorus insecticides called "systemics," when properly applied, are absorbed by the host and kill the migrating grubs in all parts of the body. Effective grub control can be obtained with these drugs, but important precautions must be taken.

Cattle, especially calves, in areas where grub numbers per animal are known to be high, should be treated as soon as possible after the adult heel-fly season is over. They should not be treated later than 8 to 12 weeks before the anticipated first appearance of grubs in the backs, as adverse reactions may develop. Migratory *H. lineatum* larvae congregate in maximum numbers at this time in the submucosal tissues of the esophagus. If rapidly killed by systemic insecticides, a massive, usually transitory, inflammatory edematous reaction will result. The swelling may partially or completely occlude the lumen, swallowing may become difficult or impossible, profuse drooling of saliva may occur, eructation may cease and the calf may become bloated. Recovery is usually rapid and complete (48 to 72 hours after treatment) but in severe cases the calf may die of bloat. Rupture of the esophagus may be caused by attempted passage of a stomach tube.

Migratory *H. bovis* larvae also may appear in maximum numbers during this period in the epidural fat of the spinal canal. If they are rapidly killed by systemic insecticides, a massive, usually transitory irritation of the spinal tissues may result. Mild to severe paraplegia may develop. Again, recovery is usually rapid and complete; rarely, a calf may become permanently paralyzed.

Six different systemic insecticides, in varied formulations, are available for treatment. Pour-on treatments using coumaphos, famophos, fenthion, phosmet or trichlorfon may be used, (℞ 282, 289, 290, 307, 337). A measured amount of the material should be poured evenly along the midline of the animal's back, making sure it runs down the sides of the animal for maximal skin wetting and absorption. Fenthion 20% may be applied (in a measured amount of ready-to-use formulation) to a single spot on the animal's midline.

Sprays containing coumaphos (℞ 278), phosmet (℞ 306) or trichlofon (℞ 337) may be applied, being especially careful that the entire surface of the skin is thoroughly wet to permit maximum absorption. Coumaphos (℞ 276) also may be used as a dip.

As an additive to the diet ronnel (℞ 315, 318) will effectively control grubs only if the treatment regimen ensures adequate intake of the drug. For example, ronnel as an additive to the mineral mix (℞ 318) is generally effective, but in some regions range cattle will not eat enough of the mineral mix to effect a complete grub kill.

No systemic insecticide should be used in conjunction with another since their actions may be synergistic. Cattle stressed by castration, overheating, vaccination, shipping, etc. should not be treated. Use of these insecticides is prohibited in lactating dairy animals as these drugs are excreted in the milk. Residues are present in all animals for varying periods after treatment.

No systemic insecticide should be used except in strict accord with the manufacturer's recommendations. THE TOXICITY OF ORGANIC INSECTICIDES AND ACARICIDES is discussed elsewhere in this MANUAL (q.v., p. 995).

Where organophosphates cannot be used, and rotenone is approved, grubs can be controlled by external applications of rotenone to the warbles after the grubs have taken up their subdermal positions in the back. Since new grubs continue to appear in the back and since rotenone kills only those with which it comes in contact through the breathing holes, it is necessary to repeat treatment every 6 weeks or oftener during the grub season. Washing or dusting by hand with crude rotenone (℞ 321, 322) gives good results. The wash or dust should be sprinkled over the animal's back and worked into the grub holes with a stiff brush or the tips of the fingers. This treatment, if properly applied, will kill 90 to 100% of the grubs present in the back.

Mechanical extraction: On small groups of tractable animals, instrument extraction or hand expulsion (by squeezing) of the individual grubs is effective. Rarely, when this procedure is carelessly performed, the grub is crushed in its cyst and an anaphylactic reaction may result.

SHEEP NOSE BOTS

The sheep nose bot fly, *Oestrus ovis,* is worldwide in distribution and is one of the most widely distributed sheep parasites in the U.S.A. Goats occasionally are affected and rarely man is attacked, mainly in the eyes. A related species is found in the nasal passages of deer.

Biology: The adult fly is grayish brown and about 12 mm in length. The female deposits larvae in and about the nostrils of sheep without alighting. These clear white larvae are very small, initially 2 mm in length. They migrate into the nasal cavity, many of them spending at least some time in the paranasal sinuses. As the larvae mature, the acquire a cream color, then darken, finally having a dark or black band on the dorsal surface of each segment. In warm climates the larval period may be as short as 1 month, but, where winters are cold it may last as long as 10 months.

When mature, the larvae leave the nasal passages, drop to the ground, burrow down a few inches and pupate. The pupal period lasts from 3 to 9 weeks, depending upon the environmental conditions. At the end of this time the flies emerge, mate, and the females begin to deposit larvae.

Clinical Findings: Once the larvae begin to move about in the nasal passages, a profuse discharge occurs, at first clear and mucoid, but later mucopurulent and frequently tinged with fine streaks of blood emanating from minute hemorrhages produced by the hooks and spines of the larvae. Continuing activity of the larvae, particularly if they are numerous, causes a thickening of the nasal mucous membrane which, together with the mucopurulent discharge, leads to impairment of respiration. Paroxysms of sneezing accompany the migrations of the larger larvae. Larvae present in the sinuses are sometimes unable to escape and die, and gradually become calcified or lead to a septic sinusitis. The purulent inflammation produced in the nasal passages may occasionally spread to the brain, via the olfactory nerve, with fatal results. However, the principal effects of the nose bot are annoyance and debilitation of the sheep. Infestations may consist of 80 or more larvae, but most commonly only 4 to 15 are found.

Adult *Oestrus ovis* do not feed, but are much feared by sheep. To avoid the fly's attempts at larvae deposition, a sheep may run about, keeping its nose close to the ground, may sneeze and stamp its feet or shake its head. Commonly, especially during the warmer hours of the day when the flies are most active, small groups of sheep gather for mutual defense, all facing to the center of a circle, heads down and close together.

Control: Ruelene given orally as a drench at the rate of 50 mg/lb (110 mg/kg) should afford good control but must not be used within 14 days of slaughter and all warnings on its label should be observed. Rafoxanide, given orally as a drench or bolus at 3.5 mg/lb (7.5 mg/kg) is effective, but not yet approved for this use in some countries.

CUTEREBRA INFESTATION (SM. AN.)

The presence of the maggot of the rodent bot fly, *Cuterebra* sp., in the subcutis.

Etiology: Adult *Cuterebra* are nonparasitic and seldom observed. Females usually deposit eggs in the burrows of wild mammals during the summer months. Tiny larvae (1 mm in length) hatch from the eggs and wait for contact with an animal in the burrow. Larvae penetrate the skin of the nose and mouth and make their way to various subcut. locations in different hosts. The route of migration is variable. The maggot may reach 25 mm in length and 10 mm in diameter. Black cuticular spines give fully developed maggots a dark color. Larval development takes approximately 1 month, after which the maggot exits from its subcut. location to pupate in the soil. They mature in about 300 days. Adult flies live approximately 2 weeks and are said to lay up to 2,000 eggs per female.

Clinical Findings: A thick-walled subcut. abscess of variable size forms around the developing larva. Pus may exude from the breathing hole made through the skin by the parasite. An aberrant larva sometimes invades the brain and causes fatal CNS disturbances.

The usual hosts are burrow-dwelling mammals such as mice, chipmunks, rabbits and squirrels. Dogs and cats sometimes become infested, presumably from investigation of such burrows. Lesions are found most often under the skin of the neck and chest during late summer and early fall. Constant licking of the chest area is frequently the most obvious clinical sign in cats.

Treatment: The lesion should not be squeezed since rupture of the parasite may result in anaphylaxis. The breathing hole through the skin should be enlarged surgically to permit careful removal of the maggot. The lesion is then treated as any abscess with flushing and instillation of antibiotic preparations.

PHYSICAL INFLUENCES

ACCIDENTS (SM. AN.)

WOUNDS

Wounds may result in loss of continuity, loss of function, pain and hemorrhage. The most frequent causes of wounds in small animals are automobile accidents, bites from other animals, broken glass and other sharp objects, and unintentional ligatures (such as a rubber band placed around the neck or leg of a pet by a child). The location, nature and extent of the lesions vary from the smallest abrasion to gross lacerations that are badly contaminated and accompanied by complicating internal or skeletal injuries.

Before proceeding with treatment of the obvious lesions, one must consider the possibility of complicating injuries. Therefore, the following routine should be followed: (1) examination of the mucous membranes for color and capillary refill; (2) observation of the nature of the animal's pulse and respiration; (3) inspection of the body orifices for blood; (4) auscultation of the thorax; (5) palpation of the abdomen for the presence of excess fluid or pain; (6) palpation of the urinary bladder; (7) testing the animal for its ability to stand, and to flex all joints without pain; and (8) a neurologic examination, especially if there is a question of head or spinal trauma.

Treatment: The following procedures are mandatory in the treatment of any accidental wound: (1) control hemorrhage; (2) relieve pain and control the patient; (3) treat shock; (4) control infection; (5) clean and close the wound; and (6) provide after-care.

To control hemorrhage, compression bandages are recommended as a first aid measure; tourniquets should be used only if pressure bandages will not control most of the bleeding. Later, bleeding vessels are sutured, ligated, or coagulated by electrocautery. If necessary, pain can be controlled with meperidine hydrochloride (℞ 380). Atropine (℞ 524) is also indicated, especially in those animals that are salivating badly; it should always be administered before general anesthesia.

Hypovolemic shock may follow blood loss to the exterior, into a body cavity, or into the tissues. The degree of shock is assessed by an estimate of blood loss, examination of pulse rate and pressure, and hemoglobin or hematocrit determinations. Hematocrit determination immediately after an episode of blood loss, however, can be misleading. It takes time for body fluids to equilibrate following severe hemorrhage, and an initial normal hematocrit reading may be significantly lowered following adequate IV fluid administration used for the treatment of shock.

Much more commonly seen than hypovolemic shock due to blood loss is traumatic shock; this is usually associated with automobile accidents. For handling of shock, *see* p. 79.

Infection is controlled mainly by adequate wound cleaning and debridement but prompt treatment of wounds also decreases the chance of infection. Follow-up care for the treatment of contaminated wounds includes the administration of oral antibiotics, such as penicillin (℞ 64), ampicillin (℞ 5), tetracyclines (℞ 77), or chloramphenicol (℞ 17), for a period of 7 to 10 days.

Successful wound management depends upon cleaning, debridement and suturing. To cleanse the wound, it is covered with a sterile dressing while the hair around it is clipped; the skin is then scrubbed with a germicidal soap. The dressing is then removed, and the wound is cleaned with mild soap and irrigated with large volumes of sterile saline. In small wounds in tractable animals, wound cleansing and repair can be done following infiltration of the periphery of the wound with a local anesthetic. To repair major wounds, general anesthesia is usually required. Thorough debridement of the wound is necessary to remove all nonviable tissue and foreign material. Debridement is minimal in incised wounds, and must be done carefully in the extremities in order to retain blood and nerve supply to the foot.

Incised wounds that are less than 24 hours old can usually be closed immediately. Dead space should be eliminated, and excess skin tension can be managed through the use of tension sutures; drains are often necessary. Puncture wounds are always infected, but overzealous local treatment of puncture wounds often does more harm than good. Flushing such wounds with nitrofurazone solution is an effective means of both cleansing and introducing antibacterial agents. These animals should always be treated with systemic antibiotics (℞ 5, 17, 64, 77), for 7 to 10 days following the accident.

The treatment of chronic, obviously infected wounds requires the removal of all foreign material and devitalized tissue by surgical, chemical, or enzymatic means. In wounds where phagocytosis and enzymatic action have accomplished self-debridement, and healthy granulation tissue is present, nothing but protection of the wound and the avoidance of exuberant granulation is necessary. This process may be assisted by the use of proteolytic enzymes (℞ 434). Most wounds heal by contraction and epithelialization; however, in some, skin grafting or reconstruction is required. The application of a well-padded, firm bandage aids in the elimination of dead space, reduces movement in the wound, and protects against self-mutilation.

THORACIC TRAUMA

Thoracic trauma is a common injury sustained either in automobile accidents or, in the case of cats and small dogs, in fights with large dogs. In many of these cases a rapid diagnosis must be made and appropriate treatment instituted if the patient is to survive. Although a thoracic radiograph can be helpful in establishing an exact diagnosis in the dyspneic patient, in some cases there is no time to make an X-ray picture.

If a dyspneic animal is presented following known trauma, the 3 primary differentials that should be considered are: pneumothorax (with or without hemothorax), pulmonary hemorrhage and diaphragmatic hernia.

Pneumothorax can be effectively treated by thoracentesis. If pneumothorax is suspected, in a critical case it may be more expedient to attempt treatment for pneumothorax before stressing the animal with radiography. The upper thorax over the 8th to 12th interspace should be rapidly clipped and prepared, a 20 or 22 gauge needle on a syringe should be gently introduced between the ribs until the tip is just into the pleural space and negative pressure applied. Most animals tolerate this procedure well, and usually a local anesthetic is unnecessary.

If free air is obtained from the chest, the diagnosis of pneumothorax is established; by withdrawing it all, the condition will be corrected. If the leakage from the lungs is severe and the pneumothorax recurs, the placement of a Heimlich one-way valve may be indicated.

If blood is obtained when thoracentesis is performed on the dyspneic trauma patient, the thoracic radiographs should be taken as rapidly as possible. The degree of hemorrhage revealed by the X-rays will determine the animal's chances of survival. Medical therapy for **pulmonary hemorrhage** consists of aminophylline (℞ 522), oxygen administration (q.v., p. 1495), and rapid and vigorous fluid therapy using a replacement-type multiple electrolyte solution. If the animal has hemorrhagic shock that does not respond to fluid therapy, or, if a relapse occurs following fluid therapy, immediate thoracotomy is indicated.

If X-rays reveal a **diaphragmatic hernia** (q.v., p. 589), surgery is essential. A left-sided diaphragmatic hernia can be an emergency situation: if the stomach is in the chest, it can rapidly dilate with air and cause fatal compression of the lungs and heart.

ELECTRIC SHOCK

Electric shock in puppies and kittens is usually a result of their chewing on electric cords. Burn wounds of the mouth, tongue and lips are consistent lesions. A striking feature of electric burns is the marked necrosis of large areas of tissue that occurs days or weeks after the burn is inflicted; this is because preferential passage of electricity along vascular channels commonly causes thrombosis.

The more common cause of emergency presentation following electric shock is dyspnea and cyanosis secondary to pulmonary edema. Stupor, unconsciousness, coma and death can also occur with electrocution.

Treatment of electrical burns is palliative; in time, necrotic tissue is replaced by granulation tissue. Antibiotic therapy (℞ 5, 17, 64, 77) should be instituted to prevent infection.

The animal that is presented with signs of pulmonary edema should be treated with IV diuretics (℞ 543), bronchial dilators (℞ 522), and steroids (℞ 148). Oxygen should also be administered.

DROWNING

Drowning is rare, since most pet animals swim instinctively and with considerable efficiency from birth. Occasionally, one hears of an animal (e.g. certain bulldogs) that apparently cannot swim. Treatment for drowning consists of establishing an open airway, drainage of the trachea by suspending the patient head down or by actual mechanical aspiration, and artificial respiration. Heart stimulants or general stimulants are of doubtful value, and are usually employed only in cases of complete or impending cardiac arrest. Restoration of body heat is also needed, although excessive heat may be harmful. Of paramount importance is the restoration of an adequate oxygen intake by any means available.

LIGHTNING STROKE AND ELECTROCUTION

Injury or death due to high-voltage electrical currents may be the result of lightning, fallen transmission wires, faulty electrical circuits or chewing on electric cord (*see also* ELECTRIC SHOCK, p.

780). Lightning stroke is seasonal, and tends to be geographically restricted.

Certain types of trees, especially those which are tall, spreading, and have well-developed root systems just beneath the ground surface, tend to be struck by lightning more often than others. Electrification of the root system charges a wide surface area, particularly when the ground is already damp; passage of roots beneath a shallow pool of water causes that pool to become electrified. A tile drain may spread an electric charge over an entire field. Fallen transmission wires may also electrify a pool of water. Differences exist in conductivity in soil, varying with geologic composition; loam, sand, clay, marble and chalk (in that order) are good conductors, while rocky soil is not.

Accidental electrocution of farm animals usually occurs as a result of faulty wiring. Electrification of a water or milk line, metal creep or guard rail can result in widespread distribution of an electric current throughout the stable.

Death from electric shock usually results from cardiac or respiratory arrest; passage of current through the heart usually produces ventricular fibrillation; involvement of the CNS may affect the respiratory or other vital centers.

Clinical Findings: Varying degrees of electrical shock may occur. In most instances of lightning stroke, death is instantaneous, the animal falling down without a struggle. Occasionally the animal becomes unconscious but may recover completely in a few minutes to several hours. Some of these latter animals have residual nervous signs, for example, depression, paraplegia, cutaneous hyperesthesia; these signs may persist for days or weeks. Singe marks on the carcass, damage to the immediate environment or both occur in about 90% of cases of lightning stroke. Singe marks tend to be linear and are more commonly found on the medial sides of the legs, although in rare instances much of the body may be affected. Beneath the singe marks, capillary congestion is common; the arboreal pattern characteristic of lightning stroke can be visualized best from the dermal side of the skin by subcut. extravasations of blood. Singe marks are difficult to find on the recovered animal.

Animals periodically receiving electric shocks while tied in stanchions are restless and nervous; they may kick at the stanchion or dividing rails; those which have received intermittent shock eat and drink with care. Smaller animals such as pigs that contact electrified water bowls or creeps may be killed instantly or, from the strength of the shock, be thrown across the pen.

Diagnosis: History of a recent storm may be confusing; finding a dead or injured animal under a tree or near a fence is significant only if one finds evidence of recent burning of bark, splitting of fence posts, welding of wire, etc. *Rigor mortis* develops and passes quickly; postmortem distension of the rumen occurs rapidly and differentiation from antemortem ruminal tympany (q.v., p. 145) must be made. In both conditions, the blood tends to clot slowly or not at all. The mucosae of the upper respiratory tract, including the turbinates and sinuses are congested and hemorrhagic; linear tracheal hemorrhages are common but the lungs are not compressed as in bloat. All other viscera are congested and petechiae and ecchymoses may be found in many organs. Due to postmortem ruminal distension, the poorly clotted blood is passively moved to the periphery of the body, resulting in postmortem extravasation of blood in muscles and superficial lymph nodes of the head, neck and thoracic limbs, and, to a lesser extent, in the hindquarters. Probably the best indication of instantaneous death is the presence of hay or other feed in the animal's mouth; the presence of normal ingesta (especially in the rumen, and lack of frothy ingesta—frothy bloat), absence of a distended gallbladder, and presence of normal feces in the lower tract, and occasionally on the ground behind the animal are supportive evidence.

Treatment: Those animals that survive may require supportive and symptomatic therapy.

BURNS

The destruction of epithelium or deeper tissues by direct heat, radiant heat, flames, friction, electricity, or corrosive chemicals.

Etiology: Thermal burns result from scalding with hot liquids, contact with hot objects or exposure to flame or radiant heat. Pigs and closely shorn sheep and dogs may suffer radiant heat burns (sunburn). Frictional burns most commonly are caused by rubbing rough ropes against the skin during restraint of large animals or by dragging or rubbing the skin along pavement in small animals hit by motor vehicles. In large animals electrical burns most commonly are caused by lightning stroke in open pastures and less frequently by contact with live electric wires (see p. 780). In small animals, electrical burns are most often caused by the animal chewing an electrical cord or by the use of a defective dryer. Corrosive chemicals include acids, phenols and strong alkalies.

Clinical Findings: Burns of animals are not strictly comparable to those of man. First-degree burns with reddening of the skin may occur but formation of vesicles and blisters is uncommon except in the pig. The usual lesions of a moderately severe burn in animals are diffuse edema of the skin and subcut. tissues, with or without formation of small vesicles and sloughs. Charring of tissue occurs in severe burns where the skin may be wholly devitalized and the injury extend into the deeper structures. Sloughing of the skin may follow, leaving large denuded areas from which constant exudation or effusion of serum can lead to considerable loss of protein and fluid. Burns of small areas of the body cause only minor discomfort. Animals with more severe burns are reluctant to move, resent handling and may be indifferent to normal stimuli. Extensive burns with loss of considerable plasma may result in shock. Later complications include infection, impaired cardiac and liver function and pneumonitis. The prognosis depends on the total area of the burn, depth of penetration, location, and age and condition of the patient.

Treatment: Chemical burns require neutralization of the irritant. Weak acetic acid solution may be applied to alkali burns, alcohol to phenol burns, solutions of sodium bicarbonate to acid burns, and for burns caused by unknown chemicals, saturated solutions of sodium bicarbonate or sodium thiosulfate may be applied. Following the neutralizing bath, the wound should be washed with mild soap and rinsed with large quantities of isotonic salt solution (ISS). A wet pack moistened with ISS or sodium thiosulfate solution should then be applied to the part.

Animals with severe burns over more than 50% of the body should be destroyed. Burns of less than 15% of the body surface can usually be treated on an ambulatory basis. Although pain may be severe initially, it most often disappears rather quickly. Systemic antibiotic treatment usually is not necessary nor is there need for special modification of fluid or food intake. The use of various dyes, local anesthetics, tannic acid, salves and oils are contraindicated. A hydrophilic ointment containing antibiotics, nitrofurazone or proteolytic enzymes (℞ 422, 434, 447, 460) should be applied and covered with a sterile bandage. Inspection of the wound for the presence of infection should be made every 2 or 3 days and the dressing changed if necessary.

Burns of more than 15% of the body surface require systemic treatment. Examination of the patient should include evaluation of the pulse, respiratory rate, temperature and packed red cell volume and sedimentation rate. The pharynx and larynx should be inspected for edema. Fluid therapy should be started immediately, with ⅓ dextrose (5%) and ⅔ lactated Ringer's solution (℞ 588) given IV at a rate of 5 to 20 ml/kg/hr. The rate and amount can be monitored by urine output and central venous pressure. Oral administration of fluids should be withheld for 48 hours to avoid inhalation and vomiting problems. Analgesics such as meperidine should be used to control pain; cool compresses will also give comfort. Local therapy may utilize the open method, the closed method, or excision of the burned area. The open method seeks to produce a dry crust over the burned area, but subjects the wound to a flow of air warm enough to prevent chilling the patient. A crust will begin to form after 1 to 2 days and will remain for about 2 weeks. The crust will slough as the epithelium regenerates. In deep burns the scab will have to be removed by surgery and skin-grafting performed.

In the closed method, a hydrophilic ointment containing silver sulfadiazine or antibiotics such as neomycin, polymyxin, bacitracin combinations or nitrofurazone with or without proteolytic enzymes (℞ 422, 434, 447, 448, 460), with or without urea is placed upon the wound and covered with a thick layer of absorbent material. The final covering is either lightly impregnated petrolatum gauze or a nylon fabric commercially prepared for this purpose. The bandage is left in place for 7 to 10 days. This form of therapy is not generally satisfactory in veterinary practice because of the difficulty of keeping the bandage in place and the probability of infection. The animal may be controlled by reasonable use of tranquilizers or other forms of chemical or physical restraint indicated during convalescence. Emphasis should be placed on maintenance of good nutrition. Healing is hastened by feeding a diet high in protein.

Small full-thickness burns should be immediately excised and treated as any other surgical wound.

The use of oils, petroleum jelly, or ointments should be avoided in chemical burns. Friction burns are treated with simple protectives such as petroleum jelly or antibiotic ointment (℞ 422) and may be further protected with sterile dressings. Electrical burns may sometimes require local therapy as described earlier. Deep infarction is a feature of electrical burns. The area should be left to demarcate in 2 to 3 weeks, when the dead tissue will slough naturally or can be removed surgically. Sunburns are best treated by removing the affected animals from the sun and limiting sun exposure in the future.

Suitable restraint to prevent biting, scratching or rubbing of burn wounds must be employed. This may require the use of Elizabethan collars in small animals, proper tying of large animals in stalls, or the ingenious use of dressings. If immobilization of the part can be accomplished, healing will be greatly facilitated. A plaster cast may be employed to effect complete immobilization of the part.

HYPERTHERMIA

(Heat exhaustion, Heat cramps, Heatstroke, Sunstroke)

Manifestations of disturbance of the heat-regulating mechanism of the body; in general, they result from high environmental temperature, high humidity and inadequate ventilation. Exposure to direct rays of the sun may be a contributory factor.

Etiology: All domestic animals are susceptible to **heatstroke.** Dogs confined to close quarters in hot weather, cattle, horses or other stock being driven in large numbers or being transported in hot weather are most commonly affected. Predisposing factors include physical effort, obesity and stagnation of the air.

Heat exhaustion occurs in draft horses, cattle and swine. It is unusual in dogs. Prolonged exposure to high environmental temperature causes the peripheral blood vessels to dilate. When dilation occurs without a compensatory increase in blood volume, circulatory collapse may ensue.

Heat cramps are commonest in animals doing hard work in intense heat. Animals with the ability to sweat are most commonly affected, e.g. draft horses. Heat cramps are rare in dogs other than those working or racing in a hot environment. Deranged electrolyte balance (acute salt loss) is the factor responsible.

Clinical Findings: The outstanding signs of heat exhaustion are weakness, muscle tremors and collapse. There may be hyperpnea and rapid pulse. The body temperature is not necessarily elevated and the onset of signs is not as sudden as heatstroke. Heat cramps are characterized by severe muscle spasm, with cessation of sweating in horses and working animals other than dogs. Clinical signs of heatstroke include hyperpnea and collapse. A staring expression of the eyes, vomiting and diarrhea are not uncommon. The oral mucosa may be bright red and the rectal temperature is greatly elevated, up to 109.5°F (43°C). Disseminated intravascular coagulation (DIC) and cerebral edema may occur as complicating factors in heatstroke in the dog.

Treatment: In cases of heat exhaustion cool water should be applied to the body and the animal moved to a cool and shaded area. Isotonic saline solution may be given IV to animals suffering from heat cramps.

Heatstroke requires immediate therapy. Animals respond best to immersion in cold water. Cold water enemas are also useful. The rectal temperatures should be checked every 10 minutes and treatment stopped as the temperature approaches normal. Cerebral edema may be prevented by the administration of dexamethasone IV at the rate of 0.5 to 1 mg/lb (1.0 to 2.0 mg/kg) body weight. If DIC is suspected, blood coagulation studies should be performed.

HYPOTHERMIA

A profound fall in body temperature resulting from exposure to external cold, drugs or failure of internal temperature regulating mechanisms. Body temperatures of 86 to 89.5°F (30 to 32°C) are classified as mild hypothermia, temperatures of 71.5 to 77°F (22 to

25°C) as moderate hypothermia and temperatures of 32 to 46.5°F (0 to 8°C) as profound hypothermia. The prognosis varies accordingly.

Rewarming and maintenance of normal body function is the aim of treatment. This is best accomplished through internal warming. Peritoneal dialysis, where the dialysate is heated to 122 to 131°F (50 to 55°C), is performed until body temperature is returned to normal.

FROSTBITE

Destruction of superficial tissues as a result of exposure to cold with secondary structural and functional disturbances of the smaller surface blood vessels. Frostbite is not uncommon in young animals, especially young, poorly nourished cattle and horses exposed to storms and extreme cold. Pigs farrowed in extreme cold may suffer from frosting of exposed parts, especially the ears and tail. Sometimes the combs of chickens are affected.

Clinical Findings: Slight frosting causes the skin to become pale and bloodless. This is soon followed by intense redness, heat, pain and swelling. In such cases, the hair may fall out and the epidermis may peel. Usually, the inflammation subsides, the swelling disappears and only an increased sensitivity to cold remains. There may be irritation and itching for some time.

If freezing is more severe, the affected part becomes swollen and very painful, remains cold and later begins to shrivel. In severe cases, patches of skin are devitalized and a line of demarcation forms between the affected and the normal parts. Finally the destroyed portion drops off, leaving a raw surface.

Treatment: Small, simple lesions caused by freezing may be treated with mild antiseptics and thoroughly covered with healing ointment. Simple frostbites are treated by rapidly warming the affected part by water bath or pack (105 to 108°F [40.5 to 42°C]) for 15 to 20 minutes, and by applying antiseptic dressing such as 5% carbolized ointment or oil, 1% solution or ointment of silver nitrate or zinc chloride. Gentle daily massage of the area may help to reduce pain and stimulate circulation.

Severe freezing may be treated by conservative means until a line of demarcation appears. The necrotic portion of severely affected tissue should then be removed surgically and the defect treated as an open wound.

MOTION SICKNESS

A systemic condition characterized by excessive salivation, nausea and vomiting brought about by continued motion, as in travel by car, sea or air. Man and many of the domestic animals are susceptible. The principal mechanism involved in motion sickness is concerned with the vestibular apparatus of the ear. Fear of the vehicle is a contributory factor in the case of dogs and cats.

Clinical Findings: The outstanding signs are salivation, nausea and vomiting. The animals may yawn and show definite signs of uneasiness. These signs disappear promptly as soon as vehicular motion ceases.

Control: Motion sickness can be overcome by having the animal become accustomed to travel. With the advent of the ataractic and antinauseant drugs, therapy for the alleviation or prevention of motion sickness is much more effective and specific. A number of these have been used with good results in dogs. Perhaps phenobarbital (℞ 552) alone or with methylatropine nitrate (℞ 484) is the commonest; the latter combination shows effectiveness in controlling salivation. Promethazine hydrochloride (℞ 486) actively inhibits both vomiting and drooling. Perphenazine (℞ 382), promazine hydrochloride (℞ 383) and mepazine (℞ 379) are all useful in control of nausea. Chlorpromazine (℞ 377) and a number of other preparations (℞ 482, 483, 487) with both psychic and antiemetic effects are also used successfully in small animals to control the signs of motion sickness. With the exception of the phenobarbital, all the above drugs are more effective if oral medication is started early, 2 doses usually being given, the first 12 hours and the second, 1 hour before the time of departure.

In cases of habitual motion sickness in small animals, the IV or IM injection of propiopromazine (℞ 385) given 1 hour before the trip will be effective for a minimum of 12 hours.

RADIATION INJURY

Radiation injury is the result of energy changes in the atomic matter of living tissues, caused by ionizing radiation. Ionizing radiation may be electromagnetic, such as gamma rays and X-rays, or particulate, such as alpha and beta particles. Electromagnetic radiation has no mass and travels at the speed of light. Particulate radiation, because of its mass, has a greater probability of ionization in tissue. Thus alpha particles are absorbed by a few layers of cells, beta particles are absorbed by a few millimeters of soft tissue and X-rays and gamma rays may pass entirely through the body of an animal without interacting. The greater the number of interactions along a given path, the greater the absorbed energy and the greater the radiation injury.

Because X-rays and gamma rays have the property of penetrating tissue, they can cause damage to organs deep within the body. However, radionuclides entering the body in food, water or air emit alpha and beta particles which are potentially injurious to tissues and internal organs. Skin and eyes exposed to beta particles may be superficially damaged. The extent of injury depends upon the absorbed dose.

Ionization which affects energy bonds within a molecule causes a change in its chemical properties. Injury follows the alteration of molecules important to normal cell functions. The direct effect of irradiation refers to the condition in which energy is absorbed by or ionization occurs in a critically important molecule. When the injury is due to secondary reaction of free radicals formed in irradiated tissue molecules or water, it is regarded as an indirect effect.

The severity of damage to a living organism depends on the amount of energy absorbed, the area of the body exposed, the specific organs within the exposure field and the rate of exposure. Total body irradiation would be expected to cause more damage than partial body irradiation.

Clinical Findings: The lethal range for total body radiation of animals with gamma or X-rays lies above 200 rads. It is difficult to detect clinically any effect of irradiation of animals with doses of less than 25 rads. If a daily dose of less than 50 rads is given over an extended period, high cumulative doses may be tolerated.

While all cellular structures are equally affected by the initial ionization, there are differences in histopathologic sensitivity to radiation. The most rapidly proliferating cells are the most sensitive to radiation. In proliferating cell systems there will be inadequate replacement of the more differentiated forms because of damage to the sensitive precursor cells. Maximum cellular destruction following irradiation is observed earliest in the hemopoietic tissues, and soon thereafter in the intestinal epithelial lining and the germinal layer of the skin. Nerve and muscle cells do not divide in adult mammals and extremely high levels of radiation are required in order to cause histopathologic evidence of damage to these tissues.

The hemopoietic tissues are very sensitive to radiation and generally their sensitivity determines the lethal dose for mammals. Although maximum damage to the hematocytoblasts may be observed in a few hours, maximum depression of circulating blood cells will not be observed for a few days. Death due to damage to hemopoietic tissues will occur around 2 weeks following irradiation because of the leukopenia with resulting antibody loss. Petechial hemorrhage may occur at about the same time because of the decrease in numbers of platelets. Septicemia develops because of the lack of defenses against bacteria normally present within the body.

Damage to the small intestines can lead to death if the doses are high enough. Although the proliferative rates of cells in the intestinal crypts are slightly less than for the precursor cells in the hemopoietic tissues, severe clinical effects are observed earlier. This is because of the rapid migration of the intestinal epithelial cells to the tips of the villi where they slough into the lumen. Deaths from intestinal damage will occur less than a week following irradiation due to loss of fluids and electrolytes and failure to reabsorb them, particularly in the first part of the small intestine. Sensitivity to radiation decreases distally, with the colon and rectum being only moderately sensitive.

Partial body irradiation may be extensive without serious injury to the whole animal. Localized exposures of 1,000 rads or greater, even if distributed over a long period may, however, initiate skin or blood neoplasms.

Acute whole-body irradiation to 10,000 rads may cause damage to the relatively resistant nervous tissue, causing severe CNS disturbances and early death.

The acute dose to the gonads required to cause permanent sterilization is greater than the lethal dose if the whole body is exposed. There will be temporary impairment of fertility with doses less than lethal. However, permanent sterilization may occur with repeated doses smaller than those required to produce severe clinical effects.

Exposure of a fetus to 5 to 25 rads during organogenesis may cause developmental defects or initiate leukemia. Genetic effects, even with higher levels of irradiation, are not a serious problem in domestic animals because of the practice of selective breeding.

Treatment and Control: Treatment for whole-body irradiation is symptomatic and aimed toward maintaining homeostasis until the body can repair itself. Blood transfusions and bone marrow implants may be used until the hemopoietic tissues repair. Antibiotics are necessary to combat infections resulting from the leukopenia. Parenteral fluids and electrolytes must be given to balance those lost in the damaged intestine. The beneficial effects of therapy are extremely limited following exposures much greater than the median lethal dose.

Radionuclide contamination of domestic animals is of concern because of the resulting food products that may enter the human biologic cycle. The radionuclides will be metabolized in the same manner as their stable isotopes. Their removal from the animal's body is dependent both on biologic removal and on the half-life of the particular radionuclide.

In veterinary practice the greatest radiation hazard is the diagnostic X-ray machine. Protection consists of judicious use of the equipment, which includes collimators, cones, diaphragms, intensifying screens and cassettes, together with approved techniques. Lead gloves and aprons should be worn by operators and assistants. Personnel should never be in the direct X-ray beam. Sedation or anesthesia should be used whenever possible. Because ionizing radiation can be detected only by its eventual biologic effects or by special detecting devices, those working with any type of ionizing radiation should wear dosimeters (film badges or ionization chambers) which should be read and recorded on a regular basis. The machine should be monitored and calibrated by qualified personnel.

REPRODUCTIVE AND URINARY SYSTEMS

REPRODUCTIVE PHENOMENA

The data presented in the following tables summarize the temporal and physiologic features of the reproductive cycle in several species. For detailed information, the reader should refer to standard texts.

BREEDING SOUNDNESS EXAMINATION OF THE MALE

The term "breeding soundness examination" describes the procedure used to estimate the potential fertility of male breeding stock. Too often the evaluation of a semen sample is the only criterion considered in an examination. The term "semen testing," commonly used by laymen and veterinarians alike, is only a part of such an examination and does not consider physical characteristics and disease that may significantly affect the fertility of the individual.

MALE FERTILITY

The only reliable measures of fertility in the male are: (a) demonstration of his ability successfully to inseminate by natural service the required number of females, in the requisite period, at the appropriate time of the year and under the prevailing conditions of husbandry, or (b) to make available an adequate supply of semen that, when properly prepared, can be used for successful artificial insemination (AI). Since these requirements obviously vary considerably, both within and between species, fertility is a relative term.

GESTATION PERIODS*

DOMESTIC ANIMALS	Days	WILD ANIMALS	Days	Months
Ass	365	Ape, Barbary	210	
Cat	59–68	Bear, black		7
Cattle, Aberdeen-Angus	281	Bison		9
Ayrshire	279	Camel	410	
Brown Swiss	290	Coyote	60–64	
Charolais	289	Deer, Virginia	197–220	
Guernsey	283	Elephant		20–22
Hereford	285	Elk, Wapiti		8½
Holstein-Friesian	279	Giraffe		14–15
Jersey	279	Hare	38	
Red Poll	285	Hippopotamus	225–250	
Shorthorn	282	Kangaroo, red	32–34**	
Simmental	289	Leopard	92–95	
Dog	56–68	Lion	108	
Goat	148–156	Llama		11
Horse, heavy	333–345	Marmoset	140–150	
light	330–337	Monkey, macaque	150–180	
Pig	112–115	Moose	240–250	
Sheep, mutton breeds	144–147	Muskox		9
wool breeds	148–151	Oppossum	12–13	
		Panther	90–93	
FUR ANIMALS		Porcupine	112	
		Pronghorn	230–240	
Chinchilla	105–115	Raccoon	63	
Ferret	42	Reindeer		7–8
Fisher	338–358	Rhinoceros, African	530–550	
Fox	49–55	Seal		11
Marten, European	236–274	Shrew	20	
Pine Marten	220–265	Skunk	62–65	
Mink	40–75	Squirrel, gray	44	
Muskrat	28–30	Tapir	390–400	
Nutria (coypu)	120–134	Tiger	105–113	
Otter	270–300	Walrus		12
Rabbit	30–35	Whale, sperm		16
Wolf	60–63	Woodchuck	31–32	

* *See also* SOME PHYSIOLOGIC DATA (Laboratory Animals), p. 1208.
** Delayed development as long as a "joey" is in the pouch.

INCUBATION PERIODS

DOMESTIC BIRDS	Days	CAGED AND GAME BIRDS	Days
Chicken	20–22	Budgerigar	17–31
Duck	26–28	Dove	12–19
Muscovy duck	33–35	Finch	11–14
Goose	30–33	Parrot	17–31
Guinea fowl	26–28	Pheasant	21–28
Turkey	26–28	Pigeon	16–18
		Quail	21–28
		Swan	21–35

FEATURES OF THE REPRODUCTIVE CYCLE

Species	Age at Puberty	Cycle Type	Cycle Length	Duration of Heat	Best Breeding Time	First Heat after Parturition	Remarks
Cattle*	4 to 18 (12) months. Usually first bred about 15 months.	Polyestrous, all year.	21 days (18 to 24).	18 hours (10 to 24).	Insemination, from mid-heat until 6 hours after end.	Varies,* best to breed at 60 to 90 days.	Ovulation 10 to 12 hours after end of heat. Uterine bleeding about 24 hours after ovulation in most.
Horse	10 to 24 (18) months.	Seasonally polyestrous. Early spring on.	Very variable, about 21 days (19-26).	6 days (2 to 10).	Last few days; should be bred at 2-day intervals.	4 to 14 days (9).	Ovulation 1 to 2 days before end of heat. Twins are usually aborted.
Sheep	7 to 12 (9) months.	Seasonally polyestrous. Early fall to winter. Prolonged seasons in Dorsets and Merinos.	16½ days (14 to 20).	24 to 48 hours.	Little significance.	Next fall.	Ovulation near end of heat.
Swine	4 to 9 (7) months.	Polyestrous, all year.	21 days (16 to 24).	2 to 3 days.	Little significance.	4 to 10 days after weaning.	Ovulation usually about 46 hours after beginning of heat.
Goat	4 to 8 (5) months.	Seasonally polyestrous from early fall to late winter.	18 to 21 days (19).	2 to 3 days.	Daily during estrus.	Next fall.	Many intersexes born in hornless strains.

* Many normal cows ovulate as early as 8 to 12 days after parturition with or without detectable external signs of estrus.

Dog	**6 to 12 months. Earlier in smaller breeds. Later in larger breeds.**	**Monestrous. All year, but mostly late winter and summer.**	**About 6 to 7 months.**	**Standing heat 4 to 14 days.**	**From day 2 of estrus, and on alternate days thereafter until end of heat.**	**Few months (3 to 5).**	**Preestrous bleeding 7 to 10 days. Ovulation usually 1 to 3 days after first acceptance. Ova shed before 1st polar body has been extruded. Pseudopregnancy (pseudocyesis) usually ends between 60 and 70 days.**
Cat	**6 to 15 months.**	**Provoked ovulation. Seasonally polyestrous spring and early fall.**	**15 to 21 days.**	**9 to 10 days in absence of male; 4 to 6 days if mated.**	**Daily from day 2 of estrus.**	**4 to 6 weeks.**	**Ovulation 24 to 56 hours after coitus. Pseudopregnancy lasts 36 days.**
Fox	**10 months.**	**Monestrous. December to March, but mostly late January to February.**		**2 to 4 days.**		**Next winter.**	**Ovulation usually on 1st or 2nd day of receptivity. Ova shed before 1st polar body has been extruded. No preestrous bleeding.**
Mink	**10 months.**	**Provoked ovulation. Seasonally polyestrous. Mid-February to early April.**	**Waves of follicles at intervals of 7 to 10 days.**	**2 days.**	**Induced ovulator.**	**Next spring.**	**Ovulation begins 36 to 48 hours after coitus which must last ½ hour at least.**

FEATURES OF THE REPRODUCTIVE CYCLE (*Continued*)

Species	Age at Puberty	Cycle Type	Cycle Length	Duration of Heat	Best Breeding Time	First Heat after Parturition	Remarks
Chinchilla	400 to 600 gm (6 to 8½ months)	Polyestrous, intense in November to May.	30 to 50 days (41).	Vagina perforated ½ to 6 days during estrus. Mate at night.	Mate on 2nd night, rarely on 3rd night.	2 to 48 hours. Ovulation on 2nd night.	
Nutria	5 to 8 months.	Polyestrous, all year.	24 to 29 days.	2 to 4 days.		48 hours.	
Rabbit	5 to 9 months. Range 4 to 12 months for most breeds.	Provoked ovulation. Breed all year, more or less. May show seasonal anestrus.	No regular estrous cycles.	To 1 month.	When vulva is enlarged and hyperemic.	Immediately, but blastocysts die if doe suckles large litter.	In United States do not breed well in summer. Ovulation 10½ hours after coitus. Pseudopregnancy lasts 14 to 16 days.
Rhesus Monkey (*Macaca mulatta*)	3 years.	Polyestrous all year; tendency to anovulatory cycles in summer in United States.	27 to 28 days (23 to 33).	Most matings near ovulation time.	Near ovulation.	After weaning of previous young.	Menstruation lasts 4 to 6 days. Ovulation usually about 13 days after onset.
Rat	37 to 67 days. Varies with strain. Body length at puberty 148 to 150 mm.	Polyestrous, all year.	4 to 5 days.	About 14 hours (12 to 18). Usually begins about 7 p.m.	Near ovulation.	Within 24 hours.	Ovulation a little after midnight. Cervical stimulation causes pseudopregnancy lasting 12 to 14 days.

Mouse	35 days (28 to 49).	Polyestrous, all year.	4 or 5 days, usually.	A few hours from 10 p.m. on.	Female most receptive during first 3 hours.	Within 24 hours.	Ovulation soon after midnight. Stimulation of cervix causes pseudopregnancy lasting 10 to 12 hours.
Guinea pig	55 to 70 days.	Polyestrous, all year.	16½ days.	6 to 11 hours. Begins usually in evening.	Mid-heat on.	Usually immediately.	Ovulation about 10 hours after onset of heat.
Hamster	7 to 8 weeks.	Polyestrous, all year. Few pregnancies in winter.	4 to 5 days.	12 hours. One night.	Mid-heat.	After weaning.	Ovulation 8 to 12 hours after onset of estrus. Pseudopregnancy lasts 7 to 13 days.
Gerbil, Mongolian	9 to 12 weeks.	Polyestrous.	4 to 6 days.	12 to 15 hours.	Mid-heat.	1 to 3 days.	Ovulation spontaneous 6 to 10 hours after mating.

The fertility of any individual animal is subject to change due to environmental influences, seasonal effects, mating frequency and disease. The more important of the environmental influences are sudden changes in feed supply and weather conditions, rapid loss of body weight, shipping from one place to another and intercurrent disease. Seasonal variation is especially important in seasonally breeding species, e.g. in stallions and rams; changes in the ratio of daylight to darkness are reflected in the quantity and quality of the semen and efficiency of breeding behavior. While in temperate zones there is little seasonal effect of temperature, in other regions, high temperatures deleteriously influence the fertility of bulls and rams. In general, high mating frequency depresses semen volume and depletes sperm reserves and if extreme, results in lowered fertility. Sexual rest, however, leads to recovery usually within one week; however, it should be noted that it takes 8 weeks for sperm to develop from the basement membranes in the seminiferous tubules to functional maturity in the semen. After prolonged inactivity, semen quality and fertility may be low for the first few services. Any objective assessment of fertility must consider these factors and relate them to the anticipated reproductive demands to be made upon the male.

In the absence of actual proof of fertility from breeding data, it becomes necessary to make an assessment of the probable fertility status by other means. This should be based on the combined information obtained from an examination of the animal itself, its desire and ability to mate, its reproductive organs and representative specimens of its semen.

Among males of the common domesticated species, there are wide differences in the nature of the semen produced, which are related to differences in the reproductive organs of the corresponding females. For all species, however, the fertilizing capacity of semen appears to be a function primarily of the morphology, number, motility and viability of the spermatozoa and, secondarily, of the volume and physical and biochemical properties of the seminal plasma. For any species, therefore, it is possible to set up average standards to which normal semen should conform under stated conditions of age of donor, frequency of service, time in relation to breeding season, and methods of collection and examination. Obvious deviations from these normal standards can then be recognized and correlated with fertility. However, as the range between what is normal and abnormal narrows, the difficulty of accurate assessment increases and, for any individual animal, the semen findings by themselves, unless abundantly obvious, must be interpreted with caution.

Since more is known about breeding soundness examination of the bull than for other species, examination of the bull will be described specifically. Equivalent standards for other species have not been as definitely established and the interpretation of findings, while necessarily somewhat arbitrary, may be useful.

The various methods of collecting semen and average semen volume and density are described under artificial insemination for each species. (q.v., p. 808 et seq.).

BREEDING SOUNDNESS EXAMINATION OF THE BULL

The following recommendations and procedures will be found useful for evaluation of the bull to be used in natural service. The examination should include the following: (1) a general physical examination; (2) a detailed examination of the external genitalia; (3) measurement of scrotal circumference; (4) rectal examination of the pelvic genital organs; (5) collection and evaluation of a semen sample or samples and (6) evaluation of serving behavior.

The Physical Examination

The physical examination should be performed prior to collection of the semen sample. In this way bulls with undesirable physical characteristics or abnormalities may be identified and eliminated before useless attempts at collection are made. Proper handling and examination of the bull avoids excitement and facilitates collection. If the artificial vagina is used, semen collection is usually attempted before interfering with the bull.

The bull should first be observed free of restraint in the pasture or corral. Its general condition is noted including nutritional status, condition of the haircoat, masculinity and conformation. Particular attention is given to locomotion; the stride should be free with no signs of lameness. Abnormal conformation of the rear limbs is especially detrimental to the bull used in natural service.

Following observation of the bull free of restraint, it is confined to a suitable chute or stock to enable completion of the physical examination and collection of the semen sample. The head and mouth are examined and identity by tattoo is verified. The feet and legs are examined closely, noting condition of hooves or any defect that may produce lameness. The external genitalia are examined with great care, the penis being palpated through the external sheath and by protruding it manually. The glans is grasped with cotton gauze. A gloved hand inserted into the rectum makes protrusion of the penis much easier. At this time any desired diagnostic preputial samples may be taken for campylobacteriosis or trichomoniasis. The scrotum and its contents are palpated, noting position and consistency. A normal testicle is firm and resilient, much like a firm rubber ball. Deviations from normal vary from extremely fibrotic testicles to a soft flaccid consistency. Conditions such as testicular degeneration or hypoplasia and orchitis affect the consistency and size of the testicles and result in abnormal spermatogenesis.

Scrotal Circumference

This is measured by encircling the neck of the scrotum with the hand and using the fingers to push the testicles ventrally to eliminate wrinkles in the scrotal skin. The operator's thumb is placed on one lateral surface and the forefinger on the other (placement on the cranial or caudal surface of the scrotum will force the testicles laterally, resulting in errors in measurement). The Colorado metal tape is passed over the scrotum and tightened snugly at the point of greatest circumference; this is recorded in centimeters. If other tapes are used the testicles are positioned ventrally, side by side in the scrotum, and both hands are used to measure the greatest scrotal circumference.

The positive relationship between scrotal circumference and testicular size and sperm production has been demonstrated in dairy and beef bulls. In addition, bulls with small testicles tend to produce a higher percentage of abnormal spermatozoa. Measurement of scrotal circumference is probably the best single method of predicting the ability of a young bull to produce spermatozoa. When properly performed, measurement of scrotal circumference is highly repeatable both by the same operator and among operators. Yearling bulls should have a scrotal circumference of at least 30 cm; however, those of *Bos indicus* breeding tend to mature at an older age and their scrotal circumference may be smaller (as yearlings).

Rectal Examination

When examining stud bulls the artificial vagina may be used, in which case rectal examination should be done after collection of semen. If massage is used then the rectal examination is done during the process of semen collection. In either case it permits examination of the pelvic reproductive organs. Abnormalities of the accessory sex organs are not uncommon and are often accompanied by poor semen quality. If an active inflammatory process is present, variable numbers (from a few to almost 100% of the sample) of white blood cells will be found in the ejaculate.

Collection of Semen

In cattle, semen may be collected by the use of an artificial vagina (AV), an electro-ejaculator or, less preferably, massage of the accessory sex glands. The artificial vagina is used universally in artificial breeding centers. Bulls are induced to serve into this instrument while it is held by an operator alongside the flank of a "teaser" cow, a bull or a phantom teaser. With experience, bulls soon become accustomed to this procedure. Stud bulls without experience with the artificial vagina may also serve that instrument, thus providing samples for diagnostic use. Reluctance or slowness can often be overcome by watching other bulls serve or by having the cow or another bull mount the slow bull. Teasing of bulls in these ways also increases the number of spermatozoa per ejaculate.

In preparing the artificial vagina for use, nonspermicidal lubricant is used and the temperature, which is a critical factor in stimulating ejaculation, is maintained between 40.5 and 42°C according to the individual preference of each bull. Temperatures up to 48°C may assist collections in the case of untrained bulls. At each collection, up to 3 services may be permitted, yielding a total of about 10 to 20 ml of semen. For the maintenance of normal fertility, collections from dairy bulls can be made, on average, about 6 times per week. Data from beef bulls are lacking. "Normal fertility" is probably maintained well after sperm concentration begins to fall.

Electrical stimulation of ejaculation is a valuable means of collecting from bulls that are unable to mount. It is now commonly used for collecting samples from large numbers of beef bulls for diagnostic purposes. A rectal probe is used, with a series of banded electrodes attached to a variable current and voltage source. The bull to be ejaculated should be restrained in a chute, because the stimulation results in vigorous contraction of various muscle groups, particularly those of the back. After emptying the rectum, the probe is placed so that it is entirely within the anus. A hand-operated rheostat permits intermittent impulses to be given as the voltage is gradually increased. The response varies considerably, but it is common to use 2- to 4-second impulses repeated at 5- to 7-second intervals. After a variable number of such stimulations, erection and protrusion of the penis occurs, followed by a flow of seminal fluid, the latter part of which is rich in spermatozoa. The semen may be collected by any convenient method; some operators use a modified artificial vagina and others an insulated bottle. In some bulls, ejaculation occurs only after a final series of momentary impulses, at 1- to 2-second intervals, is applied. Older bulls normally require a high voltage. A few bulls ejaculate within the prepuce. Semen collected by electrical stimulation is as fertile as that collected with an artifical vagina.

An alternative method is widely used in South America: The electrodes of the electro-ejaculator terminate in finger rings rather than in a solid rectal probe. A ring is placed on each of the first and third fingers of the gloved hand, the hand is inserted in the rectum, and the techniques of electro-ejaculation and massage are combined.

During collection by massage of the accessory sex glands per rectum, erection seldom occurs. If semen is to be used for artificial insemination the sheath should be cleaned by douching with 500 ml of sterile saline solution containing 1 million units of penicillin and 1 gm of streptomycin. After completely emptying the rectum, the seminal vesicles are massaged with a backward motion until a few milliliters of fluid drop from the sheath. The ampullae are then massaged, an assistant collecting the semen with a glass funnel and vial. This method is not always successful and the quality of the semen is usually lower than that collected by the other 2 procedures. Samples useful for diagnostic purposes may frequently be obtained, however, depending upon the skill of the operator and individual bull's reaction.

The volume of ejaculate varies from 4 to 8 ml and the concentration from 1 to 1.5 million per cu mm.

Evaluation of the Semen Sample

Evaluation of the quality of the semen sample should begin as soon as possible after collection. A suitable laboratory should be prepared prior to obtaining the semen sample; it may be improvised but should be clean and provide environmental control to ensure that ambient temperature does not adversely affect the semen. All surfaces with which the semen has contact must be warm (39°C) and free from water or chemicals that may be toxic to spermatozoa. Laboratory equipment required includes: (1) microscope equipped with a 1,000× oil-immersion lens, (2) slide and microscope stage heater, (3) module heater or water bath to maintain the sample at 37°C during evaluation, (4) sperm stain such as Hancock's or Blom's eosin-nigrosin stain, (5) fresh diluting solution such as physiologic saline, phosphate buffered 2.9% sodium citrate, or other suitable isotonic solution, (6) 3-place laboratory counter, and (7) microscope slides and coverslips.

Numerous criteria have been employed to evaluate bovine semen; those below are useful for clinical evaluation of bulls for breeding soundness.

Wave motion (mass activity, swirl) is a characteristic of semen observed by placing a drop on a warm glass slide and observing it under low power. It is a function of the activity of the spermatozoa and their concentration. The intensity of wave motion may be divided into 4 broad categories: (1) very good—intense swirling rapid dark and light waves (2) good—slower swirling waves not as intense (3) fair—slow movement with fewer waves (4) poor—very little or no swirl activity.

Very good wave motion is seen in samples of high concentration with a high proportion of spermatozoa moving actively forward. Sperm cells characteristically move against a current. Eddies set up in the drop create synchronous movement of groups of cells leading to dark and light bands and further eddies. Samples of lower concentration, or a lower proportion of sperm actively moving, or both, will have intense wave motion. Motility is the proportion of spermatozoa moving actively forward. It is estimated as a percentage under the high power of the microscope (400×) after placing a cover slip on a small drop. Dilution with warm fresh isotonic saline solution may be necessary to observe the individual movement. Abnormal movement such as circular, or backwards is noted. Motility may be classified as: very good—80%; good—60 to 80%; fair—40 to 60%; poor—20 to 40%; and very poor—less than 20%. Wave motion may be lowered because of a reduction in concentration, motility or both.

Density: The concentration or density of a semen sample may be estimated visually: (1) Very good—thick, creamy or white, opaque and viscid. Samples may have a yellow tinge (flavins) which is normal for some bulls; concentration ranges from 1 to 2 billion per ml. (2) Good—creamy white and opaque, but less viscid; from 500 million to 1 billion cells per ml. (3) Fair—milky in color; more dilute, approaches translucency; pours freely; from 250 to 400 million/ml. (4) Poor—watery, gray in color, pours freely; contains less than 250 million cells per ml.

While the above evaluations are given, it should be recognized that several factors can influence the characteristics observed. Concentration may be lowered as a result of poor spermatogenic function, recent intensive use, or collection technique. Motility may be lowered through poor spermatogenic function, abnormal function of the duct system, the presence of foreign material (e.g. leucocytes) recent sexual rest, poor collection technique, and environmental factors such as water in the sample or cold shock.

The presence of cells other than spermatozoa in the sample should be observed while estimating motility. Red blood cells, white blood cells, and excessive numbers of round epithelial cells are found in some samples and indicate genital tract abnormality. On initial examination of a sample, round cellular elements in the ejaculate cannot be interpreted accurately as coming from the testicles, the duct system or the accessory glands. Laboratory examination after staining will help, but may still not be conclusive. In most cases a thorough physical examination will reveal the source of foreign cells in the ejaculate.

White blood cells tend to be similar in size and are approximately the same diameter as the length of a sperm head. White blood cells are found in the ejaculate in association with active infections in the reproductive tract or accessory sex glands. Motility of the sperm cells may range from good to poor depending on the severity of the infection. Inflammation in the epididymis or ampulla of the vas deferens has a much more serious effect on motility than inflammation of the seminal vesicles. Location of the site and determination of the cause of infection is important in assessing its effect on fertility and on the future of the bull. Until this is done and the infection resolved, caution must be exercised although some bulls with leukocytes in the semen do have good fertility.

Morphology: Of all the criteria available, a careful analysis of sperm morphology has the best correlation to fertility and the highest repeatability, particularly for field evaluation of the beef bull. Increased sperm abnormalities are associated with decreased conception rates. Morphology reflects the functional condition of the testes and to some degree excurrent duct system.

Abnormalities of the head, midpiece and tail assist in identifying the site of dysfunction in the reproductive system and its severity. Normal bull semen contains some abnormal sperm cells and approximate limits are given in the table, together with an indication of the sites of formation of the defects.

TABLE OF BOVINE SPERM ABNORMALITIES

Abnormality	Upper limit of normal range (%)	Site of formation
Abnormally shaped heads, including acrisine defects, double formations and extreme undeveloped forms	20	testicle
Structural abnormalities of midpiece	2	testicle
Tightly double bent and folded tails	4	testicle
Abaxial attachment of midpiece	2	testicle
Proximal protoplasmic droplets	4	testicle or epididymal head
Distal protoplasmic droplets	4	epididymis, testicle
Tailless heads	15	testicle, duct system
Singly bent	8	testicle, duct system or after ejaculation
Coiled tails	3	testicle, duct system or after ejaculation

A stained smear is prepared by mixing a small amount of semen (the amount depending on concentration of the sample) with a suitable stain (Hancock's or Blom's eosin-nigrosin stains are most popular). A drop of stain is placed on a clean warm glass slide and the corner of a second slide is dipped into a drop of semen. The stain and semen are mixed for 7 to 10 seconds by gently rocking the second slide. The second slide is then used to spread the smear by slowly pulling it across the first slide at an angle of 30°. With practice a slide can be prepared that is not excessively stained and in which the spermatozoa are spaced to allow accurate differentiation among normal cells and those with primary and secondary abnormalities. The stained slide is allowed to dry and examined under oil immersion (1,000×). A minimum of 100 cells are evaluated from 4 or 5 randomly selected areas of the slide. If many abnormal cells are encountered, 200 or more cells should be evaluated.

Evaluation of Serving Behavior

This evaluation may be done by observing a bull serve naturally or during collection of semen with the artificial vagina. Observations are made of libido or the desire to serve, protrusion and stiffness of the penis during seeking, the seeking movements, ejaculatory thrust and body position. Such an examination establishes a bull's serving ability, i.e. that he is willing and able to serve normally. Reduced desire to serve needs to be interpreted in the light of the test conditions. Abnormalities of serving technique that are seen include deviations of the penis, filling defects, inability to protrude due to adhesions, retained frenulum, and poor seeking and thrusting referable to abnormalities of the back, limb joints or feet.

Under standardized conditions a quantitative estimate of serving capacity may be made in a 40-minute yard test with restrained heifers. When properly carried out, the number of services in this test is highly correlated with the number of services obtained in a paddock mating situation.

Classification of the Bull

Any system of classification must be based on the essential elements of a veterinarian's approach to male reproductive problems. These are: (1) observation and measurement properly recorded; (2) interpretation of these data in terms of normality or abnormality of the animal and his reproductive system; (3) a decision about the site and severity of any dysfunction; (4) a decision about the extent to which the dysfunction will interfere with fertility now or in the future; (5) a consideration of the genetic implications of abnormalities found; and (6) the formulation of a prognosis, or the basis on which a prognosis might be given, e.g. further examinations.

Where practicality precludes carrying out part of the examination then conclusions must be suitably modified.

If no abnormalities are found that could interfere with reproductive efficiency, the bull may be classed as sound for breeding purposes with the findings consistent with good fertility. If such abnormalities are found then the bull may be classed as unsound, with findings consistent with various degrees of reduced fertility.

Where the classification is in doubt further tests or examination may be necessary.

A system of scoring has been recommended by the Society for Theriogenology to assist in evaluating bulls. Scores are allotted for semen motility, sperm morphology and scrotal circumference. These are added to give a final classification into satisfactory potential breeders, questionable potential breeders, and unsatisfactory potential breeders. Such a system is useful in reporting results of a number of examinations provided all concerned are familiar with the system.

ARTIFICIAL INSEMINATION

ARTIFICIAL INSEMINATION IN CATTLE

In cattle, AI is utilized primarily as a means towards livestock improvement. Its worldwide adoption for this purpose in dairy cattle breeding has been made possible by the development of milk recording and the use of these data as an objective measure of performance on which to base the selection of superior bulls.

The development of objective measures of quality in beef cattle, such as growth rate, carcass conformation and composition, and efficiency of feed conversion, and thus the more accurate selection of sires, led to an increase in the number of beef cattle artificially bred. As control of the estrous cycle becomes practical, the use of AI in beef cattle will increase markedly.

The processing of frozen semen is a highly specialized technique that is best left to the professionals in the AI industry. Some bulls produce semen that will stand a great deal of abuse and yet others are so fragile that with only the utmost care and technique can usable semen be obtained. The basic principles will be reviewed to acquaint the reader, but it is not a process to be attempted by the novice.

Collection of the Semen Sample. (*See* p. 802). Although the semen collected with the electro-ejaculator is not a physiologic sample, there is little difference in fertility or freezability of the semen when compared to AV collections.

Extension (Dilution) and Packaging of Frozen Bull Semen: The vast majority of cattle insemination today is performed with frozen semen. Freezing has permitted semen to be collected, processed and used anywhere, for years afterwards if desired. Two or 3 times more motile cells per ml are used than in the liquid semen formerly used to compensate for the sperm that are killed in the freezing process. Once the semen specimen has been found to meet the required quality standards, it is diluted or "extended" as soon as possible. The commonest extender used for frozen semen is skim milk or homogenized milk to which is added about 10% glycerol. A successful tris-citric acid-fructose-glycerol-yolk extender is used with less than 5% glycerol. The glycerol is added to the extended semen after cooling at 5°C. The semen-extender mixture is held at this temperature for several hours before freezing to allow the sperm to equilibrate in the cold.

Bull semen is packaged in 3 ways: glass ampules of 0.5 to 1 ml of extended semen; polyvinyl chloride straws containing 0.25 to 0.5 ml; and pelleted semen of approximately 0.1 ml. Ampule packaging is still widely used, but the straw is rapidly gaining in popularity because straws require less storage space than ampules, have slightly better freezing characteristics and are thought by some to suffer less sperm loss when inseminated. Pelleted semen is not used extensively in the U.S.A. Though sperm survival is good following freezing and the pellets take little space, they are more difficult to identify as to the source.

Freezing of Bull Semen: The mechanical freezer and dry ice, liquid air, liquid oxygen, and liquid nitrogen have all been used successfully but the last is now used almost exclusively. Ampules are placed in freezers programmed to lower the temperature at a rate of 3°C per minute to −15°C, after which the temperature is rapidly lowered to −150°C, and then transferred to liquid nitrogen at −196°C. Straws are usually frozen in liquid nitrogen vapor and stored at −196°C. Semen pellets are formed by dropping the prepared liquid extender on a block of dry ice where they start to freeze in seconds. They reach −79°C in a few minutes and are rapidly transferred and immersed in nitrogen at −196°C.

Storage of Frozen Semen: Semen has been used successfully after almost 20 years of storage in liquid nitrogen. Storage containers have been developed with a wide variation of volume capabilities. It is extremely important to monitor the nitrogen level; loss of all liquid nitrogen results in damage to the sperm even though the semen may appear to be still frozen.

In case of loss of nitrogen and possible damage to the semen, the remaining vials or straws are best examined and compared to properly stored ampules or straws of the same age. It is extremely difficult to ascertain the amount of damage without a reliable comparison source and the evaluation is best left to an experienced technician.

Thawing of the Semen: Sperm do not survive for long after thawing, so that the thawed vial or straw should be used immediately. General recommendations are that ampules be thawed in a container of ice water, while straws are usually thawed in the hand or a water bath at 20 to 40°C. Different methods of thawing are recommended by frozen semen processors: The specific recommended procedure should be followed as it is based upon optimum fertility obtained using that processed semen.

Insemination Procedure: The rectovaginal method is now used almost exclusively. After thoroughly cleansing the external genitalia, one hand is introduced into the rectum and grasps the cervix. The AI pipette or straw is introduced through the vulva and vagina to the external os of the cervix. By manipulating the cervix, along with light cranial pressure on the pipette, the inseminating catheter is worked through the annular rings of the cervix and is then withdrawn until just the tip is felt slightly protruding into the body of the uterus. The semen should be expelled slowly to avoid sperm loss. Deposit of semen into one uterine horn or the other is to be avoided as lower conception rates occur. If the animal is possibly pregnant, the pipette should be passed about three-fourths of the way through the cervix and the semen expelled within the cervix. The optimum time to inseminate is during the last half of standing estrus and no later than 6 hours after going out of estrus.

If breeding problems arise when AI is being used, the semen is one of the factors to be investigated. However, most methods of evaluation of frozen semen available to the practitioner in the field cannot be highly correlated with fertility. And many factors other than semen are involved in attaining high fertility. If semen quality is suspected, the breeding records should be checked. If more than one sire is being used and one has significantly higher fertility than another, then one semen source is suspected. If all sires are of low fertility, other factors may be involved. If more than one inseminator is being used, conception rates should be compared and then semen handling and insemination techniques should be checked. These include: method of thawing, time of thawing in relation to actual insemination, temperature changes from thawing to insemination, site of deposition and method of expelling semen, heat detection procedures and the stage of estrus at insemination.

ARTIFICIAL INSEMINATION IN SHEEP

Collection of Semen: Of the 2 methods available for collection of ram semen, the artificial vagina is more commonly used. It is prepared for collection by the introduction of warm water (42 to 45°C) and air between the outer casing and inner sleeve, lubrication with petrolatum or paraffin of the end where intromission of the penis will occur, and attachment of a collecting glass at the opposite end. The rams should have been trained previously to mount a ewe, preferably in estrus, and restrained.

For collection by electro-ejaculator, the ram may be restrained on its side. The moistened bipolar electrode is inserted into the anus. The withdrawn penis may be held with a piece of gauze to facilitate insertion of the glans into a 10- to 15-cm graduated collecting tube. Ejaculation occurs after a few short electrical stimulations, and "stripping" of the urethra may be helpful when expulsion of semen is incomplete. In general, electro-ejaculation is less reliable than use of the artificial vagina and the specimens vary in quality and can be contaminated with urine.

The volume of ejaculate collected with the artificial vagina varies from 0.5 to 1.5 ml and the concentration from 2,500 to 6,000 million spermatozoa per milliliter. Semen obtained by the electrical method generally is of larger volume but of lower concentration.

Examination, Dilution and Storage of Semen: Immediately after collection the volume of semen and motility and concentration of spermatozoa are assessed. The ejaculate may be diluted up to 5-fold, depending on the initial concentration. The commonest diluents used are whole, skimmed and reconstituted cow's milk that has been heated for 8 to 10 minutes in a water bath, and egg-yolk-glucose-citrate (15% egg yolk; 0.8% glucose, anhydrous; 2.8% sodium citrate, dihydrate; in glass-distilled water). The volume of inseminate can vary from 0.5 to 0.20 ml and should contain 100 to 15 million motile spermatozoa.

The semen may be stored for up to 24 hours by cooling the diluted semen to 2 to 5°C over a 1½- to 2-hour period and by holding at this temperature. Although a proportion of the chilled spermatozoa may remain motile for up to 10 days, fertility following their use decreases rapidly after 24 hours and generally is quite low by 48 hours.

Freezing and storage of ram semen at the temperature of liquid nitrogen (−196°C) is a more difficult process than is freeze-storage of bull semen. Recently, considerable progress has been made in freezing in pellet form or in synthetic straws. Diluents used are tris- or lactose-based media that are slightly hypertonic. Use of thawed semen may result in 50% lambing after several weeks or years of frozen storage.

Insemination Technique: Estrus may be controlled in the ewe by suitable progestogen treatment preferably with associated injection of PMSG (400 to 600 IU) at cessation of treatment. If PMSG is used, estrus occurs 36 to 60 hours later and ewes may be inseminated at a fixed time, usually at 48 hours. If PMSG is not used insemination is recommended at the next estrus, 17 to 20 days after cessation. Ewes in estrus are identified by vasectomized rams carrying some suitable "marker" device on the brisket. Ewes should be inseminated while the vaginal mucus is copious, thin and clear to cloudy in appearance.

For insemination, the ewe is restrained to limit movement and to present the hindquarters at a convenient height for easy access to the vagina. After cleaning the vulvar region, the cervix is located with the aid of a speculum and suitable illumination and the insemination made as deeply as possible into the cervical canal. For this purpose a graduated 1- to 2-ml syringe, attached to a long, fine inseminating tube is preferred; alternatively, a semiautomatic inseminating device can be used. The relatively long, tortuous and firm-walled cervical canal of the ewe usually precludes penetration by the tube for more than one centimeter. In old multiparous ewes, as a consequence of distortion of the tissues, the difficulty increases and the semen can be deposited only about the posterior folds of the cervix. In maiden ewes in which insertion of the speculum and dilation of the vagina is difficult and can cause injury, the semen should be deposited into the anterior vagina. All these difficulties are minimized by experience.

Artificial Insemination in Horses

To date, few major horse breeds have registry regulations that permit the most effective utilization of artificial insemination (AI). Reproductive efficiency is lower in the horse than in any other species of farm animal, and there is at least one stallion for every 7 mares.

A successful AI program requires considerable knowledge of reproductive anatomy and physiology of both mare and stallion, familiarity with semen handling techniques and the proper equipment. However, it offers substantial benefits. It maximizes the opportunity for early recognition, selection and extended use of genetically superior sires; permits disease control; and reduces the possibility of injury to mares and stallions. Stallions with poor breeding habits or injury may be used when natural service is not possible. Semen may be evaluated at each collection, thus permitting immediate observation of minor changes in the least time, thus shortening breeding and foaling seasons. It aids in identification of reproductive problems, prevents overuse of a stallion, particularly early in breeding season, and permits more effective use of older, more valuable stallions. More mares can be bred to a young stallion providing earlier progeny evaluation, and mares can be bred more often at the most opportune time for maximum conception. Artificial insemination offers substantial benefits in the control of infectious disease such as contagious equine metritis (q.v., p. 391). Additionally, an AI program favors an accurate record keeping system.

Collection of Semen: Semen for AI should be collected with an artificial vagina designed to separate the gelatinous secretion (gel) from the remainder of the ejaculate. Since the semen must be maintained at body temperature from the moment of collection to insemination, everything that contacts it must be temperature-controlled. Immediately after collection, the gel and filter are discarded and gel-free seminal volume measured. Spermatozoa can be counted electronically or by hemocytometer. If a sperm count cannot be done on each ejaculate, it should be done at least once a week. Motility should be estimated microscopically at body temperature after the semen has been diluted 1:20 in an extender that prevents clumping of the spermatozoa. Other measurements such as pH, morphology and bacteriologic examination are not routinely essential.

Mares should be prepared for insemination prior to semen collection and inseminated as soon after collection as possible, i.e. within an hour. Between 100 and 500 million progressively motile spermatozoa should be used per insemination unit. Volume of inseminate does not appear to be important.

The use of an extender is recommended to: a) permit effective antibiotic or antibacterial treatment of semen containing pathogenic microorganisms; b) enhance viability of spermatozoa from low-fertility stallions; c) prolong survival of the spermatozoa; and d) protect the spermatozoa from unfavorable environmental conditions.

Insemination of the mare is accomplished with a 50 cm plastic catheter attached to a syringe by a rubber connector. The hand, in a sterile (or disinfected) and lubricated glove and sleeve, is inserted into the vagina and the magnitude of the cervical opening determined. If the cervix is open, the hand is withdrawn to the posterior portion of the vagina. The catheter tip is picked up, carried to the cervix, inserted through the cervix into the body of the uterus where the semen is deposited. The hand is withdrawn in a manner to prevent entry of air.

Insemination should begin on day 2 of standing heat and continue every other day until cessation of heat. If only one day must be selected, day 3 or 4 appears most appropriate. From a practical point of view, semen should be collected from the stallion every other day and all mares in standing heat for 2 days or more inseminated.

Artificial Insemination in Swine

The possibilities of prevention of spread of disease transmitted via breeding stock, and of greater use of genetically superior boars have made artificial insemination (AI) of swine attractive to producers. With careful, frequent inspection of the sow for heat, semen from fertile boars and application of presently developed techniques, AI of swine is quite feasible. Despite the labor required for accurate detection of heat (in the absence of approved ovulation control procedures), AI of swine will work using the following procedures.

Collection of Semen: Semen may be collected from a boar while he mounts a sow in heat or a dummy sow. Boars can be readily trained to mount a dummy sow, which is the preferred method of collecting semen. Grasping the corkscrew tip of the boar's penis firmly with a surgically gloved hand will provide the stimulus for ejaculation which takes 4 to 6 minutes. The semen can be collected nearly aseptically by directing the tip of the penis into a sterile widemouth 500 ml thermos bottle at 35°C. The gelatinous portion of the ejaculate can be removed by a cheesecloth over the mouth of the thermos during ejaculation. The volume of an ejaculate is 150 to 500 ml containing 30 to 100 billion sperm. Collections should not be made oftener than every 3 days.

Dilution and Storage of Semen: Semen should be handled carefully to avoid bacterial contamination and sudden drops and repeated changes in temperature. Storage of extended semen can be accomplished at 7°C for up to 30 hours in solutions of egg-yolk-glucose-sodium bicarbonate and antibiotic or heat treated milk. Boar semen stored at 15°C in sealed glass ampules in a synthetic medium saturated with CO_2 will retain fertilizing ability for at least 4 days. Longer storage periods result in a lower conception rate and reduced litter size. At least 2 billion sperm in 50 to 100 ml of volume are essential for optimum fertility.

Insemination: Ovulation occurs normally about 40 hours after the onset of heat. The optimum time for insemination occurs 12 hours before ovulation and coincides with the time during heat when most gilts and sows will tolerate heavy pressure on the loin area. Since the beginning of heat is often 12 to 24 hours prior to observation, best conception rate occurs when sows are inseminated both 12 and 24 hours after first observed in standing heat. This will result in a farrowing rate of about 75%, while inseminations at other times will result in 30 to 40% conception rate. Animals should not be restrained during insemination.

At insemination a disposable plastic pipette with a slightly bent tip is inserted into the cervix by keeping the tip of the pipette against the dorsal surface of the vagina and rotating the tip past the pads in the cervix. A rubber catheter with a corkscrew shaped tip can also be used. The semen is slowly forced into the uterus from a plastic squeeze bottle or syringe. Careful determination of the optimum time for insemination and patience during insemination are critical for success.

Farrowing rates of 40 to 70% can be expected from frozen semen. Frozen boar sperm survive for a shorter time in the sow's reproductive tract than fresh; therefore, the time of mating is critical and must occur less than 10 hours before ovulation. The thawing procedure is critical and the thaw instructions accompanying the shipment must be rigidly followed.

Artificial Insemination in Dogs

In most countries it is necessary to obtain Kennel Club permission to carry out AI if one expects to register the progeny. It may also be necessary to obtain a license from the Department of Agriculture (or like body) before one may import canine semen from abroad because of the possible danger of importing rabies.

Collection of Semen: Semen may be collected by digital manipulation or by means of an artificial vagina, the latter being preferred for both hygienic and esthetic reasons. The presence of a "teaser" bitch greatly facilitates collection.

The ejaculate of 2 to 15 ml is passed in 3 distinct fractions: the first from the urethral glands in the mucosa is a clear watery fluid devoid of spermatozoa, the second from the testicles is rich in spermatozoa, while the third and largest fraction is again devoid of spermatozoa and is prostatic secretion. From a complete ejaculate the sperm concentration should be about 125,000,000/ml.

If an "on the spot" insemination is to be carried out, the entire ejaculate may be immediately injected into the bitch, but if the semen is to be preserved for some time, only the second or sperm-bearing fraction must be used. This second fraction is isolated by changing the collecting tube on the artificial vagina between the passing of the fractions.

Dilution and Storage of Semen: Using the second or sperm-bearing fraction of the ejaculate only, canine semen may be diluted 1:8 with such extenders as heat-treated milk or egg-yolk-citrate for preservation, and will keep under such conditions at 4°C for about 6 days. Normal untreated semen will only remain viable for about 18 hours.

Canine semen may also be deep-frozen. The technique is similar to that used on bovine semen (q.v., p. 804) except that the pre-freezing glycerolization time must be reduced from 6 hours to 2 hours. The semen may also be preserved by pelleting: 0.05 ml of the diluted semen is pipetted into depressions made in a block of carbon dioxide ice and after 8 minutes is transferred into liquid nitrogen for storage. When required, thawing of the pellets is carried out in 3% sodium nitrate solution at about 30°C.

Insemination: It is important that the bitch be at the correct stage of her estrous cycle for AI. One may test the bitch with a male and observe her reactions or examine vaginal smears microscopically. Ovulation occurs about 48 hours after the commencement of true estrus, at which stage the vaginal smear contains cornified epithelial cells. This phase is usually 10 to 14 days after the proestrual bleeding begins, white blood cells will reappear in the vaginal fluid 24 to 36 hours after ovulation.

When inseminating, the plastic pipette is inserted until the tip is in the region of the cervix. It is almost impossible to inseminate directly through the cervical os. A speculum and suitable illumination may be used to facilitate passing the pipette. The pipette is connected to the glass syringe and the semen slowly injected. It is usual to elevate the bitch's hind-quarters while inseminating to avoid semen loss. After the pipette has been removed, and while the bitch is still in the elevated position, a gloved finger is inserted into the bitch's vagina for about 5 minutes. This action simulates the "tie" of natural mating and appears to enhance conception.

Artificial Insemination in Cats

Semen may be collected from toms by artificial vagina (AV) or electroejaculation. Toms of suitable temperament may be trained to ejaculate into an AV in the presence of a "teaser" queen. A 2-ml rubber bulb-pipette with the bulb end cut off makes a suitable AV. This is fitted over a 3 × 44 mm test tube, the unit is inserted into a 60 ml polyethylene bottle filled with water at 52°C, and the open end of the rubber tube is stretched over the mouth of the bottle to seal it. The AV opening is lightly lubricated, and slipped onto the penis of the tom as he mounts the teaser. Collections 3 times weekly appear most desirable.

Electroejaculation may be performed on toms under manual restraint or light surgical anesthesia. Probes 0.6 to 1.0 cm in diameter are inserted into the rectum to a depth of 7.0 to 9.0 cm. Ejaculation is usually produced by 3 to 12 five-second stimuli at 2-second intervals. Semen is collected in a warm vial. Four or 5 ejaculates may be collected in less than an hour.

The ejaculate is often less than 0.05 ml in volume but highly concentrated. Ejaculates may be diluted with isotonic saline solution. Not more than 0.1 ml of the diluted semen containing at least 10×10^6 spermatozoa is deposited at the external uterine os of a queen in full estrus with the aid of a bulb-tipped long spinal needle and a 0.25 ml syringe. Ovulation may be evoked by manual stimulation of the anterior vagina, coitus with a vasectomized tom or injections of human chorionic gonadotropin (HCG).

EMBRYO TRANSFER IN FARM ANIMALS

In farm mammals it is possible to remove pre-attachment embryos from their dam (the donor) and transfer them to other females (recipients) for development to term. The first embryo transfer was performed in rabbits in 1890, and successes in farm animals date from the 1930s for sheep and goats, the early 1950s for pigs and cattle, and the 1970s for horses. Commercial use of the technique in cattle by specialized embryo-transfer units began in the early 1970s and was largely spurred by the profitability of multiplying "exotic" (European) cattle that had been imported into North America and Australia in limited numbers under quarantine regulations. Recent technical advances in transfer procedures have been rapid.

Proliferation of selected genotypes remains the principal direct application of embryo transfer to animal production. Other useful applications include genetic improvement programs, the induction of twinning in beef cattle, importation and exportation of livestock, disease control (e.g. to introduce new bloodlines into specific-pathogen-free pig herds) and the treatment of some infertilities. Embryo transfer is also a useful research tool: to investigate the degrees to which the mother and fetus control characteristics such as gestation length, birth weight, fleece qualities and immunoglobin absorption from colostrum; to elucidate the interrelationships between the embryo, uterus and ovary that are essential to establish and maintain pregnancy; and to manipulate embryos to produce specialized experimental animals such as twins, chimeras and fetuses of known sex.

Meticulous techniques and practice are required for successful embryo transfer, particularly for cattle embryos which are now usually collected from donors nonsurgically, 5 to 10 days after insemination. Donors are induced to superovulate by treatment during the luteal phase of the cycle with gonadotropin (PMSG or FSH-LH) followed by prostaglandin to cause luteolysis and estrus. Sixty to 90% of cows will respond, and an average yield of 5 (range 0 to 20) transferable embryos can be expected from each responding donor, but variability in response to superovulatory treatments remains a problem. Induction of superovulation is particularly difficult in high-yielding, lactating dairy cows, leading some units to concentrate on repeated collections of single embryos during successive, untreated cycles.

In nonsurgical collection a Foley-type catheter is introduced, under aseptic conditions, through the cervix into the base of a uterine horn. Inflating the balloon on the catheter seals off the horn. Sterile flushing, by gravity feed or syringe with (most often) an enriched, phosphate-buffered saline medium and collection through the same catheter, is repeated several times for each horn. The medium is introduced into the horn to the point of mild uterine distension, which is checked by rectal palpation of the horn during the flushing operation. With a dissecting microscope, the embryos are easily located as they settle out in the bottom of the collection vessel.

Embryos are collected with a Pasteur pipette, transferred to a smaller volume of fresh medium, examined for morphologic normalcy, and those selected are held in medium at room temperature (or at 37°C) until they are transferred to recipients or prepared for more specialized treatment such as sex determination or freezing. Sexing of bovine embryos by chromosomal analysis of cells from a piece of trophoblast requires 12- to 15-day embryos but techniques for sexing younger embryos are being developed.

Cryoprotective agents such as dimethylsulfoxide, glycerol or ethylene glycol, and closely controlled cooling and thawing rates, enables successful long-term preservation of 7- to 8-day bovine embryos in liquid nitrogen (−196°C), and this service is now available commercially.

The nonsurgical transfer of embryos in a small volume of medium into each uterine horn is done with a Cassou AI gun threaded through the cervix. With practice, it commonly results in twinning and compares favorably with earlier (and still more widely used) methods involving flank incision in standing animals (or midline incision under general anesthesia), and the introduction of an embryo suspended in fluid medium through a puncture wound into the uterine horn.

For pregnancy to ensue the recipients and donors must have closely synchronized estrus cycles, and if fresh embryos are being transferred, a large herd of cattle is required to provide the appropriately synchronous recipients. An alternative is either to induce artificial synchronization of estrus cycles of recipients or provide cryopreserved embryos for naturally cycling recipients.

Following direct transfer of single embryos to the uterine horn adjacent to the corpus luteum, about 60% of recipients become pregnant; with twin transfers (one to each horn) pregnancy rates range from 60 to 90%, with 40 to 60% embryo survival.

Techniques and results in sheep and goats are basically similar to those described for cattle, except that surgical methods have to be used for collection and transfer. Indeed, sheep have been, and continue to be, useful models in which to develop procedures and applications.

Transfers in pigs also have to be made surgically. Within 5 days of ovulation (but not later), embryo survival rates are similar to those occurring naturally. Pigs can be readily superovulated, but methods of synchronization are more complicated than in cattle. So far, pig embryos have proved refractory in attempts to preserve them by cooling and freezing.

The mare has been especially difficult to superovulate but the easily dilated, simple cervix lends itself well to nonsurgical collection and transfer methods now most frequently used. Synchronization of ovulation is possible using prostaglandins together with human chorionic gonadotropin. Practical application of embryo transfer in horses is presently limited by the registration requirements of most breed societies.

It is unlikely that the costs of embryo transfer will ever be low enough to make it a production tool used to the same extent as artificial insemination. However, the rapid and continuing progress in its techniques have consolidated its position as a unique means of meeting certain production and many research requirements in farm species.

HORMONAL CONTROL OF ESTRUS

Hormonal control of the estrous cycle involves therapy that either delays the onset or induces estrus. Parenteral administration of progesterone and oral or parenteral administration of progestins mimic the action of the corpus luteum (CL) and therefore maintain the anestrous phase. The administration of luteolytic substances to an animal in the luteal phase destroys the CL and is thus followed by ovulatory estrus within a few days.

Estrus can be suppressed in cycling mares or mares showing prolonged estrus by daily IM administration of progesterone in oil for 7 to 10 days (℞ 195). Following the last injection, a normal fertile estrus occurs within 7 days. Fertility in animals bred following progesterone treatment is near normal. Oral administration of synthetic progestins such as chlormadinone acetate (CAP) for 18 to 20 days suppresses estrus and ovluation in mares. Fertile estrus follows within 10 days of the end of treatment.

Prostaglandin (℞ 169) or prostaglandin analogue injection into mares with functional corpora lutea induces luteolysis and estrus. Ovulatory estrus occurs within 2 to 4 days after prostaglandin treatment. Prostaglandin treatment does not influence the cycles of mares when applied during the first four days of diestrus.

Estrogen or synthetic estrogen (℞ 165, 171) injection into mares during anestrus and diestrus stimulates behavioral but infertile estrus lasting 24 to 96 hours.

The administration of human chorionic gonadotropin (HCG, ℞ 177) or gonadotropin releasing hormone (GnRH, ℞ 176) during early estrus in mares induces ovulation, reduces interval to ovulation, and may therefore shorten the duration of estrus.

Administration of progesterone or progestins is effectively used for estrus synchronization in cows. In some countries, progestin is available in the form of intravaginal sponges. The period of progesterone or progestin treatment is 10 to 14 days with estrus occurring within a few days following withdrawal of treatment. The fertility rate may be low; however, the second estrus is synchronized and the fertility rate is better at that time.

When prostaglandin or an analogue is administered to cows with functional corpora lutea, estrus occurs within 3 to 7 days. The treatment is effective in cows 5 to 16 days after ovulation and thus requires preselection of animals to be treated. Two treatments 11 to 13 days apart synchronize estrus in a large group of animals; the advantage of this method is that no prior examination of the animals is necessary.

A combination of pregnant mare serum gonadotropin (PMSG, ℞ 179) and prostaglandin or analogue (℞ 160, 169) is used to induce superovulation in cows. In order to achieve a high percentage of ovulation, HCG or GnRH (℞ 176, 177) is administered to the animals during the induced estrus.

Estrus synchronization and good conception rates have been obtained in sheep and goats by the insertion of vaginal tampons impregnated with progestin. The tampon is left *in situ* for 10 to 17 days. Estrus occurs within 2 to 3 days after removal of tampons. The fertility rate is near normal. Sequential intravaginal progestin treatment and PMSG administration appear to be successful in estrus induction in goats during the breeding and anestrus period (℞ 179). Fertility rates are normal.

In bitches, mibolerone (℞ 192) and progestins (℞ 188) are used to suppress estrus for indefinite periods of time. Progesterone treatment may induce cystic endometrial hyperplasia in dogs. Suppression of estrus for long periods in queens may be achieved by using a progestin, megestrol acetate (℞ 188). Induction of estrus in bitches and queens is achieved by administering follicle-stimulating hormone (℞ 179) for periods of 8 to 9 days, followed by administration of luteinizing hormone (℞ 185).

In swine, a combination of PMSG and HCG (℞ 180) or GnRH (℞ 176) administration is useful for induction of estrus. The methods are effective in gilts with delayed puberty and for post-weaning anestrus in sows.

CONGENITAL ANOMALIES OF THE GENITOURINARY TRACT

Congenital anomalies may be hereditary or result from the effect of some toxin or infectious agent on the embryo or fetus. Developmental accidents may also occur.

Anomalies of the urinary system are unusual. Defects of the kidneys include occurrence of cysts, horseshoe kidney, ring kidney, hypoplasia and aplasia. They are uncommon in domestic animals. In the dog and cat, they may result in signs indicative of diseases of the urinary system. Diagnosis is by urinalysis and X-ray. The penile urethra may open on the ventral surface of the penis (hypospadias) or on its dorsal surface (epispadias).

Cryptorchidism refers to the retention of one or both testicles in the abdominal cavity. It occurs most frequently in swine and horses, and is hereditary in these species. It is suspected to be hereditary in dogs and cats. Bilateral retention results in sterility due to thermal suppression of spermatogenesis. The normal temperature of the scrotum necessary for spermatogenesis is 1 to 8°F (0.5 to 3°C) below the normal body temperature. Unilateral cryptorchids have normal spermatogenesis in the scrotal testicle, are fertile, and pass the trait on to their offspring. Abdominal testicles produce male hormones, and cryptorchids have normal secondary sex characteristics and mating behavior. Animals with cryptorchid testicles should be castrated. Gonadotropic hormones administered to prepuberal animals may sometimes cause descent of the testicles.

Monorchidism, anorchidism and **hypoplasia** occur. The hereditary gonadal hypoplasia of Swedish Highland cattle has now largely been eliminated by a control breeding program. A similar gonadal hypoplasia has not been observed in the U.S.A. Idiopathic hypoplasia occurs frequently. Other anomalies of the testis and the epididymis are rare. Ovarian agenesis or the presence of supernumerary ovaries is extremely rare and hypoplasia is infrequent.

Prolapse of the prepuce in bulls occurs as a breed characteristic or may result from edema following trauma. Prolapse predisposes to further injury and if untreated results in abscessation, scarring, adhesions and phimosis. Prolapse of the prepuce can be corrected by surgical removal of redundant tissue. Secondary infection following surgery may result in adhesions and stenosis.

Deviations of the penis in the bull may result from injury but in most cases the etiology is obscure; a heritable factor has been suggested. Deviations are lateral, downward or upward, and if severe prevent copulation. Surgical correction by removing 1 or 2 pieces of tunica albuginea on the convex side has been done. Such operations are difficult because of the chance of infection and the difficulty in removing exactly the right amount of tissue.

Corkscrew penis is observed in some bulls. This is a result of extreme erection in which the dorsal and lateral tunica albuginea of the penis stretches more than does the thicker and stronger tunic around the urethral groove. Most bulls eventually overcome this difficulty without treatment. They learn to insert the penis before the corkscrew occurs, or libido may decrease so that there is a less vigorous erection. Corkscrew penis is sometimes seen when using high voltages for electro-ejaculation.

Persistent frenum in young bulls can be cut with scissors. The penis of bulls may be congenitally short. Diphallus occurs rarely in the bull.

Hermaphroditism or intersexuality may occur in all species of domestic animals. The true hermaphrodite has both ovarian and testicular tissue. Such a condition is usually bilateral and may result in anomalies of the external genitalia. The most common hermaphrodite is in fact a pseudohermaphrodite in which there are present either ovaries or testes, and there is an anomaly of the external genitalia, which resemble, to some degree, those of the opposite sex. Pseudohermaphroditism is most frequently seen in goats and swine.

The most frequent congenital disorder of the **uterus** is segmental aplasia which occurs in inbred cattle. Although often referred to as **white heifer disease** this is a misnomer as it has no connection with coat color. The portion of the uterus without outside opening may fill with fluid causing a distended cyst-like structure. Aplasia may occur at various levels including the cervix so that the description of the condition is quite variable between animals. The vagina may be involved in some cases and this may fill with mucus. These animals are sterile and there is no treatment.

Cattle frequently have a **double cervix.** In most cases this is not a complete double cervix but rather a double external os with 2 cervical canals that join before reaching the internal os. This condition is inherited. It has no effect on fertility and in most cases is found only incidentally in a genital examination. **Cystic Gartner's ducts** on the floor of the vagina are of no clinical importance. Rarely, cows may have an **imperforate hymen** that causes accumulation of fluid in the vagina.

One of the most frequent congenital anomalies of cattle is the **freemartin,** a female born co-twin with a normal male. Over 90% of such females have such extreme hypoplasia of the genital tract that the uterus and ovaries may be observed only histologically. The anterior portion of the vagina is hypoplastic, while the vulva and the posterior portion of the vagina are usually normal. Diagnosis of freemartinism based on vaginal hypoplasia can be determined in most cases by a vaginal examination of the calf with either the finger or a suitably small speculum. The fusion of the placental circulation of the twins allows interchange of embryonic cells and possibly also hormones. The interchange of cells results in a dual genetic pattern in the twins and this can be detected by the combination of 2 different blood types in a single animal. This specific blood-typing test is available through the Purebred Cattle Associations and elsewhere.

Mares may be sterile as a result of chromosome abnormalities; such mares are usually smaller than the breed average. There is no cyclic pattern of estrous behavior, and although there may be reaction to the teaser, they are usually passive to the stallion's advances. External genitalia are slightly smaller than usual. The striking abnormalities are confined to the internal genitalia. The ovaries are very small, smooth, firm and with no follicles or corpora lutea. Histologic examination reveals that these ovaries consist of undifferentiated stroma. The uterus is small and flaccid, and the cervix is flaccid with the os remaining open. The usual chromosome abnormality in these mares is an absence of one of the sex chromosomes and they are designated XO. Autosomes appear to be normal. Sometimes there is a mosaic involving a mixture of XO and XX, or XY. There is no treatment.

PROLONGED GESTATION IN CATTLE AND SHEEP

The basic cause of prolonged gestation in these species is a failure of the fetal adrenal cortex to produce sufficient adrenal corticoid hormone at the termination of gestation to initiate parturition. Two types of prolonged gestation in cattle are of genetic origin conditioned by a single autosomal recessive gene. In Holstein-Friesian cattle, an enzyme necessary for the synthesis of the appropriate glucocorticoid in the fetal adrenal cortex is lacking. These fetuses continue to grow beyond term and may weigh 150 to 200 lb (65 to 90 kg) when parturition is finally initiated by death of the fetus. If this condition is suspected, a cesarean section should be done. Hormonal and IV therapy have kept such calves alive, but it is not practical.

Aplasia of the adenohypophysis with lack of adrenocorticotropic hormone (ACTH) to stimulate the adrenal cortex is the other genetically conditioned cause of prolonged gestation in cattle. In the U.S.A., it has been observed in Guernsey cattle. The lack of the anterior pituitary appears to arrest fetal growth at about the seventh month of gestation. Fetuses may live *in utero* for long periods of time and gestations of 18 months have been recorded. Parturition occurs when the fetus finally dies. These fetuses are grossly abnormal, having hypotrichosis and marked facial anomalies such as cyclopia, which are associated with pituitary aplasia.

Veratrum californicum ingested by ewes on the 14th day of gestation, results in pituitary aplasia and a condition almost identical to the genetically induced pituitary aplasia of Guernsey cattle. *Veratrum album,* which is found in Europe, has caused pituitary aplasia in cattle and the resulting prolonged gestation, hypotrichosis and facial anomalies.

Parturition may be induced by the use of glucocorticoids (℞ 144, 173) in all cases of prolonged gestation mentioned above. Prostaglandin may also be used.

BOVINE DWARFISM

(Achondroplasia)

Achondroplasia of genetic origin occurs in most breeds of cattle. The forms range from the so-called Dexter "Bulldog" lethal, which is invariably stillborn, to those animals that are so mildly affected that diagnosis by visual inspection alone is unreliable.

Of chief concern are the **brachycephalic dwarfs** that were quite common among Hereford cattle in the 1950s. These have been largely eliminated through genetic selection. They are characterized by short faces, bulging foreheads, prognathism, large abdomens and short legs. They are approximately half the size of their normal contemporaries. The **dolichocephalic dwarf** is most commonly seen in Aberdeen Angus cattle and of the same general body conformation as the brachycephalic dwarf except that it has a long head and does not have either a bulging forehead or prognathism. The short-faced calves are frequently referred to as "Snorter" dwarfs because of their labored, audible breathing. Both types are of low viability and susceptible to bloat. Their carcasses are undesirable and they are rarely saved except for experimental purposes.

Various mating experiments indicate that brachycephalic dwarfs, dolichocephalic dwarfs and various types of "comprest" animals are all part of the same genetic complex that may also include the Dexter lethal. Analogous "dwarf types" also occur in other breeds. Few of these animals are now being used in breeding. Originally, it was believed that a single, autosomal recessive gene, with complete penetrance, would account for the brachycephalic dwarfs, and this still appears to be the case when matings are confined to compacts. However, when matings are confined to nonachondroplastic "carriers," the ratio of nondwarfs to dwarfs approximates 15:1, thereby implicating recessive genes at 2 loci. At present, however, there is no single genetic hypothesis which will account for all the various achondroplastic types.

CYSTIC OVARIAN DISEASE

COWS AND SOWS

One or more forms of cystic ovarian degeneration (cystic Graafian follicle, luteal cyst, cystic corpus luteum, atrophic cyst), which occur commonly in cattle and swine but uncommonly in other animals, and are characterized by either nymphomania or anestrus.

Etiology: The condition is caused presumably by an aberration of pituitary gonadotropic hormone release, leading to an insufficiency in the brief surge of gonadotropin necessary for ovulation. The failure to ovulate results in the formation of large cystic follicles, luteal cysts and possibly cystic corpora lutea. Some affected animals exhibit signs of increased and persistent estrogenic stimulation, reflecting the high estrogen levels in the blood plasma.

The incidence is higher in dairy than in beef cattle; high milk production appears to be a predisposing factor. The disease occurs most commonly during the first 8 weeks after parturition during the peak of lactation and more often in cows than in heifers. Among heifers, the incidence is higher in those kept many months without breeding or conceiving. In some countries, there is definite evidence of heritable predisposition.

Clinical Findings: The sexual behavior of cattle with cystic ovaries varies considerably. Short and irregular intervals between heat periods, the heat periods themselves often being prolonged, progress to marked masculine behavior, the animal pawing, bellowing and making numerous attempts to mount other cows but refusing to be mounted itself. About 25% of cows with cystic ovaries are anestrus. In many cases, the vulva is edematous. Relaxation of the sacroiliac and sacrosciatic ligaments is usually obvious. In long-standing chronic cases, thickening of the neck and shoulders occurs along with the development of a masculine appearance and an elevated tail head (sterility hump). The condition in swine is characterized by an extreme irregularity of estrous cycles and the ovaries contain multiple follicular cysts; physical body-changes similar to those seen in cattle are not observed in swine.

Lesions: Bovine follicular (or luteal) cysts, 20 to 60 mm in diameter, are usually present in one or both ovaries. The lining membrane of some of the cysts has patches of a thin layer of yellowish or amber luteal tissue. The stratum granulosum varies from a fairly normal cellular arrangement to almost complete absence of cells. The theca interna is often edematous and cellular degenerative changes are present. The cyst fluid is thin and clear or yellowish.

The uterus is frequently large, flabby and atonic with the cervix relaxed and open. Changes in the endometrium may be both marked and variable. Hyperplasia and cystic dilation of some of the glands may develop. In the sow, large multiple cysts (4 to 6 cm diameter) in numbers approximating normal follicles are seen more often than small multiple cysts (0.5 to 1.0 cm diameter) that greatly exceed the number of normal follicles.

Diagnosis: In cows, the history, unusual sexual behavior and the condition of the ovaries and pelvic ligaments form the chief basis for diagnosis. The presence of one or more cystic follicles is usually detectable by rectal palpation of the ovaries. There is an absence of normal corpora lutea. Cystic follicles are palpable rectally in larger sows. The clitoris is often enlarged in long-standing cases.

Prophylaxis and Treatment: Careful selection of bulls from families known not to be affected has reduced the occurrence of cystic ovaries in some countries. Avoidance of "forced" milk production associated with heavy feeding and milking more than twice daily, helps in prevention. A few cows may recover from cystic ovaries without treatment, but the calving interval may be unprofitably prolonged. Hormonal therapy has proved highly satisfactory. A single IV treatment of desiccated sheep pituitary gland (℞ 186) or a single IM injection of chorionic gonadotropin (℞ 159) seems equally effective. Hypothalamic gonadotropin-releasing hormone has been used experimentally (200 mcg, IM) to cause endogenous gonadotropin release, thereby avoiding antihormone formation.

Treatment induces formation of functional luteal tissue with the re-establishment of an estrous cycle. Repeated treatments may be necessary in some cows. Swine may be treated with the same gonadotropic products as are used for cattle; however, the results are poor. Estrogens should not be used for the treatment of anestrous swine.

MARES

Etiology and Clinical Findings: Cystic follicles similar to those observed in cows do not develop in mares. Early or late in the breeding season a large follicle that fails to ovulate may be detectable but generally undergoes spontaneous atresia in 10 or 12 days. Frequent and prolonged estrous behavior is often observed but a normal behavioral pattern usually occurs later in the breeding season.

Nymphomania is characterized by aggressive sexual behavior. Exaggerated signs of estrus including tail switching, urine squirting, squealing and refusal to copulate are seen. Such mares are vicious and dangerously aggressive toward man and other horses. The ovaries are small and ovulation usually does not occur. This same behavior may be seen in mares with granulosa cell tumors of the ovary that are producing testosterone.

Treatment: The prognosis is guarded. Luteinizing hormone and progesterone have been used with variable results in mares with large follicles that fail to ovulate. Many such mares will conceive if bred later in the season. Examination of the vagina and rectal examination of the genital tract and ovaries will aid in determining the time of ovulation. Tranquilization may help temporarily. Ovariectomy is the only treatment of value and even this may fail if the condition is of long duration (over 6 months) and the habits well established.

INFERTILITY (LG. AN.)

See also ARTIFICIAL INSEMINATION, p. 808 and BREEDING SOUNDNESS EXAMINATION IN THE MALE, p. 794

IRREGULARITIES OF ESTRUS AND ANESTRUS IN COWS AND MARES

COWS

Anestrus or irregular estrous cycles in the cow may result from a number of factors, including poor management, diseases or injury, or disturbances in endocrine functions. One of the most important of the management factors is failure to observe estrus. The average duration of estrus is 18 hours; in many cows it is only a few hours. A systematic program for observing cows in heat is important for getting cows bred at the right time. A husbandryman must be familiar with all signs of estrus. Aids in heat detection, such as the use of teaser bulls, or a device attached to the tailhead of the cow that reveals when other cows have been riding, are valuable adjuncts to the heat-detection program.

Accidental access of bulls to cows and failure to keep proper breeding records often result in pregnancy without a service history.

Silent heat refers to normal follicular development and ovulation without the psychic signs of estrus. Frequency decreases as lactation progresses, so that by the fourth postpartum month the incidence of silent heat is low. Some animals presumed to have silent heats have very short cycles and the observation methods mentioned above will help detect these. Those with true silent heats may be detected only through rectal palpation of the ovaries or the use of progesterone assay in milk or plasma.

The 21-day cyclic changes in the ovary, particularly in the period of 3 to 4 days prior to ovulation, at the time of ovulation, or 3 or 4 days after ovulation, generally can be recognized and the time of the cycle estimated. The corpus luteum regresses approximately 3 days before the mature follicle appears. It becomes smaller in size and changes from the diestrus, liver-like structure to a more fibrous structure. Estrus is determined by the presence of a palpable follicle, an absent or regressed corpus luteum, and firm uterine tone. The vaginal mucosa reveals edema, the cervix is relaxed and hyperemic and clear serous mucus of variable amounts is frequently observed at the vulva, which is puffy and swollen. The immediate postovulatory period is characterized by blood in the mucous discharge, and an ovary with a corpus hemorrhagicum, which on palpation is recognized as a soft area in the ovary, usually between 3 and 5 mm in diameter. The new corpus luteum is detectable by the fourth or fifth day as a small and somewhat softer structure than the mature corpus luteum, which reaches maximum size by the seventh day.

During almost half of the cycle the examiner can predict the next estrus with reasonable accuracy. With this information at hand the husbandryman can watch the cow closely for the next anticipated heat. In cows that are approaching ovulation, the appropriate time can be estimated and the cow bred, regardless of whether she shows psychic signs or not. Should the estimate be in error and the cow exhibit psychic signs a few days later, she can be rebred. These cows are normal; they lack only psychic signs of estrus, hence endocrine treatments are not indicated.

When a cow exhibits anestrus, or the interval between heats is irregular and prolonged, it usually indicates death of the embryo 14 or more days following coitus. The uterine contents may lead to pyometra or mummified fetus, which if left untreated may persist for a year or more. The common practice of removing corpora lutea has little to recommend it; retention of the corpus luteum in the presence of a normal, nongravid uterus is rare.

When circumstances dictate removal of the corpus luteum, it

should be done only in those cows in which the structure can easily be delineated and can be enucleated without rupture. The occurrence of hemorrhage and adhesion is greatly increased when the corpus luteum is fragmented during the enucleation procedure. The cow should show psychic estrus 3 to 7 days following removal and may be bred. If clinical heat is absent, the cow may be bred on the third or fourth day following removal of the corpus luteum. The corpus luteum can be chemically removed by the use of prostaglandin or prostaglandin analogues (as fluprostenol and cloprostenol), which are administered parenterally (℞ 160, 170, 174, 198) or locally in the genital tract (℞ 167, 168, 196, 197).

Regimens for the administration of prostaglandins and prostaglandin analogues for the synchronization of estrus to reduce the dependence on observation, have been developed but are not in use because these products have not yet been approved for use in food-producing animals. Prostaglandins are effective only on a functional corpus luteum. For estrus synchronization the prostaglandin or its analogue is administered to all animals. Those in the fifth to 18th day of the estrous cycle will have regression of the corpus luteum and come in heat in about 4 days. The others may either have recently been in heat or will come in heat in a few days. Ten days later all animals will be between the fifth and 18th day of the cycle and prostaglandin is administered a second time. Most animals will be in heat in 3 or 4 days and ovulate in 4 or 5 days. Breeding is done either on signs of heat or all animals are bred twice at 72 and 96 hours or once at 80 hours after the treatment.

Approximately 25% of cows with cystic ovarian follicles are anestrus. Cystic corpus luteum is not a cause of anestrus.

Under certain circumstances nonfunctioning ovaries will be encountered. They can be recognized as smooth, small bean-shaped structures on a single examination, or reveal no activity or change after several examinations over a period of 3 weeks. The commonest cause is low total energy intake during late winter.

This condition tends to correct itself when pasture becomes available, when there is sufficient supplemental feeding, or when production drops to a level commensurate with the food intake. The stress of chronic or severe disease or injury may interrupt ovarian activity and result in anestrus. Milk progesterone assays indicate that over 90% of dairy cows are cycling by 50 days post partum. Thus, lactation is not an important factor in the cause of anestrus. Congenital defects, such as freemartinism and ovarian hypoplasia, result in estrual failure. Certain ovarian tumors may cause anestrus. The treatment for the inactive ovary is correction of the basic cause. These ovaries usually do not respond to gonadotropic or steroid hormone treatment. A treatment that may be tried is to inject a combination of pregnant mare serum and chorionic gonadotropin (℞ 181).

MARES

The mare is seasonally polyestrus with the normal breeding season extending from February through the summer months in the Northern Hemisphere. Foaling mares usually come in heat on approximately the ninth day post partum and regularly thereafter at 21-day intervals. Breeding is recommended on the 30th day. Barren mares may have irregular estrous cycles characterized by long estrus, frequent short estrus, or long diestrus. The commonest abnormality is long estrus during the early spring. As the season progresses, these mares usually revert to normal by April or May. If the mare fails to show estrus or has irregular estrus as indicated by the teaser, the time of ovulation, which in many cases is at the normal 21-day interval, can be detected by rectal and vaginal examination. For many years, only the vaginal examination has been used and the mares were bred when there was extreme relaxation, hyperemia and edema of the cervix and an accumulation of clear serous mucus in vagina. Rectal examination to determine the presence and maturation of a follicle has supplemented the vaginal examination. The follicle in the mare is at least 1 in. (2.5 cm) and sometimes 3 to 4 in. (7.5 to 10 cm) in diameter, prior to ovulation. It is firm up to 24 hours before ovulation, and during the last 24 hours the internal pressure decreases so that ovulation may be anticipated and the mare bred at this time.

Normal estrus cycles may be initiated earlier in the season by placing mares in stalls with controlled lighting. Beginning in December, with lighting time the same as daylight for that time, the amount of light is uniformly increased daily to 19 hours per day on April 1. For the average stall 200 to 300 watts of incandescent light are satisfactory. A substantial number of mares will conceive in February with this system.

The most successful treatment for anestrus and estrual irregularity in mares is proper observation and examination. The use of endocrine products, including pregnant mare serum, is not indicated.

Retention of the corpus luteum, concurrent with a normal uterus, occurs in the mare. To treat this condition, as well as to induce estrus at a specified time, prostaglandins are used to cause regression of the corpus luteum (℞ 160, 170, 174, 198). Following this treatment the mare should be under regular observation so that she can be bred when the follicle matures 3 to 5 days later. Regression of the corpus luteum can be caused by the infusion of approximately 200 ml of warm sterile saline solution into the uterus between the fifth and 18th day of the estrous cycle when a functional corpus luteum is present. Intrauterine saline infusion stimulates endogenous prostaglandin production and release, which in turn causes regression of the functional corpus luteum. (*See* ABORTION, p. 832).

INFERTILITY IN SWINE

Infertility in swine may manifest itself as complete reproductive failure with no production of viable offspring or as a partial failure with reduction in numbers of live piglets born or weaned.

SOWS

Studies have indicated that the average healthy sow releases 17 ova, farrows 10 piglets and weans 7.5 piglets. Losses due to noninfectious factors tend to occur during the time from fertilization to implantation or at the time of farrowing. Principal causes are believed to be defective ova or spermatozoa, congenital anomalies or aplasia of the tubular genitalia, and inadequate progesterone production by the corpora lutea. Defects such as aplasia of the tract are seen primarily in gilts since they tend to be self-eliminating. Studies on the use of steroids such as progesterone to increase embryonic survival have not yielded positive results.

Faulty management practices can contribute to infertility and small litter size. Use of immature boars or the overuse of older boars also may be contributing factors (*see* p. 831). The sow should be mated late on the first day of estrus or early on the second day or both. Since ovulation generally occurs late on the second day of estrus, this should result in optimum fertilization rates. Breeding of the sow twice during the estrus period apparently will increase fertilization but this practice requires the use of additional boars.

Recently, there has been an apparent increase in problems of anestrus and poor conception rates, especially in confinement-type operations. Part of the problem is related to failure to detect estrus in confined or tethered sows. It may also be related to stress caused by close-confinement housing and a resultant increase in production of steroids by the adrenal cortex. ACTH or synthetic glucocorticoids can block ovulation in gilts or sows under experimental conditions.

Animals that are overly fat may have farrowing difficulties. Limited feeding of the sow during pregnancy seems to give best results, with some increase in feed allowance during severe cold weather. An average daily intake of 4 lb (2 kg) of a corn-soybean diet with vitamin and mineral supplements appears adequate in most cases. Adverse environmental factors, particularly high temperature and humidity, seem to contribute to failure of estrus and early embryonic mortality. Once the pregnancy has been established, high temperatures seem to have little or no effect on gestation.

Sows may show anovular estrus 3 to 4 days after farrowing; normal uterine physiology is re-established by 20 to 25 days post partum. On weaning of the piglets at 3 weeks of age, sows will usually exhibit estrus within 6 to 8 days. Use of exogenous follicle-stimulating hormone preparations and luteinizing hormones after weaning may help ensure good follicular development and improve the ovulation rate. The nutritional state of the sow is also very important. Restricting the energy intake of sows immediately after weaning piglets (restricted quantity of feed or because of social competition in group pens) will markedly reduce occurrence of estrus or result in failure to respond to exogenous hormone treatment. This latter effect may also occur because of an immune response due to the large molecular size of PMSG. In this regard gonadotropin releasing hormone (GnRH) appears promising as an alternate treatment (℞ 176).

Poor lactation is a significant cause of neonatal mortality in swine (*see* MMA, p. 854).

Toxins with estrogenic activity in the diet resulting from mold infestations, usually of the *Fusarium* group and commonly found in moldy corn, also cause swine infertility. (*See* FUSARIUM ESTROGENISM, p. 1042). In lactating sows, estrus may occur with almost immediate cessation of lactation.

Infectious diseases including brucellosis, leptospirosis, toxoplasmosis, pseudorabies, and those caused by miscellaneous bacteria and members of the parvovirus group and enteroviruses may result in frank abortions or early embryonic mortality and mummification of some of the fetuses. In such instances, the pregnancy will continue and the mummified fetuses will be expelled at term with the live pigs. The so-called SMEDI viruses appear to be responsible for a syndrome characterized by stillbirths, mummified fetuses, embryonic death and infertility. Serologic or other diagnostic methods are of limited usefulness in the diagnosis of these agents. Serologic tests for brucellosis and leptospirosis, however, are useful for diagnostic purposes.

Diagnosis of causes of infertility in the sow is difficult. Enlargement of the vulva or clitoris may be helpful in diagnosis of hyperestrogenic syndromes. Purulent vaginal discharges must be interpreted with caution, especially in postpartum sows. The discharge may originate from the involuting uterus or from the vagina and cervix with no involvement of the uterus. Uterine involution is usually complete 20 to 25 days after farrowing and normal fertility can be anticipated after that time.

BOARS

Infertility in the male is frequently caused by absence or malformations of the duct system. Boars should not be used until approximately 8 months of age, and should not be expected to breed more than one sow per day, if maximum litter size is to be maintained. Boars that have not been used for more than 4 weeks should be made to ejaculate once or twice before being put in use in order to remove degenerate spermatozoa present in the tract. One boar for no more than 10 to 12 sows is suggested, especially if hand-mating is not practiced.

Aids to diagnosis of male infertility are careful palpation of the scrotal contents, and collection (with an artificial vagina or by electro-ejaculation) and examination of a semen sample. Testicular biopsy should also be considered. Fertility evaluation of all new boars is strongly advised.

In testicular hypoplasia, the testes will be smaller and softer than normal but libido may be normal. Acute or chronic orchitis signals the appearance of abnormal sperm production or its complete cessation.

ABORTION (LG. AN.)

Most abortions in large animals result from infection, which reaches the fetus from the maternal circulation by way of the placenta. The primary need in such cases is to identify the cause of the abortion so that preventive measures may be taken.

The important infections that may lead to abortion are discussed under their respective headings. For cattle, see brucellosis (p. 366), leptospirosis (p. 379), listeriosis (p. 357), IBR-IPV (p. 269), bovine viral diarrhea (p. 266), epidemic bovine abortion (p. 375), campylobacteriosis (p. 385), bluetongue (p. 253) and trichomoniasis (p. 389).

Mycotic abortion is usually caused by either *Aspergillus* or *Mucor*, which reach the uterus by the hematogenous route and cause abortion in late gestation. In many of these fetuses the skin is not affected; in others the mold causes ringworm-like lesions. The placenta is frequently severely affected with necrosis of the cotyledons and thickening of the intercotyledonary areas. Diagnosis is based on identification of the mold through culture of the fetal or placental tissues, histologic examination of these tissues, or direct examination of cotyledons after clearing with potassium hydroxide solution. These abortions are almost always sporadic, and the only means of control is reducing exposure of the cows to the molds.

There are many cases of **bovine abortion** for which no diagnosis can be made. Almost certainly other infectious agents will be identified as causes of outbreaks of abortion. In addition to the specific causes of abortion mentioned above, numerous other agents such as parainfluenza 3 virus, *Pasteurella multocida*, *Pseudomonas aeruginosa*, *Corynebacterium pyogenes*, *Streptococcus bovis* and *Staphylococcus aureus* have been isolated from sporadically aborted fetuses.

In **horses**, the most common cause of abortion is the equine herpesvirus 1 (q.v., p. 308). Equine arteritis (q.v., p. 310) is an infrequent case. Bacterial infection of the placenta and the fetus probably results from ascension of the agents from the infected vagina through the cervix. The most frequently found agent is *Streptococcus zooepidemicus*. At a much lower frequency, *Escher-*

ichia coli, staphylococci, *Corynebacterium equi* and *Actinobacillus equuli* are found. The prevention of bacterial abortion in the mare is based on hygienic breeding procedures and treatment of genital disease prior to breeding. The same bacterial infections may cause disease of newborn foals, which can be successfully treated with antibiotics. *Salmonella abortivoequina* is currently not a cause of equine abortion in the U.S.A.

In sheep, in the U.S.A., the commonest cause of abortion is campylobacteriosis (q.v., p. 387). Other agents that have been associated with abortion in sheep, and which are discussed elsewhere in the MANUAL are: *Toxoplasma gondii* (p. 466), bluetongue virus (p. 253), *Brucella ovis* (p. 373), chlamydiae (p. 377), leptospires (p. 384), *L. monocytogenes* (p. 357) and *Salmonella* spp. (p. 299).

Similarly, the important infectious diseases causing abortion in swine are discussed elsewhere: brucellosis (p. 370), leptospirosis (p. 384), pseudorabies (p. 284), SMEDI viruses (p. 831) and hog cholera (p. 277).

MISCELLANEOUS CAUSES OF ABORTION

Trauma, fatigue, surgical shock, poisons, certain drugs and chemicals have been incriminated as causes of abortion but specific proof is usually lacking. Nitrate poisoning has frequently been mentioned as a cause of abortion; however, all controlled experiments and observations concerning the effects of nitrate on the fetus have failed to link this chemical with fetal disease or abortion. The above-listed factors may affect pregnancy through stress or direct effect on the fetus. In all probability most chemicals that affect the fetus do so by crossing the placenta and entering the fetus or the placenta or both. Such chemicals may cause fetal or embryonic death, and anomalies of varying severity. The resistance of the fetus to the effects of chemicals increases with the age of the fetus. Thus, a substance that is sufficiently irritating to a fetus to produce resorption, death or abortion early in gestation, may have little or no deleterious effect on the fetus at a later stage of development. Chemicals vary in their effect, depending upon the dosage, the duration of ingestion or exposure to the material, and the specific time of gestation. For example, *Veratrum californicum* produces adenohypophyseal aplasia in fetal lambs only when ingested on the 14th day of gestation.

Most equine twin pregnancies end in abortion. Twisting of the umbilical cord causes abortion in the mare. Introduction of bacterial contaminants in the uterus by an artificial-insemination pipette, or by other means, causes death of the fetus and abortion.

The vitamin A deficiency that occurs in range cattle sometimes causes abortion, retained placenta, or weak newborn calves. Many forms of malnutrition, dietary deficiency, or chronic disorders that result in severe cachexia may lead to abortion.

INDUCED ABORTION AND PARTURITION

Pregnancy may be interrupted with subsequent abortion or resorption of the fetus and its membranes by manually rupturing the amniotic vesicle or decapitating the fetus, which can be done on fetuses up to approximately 100 days of age. Decapitation is accomplished via the rectum by grasping the fetal neck and applying pressure between the thumb and forefinger. The maximum age at which this procedure can be carried out will depend on the ability of the operator to exert enough pressure on the neck to decapitate the fetus.

Heifers can be caused to abort with a repository form of diethylstilbestrol given IM in doses of 100, 125 and 150 mg during the fifth, sixth and seventh month of pregnancy, respectively. Abortion occurs within 5 to 10 days in 90% of the treated animals. (This drug is no longer available for use in livestock in the U.S.A.) In cattle, chemical removal of the corpus luteum with prostaglandin or prostaglandin analogue is effective in inducing abortion at any stage of pregnancy. (Note: These drugs are not approved for use in food-producing animals in the U.S.A.) Manual removal is only useful in terminating pregnancy during the first 21 days after breeding; beyond this time the corpus lutem becomes increasingly well imbedded in the ovary and the incidence of rupture of the corpus luteum and hemorrhage increases.

Mares can be aborted with prostaglandin analogue. After the fourth month a double dose or repeated treatment at 48-hour intervals (or both) is necessary. In late pregnancy prostaglandin will induce parturition but not a live foal. Douching the uterus with dilute antiseptic, saline or antibiotic solutions will result in abortion in the mare at any stage of pregnancy. From 200 to 500 ml of fluid, depending on the stage of pregnancy, is sufficient. During the first few weeks of pregnancy in the cow the same procedure, using dilute antiseptics, is also satisfactory. In the mare, abortion may be induced by dilating the cervix.

Induction of abortion with estrogens during late pregnancy should be avoided, because it is often complicated by retained placenta, uterine infection and vaginal prolapse. In cattle, induction of parturition to produce a live calf during the last 3 weeks of pregnancy can be accomplished by the injection of glucocorticoids (℞ 163). This procedure stimulates the onset of lactation and initiates the formation of surfactant material in the fetal lung, so that proper aeration of the lung occurs. About 50% of these animals have retained placenta but this usually does not affect future fertility. Parturition can be induced as early as the fifth month of gestation with glucocorticoids by repeating the dosage as many as 5 consecutive days.

Mares that have beginning relaxation of the cervix and colostrum in the udder may be induced by administering 40 u of oxytocin IV.

Parturition occurs in approximately 30 minutes. This is accompanied by premature release of the allantois-chorion and assistance should be available to aid in delivery of the foal and to remove the membranes from the foal. A variation of this treatment is to give 5 u of oxytocin at 15-minute intervals for 3 times, and then increase the dosage to 10 u at 15-minute intervals until parturition occurs.

PREVENTION AND TERMINATION OF PREGNANCY IN THE BITCH

The commonest and most popular method of preventing pregnancy in the bitch is ovariohysterectomy. This is unacceptable in breeding stock and has the disadvantage of subjecting the animal to the risks of surgery, as well as possibly being associated with urinary incontinence in later years. The progestagens will suppress estrus and thus pregnancy, but it is unwise to employ these agents in breeding bitches as a small percentage develop disease of the uterus. Megesterol acetate (MGA, ℞ 187) will suppress estrus as will mibolerone (℞ 192).

Pregnancy may be prevented following undesired mating by administration of estrogens. Diethylstilbestrol (℞ 164) and estradiol (℞ 171) are effective in preventing implantation if given within 5 days after mating, but the signs of estrus frequently persist for 2 to 3 weeks. It is unwise to employ estrogens in breeding bitches as infertility has occurred afterwards. Large doses of estrogens cause blood dyscrasias. The various repellents are of little value in repelling males attracted to a bitch in estrus.

Pregnancy can be terminated safely by ovariohysterectomy until the middle of the term. After this, the risks involved are unwarranted. Other methods of surgical interference are seldom performed in bitches because of the lack of knowledge about their effectiveness, complications and long-term effects.

METRITIS (LG. AN.)

Inflammation of the muscular and endometrial layers of the uterus.

Acute metritis almost always occurs following abnormal parturition. Delayed uterine involution is the major predisposing factor. It is often accompanied by retention of the fetal membranes. Contaminants enter the uterus during parturition and establish infection, especially in association with stress caused by dystocia, abortion, concurrent systemic disease, or malnutrition.

Commonly there is a fetid discharge from the uterus. In severely affected animals the uterus is atonic and in cows and horses several gallons of fluid may accumulate. The systemic signs include fever, anorexia, depression and, in horses, laminitis. The uterus may be swollen and friable so that caution should be used in examination. Manipulation of the uterus by rectal palpation may cause perimetritis.

Treatment should be both systemic and local, ℞ 31, 59, 66, 71, 76, 96, 102 (*see* treatment of laminitis in horses, p. 551). In severe cases supportive therapy should be used in addition to local treatment of the uterus. Fluid accumulation should be removed. In most cases the uterus will respond to oxytocin (50 u, IM) for several days after parturition; however, if it does not respond, siphoning must be used followed by topical application of antibiotics. Eventually the condition subsides to an endometritis and should be treated thus.

Untreated metritis in animals that survive may become chronic. The uterus in such cases becomes thick-walled and fibrotic. The disease usually has no effect on the general condition of the animal but such animals are sterile. The prognosis for reproductive efficiency is unfavorable. Treatment may be attempted with topical antibiotic infusions or an infusion of 5 to 10 ml of Lugol's solution in each uterine horn. The latter agent will cause necrosis of the superficial layers of the endometrium with the hope that functional epithelium will regenerate.

See also CONTAGIOUS EQUINE METRITIS, p. 391.

VAGINITIS AND VULVITIS (LG. AN.)

Bruising or laceration of the vagina and vulva frequently result from parturition. Infrequently, traumatic vaginitis may result from malicious injury, service from a large and vigorous bull or prolapse of the vagina. The inflamed vagina is painful, edematous, and often there is a fetid exudate indicating baterial infection. Usually vaginal lacerations are limited to the retroperitoneal area, and cellulitis with accompanying edema, necrosis and fetid discharge are common, often with an accompanying acute metritis. There may be tenesmus and swelling of the vulva. The degree of depression, loss of appetite and fever depends on the severity of the infection. Malignant edema occasionally establishes itself in the injured tissue.

Examination and treatment must be done with a clean, well-lubricated, gloved hand in order to minimize pain and straining. If the fetal membranes are retained, they should be removed if this can be done easily and quickly. Since the uterus is usually affected, it should be treated with antibiotics. Antibiotics placed in the uterus will escape through the vagina and assist in treating the infection there (℞ 31, 59, 71). Oily antibiotic preparations may be placed in the vagina with a catheter (℞ 69). Animals with severe vaginitis should be treated by parenteral administration of antibiotics or sulfa drugs (℞ 66, 76, 96, 102). Tenesmus in traumatic vaginitis is usually transitory or caused by examination. It should be controlled by epidural anesthesia. Inflammatory changes usually prevent prolapse in these cases.

Granular venereal disease (granular vaginitis): This condition is characterized by the presence of spherical nodules, about 1 mm in diameter, on the vulvar mucosa of cattle. Similar hyperplasia may occur in the lymphatic follicles of the bull's penis. This condition should be considered a response of the lymphatic tissue in this area to an irritant or an antigen. It is nonspecific and is not a disease in the classic sense. The agent stimulating the hyperplasia is usually unknown. One disease known to produce this hyperplasia after recovery from the acute infection is IPV (q.v., p. 269). Treatment of females is not indicated and the condition subsides spontaneously in several weeks to several months. Young animals are most frequently affected since these experience the most exposure to new antigens. In the female the condition is not related to fertility, although the predisposing agent may influence fertility.

The condition in bulls tends to be more persistent and affected bulls may refuse to breed. They should be treated by sexual rest, and massage of the anesthetized prolapsed penis and sheath with a suitable antibiotic ointment (℞ 69). This should be repeated sufficiently often to assure elimination of any existing infection. If the nodules persist, they should be cauterized with silver nitrate sticks. Following cautery, the penis should be washed and protected with an antibiotic ointment.

A condition characterized by hyperemia of the vagina and the accumulation of as much as 50 ml of yellow mucoid exudate, occurs as an epidemic in some herds. A virus has been isolated from some of these animals although in many instances no etiologic agent has been isolated. It is postulated that this agent is an enterovirus and gains access to the vagina either by coitus or by extension from a contaminated vulva. The effect on fertility is slight and recovery is spontaneous.

VAGINAL AND CERVICAL PROLAPSE

Eversion and prolapse of the vagina or prolapse of cervix through the vulva occurs in all species, but is most frequently observed in sheep and cattle. The bladder may be occasionally contained within the prolapsed vagina.

Etiology: The condition usually occurs in mature females in late pregnancy. A number of causes appear responsible, e.g. increasing mobility of the genital tract due to relaxation of pelvic musculature, flaccid perineum, loosely attached wall and floor of the vagina and excessive abdominal pressure. The condition may be an inherited weakness in some families and occurs in young animals without regard to pregnancy. However, most prolapses occur in multipara suggesting that stretching of the vagina predisposes to eversion. Relaxation of the vulva and the vagina in late pregnancy allows intermittent prolapse when the animal is lying down. This leads to irritation and swelling of the mucosa, which results in straining and creates a continuous complete prolapse.

In sheep, the primary etiologic factors are inheritance; distension of the digestive tract, which creates high intra-abdominal pressure; grazing on hill country; and estrogen in the feed. In cattle, a similar etiologic basis may be presumed.

Clinical Findings: The signs are obvious. Usually the floor of the vagina prolapses first and repeated prolapsing may result in a diverticulum of one or, less frequently, both sides of the vagina. Occasionally the cervix prolapses through the vulva. Usually pregnancy is not interrupted, although the external os of the cervix may be greatly enlarged and congested. The urethra may be occluded and prevent urination. Failure to treat results in uremia, vascular stasis, necrosis, infection and eventually death.

Prevention and Treatment: Elimination of families predisposed to the condition and those animals that have previously suffered from the condition will reduce the incidence. Feeding practices should be examined and estrogenic sources eliminated, if possible. Sometimes, where pasture is the source of feed, this cannot be done and treatment measures must be continuously applied. Animals should be kept on level ground during late pregnancy. Methods such as rope harnesses, Caslick's operation or a buried-purse-string suture of surgical tape above the vulva to prevent partial prolapse during recumbency in late pregnancy are useful in cows. For sheep that are pastured on estrogenic feed and chronically affected with prolapse, a commercially available plastic pessary is very useful. The pessary, in the shape of a "T" with the vertical member approximately 6 in. (15 cm) long, and the cross member approximately 8 in. (20 cm) long, is placed with the vertical part in the vagina and the ends of the cross member tied to the wool.

Treatment, to be effective, should follow these steps: (1) administer epidural anesthetic when necessary; (2) wash the organ with soap and water and rinse thoroughly; (3) empty the bladder if necessary; (4) reduce congestion by applying gentle pressure if necessary; (5) replace the vagina and apply antibiotic (℞ 69); and (6) retain the vagina in position. Only the last procedure presents serious difficulty. The irritation of the vaginal mucosa results in extreme tenesmus, and retention devices must be strong in order to prevent recurrence. Temporary or permanent retention is accomplished through various methods of suturing the vulva. If interrupted sutures are used, they are usually deeply placed about ¾ in.

(2 cm) apart and the entire vulva is closed. Metal prolapse pins with heavy buttons or similar devices have also been used. These devices are removed during parturition. Perivaginal sutures, resection and removal of some of the mucosa of the vaginal wall, or cervical or vaginal wall fixation are other methods for providing long-term solutions to recurrent prolapse. Fly control may be necessary.

UTERINE EVERSION AND PROLAPSE

Prolapse of the uterus may occur in any species; however, it is commonest in dairy cows and sows and somewhat less frequent in ewes. Etiology is unclear and occurrence is sporadic. Recumbency with the hindquarters lower than the forequarters, invagination of the uterus, and excessive traction to relieve dystocia, all have been incriminated as causes. Prolapse of the uterus can occur only within a few hours after parturition when the cervix and the uterus are open and lack tone. Prolapse is always complete, and the mass of uterus usually hangs below the hocks of the affected animal, except that in sows sometimes one horn becomes everted while unborn piglets in the other prevent further prolapse.

Treatment involves removing the placenta, if it is still attached, and thoroughly cleaning the endometrial surface. The uterus is then returned to its normal position by one of several methods. If the cow is in the standing position, epidural anesthesia should be administered, the uterus should be elevated to the level of the vulva on a tray, or by means of a hammock held by 2 assistants, and then replaced beginning at the cervical portion and gradually working toward the apex. Once the uterus is replaced, the hand should be inserted to be sure that there is no remaining invagination. If the cow is recumbent, she should be placed in a position so that the hindquarters are elevated. This can be done by moving her onto a sloping area, or elevating the hind quarters with some type of lift attached to the hind legs thus placing the cow in dorsal recumbency. Alternatively, the cow is placed in sternal recumbency with hindlegs extended backwards. With these methods of restraint epidural anesthesia is seldom necessary. The uterus is replaced as indicated above. In sows, reposition may be also achieved by manipulating the uterus from outside with one hand and through a flank incision with the other hand.

Following return of the uterus to its normal position, antibiotic is placed in the uterine cavity and oxytocin administered (℞ 31, 59, 193, 199). The prognosis depends upon the amount of injury, contamination and infection of the uterus. Prompt replacement of a clean minimally traumatized uterus results in an uneventful recovery. There is no tendency for the condition to repeat in subsequent parturitions.

Complications tend to develop when laceration, necrosis and infection occur or when treatment is delayed. Shock is an important factor in prolonged prolapse and requires supportive therapy. In some instances the bladder and the intestines may prolapse into the everted uterus; these require careful replacement before the uterus is returned. The bladder may be drained with a catheter or trocar. Elevation of the hindquarters and pressure on the uterus will aid in replacement of bladder and intestines. It may be necessary to incise the uterus in order to replace these organs.

Amputation of a badly traumatized or necrotic uterus may be the only means of saving the animal. This is accomplished by incising the dorsal side of the uterus, ligating the 2 middle uterine arteries, placing a heavy ligature around the uterus in the region of the cervix and amputating distal to the uterine and vascular ligatures. The stump is replaced in the vagina. Supportive treatment and antibiotic therapy are indicated.

MASTITIS (LG. AN.)

Mastitis is of greatest economic importance in the dairy cow, but the disease may affect any species and is handled in much the same way in all of them. Brief notes on mastitis in ewes, goats, sows and mares are given separately.

Mastitis may be defined as inflammation of the mammary gland due to the effects of infection of the gland by bacterial or mycotic pathogens. Technical factors that predispose to establishment of infection within the gland are poor milking hygiene, milking machine faults, faulty milking management, teat injuries and teat sores.

A diagnosis of mastitis is based on: (1) clinical signs, (2) culture and identification of a mastitis pathogen from a sample of milk collected aseptically and (3) results of tests designed to detect increases in the leukocyte content of milk (in subclinical cases). In clinical cases a provisional diagnosis is usually based on signs and knowledge of the predominant pathogens in the herd but it should be backed up by culture of the secretion and sensitivity tests.

The 4 clinical types of mastitis are: (1) peracute—in which swelling, heat, pain and abnormal secretion in the gland are accompanied by fever, and other signs of a systemic disturbance such as marked depression, rapid weak pulse, sunken eyes, weakness and complete anorexia; (2) acute—in which similar changes in the gland occur with only slight to moderate fever and depression; (3) subacute—in which there are no systemic changes and the changes in the gland and secretion are less marked; and (4) subclinical—where the inflammatory reaction within the gland is only detectable by tests, such as the California Mastitis Test (CMT) (q.v., p. 848), the

Wisconsin Mastitis Test, the Whiteside Test and the electronic cell count, which are used at intervals to detect a persistently high-leukocyte content in the milk.

Changes in the secretion can vary from a slight wateriness with a few flecks (e.g. subacute staphylococcal mastitis) through wateriness with large yellow clots (e.g. acute and peracute streptococcal and staphylococcal mastitis) to watery, brownish secretion with fine mealy flakes (e.g. coliform mastitis). Without treatment the affected quarter gradually loses its productive capacity and may either atrophy or slowly develop firm nodular granuloma-like masses within the parenchyma.

The bacterial pathogens most commonly responsible for bovine mastitis (in approximate decreasing order of frequency) are: *Staphylococcus aureus, Streptococcus agalactiae,* other streptococci, coliform organisms, *Corynebacterium pyogenes* and *Pseudomonas aeruginosa.* Less commonly, mastitis may be associated with infection of the gland by *Nocardia asteroides, Clostridium perfringens, Mycobacterium* spp., *Mycoplasma* spp. and yeasts.

Treatment of Mastitis: In cases of peracute mastitis systemic treatment with antibiotics, such as penicillin-streptomycin combinations (℞ 66) or oxytetracycline (℞ 50) or ampicillin (℞ 2), is indicated together with a mastitis infusion of the same antibiotic into the affected quarter every 24 hours for 3 to 4 treatments. The affected quarter is infused after the evening milking and repeatedly stripped out during the day. Single or repeated injections of an antihistamine (℞ 560) or the administration of a corticosteroid (℞ 146) with IV-administered, isotonic, balanced electrolyte solutions may be of use as supportive therapy in toxemic cases. In acute mastitis, intramammary antibiotic infusions with or without systemic antibiotics initially (depending on the severity) are usually sufficient if the organism is sensitive to the antibiotic in use. Certain antibiotics such as the penicillin ester, penethamate hydriodide (℞ 61) and erythromycin (℞ 38) reach much higher levels in the milk than in plasma after systemic administration and are useful in acute cases. Subacute infections are best treated by a 3- to 4-day course of an appropriate intramammary antibiotic infusion. Subclinical infections may preferably be treated by infusing an appropriate long-acting antibiotic preparation into the affected quarter at drying off.

Depending upon which antibiotic and base is infused into the udder and what repository form is injected, the milk collected from the cow for as long as 96 hours following treatment must not be used for human consumption.

SPECIFIC TYPES OF BOVINE MASTITIS

Streptococcal Mastitis: *Streptococcus agalactiae* requires the mammary gland for its perpetuation in nature. All other streptococci, whether saprophytes or potential pathogens, enter the mammary gland by chance and are not dependent upon it for survival. Therefore, *Str. agalactiae* mastitis is a specific infectious disease that can be completely eradicated from dairy herds. The organism enters the gland through the teat opening and resides in the milk and on the surface of the milk channels. It does not penetrate the tissue. Initially it multiplies rapidly causing an outpouring of neutrophils into the ducts and damage to the ductal and acinar epithelium leading to ductal obstruction with cells and cellular debris. Fibrosis of interalveolar tissue and involution of acini in affected lobules quickly follow leading to a loss of secretory function.

Streptococcus agalactiae spreads from cow to cow during the milking act and, therefore, shedder-cows should be milked after the noninfected portion of the herd. Calves fed on milk containing the pathogen may transmit it to the immature glands of penmates if they are permitted to suck each other's teats. Therefore, during an eradication program, it is essential that calfhood infections be prevented; otherwise, at some later date, an animal infected as a calf may reintroduce *Str. agalactiae* into the lactating herd during its first lactation.

The other streptococci that may cause mastitis are *Str. dysgalactiae, Str. uberis, Str. zooepidemicus* and Lancefield groups G and L streptococci. Both *Str. dysgalactiae* and *Str. uberis* are common to the environment of dairy farms. *Str. uberis* may contribute significantly to the bacterial count as bacterial numbers per milliliter of milk from infected glands commonly are much greater than is the case with *Str. agalactiae* or staphylococci. *Str. zooepidemicus* is a common pathogen of horses and has been found in purulent conditions of swine. Its occurrence in the mammary gland has been more or less limited to small dairy herds where cows and other farm animals are run together.

Penicillin is specific for *Str. agalactiae,* but some of the other streptococci appear to be more resistant. The antibiotic is infused into the infected gland through the teat canal (℞ 219). Chlortetracycline (℞ 211), oxytetracycline (℞ 218) or sodium cloxacillin (℞ 212) also may be used. Variable results have been reported for neomycin (℞ 217). Benzathine cloxacillin (℞ 207), penicillin-novobiocin (℞ 209) or long-acting penicillin (℞ 208) preparations may be used in dry-cow treatment.

Staphylococcal Mastitis: This is the most important type of mastitis in most dairying areas today because (1) the organism is ubiquitous and can colonize the cow's skin and teat sores, as well as the udder, (2) as a high proportion of isolates in many herds are now penicillin resistant, (3) treatment with appropriate antibiotic infusions is less successful than in *Streptococcus agalactiae* infections.

In herds in which staphylococcal mastitis is a problem, 50% or more of the cows may have subclinical infections. *Staphylococcus aureus* may cause peracute mastitis, peracute gangrenous mastitis (in which the skin of the quarter and teat becomes cold and bluish in color and eventually sloughs), as well as the acute, subacute and subclinical types. Infections of a year or more in duration are often refractory to treatment because of the development of a tissue barrier between the antibiotic and the organism.

Treatment of cows with subclinical infections during lactation is not as successful as dry-cow treatment, hence these should be treated at drying off with an appropriate long-acting infusion, e.g. penicillin-streptomycin (℞ 220) preparations or benzathine cloxacillin (℞ 207). A high proportion of staphylococci are sensitive to the penicillinase-resistant drug cloxacillin.

Peracute and acute staphylococcal mastitis may be treated systemically with an appropriate antibiotic, e.g. erythromycin (℞ 38), streptomycin (℞ 35), chlortetracycline (℞ 27). For intramammary therapy, cloxacillin (℞ 212) is recommended but sensitivity tests may reveal that others such as erythromycin (℞ 214), lincomycin (℞ 215), penicillin-streptomycin (℞ 220), chlortetracycline (℞ 211) and neomycin (℞ 216) infusions may be more effective in some instances. Staphylococcal vaccines have been recommended but their value in the control of the disease is debatable.

Coliform Mastitis: The coliform organisms most frequently encountered have been *Escherichia coli, Aerobacter aerogenes* and *Klebsiella* spp. Coliform mastitis is a disease of the normal lactating mammary gland. Coliform bacteria are prevented from multiplying by even low numbers of infiltrating leukocytes, but in cell-free milk, they multiply rapidly, producing a large pool of potential endotoxin. The inflammatory reaction that follows destroys the coliform population, thereby releasing the endotoxin. The resulting toxemia produces the local and systemic signs of peracute mastitis. The temperature ranges from 103 to 108°F (39 to 42°C), milk secretion ceases even though only one gland usually is the seat of the infective process, and anorexia, depression, dehydration and rapid loss of weight are prominent. The secretion of the affected quarters is usually brownish and watery. Diarrhea also commonly occurs and in cases due to *Klebsiella* spp. joint swellings (especially hock joints) may be present. A unique feature is that, upon recovery, the udder tissue generally returns to normal so that, in a subsequent lactation, no fibrosis is found and the gland is capable of producing to capacity.

Cows producing milk with low leukocyte counts, (i.e. $<100,000$ cells per ml) are more susceptible to attacks of acute coliform mastitis and older cows may be even more so because of increased patency of the streak canal. Acute coliform mastitis should be treated locally and parenterally with dihydrostreptomycin sulfate

(℞ 35) or ampicillin (℞ 2). Chlortetracycline (℞ 211), oxytetracycline (℞ 217) and neomycin (℞ 216) have been used in a similar manner, but with variable results. In the absence of systemic signs, the most specific therapy consists of dihydrostreptomycin sulfate in a water-in-oil vehicle (℞ 213) but other drugs may be used depending on sensitivity tests.

***Pseudomonas aeruginosa* Mastitis:** *Pseudomonas* is occasionally important as a cause of mastitis. Generally, a persistent infection occurs which may be characterized by intermittent acute or subacute exacerbations. *Ps. aeruginosa* is a soil-water organism common to the environment of dairy farms. Herd-wide infections have been reported following extensive exposure to intramammary treatments administered by milkers. The indications are that failure to employ aseptic techniques for udder therapy may lead to the establishment of *Ps. aeruginosa* infections within the mammary glands. Severe peracute mastitis with toxemia and high mortality may follow immediately in some, while subclinical infections may occur in other cows. The pathogen has been observed to persist in a gland for as long as 5 lactations, but on the other hand, spontaneous recovery may occur.

A satisfactory treatment for mastitis caused by *Ps. aeruginosa* has not been developed. The pathogen is often sensitive to streptomycin, neomycin and carbenicillin *in vitro* but variable results have been reported when these drugs have been infused into the udder. Carbenicillin (℞ 210) appears to be the drug of choice.

***Corynebacterium pyogenes* Mastitis:** This pathogen is commonly encountered in suppurative processes of cattle and swine and it produces a characteristic mastitis in dry cows. It is occasionally observed in mastitis in the lactating udder, but may be a secondary invader. The pathogen produces an inflammation typified by the formation of profuse, foul-smelling, purulent exudate. The foul smell is not caused by *C. pyogenes,* but by an anaerobic micrococcus, *Peptococcus asaccharolyticus* that commonly is found in association with the former. In the rare instances of *C. pyogenes* mastitis in which *P. asaccharolyticus* is not present, the exudate is odorless.

Corynebacterium pyogenes mastitis may occur in epidemic form among dry cows kept in small enclosures during a protracted wet period. To combat this occurrence, it is important to move the nonaffected animals to dry quarters or to pasture. Surgical removal of the teat, to establish drainage, thus far has proved to be the most satisfactory method for handling well-established clinical cases. Cows or even young heifers with multiple udder abscesses due to *C. pyogenes* or other infections should be slaughtered. Peracute and acute cases should be treated with systemic and intramammary penicillin (℞ 218). Long-acting penicillin infusions (℞ 208) at drying off and halfway through the dry period may prevent *C. pyogenes* mastitis in dry cows.

Unusual Forms of Mastitis: *Mycoplasma* mastitis, caused by pleuropneumonia-like organisms, is a severe form of mastitis that has been reported in North America, the U.K., Israel and Australia. The infection may spread rapidly through a herd with serious consequences. Typically, all quarters become involved following a rapid onset. Loss of production is often dramatic, secretion soon being replaced by a serous or purulent exudate. Initially, a fine granular or flaky sediment is characteristic of the material removed from infected glands. Despite the severe local effects on udder tissue, the cow usually does not manifest signs of systemic involvement. The infection will persist through the dry period. Since there is no satisfactory treatment, affected cows should be slaughtered and sanitary measures strictly enforced.

Nocardia asteroides causes a destructive mastitis characterized by an acute onset with high temperature, anorexia, rapid wasting and marked swelling of the udder. Pathology in the udder is typical of a granulomatous inflammation leading to extensive fibrosis and formation of palpable nodules. Herd histories suggest that infection of the udder may be associated with failure to ensure asepsis in intramammary treatment of the common forms of mastitis. Slaughter is recommended for obvious clinical cases, while intramammary infusions of a furaltadone-penicillin preparation (℞ 206) may be successful in removing latent and subclinical infections.

Mastitis due to a variety of **yeasts** has appeared in a number of dairy herds, especially following the use of penicillin in an attempt to eradicate *Str. agalactiae* or in association with prolonged repetitive use of antibiotic infusions in individual cases. Yeasts grow well in the presence of penicillin and some other antibiotics and if accidentally introduced during treatment they may be able to multiply and cause mastitis. Signs may be severe and accompanied by a high temperature followed by spontaneous recovery in about 2 weeks or by a chronic destructive mastitis. If mastitis due to yeast is suspected, antibiotic therapy must cease immediately.

A chronic indurative mastitis similar to that caused by the tubercle bacillus has been reported to be caused by **acid-fast bacilli** derived from the soil when such organisms are introduced into the gland along with antibiotics, especially penicillin, in oil or ointment vehicles. The oil is required for the organisms to become invasive for the mammary tissue.

Control of Bovine Mastitis

There are 8 related points to consider: (1) Milking machine function and milking procedures—these should be checked and corrected where necessary. The following factors have been associated with higher incidences of mastitis: (a) Excessive irregular vacuum fluctuation in the teat cup and in the vacuum or milk line. This sometimes occurs due to faulty handling of teat cups (letting excess air into the system) or to inadequate vacuum reserve. (b) Vacuum level—levels of 2 in. (5 cm) of mercury or more above and below the recommended 15 in. are undesirable. (c) Blocked air-admission holes in the claw pieces. (d) Narrow-bore milk liners (< 1 in. internal diameter are preferred to wide-bore liners). (e) Gross abnormalities in pulsation rate (normal 40 to 60/min) and ratio (40 to 50 rest:50 to 60 vacuum usual) are undesirable. (f) Clusters should be removed (correctly—by releasing the vacuum first) as soon as cow has milked out, i.e. avoid overmilking. (g) Adequate stimulation is essential prior to applying teat clusters.

(2) Milking hygiene should be observed and corrected. A recommended hygiene system is: (a) Initially remove residual milk in teat and discard. (b) Wash teats in clean running water, using antiseptic soap and disposable paper towels. (c) Dip teats of cows at end of milking in a hypochlorite solution yielding 4% available chlorine, a chlorhexidine solution, 0.5%, or an iodophor solution containing 5,000 ppm iodine. (d) Milkers should wear rubber gloves and disinfect their hands when going from cow to cow.

(3) Detect infected cows by repeat CMTs (q.v., p. 848) and cultures. Isolate infected cows and milk last. Milk clean heifers first, then clean cows, then recently treated cows and then infected cows.

(4) Treat clinical infections as they occur, but treat subclinical infections preferably at drying off (especially *Staphylococcus aureus* infections). Cows carrying *Streptococcus agalactiae* infections may be treated during lactation with a reasonable degree of success. Preferably treat all quarters at drying off with an appropriate long-acting antibiotic infusion.

(5) Cull any cows that have had 5 or more clinical attacks of mastitis during the lactation or have failed to respond to repeated therapy including dry-cow therapy.

(6) Examine all introductions to herd by udder palpation, culture and CMT of secretion from all quarters.

(7) Teat cracks, chapping and pseudo-cow pox should be controlled by appropriate measures as they may predispose to high herd levels of mastitis.

(8) Maintain client interest and awareness of the mastitis problem by furnishing regular reports of CMT results of cows, or bulk milk cell counts in his herd.

MASTITIS IN GOATS

The etiology of infectious mastitis in goats and cattle is similar. *Streptococcus agalactiae* produces a subacute mastitis, *Staphylococcus aureus* may cause either subacute or gangrenous mastitis, coliform mastitis has been encountered both sporadically and as a herd-wide infection, and *Corynebacterium pyogenes* produces multiple nodular abscesses.

Programs for diagnosis, control and treatment of mastitis in the goat should be similar to those discussed for the cow.

MASTITIS IN SHEEP

This can be quite an important disease in ewe flocks, with incidences of 2% or more. Apart from deaths from peracute infections, the disease can be a cause of lamb mortality from starvation, or of depressed weaning weights of lamb. Peracute, peracute gangrenous (usually due to *Staphylococcus aureus*), acute, subacute and probably subclinical types occur. The organisms most commonly involved are *S. aureus*, streptococci, *E. coli*, *Pasteurella haemolytica* and *Corynebacterium pyogenes*.

The principles of diagnosis and treatment used in bovine diagnosis can be applied to the ewe. Little is known about the control of ovine mastitis.

MASTITIS IN SOWS

Mastitis can be important in swine-raising units. Peracute mastitis can affect sows and gilts and is most commonly associated with coliform (*E. coli*, *Aerobacter aerogenes* and *Klebsiella*) infections. It most commonly occurs at or just following parturition, and affected sows have a moderate to severe toxemia. The sow's temperature may be elevated to 107°F (42°C) or may be subnormal. The affected glands are swollen, purple in color and have a watery secretion. Sow mortality is high and the litter will also die unless fostered or fed artificially. Recovered sows may have impaired milk production in the next lactation. The treatment of peracute coliform mastitis in sows is similar to the treatment of this condition in the cow (q.v., p. 843). Ampicillin (℞ 2), dihydrostreptomycin (℞ 35) or oxytetracycline (℞ 50) systemically have been used.

Subacute mastitis may occur in older sows and lead to induration of one or more glands and impair the sow's ability to suckle a large litter adequately. This form of mastitis is more likely to be associated with infection by streptococci or staphylococci. Granulomatous lesions in the mammae of sows have been associated with *Actinobacillus lignieresi*, *Actinomyces bovis* and *Staphylococcus aureus* infections. *Fusobacterium necrophorum* (*Sphaerophorus necrophorus*) and *Corynebacterium pyogenes* have also been incriminated in sow mastitis. A thorough examination of the mammary glands of the sow is important to diagnose any of the above peracute and subacute types of mastitis.

The control of porcine mastitis has not been extensively investigated but isolating sows in adequately disinfected farrowing pens prior to, during and for an adequate period after farrowing should help prevent the severe losses associated with coliform mastitis.

MASTITIS IN MARES

Acute mastitis occurs in one or both glands occasionally in lactating mares. The commonest organisms involved are streptococci (Group C) and staphylococci. Marked painful swelling of the affected gland and adjacent tissues occurs and the secretion is often seroflocculent. Fever and depression may be present. The mare may walk stiffly or stand with hind legs apart due to the discomfort.

Treatment is the same as in the cow, but where intramammary infusions are used, they should be inserted separately into both orifices of the teat. Without prompt treatment, abscessation or induration of the gland can occur. Little is known about the frequency and persistence of subclinical intramammary infections in mares.

CALIFORNIA MASTITIS TEST (CMT)

A kit consisting of the plastic paddle plus all the necessary reagents is available commercially. Equal quantities of reagents and milk are mixed in the depressions of the plastic paddle by a swirling motion. Negative samples are free from gel formation, positive samples show various degrees of precipitate, which is a reflection of the degree of udder inflammation. There is a high degree of correlation between the CM test and the microscopic examination for leukocytes in milk. The CMT may be used to estimate the leukocyte count of bulk herd milk, bucket milk or quarter milk.

MISCELLANEOUS DISEASES OF THE BOVINE UDDER

UDDER ACNE

A disease of dairy cows characterized by occurrence of pustules on the skin of the udder and teats, often on the udder near the base of the teat. It has a tendency to spread in some herds. Staphylococci can usually be isolated from the pustules. A predisposing factor may be excessive teat-cup "crawl" at milking associated with a prolonged interval between cessation of milk flow and teat cup removal. The affected skin should be clipped, thoroughly washed with chlorhexidine (5,000 ppm) or iodophor (10,000 ppm) and an antibacterial ointment such as chlorhexidine ointment or sulfathiazole ointment (℞ 111) applied twice daily after milking. The use of iodophor or chlorhexidine solutions as udder washes and post-milking teat dips will help prevent the spread of the disease.

BOVINE ULCERATIVE MAMMILLITIS

A severe ulcerative condition of the teats of dairy cows that can occur in outbreaks resulting in marked loss of milk production and a high incidence of secondary mastitis in affected herds. Initially reported from Great Britain, it also occurs in other countries including the U.S.A. It is caused by a herpesvirus very similar to the Allerton strain of Group II lumpy-skin-disease viruses. (*See* LUMPY SKIN DISEASE, p. 246.)

The lesions commence as one or more thickened plaques of varying size on the skin of one or more teats. Vesiculation quickly occurs within these plaques and the surface sloughs leaving a raw ulcerated area that becomes covered with a dark black-brown scab. The scabs tend to crack and bleed especially if milking is attempted. In some cases a large proportion of the teat wall is involved and often the lesion includes the teat orifice, predisposing to mastitis and obstruction of the streak canal. In the early stages of the lesions before vesiculation is marked, intranuclear inclusions may be detected in the cells of the dermis. The disease is more severe in cows that have recently calved, especially those with udder edema. Severe lesions may take several weeks to heal.

Diagnosis is based on the signs and confirmed by histopathology or by virus isolation from early lesions. Serum virus neutralization titers rise quickly and the first sample must be taken very early in the course of the disease.

Affected cows should be isolated and separate milking utensils used. Emollient ointments used before milking may reduce trauma and hemorrhage. Prophylactic infusions for mastitis should be considered if the teat orifice is involved. Iodophor solutions (V/V 1:320) may be useful as teat and udder disinfectants to aid control in infected herds.

Traumatic Diseases

Superficial wounds to the udder and teats may be cleaned with suitable antiseptic solutions and treated as open wounds with the frequent application of antiseptic powders or sprays. Those of the teats may, in addition, be bound with adhesive tape to hasten healing. Those involving the teat orifice should be dressed with antiseptic creams and bound twice a day to prevent udder infections. Severe hemorrhage necessitating prompt compression and ligation may result from some wounds to the udder due to severance of a large milk vein.

Deeper wounds of the udder and teats should be promptly (within 6 hours) cleansed and sutured under local anesthesia with physical or chemical restraint, to promote first-intention healing. Where the wound involves the teat cistern, it may be necessary to insert a self-retaining teat cannula with removable cap into the teat for the first 24 hours to prevent milk seeping through the wound (which would delay or prevent healing) and to aid in milking. Aftercare should include the infusion of the affected quarter with antibiotic preparations and the maintenance of high antibiotic blood levels by parenteral therapy, especially with deep udder wounds.

Permanent fistulae into teat or gland cisterns are best repaired when the cow is dry by making an elliptical incision around the fistula and then suturing.

Teat chapping and cracking can occur due to exposure of teats to frequent washing and drying, cold wet winds or irritant solutions. In some countries, teat chapping and pseudo-cowpox (q.v., p. 243) may occur simultaneously, leading to severe lesions. Both conditions can be treated with antiseptic udder ointments such as those containing chlorhexidine or iodophors. Teat dips containing the latter plus 5% glycerin may help prevent teat chapping and aid in mastitis control.

Contusions and hematomas of the udder and teats produce painful swellings and frequently result in bloody milk. **Temporary stenosis** of the teat canal or orifice may occur. Cold applications applied regularly at intervals over several days, are indicated in the early treatment of this condition to control swelling and pain. Later, warm applications, hot packs, liniments and gentle massage may hasten the resolution of the swelling. In these conditions machine milking should be replaced by gentle hand milking until recovery is complete. Rarely, large hematomas may interfere with the circulation of blood in the skin of the udder and necrosis and infection may occur. Hematomas should not be incised or drained unless they become infected, as they will disappear in time.

Bloody milk is frequently seen following calving when the udder usually is severely congested and edematous, as well as following udder trauma (see above). This condition is observed most commonly at the first to third parturitions. Most cows with bloody milk recover without treatment in 4 to 14 days providing the gland is milked out regularly.

Abscesses of the udder may be secondary to wounds, advanced mastitis, infected hematomas, or severe contusions. These abscesses should be incised and drained when they are chronic and near the surface of the udder. The wound should be packed for 2 days with gauze containing a counterirritant and washed daily thereafter with an antiseptic solution.

Teat stenosis is characterized by a marked narrowing of the teat sphincter and orifice or canal and occasionally is observed as a hereditary condition, affecting all teats and making milking very difficult. More often, however, it is the result of a contusion or wound of the teat that produces swelling or formation of a blood clot or scab causing an acute stricture. In these acute cases, conservative treatment as outlined for wounds and contusions is indicated. The use of the milking machine should be temporarily discontinued in favor of hand milking of the affected teats. In rare cases, a teat cannula taped in place may be used, with proper aseptic precautions, for withdrawing the milk. Many acute cases of stenosis progress to the more chronic form, characterized by a fibrous thickening of the canal lining and sphincter muscle, if teat dilators are used routinely or a wound is present in or around the teat orifice, or if the milking machine is applied for excessive periods over the course of several weeks. In these chronic cases, surgical intervention may be necessary to correct the stenosis. All injuries to, or surgical procedures on, the teat should be handled carefully to prevent the introduction of infection. Prophylactic antibiotic infusions of the quarter are indicated in all surgical procedures or wounds involving the teat or teat orifice. The disorders of teat "spider" and "black spot" or "black scab" may cause necrosis, scab formation and a fibrous thickening of the teat orifice and sphincter and may lead to teat stenosis (as above). They frequently respond to the regular application of antibiotic-corticosteroid ointments.

Complete teat obstruction is caused by the same factors that cause teat stenosis, or by a congenital membranous obstruction. Treatment is similar to that for stenosis, but the prognosis usually is more guarded. Occasionally, if the injury is severe enough, milking of the quarter should be discontinued for the remainder of that lactation period or permanently. Occasionally, teat obstructions may be due to corpora amylacea, firm blood clots, small pedunculated tumors of the teat lining or foreign bodies, such as teat dilators in the teat cistern, that cause an intermittent obstruction of the teat orifice. These may be removed by massage or by dilation or incision of the teat orifice and grasping and removing the object with a fine pair of forceps.

"Leakers" is a term referring to cows with teats that drip milk continuously or after the stimulus causing milk letdown. These animals usually have sustained a severe teat injury or have a large streak canal. In general, little can be done to correct this condition satisfactorily. Injecting small amounts of Lugol's solution around the teat sphincter with an intradermal syringe or cauterizing the external teat orifice or teat end as well as surgical correction have been tried with limited success.

Eversions and vegetative growths on the external teat orifice are usually due to the use of a milking machine with too high a vacuum, or to leaving the machine on the cow for an excessive period at each milking. Residual milk at the site of vegetative lesions after milking favors bacterial growth at the external teat orifice, an undesirable condition often resulting in the development of local infection, ulcers ("black scab") and mastitis.

"Blind" or nonfunctional quarters usually are the result of a severe infection, which may occur either in the dry or lactating cow or in the heifer, due to sucking by other heifers or calves. If treated, the infection may be overcome and the quarters milk fairly satisfactorily during the next lactation if fibrosis is not extensive. Blind quarters that still contain a small amount of pus may be dried up permanently by the injection of silver nitrate (℞ 642). Rarely, blind or nonfunctional quarters may be congenital.

Congenital or Physiologic Diseases

Congenital aberrations in the bovine udder include many structural defects, such as fusion of the front and hind teats, large-base or funnel-shaped teats, very small short teats, improperly placed teats, "cut-up" udders, predisposition to pendulous or swinging udders, hypoplasia of front- or hind-quarters of an udder and supernumerary teats. With the exception of the latter condition, there is no treatment. These defects should be eliminated by breeding.

Supernumerary teats may be located on the udder behind the posterior teats, between the front and hind teats, or attached to either the front or hind teats. They are easily removed with a pair of sharp scissors when the animal is from 1 week to 12 months of age. Removal just prior to lactation or during lactation is undesirable as a teat fistula often forms that is difficult to correct. The practice of removing supernumerary teats from dairy heifers is desirable in order to make the udder look better, to eliminate the possibility of mastitis in the gland above the extra teats and to facilitate milking. It is best done at 3 to 8 months of age.

Inversion of the teat orifice is a congenital condition that may be hereditary. It is not desirable, even though usually associated with ease in milking, because the teats frequently spray. This type of teat orifice favors udder infection.

Agalactia is occasionally observed in heifers and probably is a hereditary condition associated with an imbalance of the hormones controlling either udder growth and development, or lactation. No treatment has yet proved of definite value. Occasionally, this condition is due to a severe systemic disease in the recently fresh animal, or it may be associated with advanced chronic mastitis with extensive fibrosis of the mammary gland. Animals affected with the latter condition will never produce a normal supply of milk.

Failure of "letdown" of milk is observed occasionally after parturition in young dairy cattle. This condition may be caused by the pain and discomfort of a large and edematous udder. If usual methods of massage, use of warm compresses, calves sucking and frequent milking fail to result in proper letdown of milk, the administration of posterior pituitary extract (℞ 199) or oxytocin (℞ 193) may be successful. This treatment may have to be repeated for several milkings or even for several days. Development of letdown failure may be prevented by using a milking machine from the very start, i.e. never milking by hand. An exact milking and feeding routine is important in training heifers to develop a proper letdown habit.

Physiologic udder edema and congestion is commonly observed in high-producing dairy cattle prior to and after parturition. This problem cannot be controlled satisfactorily, but several practices may help. Some veterinarians advise milking cows before parturition as a means of reducing the congestion and edema. Frequent milkings may be helpful. Massage and the use of hot compresses and udder ointments and liniments stimulate circulation and promote reduction of the edema in the udder tissues. This massage should be repeated as often as possible. When milk letdown fails, udder edema and congestion will appear to increase. In severely affected cows, the udder will often "break down" and become pendulous. The use of diuretics, such as chlorothiazide (℞ 541), or similar preparations (℞ 533, 544), have proved highly beneficial in reducing udder edema, especially in young cattle.

Necrotic dermatitis is observed in cows or first-calf heifers with large edematous udders several weeks after calving. In heifers, the area involved is usually the lateral aspect of the udder and medial aspect of the thigh as the udder is pressed tightly against the leg causing chafing, dermatitis and finally necrosis. In cows, it usually is observed at the anterior portion of the udder between the 2 forequarters. Possibly, poor circulation or ischemia due to the extensive edema is the cause of the necrosis at this site. In heifers, treatment consists of reducing udder congestion as rapidly as possible (℞ 541, 544, 547), limiting movement, daily cleansing of inflamed skin and application of soothing powders, antiseptic oils, or astringents. In cows, the swollen necrotic area at the front of the udder should be washed daily to control the objectionable odor, and astringent and drying powders should be applied along with fly repellents during the summer months. There is no specific treatment to hasten the normal tissue sloughing and repair in this area.

Urticaria or allergic swelling of the udder and teats is observed in association with generalized urticaria (q.v., p. 949), and occasionally, it may be a localized condition where cows are bedded on buckwheat straw or other allergenic plants.

Rupture of the suspensory ligaments of the udder (mainly the medial ligaments) occurs gradually in some older cows over several lactations leading to a dropping of the udder and causing the teats to point somewhat laterally. Occasionally acute rupture can occur at or just after parturition and is characterized by a sudden dropping of the udder, hardness and swelling and by marked edema with serous exudation at the base of the udder especially anteriorly. There are no satisfactory remedies; supportive trusses are not generally satisfactory.

MASTITIS (SM. AN.)

Acute or chronic inflammatory change in one or more mammary glands, often accompanied by abscessation.

Etiology: Acute mastitis usually occurs from traumatic injury to the mammary gland, in association with acute metritis, or following weaning. Failure of the glands to empty (galactostasis) may be a contributing factor. Infection, usually with streptococci or staphylococci may occur. Metritis may result in metastatic mammary infection. Galactostasis may be promoted by malformations of the nipples. Chronic mastitis (cystic hyperplasia, polycystic disease) is more common in older animals and its occurrence is probably hormone-influenced.

Clinical Findings: The initial signs are swelling and inflammation of the involved mammary glands. Discoloration and abscessation may occur. As the infection progresses, pyrexia, lethargy, dehydration and bacteremia follow. Metritis may be present. Young nursing an affected female may die unless weaned and hand-fed. Chronic mastitis is characterized by cyst formation in mammary tissue. These cystic enlargements can be confused with neoplasia and may, in fact, coexist with neoplasia.

Treatment: The litter should be weaned and hand-fed. Antibiotic therapy should be instituted as early as possible (℞ 1, 27, 43, 56). Abscesses should be lanced and drained. This may be followed by flushing with hydrogen peroxide and local instillation of antibacterial medicaments. Abscesses that are not lanced will rupture spontaneously. These should be treated as above. In either case, the area will heal rapidly by second intention, usually with no future impairment of mammary function. Estrogens should be used with caution in the luteal phase of the canine estrus cycle. Suppression of milk flow may be accomplished by the administration of hormones (estrogen or testosterone) or by restriction of food intake. Judicious use of corticosteroids should be considered to relieve inflammation. In cases where galactostasis is pronounced, a breast pump may be used 2 to 3 times daily. Hot followed by cold compresses, applied to the glands 2 to 3 times daily, may be helpful. If the animal shows signs of toxemia, supportive fluid therapy, such as 5% dextrose in lactated Ringer's solution (℞ 578) should be employed. In chronic mastitis, excision of the mammary cysts and, in some cases, ovariohysterectomy should be recommended.

LACTATION FAILURE IN THE SOW

(Mastitis-agalactia syndrome, Metritis-mastitis-agalactia syndrome, MMA)

A prevalent syndrome of the gilt or sow that becomes apparent at parturition or within 2 to 3 days later. It occurs throughout the year, frequently after such stresses as drastic feed changes, sow confinement in a new or remodeled facility or extremely variant temperatures. It is characterized by a decrease in or absence of milk with resultant starvation of pigs and increased susceptibility to other neonatal diseases. Death of the affected sow is rare and most will recover in 3 to 5 days without treatment although some remain in poor health. Neither large litter size nor prolonged parturition are constant features. It is more prevalent in second- or third-litter sows.

Etiology: The cause is unknown although various microbial agents are suspect. Coliform bacteria are frequently isolated from affected mammary glands and uteri. Microbial endotoxins, hormone imbalance, and poor management practices such as improper housing, bedding, feeding and temperature control have all been suggested as causes; however, the disease does occur under ideal management systems. No infectious agent seems uniformly present, although possibly the syndrome is infectious in some herds. Bacterial invasion of mammary gland tissue frequently occurs but often appears to be a secondary factor that prolongs the course of the disease. Hormonal imbalance or insufficiency (possibly stress induced) can result in mammary gland failure. Adrenocortical function increase in affected sows has been demonstrated.

Clinical Findings: Listlessness and anorexia several days before farrowing is sometimes seen. Signs usually appear at the time of parturition or within 2 or 3 days (the disease has not been reported after the first few days of lactation). Hunger in piglets is often the first manifestation. Close observation of the affected sow will often reveal: reluctance to rise or to allow nursing, presence of one or several firm, warm mammary glands, refusal to eat, increased heart and respiratory rates, febrile response and viciousness. The sow may be comatose or normal in attitude. Signs may appear in one sow or many or in a progressive manner suggesting contagion. The sign most frequently seen is involvement (edema, congestion and frequently small foci of mastitis due to bacterial invasion) of one or several mammary glands, rarely all glands. The milk is more alkaline than normal. Cyanotic splotches in the skin covering the mammary glands are seen occasionally in white sows. Vaginal discharge is frequently seen and may be of a different character than the discharge from normal sows.

Lesions: Uterine examinations reveal no differences between affected and normal sows. Mastitic foci and nonfunctional tissue are interspersed with normal mammary gland tissue in most cases. Edema and possibly hemorrhage are present in and around the mammary glands, associated lymph glands, kidneys, synovial membranes, adrenal glands and in some instances the pituitary gland.

Treatment: Immediate relief from unusual stress factors such as extreme heat or cold, poor-quality feed or rough handling is indicated. Trials with various hormones suggest that desirable results can be obtained without multiple drug therapy but conventional treatment includes oxytocin (℞ 193), antibacterial (℞ 66) and corticosteroid (℞ 146) medication repeated at 12- or 24-hour intervals. Oxytocin should be given more frequently if the pigs require feeding.

It may be necessary to remove the pigs to other sows for supplemental feeding or to use milk replacer or fresh cow's milk warmed to body temperature and placed in a shallow pan. Corn syrup (1 tablespoon per pint) improves acceptability; antibacterials can be added. Baby pigs should be fed 6 times daily during days 1 and 2; 4 times daily during days 3 and 4; and 3 times daily during days 5 through 7. Ten-minute feedings are satisfactory. A dry commercial pig starter can be gradually substituted for the milk. If signs in the sow are recognized before the pigs are hungry, early treatment improves pig survival.

Prevention: Stress should be minimized. Phosphorus, calcium, vitamin E and selenium deficiencies have been incriminated and should be avoided. A well-balanced bulky gestation diet should be fed. After farrowing the amount fed should be gradually increased. Radical dietary changes immediately before or after farrowing should be avoided. Batch farrowing with an all in, all out system and strict attention to clean-up, disinfection and a period when a farrowing unit is kept empty (for 1 week) will assist in reducing the incidence of lactation failure in some herds. More specific suggestions await better understanding of the disease.

CONTAGIOUS AGALACTIA

A mycoplasmal disease of goats and sheep occurring in Mediterranean countries, Portugal, Switzerland, Iran, U.S.S.R., Pakistan, India, Mongolia and parts of Africa. A febrile illness with a seasonal incidence coinciding with the onset of lactation, the mortality is low but morbidity of 25% is common. Mastitis is predominant, the milk is reduced in amount and is either viscous and purulent or watery, separating on standing into a yellow deposit and a gray supernatant; the udder may atrophy. Arthritis often occurs with pain, inflammation of periarticular tissue and tenosynovitis; abscessation and ankylosis can take place. Sometimes there is keratoconjunctivitis but eye lesions can vary from conjunctivitis to hypopyon and even perforation of the eyeball.

Diagnosis made on the history and clinical signs may be confirmed by isolation of *Mycoplasma agalactiae* from infected milk, eye or joint fluid, or a complement fixation test.

The organism may be transferred from apparently healthy recovered animals during milking so that control measures should include removal of infected animals from the flock and attention to milking hygiene. Treatment with tylosin (2 to 5 mg/lb [4 to 10 mg/kg] body wt daily, IM) instituted early may be beneficial. Live attenuated or killed vaccines have been used with apparent success in several countries.

BACTERIAL POSTHITIS AND VULVITIS

(Enzootic balanoposthitis)

A spreading ulceration of the epithelium of the prepuce sometimes involving the penis (balanoposthitis), and also the vulva of sheep.

Etiology: The disease is associated with protein rich diets and castration but caused by a bacterium indistinguishable from *Corynebacterium renale* (q.v., p. 858) which hydrolyses urinary urea and initiates ulceration. Lesions of similar appearance are produced by venereal transmission of the virus of ulcerative dermatosis (q.v., p. 249).

Epidemiology: Posthitis (sheathrot, pizzle rot) is common in wethers in Australia and New Zealand; rams are sometimes affected and ewes show analogous vulval ulceration. Posthitis is also seen in steers, sometimes in bulls, and has been reported from wether goats. Contagion occurs from sheep to sheep and between sheep and cattle. Venereal transmission occurs in sheep, and flies may assist in spread of the disease. The disease shows well-marked seasonal fluctuations in grazing sheep where an increase in the clover and protein content of pasture and the urea content of the urine, as occurs in spring and autumn, results in a higher incidence.

Clinical Findings: The early stage, characterized by external lesions only, is unimportant clinically and does not affect productivity. Ulcers a few millimeters in diameter first appear adjacent to the preputial orifice in areas which become wet during urination. Individual ulcers may extend and coalesce with others producing a confluent lesion surrounding the opening and covered with scab. Later, the phagedenic process may extend to the interior of the prepuce and in advanced cases can involve the urethral process and glans penis. Associated external scabbing and stenosis may block the preputial opening and the sheath become distended with foul-smelling urine, pus and necrotic detritis. Affected wethers, especially where urination is difficult, rapidly lose condition. They may be humped, walk stiffly and the hind fetlocks show staining from kicking at the swollen sheath. Stained wool around the prepuce is liable to flystrike. Untreated sheep may die. Advanced lesions are seldom seen in rams, but when they occur are of more consequence than in wethers. In ewes repeated vulval ulceration and scabbing leads to foreshortening of the ventral commissure and misdirection of urine and predisposes to flystrike. Involvement of the vagina is not frequent but serious when it occurs.

Diagnosis: The history and clinical signs provide the basis for diagnosis. Differentiation between bacterial posthitis and the infectious venereal form of ulcerative dermatosis requires transmission experiments to show that contagion from the former only produces lesions on the prepuce and vulva and not on other parts of the body.

Prophylaxis and Treatment: For prevention, wethers are treated with testosterone implants (e.g. 60 to 90 mg testosterone propionate) before spring and autumn growth of pasture. (Testosterone implants are not available in the U.S.A.) Application of antiseptics (e.g. chlorhexidine digluconate solution) to the prepuce at the same time or when the risk is high, also aids in prophylaxis. Affected sheep should be isolated and the wool removed from around the sheath before treatment is started. Dietary restriction (low-quality pasture or cereal hay) with free access to water for about 10 days assists in cure, especially of early external lesions. Healing can be hastened by testosterone implantation (e.g. 100 to 150 mg testosterone propionate) and application of antiseptics such as 5 to 10% copper sulfate ointment, solutions of quarternary ammonium compounds (e.g. 20% alcoholic cetyltrimethylammonium bromide), chlorhexidine digluconate solutions or antiseptic aluminum silicone pastes. Any scabs, urine, pus and debris should be removed from the sheath as thoroughly as possible at the time of treatment. Chronic infections not responding to treatment can be resolved by incising the full ventral aspect of the sheath to allow drainage. Surgical interference may be combined with testosterone implantation, antiseptic treatment and IM injection of procaine penicillin. Treated wethers can be fattened for disposal.

BOVINE CYSTITIS AND PYELONEPHRITIS

A sporadic inflammatory disease of the urinary tract of cattle, and sometimes other species, caused generally by *Corynebacterium renale.*

Etiology: The causative agent in the vast majority of cases of bovine cystitis and pyelonephritis is *C. renale*. The organism has a predilection for the urinary tract and rarely produces pathologic changes in other tissues. *Escherichia coli, C. pyogenes,* streptococci and unidentified diphtheroid bacilli also have produced urinary-tract infections, either as the sole agent involved or in a mixed infection with *C. renale.*

Epidemiology: Aberrant *C. renale* infections have been reported in the horse, sheep and dog. The disease is of economic importance in cattle and occasionally in swine. Cows are affected more commonly than are bulls. The short, wide and often traumatized urethra of the female probably offers a predisposition to infection by allowing the entrance of the organism into the bladder.

C. renale has been cultured from the vulva, vagina and penile sheath of apparently normal cattle. It is now recognized as the cause of enzootic balanophosthitis (q.v., p. 857) of sheep. The bacteria that have been isolated produce experimental pyelonephritis in laboratory albino mice. The incidence of carrier cows has been found to be significantly higher in herds with clinical cases than in herds with no clinical signs of pyelonephritis before a sporadic case appears. The transmission of bovine pyelonephritis is possibly favored by grooming animals with contaminated brushes, vulvar contact with urine-soiled bedding, tail switching and the use of improperly sterilized obstetric instruments and particularly urinary catheters. Venereal transmission seems to be a likely means of spread in animals bred by natural service.

Susceptibility to the disease appears to be increased by the stress of heavy feeding, high production, advanced pregnancy, or cold, uncomfortable weather.

Clinical Findings: A gradual loss in condition occurs over a period of weeks or months. Animals in the advanced stages of infection are emaciated and dehydrated. The appetite is often poor. Generally, the temperature, pulse and respiratory rates are normal.

Restlessness, kicking the abdomen, switching the tail, frequent urination and straining are common signs. The passing of bloody urine containing clots of blood is considered to be almost pathognomonic of pyelonephritis. By careful rectal palpation it is possible to detect the enlarged painful kidney, ureter and thick-walled bladder in advanced cases. In cows with early cases showing severe signs, all palpation findings may be normal. Palpation of the ureters by the vaginal route in mature cows or mares reveals a cordlike ureter often containing crepitating blood clots. The ureters are most easily located several inches proximal to their entrance into the neck of the bladder. The animal's stance may resemble that associated with traumatic pericarditis, gastritis, or indigestion.

Lesions: The urethra of infected cattle is inflamed, edematous and streaked with submucosal ecchymoses. The bladder contains considerable cellular debris, clotted and free blood, and a characteristic "sandy" deposit. The bladder wall is greatly thickened and edematous. Its mucosa is hemorrhagic, may show ulceration, and large vesicle-like swellings usually are present over most of the epithelial surface. The ureters are usually greatly enlarged, from several times their normal diameter up to 2.5 cm. The walls are thickened, edematous and hemorrhages are present. The lumina often are filled with clots of blood, pus and necrotic kidney tissue.

Although the infection may be unilateral, both kidneys are generally involved. The kidneys may be 2 to 3 times their normal size and weight. The external cortical lobulations frequently are ill-defined and the surface may be almost smooth. The capsule may be adherent. The calices are filled with a gray, slimy exudate, shreds of necrotic tissue, clotted blood and urine. Calculi and sand-like precipitate are present. A strong odor of ammonia is emitted. Numerous abscesses and hemorrhages occur throughout the medullary and cortical areas. Atrophy of the parenchyma and considerable fibrosis occur in advanced cases. In general, the infection is characterized by an active, extensive and diffuse necrotizing inflammatory process.

Diagnosis: The signs of the disease are most helpful in establishing a diagnosis. Generally, there are only 1 or 2 animals with pyelonephritis in the herd at any one time. Herd history may indicate that sporadic infections have occurred in the past. Pyelonephritis should be differentiated from other diseases such as leptospirosis and bacillary or postparturient hemoglobinuria, in which hematuria or hemoglobinuria are constant findings.

The sediment of a centrifuged urine sample from an animal with pyelonephritis will contain numerous *C. renale.* A smear of this sediment stained by the Gram method will show clumps and parallel arrangements of gram-positive, pleomorphic bacterial rods. Urine from suspected cases may be cultured on bacteriologic media for the presence of *C. renale.*

Prognosis depends principally upon amount of functional kidney tissue present, virulence of the microorganism, and its susceptibility to therapy. The increased functional demand on the kidney during pregnancy may mean that cows with a marginal amount of functional kidney tissue (approximately 30%) will die when the metabolic load is greater than can be handled.

In advanced cases, the outcome is usually unfavorable. If the clinician can detect the enlargement of the ureters before they exceed 10 mm in diameter, the prognosis may be favorable. Relapses are not uncommon, even after the animal appears to have recovered. In general, a guarded prognosis should be given.

Treatment: *C. renale*-infected animals usually respond dramatically to penicillin therapy (℞ 63, 66) for 8 to 15 days, while those infected with *E. coli* do not. The effectiveness of the therapeutic agent may be reduced in the presence of necrotic tissue debris. Therefore, the effects of therapy should be checked by bacteriologic examination of the urine sediment. Relapse is common especially in advanced cases. To avoid it the course of treatment must be at least 7 days and treatment should be repeated if the organism is present in urine sediment a month after cessation of therapy. Other antibiotics may be of value, but critical studies of their efficacy have not been reported. In general, the sulfonamides have not proved as valuable as penicillin products in the treatment of pyelonephritis.

URINARY CALCULI

(Urolithiasis)

The calculi of all species of animals are similar in composition, comprising some 20 crystalline substances representing different mineral forms of phosphate, oxalate, urate, cystine, carbonate and silica. The constituent elements and radicals can be identified by chemical analysis and the precise crystalline compounds by optical and X-ray crystallography. Chemical analysis is usually all that is required for routine clinical purposes and is simple and inexpensive to perform.

The mechanisms involved in the actual stone formation are not well understood; 3 main theories exist: **the matrix hypothesis** in which the inorganic protein matrix is emphasized as initiating urolith formation; **the crystallization inhibitor hypothesis** in which the importance of organic and inorganic inhibitors of crystallization is emphasized, and **the precipitation-crystallization hypothesis** in which the importance of salt supersaturation receives emphasis.

The factors involved in urolithiasis of some species for some calculi are well documented. It has been known that the organic stones of the dog (cystine, urate) are metabolic in origin; that the inorganic phosphate calculi of dogs are associated mainly with urinary tract infections with urease producing bacteria; and that ruminant urolithiasis is largely nutritional in origin, being associated with diets high in cereal grains or grazing on the silica rich soil of the northwest plains of Canada and the U.S.A. However, not all factors responsible are known and it is probable that urolithiasis is a problem with a multifactorial etiology.

The basis of prevention is identification of the chemical composition of the calculi so that appropriate steps can be taken to reduce the concentration of the particular chemicals in the urine by increasing urine volume, eliminating infection, changing urine pH or altering the metabolism with drugs.

UROLITHIASIS IN RUMINANTS

Urolithiasis is one of the most important diseases in feeder cattle and sheep and a significant number of cases also occur in mature breeding males. Clinical urolithiasis is seen most frequently during the winter months and particularly in steers and wethers on full feed. Affected animals are usually 5 to 10 months old but it may occur much earlier or later.

Although formation is probably equal in both sexes, the short, large urethra of the female affords little opportunity for obstruction, hence the greater clinical incidence of obstruction is in males. Renal or cystic calculi are usually without noticeable clinical effect in ruminants in the absence of obstruction. Calculi originating in the kidney or bladder lodge at points where the urethra changes direction or is limited in dilatability, commonly the ischial arch and the sigmoid flexure in cattle and sheep and the urethral process in sheep. A single calculus is usually responsible for obstruction in cattle, but sheep are commonly affected with multiple calculi blocking the urethra for several centimeters. Occlusion of the urethra may lead to rupture of the urethra due to pressure necrosis or to rupture of the bladder due to the accumulating urine.

Urethral obstruction: Early urethral blockage in ruminants is expressed by restlessness, twitching of the tail and straining. Partial obstruction results in dribbling blood-stained urine. In complete obstruction, the preputial hairs are dry. Minerals may be precipitated on the preputial hairs. As blockage persists, colic-like signs develop, and the animal kicks at its abdomen, rolls on the ground, and may lie down and rise frequently. The tail is held away from the body and secondary rectal prolapse is common. A pulsating urethra is frequently observed, but is not pathognomonic. Hypersensitivity in the region of the sigmoid flexure of cattle may be evident, and deep palpation may locate the swelling resulting from the obstructing calculus. The urethral process of sheep can be prolapsed and the obstruction visualized. The bladder may be in various stages of distension, with severe distension developing 24 to 36 hours after complete blockage.

Other conditions causing signs of abdominal pain are indigestion, consumption of large quantities of cold water, digestive tract stasis or obstruction, primary enteritis, coccidiosis, rabies and rectal prolapse. Urinary tract infection often causes straining along with frequent attempts to urinate.

In sheep, amputation of the urethral process is simple and allows the immediate passage of urine. Such surgery does not interfere with the ram's breeding capability. Several other techniques for urethrostomy, which by-pass the obstruction via an incision proximal to the occlusion, are successful except that they end breeding capabilities. In breeding animals a urinary calculi retriever may be tried; a urethrostomy can still be performed if results are not successful. Postoperative antibiotics are recommended to prevent infection (℞ 66).

Ruptured urethra: Pressure necrosis and perforation of the urethral wall is common if urethral obstruction is not relieved. Urine then collects subcut. along the sheath and umbilicus to cause the characteristic swelling called water belly. This swelling is cold and edematous; aspiration yields a clear fluid, frequently without the smell of urine. Urine may still dribble from the sheath, but signs of abdominal pain and colic are no longer seen, and appetite and bowel function are normal. The BUN concentration begins to rise following rupture of the urethra. While complete skin necrosis is rare, sloughing may be seen due to delayed or incomplete treatment.

Instances of ruptured urethra resemble traumatic injury, subcut. abscesses, and umbilical or ventral hernias. In breeding animals, laceration of the prepuce, with resultant prolapse and infection of the sheath and subcut. tissue, may resemble the urine accumulation following urethral rupture. Hematoma of the penis must also be differentiated.

Treatment of urethral rupture is by urethrostomy and drainage of the subcut. urine. Urethrostomy is performed slightly dorsal to the site employed for relief of urethral obstruction, since hemorrhage and edema are present due to the rupture. The skin over the subcut. urine accumulation is lanced in numerous places to permit drainage for several days. Topical antiseptics (℞ 428) and fly repellents (℞ 285, 311) may be applied to these ventral wounds. Parenteral antibiotics (℞ 66) are administered postoperatively as for uncomplicated obstructions. Electrolyte (℞ 579) or dextrose solutions (℞ 577) are given to correct dehydration and promote urine flow if necessary.

Rupture of the bladder: The most serious sequela to untreated urolithiasis is rupture of the bladder. Sudden relief from the signs of urethral obstruction and pain occur at the time of rupture. The animal may then appear improved for several days before signs of uremia develop. However, dry preputial hairs indicate an absence of recent urination, and the BUN concentration will be greater than 50 mg/100 ml of blood. As urine accumulates in the peritoneal cavity, feed and water consumption decrease and the animal's abdomen becomes progressively swollen. Ballottement allows detection of the fluid, and from behind the animal the abdomen appears pear-shaped. A collapsed bladder and other abdominal organs are felt floating or partially submerged in the urine by rectal examination. Confirmation is obtained by paracentesis through the ventral abdominal wall. Urine is very irritating and will cause peritonitis. The animal is weak and depressed, and the fluid in the peritoneal cavity is red and has a strong odor of urine.

A recently ruptured bladder may be diagnosed by dry preputial hairs, collapsed bladder, a history of abdominal pain and colic-like signs. Once abdominal distension is present, rupture of the bladder must be differentiated from rumen tympany, diffuse peritonitis, tumors of the peritoneal cavity and digestive tract obstructions.

Treatment requires the establishment of ability to urinate, providing for healing of the bladder, and assisting in the correction of uremia. The use of a trocar to drain the urine from the peritoneal cavity will help relieve the uremia. A urethrostomy should be performed to provide free passage of urine. Attempts to repair the ruptured bladder have largely been unsuccessful. Spontaneous healing of the bladder frequently occurs following urethrostomy and removal of the abdominal fluid, although these animals are best salvaged within 3 to 4 months to avoid further complications. Some cases of bladder rupture treated by paracentesis and urethrostomy will fail to pass urine within 48 hours following surgery. Urine will again accumulate in the peritoneal cavity due to lack of bladder healing. Such animals may be treated by performing a cystotomy, suturing a plastic drain into the bladder, and then exteriorizing the other end of the tube through the posterior ventral abdominal wall. Antibiotic (℞ 76) and fluid therapy (℞ 577, 578) may be employed following the procedure since infection and shock are potential complications. These animals should be salvaged within a few months. Occasionally, neglected animals are examined that have a ruptured bladder and severe uremia. Treatment as outlined above may be attempted, but the prognosis is poor.

Prevention: Since the specific cause of urolithiasis is still unclear, no specific prevention is available. Management practices intended to reduce predisposing factors for calculi formation vary widely. In all cases, abundant water should constantly be available and should be heated in cold weather. It is useful to further increase water consumption by including 5 to 10% sodium chloride in the ration. The addition of a broad-spectrum antibiotic (℞ 27) to the ration has also been useful to control urolithiasis in certain instances. Compounds, such as ammonium chloride (℞ 562), to alter urinary pH are available, but have not been widely successful. Careful observation of susceptible animals by experienced persons several times daily will allow early detection and more successful treatment.

UROLITHIASIS IN DOGS AND CATS

Calculi are common in the urinary tract of the dog, the reported incidence being as high as 2.8% of hospitalized dogs. Male cats commonly suffer from obstruction of the urethra due to an accumulation of crystals and mucus, the general incidence being estimated at 1%, but the presence of large uroliths is relatively uncommon in cats of either sex.

Urolithiasis in Dogs

Breeds predisposed are the miniature schnauzer, dachshund, Dalmatian, pug, bulldog, Welsh corgi, basset hound, beagle and terriers. Sex is not a predisposing factor in the overall incidence but bladder stones are found more commonly in females and urethral stones in males. Most affected dogs are between 3 and 7 years of age, although calculi have been found in the very young and the very old. Renal lithiasis accounts for only 5 to 10% of cases and ureteral calculi are rare. Recurrence after treatment has been estimated to be between 12 and 53% but this varies considerably with the breed, type of stone and therapy. The uroliths of dogs are composed of organic matrix and organic or inorganic crystalloids, the former being mucoprotein and the latter mixed substances but with a predominant chemical that usually identifies the stone as 1 of 4 types: 1) phosphate calculi, composed of calcium, magnesium and ammonium phosphate (sometimes called triple phosphate), 2) urate calculi, composed of ammonium urate, 3) cystine calculi, consisting of the amino acid cystine, and 4) oxalate calculi, consisting of calcium, magnesium or ammonium oxalate. Other, rare types consist of silicon dioxide, calcium phosphate and xanthine.

Phosphate calculi account for 60% or more of the total incidence and have been found in most breeds, often in the females and usually in the bladder. In some cases, phosphate calculi can be found in the kidney in addition to the bladder and urethra of male dogs. They are often large, spherical or tetrahedral, sometimes single, but frequently multiple, and most are radiopaque. Infection of the urinary tract with urease producing bacteria (*Staphylococcus* and *Proteus* spp.) is associated with phosphate urolithiasis and the urine in such cases contains protein, pus cells, red blood cells, epithelial cells, bacteria, phosphate crystals and the pH is 7.0 to 8.5. Urea-splitting bacteria may also be isolated from the center of phosphate calculi.

Urate calculi account for about 6% of the incidence and occur almost exclusively in male Dalmatian dogs due to a unique ability to excrete most of their purines as uric acid rather than allantoin. Miniature schnauzers and a few other breeds have been reported to have urate stones as well but the frequency of the problem in these breeds has not been great enough to warrant investigation. The urine of Dalmatian stone-formers may contain blood and may become infected if obstruction of the urethra persists, but otherwise, infection of the urinary tract is not a feature of urate urolithiasis. The stones are small and are found in great numbers in the bladder and urethra of males. Urethral obstruction is the presenting problem and as these stones are the most radiolucent of all calculi, radiographic location of them can be difficult without contrast studies.

Cystine calculi are found in 20% of dogs with urolithiasis, almost exclusively in young males of a variety of breeds, due to a defective tubular reabsorption of cystine and other amino acids. The stones are small, located in the bladder and urethra, causing obstruction of the urethra and like urate stones; they are radiolucent. Bacterial infection of the urine is not usually present.

Oxalate calculi are found in 14% of urolithiasis in dogs and are always small. The stones, composed of the dihydrate of calcium oxalate, are rough, bloodstained and have sharp shelflike crystals projecting from the surface, while those composed of the monohydrate of calcium oxalate have a smooth surface and are brittle. These calculi are radiopaque and little is known about their cause or prevention.

Clinical Findings: The usual problems relate to (a) obstruction of the outflow tract, (b) presence of a large calculus or many calculi in the bladder, (c) loss of kidney function due to nephrolithiasis. Obstructive urolithiasis is a medical emergency as death can occur after 48 to 72 hours. Obstructed dogs will strain frequently but pass small volumes or only drops of urine. The urine may be bloody. The bladder will be distended, reaching the rib cage in severe cases. Signs of uremia will be present. The location of the calculus or calculi in the urethra may be determined by attempting to pass a catheter; the extent of the block can be determined by radiographs of the urethra and bladder.

Bladder uroliths cause dogs to urinate frequently and have hematuria at the end of urination. If bacterial infection exists, the urine may have a strong odor of ammonia and the dog may be inactive and have a poor appetite. Calculi of a significant size can usually be palpated and detected by radiology. Small radiolucent calculi can be located by use of double-contrast radiology.

Renal uroliths cause hematuria and if severe injury to kidney tissue has occurred signs of uremia will be present. A simultaneous bacterial infection will be manifested by cloudy urine that contains bacteria, pus cells, red blood cells and renal tubular epithelial cells. The only means of detecting renal stones is the radiograph.

The signs of **ureteral calculi** are few but evidence of abdominal pain, such as biting at a flank, has been observed.

Diagnosis: The presence of uroliths is often suspected from the history and physical examination results. It can be confirmed by palpation of the urethra and bladder and by radiology. Radiographs should be taken of the entire urinary tract.

Treatment and Prevention: The aim of treatment of **obstructive urolithiasis** is to establish the excretion of urine as quickly as possible. This can be done by (a) passing a small diameter catheter into the bladder, bypassing the stone or by pushing the calculi into the bladder, (b) removing the calculi from the urethra with alligator forceps so that the dog can void spontaneously or so that a catheter can be passed and, (c) using hydraulic pressure to dilate the urethra of the male so that the sudden release of pressure will flush the calculi from the urethra. This is done with the animal anesthetized by compressing the urethra in the pelvis by digital pressure and by compressing the penile urethra around a catheter while saline is infused vigorously into the urethra through a catheter. Sudden release of either compressed area may move the obstructing stone. If none of these methods is effective, the only alternative is (d) urethrostomy, which is the surgical opening of the urethra at a site close to the obstruction. This is necessary when the calculi are adherent to the mucosa of the urethra or when a diverticulum has formed and is filled with calculi.

The main treatment of **bladder calculi** is to remove them by performing a cystotomy. Small calculi in the bladder of females will often pass spontaneously, especially if urine volume is high and infection is eliminated (℞ 6, 16, 115, 121).

Kidney stones that are only a few mm in diameter should be treated conservatively. They are often soft phosphate concretions that will disappear when the predisposing bacterial urinary infection is eliminated with long term antibacterial treatment (℞ 6, 115, 121) or when preventive measures are instituted. Large kidney stones can be removed surgically. Care must be taken to ensure that adequate kidney function exists and that bacterial infections are controlled prior to surgery.

The dissolution of existing uroliths *in situ* may be accomplished by undersaturating the solution of the salt concerned in the urine for a sufficiently long period of time. This same principle is applied to the prevention of uroliths, which is important as recurrence is found in 17% of dogs with phosphate uroliths, 33% of those with urate uroliths, 47% with cystine uroliths and 25% with oxalate uroliths. Thus it is essential to perform an analysis of the calculi found and to understand the role of bacterial infection; that infection with urease producing organisms leads to phosphate urolithiasis but that nonphosphate urolithiasis may predispose to infection which subsequently may cause the primary calculus or calculi to be covered with layers of phosphate stone. Likewise the first stone found and removed may be of cystine, urate or oxalate, but the subsequent stones found may be phosphates and caused by persistent infection initiated by the presence of the original urolith.

Prevention: The prevention of phosphate urolithiasis may be accomplished by identifying the urease producing bacteria present in the urine or the calculus and eliminating them with treatment of 1 to 2 months duration (℞ 6, 115, 121) and by acidifying the urine (℞ 564). Specific antibacterial treatment is more important than acidifying the urine as the quantity of ureases present may make acidification impossible without inducing a state of acidosis. The addition of salt to the diet may also be of benefit by increasing the volume of water drunk and thus the volume of urine excreted. The above treatment plus removal of all calculi (except the small ones) is the current method of managing a dog with phosphate urolithiasis.

The prevention of urate calculi in Dalmatian dogs consists of administering sodium bicarbonate (℞ 498) to maintain a urine pH between 6.5 and 7, providing as much water as the dog will drink and administering allopurinol (10 mg/kg), a xanthine oxidase inhibitor which reduces the quantity of uric acid in the urine.

Cystine calculi may be prevented by maintaining a dilute urine of pH greater than 7.5 by administering sodium bicarbonate (℞ 498). The drug D-penicillamine (℞ 664) combines *in vivo* with cystine to form penicillamine-cysteine which is 50 times more soluble than cystine in urine and may be used to control cystine urolithiasis. As this problem is hereditary, affected dogs should not be used in breeding programs.

Oxalate calculi are less well understood and methods of prevention are general. The urine should be kept diluted if possible and measures taken to reduce the calcium and oxalate salts in the urine. Bacterial infections of the tract should be treated. Thiazide diuretics (℞ 541, 544) which reduce the concentration of calcium in the urine may be of value and allopurinol has been used for humans with oxalate urolithiasis.

In summary, urolithiasis in dogs may be prevented and some uroliths may be dissolved *in vivo* if their size, location and number are determined, if the chemical composition is determined (by chemical analysis or by knowledge of breed, incidence and stone characteristics), and if urinary infection is eradicated and a plan of management is devised that includes appropriate drug therapy to alter metabolism as well as scheduled evaluations.

UROLITHIASIS IN CATS

The feline cystitis, urethritis, urethral obstruction complex (feline urological syndrome) is the most important disease of the urinary system in cats. It occurs in cats 1 to 5 years of age and although both males and females are affected, the male suffers more because of obstruction of the penile urethra with a plug consisting of struvite (magnesium ammonium phosphate) crystals and mucoid material. An actual urolith is rarely found in the urethra of the male cat. The feline cystitis, urethritis, urethral obstruction complex is more common in the colder months, and in inactive obese indoor cats and in cats eating dry food as more than half their diet. Cats living in the same household with an affected cat do not have a greater incidence of the disease than other cats. Mortality of 22% is reported and a recurrence rate of 32%.

Etiology: The etiology is unknown and apparently complex. Bacterial infection is not associated with most cases, and no virus has been found in the urine of affected cats. Castration and the complex are related, although not necessarily directly; the castrated male may be predisposed to the problem because of inactivity and obesity. A recent study failed to show any relationship between age at the time of castration and urethral obstruction. The struvite crystals in the urethra are more likely secondary to the obstruction rather than the cause of it.

Clinical Findings: Male cats with the syndrome usually are found sitting in a litter box straining as if to defecate. The owner may suspect that the cat is constipated or report the finding of blood-tinged urine in the house or blood-tinged urine dripping from the penis. A painful distended bladder will be palpable within the abdomen of obstructed males and the penis is often erect, sometimes with a plug visible in the urethra. Licking of the penis is common. Females with the syndrome exhibit signs of cystitis (frequent urination of a small volume of bloody urine, straining) and urinate in abnormal sites in the house. Obstructed male cats become obviously ill because of uremia, dehydration and pain within 24 to 72 hours of the onset of obstruction. Anorexia, vomiting, inactivity and severe weight loss are the associated signs.

Diagnosis: The diagnosis of the complex is based on the history and the clinical findings. Radiology of affected cats adds little information as large uroliths are seldom present.

Treatment: Cats with obstruction of the urethra should be treated as medical emergencies; removal of the obstruction and the restoration of urine flow is imperative. This can be accomplished in mildly obstructed males by gently compressing the bladder or by milking the penile urethra to force the plug out of the urethra. More firmly obstructed cases require the use of a general anesthetic so that a catheter can be passed into the bladder. The catheter can be used to dislodge the obstruction by simply pushing the plug into the bladder, or by flushing saline through it into the urethra so as to flush the particles of sand away, either into the bladder or to the exterior. Care should be taken during catheterization to not cause undue trauma to the urethra. In more difficult obstructions alternate flushing and compressing of the bladder may relieve the obstruction. Once past the obstruction, the catheter should be advanced to the point where urine begins to flow. The catheter is then sutured to the urethra and the bladder allowed to empty. Additional flushing may be necessary to maintain the flow of urine. Once the bladder is empty it can be partially filled with saline and allowed to drain again. If the cat cannot be catheterized, cystocentesis will have to be performed. After emptying the bladder it is often possible to pass a catheter. If this is not possible it is worthwhile to perform a cystotomy as it may be possible to pass a catheter from the bladder to the exterior through the urethra. Sometimes small uroliths are found when the cystotomy is done.

Prior to the cat recovering from the anesthetic, an Elizabethan collar should be placed on the cat to prevent the catheter from being pulled out or bitten in two.

Since obstructed cats are often severely dehydrated and in a state of acidosis when presented, it is advisable to begin fluid therapy (℞ 588) prior to administering anesthetic agents. Urinary acidifiers should be avoided during this acute phase as they will increase the acidosis. The fluid therapy should be continued until the cat will maintain a hydrated state by eating or drinking. The catheter may be left in place for 48 to 72 hours or until the urine is clear and flowing freely. Antibiotic (℞ 6) is usually administered during the time the catheter is in place.

Prevention of recurrence: Since recurrence is frequent it is important to institute preventive measures. These consist of increasing the volume of and acidifying the urine (℞ 563, 625) to increase the solubility of struvite crystals in the urine. The urine volume can be increased by feeding wet foods, by giving the cat milk to drink and by adding salt to the food; however, salting the food tends to cause diarrhea in cats. Increasing the amount of meat in the diet may also be beneficial. Females are treated with antibiotic (℞ 6) after being examined carefully and radiographed to rule out bladder stones.

UROLITHIASIS IN HORSES

The horse generally suffers from fewer urinary tract diseases than other species of domestic animals. However, of the renal diseases, urinary calculi are most frequent. The presence of mucus and epithelial debris in equine urine leads not only to viscous and turbid appearing urine, but also may serve as nuclei for calculi. Two types of equine calculi are commonly found. The first occurs in horses fed hay or pasture grasses, is yellow-brown and crystalline, and composed principally of calcium carbonate. The second forms in horses being fed grain rations; this type is smooth, white and composed of phosphates. The calculi may occur anywhere in the urinary tract, but are found principally in the bladder or urethra.

Urethral calculi: Urethral calculi produce restlessness, abdominal pain, and frequent urinary attempts. The bladder is found distended on rectal examination. The stone may be located in the urethra by use of a metal catheter. The obstruction may occur anywhere in the urethra, but is more commonly found at the turn at the pelvic inlet.

Passage of a catheter may occasionally dislodge the stone with subsequent expulsion. A smooth-muscle relaxant may also help passage of the stone through the urethra, otherwise surgery is indicated.

Bladder calculi: The commonest site for equine urinary calculi is the bladder. It is thought that the initial calculi form in the renal pelvis and pass to the bladder where they increase in size by mineral deposition around the initiating nuclei of white or red blood cells, albumin, fibrin or epithelial cells. Usually one large stone is found in the bladder; it may be accompanied by several smaller granules.

Clinical Findings: The signs of a bladder calculus in the horse vary with the specific size and composition of the stone. The horse may merely exhibit signs of abdominal discomfort when exercised, or may void urine frequently accompanied by straining and occasional blood in the urine. In advanced cases severe abdominal pain may be seen, the horse may walk with a stilted gait, and it may refuse heavy exercise. Bloody urine is common following strenuous work. Rectal examination facilitates identifying the calculus in the bladder, but epidural anesthesia or tranquilization may be required during this procedure. The calculus is palpated most easily when the bladder is empty. If the animal exhibits strangury and the bladder is distended, the neck of the bladder and proximal urethra should be examined carefully for an obstructing calculus.

Treatment: Bladder calculi must be removed surgically. Postoperative antibiotics (℞ 66) and adequate available drinking water help reduce postoperative complications. Electrolytes and fluid therapy (℞ 577, 579) assist to promote urine flow.

DISEASES OF THE REPRODUCTIVE TRACT (SM. AN.)

METRITIS

An acute or chronic inflammation of the uterus.

Etiology: Metritis usually results from infection acquired at the time of parturition or estrus, or shortly thereafter. Retained fetal membranes, dead fetuses, blood and exudate provide suitable substrates for bacteria, which gain entry through the open cervix. Sometimes, infection is introduced by careless use of instruments, and it may also occur at the time of breeding, being introduced either by the stud or attempts to dilate a small vagina. The organisms causing the infection are the common gram-negative bacteria found in the feces, plus streptococci and staphylococci. Hyperplastic endometritis is discussed under the heading PYOMETRA IN DOGS (q.v., p. 872).

Clinical Findings: Acutely ill animals exhibit fever, polydipsia, depression, vomiting and sometimes diarrhea. Occasionally there is a uterine discharge which may be mucopurulent or bloody.

The signs of chronic metritis are not constant. A persistent or intermittent uterine discharge may be apparent. Failure to conceive or the delivery of dead or weak pups, which die soon after birth, is suggestive. Sometimes the condition is asymptomatic.

Diagnosis: A history of abortion, dystocia, or resorption of fetuses may accompany cases of acute metritis. Occasionally, a thickened, indurated uterus can be palpated through the abdominal wall. Radiography may reveal a uterus of abnormal size or density. A leukocytosis is usually found, especially in acute metritis. Repeated failure to conceive or the delivery of weak or dead pups suggests chronic metritis. A history of frequent or prolonged estrual bleeding indicates endometrial changes that can be regarded as chronic metritis.

Treatment: Treatment of acute metritis includes supportive therapy, such as parenteral fluids, and a prolonged course of antibiotic therapy. Very small repeated doses of posterior pituitary hormone (℞ 199) may increase uterine tone and help it to discharge the contents. This is, however, contraindicated if the uterus is grossly distended. Introduction of 5 to 15 ml of 0.2% nitrofurazone into the uterus with a sterile metal bitch catheter may be useful. A helpful procedure in acute metritis when hemorrhage is not excessive is to combine an antibiotic with estrogen (℞ 166): the antibiotic may be penicillin (℞ 63), chloramphenicol (℞ 22), or tetracycline (℞ 80); the estrogen is given until signs of estrus appear. This increases the antibiotic concentration in the uterus and facilitates a more rapid debridement of the endometrium. Intensive antibiotic therapy is most effective when used at the beginning of estrus. The treatment of chronic metritis is the same except that hormone therapy is contraindicated and prolonged treatment with antibiotics is often necessary. Ovariohysterectomy is indicated if resistance to chemotherapy is encountered.

PYOMETRA IN DOGS
(Hyperplastic endometritis)

An accumulation of pus within the uterus accompanied by hyperplastic changes in the uterine mucosa.

Etiology: This condition most frequently is encountered in bitches over 5 years of age. The disease is attributed to ovarian dysfunction with increased progesterone secretion. The contents of the affected uterus may be sterile though in some cases there is gross bacterial contamination. The organisms most commonly found are *Escherichia coli* and *Streptococcus*. *E. coli* is seldom to be found in the purulent material, but can usually be isolated from the hyperplastic endometrium. Most evidence suggests metritis to be most commonly a bacterial infection while pyometra appears to be of endocrine origin. Pyometra is less common in cats, which can remain asymptomatic for long periods.

Clinical Findings: Anorexia is usually the first sign followed by depression, polydipsia and polyuria. Vomiting frequently follows drinking, and the animal will drink and then vomit as long as water is provided. At this stage, the respiratory rate is increased and the temperature may be elevated, but, as the condition progresses, the temperature falls and finally becomes subnormal. Progressive weakness develops and eventually the animal is unable to stand. The abdomen is distended and pain may be manifested on palpation. Discharges often have a characteristic "sickly sweet" odor and small quantities may accumulate on the hair around the vulva and on the tail. The vulva is often enlarged and occasionally a persistent diarrhea accompanies the disease. Neglected or untreated animals commonly die.

Diagnosis: There is usually a moderate to severe neutrophilic leukocytosis with immature cells being common. The distended uterine horns are easily detected by palpation. Radiographic confirmation is a simple procedure, the pus-filled cornua being clearly evident. Many animals with pyometra also have renal failure and its associated biochemical changes. These findings, together with a history of nonpregnancy or pseudocyesis and the clinical signs, point to a fairly positive diagnosis. A salient point in the history is the occurrence of signs 2 to 8 weeks after estrus.

Treatment: Ovariohysterectomy should be undertaken as soon as the electrolyte and fluid imbalance is corrected. During the delay occasioned by the replacement of fluids and electrolytes, antibiotics should be administered in heavy dosage. The extent of dehydration should be estimated (mild—5% of body weight, moderate—8 to 10%, severe—12%) and that quantity of replacement fluid (lactated Ringer's solution, ℞ 588) should be administered over a period of several hours. A maintenance dose of 45 ml/kg daily should be given during the remainder of the time parenteral fluids are needed. If excess fluid losses occur such as in polyuria, vomiting or diarrhea, additional fluids should be given. After surgery all patients should be monitored for signs of renal failure. If this occurs it should be treated as other forms of acute renal failure (q.v., p. 883). Antibiotics, such as penicillin and streptomycin combinations (℞ 66) or chloramphenicol (℞ 16), should be given. Medical treatment alone may be attempted on selected patients; satisfactory results, however, are rare. Hormones, such as diethylstilbestrol (℞ 166), followed by posterior pituitary hormone (℞ 199) 3 or 4 days later, may be administered in an attempt to evacuate the uterus.

HYPERESTRINISM
(Nymphomania)

A condition arising from the excessive production of estrogenic hormones in which the female is attractive to males, but may lack sexual desire herself. Active ovarian cysts are usually the source of the estrogen. The primary cause, however, may be in pituitary or adrenal dysfunction.

The bitch or queen suffering from hyperestrinism is usually nervous, irritable and sometimes vicious. The bitch will mount and ride males, toys and members of the family, but will rarely permit copulation. The queen shows intense and exaggerated manifestations of estrus and copulates freely. The vulva is usually swollen, reddened and occasionally there may be a bloody discharge. Such animals are commonly sterile.

Prolonged periods of excessive sexual desire, usually without copulation, and without conception if breeding is permitted, together with the swollen appearance of the vulva, indicate nymphomania. Since infection of the vulva, vagina and cervix can produce discharges having an odor that excites males sexually, careful examination of these structures is necessary in arriving at a diagnosis.

Injection of chorionic gonadotropin, 100 to 500 IU to luteinize the cysts and establish a regular estrual cycle, has been tried with variable results. Ovariectomy is the most satisfactory treatment. In valuable breeding animals one may perform a unilateral ovariectomy if the cysts are confined to one ovary. Successful pregnancies have been reported following this procedure. If vulvitis, vaginitis, or cervicitis is the etiologic factor, treatment is as indicated for these diseases (q.v., p. 889). The use of 17α-hydroxyprogesterone will often suppress the signs but does not effect a cure.

Satyriasis: The comparable problem in the male, exaggerated sexual desire, can occasionally be troublesome in dogs because the frequent attempts to mount other animals, objects or persons are annoying. Administration of an estrogen, obedience training or, ultimately, castration, may result in alleviation of signs.

VAGINAL HYPERPLASIA ASSOCIATED WITH ESTRUS

Enlargement of the mucosa of part of the vaginal floor or wall in bitches during estrus, believed to be due to estrogen overstimulation. The condition occurs in all breeds, but is most commonly seen in brachycephalic types, particularly boxers.

The excessive hyperplastic reaction usually involves a small portion of the vaginal mucosa, other areas showing only the normal changes of estrus. Difficulty in breeding or in urination often calls attention to the hyperplasia. Frequently, the mass protrudes through the vulvar orifice.

The coexistence or recent history of estrus and the appearance of the swelling are diagnostic. Examination reveals that the mass originates from the vaginal floor or wall, usually between the cervix and urethra. The condition may be confused with tumor or prolapse of the uterus or vagina. In hyperplasia, however, the mass is dome-shaped and often pedunculated, while in prolapse of the vagina or uterus the protruding tissue is more voluminous and broadly based.

The swelling usually subsides soon after estrus. Spaying will hasten involution of the residual hypertrophy and prevent its recurrence. Both spaying and surgical removal of the tissue may be necessary with massive hypertrophy. Surgical removal is always indicated when a large, protruding mass becomes abraded, ulcerated or infected. In the brood bitch, surgical removal is usually practiced, but the owner should be cautioned that the condition may recur at subsequent estrous periods. Such patients may be bred by artificial insemination.

STERILITY IN DOGS

In the study of infertility, the dog has been largely neglected and little information is available. Even less appears to be known about anomalies of reproduction in the cat.

The nature of the estrous cycle in the bitch, gonadal malfunctions and certain more or less well-defined anomalies in sexual behavior in both sexes, are referred to in REPRODUCTIVE PHENOMENA, p. 794, FALSE PREGNANCY, p. 876, ARTIFICIAL INSEMINATION IN DOGS, p. 814, and other headings in this chapter. In the bitch, endocrine disturbances resulting in infertility may be of several varieties and it is impossible to make sharp distinctions between them. The prolonged and excessive production of estrogen usually coincides with the presence of ovarian cysts. Ovariohysterectomy is the best method of treatment, but chorionic gonadotropin (℞ 159) or progesterone (℞ 194) therapy may be attempted.

Hypoestrinism sometimes results in continuous anestrus, or in "silent heat" with absence of gross proestrual bleeding. For this condition, estrogens (℞ 166) may be helpful. However, they should be used with care or serious repression of ovarian function may result. Some bitches have an abnormally long anestrus and may respond to equine gonadotropin (℞ 175).

Hypoprogesteronism, leading to failure of implantation or early abortion, is believed to be the cause of infertility in some instances. In these, progesterone, in doses of 5 to 25 mg, IM, 2 or 3 times weekly during the early stages of pregnancy, may be helpful.

Hypoandrogenism in males may result in impotence. The desire for coitus may be increased by the administration of testosterone (℞ 200) 1 or 2 days before breeding.

Congenital defects or **tumors** of the reproductive system of either sex may result in breeding failures. **Infections** of the female genital system, such as vaginitis, acute and chronic metritis and pyometra, may result in infertility. Similarly, in the male, balanitis, orchitis, epididymitis and prostatitis may result in reduced fertility. Brucellosis (q.v., p. 370) has been shown to produce sterility following orchitis.

Psychologic and environmental factors also influence fertility. House pets may be reluctant to breed and rough handling or distractions during supervised breeding may affect the conception rates. Close confinement of male dogs may result in temporary sterility. Inanition and obesity may affect reproduction, but the influence of nutrition is apparently not great. Senile changes affect the reproductive capacity of both sexes. The senile dog may be completely infertile.

The following suggestions may be helpful in improving fertility in dogs: (1) Both male and female should be in a good state of health and in good, lean physical condition. (2) The breeding should take place in an atmosphere free from unnecessary distractions. (3) The correct breeding time should be accurately determined. The best conception rates usually occur when bitches are bred twice, within 48 hours, during the first 4 days of true estrus. The examination of daily vaginal smears may help to define more accurately the optimum time for breeding (*see* ARTIFICIAL INSEMINATION IN DOGS, p. 814). (4) The reproductive organs of the male should be examined and, if necessary, a specimen of semen collected for assessment of quality (*see* EVALUATION OF SEMEN SAMPLE, p. 804). (5) Artificial insemination may be used when physical or psychic abnormalities preclude successful natural mating.

FALSE PREGNANCY IN DOGS

(Pseudopregnancy, Pseudocyesis)

The appearance of the signs of pregnancy and lactation in the bitch at approximately 60 days after estrus. The syndrome can follow the first or any estrus and tends to recur during subsequent estrus cycles. It may be complicated by uterine lesions. False pregnancy is associated with persistent corpora lutea but the mechanisms responsible are unknown. The role of the hypothalamus and pituitary is uncertain. Prolonged activity of the corpora lutea is thought to be responsible for the clinical signs.

The signs are those of intensified and prolonged metestrus and vary in intensity from slight distension of the abdomen and hyperplasia of the mammary glands to those of impending parturition. A serous secretion may appear at the nipples or lactation may begin, sometimes complicated by mastitis. Changes in temperament are frequent. Some bitches make a nest in a dark area, "mother" a toy or shoe, etc., and refuse to eat or come when called. Digestive disturbances and mild hypothermia or hyperthermia may also occur. The history, abdominal palpation and radiographs can serve to exclude the possibility of true pregnancy.

Mildly affected bitches need not be treated. Pregnancy may lessen the intensity of subsequent episodes. Ovariohysterectomy can be performed once lactation ceases. Testosterone (℞ 200), or estrogens, particularly diethylstilbestrol (℞ 166) or a combination of both have been employed with variable results. Hormones should not be used in breeding bitches as they probably increase the severity of concurrent endometrial pathology. Progesterone (℞ 194) has also been used. Self-nursing should be prevented through the use of suitable restraints.

INCONTINENCE OF URINE DUE TO HYPOESTRINISM

Inasmuch as the disease is seen principally in spayed bitches, the cause is thought to be hypoestrinism.

Clinical Findings and Diagnosis: Involuntary urination usually occurs when the family is relaxed or asleep. Urine is frequently found where the animal has been sitting, or the animal may unconsciously dribble urine when in motion. The perineal hair often is urine-soaked and the skin scalded. In addition to intermittent incontinence, the animals will urinate normally.

That the animal is a spayed female and that the passage of urine is an unconscious act are important. Differential diagnosis includes unilateral ureterovaginal fistula, neoplasm of the bladder neck and bladder atony. The mechanism of this condition is unknown. Other causes of incontinence such as ectopic ureters and neurologic causes of incontinence must be eliminated.

Treatment: Diethylstilbestrol is administered at the rate of 0.1 to 1.0 mg daily to effect. Large dogs may be started on a high initial oral or parenteral dose of up to 2 mg the first day or two. Oral dosage is as effective as parenteral and has the advantage of being adaptable to home administration. When the animal is no longer incontinent, the dose is gradually reduced to the minimum maintenance dose. It is important that the clinician take time to explain to the owner that the disease will require lifelong treatment, that the animal can be a pleasant house pet with the cooperation of the owner, and that signs of estrus and a bleeding tendency can result from prolonged or unnecessarily high doses of diethylstilbestrol. Also, excessive doses of estrogens will cause depression of bone marrow activity and possibly an aplastic anemia.

In a few instances the dosage required to control incontinence may be great enough to produce estrus. In such cases, combining stilbestrol with testosterone may control the incontinence and suppress the signs of estrus. In some spayed females, stilbestrol does not control the incontinence. In rare cases, a postoperative adhesion between the uterine stump and the bladder may be responsible for the incontinence.

DISEASES OF THE PROSTATE GLAND

BENIGN OR CYSTIC HYPERPLASIA

This is the commonest disease of the prostate gland of dogs. Sixty percent of all dogs over 6 years of age have some degree of prostatic hyperplasia, although the majority of these animals show no signs. Prostatic hyperplasia in dogs is usually of a cystic type; these cysts may reach an enormous size. The etiology of the condition is unknown, but it may be the result of endocrine imbalance.

Clinical Findings: The principal signs are tenesmus and constipation. Urinary signs, such as frequent attempts to urinate, hematuria, distension and atony of the bladder occur infrequently. Alteration of the gait of the animal frequently accompanies prostatic enlargement. There may be a definite lameness in a hind leg, or weakness may be evident in the hindquarters.

Perineal hernia may occur in association with prostatic enlargement. Although all dogs with perineal hernia do not have enlarged prostates and vice versa, the association between the 2 conditions is so frequent that prostatic enlargement should always be suspected in cases of perineal hernia.

Diagnosis: While the size of the prostate can be estimated by simultaneous rectal and abdominal palpation, the only accurate determination of its size is by radiography. The introduction of contrast material (radiopaque substance or air) into the bladder will provide sufficient contrast to outline the prostate. Radiographs, while showing definite abnormalities of size and shape of the gland, cannot differentiate all the disease conditions of the prostate.

Treatment: Castration is the most simple and direct treatment but may be unnecessary in many cases of hypertrophy. Prostatic atrophy may be induced by the administration of small (0.1 mg) doses of diethylstilbestrol, given intermittently. Continuous administration of large doses of synthetic estrogens in dogs may result in squamous metaplasia or cystic enlargement of the prostate.

Benign hyperplasia with large cyst formation is not likely to respond to diethylstilbestrol. In these cases surgical drainage of the cyst or castration or both are indicated.

SUPPURATIVE PROSTATITIS
(Prostatic abscess)

Inflammation following infection of the prostate is not uncommon in dogs. Whether suppuration occurs will depend upon the type of organism involved. The infection may be ascending or descending. It is presumed that most prostatic infections are secondary to urinary-tract infections.

The signs of prostatitis are similar to those previously described for benign prostatic hyperplasia. In addition, however, these animals show an elevation of temperature and pain upon abdominal or rectal palpation of the prostate. If the finger can reach the inflamed gland, the prostate is found to be warm, sensitive and fluctuant. A blood count may reveal leukocytosis, and white blood cells as well as bacteria are found in the urine. By rectal massage of the prostate, exudate can usually be collected for microscopic examination. Not only does this procedure confirm the site of the inflammatory reaction, but it allows one to characterize the exudate.

The diagnosis is based upon the clinical signs and upon radiographic evidence of prostatic enlargement.

Prostatic Cysts

Blockage of prostatic ducts may result in accumulation of secretions and cyst formation.

The development of clinical signs usually occurs when the cyst is of sufficient size to cause pressure on adjacent organs. The syndrome may resemble benign prostatic hyperplasia or, if the cyst becomes infected, the signs may be similar to those of prostatic abscess. Some cysts attain a huge size and are readily detected by abdominal palpation in the posterior abdomen. They must then be distinguished, both by palpation and by radiography, from the urinary bladder. A pneumocystogram or the use of a radiopaque catheter may be helpful in making this distinction.

Aspiration of the contents of the cyst has been recommended, but this technique is frequently followed by recurrence. Some cysts are attached to the prostate gland by a relatively small stalk, making surgical removal easier. Marsupialization of the cyst has been reported to be of benefit in a few instances. Castration may be of some benefit. If the cyst is infected, antibiotics should be used as indicated by culture and sensitivity testing.

Prostatic Neoplasms

Several types of primary neoplasms have been encountered in the prostate gland. The prostate may also be the site of metastatic tumors, e.g. lymphosarcoma. Primary carcinoma of the prostate is not rare and it is to be expected that with increasing numbers of older dogs there will be a corresponding increase in prostatic neoplasms.

The signs of prostatic neoplasm parallel those of the other prostatic diseases. True urinary incontinence may be present. Together with the usual signs of prostatic disease, radiographic studies give the best diagnostic evidence. Prostatic carcinomas frequently spread to the bony pelvis and extend into the bladder or ureters. Metastasis has usually occurred before a diagnosis is established. The animal should be examined very carefully for metastasis before surgery is attempted. Castration and treatment with estrogens has been recommended as a palliative treatment for prostatic carcinoma.

Prostatic Calculi

This condition is relatively rare. The cause of primary prostatic calculi is poorly understood. The calculi consist of bacteria, tissue debris and mineral deposits. The signs are those common to other prostatic and urinary-tract diseases, e.g. hematuria, pain, frequent urination and constipation. Radiography provides diagnostic confirmation since the calculi are obvious. Surgical removal of the calculi from the prostatic parenchyma, followed by suitable antibiotic or chemotherapeutic measures, is the only treatment.

Cystic Uterus Masculinus

This condition is part of the complex of conditions that result in enlargement of the prostate gland.

The size of these cysts, which often exceeds 5 cm, suggests that they are not merely dilations or confluency of smaller cysts but vestiges of the mullerian ducts, the uterus masculinus, that have become activated to secrete. Unlike the reaction of the enlarged acini of cystic hyperplasia to estrogens, i.e. to become smaller, these cysts of the uterus masculinus enlarge and may become massive. It is imperative, therefore, if estrogen therapy is employed to reduce the size of a hyperplastic gland, that the dosage be minimal and that the patient be closely observed for untoward reaction.

The cyst is most easily identified radiographically. The urine should be cultured to determine the sensitivity of any organisms. The urine should also be examined for the presence of malignant epithelial cells.

The treatment is surgical. Estrogen therapy is contraindicated.

CANINE TRANSMISSIBLE VENEREAL TUMOR

Tumors are usually found on or near the genitalia. Occasionally they occur on the face, shoulders and other regions. It is a venereal disease, with most evidence suggesting that the transmission is by cell transplantation. There is little evidence to date to support the viral etiology that has been proposed.

Spontaneous regression of the tumor may occur. Metastasis is occasionally reported, most often to the regional lymph nodes, but infrequently to internal organs and to the eye. Transmission readily occurs through coitus, and dogs of all ages are susceptible. The tumors are first noted as small hyperemic nodules, which gradually increase in size. There is usually a broad base of attachment with the surface being lobulated or ulcerated. During rapid growth, the tumor is bright red. Later when ulceration occurs, a serosanguineous discharge, possibly accompanied by some suppuration, is present. In the male, the tumors are located most frequently on the penis or prepuce, less often on the scrotum or perineum. The vulva and vagina are the usual sites of the tumor in the female.

Radiotherapy has been used with apparent benefit at doses of 1,000 to 2,000 r in 2 to 4 divided doses. Additional evaluation of this approach to treatment is needed.

Surgical removal is successful in cases where vital structures are not extensively involved. Chemotherapeutic agents, particularly cyclophosphamide (℞ 657), induce regression and involution of the tumor. Indeed, chemotherapeutic agents may become the treatment of choice as more data become available.

DISEASES OF THE URINARY SYSTEM (SM. AN.)

CHRONIC RENAL FAILURE

A condition resulting from prolonged, significant, and usually progressive loss of functional renal tissue. Its causes include: pyelonephritis, renal amyloidosis, chronic obstructive uropathy, congenital lesions, glomerulonephritis and genetic renal diseases as well as unknown causes. The term **chronic interstitial nephritis** has been used to describe this condition but since this term is essentially a pathologist's term to describe the morphologic appearance of kidneys of dogs and cats affected with chronic, progressive and irreversible renal disease, it does not contribute to the understanding of the underlying cause.

Clinical Findings: Polydipsia, polyuria and occasional vomiting are the early signs. As renal failure ensues over a period of weeks or months, anorexia, dehydration, nonregenerative anemia, renal osteodystrophy, depression and weight loss are commonly seen. In the terminal stages, oral ulcerations, diarrhea or constipation, severe dehydration, continual vomiting, convulsions and coma lead to death.

Diagnosis: The animal is unable to alter urine specific gravity from a range of 1.008 to 1.012; there may occasionally be abnormal elements in the urine sediment, including white cells and casts. The BUN, plasma creatinine and inorganic phosphorus are elevated. A moderate to severe nonregenerative anemia is commonly present in the late stages of the disease. In terminal uremia, hyperkalemia and acidosis may occur. In order to determine the cause and severity of renal failure, IV pyelograms, renal biopsy, urine culture and specific renal-function tests are generally required, though in the advanced stages it is frequently impossible to determine the underlying cause and the term "end stage renal disease" is used to describe the kidney disease present.

Differential Diagnosis: This condition must be distinguished from acute nephritis and renal failure, which is potentially reversible. This can usually be accomplished with a very careful history and the laboratory findings listed above. The polydipsia and polyuria of chronic renal failure may be confused with diabetes insipidus, diabetes mellitus, pyometra, pyelonephritis without renal failure, and several other obscure polyuric states. Adrenal insufficiency may be confused with renal failure, since many of these animals are vomiting and azotemic. The prevalence of chronic renal failure is equally high in dogs and cats.

Prognosis: Severe loss of renal tissue is a permanently disabling condition. However, animals can survive for long periods with a small fraction of their renal tissue, due to compensatory hypertrophy and hyperplasia. The prognosis of an individual animal depends upon the severity of the metabolic defects associated with uremia, cause of the renal failure, number of surviving nephrons and concurrent infections.

Treatment: The first step in therapy is to break the vomiting-dehydration cycle that further diminishes renal function. All fluid and some caloric requirements are met by parenteral fluid administration, either subcut. or IV. The severity of dehydration should be estimated (mild—5% of body wt, moderate—6 to 8%, severe—12%) and a quantity of a balanced electrolyte solution, based on this estimate, should be administered. The response of the patient should be monitored by frequent clinical evaluations, rate of urine flow, frequent weighing and repeated measurements of the BUN or plasma creatinine concentration. Lactated Ringer's solution (℞ 588) should be used if hyperkalemia is not present. Sodium bicarbonate infusion or tablets (℞ 498) may be given to correct acidosis. Vomiting may be eased by treating the gastritis with protectants such as aluminum hydroxide (℞ 489). Aluminum hydroxide also reduces intestinal absorption of phosphate and helps control hyperphosphatemia. Vomiting may be suppressed with specific antiemetic drugs, antihistamines, or one of the tranquilizers (℞ 377). Under no circumstances should fluid restriction be imposed.

Dietary therapy that restricts protein intake will sometimes relieve the uremic signs. A very low-protein intake of only high-quality proteins such as egg and meat is used. Commercial low protein diets are now available. Major changes in diet usually require considerable change in the animal's dietary habits. A high-caloric intake should always be encouraged. Cats are notoriously adverse to dietary change and must be induced to eat a variety of nonprotein foods.

Additional therapeutic considerations include: multiple B-vitamin preparations; a high-calcium intake; vitamin D; sodium chloride, 2 to 10 gm/day in divided doses; sodium bicarbonate, 1 to 6 gm daily; bone-marrow stimulants; and in some cases periodic blood transfusions. Animals in chronic renal failure require additional sodium chloride and sodium bicarbonate for the remainder of their lives.

Acute Tubular Necrosis

Acute tubular necrosis is the result of a major insult to the kidney parenchyma that results in acute renal failure. In general, 2 broad groups of etiologic factors may be identified. The first group of etiologic factors are situations associated with vascular collapse and hypotension with resultant ischemia of renal tissue: severe hemorrhage, burns, major surgery, overwhelming infections, hypersensitivity, shock, and severe water and electrolyte depletion. The second etiologic group is nephrotoxic substances. Mercuric chloride, phosphorus, carbon tetrachloride, arsenicals and ethylene glycol are the most common nephrotoxins. Amphotericin B, gentamicin, kanamycin and other antibiotics may cause acute renal failure.

The signs of acute renal failure include: vomiting, anorexia, dehydration, oral ulceration, hypothermia and oliguria or anuria. Laboratory results are similar to those found in chronic renal failure, except anemia is not commonly present and hyperkalemia is usually found. A renal biopsy is most useful in confirming a diagnosis and in helping to establish a prognosis.

Immediate and adequate attention must be given to the restoration of deficits of blood volume, extracellular fluid and electrolytes. This must be done with some caution in the oliguric animal and with awareness that correction of the fluid deficit itself may not correct the renal dysfunction. Repeated blood chemistry determinations and measurement of urine flow must be monitored for several days. The use of mannitol (℞ 545) or a potent diuretic (℞ 543) to stimulate diuresis may be helpful if the animal is treated early in the course of acute renal failure.

Metabolic acidosis may be a life-threatening factor in this situation and is treated with sodium bicarbonate infusions. If renal function is not improved within 48 to 72 hours, peritoneal dialysis may be used to maintain the animal until the extent of renal injury is known.

CONGENITAL RENAL DEFECTS

Renal Dysplasia and Hypoplasia: These defects are present most commonly in the dog. The kidneys may be unilaterally or bilaterally small, firm and pale. Some kidneys have a uniformly diminished renal cortex. At histologic examination such kidneys demonstrate primitive and bizarre tubules and glomerular structures, and excessive fibrous tissue.

Affected animals usually have signs of polydipsia and polyuria, which precede signs of uremia. Dwarfing will occur if the onset of renal failure occurs within the first few months of life. Changes in the urinalysis, hemogram and blood chemistry are the same as in other chronic, progressive renal diseases. Severe renal failure is usually present at 6 months to 2 years of age. The diagnosis can be suspected on the basis of breed and age of onset. A renal biopsy may be helpful in confirming the diagnosis. Treatment is the same as for any other chronic renal failure.

Ectopic Ureter: This defect has been most commonly reported in the dog (usually females) and is usually first noticed at 3 to 6 months of age. Urinary incontinence with continual dripping of urine is the classic sign. A low-grade vaginitis or vulvitis may be present due to urine scalding. The ureter or ureters involved may open into the urethra, prostate, or vagina. Diagnosis may be confirmed by an IV pyelogram that traces the course of the ureter. The most successful treatment is transplanting the affected ureters into the bladder when the disease is bilateral, when the opposite kidney is abnormal, or when the kidney with an ectopic ureter is normal or near normal. Animals with ectopic ureters terminating in the urethra often remain incontinent at a reduced level following surgery.

Unilateral Renal Agenesis: This is relatively common in the cat and quite rare in the dog. One kidney and its associated ureter are usually absent. This is usually an incidental finding in the cat and renal function is usually normal.

Polycystic Kidneys or Solitary Cysts: Also known as congenital cystic kidneys, the term polycystic kidney applies when the renal parenchyma is largely replaced by multiple-cyst formation. It is relatively uncommon in both dog and cat. Such kidneys are usually found to be grossly enlarged by palpation. Polycystic kidneys may cause no clinical signs or may lead to progressive renal failure. The diagnosis is usually made on the basis of physical and radiographic findings or by exploratory laparotomy. Pyelonephritis is a common finding in such kidneys and may precipitate renal insufficiency.

Miscellaneous Anomalies: Double or multiple renal arteries are seen in approximately 5% of dogs. Other congenital defects, including renal fusion, persistent urachus, congenital changes in position, and congenital hydronephrosis and hydro-ureter, are relatively infrequent in both the dog and cat.

GLOMERULONEPHRITIS

An inflammatory lesion of the glomerulus and associated vasculature, some forms of which may be immune mediated. The exact mechanism through which injury to the glomerulus occurs remains obscure. Histologically it is characterized by diffuse inflammation and thickening of the glomerular capillary basement membranes. This condition commonly leads to progressive renal failure.

Glomerulonephritis may be asymptomatic until severe proteinuria or renal failure develop. Classical signs, when associated with the nephrotic syndrome, include loss of lean body mass, edema, ascites and anorexia. Laboratory findings may include massive proteinuria, hypoalbuminemia, lipemia and anemia. In the later stages, all the signs and laboratory findings of chronic renal failure may be present. The nephrotic syndrome is not always associated with glomerulonephritis. Urine specific gravity is usually normal early in the disease; in late stages, it is usually low. The finding of massive proteinuria should suggest the possibility of a glomerular lesion. A renal biopsy is necessary to determine the cause.

Treatment is aimed at relieving the nephrotic syndrome by correcting the fluid balance and elevating plasma-protein concentrations. In the absence of severe renal failure a high-protein diet should be fed. A low-sodium diet and intermittent diuretic therapy (℞ 541, 543, 546) is helpful to control the edema and ascites.

PYELONEPHRITIS

An inflammatory disease of the renal pelvis and parenchyma. It may be acute or chronic, focal or diffuse, arrested or active. The most common bacterial organisms associated with this infection are staphylococci, *E. coli* and *Proteus*. It is usually considered an ascending urinary-tract infection and may be associated with chronic obstruction, calculi, cystitis or congenital defects. Also, it may occur in the absence of any other urinary-tract infection.

Because pyelonephritis may be subclinical, the incidence is unknown. Its presence should always be considered in cases of calculi and lower urinary-tract infection. Signs may include obstruction, depression, anorexia, polydipsia and polyuria. When the condition is advanced, renal pain, intermittent fever and vomiting may be seen in cases associated with renal calculi. Examination of the urinary sediment usually reveals many white blood cells, bacteria, microscopic hematuria and cellular casts.

Urinary culture and antibiotic sensitivity tests are essential; long-term antibiotic therapy, several months in duration, is usually necessary. In addition, urinary acidifiers, as ammonium chloride (℞ 562), and urinary antiseptics (℞ 564) are helpful. High-protein diets and high-fluid intake should also be encouraged. Eradication of the infection can be confirmed by repeated negative urine cultures.

ACUTE INTERSTITIAL NEPHRITIS

This disease in dogs is attributable to a number of infectious disorders, including *Leptospira canicola* or *L. icterohaemorrhagiae.* It has, therefore, been classified as an infectious bacterial disease and is discussed under LEPTOSPIROSIS IN DOGS (q.v., p. 380).

RENAL AMYLOIDOSIS

An idiopathic disease characterized by intercellular deposition of an amorphous, eosinophilic, hyaline-appearing substance in many organs and body tissues. In dogs and cats the kidneys are sites where amyloid deposition frequently assumes major clinical importance. While this condition occurs in many species, it has been most frequently reported in the dog.

Early signs usually include severe proteinuria, weight loss, polydipsia and polyuria. As the condition progresses, azotemia, anemia, and the classic signs of renal failure are seen. In some cases, renal failure appears very late following the chronic debilitating course. The nephrotic syndrome may be present with ascites and peripheral edema.

Diagnosis is made on the basis of progressive renal failure, hypercholesteremia and persistent proteinuria. The 24-hour urine-protein excretion may range from 0.5 to 15.0 gm in the dog and lead to hypoproteinemia. A renal biopsy is necessary to confirm the presence of amyloid deposition in the glomeruli.

There is no known treatment; however, symptomatic and supportive treatment of the accompanying progressive renal failure may be beneficial. A high-protein diet may be used before severe renal failure is present and may retard hypoproteinemia and the nephrotic syndrome. A diuretic (℞ 542, 543) may be used in alleviating signs associated with excessive fluid accumulation in the nephrotic syndrome.

HYDRONEPHROSIS

Hydronephrosis is characterized by a dilatation of the renal pelvis caused by partial or complete obstruction to outflow of urine in one or both kidneys. When the obstruction is acute, complete and bilateral, less extensive changes in the kidneys occur because the period of survival is too short. In unilateral or partial obstruction the animal survives long enough to have severe pressure atrophy of the renal parenchyma and cystic enlargement of the kidney. Hydro-ureter is a common accompaniment and is seen when the obstruction occurs lower in the tract. The condition is not infrequent and occurs in all species.

Urinary outflow obstruction may result from infections with inflammation of the pelvis, ureter, bladder or less often the urethra. Mechanical obstruction of the urinary tract may be produced by calculi or tumors, or by external pressure on the ureters, urethra, or neck of the bladder by an abdominal tumor, a gravid uterus, or by prostatic enlargement.

Swine may be predisposed to hydronephrosis by the conformation of the bladder. In cattle, a distended rumen may displace the left kidney and cause sharp curvature of, or pressure on, the corresponding ureter. Calculi are important etiologically.

The condition that is unilateral commonly goes undiagnosed by virtue of compensatory hypertrophy of the other kidney, which maintains renal function. Signs of vomiting, pain upon palpation and anorexia may be seen in cases of acute and complete obstruction. Infection may supervene and complicate the diagnosis. The fluid pressure produces atrophy of the functional kidney tissue and there is chronic inflammation of the interstitial tissue with fibrosis and lymphocytic infiltration. The papillae of the medulla disappear first; later, even the cortex may atrophy, leaving only interlobular connective tissue, persistent glomeruli and blood vessels. The affected kidney eventually becomes a grossly enlarged, functionless sac filled with urine or serous fluid. The enlarged kidney may become palpable through the abdominal wall in small animals or per rectum in large animals. Bilateral hydronephrosis produces renal insufficiency and terminal uremia. X-ray examination and IV pyelograms are useful to grossly determine the residual renal mass.

The primary objective is to re-establish the flow of urine by removing the obstruction or alleviating its cause.

CYSTITIS

This common bladder disease is usually caused by bacterial infection, most commonly by ascension of *E. coli*, staphylococci or *Proteus* from the urethra. In cats, the disease has been transmitted by inoculating other cats with a bacteria-free filtrate of urine from affected cats and also by the inoculation of a virus isolated from affected animals. Urinary stasis, neurologic derangements of micturition and acquired or congenital defects of the bladder wall are often predisposing factors. Iatrogenic infection by catheterization is not unknown.

Clinical Findings: Cystitis is characterized by frequent urination, hematuria, dysuria, straining and unproductive attempts to urinate. Frequency is less obvious to the owner of the male dog because of its natural tendency to urinate often. House-trained pets often will signal their desire to go out more frequently than before. However, mild chronic cystitis frequently causes a housebroken animal to violate its training without showing urgency. Hematuria is most evident in the last part of the voided sample. The bladder often is in a state of spasm, or the wall may be thickened.

In chronic cystitis, the signs are similar, but not as pronounced except that the incidence of hematuria is greater and the bladder wall thicker.

Diagnosis: The history usually is revealing, although an owner may confuse the animal's attempts to urinate with attempts to defecate, and hence interpret the condition as constipation or diarrhea. Palpation disclosing a distended bladder suggests urethral obstruction. Palpation of a thickened, or a small, firm contracted bladder suggests cystitis. Examination of the prostate in male dogs should be routine to eliminate or confirm the possibility of complicating prostatic disease. The prostate may be examined by digital and abdominal palpation; however, radiographic studies are necessary for accurate diagnosis. A pneumocystogram or injection of a 5% solution of a contrast medium into the bladder is particularly helpful in detecting abnormalities of the bladder. The passage of catheters may reveal the presence of urethral calculi or strictures. It is especially important to search for predisposing factors such as neoplasms, calculi, persistent urachus, prostatic disease and upper urinary tract infection when early attempts at therapy fail. Urine sediment contains white blood cells, red blood cells, bacteria and transitional epithelial cells. Common invading organisms are *E. coli*, *Pseudomonas aeruginosa*, *Proteus* spp., streptococci and staphylococci.

Treatment: Urinalysis, especially pH determination, is a prerequisite to rational therapy. In cystitis, the urine is frequently alkaline. Altering the pH to acid has a useful bacteriostatic effect and also tends to halt precipitation of crystalline sediment. Acidification is usually attempted with any one of several agents (℞ 562, 563, 622, 625), the dose to be increased until urine tests by litmus or nitrazine paper indicate a constantly acid urine. A high-protein (meat) diet will assist in keeping the urine acid. In the absence of antibiotic sensitivity tests, a fairly successful empirical procedure is to treat the patient with one of the proven urinary bacteriostatic agents, such as sulfisoxazole (℞ 112) or nitrofurantoin (℞ 121) and to change the treatment, if necessary, after a few days' trial. Chemotherapeutic agents, such as the sulfonamides, nitrofurantoin, and the antibiotics, such as streptomycin (℞ 73), chlortetracycline (℞ 27) and chloramphenicol (℞ 16) that are eliminated by way of the urinary tract, may have therapeutic value. Chloramphenicol appears to be particularly effective. Some of the semisynthetic penicillins such as ampicillin (℞ 6) are highly effective against gram-negative bacteria.

If additional bacteriostatic therapy is desirable, a urinary antiseptic that functions in an acid medium, such as methenamine mandelate (℞ 564), may be administered. In all cases of cystitis, the treatment should be continued for at least a few days after signs subside; animals with persistent cases may require several weeks of therapy, and therapy should be discontinued only after normal urinalyses and negative cultures.

Urethritis: This is rarely diagnosed as a separate entity: it is usually a complication of other diseases. These include urethral stricture, urethral calculi or other trauma.

ATONY OF THE BLADDER

Loss of tone of the muscular coat of the bladder wall is common in male dogs and cats, usually as a sequela to interference with urination by urethral obstruction. Urine retention with distension and atonicity of the bladder is a common and grave sequela to posterior paralysis (q.v., p. 651) (trauma of the spinal cord). Acute or chronic distension of the bladder separates the tight junctions of the bladder wall so muscle contractility is lost for varying periods or permanently.

Frequent, and mostly unsuccessful, attempts to urinate characterize a recently developed case of atony and may be misinterpreted as a sign of cystitis. More commonly, there are few if any attempts to urinate, but a more or less constant dribbling from an inert, overloaded bladder.

Diagnosis is based on the presence of a large, distended bladder from which the urine can be easily expressed. When empty, the organ feels like a collapsed balloon, the walls failing to contract as in a normal bladder. The diagnosis is easily confirmed by radiography.

Constant or, at least, frequent emptying of the bladder is required and the primary cause of the condition (urethral obstruction) must be eliminated if possible. Existing bladder infection should be appropriately treated. Distension of the bladder must be prevented for a period sufficient to allow the bladder to regain tone (usually 5 to 10 days). Bethanechol chloride (℞ 655) may be useful. In refractory cases where muscle tone does not return, frequent manual expression is necessary or surgical urinary diversion is used.

MISCELLANEOUS GENITOURINARY DISEASES (SM. AN.)

VULVITIS AND VAGINITIS

Although common, inflammation and infection of the vulva or vagina are often overlooked. Entire adult, adolescent or spayed females may be affected. Contamination of the perineal area may result in ascending infection. Foreign bodies, congenital anomalies of the vulva, and perivulvar folds are the most common causes in the dog. Chronic vulvovaginitis may be of endocrine origin, e.g. in the hyperestrinism of cystic ovaries. Many cases are associated with urethritis (bacterial) or a chronically infected or inflamed cervix after ovariohysterectomy for pyometra.

Clinical Findings: The common signs are increased licking of the vulva, blood-tinged mucoid discharge, or yellowish purulent discharge. The labia may or may not be swollen. Spayed females may attract males as the discharge emits an odor attractive to them. This condition is often inaccurately described as constant heat. (*See* HYPERESTRINISM, p. 874.)

Diagnosis: Diagnosis is made on the finding of a persistent discharge emanating from a reddened and sometimes swollen vaginal mucosa. Close examination, with good light and magnification (an electric otoscope with a large ear speculum makes a convenient and efficient instrument for examining the vagina) discloses small red nodules, pustules or hypertrophied lymph follicles covering the mucous membrane. The area most commonly affected and most apt to be overlooked is the small cul-de-sac on the floor of the vagina formed by the folding of its walls. In severe cases, the entire vaginal mucosa may be affected. The clitoris is often engorged and sensitive. After ovariohysterectomy, granulomas of the stump of the uterus occur on rare occasions and will present similar signs.

Treatment: Good hygiene, clipping of the perineal hair, bathing, douching with isotonic saline or antibiotic solutions, or introduction of antibiotic suppositories is often effective.

Antibiotic sensitivity tests are needed in persistent and chronic infections. Good results usually follow oral administration of antibiotics, e.g. potassium penicillin V, 40,000 u/kg of body wt daily in 3 divided doses; chloramphenicol 30 to 60 mg/kg daily in 3 doses or sulfisoxazole, 60 to 130 mg/kg daily in 3 divided doses. Treatment should be continued for several days after the visible signs subside. Adolescent puppies may be treated conservatively inasmuch as the vaginal infection often subsides spontaneously after estrus.

FISTULA

Genitourinary fistulas in small animals vary from urethrocutaneous fistulas in male animals to rectovaginal, ureterovaginal, vesiculoureterocervical, vaginal and vesiculorectal fistulas in females. Except for the few cases of congenital fistulas, the condition is acquired. Penetrating wounds, particularly bite wounds into the urethra, are seen only occasionally in the male, and rectovaginal fistulas from the same cause rarely are seen in the female. The commonest cause of acquired fistulas is surgical error. The persistence of the fistula usually is due to the presence of a foreign body, such as a calculus or suture that has remained in the surgical wound. The presence of a stricture below the wound will help perpetuate the fistula. The uncomplicated wound or fistula usually will heal spontaneously. Treatment consists of removing the obstruction to healing, e.g. calculus or suture, whereupon the fistula usually heals.

STRICTURE

Aside from stricture of the urethra, the only other genitourinary stricture, rarely seen in small-animal practice, is that of the ureter. It is discussed under HYDRONEPHROSIS (q.v., p. 886). Some narrowing or lack of distension of the urethra normally occurs in male dogs and cats: in dogs (1) proximal to the os penis, (2) at the ischial arch and (3) sometimes at the prostatic groove; in cats (1) at the tip of the penis and (2) at the ischial arch. Most cases of urethral stricture occur as a result of surgery or trauma to the extrapelvic part of the urethra. In the pelvic part of the urethra, strictures arise from trauma caused by pelvic fractures, neoplasm, urinary calculi, or prostatic disease. Urethral strictures develop in cats from the inflammation caused by the passage of calculi or repeated or unskilled catheterization.

Signs consist of frequent attempts to urinate, diminished stream, dribbling, straining to urinate, hematuria and licking of the external urethral orifice. If the urethra is occluded, retention of urine and distension of the bladder result. Strictures commonly cause atony of the urinary bladder (q.v., p. 889).

Relief of the obstruction caused by the stricture is imperative. Catheterization is the simplest procedure, with use of successively larger sounds to distend the constricted area after the bladder distension has been relieved. Placement of an indwelling catheter is sometimes successful, although dogs and cats are adept at removing catheters no matter how carefully restrained. When passage of a catheter is not advisable or possible, temporary relief may be provided by cannulating the bladder through the abdominal wall with a small-bore (22-gauge) hypodermic needle and withdrawing the urine by means of an attached syringe. Surgery may be necessary to relieve the stricture, depending on the site and etiology of the lesion.

PHIMOSIS

An abnormally small preputial orifice that prevents extrusion of the penis and in its most severe form may interfere with micturition. This may be congenital, but often results from or accompanies balanitis, especially in adolescent puppies. Dysuria or a preputial discharge and licking of the part will call attention to the difficulty.

In congenital phimosis, the orifice may be so small that urine is expressed only with difficulty and sheath in such cases often is distended with urine. The phimosis occurring in adolescent puppies may correct itself as the dog becomes sexually mature. If balanitis is the cause, and does not respond to therapy, surgery is required. Prompt surgical relief is imperative if dysuria is present.

PARAPHIMOSIS

Constriction of the prepuce posterior to the glans penis. The usual cause is partial phimosis that prevents retraction of the engorged glans into the sheath following erection. The venous circulation in the organ is impaired by the constricting prepuce. The edematous glans then cannot be withdrawn into the sheath. Cold packs may aid in reducing the edema. Liberal lubrication may then facilitate reduction of the prolapsed organ by manipulation. Severe paraphimosis is treated surgically. Usually the erection will subside when the animal is sedated or anesthetized. If this does not happen, one of the veins draining the penis may be thrombosed. Prolonged strangulation of the penis may result in necrosis.

FANCONI SYNDROME IN THE DOG

A constellation of renal tubular defects leading to excessive loss of many solutes in the urine resulting in metabolic disturbances and in some cases renal failure. This newly described syndrome, apparently an inherited metabolic defect, has been reported in several breeds, most commonly in the basenji. It is seen in adults of both sexes. Clinical signs include polydipsia, polyuria, weight loss, gradual debilitation and development of renal failure after months or years. The urine is generally dilute and contains glucose. There is no evidence of diabetes mellitus. Plasma electrolytes (until the terminal stages) and enzymes are usually normal. Renal function studies indicate excessive urinary loss of glucose, sodium, potassium, phosphorus, uric acid and amino acids. Moderate proteinuria is seen in some cases and moderate acidosis may also be present.

The microscopic renal changes are not remarkable. Some dogs have normal kidneys and others have nonspecific changes. Death follows dehydration, debilitation and acidosis associated with acute renal failure. A successful treatment regimen has not been devised.

HYPERCALCEMIC NEPHROPATHY

The renal injury secondary to hypercalcemia has been described in many species. Hypercalcemia may be caused by many diseases including hyperparathyroidism, pseudohyperparathyroidism, vitaminosis D and the excessive administration of parenteral calcium. Abnormally high calcium concentrations, sometimes in excess of 20 mg/dl, may occur. This leads to polydipsia, polyuria, constipation, lethargy and renal failure. The kidney is particularly sensitive; renal calcification and acute tubular necrosis leading to renal failure occur within a few weeks. The inability to produce concentrated urine is usually the first clinical sign.

In the dog, the commonest cause of hypercalcemia is malignancy, e.g. malignant lymphoma, where the neoplasm produces a parathyroid hormone-like substance. Therapy consists of the usual chemotherapy regimens recommended for the tumor type and appropriate supportive therapy for acute renal failure if present (*see* ACUTE TUBULAR NECROSIS, p. 883).

Hypercalcemia associated with nephrocalcinosis has been reported in horses and cattle that consume plants containing a substance similar to vitamin D. (*See* ENZOOTIC CALCINOSIS, p. 1032.)

RESPIRATORY SYSTEM

EPISTAXIS IN THE HORSE

Hemorrhage from the nostrils occurring in the horse as the result of hemorrhage arising from anywhere in the respiratory tract or guttural pouch. The commoner sites of hemorrhage are lung, guttural pouch and nasal cavity, in that order. Epistaxis precipitated by exercise (in most cases by the stress of racing) is, in almost every instance, the result of pulmonary hemorrhage. Episodes of epistaxis that occur spontaneously in a resting horse are nearly always the result of hemorrhage from the guttural pouch or nasal cavity. Epistaxis that is strictly unilateral is likely to have arisen from the nasal cavity; that which is predominantly from one nostril is likely to have arisen from the pharynx or ipsilateral guttural pouch; that which is bilateral and equally distributed at both nostrils is likely to have arisen from the lungs. In man, blood of pulmonary origin is admixed with air and the frothy nature of the blood is a diagnostic guide which helps to differentiate between hemorrhage from the upper respiratory tract and hemorrhage from the lungs; in the horse this guide is not applicable and nonfrothy blood of pulmonary origin escapes freely at the nostril by gravity and does not have to be ejected by coughing.

Epistaxis is a sign and not a disease *per se.* In order of occurrence the following diseases are most commonly associated with epistaxis: alveolar emphysema (chronic obstructive pulmonary disease); guttural pouch mycosis (aneurysm of the internal or external carotid artery); fractures of the skull; contusion of the nasal cavity, and progressive ethmoidal hematoma (vascular nasal polyps). The following diseases are occasionally associated with epistaxis: foreign bodies in the nasal cavity, nasopharynx, laryngopharynx or esophageal pharynx; neoplasms of the respiratory tract and guttural pouch; ulcerative rhinitis (sequel to a respiratory virus infection); abscesses in the lung, and some specific diseases such as anthrax and glanders. The problem most commonly associated with epistaxis is the "broken blood vessels" problem in the racehorse. This is a pulmonary hemorrhage and may be a sign of the early stages of chronic obstructive pulmonary disease (*see* HEAVES, p. 921). Horses that break blood vessels are often referred to as "bleeders" but this is a confusing synonym as the problem has nothing to do with hemophilia in the horse. Treatment will depend on the etiology of the epistaxis.

RHINITIS

An inflammation of the nasal mucous membrane, producing a serous, mucoid, blood-tinged or mucopurulent discharge.

Etiology: The most frequent cause of a bilateral nasal discharge in domestic animals is infection. In dogs, the cause is often canine distemper (q.v., p. 332); in swine, atrophic rhinitis (q.v., p. 899); in cattle, IBR (q.v., p. 269); while in cats it may be panleukopenia (q.v., p. 330) or other respiratory diseases (q.v., p. 324). Other causes are extensions of oral infections via the nasopharynx; traumatic or congenital palate defects; poor nutrition, often accompanied by severe parasitism; projectile vomiting, with resulting nasal contamination; and sinusitis. Chronic rhinitis may result from mycotic infections such as aspergillosis or cryptococcosis (*see* p. 445 et seq.). Rhinitis accompanied by serous nasal discharge is often seen with acute allergic reactions, but its role is difficult to evaluate.

The commonest causes of unilateral rhinitis are nasal foreign bodies (most often plant matter); extension of an alveolar infection; and nasal or sinus tumors (especially in horses), with secondary infection.

Clinical Findings and Diagnosis: The nasal mucosa first becomes dry and hyperemic. This is followed by a serous discharge which later becomes mucoid and mucopurulent. In simple rhinitis, there are no other signs and the animal appears to be in good condition generally. There may be some sneezing or a slight cough. Excoriation of the skin about the nose may occur. Later, encrustation of the discharge around the nose may lead to difficulty in breathing. Epithelial hyperplasia and submucosal proliferation are common.

Treatment: An effort should be made to find and eliminate the primary cause. Foreign bodies must be removed. Identification of the infectious agent is of value in treating chronic bacterial rhinitis, which is often accompanied by sinusitis. The proper drug should be used in high doses. It may be necessary to trephine the affected sinuses in chronic infections. Culture, sensitivity testing and experience will assist the selection of appropriate antibacterial agents. Other medications may be of value (℞ 78, 81, 91, 476, 556).

Infections caused by gram-positive bacteria often respond to penicillin parenterally administered (℞ 63); gram-negative organisms usually respond to streptomycin (℞ 73); a penicillin-streptomycin combination (℞ 66), administered parenterally, may be helpful in controlling secondary bacterial infection when the organism is not identified.

The nose should be cleaned daily with a warm boric acid solution and the nostrils and surrounding areas coated with petrolatum to prevent excoriation. Proper care and hygiene are essential.

NECROBACILLOSIS

The term necrobacillosis is used to describe any disease or lesion with which *Fusobacterium necrophorum* (*Sphaerophorus necro-*

phorus) is associated. It includes calf diphtheria, necrotic rhinitis of pigs, foot rot of cattle, foot abscess of sheep, postparturient necrosis of the vagina and uterus, and focal necrosis of the liver of cattle and sheep, quittor of horses, and numerous other necrotic lesions in ruminants and, less commonly, pigs, horses, fowls and rabbits. It is probably a secondary invader rather than a primary cause and is usually part of a mixed infection. However, its necrotizing endotoxin undoubtedly plays a role in the production of characteristic lesions.

F. necrophorum is part of the normal flora of the mouth, intestine and genital tracts of many herbivores and omnivores, and is widespread in the environment. It is thought to gain entry to the body through wounds in the skin or mucous membranes.

CALF DIPHTHERIA

An infectious disease of calves affecting the larynx (necrotic laryngitis) or the oral cavity (necrotic stomatitis) characterized by fever and ulceration and swelling of the affected structures.

Etiology: *F. necrophorum* has long been considered the cause of this disease. However, traumatic injury of the mucous membranes of the oral cavity by coarse feed or feed containing an excessive quantity of thistles or tough stems is a common predisposing factor.

Clinical Findings: Calf diphtheria usually occurs as necrotic stomatitis in calves less than 3 months of age and as necrotic laryngitis in older calves. The calf with necrotic stomatitis has difficulty in nursing, the appetite is depressed and temperature may rise to 104°F (40°C). In calves with necrotic laryngitis, the most prominent sign in severe cases is loud wheezing. The early signs may include a rise in body temperature to 106°F (41°C), rapid respiration and salivation. Later, protrusion of the tongue and a nasal discharge may be noted. Calves may develop both necrotic stomatitis and necrotic laryngitis, and may develop a cough as the lungs often become involved. Dehydration and emaciation are also prominent signs. The course of the disease usually is short, the untreated patient succumbing to toxemia and pneumonia within 2 to 7 days.

Lesions: The chief lesions are necrotic ulcers of varying depth on the oral and pharyngeal mucous membranes. The occurrence of croupous or diphtheritic membranes is common. The parts most often involved are the tongue, particularly its borders, the inner surface of the cheeks and the lining of the pharynx. In the more severe cases, the lesions extend into the nasal cavity, the larynx, the trachea and even the lungs.

Diagnosis: The signs are usually sufficient for establishing a prompt and accurate diagnosis. Difficulties may be encountered in outbreaks where an older calf is the first to become ill, or in herds where the disease affects only 1 or 2 calves. A careful study of the signs and the lesions should be made under all circumstances. Contributing etiologic factors include excessive moisture, dirty barns and feedlots, and warm weather.

Prophylaxis and Treatment: Affected animals must be isolated from healthy ones. Cleaning and disinfecting the stables and sheds are important steps in preventing spread of the disease. Daily physical examination of all young calves is recommended for early recognition of new cases. Sulfonamide and antibiotic therapy is recommended. The sulfonamides of choice are sulfamerazine (℞ 96) and sulfamethazine (℞ 100). Penicillin (℞ 63), or penicillin and streptomycin (℞ 66) may prove beneficial, and also chloramphenicol (℞ 18) where its use is permitted. Supplemental feeding with milk, eggs and nutritious gruel is advisable.

NECROTIC RHINITIS OF PIGS

(Bull-nose)

A disease of young growing pigs characterized by suppuration and necrosis, arising from wounds of the oral or nasal mucosa. Confusion exists in the literature because of the use of the misnomer "bull-nose" to also describe atrophic rhinitis (*see* below).

Etiology: *Fusobacterium necrophorum* is commonly isolated from the lesion and undoubtedly contributes to the disease, but many other types of organisms are frequently present. They gain entry through damage to the roof of the mouth, often as a result of clipping the needle teeth too short.

Clinical Findings: Swelling and deformity of the face, occasionally hemorrhage, snuffling, sneezing, foul-smelling nasal discharge, sometimes involvement of the eyes with lacrimation and purulent discharge, loss of appetite and emaciation are signs of bull-nose. Generally, only 1 or 2 pigs are affected in the herd.

Lesions: The facial swelling usually is hard, but incision reveals a mass of pinkish gray, foul-smelling, necrotic tissue or greenish gray tissue debris, depending on the age of the lesion. The nasal and facial bones become involved in the process and as a consequence the facial deformity may be marked.

Diagnosis: Necrotic rhinitis is readily differentiated from atrophic rhinitis by the bulging type of facial distortion observed in bull-nose. Atrophic rhinitis causes no swelling other than that due to the upward or lateral deviation of the snout. The character of the exudate and its location within the tissue of the snout or face are distinctive of bull-nose.

Prophylaxis and Treatment: Prevention is directed towards avoiding injuries to the mouth and snout and improved sanitation. Where the disease occurs repeatedly, great care should be taken in clipping needle teeth.

If the condition is advanced, it is doubtful whether treatment is advisable. Early surgical intervention and packing the cavity with sulfonamide or tincture of iodine may be useful. In young pigs, sulfamethazine (℞ 100) given orally is of value.

ATROPHIC RHINITIS OF SWINE

A disease characterized by sneezing followed by atrophy of the turbinate bones and distortion of the nasal septum which may be accompanied by shortening or twisting of the upper jaw.

Etiology: A variety of infectious and noninfectious agents can cause enough inflammation of the upper respiratory tract to stimulate sneezing. An important primary cause of atrophic rhinitis in the U.S.A. and other parts of the world appears to be *Bordetella bronchiseptica.* This bacterium is not host-specific and dogs, cats, rodents and other species may harbor the organism for long periods but their role in the spread of the disease to pigs is uncertain. The viruses of inclusion-body rhinitis and of pseudorabies cause a very acute transient rhinitis in young pigs, but in uncomplicated infections, do not usually lead to atrophy and distortion. The disease is usually introduced by the purchase of affected pigs that are shedding *B. bronchiseptica.* Piglets may be infected at any age but those infected early in life usually develop the most severe disease. The carrier sow is the usual source of the infection.

Turbinate atrophy has also been associated with and experimentally reproduced by the intranasal inoculation of young piglets with pure cultures of *Pasteurella multocida* but such infected pigs have not been adequate transmitters of the disease to contact pigs.

Crowding, inadequate ventilation, continuous farrowing systems, other concurrent diseases and inadequate sanitation are considered to be important predisposing factors in intensification of the disease. Dietary imbalance of calcium and phosphorus does not appear to be a major factor in the disease.

Clinical Findings: Acute signs usually appear between 3 and 8 weeks of age, and in severe cases, nasal hemorrhage may occur. The lacrimal ducts may become occluded and tear stains then appear below the medial canthus of the eyes. As the disease progresses, some affected pigs may develop lateral deviation or shortening of the upper jaw but others may suffer some degree of atrophy of the turbinates with no outward distortion apparent. The degree of distortion can be judged from the relationship of the upper and lower incisors if breed variations are taken into account.

The severity of *Bordetella*-caused rhinitis in a herd depends largely on: (1) the age of the pig when infected (severe turbinate damage most frequently results when infection occurs before 3 weeks of age); (2) the virulence of the infecting strain; (3) the presence of other infectious agents (e.g. simultaneous infection with *Pasteurella multocida* results in increased turbinate atrophy); and (4) the immune status of the pigs.

The effects of the disease on production are dependent on the virulence of the infection and on the level of management.

Lesions: The degree of atrophy and distortion is best assessed by examining a transverse section made with a saw at the level of the second premolar tooth (the first cheek tooth up to 7 to 9 months of age); additional parallel sections are recommended in some areas. In the active stages of inflammation, the mucosa will have a blanched appearance and there may be purulent material present on the surface. In later stages the nasal cavities may be clear, but there may be variable degrees of softening, atrophy, or grooving of the turbinates, deviation of the nasal septum, and asymmetric distortion of the surrounding bone structure.

Diagnosis: The characteristic signs and lesions are commonly used as the basis for diagnosis. A specific diagnosis of *B. bronchiseptica* infection can only be made by laboratory culture. Culture of nasal swabs from 6- to 8-week-old pigs is an effective method of determining infection in a herd. Atrophic rhinitis must be differentiated from necrotic rhinitis (q.v., p. 898).

Prophylaxis: The control of rhinitis due to *B. bronchiseptica* may be attempted by a total eradication program or minimization of the infection with chemoprophylaxis or vaccination. The maintenance of a closed herd helps to reduce the chances of exacerbation through the introduction of additional agents. When pigs are introduced into a rhinitis-free herd, the health status of the donor herd should be checked. Repopulation with specific-pathogen-free pigs is usually an effective method of establishing herds free from serious forms of atrophic rhinitis. It is rarely possible, however, to keep herds entirely free from mild outbreaks of sneezing, and a low level of aberrant turbinates and nasal bones at necropsy is common even in herds that show no clinical signs of rhinitis.

The incidence and severity of rhinitis may be reduced by good sanitation, adequate ventilation and nutrition and the strategic use of sulfonamides at 0.01% in the feed. The sulfonamide therapy is usually given for 3 to 5 weeks following the recognition of atrophic rhinitis. All pigs in a breeding herd, including the sows and the piglets, should receive a course of the sulfonamide. Adequate withdrawal time must be observed prior to marketing. The culturing of nasal swabs from the sows and piglets following therapy will indicate the level of infection and the efficacy of the treatment. Failure to reduce the level of infection occurs commonly due to sulfonamide resistance of the bacteria. Other antimicrobials are usually not effective even though the *B. bronchiseptica* isolated is found sensitive to them.

A *B. bronchiseptica* bacterin is available that will reduce the level of infection and clinical disease in pigs of all ages. The sows are vaccinated at 4 and 2 weeks before farrowing and the young pigs at 7 and 28 days of age. A high level of colostral immunity develops in pigs that suck vaccinated sows and this prevents the development of significant lesions even though *B. bronchiseptica* may become established in their nasal cavity.

LARYNGITIS

An inflammation of the larynx. Although laryngitis may be caused by irritation of the larynx by the inhalation of dust, smoke, irritant gases, the lodging of a foreign body or excessive vocalization, more often it is caused by one of the upper respiratory tract diseases. Laryngitis may accompany infectious tracheobronchitis and distemper in dogs, infectious rhinotracheitis and calicivirus infection of cats, infectious rhinotracheitis and calf diphtheria in cattle, strangles, infectious viral rhinopneumonitis, viral arteritis and infectious bronchitis in horses, *Fusobacterium necrophorum* or *Corynebacterium pyogenes* infections in sheep and influenza in pigs.

Clinical Findings: A cough is the principal sign. It is at first harsh, dry and short but later becomes soft and moist and may be very painful. It may be induced by pressure on the larynx, exposure to cold or dusty air, the swallowing of coarse food or by attempts to administer medicines. A fetid odor may be detected on the breath. Difficult noisy breathing may be evident and the animal may stand with head lowered and mouth open. Swallowing is difficult and painful. Cats may have vocal changes. Systemic signs are usually attributable to the primary disease as in calf diphtheria where temperatures of 105°F (40.5°C) may occur. Death due to asphyxiation may occur especially if the animals are exerted.

Diagnosis: Diagnosis is made on the clinical signs and may be confirmed by examination of the larynx through a speculum or an endoscope. In dogs and cats it may be possible to examine the larynx, but the pain will make this difficult unless anesthesia or analgesia is first induced. The history and signs of the primary disease will usually quickly identify the cause of the laryngeal problem.

Treatment: Identification and treatment of the primary disease is essential. In addition, certain palliative procedures such as the inhalation of steam, the confining of the animal to a warm, clean environment, the feeding of soft or liquid foods and the avoidance of dust will speed recovery and give comfort to the animal. The cough may be suppressed with antitussive preparations (℞ 416, 418) and bacterial infections controlled with antibiotics (℞ 78) or sulfonamides (℞ 96, 102). Control of pain with judicious use of an analgesic (℞ 612), especially in cats, will allow the animal to eat and thus speed recovery. Tracheotomy may be necessary if obstruction of the larynx is severe enough to cause cyanosis.

LARYNGEAL EDEMA

Edema of the mucosa and submucosa of the larynx, particularly the aryepiglottic folds and vocal cords. The course is acute or peracute, depending on the cause and severity of the disease. Obstruction of the larynx may result.

Etiology: Laryngeal edema may result from allergy, inhalation of irritants, or trauma from endotracheal tubes or surgery. Brachycephalic dogs and obese dogs develop laryngeal edema during severe panting due to hyperthermia or excitement. In cattle, laryngeal edema has been observed in the course of blackleg, respiratory infections, urticaria and serum sickness. In swine, it may occur as a part of edema disease.

Clinical Findings: Edema of the larynx may develop within hours. It is characterized by a rapidly increasing, predominantly inspiratory, dyspnea accompanied by roaring, whistling or rattling sounds from the larynx. There is a severe cough, the visible mucous membranes are cyanotic and the pulse rate is increased. In severe cases in horses, there is profuse sweating. The temperature is increased. Laryngoscopic examination reveals a severe swelling of the laryngeal mucosa, with little space between the vocal cords.

Treatment: In severe cases, a tracheotomy should be done immediately. Systemic treatment depends on the cause. In cases of infectious and inflammatory laryngeal edemas, antibiotics should be administered systemically. In allergic laryngeal edema, epinephrine (℞ 528) and corticosteroids (℞ 143, 148) are administered. Prognosis is favorable if treatment, particularly surgical intervention, is performed in the early stage; otherwise it should be guarded.

LARYNGEAL HEMIPLEGIA

(Roaring)

A chronic, unilateral or occasionally bilateral paralysis of the intrinsic muscles of the larynx causing audible inspiratory dyspnea. The condition is commonest in thoroughbred and other light horses and occurs less frequently in draft horses. It is rare in other species, occurring occasionally as a bilateral condition in large breeds of dogs.

Etiology: The immediate cause is degeneration of one or both of the recurrent laryngeal nerves producing paresis and eventually paralysis of the intrinsic muscles of the larynx. As a result, the arytenoid cartilages and the corresponding vocal cords fail to rotate outward (abduct) on inspiration, causing reduction in the size of the lumen of the larynx with consequent inspiratory dyspnea. Paralysis occurs on the left side in 92% of the recorded cases, on the right side in 6% and on both sides in 2%; this observation has led to the theory that the degeneration is related in some way to constant irritation produced by the pulsations of the aorta as the left recurrent laryngeal nerve passes around it. Accidental injury to the nerve by overextension of the head and perivascular injection of irritating substances are other causes. Some cases of roaring presumably can be traced to previous infectious or debilitating diseases, ingestion of lead or certain plants. Hereditary predisposition to the disease is recognized.

Clinical Findings and Diagnosis: The obvious sign is a whistling or roaring sound heard on inspiration and produced by the poorly abducted vocal cord and arytenoid cartilage. In mild or recent cases, the sound may be produced only after strenuous exercise, while in advanced cases, it may become obvious after light exercise or even in the resting animal. The roaring usually subsides within 10 minutes after exercise is stopped. Badly affected animals are unfit for work and tire quickly as a result of the dyspnea. Many horses in the early stages of the disease because of adductor paralysis may emit a characteristic grunt when frightened or when struck a sudden blow over the ribs. Experienced clinicians may be able to detect a pit between the arytenoid and thyroid cartilages on laryngeal palpation. Some animals show respiratory difficulty when the head is pulled to the side or when eating grain.

The characteristic respiratory signs may be sufficient for diagnosis; it may be confirmed by endoscopic examination of the larynx.

Treatment: Spontaneous remissions are rare. Extirpation of the laryngeal ventricles is successful in restoring about 60% of affected horses to usefulness. Surgical retraction of the arytenoid cartilages by means of a heavy tension suture from the muscular process of the arytenoid cartilage to the cricoid cartilage has proven effective in some cases that have not responded to ventriculectomy. Removal of the left arytenoid cartilage may also be useful.

INFECTIOUS TRACHEOBRONCHITIS OF DOGS

(Kennel cough)

A mild, self-limiting disease, involving the trachea and bronchi of dogs of any age. It spreads rapidly among animals that are closely confined as in hospitals or kennels.

Etiology: There is no single cause. *Bordetella bronchiseptica*, canine adenovirus type 2 (CAV-2) and parainfluenza (SV-5) are frequently involved either alone or in combination. Less frequently implicated are canine adenovirus type 1 (CAV-1 [infectious hepatitis virus]), canine distemper, reovirus and canine herpesvirus. Bacteria other than *Bordetella* play a secondary role. Environmental factors such as cold, drafts and high humidity apparently increase susceptibility to the disease.

Clinical Findings: The incubation period is 5 to 10 days. The outstanding sign is a harsh, dry cough, which is aggravated by activity or excitement. The coughing occurs in paroxysms, followed by retching or gagging in attempts to clear small amounts of mucus from the throat. Paroxysms of inspiratory dyspnea (reverse sneeze) are noted in some cases. The cough is easily induced by gentle pressure over the larynx or trachea.

The body temperature is normal in the early stages, but may be moderately elevated as secondary bacterial invasion takes place. Blood cell counts are normal initially, but may show slight neutrophilia with a left shift in the later stages.

Diagnosis: A history of exposure to other dogs, a profound cough in the absence of other findings, and apparent localization of the condition in the trachea and bronchi should lead to a tentative diagnosis of infectious tracheobronchitis. Trauma to the trachea produces somewhat the same clinical picture, but signs are generally not as severe as in infectious tracheobronchitis.

The primary disease is self-limiting. The most severe signs are noted during the first 5 days, but continue in some degree for 10 to 20 days. A longer course suggests secondary bacterial complications. Stress, particularly of adverse environmental conditions, may cause relapse during the later stages.

Treatment: Because of the highly contagious nature of the disease, animals should be treated as out-patients if possible. Individual cases are best treated with mild expectorants containing codeine (℞ 420). Expectorants containing antihistamines may also be used (℞ 561). While antibiotics have no effect on the primary disease, they may be used to good effect in controlling secondary bacterial infection (℞ 16, 76). Corticosteroids (℞ 142, 152) may alleviate signs but should not be used in the absence of an antibacterial agent. The use of nitrofurantoin (℞ 121) is reported to provide relief from the clinical signs. Proper hygienic measures, good nutrition and good nursing all contribute to recovery.

Protection against some elements of the tracheobronchitis complex (distemper and CAV-1) is provided by traditional vaccines, with adenovirus 1 being cross protective with adenovirus 2. Canine parainfluenza vaccines have recently become available and these increase the range of protection.

BRONCHITIS (SM. AN.)

Acute or chronic inflammation of the bronchi. The primary site most commonly is in the bronchioles, but may extend to the lung parenchyma.

Etiology: Bronchitis frequently is secondary to other disease, such as heart disease, enteritis and parasitism. Initiating factors include bacterial and viral infections, allergens, aspiration of smoke, irritating gases or other chemicals and sudden changes in atmospheric temperature. Foreign bodies in the airway and developmental abnormalities such as laryngeal deformities may lead to bronchitis.

Clinical Findings: Spasms of coughing are the outstanding sign. These are most severe following rest, beginning exercise or after a change of environment. On auscultation, the respiratory sounds may be essentially normal. In advanced cases, sonorous rales are heard. The temperature is slightly elevated. The acute stage of bronchitis passes quickly—in 2 or 3 days. The cough, however, may persist for 2 or 3 weeks. In severe cases, it is difficult to differentiate bronchitis from pneumonia and the process frequently extends into the lung parenchyma, resulting in pneumonia. A chronic form of bronchitis is seen commonly in middle aged dogs and is often exacerbated during inclement weather and other environmental stresses.

Lesions: The mucous membranes of the bronchi and bronchioles are inflamed. Their lumina contain frothy serous or mucopurulent exudate. The act of coughing is an attempt to remove the exudate from the respiratory passages.

Diagnosis: The diagnosis is made from the history, clinical signs and consideration and elimination of other causes of coughing in small animals. In chronic bronchitis, chest radiographs may show an increase in linear markings and peribronchial densities. Bronchoscopy will reveal the inflamed endothelium and tacky, often mucopurulent mucus in the bronchi. In addition the procedure allows biopsies and swabs for microbiologic culture to be obtained. Bronchial washing is a further useful diagnostic aid that may demonstrate significant cells (eosinophils).

Treatment: In mild or acute cases palliative treatment may be effective, however treatment of concurrent disease is indicated. Rest, warmth and proper hygiene are important. The persistent cough is best controlled by expectorants containing codeine (℞ 420), or similar antitussives. Some relief may be afforded by medicated inhalants (℞ 417). Antibiotics, such as penicillin (℞ 66), tetracycline (℞ 76) or chloramphenicol (℞ 16) are indicated if the fever persists for more than 3 days or if the infection extends to the lung parenchyma. The use of oxygen may be considered in severe cases. Established cases of chronic bronchitis are refractive to treatment and complete resolution rarely, if ever, occurs. Therefore once the diagnosis is established, owner education and enlightenment as to the management of the disorder forms an important part of treatment. Periodic therapy of combined broad-spectrum antibiotics and steroids is useful. Alternatively continuous steroid therapy at low doses has been advocated.

MISCELLANEOUS RESPIRATORY PROBLEMS

Bronchiectasis: A chronic disease of the bronchi and bronchioles characterized by irreversible cylindrical or saccular dilatation and complicated by secondary infection. Clinically, it is difficult to differentiate from chronic bronchitis. The differential diagnosis can only be accomplished reliably by bronchography, although a diagnosis may usually be made from plain radiographs in chronic cases. Animals with early cases may respond to surgical intervention, i.e. resection of the affected lobe; however most, when seen by the practitioner, are too far advanced for this. Treatment as for chronic bronchitis offers the best chance of a comfortable existence.

Lung Hemorrhage: Hemorrhage from the respiratory tract beyond the larynx, but usually from the lungs. Causes include trauma, warfarin poisoning, parasites, neoplasms, infectious processes that erode capillaries, pulmonary infarction and cardiac dilatation in the horse. Diagnosis is made from the appearance of blood-tinged saliva or nasal discharge or free blood coming from the nostrils. There may or may not be respiratory embarrassment. Treatment consists of enforced rest and treatment of any cause such as trauma, parasites or an infectious disease. Blood transfusions may be helpful.

Pulmonary Edema: An abnormal accumulation of serous fluid in the interstitial tissue, airways and alveoli of the lung. Edema of the lungs may occur in conjunction with circulatory disorders, occasionally in anaphylaxis and allergies, and in some infectious diseases. Brain injury in dogs may cause pulmonary edema.

Discomfort, respiratory embarrassment, dyspnea and open-mouth breathing are evident. Animals will stand in preference to lying down or will lie only in sternal recumbency or may assume a sitting position. Auscultation of the chest may reveal wheezing and fluid sounds. Radiographs will reveal increased density. If the cause is removed, the fluid will be resorbed. If not, the course may be fatal.

The lungs are pale, heavy, doughy in consistency, pit on pressure and do not collapse. Fluid oozes from the cut surface and foam fills the bronchioles and bronchi. The interlobular septa are widened.

The cause should be removed and the animal kept quiet. Antihistamines (℞ 560) may be useful for allergies, digitalis (℞ 526) for cardiac insufficiency and antibiotics and sulfonamides for infections. A diuretic (℞ 541) may be indicated.

Pleuritis (Pleurisy) (Sm. An.): Inflammation of the pleura, which may be caused by any pathogenic organism that gains entrance to the pleural cavity but often is an extension of other respiratory infections. Rapid, shallow breathing, elevated temperature and thoracic pain are suggestive of pleuritis. Auscultation will reveal friction sounds and radiographs will reveal the line of effusion along the chest wall.

Acute pleuritis is characterized by hyperemia and swelling of the membrane. After about 48 hours serous exudate appears, which may progress to a fibrinous or purulent state. Fibrin attaches to the surface in the form of threads or bands or elevated patches. The fibrin may form an attachment between the visceral and parietal surfaces of the pleura and if it is not resorbed it becomes organized by fibroblasts and permanently ties the 2 surfaces together. If the inflammatory process heals early, no adhesions form and no permanent damage is done.

Rest and relief of cough, if present, are important. Meperidine (℞ 617) repeated every 8 hours will control the pain. Fluid may be aspirated by thoracocentesis to relieve respiratory distress. Antibiotics (℞ 27, 66) should be given to control the infection. An enzyme (℞ 594) may be mixed with the antibiotic or injected IM.

Empyema (Purulent pleuritis, Pyothorax): Pus in the pleural cavity.

It is caused by pyogenic bacteria, fungi reaching the thoracic cavity by way of the blood, extension of a pneumonic infection, traumatic gastritis or penetrating wounds of the chest. In dogs with empyema, nocardiosis (*Nocardia asteroides*) should be suspected.

Empyema usually is a secondary infection and the signs may be masked by the primary disease. Cough, fever, pain and dyspnea in combination may be present. Lung sounds will be heard above the fluid line and percussion will reveal loss of resonance in the lower chest cavity. Thoracocentesis and radiographs are useful diagnostic aids.

Prognosis is guarded. All pus should be aspirated from the pleural cavity, cultured for bacteria and the bacteria checked for drug sensitivity. One half of the calculated dose of antibiotic (℞ 27, 66) dissolved in sterile water should be given through the same (aspirating) needle, and the other half given IM. (**Caution:** The antibiotic mixture should not contain potassium salts.) This is repeated daily until the animal is afebrile and the exudate sterile. Proteolytic enzymes (℞ 594) mixed with the antibiotic and given IM or injected in the pleural cavity may hasten lysis and resorption of pus. Prolonged treatment may be essential and some forms, e.g. infectious feline peritonitis and pleuritis, q.v., p. 327, do not respond. Sulfonamides are useful for nocardiosis.

Hemothorax, Hydrothorax and Chylothorax: Hemothorax is the accumulation of blood in the pleural cavity and is most commonly caused by trauma to the thorax. Hydrothorax is the accumulation of transudate in the pleural cavity and in nearly every instance is caused by some interference with blood flow or lymph drainage. Chylothorax, a relatively rare condition, is the accumulation of chyle in the pleural cavity and is caused by the rupture of the thoracic duct, or leakage from thoracic lymphatics.

The signs of all 3 conditions include respiratory embarrassment and weakness, if severe. Diagnostic aids include examination of fluids, radiographs and auscultation. Treatment is directed toward removing or correcting the cause. Surgery may be indicated in hemothorax and chylothorax.

Pneumothorax (Sm. An.): Air in the pleural cavity. This may be traumatic or spontaneous in origin. Air enters the pleural cavity through penetrating wounds of the thoracic wall or by traumatic or spontaneous rupture of the lung or airways. If the body of air is large, the lung will collapse. Respirations are painful, dyspneic and abdominal. The animal may be in a stage of collapse. Mucous membranes may be cyanotic. There may be puncture wounds of the chest or evidence of fractured ribs. Radiographs reveal a pocket of air in the dorsal thoracic cavity and rib fractures if present. Traumatic wounds of the chest wall may be evident.

Any penetrating wound or tear in the trachea or major bronchus must be closed. In severe cases air can be removed by thoracocentesis and use of a 3-way valve. However, the latter may be useful only if the air leak has been closed. It is advisable not to search for small leaks but large openings may have to be located and closure attempted. Mildly affected animals recover with cage rest as the air is slowly absorbed and lung function gradually returns. Oxygen therapy may be indicated if the hemoglobin is not being saturated. If wound infection is a possibility, antibiotics (℞ 66) should be administered.

PNEUMONIA (SM. AN.)

Acute or chronic inflammatory change of the lungs and bronchi, characterized by disturbance in respiration and hypoxemia, and complicated by the systemic effects of toxins absorbed from the involved area.

Etiology: This condition usually results from primary viral involvement of the respiratory tract followed by secondary bacterial invasion. Components of the feline respiratory complex, canine distemper and infectious tracheobronchitis may predispose to it. Canine and feline herpesvirus may cause severe reactions, especially in young animals. Classical pneumonia is usually the disease noted in the bacterial invasion phase. Any interference with immune and protective mechanisms may predispose to pneumonia. Many different bacteria have been isolated from animals with this disease. Parasitic invasion of the bronchi, as by *Filaroides*, *Aelurostrongylus* or *Paragonimus*, may cause pneumonia. Protozoan involvement, usually caused by *Toxoplasma* (q.v., p. 466) is seen rarely. Mycotic bronchopneumonia may result from *Aspergillus*, *Histoplasma* (q.v., p. 446) or *Coccidioides* (q.v., p. 447) invasion. *Cryptococcus* pneumonia has been described in cats.

Injury to the bronchial mucosa and the inhalation or aspiration of irritating materials may cause pneumonia directly and predispose the tissues to secondary bacterial invasion.

Clinical Findings: The initial signs are usually those of the primary disease. Lethargy and anorexia are usual. A deep cough of low amplitude is noted. Progressive dyspnea, "blowing" of the lips and cyanosis may be evident. Body temperature is usually increased moderately and blood counts show a leukocytosis. Auscultation of the thorax usually reveals consolidation, which may be patchy but usually is diffuse. Radiographic examination reveals very little early in the disease, but as inflammation progresses there is evidence of increased density and peribronchial consolidation. Complications such as pleuritis, mediastinitis, or perhaps invasion by opportunist organisms such as *Nocardia* may occur.

Diagnosis: Diagnosis of pneumonia may not be difficult but determination of the specific cause will require laboratory examination of exudate, mucus, etc. Viral involvement usually results in an initially high body temperature of 104 to 106°F (40 to 41°C). Leukopenia is usual except in infectious tracheobronchitis. Mycotic pneumonias are usually chronic in nature and respond poorly or not at all to routine antibacterial therapy. Protozoan pneumonia may be acute or chronic. Acutely affected animals may die within 24 to 48 hours of the onset. Miliary nodules in the lungs may lead to a suspicion of protozoan pneumonia on necropsy. Those chronically affected typically fail to respond to antibacterial therapy. A history of recent anesthesia or severe vomiting might lead one to suspect aspiration pneumonia.

Treatment: The animal should be placed in warm, dry quarters. Anemia should be corrected if it is present. Oxygen therapy may be used if cyanosis is severe and is best applied by means of a tent, using an oxygen concentration of 30 to 50%. Antibiotic therapy (℞ 2, 65, 76) should be instituted as early as possible. Expectorants should be employed only with extreme caution, and probably never in the acute case. Supportive therapy should be used where indicated. Fluid infusion, particularly when administered IV, can be dangerous in the pneumonia patient and should be used with caution.

Animals treated as outpatients should be re-examined 4 to 6 days later. The chest should be radiographed again even though the animal may have improved clinically since consolidation of the lungs may still be present.

PULMONARY EMPHYSEMA

Two distinct forms of pulmonary emphysema occur in animals, alveolar and interstitial. **Alveolar emphysema** is abnormal enlargement of air spaces distal to the terminal bronchioles, with evidence of destruction of their walls. The lesion is similar to the more frequent and severe one causing pulmonary emphysema in man. Unless otherwise stated, pulmonary emphysema is understood to mean alveolar emphysema. Clinically, pulmonary emphysema in animals is recognized to be of significance only in the horse, where it has variable expression as part of the bronchiolitis-emphysema complex associated with "heaves," (q.v., p. 921). Small amounts of emphysema can be found at necropsy in the apices and along the narrow ventral borders of the lungs of old animals such as dogs and cats. Failure of lungs to collapse when the pleural cavity is opened, as when there is blockage of major airways, must not be confused with emphysema.

The pathogenesis of alveolar emphysema is incompletely understood. There is believed to be involvement of one or more of: genetic predisposition; inflammatory destruction of walls of airspaces; atrophy of alveolar walls; or mechanical overstretching of alveolar connective tissues. Currently, the favored hypothesis is that there is excessive release of proteolytic enzymes, particularly elastase, by inflammatory cells within airspaces. Breakdown of elastin and other connective tissue fibers then leads to enlargement and remodeling of the airspaces.

Interstitial emphysema is the accumulation of air within major interstitial compartments of the lung: interlobular septa, perivascular and peribronchial sheaths, and subpleural zone. It occurs in species with complete lobular septation, notably the cow and much less commonly the pig, sheep and horse. In cattle, severe interstitial emphysema can be accompanied by subcutaneous emphysema over the back because air has dissected a pathway from the lung into the mediastinum and from there through the thoracic inlet to the skin of the back.

Interstitial emphysema is mostly seen as a result of severe expiratory distress in cattle, usually in association with acute (atypical) interstitial pneumonia (q.v., p. 914). In cattle, minor degrees can be seen following any bout of severe agonal struggle preceding death.

BOVINE RESPIRATORY DISEASES

Bovine respiratory diseases cause serious economic losses. Several distinct clinicopathologic entities are now recognized. The etiologic factors responsible for some of these are understood fairly clearly but there still remains considerable disagreement about others, particularly the pneumonias of calves. The following discussions cover the commoner of the recognized entities. *See also* LUNGWORM INFECTION, p. 715. Acute respiratory involvement can also be present in IBR (q.v., p. 269), malignant catarrhal fever (q.v., p. 264), pleurisy accompanying traumatic reticulitis (q.v., p. 138), and occasionally results from milk allergy (q.v., p. 6).

BOVINE PNEUMONIC PASTEURELLOSIS
(Shipping fever)

An entity usually distinguishable from other bovine respiratory diseases by clinical signs and the distinctive fibrinous pneumonia evident at necropsy. The term "shipping fever" is losing favor because it is misleading and the term "hemorrhagic septicemia" is best reserved for the septicemic *Pasteurella* infections seen in cattle, swine and beasts of burden in Southern Asia.

Etiology and Epidemiology: Although the details of the pathogenesis remain obscure, infection with the bovine paramyxovirus, parainfluenza 3 (PI3) or one of several other respiratory viruses followed by either *Pasteurella multocida* or *P. haemolytica* is considered to be responsible for most cases. These bacteria can be cultured from the upper respiratory tracts of healthy cattle, but the frequency of isolation is greater from shipped cattle. The argument persists about whether their role is as primary pathogens or as opportunists colonizing tissues weakened by viral-infection stress and due to transportation or to other environmental factors such as a sudden change in the weather. Affected animals have often been shipped or exposed to cattle recently transported.

Clinical Findings: Affected cattle have depression, anorexia, a serous nasal discharge, cough, fever (104 to 108°F [40 to 42°C]), increased pulse rate and rapid, shallow respirations. Lung auscultation may reveal moist rales, pleuritic friction rubs or crackling associated with interstitial emphysema. As the disease progresses absence of lung sounds may indicate areas of consolidation.

Lesions: The cranioventral portions of the lungs are frequently swollen and firm with red and purple discoloration of lobules separated by thickened yellow interlobular septae containing fibrin and inflammatory cells. Discrete lobular or sublobular zones of necrosis with pale margins are sometimes present. Fibrinous pleuritis is usually present and may be extensive. Microscopically the lesions are typical of an acute exudative fibrinous bronchopneumonia.

Treatment: Affected cattle should be isolated if possible. Dihydrostreptomycin in combination with penicillin (℞ 66) is effective in the treatment of early cases. The sulfonamides and particularly sulfamethazine (℞ 101) are quite effective, as are the broad-spectrum antibiotics, e.g. oxytetracycline (℞ 53). Regardless of the initial antibiotic or sulfonamide used, the same drug should be used for 3 to 4 days, beginning as early as possible.

Control: Where control by preventing stress or contact with transported animals is impossible, vaccination against PI3 and pasteurellae, or the feeding of antibiotics may be tried. The value of these various measures is still debated.

ENZOOTIC PNEUMONIA OF CALVES

Any pulmonary disease, excluding pneumonic pasteurellosis, of calves or young cattle housed together in groups either indoors or in yards. At least several animals in the group are affected and the morbidity may approach 100%. It is primarily a problem in calves 2 to 6 months of age although pneumonias occurring in groups of young cattle up to a year old have also been given this designation. The term does not signify one specific entity defined on either an etiologic or pathologic basis.

Etiology: The causes of the calf pneumonias are the subject of much debate. Some mycoplasmas and viruses are thought to act as primary agents, with bacteria as secondary invaders exacerbating the initial infection. *Mycoplasma dispar, M. bovis* and *Ureaplasma* spp. (T-mycoplasmas) are probably the most significant mycoplasmas involved. Parainfluenza 3 (PI3) virus, bovine respiratory syncytial (RS) virus and in some areas bovine adenovirus 3 may be the most important viruses associated with calf pneumonias. The relative importance of various viruses is uncertain, but the evidence indicates broad geographic variations.

Clinical Findings: The clinical signs vary in frequency of occurrence and in severity. On the one hand there are acute outbreaks of pneumonia in which many of the calves have fever ranging from 103 to 105°F (39.5 to 40.5°C) and increased respiratory rates accompanied by some coughing. Recovery is usually gradual unless a more severe pneumonia develops from bacterial secondary infection. Some of these acute incidents may be true viral pneumonias. On the other hand there are episodes in which the disease appears to be more insidious in onset. Many of the calves cough frequently, some have increased respiratory rates and there is poor productivity. It is likely that mycoplasmas are more important in the pathogenesis of this manifestation. During these less acute outbreaks, calves might develop severe respiratory signs from superimposed acute exudative bacterial pneumonias or other complicating lesions.

Lesions: In most cases the lesions are confined to the cranioventral part of the lung and are fawn or gray-purple. A proportion of them, particularly those associated with long-standing disease of insidious onset, have microscopic lesions of cuffing pneumonia. In these animals the bronchioles are surrounded by follicular masses of lymphocytic accumulations.

Treatment: Calves that are severely ill should be treated with broad-spectrum antibiotics such as oxytetracycline given IV. A combination of penicillin and streptomycin is sometimes effective. A combination of antibiotics and a steroidal anti-inflammatory agent may be appropriate for severe cases.

Control: Control of calf pneumonias is difficult even with good housing. At present there are no useful vaccines. It is important that calves should receive colostrum at birth and then be housed in comfortable conditions, ideally individually, for the first 4 to 6 weeks of life. When calves are grouped this should be done by age and they should be kept in these groups as long as possible. Overcrowding should be avoided and young calves should not be allowed to share the same air space as older animals.

ACUTE BOVINE PULMONARY EMPHYSEMA AND EDEMA (ABPE)

(Fog fever, Bovine atypical interstitial pneumonia)

One of the commoner causes of acute respiratory distress in cattle, particularly adult beef cattle, characterized by sudden onset, minimal coughing and a course that terminates fatally or goes on to dramatic improvement within a very few days. It is a disease of groups; morbidity ranges to over 50% although usually only a small minority develop severe respiratory distress. Typically it occurs in autumn, 5 to 10 days after a change to a better, often a lush, pasture. The term fog fever derives from its association with "fog" pastures, i.e. foggage or aftermath.

Etiology: Although some uncertainty still exists, it appears probable that ingestion of the naturally occurring amino acid L-tryptophan and its conversion in the rumen to the toxic 3-methylindole is responsible in many instances. Apparently the L-tryptophan level of crops is most likely to be high in lush, rapidly growing pastures, particularly but not exclusively in the fall. Indistinguishable clinicopathologic syndromes may follow ingestion of moldy cornstalks or sweet potatoes, or wild mint (*Perilla frutescens*). Whether the respiratory disease that sometimes occurs on rape pasture is identical to ABPE has still to be determined.

Clinical Findings: ABPE is commonest in heavy beef cows, but may occur in either sex and in dairy as well as beef cattle. It may also occur in sheep. Outbreaks usually develop within 5 to 10 days of a change to better grazing, and rarely occur in animals that have been on a field for more than 3 weeks. Morbidity ranges up to 50% or even to 100% but usually only a few are severely affected.

Cattle with mild cases may go unnoticed: they are subdued but still alert; there is tachypnea and hyperpnea but auscultation is usually unrewarding. Such cows usually recover spontaneously within days. Severely affected cattle show extensive respiratory distress with mouth-breathing, extension of the tongue and drooling of saliva. A loud expiratory grunt is common but coughing is unusual. In the early stages, auscultation reveals surprisingly soft respiratory sounds; rales are rare. If death does not supervene (up to a third will die) there is dramatic improvement on the third day and the animals resume eating. At this stage, auscultation reveals harsh respiratory sounds and in some animals, dorsal (emphysematous) crackles. Some cows have subcut. emphysema extending along the back from the withers. Full clinical recovery may take up to 3 weeks.

Lesions: Significant lesions are limited to the respiratory tract. In affected cattle that have died or have been slaughtered *in extremis* the lungs are heavy and distorted and do not collapse normally. They are widely affected with various degrees of rubbery firmness; there is extensive interstitial edema and emphysema, often with the formation of large air-filled bullae in interlobular and subpleural regions. Submucosal hemorrhages are often present on the larynx and in the trachea and larger bronchi. Histologically, the lesion is an acute interstitial pneumonia with alveolar edema, hyaline membrane formation and areas of early alveolar epithelial hyperplasia producing what is commonly called epithelialization; occasionally, areas of bronchiolar necrosis may be found. The emphysema is often dramatic and is limited to interstitial fascia where it is accompanied by edema.

In animals that are slaughtered after 3 days of illness the pathologic findings are less dramatic. The lungs are still heavy and do not collapse normally; they are a pinkish gray and of increased firmness; edema and emphysema are inconspicuous or absent. Histologically, these animals show widespread alveolar epithelialization and early interstitial fibrosis.

Diagnosis: Diagnosis is based on history, signs and lesions. Since the syndrome is not specific with regard to cause, clues to this must be obtained from management factors such as change in pasture, or exposure to perilla mint or moldy sweet potatoes.

Treatment and Prophylaxis: Severely affected animals have so little reserve that any driving or handling must be cautious to prevent immediate deaths. No drug has been proved effective in controlled trials but epinephrine, aminophylline and corticosteroids are widely used. Even severely affected animals can recover if removed from the offending pasture and handled quietly. After a week the cattle may be gradually reintroduced to the pasture.

FARMER'S LUNG DISEASE IN CATTLE

A condition that appears to be identical to farmer's lung disease in man occurs in both acute and chronic forms in adult cattle. For obvious reasons, the human and bovine forms of the disease may often coexist on problem farms.

Etiology: The basis of the pulmonary reaction is predominantly an Arthus's (type III) hypersensitivity reaction (q.v., p. 4) that occurs in the peripheral parts of the bronchopulmonary system when sensitized individuals inhale the spores of thermophilic actinomycetes, in particular the spores of *Micropolyspora faeni*. The actinomycetes proliferate in vast numbers in hay that has overheated as the result of having been stored in a damp state; the spores are released when moldy hay is shaken, and their small size (1 μ) allows them to enter the smallest airways, even to the alveolar level. The reaction they provoke may be termed an "extrinsic allergic alveolitis."

Farmer's lung herds exist in areas where significant rainfall occurs during the haymaking season in most years, suggesting that a clinical problem may arise only after repeated sensitization and challenge from the spores. Clinical disease tends to arise during the latter half of the winter feeding period and usually only where moldy hay is fed indoors. Under such circumstances, precipitating antibodies to *M. faeni* are widespread among the adult cattle by the end of each winter feeding period and many apparently normal cattle are seropositive. By contrast, few adult cattle are seropositive on other farms where "good" hay is the norm or where grass silage is fed.

Clinical Findings: Individuals may succumb to the acute form of the disease over a period of weeks and it is unusual to get several severe cases occurring simultaneously although background coughing is common. The presenting sign is a variable degree of respiratory distress in an animal aged 5 years or more; deaths are rare. Coughing occurs but is not a prominent feature of acute cases; marked depression and anorexia are common but fever is rare. Tachypnea and hyperpnea occur but dyspnea is only occasionally seen; auscultation hardly ever reveals adventitious sounds but when present they occur as crackles in the anteroventral thorax.

The **chronic** disease usually has a higher morbidity and in most instances the presenting signs are weight loss, poor production and persistent coughing. On closer examination, affected individuals are fairly bright and eat reasonably well but tachypnea, hyperpnea and coughing are widespread in the group. Auscultation may reveal anteroventral crackles and sometimes, in more severe cases, scattered rhonchi. **Cor pulmonale** (q.v., p. 63) may occur in some acute and chronic cases.

Lesions: The macroscopic lesions are often unremarkable, being in most cases very mild peripheral lobular overinflation with diffusely scattered small gray subpleural spots. Although there is some suggestion that a transient pulmonary edema may be a feature of severe acute cases, the histopathologic lesions that are consistently found after a day or two's illness are interalveolar cellular infiltration, epithelioid granulomata and bronchiolitis obliterans. In some chronic cases, small foci of alveolar epithelial hyperplasia and metaplasia with interstitial fibrosis may be found and occasionally these areas may extend to include most, if not all, of the lung substance. These latter cases are clinically indistinguishable from diffuse fibrosing alveolitis (DFA); indeed the relationship, if any, between this latter disease and farmer's lung in cattle is unclear although circumstantial evidence would suggest that many cases of DFA are individuals with end-stage chronic farmer's lung.

Treatment and Control: Since it is often impossible to completely shield them from further challenge, most cattle, even acutely affected ones, make only a partial recovery following corticosteroid therapy. However, there is usually a marked improvement when they are turned out in the spring. Prevention is difficult in areas where hay is likely to be wet during the curing process.

PARASITIC BRONCHITIS IN ADULT CATTLE

In certain areas, parasitic bronchitis (i.e. *Dictyocaulus viviparus* infection) in adult stock is common. It may occur in either of 2 forms, viz. the patent disease or the reinfection phenomenon. *See also* LUNGWORM INFECTION, p. 715.

The patent disease occurs in individuals, groups or herds which have been shielded from earlier exposure or vaccination, there being no age-immunity in this infection. It arises in the autumn, usually in dairy cattle and the presenting signs are widespread coughing and tachypnea. A severe drop in milk yield may occur. Clinical signs vary considerably in severity but quite often animals are dull and anorectic, and deaths or subsequent culling are common. Auscultation in severe cases usually reveals widespread ronchi and crackling, particularly over the dorsal (diaphragmatic lobe) areas. Larvae can usually be detected without difficulty in feces. Postmortem features are as for immature cattle. Conventional therapy may produce a marked response if administered early in the course of the problem but recovery is often prolonged and coughing may remain throughout the following winter.

The reinfection phenomenon (reinfection husk) occurs when immunity has waned and cattle are suddenly faced with a high challenge. Again, it arises in the autumn, usually in dairy herds. The presenting signs are widespread coughing and tachypnea, with marked drop in milk yield. Cattle tend to be less severely affected than with the patent disease and deaths are not a feature. Auscultation of representatively sick cattle reveals no adventitious sounds and larvae are not usually found in feces or if present are in very small numbers. Postmortem signs are not dramatic, merely consisting of scattered gray-green subpleural nodules about 2 to 4 mm in diameter, made up of plasma cell and lymphocyte nodules surrounding lungworm larvae that have been killed in terminal bronchioles. There is usually an associated eosinophilic bronchitis and bronchiolitis that no doubt accounts for the clinical signs. If live worms are found they are generally stunted. Early therapy with diethylcarbamazine or levamisole seems to be effective and milk yields are largely recovered, presumably because the drug kills invading larvae quicker than the host's immune apparatus; however, if treatment is delayed or if challenge continues, prolonged coughing may result and production may be depressed over an extended period.

MYCOTIC PNEUMONIA

A chronic inflammation of the lungs caused by fungi and yeasts. (It has been customary to include the lung infections caused by *Actinomyces* and *Actinobacillus*.)

Etiology: *Cryptococcus*, *Histoplasma*, *Coccidioides*, *Blastomyces* and *Aspergillus*, along with other fungi and yeasts have been incriminated as causative agents in this condition in domestic animals (*see* SYSTEMIC FUNGUS INFECTIONS, p. 445). The tissues and secretions of the respiratory passages are an excellent environment for the multiplication of these organisms. Fungal infections are often concurrent with bacterial infections.

Clinical Findings: A short, moist cough is characteristic. As in other types of pneumonia, a thick mucoid nasal discharge may be present. As the disease progresses, dyspnea, emaciation and generalized weakness become increasingly evident. Respiration becomes abdominal, resembling that seen in diaphragmatic hernia. On auscultation, harsh respiratory sounds are heard. In advanced cases, the normal sounds of breathing are decreased or almost inaudible. Leukocytosis and periodic elevation of the temperature occur, probably in conjunction with aggravation of the bacterial infection. Pathologic changes in the eyes, e.g. corneal ulcer, blindness and purulent discharge, are not uncommon in cases of blastomycosis.

Lesions: Focal lesions of chronic inflammation are present in the lungs. Abscess formation and cavitation may be seen in conjunction with yellow or gray areas of necrosis. Some animals show numerous miliary nodules which can be seen on roentgenograms.

Diagnosis: A tentative diagnosis of mycotic pneumonia may be made if an animal with chronic pneumonia exhibits the signs described and does not respond to antibiotic therapy. However, a positive diagnosis will require laboratory assistance, and radiography may be useful. Some antigens, e.g. histoplasmin and blastomycin, have been developed and are an aid to diagnosis. Culture of the sputum which is expelled in spasms of coughing may reveal the infective organism. The clinical diagnosis can be confirmed at necropsy by appropriate cultural and histopathologic techniques.

Treatment: There is no entirely satisfactory method of treating systemic mycotic infections, but amphotericin (℞ 364) may be helpful although undesirably toxic. (*See also* p. 445.)

ASPIRATION PNEUMONIA

(Foreign-body pneumonia, Inhalation pneumonia, Gangrenous pneumonia)

A form of pneumonia characterized by pulmonary necrosis and caused by the entry of foreign material into the lungs.

Etiology: Faulty administration of medicines is the commonest cause of aspiration pneumonia. Liquids administered by drench or dose syringe must not be given faster than the animal can swallow, and drenching is particularly dangerous when conducted with the animal's tongue drawn out, when the head is held high, or when the animal is coughing or bellowing. Administration of liquids by nasal intubation is not without risk, and careful technique is especially necessary in debilitated animals. Cats are particularly susceptible to pneumonia caused by aspiration of mineral oil. Inhalation of food sometimes occurs in calves and swine. Attempts by animals to eat or drink while partly choked may result in aspiration pneumonia. Disturbances of deglutition, as in anesthetized or comatose animals (e.g. mature cattle under a general anesthetic and cows in lateral recumbency with milk fever) or in those suffering from vagal paralysis, acute pharyngitis, abscesses or tumors of the pharyngeal region, esophageal diverticula and encephalitis, are frequent predisposing causes. In sheep, inexpert dipping may cause aspiration of fluid. Inhalation of irritant gases or smoke is an infrequent cause.

Some anesthetics, such as the thiobarbiturates, stimulate salivation. Atropine sulfate (℞ 511) will help to control salivation, while the use of an endotracheal catheter with an inflatable cuff will prevent fluid aspiration during surgery.

Clinical Findings: A history disclosing an event within the previous 1 to 3 days when foreign-body aspiration could have occurred, is of great diagnostic value. In the horse, the temperature usually rises to 104 to 105°F (40 to 40.5°C) during the first few days and then becomes remittent. Pyrexia is also observed in cats, dogs and cattle, but sometimes cattle develop little or no fever. The pulse is accelerated and respiration rapid and labored. A sweetish, fetid breath characteristic of gangrene may be detected, the intensity of which increases as the disease progresses. This is often associated with a purulent nasal discharge that sometimes is reddish brown or green. Occasionally, evidence of the aspirated material can be seen in the nasal discharge or in expectorated material, e.g. oil droplets. On auscultation, moist rales over one or both sides of the chest are heard early in the condition, followed by dry rales, pleuritic friction rubs and sometimes the crackling sounds of emphysema. A course of 1 to 5 days is usual. Cattle and swine recover more frequently than horses, but in all species the mortality is high. In outbreaks following dipping of sheep, losses rise from the second day to about the seventh and then decrease gradually.

Lesions: The pneumonia is usually in the anterior ventral parts of the lungs and may be unilateral or bilateral. In the early stages, the lungs are markedly congested, with areas of interlobular edema. The bronchi are hyperemic and full of froth. The pneumonic areas tend to be cone-shaped with the base toward the pleura. Suppuration and necrosis follow, the foci becoming soft or liquefied, reddish brown and foul smelling. There usually is an acute fibrinous pleuritis, often with pleural exudate.

Treatment: The animal should be kept quiet. A productive cough should not be suppressed. Broad-spectrum antibiotics should be used in animals known to have inhaled a foreign substance, whether it be a liquid or an irritant vapor, without waiting for signs of pneumonia to appear. Care and supportive treatment are the same as for infectious pneumonia. In small animals, oxygen therapy may be beneficial. Despite all treatments prognosis is poor.

HYPOSTATIC PNEUMONIA

A condition arising from failure of the blood to pass readily through the vascular structures of the lungs.

Etiology: This condition is a result of passive congestion of the lungs and is seen most commonly in old or debilitated animals. It is usually secondary to some other disease process, e.g. congestive heart failure. Paralyzed dogs or animals recovering from anesthesia sometimes develop hypostatic pneumonia if they are not moved regularly.

Diagnosis: Any primary disease must be determined and treated. Coughing is not always a prominent sign, but as the condition progresses, dyspnea and cyanosis become apparent. Secondary bacterial infection is common. A roentgenogram will reveal increased density of the long and the mediastinal space may be shifted to the atalectic side.

Treatment: The position in which the patient lies must be changed regularly, at least once every hour. Exercise must be encouraged insofar as it is compatible with the condition of the patient. If a primary cause can be determined, specific therapy, e.g. digitalis (℞ 526) for congestive heart failure or chlorothiazide (℞ 541) for edema, may be instituted.

Narcotics and sedatives should be kept to a minimum to encourage mobilization and to avoid depression of the cough reflex. Maintenance of proper hydration is also important.

CHRONIC ALVEOLAR EMPHYSEMA
(Heaves)

A respiratory disease of horses characterized by labored expiration, chronic cough, unthriftiness and lack of stamina. Alveolar emphysema is an anatomic disease of the lung characterized by an enlargement of air-spaces associated with a loss of tissue distal to the terminal bronchioles. The signs may be aggravated by exercise, dusty surroundings and feeding of certain roughages, particularly dusty or moldy alfalfa hay.

Etiology: The primary cause of the disease is unknown; the cause of the expiratory distress is rupture of the alveolar walls associated with narrowing or collapse of airways during exhalation. Possible exciting causes are: pulmonary allergic reaction, exposure to dust, molds, or other air pollutants, infections of the respiratory tract, hereditary predisposition. Extreme exertion, particularly if the animal has coexisting respiratory disease, may be a cause.

Clinical Findings: The disease is long standing, usually progressive in nature and may appear to be periodic. In most cases, respiratory distress is greater during hot and dry weather, or when the animal is exposed to dusty surroundings. Inspiration is hurried with the nostrils dilated. In advanced cases the elbows may be abducted. The expiratory phase of the respiratory cycle is prolonged with forcible contraction of the abdominal muscles resulting in the formation of a ridge (heave line) along the costal arch. In severe cases, the anus may protrude, the ribs are permanently rolled forward, and the animal may appear to have an enlarged chest cavity. A short, weak, persistent cough and a nasal discharge commonly are present. The cough often occurs on or following feeding of a grain ration. High pitched, end-expiratory rales are usually present. Percussion may reveal hyperresonance in advanced cases.

Lesions: The lungs are pale and fail to collapse when the thorax is opened. Imprints of the ribs upon the lungs may be noted. Microscopic examination reveals alveolar and interstitial emphysema. The normal pulmonary architecture is lost, the alveolar walls being disrupted and thinner than normal. Rupture of alveoli results in formation of large and irregular air sacs. A diffuse bronchiolitis is usually present.

Diagnosis: The diagnosis of alveolar emphysema is made from the signs and history. The early stages may present some difficulty because of similarity of signs accompanying other respiratory diseases such as bronchitis and pharyngitis. Alveolar emphysema is longstanding and resists various treatments.

Treatment: There is no specific cure; treatment is palliative. The affected animal should be kept in dust-free surroundings. Moldy hays should be avoided. Keeping the animal on green pasture may be of considerable benefit. Complete pelleted feeds, particularly those containing beet pulp as the roughage, may be quite effective in certain cases. Avoidance of respiratory infections and prompt appropriate treatment of infectious bronchial disease are indicated. Those cases due to allergic causes may respond to bronchial dilators (℞ 522, 659) or to the steroids.

PROGRESSIVE PNEUMONIA OF SHEEP

(Maedi-Visna, Laikipia disease, Zwoegersiekte)

Progressive pneumonia of sheep is a chronic viral disease of sheep and goats involving either the respiratory tract, the CNS, or both. It has been reported from North America, Europe, Africa and Asia. A distinction should be made between progressive pneumonia and pulmonary adenomatosis (q.v., p. 923).

Etiology: The disease is caused by an RNA virus, which persists in infected animals in the presence of complement-fixing and neutralizing antibodies. Complement fixing, precipitating and indirect immunofluorescent antibodies are usually present before neutralizing antibodies. Experimental inoculation can result in pulmonary or CNS lesions or both. Transmission is thought to occur by the aerosol-droplet route and perhaps by ingestion of feces or colostrum from infected sheep. All breeds of sheep appear to be susceptible but management practices may influence morbidity and mortality rates.

Clinical Findings: Clinical signs rarely occur in sheep under 2 years and are commonest in sheep more than 4 years old. The disease may last from 2 to 18 months. Affected animals have a progressively increasing dyspnea and a double expiratory effort. There is progressive loss of condition and, surprisingly, no significant bronchial exudate and little coughing. Under natural conditions affected sheep often succumb to a secondary *Pasteurella* pneumonia. In the neurologic form, there is progressive weakness of the hind legs.

Other signs may include deviation of the head, circling or a fine trembling of the lower jaw. Following recumbency, animals remain alert and continue to eat.

Lesions: The macroscopic lesions are confined to the lungs and the associated lymph nodes. The lungs do not collapse normally when the thorax is opened, and they weigh 2 or 3 times the normal weight. They are a dull-beige color. The basic changes are typically diffuse, involving the entire lung. On palpation the tissue is firmer than normal, but retains some elasticity. In advanced cases there are consolidated areas in which secondary infections are usually involved. The mediastinal lymph nodes are enlarged and somewhat edematous. Microscopically the primary lesions are interstitial pneumonia, perivascular and peribronchial lymphoid hyperplasia and hypertrophy of smooth muscle surrounding bronchioles and alveolar ducts. This distinguishes progressive pneumonia from pulmonary adenomatosis (*see* below) in which the primary lesion is papilliform epithelial proliferation. The lesions in the brain are those of a meningoleukoencephalitis with secondary demyelination.

Diagnosis: The clinical diagnosis of progressive pneumonia cannot be made with certainty. In pulmonary adenomatosis there is often a copious mucous nasal exudate but in some instances this sign may be absent. Verminous pneumonia and pulmonary caseous lymphadenitis are other conditions requiring differentiation. Necropsy will rule out the latter 2 and, in most cases, pulmonary adenomatosis also. Rabies, listeriosis, scrapie, louping ill and space-occupying lesions should be considered when neurological signs are observed. In flocks experiencing progressive pneumonia for the first time, the diagnosis should be confirmed by histopathology, serology or isolation of the virus.

Control: There is no effective treatment. Three methods of control are possible: (1) slaughter of all suspects as soon as they are detected; (2) slaughter of the entire flock and replacement with serologically negative sheep after a suitable interval; and (3) a 2-flock system whereby serologically positive sheep from the affected flock are slaughtered as soon as possible and serologically negative sheep are purchased and kept strictly isolated from the affected flock.

PULMONARY ADENOMATOSIS

(Jaagsiekte)

A contagious neoplastic viral disease of adult sheep and goats. The disease has been reported from Europe, Asia, Africa, South America and the U.S.A.

Crowding enhances the spread of the disease, which is thought to be by inhalation of infected droplets by susceptible sheep. Inhaled virus apparently enters epithelial cells of the lungs and establishes foci of infection throughout them. Affected cells proliferate and form neoplastic areas which, over periods of months to years, eventually result in decreased pulmonary function.

The incubation period is long (4 months to several years) and the course chronic but relentless. Early signs of panting after exercise and occasional coughing are followed by progressive emaciation, dyspnea and nasal discharge. In advanced cases, moist rales can be heard at a distance from affected sheep. Forcible lowering of the head is followed by discharge of copious watery mucus from the nostrils, a sign considered to be pathognomonic. Appetite and body temperature are unaffected unless complicated by a secondary bacterial infection, which is common in the terminal stages.

Lesions are confined to the thorax, and consist of pulmonary consolidation, excessive bronchial fluid and sometimes abscesses and pleuritis.The characteristic alveolar adenomata are seen histologically.

There is no treatment. Field trials of a formalized vaccine have yielded conflicting results. Incidence can be lowered by slaughter of clinically affected sheep; eradication requires slaughter of all sheep in affected areas.

SKIN AND CONNECTIVE TISSUE

DERMATITIS

Dermatitis can be produced by a myriad of agents, including external irritants, burns, allergens, trauma, and bacterial, parasitic or fungal infections. Dermatitis can be associated with a concurrent internal or systemic disease and hereditary factors also may be related to the development of the cutaneous disorder. Allergies form an important group of etiologic factors, especially in small animals (q.v., p. 5).

Clinical Findings: The most common sign is scratching, followed by the appearance of the skin lesions which progress from edema and erythema to papules, vesicles, oozing and crusting or scaling. Secondary infection is common, with pustules or purulent lesions. As the disease becomes chronic, the erythema decreases and there are fewer vesicles or papules, but as infiltration and thickening of the skin increases, the lesions are dryer and the skin may crack. The clinical picture may vary considerably with the species affected and with the causal agent of the skin lesions.

Treatment: If the underlying cause is determined, its elimination will effect a prompt recovery. However, the numerous possible origins of dermatitis can at first necessitate establishing therapy on an empirical basis. In the choice and application of local treatment, certain general principles should be observed. Treatments of moist skin areas will differ from those of dry lesions. The former are best treated with wet dressings and the latter with ointments. Systemic as well as topical therapy may be indicated. The corticosteroids are often of great value in reducing the acute phase of dermatitis and in relieving pruritus. The systemic dosage of adrenocortical steroids must be established individually. Corticosteroids, at times with antibiotics, can be used as topical ointments or lotions in erythematous, edematous and pruritic dermatitis and are usually effective (℞ 431, 449).

Local treatment of each type of lesion should be considered individually. Clipping of the haircoat of the affected area and surrounding the lesion is highly advantageous. To prevent scratching and licking, sedatives and various protective devices (as stuffed, pneumatic or cardboard collars, hobbles, or, when necessary, bandages) should be employed in conjunction with antipruritic medication. Preparations with a salicylic acid or tar base (℞ 440, 451) are commonly used in the local treatment of dry, scaly, or crusted dermatitis; wet dressings (℞ 425) and astringents (℞ 645) are useful in weeping or moist lesions. An iodochlorhydroxyquin steroid ointment (℞ 443) can be used for local treatment of chronic dermatitis. Where it is desirable to remove scurf and epithelial debris thoroughly, a selenium sulfide shampoo (℞ 454), or nonirritating oily preparations are quite effective. Indirect causes of dermatitis, e.g. imbalanced nutrition, concurrent disease or infections, must be treated accordingly.

PYODERMA

(Pyogenic dermatitis, Acne, Secondary pyoderma)

A pyogenic infection of skin, which can be primary or secondary, superficial or deep. Microorganisms commonly isolated from pyodermas include *Staphylococcus aureus*, coagulase-positive (found most often); *Staph. epidermis*, coagulase-negative; streptococci (both hemolytic and nonhemolytic); corynebacteria; pseudomonas and *Proteus vulgaris*. Short-haired breeds and young animals are more often affected. Metabolic disorders, immune deficiencies, endocrine imbalance or various intoxications may, in some cases, predispose to the development of pyogenic dermatitis.

Clinical Findings: In horses, folliculitis often develops in the saddle and lumbar region (*see also* SADDLE SORES, p. 951), particularly in summer. The affected area initially may be swollen and very sensitive. This is followed by formation of follicular papules and pustules. These may become confluent or rupture, forming plaques and crusts. Deep folliculitis followed by ulceration may develop over large areas of the body, especially on the neck, sides of the thorax, inner surface of the thighs or on the prepuce. In cattle, folliculitis, which may proceed to necrosis, develops mostly on the abdomen, groin and medial surfaces of the thighs. Other primary pyodermas frequently occur on thin-skinned or frictional areas.

Deep pyogenic dermatitis is characterized by a penetrating suppurative inflammation of skin, hair follicles, sebaceous glands and deeper parts of the cutaneous and subcut. tissues. Thus, folliculitis, furunculosis and abscesses are successive stages. Deep suppurative lesions may fuse, especially in the subcutis, forming ulcerated fistulous tracts discharging pus. These involvements are most commonly noted on the extremities and rump. In dogs, deep pyogenic dermatitis involves the trunk, lips, dorsal aspect of the nose, interdigital skin and the posterior portion of the abdomen and axillae. Animals suffering from extensive deep pyoderma may have elevated temperature, anemia, leukocytosis and enlargement of the regional lymph nodes.

Prognosis: The prognosis for pyoderma is more favorable in horses than in other animals. In horses, the lesions may disappear spontaneously within several weeks. The prognosis for secondary pyoderma in severely affected animals, particularly dogs, may be unfavorable unless the predisposing primary factor(s) favoring the infection can be determined and corrected.

Treatment: Irritation of the affected areas should be avoided. In the early stage, bathing in warm antiseptic solutions such as hexachlorophene or povidone-iodine (℞ 439, 602) is useful. Choice of therapy depends upon the type of the lesions. Superficial pyogenic dermatitis is relatively easy to treat. Among the topical preparations for superficial conditions are: STA (salicylic acid 8, tannic acid 8, 70% alcohol 100 parts); 5% alcoholic solution of crystal violet (gentian violet) and a variety of proprietary antibacterial agents (℞ 422, 449, 458).

It is essential to treat deep pyogenic dermatitis both topically and systemically. Deep pyodermas should be incised for drainage before local application of antibiotic ointments (℞ 422, 446). In undetermined cases, nitrofurans or antibiotics along with enzyme preparations may be injected through a blunt needle directly into the fistulous tracts. If possible, cultures should be made and sensitivity tests done to determine the most effective antibiotic. Pyoderma of lip or vulvar folds is treated topically by antiseptic drying preparations such as 10% silver nitrate. When the lesions become dry, an antiseptic ointment is rubbed into the affected areas, which are then dusted with a powder (antibiotic, sulfonamide, iodoform, tannoform). Surgical correction of predisposing skin folds may be necessary for a permanent cure.

Juvenile pyoderma lesions are cleansed with a mild antiseptic solution. Crusts covering the skin are softened with lukewarm mineral oil or with antibiotic compresses (neomycin 1:1,000) and gently removed. Mild antiseptics are then applied.

For systemic treatment, antibiotics (℞ 12, 23, 42, 50, 115), autogenous bacterins and enzymes may be used.

RHABDITIC DERMATITIS

An acute dermatitis of dogs and cattle caused by the nematode *Rhabditis (Pelodera) strongyloides*. *R. strongyloides* is saprophytic, living in moist soil and decaying organic matter. Lesions are confined to areas of the body soiled by urine and feces, or in contact with moist, filthy bedding.

The condition is infrequent and occurs sporadically in dogs but may assume epidemic proportions in cattle. It is characterized by alopecia and varying degrees of pruritus, or an acute dermatitis followed by pustules, crusts and alopecia. The worms can be found in skin scrapings or expressed from pustules. The larva is cylindrical, approximately 600 μ long and 38 μ wide.

Rhabditic dermatitis can be prevented and controlled by providing clean dry bedding and disinfecting the surroundings. Improving the hygiene usually results in spontaneous recovery. Exposure to sunshine is also beneficial. Recovery may be hastened by cleaning the areas involved and applying rotenone or an astringent and disinfectant preparation (℞ 324, 645).

DERMATOPHILOSIS

(Dermatophilus infection, Cutaneous streptotrichosis, Lumpy-wool, Strawberry foot-rot)

Dermatophilosis is an epidermal infection due to the aerobic actinomycete *Dermatophilus congolensis*. It is characterized by the formation of horny crusts that adhere firmly to the infected skin. The disease is world-wide in distribution, affecting many wild and domestic animal species, mainly herbivores. Related but separate organisms were once thought to cause several clinical forms including streptotrichosis in cattle, horses and goats, lumpy-wool in sheep, and strawberry foot-rot in sheep; all are presently considered to be one species.

Etiology: *Dermatophilus congolensis* currently shares the family Dermatophilaceae with the nonpathogenic soil inhabitant *Geodermatophilus obscurus*. *D. congolensis* forms a branched mycelium that divides transversely and then longitudinally to produce thick bundles of small cocci. These enlarge and mature into flagellated ovoid zoospores, 0.6 to 1 μ in diameter. When the crusts are wetted, the zoospores emerge to the surface where they are available for the transmission of infection. The organism has no resistant stage and transmission is presumably direct although plants and insects probably serve as mechanical vectors. In some cases spiny plants and insects also disrupt the lipid and keratinous covering of the skin, thus providing the zoospores with access to the living epidermal layer. Infection may also be associated with skin damage by other agents including heavy rain.

The distribution of lesions usually corresponds to the predisposing skin damage. Thus, in the presence of spiny plants, sheep may be infected on the lips or brisket, or on the legs and feet (strawberry foot rot) whereas infections following heavy rain are mainly on the dorsal areas of the body (lumpy-wool). In infected cattle (cutaneous streptotrichosis) the lesions are often generally distributed suggesting the possible involvement of insects that attack all parts of the body surface.

Clinical Findings: The hyphae of *D. congolensis* invade the living epidermal cells, especially in the hair- or wool-follicle sheaths, inducing acute inflammation and rapid cornification of the infected epidermis. Alternate layers of dried exudate and cornified epidermis accumulate on the skin where they are bound by the hair or wool fibers into a compact amber crust.

The lesions vary in 2 important qualities—extent and persistence. The extensive confluent infection sometimes seen in lambs and calves often proves fatal. Less extensive infections usually have little effect on the general health of the animal, apart from severe lesions on the lips, which may lead to death from starvation. Death may also follow secondary blow-fly strike or screwworm infestation.

In most individual animals the infection is overcome and the crusts are separable from the skin within about 3 weeks. However, in a number of sheep (particularly Merinos) and cattle the infection becomes chronic and the crusts are built up into large horny masses. In sheep this produces the typical lumpy-wool condition. Chronic infection prevents the shearing of sheep and detracts seriously from the value of the hides of cattle.

Diagnosis: *D. congolensis* is usually demonstrable in stained smears and cultures made from finely chopped macerated crusts. It is gram-positive and grows well on nutrient agar at 37°C, especially in an atmosphere of 10% carbon dioxide. There is complete hemolysis around colonies on sheep- but not horse-blood agar. Isolation from material that is heavily contaminated or poor in viable *D. congolensis*, is facilitated by passage in sheep or guinea pigs. The material should be wetted and applied to lightly scarified skin.

In sheep, dermatophilosis may be distinguished from contagious ecthyma by the lack of infectivity of bacteria-free filtrates made from suspensions of crust material. The lesions usually differ from those of ringworm and scabies in their greater tendency to accumulate hard crust, but must sometimes be differentiated by microscopic and cultural examination.

Prophylaxis: Because small, almost inapparent lesions are widespread among wild and domestic animals, quarantine measures are of little or no value. Vaccination induces a good immunologic response but has little effect on the extent or duration of infection. The application of disinfectants should decrease the spread of infection if applied at times when transmission is likely; in sheep, shear-cut infections have been successfully prevented by spraying with

0.5% zinc sulfate within 1 to 2 hours of shearing. In other circumstances the time to spray is difficult to predict.

Treatment: In acute cases the duration of infection is short and treatment is usually unwarranted. Healed lesions, in which the crusts are held in place by the hair fibers, are sometimes mistaken for active infection and treated. This has led to erroneous claims for local treatments involving the removal of crusts prior to disinfectant applications. External treatments are of questionable value because many hyphae are inaccessible in the follicle sheaths.

Persistent infections may be rapidly and effectively cured with a single large injection of streptomycin and procaine penicillin combined. Although ineffective alone, penicillin greatly potentiates the action of streptomycin. A dose rate of 20 mg streptomycin plus 20,000 u procaine penicillin per pound of body weight (44 mg + 44,000 u/kg) IM is recommended. Sheep with lumpy-wool can be shorn 2 months after treatment. An insecticide may have to be applied to control secondary blow-fly strike.

DERMATOMYCOSES

(Ringworm)

Infections of keratin-bearing tissues (skin, hair and nails) caused by fungi called dermatophytes. Most domestic animals are susceptible although swine and sheep seem to be less commonly infected than other animals. Some dermatophytes infect man primarily and lower animals only rarely, others are animal pathogens mainly but can cause disease in man, still others are free-living soil fungi that parasitize man or animals under certain conditions. The infection starts in the stratum corneum where thread-like hyphae develop from spores. The hyphae grow about halfway down the hair follicles and then enter the hairs. They grow down the hair to the first layer of keratinized cells where growth stops. The hyphae may produce spores within the hair (endothrix type) or produce spores in rows or mosaics along the outer surface of the hairs (ectothrix type). The lesion usually spreads in a circular manner from the original point of infection giving rise to the term "ringworm."

The clinical signs of ringworm are not pathognomonic. Diagnosis must be achieved by (1) examination using Wood's lamp (cobalt-filtered ultraviolet), (2) direct microscopic examination of hairs or scrapings, or (3) culture.

1. The Wood's lamp is useful for the diagnosis of *Microsporum canis* (*Nannizia otae*) infections in animals and *M. audouinii* infections in man. Infected hairs or lesions fluoresce with a yellowish green color. However, most dermatophyte infections are nonfluorescent and thus this procedure has limited application. The examination should be made before medication is started because certain

medicaments, mineral oil for example, will cause pseudofluorescence, while others, such as iodine, may block fluorescence in infected hairs.

2. Direct microscopic examination of hairs or skin scrapings is an effective office or field procedure for the rapid diagnosis of ringworm infection. Hairs or scrapings from the periphery of a suspected area of infection are put on a slide in a drop of 5% potassium hydroxide and 20% glycerin in distilled water and covered with a cover slip. After gentle heating to clear the specimen, and a wait of about one hour, it is examined for the presence of hyphae or spores.

3. Culture on Sabouraud's agar plates takes the longest time but is the most effective and specific means of diagnosis. It frequently shows infections that may have been missed by the first 2 procedures, and also aids in the identification of the specific etiologic agents. Hairs or scrapings are placed on the agar and the Petri dish is sealed with adhesive tape to reduce evaporation. Addition of 0.5 mg of cycloheximide per milliliter of agar is necessary to prevent rapid growth of other contaminating molds. The plate can be kept at room temperature. It should be incubated at least one week and may require as much as 4 weeks to produce sufficient growth for identification. A faster diagnosis may be accomplished by culturing suspected material on Dermatophyte Test Medium (DTM) in which dermatophytes change the medium from yellow to red within 3 or 4 days.

RINGWORM IN CATTLE

Trichophyton verrucosum is the most frequent cause of ringworm in cattle, but *T. mentagrophytes* (*Arthroderma benhamiae*) is occasionally isolated. Although cattle of all ages may be affected, the disease is commonest in calves. After an incubation period of 2 to 4 weeks, the hair in the infected area breaks off or falls out and, by 2 to 3 months, round, sharply circumscribed, thick, asbestos-like plaques are seen. Lesions expand at the periphery and frequently are 12 to 75 mm in diameter. Sites of predilection include the skin around the eyes, ears, muzzle and neck; but few areas escape infection if the condition is left untreated. The disease is more commonly seen during the winter months in stabled animals, but may occur at any time. The fungus is resistant and may survive for up to 4 years in dry scales shed by the animal. Infection is transmitted readily from animal to animal and from animal to man by direct or indirect contact.

Diagnosis: The appearance of round, scaly or encrusted, alopecic patches or plaques strongly favors a diagnosis of ringworm. The diagnosis can be readily confirmed by demonstration of the fungus on the affected hairs by microscopic examination of specimens cleared by potassium hydroxide. Chains of spherical, rather large (4 to 6 μ) spores surround the hair shaft.

Treatment: When thick crusts are first removed with a brush and mild soap, ringworm usually responds to local application of fungicidal drugs, but persistent treatment may be required. Daily applications of a mixture of equal parts tincture of iodine and glycerin or a 20% solution of sodium caprylate to the lesion until it disappears often is effective. All parts of the lesion should be soaked thoroughly at each application. Tincture of iodine or Lugol's solution applied every other day also is effective. Cattle with widespread infection may be given 2 IV treatments one week apart consisting of 30 gm of sodium iodide in 250 ml of water. Oral administration of griseofulvin has given good results, but may not be used in animals kept for food purposes, and is not economically feasible for most large animals. Total body sprays of a formulation of pimaricin are effective and also sterilize lesions, preventing spread of infection to other animals. The antifungal activity of topically applied 75% thiabendazole may provide a useful treatment. The preparation should be applied at least 3 times over a period of 7 to 9 days.

RINGWORM IN HORSES

Trichophyton equinum is the primary cause of ringworm in horses. *T. mentagrophytes* is found occasionally. The infection is characterized by a focal edematous lesion with piloerection and finally alopecia and formation of a thick crust. Microscopic examination of cleared hairs reveals spores arranged in chains around the hair.

Ringworm in horses usually occurs at sites where the skin comes in contact with infected animals or contaminated saddle blankets, harness and grooming tools.

Treatment: After working, the horse should be washed with a solution of 30 gm of captan (Vangard 45) in 3 gal. (11 L) of water. This should be repeated every 4 days until clinical cure is obtained. A mixture of equal parts of iodine and glycerin applied daily to the lesion is effective.

RINGWORM IN DOGS AND CATS

Approximately 70% of ringworm in dogs is caused by *Microsporum canis*, 20% by *M. gypseum* and 10% by *Trichophyton mentagrophytes*. In cats, 98% is caused by *M. canis*, while the *M. gypseum* complex and *T. mentagrophytes* each account for about 1%. Because of the high percentage of *M. canis* infections, the Wood's lamp becomes a valuable diagnostic tool when examining these species. However, *M. gypseum* and *T. mentagrophytes* do not fluoresce and a negative Wood's lamp examination does not rule out ringworm.

The clinical appearance of ringworm is more variable in cats than in dogs. There may be no clinically apparent lesions or there may be only a few broken hairs around the face and ears. Other lesions may be scaly and alopecic, or, in more severe cases, there may be alopecic crusted lesions involving a large part of the body. In general, older rather than younger cats are more likely to be carriers with clinically inapparent infections. The clinically normal carrier dog is seen less frequently.

Lesions in dogs usually appear as circular scaly patches with broken stubs of hair within the lesions or they may be completely alopecic inside the ring. The lesion is most active at the periphery where there may be vesicles and pustules. In severe infections, large areas of the dog's body may show alopecia, scaling, erythema or crust formation. *M. canis* is transmissible to man and it is not uncommon for the owner and the animal to have similar lesions.

Treatment: Both systemic treatment with griseofulvin (℞ 365) and topical applications of antifungal agents are necessary. Spread of the infection to other parts of the body or other animals or man can be reduced or eliminated by the use of antifungal dips, such as a 1:200 solution of 45% captan, or iodine shampoos applied to the whole body on the 7th and 14th days of griseofulvin therapy. After clinical recovery there may still be fungal elements in the portions of the hairs above the skin surface and therefore a healed lesion should be recultured to ensure that no viable spores remain to reinfect the skin later.

Lesions that become infected secondarily should be treated with suitable antimicrobial agents (℞ 429).

RINGWORM IN PIGS

Microsporum nanum (*Nannizia obtusa*), *M. canis*, *Trichophyton mentagrophytes*, *T. verrucosum* var. *diskoides* and *T. rubrum* have all been incriminated, as have *Alternaria* and *Candida albicans.* The lesion caused by *M. nanum* is superficial and loss of hair unusual. In all forms the lesion spreads centrifrugally, leaving a brown, flaky or crusty center. These "rings" may become quite large, but more commonly are about 4 to 6 cm in diameter. Affected pigs should be isolated until the lesions heal, and their pens, especially any rubbing posts, cleaned and disinfected. For treatment *see* RINGWORM IN CATTLE, p. 933.

PITYRIASIS ROSEA IN PIGS

A sporadic disease of uncertain etiology of the skin of young growing pigs from 8 to 12 weeks old and occasionally in suckling pigs as young as 3 weeks old. One pig or several pigs of a litter may be affected. The disease is usually mild but a slight anorexia and diarrhea may occur for a few days. The lesions are characterized by erythematous ringlike swellings with distinct borders. The lesions usually enlarge at their periphery and adjacent lesions coalesce resulting in a mosaic pattern. The center of the lesion is flat and covered with a branlike scale that usually dries off leaving normal skin. The lesions occur predominantly on the abdomen and may appear symmetrically over the back and down the sides of the leg. There is usually no pruritus. Spontaneous recovery usually occurs in a few weeks and treatment is unnecessary. The lesions must be differentiated from swine pox, parakeratosis, ringworm, sarcoptic mange and allergic dermatoses.

The disease is considered to be heritable but the mode of inheritance is uncertain. A viral infection is a possibility (because of a similar disease in man). Affected pigs should be isolated from the remainder of the herd, identified and not used for breeding purposes.

PARAKERATOSIS IN SWINE

A nutritional deficiency disease, characterized by skin lesions involving the superficial layers of the epidermis, frequently affecting young pigs between the ages of 6 and 16 weeks. The incidence may reach 60% in some herds.

Etiology: Parakeratosis is a metabolic disturbance resulting from a relative deficiency of zinc (q.v., p. 1409) and an excess of calcium in the diet. The disease is most prevalent in pigs receiving diets containing mainly vegetable proteins and excess calcium supplements.

Clinical Findings: Signs are limited to the changes in the skin; mild lethargy and slight anorexia may be associated with increased severity of the lesions.

Lesions: Excessive growth and keratinization of skin epithelium with the formation of horny crusts and fissures are the outstanding lesions. Brown spots or papules are first seen on the ventrolateral areas of the abdomen, and on the pastern, fetlock, hock and tail, coalescing to involve larger areas until the entire body may be covered. The crusts are horny and dry on exposed surfaces and are usually easily removed. Occasionally, secondary infection of the cracks and fissures causes them to fill with a dark, sticky exudate and debris which may tend to confuse the condition with exudative dermatitis of an infectious nature.

Treatment: Highly satisfactory results can be obtained by adjusting the intake of calcium and zinc. The calcium level in the diet should be maintained between 0.65 and 0.75% and supplemental zinc added at the rate of 25 to 50 ppm (equivalent to an addition of 0.4 lb

[181 gm] of zinc sulfate or carbonate per ton of feed). For pigs that have developed the disease as a result of improper diets, access to succulent, green pasture forage will shorten their convalescence and hasten recovery.

EXUDATIVE EPIDERMITIS (XE)

(Greasy pig disease)

An acute, generalized dermatitis of pigs which occurs from 5 to 35 days of age, characterized by sudden onset, with morbidity of 10 to 90% and mortality of 5 to 90%.

Etiology: The lesions of XE are caused by *Staphylococcus hyos* but the bacterial agent is unable to penetrate the intact skin. Abrasions on the feet and legs or lacerations on the body frequently precede infection. In acute cases a vesicular-type virus may be the predisposing factor.

Clinical Findings: The first signs are listlessness, apathy, and dullness of the skin and hair coat, followed by a dandruff-like condition. Later the pig becomes more depressed and refuses to eat. The body temperature remains near normal. The skin thickens and reddish-brown spots appear from which serum exudes. There is often purulent inflammation of the external ear, and catarrhal inflammation of the eyes.

Vesicles, possibly caused by a virus, develop on the skin, burst, and become infected. The body is rapidly covered with a moist, greasy exudate of sebum and serum, which becomes crusty, and an obnoxious odor develops. Vesicles and ulcers also form on the nasal disk and tongue. The feet are nearly always involved with erosion of the coronary bands and heel, and the hoof may be lost. Death occurs within 3 to 5 days.

In some animals the disease may be milder with lesions developing slowly. The mortality usually is low but many affected pigs recover slowly and growth is retarded.

Lesions: Necropsy of severely affected pigs reveals marked dehydration, congestion of the lungs and inflammation of the peripheral lymph nodes. Distension of the kidneys and ureters with mucus, cellular casts and debris is a constant lesion noted in peracute and acute forms of the disease. Other lesions that may be present usually do not have specific diagnostic value.

Treatment: The causative organism is inhibited by most antibiotics. Early treatment may reduce the severity of the disease, but treatment is less effective as the disease progresses. Treatment should include isolation of infected litters and administration of a broad-spectrum antibiotic to infected pigs, as well as to those not yet showing clinical signs. The treatment of pigs with no signs should be continued for several days. Pigs gain resistance with increasing age. Litters farrowed for some time after clinical signs have subsided should receive antibiotics prophylactically. The farrowing areas should be disinfected.

MANGE (LG. AN.)

A contagious skin disease caused by one of several species of mites that may spread by contact with diseased animals or their attendants or from various objects that have been in contact with diseased animals, e.g. harness, blankets, grooming utensils, bedding or stables. The incubation period for the development of clinical mange depends on the mode and the place of the infestation and the susceptibility of the host. Usually, 2 to 6 weeks elapse before the first visible skin lesions develop. Mites of similar appearance occurring in different host species are regarded as being different species or as varieties of the same species; they tend to be specific to their respective hosts.

MANGE IN HORSES

Sarcoptic mange (*Sarcoptes scabiei* var. *equi*) is the most severe type. It spreads very quickly on an infested horse as well as to other animals. Early lesions appear on the head, neck and shoulders. Regions protected by long hair and lower parts of the extremities usually are not involved.

The disease is first characterized by intense itching. Small papules and vesicles develop into an acute dermatitis, scaling increases rapidly and later crusts form. The bald and encrusted patches enlarge and the skin thickens, forming folds, particularly in the neck region. In advanced cases, the lesions may extend over the entire body, leading to emaciation, general weakness and loss of appetite. The course is always chronic. The prognosis is the most unfavorable of all the types of horse mange, particularly in severe infestations and in animals in poor condition.

For treating infested individuals, acaricidal preparations are applied by spraying, rubbing, or dipping. For groups of animals, dipping is the most convenient and effective method of treatment. Lime-sulfur (℞ 292) can be used if the dip is heated and the animals are dipped 4 to 6 times at intervals of 10 to 12 days. Toxaphene dip at 0.5% usually gives control with one application. Lindane at 0.06% concentration can be used as a spray or dip, where local laws permit its use.

Psoroptic scabies (caused by *Psoroptes ovis*) is a notifiable and quarantinable disease wherever it is found, but it has not been reported in horses in the U.S.A. in 30 or 40 years. It produces lesions on sheltered parts of the body, such as, under the forelock and mane, at the root of the tail, under the chin, between the hind legs, and in the axillae. Mites sometimes may be found in the ears. The lesions are similar to the sarcoptic type, but the crusts are larger and thicker, the skin is less folded, the itching is less severe, and the mites are more easily found in the crusts since they are surface dwellers and do not burrow. The course is chronic and the prognosis favorable. The treatment corresponds to that for the sarcoptic type or for psoroptic scabies of cattle (*see* below).

Chorioptic mange, often known as "leg mange," is caused by *Chorioptes bovis.* Cutaneous lesions are found chiefly on the lower parts of the hind legs. In severe cases, skin lesions may spread to the flanks, shoulders and neck. The disease is characterized by intense itching, scales, crusts, thickening of the skin and, in neglected cases, a moist dermatitis in the fetlock region. The signs subside in summer; however, with the return of cold weather, they develop again. The chorioptic mites are easily found in scrapings collected from the affected area. The course as a rule is chronic; the prognosis for "leg mange" is favorable. Treatments recommended for other mange mites also are effective against chorioptic mange.

Demodectic mange is seldom diagnosed in horses. The mites live in the hair follicles and in the sebaceous glands and produce papules and ulcers, particularly around the eyes and on the forehead. Subsequently the lesions spread to the shoulders and finally over the entire body. The affected skin is covered with scales. Pruritus is absent. There is no satisfactory treatment.

MANGE IN CATTLE
(Barn itch)

All types of mange occur in cattle, but the chorioptic type usually is predominant. Identification of the type of mange present and its differentiation from other dermatoses can only be achieved microscopically. At times mange and ringworm occur simultaneously or as intercurrent infections in herds and individual animals.

Scabies (*Sarcoptes scabiei* var. *bovis*) lesions first appear on the head and neck and then spread to other parts. Sometimes, the lesions appear in the perineal region and between the thighs. The skin eruptions are similar to those in horses. They are characterized by a squamous, crusted appearance; the skin itself thickens, forming large folds. The lesions may heal spontaneously during the summer, particularly when the animals are kept on pasture.

Common scabies of cattle (psoroptic mange) is caused by *Psoroptes ovis* which also attacks horses, sheep, and Rocky Mountain bighorns in the U.S.A., Canada and Mexico. It is a notifiable and quarantinable disease, and when suspected should be reported immediately to regulatory officials. The disease is now appearing in epidemic proportions in range and feedlot beef cattle in the Central States of the U.S.A. with the largest numbers of outbreaks reported from Texas, New Mexico, Oklahoma, Kansas, Colorado and Nebraska. It appears first on the withers and soon spreads along the neck and back, over the shoulders and brisket to the belly and flanks. In severe cases, lesions may cover almost the entire body and deaths in untreated calves and yearlings are not uncommon. The course is usually chronic, but may be acute in younger animals during the winter months; the prognosis is favorable if treatment is applied regardless of the weather. Four permitted dips are listed by the USDA: toxaphene 0.50 to 0.60% (28-day withholding period before slaughter required), coumaphos 0.30% (no withholding period required), phosmet 0.20 to 0.25% (21-day withholding period before slaughter required), and hot lime-sulfur (2% calcium polysulfides heated to 95 to 105°F [35 to 40.5°C]). Only hot lime-sulfur is registered for use on lactating dairy cows. The regulations call for 2 dippings of known infested animals in any of the permitted dips at intervals of 7 to 14 days, depending upon the product used. Exposed cattle must also be dipped twice in coumaphos or phosmet, but only a single dipping is required in toxaphene or hot lime-sulfur. Owners should not attempt to treat cattle infested with psoroptic scabies on their own. The present widespread occurrence of scabies in cattle is thought to be due, in large part, to the frequent use of ineffective or partially effective acaricides on cattle moving in the market channels. Infested cattle should be dipped, not sprayed.

Chorioptic mange caused by *Chorioptes bovis* is the commonest type of mange in cattle. The skin lesions develop chiefly in the tail region and spread to other parts of the body. Sometimes, the lesions start on the legs and the disease is called "leg mange." The treatment of cattle mange is similar to that described for horses. Lime-sulfur dips (℞ 292) are effective, if the full course of 6 treatments is given—one treatment every 7 to 10 days. Dips or sprays containing 0.06% lindane are effective where use of this drug is permitted. All of the permitted dips for psoroptic scabies are effective against *Chorioptes*.

Demodectic mange is transferred from cow to calf while nursing and causes considerable damage to hides. The disease is rarely found in cattle less than 1 year of age. The lesions generally appear on the neck, shoulder and face of dairy cattle and are rarely visible or palpable on beef cattle. In rare instances lesions may appear over the entire body surface. Approximately 90% of hides that have been dehaired prior to tanning are found to contain blemishes due to demodectic mites. First, small papules and nodules develop. Sometimes, they have a red color and a thick, white material, having a waxy consistency, can be expressed from them. This caseous and greasy material contains numerous mites. In rare cases, the nodules are filled with pus and may coalesce, forming abscesses covered with small scales. In some cases, cutaneous lesions consist of thick crusts and the skin thickens forming heavy folds. The course of bovine demodectic mange generally is mild, but may extend over many months. Recovery is usually spontaneous. There is no satisfactory treatment. In valuable animals the best therapeutic results have been achieved with incisions of the nodules and painting with tincture of iodine.

MANGE AND SCABIES IN SHEEP AND GOATS

In sheep, these diseases are caused by *Sarcoptes scabiei* var. *ovis* (*megnini*), *Chorioptes bovis* and *Psoroptes ovis*.

Sarcoptic mange in sheep occurs only on the nonwooly skin, starting, as a rule, on the head and face; it is very rare.

Chorioptic mange is the most frequent type in sheep. It is most often found on the hind legs and between the toes, or on the scrotum of rams. It is commonly called "leg" or "foot mange."

Psoroptic scabies (sheep scab) is a notifiable disease and affected flocks are subject to quarantine and dipping regulations. No psoroptic scabies of sheep has been reported from the U.S.A. since 1970, but it still exists in cattle. Countries where sheep scabies (scab) is still a problem include Great Britain, Eire, France, West Germany, Lebanon, Israel, Egypt, South Africa, Kenya, Argentina, Brazil and Mexico. It occurs almost exclusively on the wooled parts of the body where it produces large, scaly, crusted lesions. Biting and scratching brought on by intense itching are generally the first signs. When large skin areas are involved, animals gradually become emaciated and suffer from anemia and cachectic hydremia. Psoroptic mites are sometimes found in the ears of sheep, but not in the absence of mites on other parts of the body.

Since large numbers of animals usually are affected, dips are the most suitable, and in the case of psoroptic scabies, the only approved method of treatment. A single dipping in 0.50 to 0.60% toxaphene will eliminate all of the mites that attack sheep except *Psorobia* (*Psorergates*) *ovis*. Other dips approved for use against *Psoroptes*, viz. coumaphos (0.30%) and phosmet (0.20 to 0.25%) will also control chorioptic mites, but their efficacy against *Sarcoptes* has not been tested. Lindane is the only approved dip allowed against *Psoroptes* in Great Britain; diazinon is used in South Africa.

Demodectic mange has also been reported in sheep, causing skin lesions similar to those in other large animals.

Psoroptic ear mange in goats is caused by *Psoroptes cuniculi*, which also attacks domestic rabbits. The condition is usually much more severe in Angora goats than in milk goats, and sometimes spreads to the head, neck, and body causing much irritation and damage to the mohair. It is a notifiable disease of Angora goats in Texas where it is less common than in adjacent areas. The course is chronic and the prognosis is good. Any of the acaricides approved for use as sheep dips will eliminate ear mange from goats. Lactating dairy goats should not be treated with anything but lime-sulfur solution (℞ 292).

In **goats, demodectic mange** is similar to that described for dairy cattle. The cutaneous lesions are found on the skin of the neck, shoulder, thorax and flank. The nodules, ranging in size from pinhead to hazelnut, contain a thick, grayish material of waxy consistency, which can be easily expressed. Numerous demodectic mites are found in this material. The nodules of demodectic mange in goats appear as cysts with mild inflammation in the surrounding tissue. This infection in goats may be a very stubborn condition causing, in some countries, great damage to the hides. There is no satisfactory treatment. In valuable goats, incision of the nodules and painting with tincture of iodine gives the best therapeutic results.

"ITCH MITE" INFESTATION

An infestation of sheep by *Psorobia* (*Psorergates*) *ovis* in which the pruritus induced by the mite caused the host to bite and rub the affected areas damaging the fleece. The disease has been reported from Australia, New Zealand, South Africa, the U.S.A., Argentina and Chile. As control measures can be carried out before the infestation becomes serious, the disease is not regarded as of major economic importance.

The life cycle (6 stages—egg, larval, 3 nymphal and male and female adult) is completed in 4 to 5 weeks. The development of all stages occurs in the stratum malpighii of the epidermis, where the mites are considered to feed on cell fluids.

The first signs often occur about 2 to 3 years after arsenical dips are abandoned in favor of the newer insecticides. The incidence increases slowly in the flock until, after 3 or 4 years, 10% of the older sheep may be actively biting or rubbing. Characteristic signs are few. A damaged fleece, alopecia, crusting or chronic dermatitis resulting mainly from self-inflicted trauma (in the absence of *Psoroptes*, lice, keds, mycotic dermatitis, fleece rot or grass seeds) are suspicious signs. The withers and sides of the trunk are usual sites of involvement.

Demonstration of the mites in skin scrapings is the only positive diagnosis (*see* CLEARED, UNSTAINED SMEAR METHOD, p. 1478). Several skin scrapings may be necessary.

Dipping in 1% lime-sulfur or 0.2% arsenic is considered to give satisfactory results. This need not be done annually, but only as the incidence in the flock warrants.

MANGE IN SWINE

The **sarcoptic type** caused by *Sarcoptes scabiei* var. *suis* is the only form of any importance in swine. The lesions usually start on the head, spread over the body, the tail and the legs. The skin is thickened, rough and dry, covered with grayish crusts and thrown into large folds. Itching is intense, and growth is stunted. Deep skin scrapings should be examined as swine also suffer from other kinds of skin disease, including ringworm. Spraying with lindane at a concentration of 0.05 to 0.1% or malathion at 0.05% is effective; 0.25% chlordane solution also has been used. (Use of some or all of these on food-producing animals is prohibited in some countries.)

Demodectic mange occurs also in swine, causing skin lesions similar to those seen in other large animals. Treatment with remedies used in sarcoptic mange has been attempted, but the results appear unreliable.

MANGE (SM. AN.)

CUTANEOUS ACARIASIS

A skin disease caused by parasitic mites of either the sarcoptic or demodectic type. Sarcoptic mange is highly contagious while demodectic mange is normally noncontagious.

Etiology: Sarcoptic mange of dogs is caused by *Sarcoptes scabiei* var. *canis*. The body of the mite is almost circular with 4 pairs of legs, all except the posterior pair extending beyond the margin of the body. Eggs are laid in tunnels as the female burrows into the skin. Eggs hatch in the tunnels and become larvae, which have only 3 pairs of legs. Sarcoptic mange of cats is caused by *Notoedres cati*, which is smaller and more circular than the mite that attacks dogs. The transition from ova to adult usually takes 10 to 14 days.

Canine **demodectic mange** is caused by *Demodex canis*. The mites have vermiform bodies and the elongated abdomen is marked with transverse striations. Adults and nymphs have, on the anterior portion of the body, 8 legs, each divided in 5 segments, while larvae have only 6 legs. All stages of the mite: eggs, larvae, nymphs and adults inhabit the hair follicles and sebaceous glands in the skin of mangy as well as normal dogs. The complete life cycle is not known. *D. cati* is occasionally found on cats and may cause lesions similar to those in the dog.

Clinical Findings: The sarcoptic mite causes intense itching as it burrows in the skin and the animal scratches and rubs persistently. The skin becomes dry, thickened and wrinkled. Crusts are formed in the involved areas. Usually, the lesions first appear on the head around the eyes, ears or muzzle and then spread to the neck, abdomen and extremities.

In cats, mange usually starts at the tips of the ears, spreads to the face and then to the whole head. It also may extend to involve the rest of the body and legs.

The *Demodex*-infested animal may have a variety of lesions from small patches of hairlessness around the eyes or over the body to extensive bloody or purulent lesions completely covering the body. Skin lesions can be classified as squamous or pustular. In the squamous type, there is only a mild inflammatory change with absence of hair in the affected region and a slightly thickened skin with fine scales. The skin may be reddened or darkly pigmented to varying degrees.

In the pustular type, the skin is highly reddened, with blood and serum oozing from affected areas, along with purulent material resulting from bacterial invasion (usually *Staphylococcus aureus*). The skin may be thickened and often appears to have been worn away. Lesions may cover the entire body. Occasionally, the entire skin is markedly reddened with little or no pustule formation ("red mange"). In severe cases, the mites may invade the lymph nodes and other tissues.

Diagnosis: The mites should be demonstrated in skin scrapings. Since the demodectic mites are in the hair follicles and sebaceous glands and the sarcoptic mites are in burrows, deep scrapings of infested areas are best. A 6 to 10% solution of potassium hydroxide, placed on the slide with the skin scraping, dissolves the debris and the mites are seen more easily under the low power of the microscope.

Treatment: Clipping the hair, especially if the dog has a long coat, is important, for many lesions will be uncovered. A soap and water or mineral oil bath to soften and remove crusts and scurf assists the acaricide in reaching the mites. In treating sarcoptic mange, lime and sulfur dips and washes (℞ 292) have been successful, but several treatments always are necessary before all of the mites are destroyed. This is the safest treatment for puppies. Sulfur ointments (℞ 333) are useful, especially in localized lesions or in cases where dipping would not be practical. Benzyl benzoate emulsions or solutions also are practical; either a 25 or 50% emulsion (℞ 270) is excellent for topical application. Benzyl benzoate in combination with other acaricides (℞ 269) also gives excellent results. Dips containing 0.1% lindane have been widely used. A single and thorough dipping and scrubbing is often all that is necessary. Chlordane dips (℞ 273) given 7 days apart also are used successfully. Since the disease is so often generalized, dips are usually far more practical than the use of ointments.

The chlorinated hydrocarbon acaricides are toxic for cats. Lime and sulfur washes (℞ 292), sulfur ointments or rotenone compounds are successfully used. Good results can be obtained by using an ointment of sulfur (℞ 233) applied to affected areas.

Demodectic mange, particularly the generalized form, may be one of the most persistent of diseases and often responds poorly to treatment. The squamous or localized form often heals spontaneously. Benzyl benzoate emulsions (℞ 270), or an emulsion of lindane and benzyl benzoate (℞ 269), have been used successfully. These emulsions should be thoroughly massaged into the skin daily for a week and the animal then should be rested for another week before further applications are made, or treatment can be carried out every third day until the lesions heal. Not more than 30% of the body should be treated at any one time. Rotenone preparations, such as Canex (℞ 271), also are very useful. The use of organophosphates both orally and topically has given good results (℞ 319). In the generalized form of the disease, a 4% ronnel solution in propylene glycol applied to one-third of the body daily until no more mites can be demonstrated has given excellent results. Great care should be used when employing organophosphates; and in the latter treatment program, legal responsibility must be assumed by the veterinarian as the drug is not officially approved for this use. Demodectic mange in cats can be treated locally with Canex (℞ 271).

In cases where secondary infection has become established, vigorous antibiotic therapy is recommended, especially chloramphenicol, lincomycin, or erythromycin. Reports indicate that griseofulvin (℞ 365) may be used successfully as systemic therapy.

NASAL ACARIASIS

(Nasal mites)

An infestation of the nasal cavity and paranasal sinuses of dogs by the mite *Pneumonyssus (Pneumonyssoides) caninum* usually without, or with only mild, signs. The adult mite has a pale-yellow body. The gravid female contains a fully developed embryo that almost fills the abdomen. The method of transmission of the parasite is unknown.

Except for an accumulation of mucus and a mild hyperemia of the mucous membranes, no signs or lesions are usually attributed to the infestation. Signs of a severe rhinitis may occasionally be seen. Most infestations are found on postmortem examination. A few cases have been reported where the mite was found on the nose of sleeping dogs. Treatment has not been attempted.

OTOACARIASIS

(Otodectic mange, Ear mange, Parasitic otitis externa)

An infestation of the ears with parasitic mites, e.g. *Otodectes cynotis* in dogs and cats. (*See* PARASITIC OTITIS EXTERNA, p. 231. *See also* DISEASES OF RABBITS: EAR MITE INFESTATION, p. 1184).

CHEYLETIELLA INFESTATIONS

Mite infestations by *Cheyletiella parasitivorox* and related species on rabbits, cats, and foxes, and by *C. yasguri* on dogs have occasionally been reported to extend to humans if they are closely associated with infested animals. Most human infestations can be traced to infested cats that are allowed to sleep on a person's bed. The disease is highly contagious and cross-infestations between species occur. The causative agent, commonly known as the rabbit fur mite, inhabits the pelage and skin surface of animals; it also can live free in nature. It is a large mite (388 by 266 μ) easily identified microscopically by its large palpal claws, numerous feathered bristles and cones on the tarsi.

Two clinical forms, exfoliative and crustose, have been recognized in the dog. In the first, a scaling process (mimicking dandruff) occurs primarily on the dorsal trunk, and is most evident on the skin, with a few scales in the pelage. Alopecia and inflammatory changes are usually present only secondary to scratching. The degree of pruritus varies from moderate to intense. In the second form, multiple discrete, circular, alopecic crusts (2 to 5 cm in diameter) are observed on the dorsal and lateral trunk. The lesions may expand or enlarge and appear similar to ringworm; however, no inflammatory border is evident and no dermatophytes can be demonstrated. The lesion also resembles the crustose form of seborrhea that occurs so commonly in cocker spaniels.

Though cats may have the exfoliative form, most have the crustose variety. The lesions strongly resemble ringworm except that most of them occur on the neck and trunk.

Diagnosis depends upon identification of the organism in skin brushings. Deep scrapings are unnecessary. Material removed for microscopic examinations should be placed in 10% potassium hydroxide and viewed under 25X magnification.

Successful **treatment** may be achieved with derris washes or dustings, or the topical application of a variety of insecticides including 0.02% lindane (℞ 293), organophosphorus compounds (℞ 374), benzyl benzoate-lindane solution (℞ 303) or potassium tetrathionate shampoo with lindane (℞ 334). Topical applications should be repeated until clinical cure is achieved and neither the organism nor its eggs can be demonstrated by microscopic examination.

ACANTHOSIS NIGRICANS

Dermatosis characterized by acanthosis, hyperkeratosis and increased pigmentation. It occurs in dogs, particularly dachshunds.

Etiology: The cause of the disease is unknown, but some dogs have a significant decrease in thyroid activity. The pituitary, gonads and adrenal cortex also may be involved in the development of this condition. The frequent appearance of lesions in friction areas suggests that mechanical influence may also play a role.

Clinical Findings: Lesions occur with bilateral symmetry, consistently appearing first in the axillae and often in the inguinal region. Initially the skin is swollen, the hair thins and brown, gray-blue or black pigmentation appears. As the disease progresses, lesions may extend to the anterior and medial surfaces of the legs, flanks, ear flaps and ventral surface of the body, i.e. ventral thorax, abdomen, neck, chin and perineum. The skin thickens, forming deep folds, and becomes black. Greasy seborrheic secretions, scales and crusts accumulate. Although the primary disease is nonpruritic, seborrhea and secondary infection may cause moderate to severe itching.

The course of the disease is usually chronic. Since the advent of hormone therapy the prognosis has become more favorable, and many cases of acanthosis nigricans can be controlled, but permanent cure is rare.

Treatment: If possible, a definitive etiologic diagnosis should be made to serve as the basis for therapy. If hypothyroidism is diagnosed, L-thyroxin (℞ 202) should be administered. Triiodothyronine also may be effective as thyroid replacement therapy. The dose is 0.5 mcg/lb (1.1 mcg/kg) of body wt daily for 28 days. It can be repeated after 2 weeks of rest. Thyrotropic hormone, 1 to 2 USP units daily for 5 days, also is beneficial in some patients. Sex hormones may be used, especially, in aged dogs, in the same way as described in hormonal eczema (*see* MISCELLANEOUS DERMATOSES, below). Corticosteroids (℞ 154) are especially useful in dogs with severe hyperpigmentation. For topical therapy, sulfur ointment (℞ 452), antiseborrheic shampoos, ichthammol ointment (℞ 440) and corticosteroids in propylene glycol have been used. In obese animals, weight reduction may be beneficial.

MISCELLANEOUS DERMATOSES

A number of systemic diseases produce varying lesions in the skin as part of their clinical manifestation. These are most often noninflammatory and commonly display alopecia as part of their syndrome. In some instances the cutaneous changes are characteristic of the particular disease. Often, however, the dermatosis is not obviously associated with the underlying condition and careful differentiation must be made to separate a primary skin disorder from the secondary signs of an apparently unrelated or undiagnosed ailment. Some of these are mentioned briefly below, and are also described in the chapter on the specific disorder.

Dermatosis may be associated with nutritional deficiencies, especially those of proteins, fats, minerals, some vitamins, and trace elements. Dermatitis is sometimes observed in the course of chronic disorders of internal organs, such as nephritis, hepatitis or pyometra and with diseased anal glands. A variety of skin changes also may develop in the course of poisoning, e.g. hyperkeratosis in cattle, poisoning by thallium sulfate (rat poisons), ergot, mercury and iodides.

In dogs, dermatosis can develop as a result of endocrine dysfunction. In males, dermatoses may be associated with underdevelopment of the testicles and especially Stertoli cell tumors. Skin disorders caused by imbalance of sexual hormones are commoner in female than in male dogs. Skin lesions may also develop in dogs and cats after spaying and castration. These dermatoses assume, as a rule, a special location and character. Alopecia or a squamous eczema with crusted accumulations of skin debris characteristically develops around the base of the tail, perineum, thighs and posterior abdomen. In advanced cases, the lesions may spread to other parts of the body.

Dermatoses have also been observed in hypofunction of the thyroid gland. The skin lesions are characterized by diminished hair growth and bilaterally symmetrical alopecia. In rare cases, cutaneous signs of myxedema develop. The skin of the hypothyroid patient is dry, scaly, thickened and folded. Acanthosis nigricans and seborrheic disorders also may be found in association with the hypothyroidal state.

Faulty production of hypophyseal hormones also may cause dermatoses. Hypopituitarism is characterized by loss of hair, especially in the axillary region and on the sides of the thorax and abdomen. Hyperfunction of the adrenal glands also is manifested by skin changes. In diabetes mellitus, pruritus and secondary infection may occur.

The treatment of all these conditions depends on a specific etiologic diagnosis. Once this is established and dealt with, the skin lesions usually need only symptomatic care (e.g. control of scratching) until they disappear with the resolution of the primary disease.

If a hormonal deficiency is present replacement therapy is indicated. In gonadal hormone deficiencies, androgens and estrogens are used. In male dogs 0.25 mg/lb (0.5 mg/kg) of body wt is given orally daily. Where skin lesions are caused by testicular tumors, castration is indicated. In females with eczema associated with hypoestrinism, 0.1 to 0.5 mg of diethylstilbestrol is given daily. For treatment of hypothyroidism L-thyroxine (℞ 202) is given orally.

ALOPECIA

(Baldness, Atrichia)

Local or general loss of hair, fur or wool. True alopecia is baldness without other visible skin disease. However, the term alopecia is also associated with many inflammatory skin disorders.

Etiology: Congenital alopecia has been described in cow, horse, dog and cat. Hairlessness invariably accompanies congenital goiter in pigs farrowed by iodine-deficient sows. Acquired alopecia is due to a variety of diseases and intoxications, e.g. gastroenteritis, pneumonia, dietary deficiencies, infectious diseases, particularly those causing febrile reactions or epithelial destruction, and poisoning as by mercury, thallium, iodine or formaldehyde. Disorders of the thyroid, pituitary and gonads have caused hair loss, especially in dogs, as have large doses of estrogens. Temporary alopecia in horses, sheep and dogs is sometimes seen in advanced pregnancy or lactation. Localized hair loss may result from repeated local friction, the continued application of chemicals or irritants, the presence of ectoparasites and X-rays.

Clinical Findings: Alopecia in veterinary medicine is a frequent sign of a specific skin disease, e.g. ringworm and mange. The loss of hair in acquired alopecia usually starts as localized areas of baldness, which then may increase in size, coalesce with adjacent lesions, or remain static. Pruritus is variable, depending on the primary cause. In neurogenic and endocrine alopecia, the lesions are confined to local areas or show a symmetric pattern of development. The course of alopecia is chronic and the prognosis unfavorable, unless the primary cause is identified and treated.

Treatment: The primary cause of the alopecia must be diagnosed and treated for satisfactory recovery to take place. The extent of recovery depends on the duration of the disease and the amount of damage to the hair follicles. Particular attention should be given to diet and skin cleanliness. In alopecia arising from endocrine hypofunction, substitution therapy is indicated. In other cases removal of obviously diseased glands may be helpful. Dogs affected with a hypothyroidism characterized by alopecia respond well to thyroid therapy (℞ 202). Local treatment of alopecia is of questionable value.

ECZEMA NASI OF DOGS

(Collie nose, Nasal solar dermatitis)

A congenital, abnormal reaction of the skin to sunlight, mostly in collies, Shetland sheepdogs, German shepherd dogs and mixed breeds closely related to these. The disease primarily affects the nose, the eyes and the adjacent areas.

Clinical Findings: The disease runs a slow, insidious course. The onset is mild; as the condition progresses, the skin on the bridge of the nose becomes markedly irritated and the lesion may extend from the dorsum of the nose to the periorbital skin, with an associated conjunctivitis and blepharitis. Exfoliation of the skin of the nose becomes progressive with encrustation, ulceration and bleeding. Depigmentation occurs and the skin becomes pink to bright red and sore. The lesions are most intense in the summer months and subside during the winter.

Treatment and Prophylaxis: The condition may greatly improve merely by keeping the dog away from sunlight or by the application of PABA-containing topical preparations. Local application of an antibiotic corticosteroid ointment also is beneficial in resolving the lesion (e.g. ℞ 471). Unfortunately, on cessation of treatment, the signs often reappear, so the therapy must be more or less continuous during the season in which signs are obvious. Tattooing the nose with a mechanical device manufactured for that purpose has been reported to be helpful in many animals.

URTICARIA

(Nettle rash, Hives)

A skin disorder characterized by multiple plaque-like eruptions, which are rounded in outline, elevated and flat-topped. The urticarial skin eruptions, formed by a localized edema in the dermis, often develop and disappear suddenly.

The disease occurs in all domestic animals, but most often in horses (*see also* SWEET ITCH, p. 962) and pigs. Allergic urticaria may be either exogenous or endogenous. Exogenous hives may be produced by toxic, irritating products of the stinging nettle or by the stings or bites of insects, and can occur most during the summer season, in horses, dogs and swine. Some chemicals such as carbolic acid, turpentine, carbon disulfide, or crude oil also may cause the condition.

Sensitive animals, particularly short-haired dogs and purebred horses, also may exhibit a phenomenon called **dermographism,** wherein rubbing or whipping produces urticaria-like skin lesions. It is of no clinical significance.

Endogenous or "symptomatic" urticaria may develop after inhalation or absorption of ingested allergens and has been mostly seen in horses and dogs (*see* ATOPIC DERMATITIS, p. 8). In horses, it has been noted in the course of gastrointestinal conditions, particularly severe constipation or inflammation of the intestinal mucosa. Sensitive animals may develop urticaria as an allergic reaction after feeding on various plants, foodstuffs, or after parenteral administration of foreign proteins, particularly serums, vaccines, antibiotics, especially penicillin, and bacterins (*see* URTICARIAL REACTIONS, p. 6). Urticaria has been observed in cows being dried off and in bitches during estrus. In young horses, dogs and pigs, urticaria has been associated with intestinal parasites. **Angioneurotic edema** is a variant of urticaria in which there is diffuse subcut. edema, often localized to the head, limbs or perineum.

Clinical Findings: The wheals or plaques appear within a few minutes or hours of exposure to the causative agent. In severe cases, the cutaneous eruptions are preceded by fever, loss of appetite, or dullness. Horses often become excited and restless. The skin lesions are of a rounded shape, flat-topped, varying in diameter from ½ to 8 in. (1 to 20 cm), and may be slightly depressed in the center. They can develop on any part of the body, but mainly on the back, flanks, neck, eyelids and the legs. In advanced cases, they may be found on the mucous membranes of the mouth, nose, conjunctiva, rectum and vagina. As a rule, the lesions disappear as rapidly as they arise, usually within a few hours.

In sheep, the urticarial skin lesions usually are observed only on the udder and on the hairless parts of the abdomen. In pigs, the eruptions have been observed around the eyes, on the snout, the abdomen and between the hind legs, as well as on the back.

In general, the prognosis for urticaria in animals is favorable. A fatal outcome is rare and then probably due to anaphylactoid effects.

Treatment: Acute urticaria usually disappears spontaneously without treatment. In especially severe cases, epinephrine (℞ 529) or antihistamines (℞ 556, 560) should be given IV. The rapid acting forms of adrenocorticosteroids, hydrocortisone sodium succinate 100 to 500 mg IV or prednisolone sodium succinate or hemisuccinate 50 to 200 mg IV, are useful in dogs and cats. The lesions promptly disappear, but will return rapidly if the allergen is not eliminated. Usually local treatment of the urticarial skin lesions is not necessary. In especially severe cases, cold packs of water, vinegar or alcohol (70%) may be applied.

INTERDIGITAL "CYSTS"

Inflamed, multiform nodules (not true cysts) involving the interdigital webs of dogs. Opinions differ on their etiology; the most probable main causes are: (1) foreign bodies, ingrowing hairs, awns and grains of sand, which cause granulomatous reactions, and (2) bacterial infections, mainly staphylococcal, which cause suppurative reactions. Hypersensitivity to contact or bacterial allergens may also play a role.

Clinical Findings: In its early stage, the interdigital lesion appears as a small papule, but later it progresses to a nodule. The latter usually is between 1 and 2 cm in diameter, reddish purple, shiny, fluctuant, and may rupture when palpated to exude a bloody material. There may be single or multiple nodules on one or more feet. Those caused by foreign bodies are usually solitary and often occur on a front foot. Recurrence is not common in these cases. If caused by bacterial infection, there may be several nodules with new lesions developing as others dry up. Pain may or may not be apparent, but is more common in nodules that are about to rupture and which contain foreign bodies.

Treatment: Foreign-body granulomas may respond to application of moist heat for 15 to 20 minutes 3 to 4 times a day, and removal of the foreign object. One or 2 weeks are required for the lesion to resolve. If hot foot baths are not effective, surgical excision is the most practical approach.

Bacterial lesions are treated systemically with antibiotics selected according to culture and sensitivity results. High doses and prolonged treatment may be required. Lesions should be surgically incised and debrided. Antibiotic dressings may then be applied for several days followed by daily soaking or washing with antiseptic solutions (℞ 439, 602). Therapy with staphylococcal bacterins and toxoids also has been used successfully.

SADDLE SORES

(Collar galls)

The saddle region of riding horses (or shoulder area of those driven in harness) frequently is the site of injuries to the skin and deeper soft and bony tissues. Clinical signs vary according to the depth of injury and the complications caused by secondary infection. Sores affecting only the skin are characterized by inflammatory changes that may range from erythematous through papular, vesicular, pustular and finally necrotic. Frequently the condition starts as an acute inflammation of the hair follicles and progresses to a purulent folliculitis. The affected areas show loss of hair and are swollen, hot and painful. The serous or purulent exudate dries, forming crusts. Advanced lesions are termed "galls." In cases of more serious damage of the skin and underlying tissues, abscesses may develop. They are characterized by hot, fluctuating, painful swellings from which purulent and serosanguineous fluid can be aspirated. Severe damage to the skin and subcutis or deeper tissues results in dry or moist necrosis. Chronic saddle sores are characterized by a deep folliculitis (hard nodules) or a localized indurative and proliferative dermatitis.

Treatment: Excoriations and inflammations of the skin of the saddle and harness regions are treated as any other dermatosis. Absolute rest of the affected parts is necessary. During the early or acute stages, astringent packs (Burrow's solution or 2% lead acetate) are indicated. Chronic lesions and those superficially infected may be treated by warm applications and massage with stimulating ointments (iodine), or antibiotic ointment (℞ 446). Hematomas should be aspirated or incised. If tissue necrosis occurs, the devitalized tissue should be surgically removed. A skin astringent and antiseptic of value in some cases consists of 500 ml of 0.1% alcoholic sublimate, 30 gm tannic acid and 1 gm gentian violet.

LAMINITIS OF CATTLE

An aseptic inflammation of the tissues of the digits primarily involving the hoof laminae. It commonly occurs as an acute syndrome and some animals will go on to develop the chronic form of the disease. The acute form is often a sequela to the over-feeding of grain (q.v., p. 143). Acute laminitis also occurs in cows shortly after calving, usually related to cases of acute metritis or acute mastitis in these animals.

Clinical Findings: Acutely affected animals tend to move stiffly with an arched back, the hind limbs under the body and the forelimbs placed well in front. Those most severely involved are often reluctant to move, prefer to lie, and exhibit difficulty in getting up. Local signs such as tenderness of the skin above the coronet, sensitivity of the hoof wall to pressure from hoof pincers and increased pulsation in the arteries over the fetlock have been reported but are difficult to appreciate on clinical examination in cattle.

Acute laminitis that does not respond to treatment or recover spontaneously in 5 to 10 days may develop into the chronic form. These animals are also stiff, reluctant to move and in cases of a long duration often show a marked change in the hoof. These changes include an elongation of the foot, curling up of the toe (slipper foot), concavity and prominent ridges of the wall.

Both acute and chronic cases of laminitis can lead to vascular damage in the foot sometimes resulting in sole ulcers. Septic laminitis may be a complication of sole ulcers, foreign body penetration and stable foot rot (q.v., p. 955).

Diagnosis: A complete history and careful clinical examination will usually allow a diagnosis of acute laminitis and differentiate it from interdigital necrobacillosis, stable foot rot and injuries to the foot. Clinical signs will commonly permit a diagnosis of chronic laminitis, which can be confirmed by a lateral radiograph of one hoof to demonstrate the tilting of the distal phalanx that brings this phalanx closer to the bearing surface at the toe than in the normal foot.

Treatment: In the treatment of acute laminitis, the existing cause should, if possible, be removed (excess grain). The main methods of treatment have been corticosteroids and antihistamines; the old-fashioned remedy of standing cattle in cold running water is still considered useful. There is no practical treatment for chronic laminitis and affected feeder cattle should be sent to slaughter as soon as possible. Valuable breeding cattle can be maintained for a time by frequent paring of excessive wall and heel growth.

Prevention: Careful management practices related to grain feeding will prevent many cases. Conditions which can cause a severe inflammatory reaction leading to acute laminitis, e.g. acute mastitis and metritis, should be treated promptly and adequately. The prevention of chronic laminitis can only be directed to the prevention of the acute form, and if it occurs, attempting to obtain a rapid cure.

FOOT ROT OF CATTLE

(Interdigital necrobacillosis, Foul of the foot)

An acute or subacute necrotizing infection involving the skin and the immediately adjacent soft tissues of the interdigital spaces. The disease is worldwide and all breeds of cattle are susceptible. Throughout the U.S.A., it is common in cattle confined in pens or on pasture.

Etiology: *Fusobacterium necrophorum (Sphaerophorus necrophorus)* is the only organism that may be recovered consistently from the lesion. (*See also* FOOT ROT IN SHEEP, p. 956.) Before the infectious agent can gain entry, some break in the continuity of the skin or horn of the foot must occur. Injury to the skin in the interdigital space and around the coronet is commonly caused by sharp objects, by maceration from continuous exposure to mud or manure, and possibly by other primary infectious agents. Cracks in the horny integument may also permit entry of infection.

Clinical Findings: Once established in the injured epithelium, the organisms invade connective tissue, causing a coagulative necrosis. Rarely, the infection may spread proximally in the limb and metastasize to the lungs and other viscera and to joints other than those of the foot. One or more feet may be infected. In the acute stage, inflammation usually extends to the fetlock joint. Interdigital tissues are necrotic and covered with a dry exudate; the surrounding tissue is edematous and hyperemic. The necrotic process may extend deep into connective tissue and occasionally into the interphalangeal joints; such chronically infected joints discharge exudate continuously through tracts that open into the interdigital space or around the coronet. Healed feet show thickening from scar tissue, which may bulge into the interdigital space. Healed coffin joints usually exhibit ankylosis and exostoses of the second and third phalanges.

The patient is acutely lame. In severe cases, anorexia and fever are present, weight is lost and milk yield falls. Deaths are extremely rare but may occur as a result of the spread of infection to internal organs. The course is short for uncomplicated cases and prolonged if joints become arthritic or other complications develop.

Diagnosis: This is based on history and the presence of the typical signs and lesions. Thorough cleaning and trimming of the hoof is essential to permit a complete inspection. The disease is to be differentiated from deep penetration of the foot by foreign bodies, mechanical injuries and sprains of various kinds, vesicular lesions from viral diseases and hematogenous infections of the feet. Radiographs occasionally are of value in identifying foreign bodies, arthritis, exostoses and other skeletal changes. Careful clinical examination will also differentiate this condition from sole ulcers, stable foot rot and interdigital fibromas.

Treatment: Early treatment is essential to shorten the course of the disease and prevent sequelae such as suppurative arthritis. The kind of treatment is usually determined by the class of cattle affected, housing method and stage of the disease. Valuable breeding stock are usually treated individually. The animal is closely confined and the foot is cleaned, trimmed and debrided if necessary. When an open lesion is present an antibacterial ointment (℞ 457) or 5% copper sulfate is applied and the foot is bandaged. If given early in the course of the disease, a single therapeutic dose of either penicillin (℞ 63) or sulfonamide (℞ 96, 102) is usually curative.

Commercial cattle of lesser value are usually treated orally. Individual treatment with a long-acting sulfonamide such as sulfabromomethazine (℞ 87) is satisfactory when only a few animals are affected. When numerous animals are affected, sulfonamides (e.g. ℞ 87) placed in the feed and copper sulfate foot baths (2 to 5%) are frequently used. The whole herd is driven through a foot bath once or twice daily for several days. Walking animals through a 1:20 mixture of powdered copper sulfate and slaked lime is useful around water holes or where a foot bath is not practical.

When suppurative arthritis occurs, the affected claw may be amputated through the first phalanx or by disarticulation of the pastern joint with curettage of the distal end of the first phalanx to destroy the secreting joint surface. A third method, disarticulation through the infected coffin joint distal to the coronary band is less commonly performed. Animals can usually function well with one claw removed, if a sound claw and strong pastern remains.

Prophylaxis: Avoidance of sources of injury to the feet is of primary importance. Barn lots should be cleaned frequently and be smooth, level and free of sharp objects, especially cinders. Mud holes and stagnant pools that act as reservoirs for the infective organisms should be eliminated. Routine foot trimming should be practiced when cattle are confined on soft footing. If concrete is so rough that it will cause excessive hoof wear, generous amounts of bedding should be provided. Foot injuries should be treated promptly. Ethylenediamine dihydroiodide is commonly added to salt in an attempt to prevent foot rot; although controlled experimental evidence of its effectiveness is lacking, the practice finds wide support among cattlemen.

STABLE FOOT ROT OF CATTLE

A condition occurring primarily in mature dairy cows stabled over the winter feeding period. It is the commonest condition affecting cows' feet during this time. The hind feet are more commonly involved and usually the medial rather than the lateral claws.

Etiology: Predisposing factors include wet, dirty stables and overgrown feet. Some cattle may have inherited poor horn quality or deformities of the feet leading to the problem. The condition begins with an infection that primarily involves the heels with necrosis of horn in this region. Both *Fusobacterium necrophorum (Sphaerophorus necrophorus)* and *Bacteroides (Fusiformis) nodusus* have been isolated from these necrotic areas.

Clinical Findings: The necrosis develops gradually and treatment early in the condition will arrest the process before lameness develops. If untreated, the necrosis will lead to deep, black grooves in the sole, adjacent to the necrotic heels. This can lead to severe lameness caused by such complications as undermining of the sole or severe infections along the axial and abaxial grooves and leading to the sensitive laminae and deeper structures of the foot.

Treatment: It is most important to remove all necrotic horn. Uncomplicated cases should then be kept in a clean, dry area and affected feet placed in a 5% copper sulfate foot bath for 20 min. daily for 4 to 5 days. Parenteral antibiotics are not required. Complicated cases may require extensive hoof trimming, bandaging, a wooden block applied to the sound claw and in some cases even claw amputation.

Prevention: Control measures include regular foot trimming, improved housing conditions and regular exercise (cows turned outside most days during the winter). The condition has been controlled in herds with a severe problem by having the cattle pass through foot baths of 5% copper sulfate or 5% formaldehyde twice weekly. Where freezing of these solutions would occur, a mixture of one part copper sulfate to 9 parts of slaked lime can be used as a dry foot bath.

INFECTIOUS FOOT DISEASES OF SHEEP

(Foot Rot)

Apart from the diseases that also affect other parts of the body (e.g. foot-and-mouth disease, contagious ecthyma, bluetongue and dermatophilosis) there is a group of infections specific to the feet. These diseases are all due to mixed infections with combinations of bacteria including the gram-negative anaerobe *Fusobacterium necrophorum (Sphaerophorus necrophorus).* The skin between the claws is the primary site of invasion but this does not occur when the stratum corneum is dry and intact. Prior damage by water maceration, frostbite or mechanical trauma is necessary. Epidermal penetration by *F. necrophorum* and *Corynebacterium pyogenes* induces a transient condition, ovine interdigital dermatitis (OID). Where there is a concurrent invasion by *Bacteroides (Fusiformis) nodosus,* foot rot results. This may be benign or virulent depending on the strain of *B. nodosus* involved. When dermal and subdermal invasion by *F. necrophorum* and *C. pyogenes* occurs the disease is infective bulbar necrosis (IBN) or heel abscess. These 3 distinct but related conditions are described in turn.

OVINE INTERDIGITAL DERMATITIS (OID)

A necrotizing condition of the interdigital skin due to a mixed infection with *F. necrophorum* and *Corynebacterium pyogenes.* Cold weather and damp pastures are considered to be predisposing causes. A similar condition in sheep grazing on stubble has been attributed to mechanical damage inflicted by the short, stiff stubble; similarly, injuries to the interdigital epithelium frequently result from "clay balling," a condition in which hardened balls of clay mold themselves into the shape of the interdigital space, and become difficult to dislodge causing constant irritation and great lameness.

Clinical Findings: Lameness may be seen in more severe cases. The interdigital skin is usually red and swollen. The necrotic epidermis tends to erode in patches. At the skin-horn junction the hoof may be separated slightly from the underlying tissue. The disease is often transient but may persist, or recur, while pastures remain wet; most lesions heal rapidly with the advent of dry conditions. Where the disease is associated with stubble, there is usually improvement on removal to ordinary pastures.

Diagnosis: The clinical appearance is characteristic but similar conditions involving other organisms must be excluded. In the case of foot rot (*see* below) microscopic examination of stained smears will reveal the presence of *Bacteroides (Fusiformis) nodosus*. Strawberry foot rot (q.v., p. 929) affects the hairy skin of the coronet and pastern. Virus diseases such as contagious ecthyma and foot-and-mouth disease must be diagnosed by reference to flock history and appropriate virologic methods but *F. necrophorum* may infect these also.

Control and Treatment: Healing may be assisted by the external application of disinfectants such as 5% formalin (℞ 435), and by removal to drier pastures if available. Sheep on stubble should be transferred to ordinary pasture.

VIRULENT FOOT ROT (VFR)

A specific chronic necrotizing disease affecting the epidermis of the interdigital skin and hoof matrix. It commences as an interdigital dermatitis and extends to involve large areas of the hoof matrix. The infected tissue is destroyed so that the hoof loses its anchorage and becomes detached. Foot rot is contagious and under suitable conditions the morbidity may approach 100%. The infection is also found in cattle, goats and deer.

Etiology: Foot rot is due to a mixed infection in which 2 gram-negative anaerobic bacteria, *B. nodosus* and *F. necrophorum*, are essential. The latter is a normal resident of the sheep's environment and is thus always available. Infection, therefore, depends on the presence of *B. nodosus*, a strict parasite that does not survive for more than a few days in the soil or pastures; hence its availability depends on the presence of infected animals. *B. nodosus* is accordingly regarded as the transmissible and specific causal agent of foot rot, although its contribution to the disease process is not necessarily greater than that of *F. necrophorum*.

The transmission of foot rot to healthy animals requires a warm, moist environment. Under these conditions the interdigital stratum corneum becomes macerated; filaments of *F. necrophorum* superficially invade the epidermis and induce OID (q.v., p. 956). If *B. nodosus* makes contact with the skin at this stage foot rot results.

Clinical Findings: The most obvious sign is lameness, which may be very severe. Some animals remain recumbent or on their brisket and knees, which tend to become depilated and ulcerated. Affected animals lose condition. Rams infected in the hind feet may be unable to serve and similarly ewes with hind-feet lesions may be unable to bear the weight of a ram at service. Wool production is reduced. In early cases, examination of the feet may reveal nothing more than dermatitis similar to OID. In slightly more advanced cases, where the infection has begun to extend into the hoof matrix, there is slight detachment of the hoof at the skin-horn junction. As the disease progresses the epidermal necrosis and separation of horn spread to the heel and sole, and finally the outer wall, so that the hoof is eventually attached only at the coronet. The necrotic tissue has a very characteristic unpleasant odor. Myiasis is a common sequela.

The disease persists for years in some sheep. Under dry conditions the infection may be hidden in small pockets within the foot where it is detectable only on paring. Sheep so affected act as subclinical carriers. Recovery from foot rot occurs but is not followed by appreciable immunity.

Diagnosis: Early cases confined to the interdigital space may be confused with OID or benign foot rot, advanced ones with infective bulbar necrosis (q.v., p. 959). In affected flocks with VFR, underrunning and separation of the hard horn of the hoof, usually of more than one foot, is characteristic. In IBN there is a deeper invasion and discharge of necrotic material; one foot only is normally affected. *B. nodosus*, a large gram-negative rod with swollen ends, is present in smears of stained necrotic material from foot rot although other bacteria predominate.

Treatment: Two methods are available but the success of both is dependent on sheep being kept in dry surroundings for the next 24 hours. In groups of sheep, optimum cure rates of 90 to 95% can be achieved by either. *Topical* treatment requires prior efficient surgical removal of all underrun horn to expose necrotic tissue. Bactericidal solutions such as 5% formaldehyde solution (℞ 435), 20% cetrimide, or 10% chloramphenicol in alcohol are then applied. *Parenteral* treatment consists of combined IM injections of procaine penicillin G and dihydrostreptomycin at dose rates of 50,000 to 70,000 IU/kg and 50 to 70 mg/kg, respectively. Detailed paring is unnecessary if parenteral treatment is used. Treated sheep should be re-examined in 2 to 3 weeks to identify those not responding.

Control: Some control may be achieved by walking affected flocks through formaldehyde foot baths during periods of the year that favor transmission. Intensive treatment of individual sheep should be restricted to dry periods that are more likely to result in a high cure rate.

B. nodosus vaccines are available that accelerate healing in affected animals and protect unaffected ones. Alum precipitated vaccines require 2 doses 4 to 6 weeks apart to establish effective immunity (regardless of weather) and this persists for about 2 months. Most affected sheep heal 4 to 6 weeks after immunity is established. Oil-emulsion vaccines induce immunity within 3 weeks of the initial dose and this may persist for 3 to 4 months. Revaccination is recommended at appropriate intervals in endemic areas. Vaccination alone should achieve a high degree but not complete control.

Eradication: Where desirable, eradication may be achieved by eliminating all cases of *B. nodosus* infection. Methods available are (a) replacement of the affected flock with disease-free sheep, (b) disposal of affected animals, and (c) rigorous treatment of all infections. Identification and elimination of all affected animals is achieved by clinical examination; no other diagnostic tests are available. Subclinical cases constitute a major problem since they may relapse and transmit infection at the next favorable season. Other ruminants (goats, deer and cattle) are potential sources of *B. nodosus* and should be considered in eradication programs.

Success in control or eradication is more likely if intensive individual treatments and inspections are done when the environment is dry and least favors the disease. At other times flock treatments—either foot bathing without paring or immunization—should be used.

BENIGN FOOT ROT (BFR)

A form of foot rot in which the infection is confined largely to the interdigital skin, with minimal underrunning of the adjacent horn. Lameness is common but less severe than in VFR. The etiology and pathogenesis are the same as in the virulent disease but the causal strains of *B. nodosus* are less virulent. *B. nodosus* isolated from cattle is usually benign for sheep. The economic effect of BFR (other than in lambs) is much less than in VFR. Topical treatment with 5% formaldehyde solution applied by foot bathing is adequate.

INFECTIVE BULBAR NECROSIS (IBN)

(Heel abscess, Digital suppuration)

A necrotizing disease of the deeper connective tissues of the foot, IBN usually has a sporadic incidence but may affect up to 15% of ewes in late pregnancy. IBN develops as a complication of OID and is not itself communicable.

Etiology: IBN is due to a mixed infection with *F. necrophorum* and *C. pyogenes*. These 2 organisms invade the deeper tissues of the foot as an extension of infection from the epidermal lesions of OID. The joints, joint capsules and ligaments all may be damaged. Hypoxia, due to an interference with blood supply to the foot, may be a factor facilitating invasions of deeper tissues but body weight seems also to be involved.

Clinical Findings: IBN develops most often in cool weather when the soil and pastures are wet. It appears during or following outbreaks of the interdigital infections from which it arises. The disease may affect any foot of any sheep but is commonest in the medial digits of the hind feet of ewes in late pregnancy. It is commoner in fat rams than in other dry sheep.

IBN causes severe lameness. The infected digit is usually carried and the bulb of the heel swollen. In the early stages it may be possible to express necrotic material through an opening in the interdigital skin via the channel left by the bacterial invasion. With healing of the interdigital lesions this opening usually closes to be replaced by one or more sinuses opening through the skin above the coronet. The lesions usually heal spontaneously, but slowly. This may leave the foot deformed or with its function affected and the sheep permanently lame, especially in cases where the necrotizing process has extended from the digital cushion into joints and in which ankylosis has occurred.

Diagnosis: Acute lameness, swelling of the digit and discharging sinuses distinguish IBN from foot rot. Characteristic filaments of *F. necrophorum* are seen in smears.

Control and Treatment: There is no known surgical or chemotherapeutic treatment of any value. The incidence may be limited by measures to control the initial cause of interdigital dermatitis and by controlling body weight in late pregnancy.

LAMELLAR SUPPURATION
(Toe abscess)

An acute infection of the laminar matrix of the hoof, usually restricted to the toe and abaxial wall. The disease is sporadic and the bacterial etiology variable, but cases due to *F. necrophorum* and *C. pyogenes* are usually more severe and extensive than those involving streptococci or other organisms. Infection probably enters through fissures in the bearing surface between the wall and sole and through vertical and horizontal fractures of horn. It is sometimes, but not always, assisted by impaction with mud and feces where there is overgrowth of the hoof or where there is separation of the wall following laminitis.

Front feet are more commonly affected. Lameness is severe and the affected digit hot and tender. There may be a sinus above the lesion at the coronet. Affected sheep recover rapidly after paring of the horn to provide dependent drainage.

FOOT ROT OF SWINE

Although the etiology remains uncertain this is an important disease in swine. Now reported from many countries, it is a disease of intensification and thus increasing in frequency. It affects pigs of all ages: perhaps the most severe economic loss is in breeders and suckers. In individual herds up to 60 to 70% of fatteners and 100% of breeders have lesions, and as many as 20% of a farm herd may be culled annually.

Etiology: Recognized or suspected precipitating factors include: trauma from abrasive concrete (particularly new "green" concrete), and metal floors, badly finished slats, lack of bedding, alternately housing on concrete and "dirt," wet unhygienic floors, and possibly nutritional factors such as lack of biotin, certain minerals, and excessive whey or skim-milk feeding. Infection with fusiform organisms, spirochetes and *Corynebacterium pyogenes* then occurs through breaches in the hoof horn. Hereditary factors, unequal claw size (medial claw smaller than lateral particularly in hind feet) and level of mineralization of horn, possibly associated with horn color or breed, may cause uneven wear or excessive wear of horn.

Clinical Findings: Severity of lameness depends on the site and extent of the lesions. Primary lesions are mainly erosions of, or cracks in, the horn. Erosions occur at the heel bulb, the heel-sole junction and the axial groove. Lesions rapidly coalesce to involve most of the volar surface. A white-line lesion can develop anywhere along the junction of the horn of the abaxial and volar surfaces. False sand-cracks occur in the wall usually towards the bulb of the heel. Localized hemorrhage into, or bruising of, the heel, sole or wall may be seen (attributed by some to biotin deficiency) and erosions may speedily follow.

The lateral hind claw is the most frequently affected, followed by the lateral and medial front claws; the medial hind is rarely involved.

Secondary Lesions: Any of the above may progress to penetration of the hoof and infection. This tunnels up the wall and pus escapes via a circumscribed sinus or a slit-like separation varying in length at the coronary band (a "bush" or "bumblefoot"). The resulting lesion may heal slowly, or bones and joints or the tendon sheaths may become involved thus leading to tendinitis, abscessation or septic arthritis higher up the leg. The claw may be shed. Other sequelae include pyemia with resultant abscess formation in lungs, brain and spinal vertebrae. Excess horn production can develop at the heel and the resultant "corn" may cause severe lameness, and if bilateral, a goose-stepping gait.

Diagnosis: Clinical examination will usually establish the diagnosis in the advanced case but care must be exercised with swine vesicular disease (q.v., p. 258) and the other vesicular viruses. The claw distribution of foot rot should help here but serology should resolve any doubt. The various causes of arthritis must also be eliminated and it must be appreciated that more than one condition may occur in the same animal.

Treatment: Complete prevention is impossible because of the continuing trend towards intensification. New concrete should be well-washed before contact with pigs and more care should be taken over the laying of concrete floors. The cardinal rules are: Natural aggregates are usually best and very hard crushed aggregates should not be used. The correct "mix" is important (do not add extra water) and overuse of tamp or trowel is to be avoided. Slats should be individually cast and pencil-edged, metal floors should be well-finished and bedding should be used when possible, particularly for the period from selection for breeding to service. Floors should be kept as dry as possible.

The routine use of a 2-in (5-cm) deep foot bath containing 5% copper sulfate or formaldehyde solution, once a day for 5 to 10 days and for prevention at 2- to 4-week intervals, will help. Careful paring of excess or necrotic horn, and surgical drainage is useful in valuable animals, and they may be turned out.

Treatment with antibiotics alone is rarely successful, but may help to prevent pyemia if osteomyelitis of the pedal bones occurs. Claw amputation (with a wire saw) can be tried but topical treatment with astringents usually gives as good, if not better, results. Heavy biotin supplementation is currently used, but with mixed results.

Foot Trauma in Suckling Piglets: Severe outbreaks of foot damage have been seen in piglets housed on badly laid concrete floors or badly designed and finished metal floors. Bruising of the sole is present soon after birth and further trauma leads to infection of the foot. Claws may be lost or ascending tendinitis and cellulitis may develop. There is marked lameness, severe growth retardation and even death.

Treatment should be aimed at preventing further trauma and controlling the infection with injections of antibiotics such as penicillin and streptomycin. Painting the floors with epoxy- or resin-based paints has given a measure of control.

SWEET ITCH IN HORSES

An annually recurring seasonal disease manifest as an acute irritating dermatitis along the mane and tail of horses during the warmer months of the year. In some countries the disease can spread ventrally to cover most of the body. It occurs widely and is known by various names such as "Queensland Itch" in Australia, "Microfilariaepityriasis" in the U.S.A., "Kasen disease" in Japan and "Allergic urticaria" in Israel. The lesions are intensely itchy and the horse scratches itself against fixed objects continuously. This causes loss of hair, crusting, thickening of the skin and occasionally secondary infection.

In England the disease starts about April each year and ends about October, after the first frosts, with 2 peaks of severity in May and September. There is commonly a history that one or both parents or grandparents also suffered from the disease, which is especially common in the hackney breeds. About 2.8% of ponies are affected in the U.K., 4.5% in Japan and up to a third of horses in Queensland.

The disease is rare in larger horses and thoroughbreds. It appears at any age above 18 months, with a peak at 4 or 5 years. Once it has appeared it will recur each summer with few horses recovering completely. The incidence is lower at higher altitudes, particularly in India, where it occurs on the plains, but not in the hills.

Infestation of the skin by the microfilariae of *Onchocerca cervicalis* has been suspected as the cause but it now appears to result from an allergy to the bites of various species of insects, particularly midges, e.g. in England, *Culicoides pulicaris*. (*See also* URTICARIA, p. 949.)

Treatment consists of reducing the irritation either locally or parenterally. Antihistamines are of some use as are corticosteroids with antibiotics, applied to the affected parts, but the injection of long acting corticosteroids is considerably better and longer lasting. Prevention is ideal but fly repellents have a short active life on the horse and should be applied daily in the late afternoon to have the maximum effect. The various experimental pyrethrin-piperonyl butoxide compounds give hope for a much longer repellent action of up to 3 or 4 days in dry weather.

Since the midge rarely enters buildings the best method of prevention is a combination of stabling the ponies and removing the midges from the area. The ponies are brought in some 3 hours before dusk to a stable where an insecticide strip is hanging. If feed is required then this is given at the time of stabling, no feed being left inside for any length of time.

PART II
TOXICOLOGY

ARSENIC POISONING

In describing arsenic poisoning and its treatment, distinction must be made between the effects produced by inorganic and organic compounds.

Inorganic Arsenicals

These include arsenic trioxide, arsenic pentoxide, sodium and potassium arsenate, sodium and potassium arsenite, and calcium and lead arsenate.

Etiology: Due to the diminishing use of these substances, poisoning is now relatively infrequent. Sources are preparations used as rodenticides, weed killers, baits and insecticides. Arsenites are used to some extent as dips for the eradication of ticks. Lead arsenate is sometimes used as a taeniacide in sheep.

Clinical Findings: Inorganic arsenic poisoning is an acute disease whose major action is on the gastrointestinal tract. Profuse, watery diarrhea, sometimes tinged with blood is characteristic. This condition is accompanied by severe colic, dehydration, weakness and depression. The pulse is weak and abdominal pain is evident. The underlying cause of these effects is increased capillary permeability and cellular necrosis. Animals inadvertently sprayed with soluble arsenites may exhibit massive skin necrosis. The onset is rapid and the course from hours to several weeks. In peracute poisoning, death may occur so rapidly that the animal is simply found dead.

Lesions: Principal effects are observed in the gastrointestinal tract. Inflammation of the intestine is followed by edema, rupture of the blood vessels, and necrosis of epithelial and subepithelial tissue. The necrosis may progress to perforation of the gastric or intestinal wall. The contents of the gut are fluid, tinged with blood, and may contain shreds of epithelial tissue. There is a diffuse inflammation of the liver and other abdominal viscera.

Laboratory Diagnosis: The chemical determination of arsenic in tissues and ingesta provides confirmation. Liver and kidney of normal animals rarely contain more than 1 ppm arsenic (wet weight); poisoning is associated with concentrations in excess of 3 ppm in these organs. The determination of arsenic in ingesta is of value if exposure occurred within the previous 24 to 48 hours. High concentrations of arsenic can be found in the urine for up to 14 days following ingestion.

Treatment: The only specific antidote of proven value is dimercaprol (℞ 628). The water-soluble derivative 2, 3-dimercaptopropane-1-sulfonate (DMPS) is stated to be superior to dimercaprol, but it is unavailable for clinical use in the U.S.A. Supportive therapy may be of even greater value, particularly where cardiovascular collapse is imminent, and should be directed toward restoration of blood volume and correction of the massive dehydration. Electrolyte solutions of the extracellular type are indicated for this purpose.

Organic Arsenicals

These include several phenylarsonic acid derivatives used in swine and poultry for the purpose of improving production and, in the case of swine, to treat dysentery. The major compounds in this class are arsanilic acid, roxarsone and carbarsone.

Etiology: This form of poisoning results from the use of excessive amounts of arsenic containing additives in the diet of swine and poultry. Severity and rapidity of onset are dose-related. Visible signs of poisoning may be delayed for weeks following incorporation of 2 to 3 times the recommended levels or may occur within days when the excess is tenfold or more over recommended levels.

Clinical Findings: The earliest sign is reduction in weight gains. This is followed by motor incoordination and posterior paralysis in swine and by convulsions in lambs. Animals remain alert and retain good appetites. Blindness is characteristic of arsanilic acid intoxication, but this property is not shared by the other organic arsenicals.

Laboratory Diagnosis: An analysis of the feed for either total arsenic content or the suspect compound is indicated if doubt exists.

Treatment: There is no specific treatment of demonstrated value, but the neurotoxic effects of these compounds are usually reversible. Blindness due to arsanilic acid is often irreversible, but the animals still retain good appetites and make good weight gains if competition for food is eliminated. Doubt exists as to the reversibility of the other neurotoxic effects when the onset of intoxication is slow and the exposure is prolonged.

LEAD POISONING

Lead poisoning is the most frequently diagnosed toxicologic problem in veterinary medicine. Its occurrence has been reported in all domestic species and in several species of zoo animals. It occurs most commonly in cattle and dogs, probably because of their indiscriminate eating habits and relative susceptibility to lead. Swine, goats, and chickens are relatively resistant. The occurrence of clinical lead poisoning may decline in the future because lead is now used sparingly in paint and there is a growing tendency toward the use of nonleaded gasoline.

Etiology: Exposure may be acute or chronic. Examples of acute exposure include cattle ingesting paint, plates from storage batteries, grease, or used motor oil. Dogs may receive an acute exposure by ingesting a large lead object, such as a curtain weight or a shotgun slug, that remains in the stomach. Chronic exposures culminating in clinical lead poisoning have occurred in cattle, horses and sheep ingesting vegetation and soil contaminated by atmospheric fallout from smelters and mining operations. (This has been the only source documented for clinical lead poisoning in horses.) Dogs may be chronically exposed by ingesting materials found in the home such as linoleum, crumbling plaster and peeling paint. A veterinarian diagnosing lead poisoning in a dog should advise an examination of any young children in the same dwelling since the sources of lead for dogs would also be available to children. Lead poisoning is rare in cats, probably because of their fastidious eating habits. Wild ducks frequently are poisoned by ingested lead pellets (q.v., p. 1147).

Clinical Findings: Young animals usually are more severely affected than older animals. Although the hemopoietic systems of some species are highly sensitive to lead, the major clinical signs are neurologic or abdominal in origin. Signs in cattle usually commence 2 to 3 days following ingestion of a fatal dose. The animal may bellow, stagger, show maniacal excitement, crash into objects and appear blind. Death occurs within 2 hours, or these convulsive episodes may be interspersed with periods of depression, ataxia, circling, and leaning and pushing on objects. Muscle twitching, "snapping" of the eyelids, and grinding of the teeth are commonly observed. In some cases dullness and anorexia are predominant with signs of colic. Often constipation, and occasionally diarrhea, persists for several days. The latter syndrome occurs more frequently in older cattle and sheep.

The chronic ingestion of contaminated forage for a period of weeks or months, during which cattle are asymptomatic, may suddenly culminate in a convulsive seizure and death. Thus the clinical manifestations of acute or chronic ingestion of lead in cattle are similar.

A chronic syndrome is characteristic of lead poisoning in horses. Clinical signs include loss of appetite, weight loss, depression, muscular weakness, stiffness of the joints, colic, diarrhea, laryngeal paralysis that causes the horse to "roar," and often anemia.

The initial signs in dogs may consist of anorexia, emesis, colic and diarrhea or constipation. The occurrence of neurologic signs, which may be expressed as either depression or excitation, usually alert the owner to seek veterinary assistance. Excitatory signs include hyperesthesia, hysterical barking, champing fits, short convulsive seizures and muscular spasms.

Lesions: Animals may die of lead poisoning with no observable gross lesions. Evidence of ingested lead-containing material may be found in the gastrointestinal tract. There may be gastritis, hyperemia, petechial or ecchymotic hemorrhages in various organs, and brain edema. Horses often die as a result of aspiration pneumonia secondary to the laryngeal paralysis.

Laboratory Diagnosis: The concentration of lead in the kidney cortex and liver or in unclotted blood provides adequate confirmation of lead toxicity; values greater than 4, 4 and 0.2 ppm (wet weight) for these tissues, respectively, indicate abnormal lead accumulation. Levels at least twice those indicated are usually found in patients with frank clinical signs of dying from lead poisoning. The presence of nucleated red blood cells and basophilic stippling is associated with canine lead poisoning.

Treatment: Effectiveness of treatment depends on the extent of injury to tissues, especially nervous tissue. Extensive and prolonged injury makes treatment of little value. Intestinal lavage or a cathartic, such as magnesium sulfate (℞ 632), may be employed to remove lead remaining in the digestive tract. Administration of CaEDTA (℞ 626) is indicated since it will mobilize lead from tissues and enhance its urinary excretion. Calcium (℞ 627) may be of some benefit when given IV because it relieves intestinal spasm. Good nursing and supportive care is necessary.

STRYCHNINE POISONING

Strychnine poisoning of a deliberate or malicious nature occurs occasionally. Accidental poisoning from rodenticides occurs frequently in dogs and occasionally in cats. Rarely, problems are encountered in livestock from excessive or continuous intake of nux vomica or other strychnine-containing medicaments.

Clinical Findings: Liquid strychnine sulfate may produce a response within a few minutes after ingestion, but often signs are delayed for at least an hour. The specific interval varies with the type of compound ingested, the dose, and the nature and amount of the stomach contents. Strychnine is usually oxidized and excreted from the body within 10 hours after absorption. Clinical signs appear within a few minutes to hours after ingestion of the strychnine. Early signs are apprehension, nervousness, tenseness and muscle stiffness. Severe tetanic seizures may appear spontaneously or be initiated by stimuli such as touch, sound, or a sudden bright light. The extreme and often overpowering extensor rigidity causes the animal to assume a "saw horse" stance. The violence of the spasm may throw an animal off its feet. Breathing may cease momentarily. The tetanic convulsion lasts from a few seconds to a minute or more. Periods of relaxation are intermittent and become less frequent as the clinical course progresses. During convulsions the pupils are dilated and the mucous membranes cyanotic. Frequency of the seizures increases and death eventually occurs from exhaustion or anoxia during a seizure. The entire syndrome, if untreated, may be less than 1 or 2 hours. There are no characteristic lesions.

Treatment: Prior to the appearance of signs, the stomach may be evacuated through the use of apomorphine (℞ 481). Gastric lavage, using warm hypertonic saline solution, 1:1,000 potassium permanganate, strong tea or a 2% tannic acid solution, should be attempted. A high enema with warm saline may be advantageous.

If convulsions are present or imminent, pentobarbital sodium IV is the drug of choice in small animals; chloral hydrate may be used in larger animals, but either must be given to effect and repeated as often as necessary. At this stage, morphine or apomorphine are contraindicated as they further depress medullary center activity and may cause early death of the patient. The administration of 5% dextrose in isotonic saline solution helps to maintain kidney function. Throughout, it is important to minimize stimulation of the patient and otherwise to maintain relaxation and prevent asphyxia through respiratory assistance.

CYANIDE POISONING

Cyanide inhibits oxidative enzyme systems and causes death from anoxia. *See also* SORGHUM POISONING OF HORSES, p. 1019.

Etiology: Cyanides are used in fumigants, soil sterilizers, fertilizers and rodenticides. Livestock loss may occur as a result of improper or malicious use of these compounds. The most important cause of cyanide poisoning among domestic animals is ingestion of such plants as arrow grass (*Triglochin* sp.), Johnson grass (*Sorghum halepense*), Sudan grass (*Sorghum sudanense*), common sorghum (*Sorghum bicolor* [*vulgare*]), wild black cherry (*Prunus serotina*), chokecherry (*Prunus virginiana*), pincherry (*Prunus pensylvanica*) and flax (*Linum usitatissimum*). These plants contain cyanogenetic glycosides that, when hydrolyzed by enzymes during digestion, yield hydrocyanic (prussic) acid. The cyanogenetic glycoside content is increased by heavy nitrate fertilization, wilting, trampling and plant disease. Very young, rapidly growing plants contain greater quantities of the glycoside. Spraying of cyanogenetic plants with a herbicide may increase the toxic hazard.

Clinical Findings: Clinical signs are caused by vital tissue hypoxia since hydrocyanic acid reacts with cytochrome oxidase in mitochondria, inhibiting cellular respiration. If large doses are consumed rapidly, muscle tremors develop and animals die within a few minutes. If smaller doses are consumed over a longer period, a commoner course is observed: the onset is sudden and characterized by salivation and a brief increase in respiratory rate. Dyspnea develops in 5 to 15 minutes. Muscle fasciculation occurs and progresses to generalized spasms just prior to death. Animals stagger and struggle before collapse. Mucous membranes are bright red, but may become cyanotic at terminus. Death occurs during severe asphyxial convulsions. The heart continues to beat for several minutes after struggling ceases and breathing stops. The course usually does not exceed 30 to 45 minutes; most animals that live 2 hours after the onset of signs will recover.

Lesions: In acute intoxication, blood is bright red and clots slowly. The rumen may be distended with gas, and the odor of "bitter almonds" may be detected when the cadaver is opened.

Diagnosis: The history, signs, postmortem findings and demonstration of the presence of hydrocyanic acid in the stomach contents permits a diagnosis. Tests for hydrocyanic acid should be made at the time of necropsy. For laboratory analysis, 150 to 250 gm of stomach contents should be collected soon after death, sealed and refrigerated in an airtight container and submitted immediately. Suspect plant material can also be tested.

Prophylaxis: Grazing cyanogenetic plants must be avoided when conditions that increase the potential toxic hazard are present. There is little danger from feeding well-cured hay. The risk of cyanide poisoning may be decreased by feeding of ground cereal grains or other feed before animals are turned out to graze.

Treatment: Since hydrocyanic acid combines readily with methemoglobin, methemoglobinemia is produced by the IV administration of sodium nitrite. Methemoglobin competes with cytochrome oxidase for the cyanide and functional cytochrome oxidase is restored. Cyanide then reacts with thiosulfate, a sulfur donor, to form thiocyanate, a relatively nontoxic substance excreted by the kidneys. Sodium nitrite and sodium thiosulfate usually are administered together (℞ 637), although treatment is most effective when nitrite is injected just before thiosulfate. It may be repeated with caution (because of the danger of excessive methemoglobinemia). Sodium thiosulfate alone (℞ 638) is relatively free from toxic effects. Methylene blue (℞ 634) is also an effective and safe therapy.

CHRONIC FLUORIDE POISONING

(Fluorosis)

Toxic quantities of fluorides occur naturally in a few products used in feeding animals, e.g. certain raw rock phosphates, the superphosphates produced from them, partially defluorinated phosphates and the phosphatic limestones. In certain areas, the drinking water, usually from deep wells, contains high levels of fluorides. Fluorine-containing gases and dusts from some chemical factories have contaminated forage crops. Among such factories are those engaged in producing acid phosphate from rock phosphates, the electrolytic production of aluminum, the manufacture of bricks from fluorine-bearing clays, the calcining of ironstone and certain enameling processes. Contamination of the surrounding area, particularly in the direction of the prevailing wind, may extend 5 to 6 miles. Furthermore, forage crops grown on high-fluorine soils have elevated values due to mechanical contamination with soil particles.

Sodium fluoride is the most toxic, and calcium fluoride the least toxic of the common fluorides. The fluorides of rock phosphates and most cryolites are intermediate between these two, whereas those in hay contaminated by industrial residues approach sodium fluoride in toxicity. A re-evaluation of the fluorine hazard suggests 50 to 100 ppm of fluorine in the total dry ration as maximal safe level for dairy and beef cattle, 100 to 200 ppm for sheep and swine, and 300 to 400 ppm for chickens. These data are based on fluorides as they exist in rock phosphates. Where the fluorides are in the form of soluble fluoride or originate from industrial fumes or dusts, the tolerance levels are approximately two-thirds these values. In the case of breeding animals whose usefulness exceeds 5 to 8 years, the lower figure given in each range should be used.

Clinical Findings: As teeth are seldom examined, the first sign of clinical fluorosis may be lameness caused by bony exostoses. Other variable clinical signs are: dryness and stiffness of the hide, poor condition, decreased appetite and lowered milk yield. Diarrhea occurs with high levels of inorganic fluoride.

Lesions: The most sensitive index of fluoride effect is the mottling, staining and excessive wearing of permanent teeth (*see* above) formed during the time of excessive fluoride ingestion. Teeth that are fully formed before exposure to fluorides are unaffected. A more advanced stage of fluorosis is marked by abnormalities of the skeletal system. The bones become chalky white, soft, thickened and, in the extreme, develop exostoses that may be palpated, especially along the long bones and on the mandible. These osseous lesions can develop in animals exposed at any age. Degenerative changes in the kidneys, liver and several endocrine organs, and anemia, have been reported, but are not pathognomonic.

Most of the fluoride retained by the body is deposited in the bones and teeth, the fluoride content of which increases in proportion to the amount and duration of the intake. Normal, dry, fat-free bone may contain up to approximately 1,000 ppm of fluorine. Fluorine contents of bones as high as 3,000 ppm are encountered in animals in which effects of fluorosis are slight and limited to mottling of the teeth. In chronic fluorosis, bone values may run as high as the "saturation" point of some 15,000 to 20,000 ppm. Urine from clinically normal animals contains less than 5 ppm of fluorine, whereas increased fluoride intakes produce values in excess of 10 ppm.

Diagnosis: Casual observation of animals suffering from fluorosis may suggest osteoporosis or deficiency of calcium, phosphorus or vitamin D. The lameness, in advanced cases, may be wrongly attributed to any number of accidents. The nonspecific staining often seen in cattle teeth may be confused with incipient fluorosis. Accurate diagnosis depends on demonstrating elevated fluorine content in urine and bone and ultimately discovering the source of the element.

Treatment and Control: Control, other than by the removal of animals from affected areas, is difficult. It has been suggested that affected areas may be utilized for the production of animals having a relatively short economic life, e.g. pigs, poultry or finishing cattle and sheep. The feeding of aluminum sulfate reduces fluorine absorption by about a third and thus offers some control of chronic fluorosis.

MERCURY POISONING

The toxic effects of organic and inorganic compounds of mercury are sufficiently dissimilar that they require separate discussions.

Inorganic Mercurials

These include mercuric chloride (corrosive sublimate), a disinfectant; mercurous chloride (calomel), a cathartic; and elemental mercury. Poisoning in animals is usually due to the accidental ingestion of mercuric chloride or its solutions. Elemental mercury may cause poisoning by inhalation of its vapor. Mercurous chloride may be toxic when retained in the gastrointestinal tract for prolonged periods.

Clinical Findings: In overwhelming doses, death may occur rapidly due to ventricular fibrillation. More commonly, the severe corrosive gastrointestinal effects, such as vomiting, bloody diarrhea and necrosis of the alimentary mucosa, are evident. In such cases severe renal damage also occurs, with anuria, or polyuria in less severe cases. In the rare case of chronic poisoning due to inorganic mercury the major action is on the CNS and resembles organic mercury poisoning (*see* below).

Lesions: In acute poisoning due to oral intake of inorganic salts of mercury, severe degenerative and inflammatory lesions of the gastrointestinal tract are observed.

Laboratory Diagnosis: Laboratory analysis should differentiate between normal concentrations of mercury in tissues and feed (less than 1 ppm) and concentrations associated with acute poisoning. The organ of choice for toxicologic examination is the kidney, which selectively accumulates mercury.

Treatment: The specific antidote for mercury is dimercaprol (℞ 628). Binding of mercury still in the gastrointestinal tract with proteins, such as eggs and milk, is advisable. A gastric lavage with sodium formaldehyde sulfoxalate (100 to 250 ml, 5% solution) also is useful. This serves to reduce divalent mercury to the less toxic monovalent form. The use of electrolyte solutions to combat dehydration should be monitored carefully to avoid overhydration in the presence of anuria.

Organic Mercurials

These include various phenyl or alkyl mercurial fungicides used to treat seeds stored for planting and mercurial diuretic drugs. Poisoning results from the inadvertent use of treated seed as livestock feed. Contaminated fish are a concern where mercury pollutes the waters; methylmercury is readily formed from inorganic mercury by aquatic microorganisms and fish accumulate the methylmercury. Commercial cat tuna has been shown to contain concentrations of 5 to 6 ppm of mercury, which raises the question of its safety to cats. Neurologic disturbances have been reported in cats following an exclusive tuna diet for 7 to 11 months. However, it is unlikely that the entire diet of domestic cats would consist of tuna.

Treatment: The neurologic signs associated with alkyl mercurials are accompanied by degenerative lesions of the CNS. Treatment in such circumstances is useless. In the case of poisoning by phenylmercurials, dimercaprol (℞ 628) may be of benefit if neurologic signs are absent. The water-soluble derivative 2,3-dimercaptopropane-1-sulfonate (DMPS) has proven superior to dimercaprol in promoting the excretion of inorganic or organic mercury, but this drug is unavailable for clinical use in the U.S.A. Dimercaprol is an effective antidote for mercurial diuretics.

MOLYBDENUM POISONING

(Molybdenosis)

In ruminants the dietary intake of excessive amounts of molybdenum causes secondary hypocuprosis, manifested clinically by persistent diarrhea and fading of haircoat color. Nonruminants are much more resistant to molybdenum toxicity.

Etiology: The tolerance of ruminants to a high intake of molybdenum depends upon a number of factors: (1) the copper content and intake of the animal—the tolerance decreases as the content and intake fall (*see* NUTRITIONAL DEFICIENCIES IN CATTLE AND SHEEP: COPPER, p. 1398), (2) the inorganic sulfate content of the diet—increasing levels of sulfate intensify toxicity associated with low copper intakes, (3) the chemical form of the molybdenum, (4) the presence of certain sulfur-containing amino acids, (5) the species of animal—cattle are less tolerant than sheep, (6) the age—young animals are most susceptible, (7) the season of the year—the plant concentration of molybdenum is highest in spring and autumn, and (8) the botanic composition of the pasture, legumes taking up more of the element than other plant species.

Molybdenum poisoning associated with copper deficiency has been observed in regions having peat or muck soils. In parts of the San Joaquin Valley of California and on some of the Eocene shales of the Western U.S.A., the forage may contain up to 100 ppm of molybdenum. In other areas the metal is used in fertilization and while normal applications of molybdenum for this purpose do not ordinarily increase the level in the forage above 1 ppm, extra quantities may result in forage with 4 or 5 ppm or more. Aerial contamination from industrial plants may result in very high levels of intake.

In the presence of high molybdenum and low copper intakes, liver copper in cattle, sheep and goats may decrease to 30 ppm or less of the dry weight. The blood copper may reach levels as low as 0.06 ppm. The presence of molybdenum in the liver at levels of 5 to 100 ppm is indicative of an abnormal molybdenum intake. A hypochromic anemia, with hemoglobin concentrations as low as 6 gm per 100 ml of blood, is observed in severe cases. Serum calcium and inorganic phosphorus values usually remain normal, even when rarefaction is present in the bones.

If the copper content is below 5 ppm in rapidly growing pastures, 1 ppm molybdenum on a dry-weight basis may be hazardous. Levels of 100 ppm copper and 0.05% sulfur and above usually prevent toxic signs with molybdenum concentrations as high as 3 to 4 ppm. With extremely high levels of molybdenum, up to 150 ppm in the dry matter, a total daily intake of copper, equivalent to between 0.5 to 2.0 gm of copper sulfate, $CuSO_4 \cdot 5H_2O$, may be required to protect cattle.

Clinical Findings: The signs of molybdenum toxicity are nonspecific and vary from an apparently poor performance, particularly in young animals, to serious conditions which include severe diarrhea ("peat scours"), anemia, emaciation, joint-pain and fading of the haircoat. Depigmentation of the hair is most noticeable in black animals and especially around the eyes, giving a bespectacled appearance. The joint pain causes difficulty in rising, disinclination to move and a stiff gait. These signs appear within 1 to 2 weeks of going onto affected pasture. Emaciation and anemia are the only conditions observed at necropsy. Diagnosis may be established on the basis of abnormal concentrations of molybdenum and copper in blood or liver. It is also customary to establish that the dietary intake of molybdenum is high. A provisional diagnosis can be made by oral dosing with copper sulfate, the diarrhea stopping within a few days.

The disease may be confused with many other enteritides but it is commonly mistaken for internal parasitism, especially in young cattle. In pastured animals it is not uncommon for the 2 diseases to occur simultaneously.

Prophylaxis and Treatment: In areas where the molybdenum content of the forage is below 5 ppm, the use of 1% copper sulfate ($CuSO_4 \cdot 5H_2O$) in salt has provided satisfactory control of molybdenosis. With higher levels of molybdenum, 2% copper sulfate has been successful. Up to 5% has been used in a few regions where the molybdenum levels are very high. In areas where, for various reasons, cattle do not consume mineral supplements, the required copper may be supplied as a drench given weekly, as parenterally administered repository copper preparations, or as a top-dressing to the pasture. These measures are listed in the section on nutritional deficiency of copper, q.v., p. 1398.

COPPER POISONING

The condition occurs most commonly in sheep, but also in cattle and swine, although these are more resistant. Acute poisoning is straightforward and follows more or less immediately upon the accidental intake of excess copper in salt mixes, improperly compounded feeds, anthelmintic treatments and injectable copper preparations. Chronic poisoning, whether primary or secondary, is complicated by interacting factors, of which the most important are intakes of molybdenum and sulfate. **Primary chronic poisoning,** due to extended exposure to excess copper in herbage, salt licks or mineral mixes, remains subclinical until storage sites—principally the liver—are overloaded; then, blood levels of copper are markedly increased and the animal dies of acute intravascular hemolysis. Chronic poisoning may be precipitated by certain "stresses" such as a falling plane of nutrition, reduced feed intake, excessive exercise and transport.

Secondary chronic poisoning is phytogenous or hepatogenous. The phytogenous condition is endemic, occurs in animals, usually sheep, grazing subterranean clover (*Trifolium subterraneum*), and is associated with normal levels of copper, low levels of molybdenum and no apparent hepatic damage. Hepatogenous chronic poisoning results from increased storage of copper in the liver damaged by plant toxins, particularly the alkaloids of *Heliotropium* and *Senecio*.

Acute poisoning may follow intakes of 20 to 100 mg of copper per kg of body weight in sheep and young calves, and 200 to 800 mg/kg in mature cattle. Daily intakes of 3.5 mg/kg, pasture containing 15 to 20 ppm, (dry matter), and pelleted feeds containing 50 ppm have caused chronic poisoning of sheep. Copper is used as a feed additive for swine at concentration of 125 to 250 ppm; levels greater than 250 ppm are dangerous—although as for sheep, other factors may be protective, e.g. high levels of protein, zinc or iron.

Clinical Findings: Most animals that develop clinical signs will die. **Acute poisoning:** Severe gastroenteritis is marked by abdominal pain, nausea, salivation and diarrhea. Monogastric animals may vomit. Feces and vomitus are bluish green. Shock, prostration and death follow a short clinical course. Icterus becomes apparent in animals that live more than 24 hours. **Chronic poisoning:** The manifestations are acute and due to the hemolytic crisis. Anorexia is accompanied by thirst and marked depression. There is severe hemoglobinemia, hemoglobinuria, anemia, icterus and methemoglobinemia. Most animals die within 1 to 2 days of the onset of signs.

Lesions: In the acute disease, gastroenteritis predominates; a hemorrhagic and edematous abomasum may be ulcerated and contain bluish green contents. In the chronic disease, the tissues are discolored by icterus and methemoglobinemia, the bladder contains port-wine colored urine; the kidneys are bluish black due to their content of hemoglobin; the spleen is enlarged, mushy and dark red; and the liver is smaller, discolored and firm (may be enlarged, friable and yellow).

Diagnosis: The signs and lesions, especially the blue-green ingesta and the gun-metal discolored kidneys are quite suggestive, but require laboratory confirmation. Levels of copper in the blood and liver are markedly increased in chronic copper poisoning. During the hemolytic crisis, blood levels of copper are of the order of 500 to 2,000 mcg/100 ml compared to about 100 mcg/100 ml in normal animals. Normal liver levels, usually less than 350 ppm dry matter, are increased to levels about 1,000 ppm in chronic poisoning. In acute cases, feces may contain as much as 8,000 to 10,000 ppm of copper.

Treatment: The prognosis is grave. In acute cases, gastrointestinal sedatives and symptomatic treatment for shock are recommended. Calcium versenate and penicillamine may be worth trying for valuable animals. Daily oral treatment with 100 mg ammonium molybdate and 1 gm anhydrous sodium sulfate appears to prevent death of lambs known to have ingested toxic amounts of copper.

Control: For phytogenous and hepatogenous outbreaks, ingestion of the plants involved must be prevented. When the problem is related to grazing of subterranean clover, encouragement of grass growth and top-dressing with molybdenized superphosphate (4 oz molybdenum per acre [300 mg/hectare]) to increase molybdenum content of the pasture and reduce the retention of copper are useful. A molybdenized mineral mixture (90 kg salt, 70 kg finely ground gypsum, 500 gm sodium molybdate) is also protective.

SELENIUM POISONING

Although selenium is highly toxic in overdoses, the element is required in trace amounts to maintain life and to prevent such conditions as exudative diathesis in chicks (q.v., p. 1429) and muscular dystrophies in many species (*see* MYOPATHIES AND RELATED CONDITIONS IN DOMESTIC ANIMALS, p. 590).

Etiology: Chronic selenium poisoning ("alkali disease") results when animals consume naturally seleniferous forages and grains that contain 5 to 40 ppm of selenium. Soils capable of supporting seleniferous plants have been found only in regions where the mean annual rainfall is less than 20 in. (50 cm). Certain plants known as "accumulators" require selenium for growth and often contain several thousand ppm of selenium. When consumed by animals, these accumulator plants may produce an acute type of poisoning called "blind staggers." Seleniferous plants that are not removed from the land may decay, be incorporated in the topsoil and become a source of selenium for nonseleniferous plants, which may then be a toxic hazard. Seleniferous *Astragalus* plants may contain other toxic substances and many nonseleniferous *Astragalus* spp. contain toxins.

Seleniferous vegetation containing over 50 ppm of selenium has been found growing in all of the states west of the Mississippi River except those adjoining the river and the State of Washington. Such vegetation also has been found in Alberta, Saskatchewan and Manitoba in Canada, and in Mexico. Since the selenium in soils comes from certain geologic formations, the areas producing highly seleniferous vegetation are spotty and localized. Most of the selenium poisoning in livestock has been reported from Colorado, Nebraska, South Dakota and Wyoming. It has also been reported from Ireland, Israel and northern Queensland in Australia. Occasionally, the condition develops in dogs following the use of selenium-containing shampoos.

CHRONIC SELENIUM POISONING

"Alkali Disease" Type

Gross lesions in chronic selenium poisoning of the "alkali disease" type usually include erosion of the joints of the long bones, atrophy and cirrhosis of the liver, atrophy of the heart, anemia and ascites. Hemoglobin concentrations decrease in the early stages and can be an aid in early diagnosis. The selenium in hair may be used as an indication of previous intake of this element.

Clinical Findings: Chronic selenium poisoning in cattle, horses and swine develops within a few weeks when seleniferous grains or forages are consumed. The signs common to these species include cracking of the hoofs, lameness, stiffness of joints, dullness and lack of vitality, emaciation and loss of hair. In horses, the loss of long hair from the mane and tail usually is the first clinical sign and is followed by cracking of the hoof at the coronary band. New growth of the hoof pushes the dead tissue downward and, if the growth interruption has been prolonged, the old portion of the hoof may separate and slough. In cattle, a series of interruptions of growth may result in deformed hoofs, 6 to 7 in. (15 to 18 cm) long and turned upward at the ends. Swine fed seleniferous feeds show breaks in the hoof similar to those in cattle. Sows have a lowered conception rate and an increase in the number of pigs born dead. Chronic selenium poisoning of the "alkali disease" type is not common in sheep. Death losses occur from acute poisoning soon after sheep are moved onto seleniferous range forage.

Control: A high-protein ration will help to control this type of selenium poisoning. The use of salt containing arsenic at 0.00375% may reduce the incidence of chronic selenium poisoning in cattle on seleniferous range. The use of arsanilic acid (0.005 to 0.01%) in the ration also seems to reduce the effects of high-selenium intake in calves and pigs. Stiffness in cattle and horses may be relieved by the oral administration of compounds, such as naphthalene and bromobenzene, which form mercapturic acids. The usual treatment is to give 4 or 5 gm of naphthalene daily for 5 days and to repeat the dosage after a 5-day interval.

"Blind Staggers" Type

This develops in animals grazing on ranges where highly seleniferous plants are growing. In cattle, blind staggers is manifested in 3 stages: First, there is a tendency to wander and the animal may walk into objects in its path. The temperature is normal, but there is impairment of vision and poor appetite. In the second stage, the wandering increases and the front legs become weak. Vision becomes further impaired. Third, the throat and tongue become paralyzed, temperature is subnormal, and death follows from respiratory failure. In sheep, the 3 stages are not as clearly differentiated as in cattle. Congestion and necrosis of the liver, congestion of the renal medulla, epicardial petechiae, hyperemia and ulceration in the abomasum and small intestine, and erosion of the articular surfaces, particularly of the tibia, are the usual lesions observed at necropsy.

There is no specific antidote; supportive therapy (e.g. forced fluids) may be useful.

ACUTE SELENIUM POISONING

Acute selenium poisoning occurs in cattle and sheep as a result of consuming, at one time, sufficient highly seleniferous (accumulator) plants to cause severe intoxication. Death usually occurs within a few hours. The gait is uncertain, the temperature elevated, the respiration labored with frothing from the nostrils, and the pupils dilated. Prostration occurs before death from respiratory failure. Losses in sheep grazing on seleniferous vegetation may be high. One outbreak is recorded in which 340 mature sheep died within 24 hours of consuming highly seleniferous *Astragalus bisulcatus*.

There is no known treatment for acute selenium poisoning.

IRON DEXTRAN TOXICITY IN NEWBORN PIGS

The oral or parenteral administration of prophylactic levels of iron dextran to newborn pigs, born from sows or gilts that were deficient in vitamin E or selenium during pregnancy, may result in acute deaths, usually within a few hours of the administration of iron. Affected pigs are depressed, stagger and become recumbent quickly. At necropsy there is widespread waxy degeneration of skeletal muscles and diffuse hepatic degeneration. Supplementation of the diet of the pregnant female with vitamin E and selenium will prevent the iron hypersensitivity in the piglets. The injection of deficient sows with vitamin E and selenium or the deficient piglets at least 3 days before the administration of the iron dextran will also prevent the disease. (*See also* ANEMIAS OF DEFICIENT HEMOGLOBIN PRODUCTION, p. 24.)

METALDEHYDE POISONING

Metaldehyde is in common use in domestic gardens as a molluscacide, a snail bait. It is usually used combined with bran, either as flakes or pellets and is palatable to dogs and farm animals. Clinical signs in affected animals are principally nervous and include incoordination, muscle tremor and hyperesthesia. Salivation, diarrhea and dyspnea are also seen and terminally there is unconsciousness; death is due to respiratory failure. Lethal doses vary from 0.1 gm/kg body wt in horses to 0.2 gm/kg in adult cattle. Evacuation of the swallowed material should be attempted. In horses, mineral oil by stomach tube is used to prevent absorption of the metaldehyde. A sedative or tranquilizer is usually necessary to reduce excitement.

SALT POISONING

Salt (sodium chloride) may be toxic when excessive quantities are ingested with limited water intake. "Salt poisoning" is a misnomer for the condition occurs only with concomitant water deprivation. Deaths have been attributed to salt poisoning in cattle, swine, sheep, horses, dogs and poultry in various parts of the world. In the U.S.A., swine, cattle and chickens are most frequently affected.

Etiology: Toxicity of the sodium ion is directly related to water consumption. With water deprivation, sodium propionate, acetate, carbonate, etc., will produce the same toxicosis as does sodium chloride.

Feeder pigs on feed containing only 0.25% salt show sodium ion toxicosis when water intake is limited, yet even 13% salt in the feed may not produce poisoning if adequate fresh water is consumed. Optimally, with fresh water fully available, swine feeds should contain 0.5 to 1.0% salt.

Chickens are susceptible to sodium ion toxicosis when water intake is restricted in hot weather or in cold weather when the water supply freezes. Chickens tolerate up to 0.25% sodium chloride in drinking water regardless of its level in the feed. Wet mash containing 2% sodium chloride has caused poisoning in ducklings. Salt in wet mash seems more toxic than it is in dry feeds, probably because birds eat more wet mash and caretakers then are less careful to provide another source of water.

Cattle and sheep on range, where a high percentage of mineral feed supplement is provided with limited or saline water intake, may develop salt poisoning. Sheep tolerate 1% salt in drinking water but 1.5% may be toxic. Some authorities recommend that drinking water should contain no more than 0.5% total salts for any species of livestock. High concentrations of salt can cause gastroenteritis and dehydration.

Clinical Findings: In swine, rarely observed early signs may be increased thirst, pruritus and constipation. Affected animals may be blind, deaf and oblivious to their surroundings, will not eat, drink or respond to external stimuli, may wander aimlessly, push against objects, circle or pivot around a single front or rear limb. After 1 to 5 days of limited water intake, intermittent convulsive seizures occur with the pig sitting on its haunches, jerkily drawing his head backward and upward, finally falling on its side in clonic-tonic seizures and opisthotonos; terminally, pigs lie on their sides, paddling in a coma and die within a few to 48 hours.

In swine (but not other species) during the first 48 hours, circulating eosinophils disappear from the blood vascular system and are attracted to the cerebrovascular and meningeal areas, collecting around the vessels within the cerebral cortex and adjacent meninges. After 3 to 4 days the eosinophils leave the cerebral area and are replaced by round cells; cortical laminar necrosis and even cavitation may follow if the animal survives.

Cattle show alimentary signs as vomiting, diarrhea, abdominal pain, anorexia and mucus in the feces; there may be continuous polyuria and a nasal discharge. Neurologic signs include blindness and convulsive seizures followed by partial paralysis. A sequela to salt poisoning in cattle is characteristic dragging of the rear feet while walking and, in more severe cases, knuckling of the fetlock joints.

Lesions: Grossly in swine, blood-filled pinpoint ulcers are found on a markedly congested and inflamed gastric mucosa. Cattle show gastric inflammation or ulceration or both, edema of the skeletal muscles and hydropericardium. Sometimes no gross necropsy lesions are evident.

Treatment: Immediate removal of the offending feed is imperative. Fresh water must be provided to all animals, initially in small amounts at frequent intervals. Those that drink seldom need additional treatment. Severely affected animals unable to find water or to drink it should be given water via stomach tube.

NITRATE AND NITRITE POISONING

Nitrates are reduced by the microflora in the alimentary tract, especially the rumen, to nitrite, hydroxylamine and finally to ammonia. The rate at which this reduction takes place is an important factor affecting toxicity.

Etiology: Some nitrate may be absorbed but has little toxic effect. Nitrites are rapidly absorbed and may cause poisoning in any species by oxidizing hemoglobin to methemoglobin and by vasodilation. Nitrite poisoning is seen occasionally in dogs following accidental consumption of antirust tablets, or the ingestion of dog foods containing excessive quantities of nitrite. Nitrite poisoning in ruminants usually occurs as a result of consumption of nitrate fertilizer or of forages of high nitrate or nitrite content. A few plants commonly have high nitrate content but under certain conditions, many plants have the ability to accumulate large quantities of nitrates. Toxic levels of nitrate are sometimes found in common pasture species, such as the rye grasses, during rapid growth. Crops grown on summer fallow may have a nitrate content in excess of crops grown on land in continuous crop production. Corn growing under hot dry conditions may concentrate nitrate in the lower parts of the stalk. Most losses occur in the Great Plains States when oats, barley or wheat are fed as hay, particularly if the hay is fed several days after it has been moistened by rain, snow or excessive dampness. A variety of common weeds growing on marshy or muck soils that have high nitrogen and relatively low phosphorus and potassium contents accumulate abnormal quantities of nitrates. Low temperatures, limited sunlight, poor mineral sources and applications of plant hormone herbicides contribute to increased nitrate levels. The most commonly incriminated plants have been the redroot pigweed (*Amaranthus retroflexus*) and lamb's-quarters (*Chenopodium album*), although many other plants can accumulate nitrates. Ruminants fed rations containing grains or concentrates can metabolize and utilize considerably more nitrate than ruminants maintained on roughage alone.

Water from shallow wells in certain areas of the Great Plains may contain nitrates in concentrations toxic for cattle. Losses have occurred during freezing weather due to an increase in nitrate concentration in the stock tanks.

Clinical Findings: The nitrite ion in blood converts hemoglobin to methemoglobin, and is a vasodilator. The signs of nitrite poisoning appear suddenly due to the tissue hypoxia and low blood pressure resulting from the vasodilation. Rapid, weak heart beat, subnormal body temperature, muscular weakness, ataxia and cyanosis rapidly develop. Respiratory embarrassment is seen in animals that are exercised. The patient may die in convulsions within an hour but in the usual case, death results after a clinical course of 3 to 4 hours. Of the animals that develop marked dyspnea but recover, some develop interstitial pulmonary emphysema and continue to suffer respiratory distress after disappearance of the methemoglobinemia. Most of these animals fully recover within 10 to 14 days. Nitrite readily passes through the placenta causing methemoglobinemia in the fetus. Pregnant females frequently abort following recovery from nitrite poisoning. Chronic nitrate poisoning has been difficult to demonstrate but is thought to cause reduced weight gain, lowered fertility, abortion and possibly avitaminosis A. Consumption of large doses of nitrate may result in severe gastroenteritis and death in any of the domestic animals.

Lesions: The blood is chocolate brown because of its methemoglobin content. The submucosa of the rumen, reticulum and omasum, and the mucosa of the abomasum usually are congested. Petechial hemorrhages on the serous surfaces are commonly observed.

Diagnosis: Methemoglobinemia is sometimes difficult to detect, especially if the necropsy is delayed. On the other hand, unless samples of blood sent for laboratory diagnosis are assayed within a few hours of being drawn, they are likely to contain a large proportion of spontaneously formed methemoglobin.

Perhaps the most sensitive and reliable simple test is the diphenylamine blue (DPB) test: to test for nitrate and nitrite, 0.5 to 1.0 ml of a 1% solution of diphenylamine in concentrated sulfuric acid is placed on a glass or porcelain plate and 1 or 2 drops of a solution or suspension of the suspect material is placed to one side, but in contact with the reagent. A blue color diffusing from the test material into the reagent indicates the presence of nitrate or nitrite. The 2 solutions should not be mixed, as faint reactions may be obscured. Water used to suspend materials to be tested should be free of all metallic salts. The DPB test can be readily used in the field for testing drinking water, plant material, stomach contents and urine. While it is not specific, a positive reaction can be very helpful.

Treatment: Administration of a 2% solution of methylene blue (℞ 633) aids in the reduction of methemoglobin to hemoglobin. Mineral oil or mucilaginous substances may be given orally to protect the irritated mucous membranes.

COAL TAR POISONING

The distillation of coal tar yields a variety of compounds, 3 of which are notably toxic: cresols (phenolic compounds); crude creosote (composed of cresols, heavy oils and anthracene); and pitch.

Etiology: Cresols, which are used as disinfectants, are readily absorbed through the skin. The lethal dose is 100 to 200 mg/kg of body weight, except in cats which are much more susceptible. Because coal-tar derived creosote is very toxic to wood-destroying fungi and insects, it is used as a wood preserver. Sows confined to wood farrowing crates treated with 3 brush applications of creosote were reported to have stillborn pigs and the surviving pigs grew slowly. Other species are less susceptible; e.g. the lethal dose of creosote in calves is 4 gm/kg of body wt. Pitch is used as a binder in clay pigeons, in road asphalt, insulation, tar paper and roofing compounds, and to cover iron pipes and line wooden water tanks. Fifteen grams of clay pigeons consumed over a 5-day period will kill swine. Other species are much more tolerant.

Clinical Findings: The cresols are locally corrosive. They stimulate the CNS; followed by depression of the heart which results in vascular collapse. Death may occur from 15 minutes to several days after exposure. The first sign of pitch poisoning often is several dead pigs. Other pigs are depressed, which may progress to weakness, ataxia, sternal recumbency, icterus, coma and death.

Lesions: Except for contact irritation, cresols and creosote do not produce distinctive morphologic lesions. Pitch poisoning causes a markedly swollen liver that has a diffuse mottled appearance. The lobules are clearly outlined by a light-colored zone and their centers contain deep-red dots the size of a pinhead. The blood clots slowly or not at all. The carcass is icteric. Excessive quantities of fluid are found in the peritoneal cavity.

Treatment: There is no known treatment for animals with frank signs.

BOVINE HYPERKERATOSIS

(X-disease)

A toxicosis resulting from the ingestion of, or contact with, highly chlorinated naphthalenes, which were found in certain lubricants and wood preservatives. An early sign is a watery discharge from the eyes and nose. This is followed by depression, anorexia, salivation, intermittent diarrhea and a loss of condition. Prior to the appearance of the visible signs, there is a rapid fall in the plasma vitamin-A concentration due to the effect of the toxic agent in inhibiting the conversion of carotene to vitamin A. As the disease progresses, there is an accumulation of hard keratin-like material on the skin, which makes it thick, inelastic and wrinkled.

Because of their known toxic effects the napthalenes are now rarely used in industry and at the present time bovine hyperkeratosis is primarily of historic interest. However attention has now been diverted to a similar disease caused by **polybrominated,** and possibly **polychlorinated, biphenyls.** These substances are in common use in industry, and by virtue of environmental contamination, enter the food chain of farm animals and man. A much publicized incident in the U.S.A. in recent years has focused a great deal of interest on industrial procedures likely to affect animal and human health. Poisoning with polybrominated biphenyls causes anorexia, diarrhea, lacrimation, salivation, depression, abortion, loss of weight and extensive subcutaneous hyperkeratosis. Necropsy lesions include mucoid enteritis, nephrosis and hyperkeratosis of glandular epithelium. Ordinarily, if the toxic substance is removed while the appetite is good, many animals will recover. There is no specific treatment.

POISONING BY HERBICIDES

Many of the chemicals used to control undesirable plants are highly toxic to domestic animals, while others are relatively nontoxic. The majority of livestock losses associated with herbicides are directly related to their improper or careless use. Very few losses occur when these chemicals are used properly. This discussion includes some of the more commonly used herbicides and those with which livestock losses most frequently have been associated.

Ammonium Sulfamate (Ammate): This has not been found to be toxic to many animals when it is fed experimentally. Ruminants, including deer, apparently can metabolize this chemical to some extent and, in some experiments, have made better gains than control animals. Reports have appeared from various parts of the country, however, which indicate that sudden deaths have occurred among cattle and deer gaining access to plants treated with ammonium sulfamate. Large doses (1.5 gm/kg) of ammonium sulfamate have been shown to induce ammonia poisoning in ruminants. Treatment is designed to lower rumen pH by dilution with copious amounts of water to which weak acetic acid (vinegar) has been added.

Borax is used as a herbicide, an insecticide and as a soil sterilant, and is toxic to animals if it is consumed in moderate to large doses. No poisonings are known to have occurred when this chemical has been used properly but cases have occurred when borax has been accidentally included in rations for livestock and when borax powder is scattered around for cockroach control. The chief signs of acute boron poisoning are diarrhea, rapid prostration and convulsions. There is no known effective treatment. The IV injection of large quantities of balanced electrolyte solutions may be beneficial.

Dinitro Compounds: The dinitrophenol and dinitrocresol compounds are highly toxic to all classes of animals. They are readily absorbed through the skin and lungs and, therefore, poisoning can occur if animals are sprayed accidentally or have immediate access to herbage that has been sprayed. Dinitro compounds produce a marked increase in oxygen consumption and depletion of glycogen reserves. The chief signs are fever, dyspnea, acidosis, tachycardia and convulsions, followed by coma and death with a rapid onset of rigor mortis. Cataracts may occur in animals with chronic dinitrophenol intoxication. Exposure to dinitro compounds can often be recognized by yellowing of the skin around the mouth and of the hair around the nose and hoofs. No effective antidote is known. Affected animals should be sheltered in a shady place and cooled with water. Chlorpromazine may help control the hyperthermia if the animals are placed in a cool environment. Infusion of large quantities of carbohydrate solutions and parenteral administration of vitamin A may also be useful. Residues of the dinitro compounds that remain on foliage that has been properly treated with these chemicals are not dangerous to livestock.

Pentachlorophenol (PCP, penta) is used as a herbicide, fungicide, molluscacide, insecticide, and as a wood preservative. It is highly toxic when ingested and, like the dinitro compounds, it can be absorbed through the intact skin and by way of the lungs. It is an intense irritant to the skin and mucous membranes. Animals fed in troughs made of lumber treated with pentachlorophenol may show salivation and irritation of the oral mucosa. Wood that has been treated with penta should be avoided. Vaporization or leaching of PCP in pens, enclosures, homes and dairy barns has caused death. The chief signs of pentachlorophenol poisoning are nervousness, restlessness, rapid pulse and respiratory rates, weakness, muscle tremors and clonic convulsions, followed by death. No effective treatment or antidote is known. Pentachlorophenol-treated foliage is not dangerous to animals when the herbicide has been used correctly.

The plant-hormone herbicides: 2,4-D (2,4-dichlorophenoxyacetic acid), **2,4,5-T** (2,4,5-trichlorophenoxyacetic acid), **MCP** (2-methyl-4-chlorophenoxyacetic acid), **silvex** (2-[2,4,5-trichlorophenoxy] propionic acid), **dalapon** (2,2 dichloropropionic acid) and their salts and esters, are the commonest chemicals used to control undesirable plants; many millions of acres of field crops and pasture have been treated. Livestock have grazed most of these pastures and have been fed feeds produced from many additional acres of field crops so treated with few if any authenticated instances of poisoning. As a group, these chemicals, themselves, have been shown to be nontoxic to experimental and farm animals under practical conditions. When large doses are fed experimentally, general depression with loss of appetite, accompanied by loss of weight, general tenseness and muscular weakness, particularly of the hindquarters, are noted. Large doses in cattle may interfere with rumen function. Even very large doses, up to 2 gm/kg, have not been shown to leave chemical residues in the fat of animals. Certain hazards to livestock may, however, arise as a sequence of an alteration in the chemical composition of the plant induced by these herbicides (*see* NITRATE AND NITRITE POISONING, p. 983). Use of these compounds may not only increase palatability of some poisonous plants but also increased the toxic ingredient.

Currently the use of the chlorophenoxy herbicides is curtailed, especially 2,4,5-T. Recent studies have shown that some extremely toxic contaminants (2,3,7,8-tetrachloro-dibenzo-*p*-dioxin or **TCDD**; hexachloro-dibenzo-*p*-dioxin or **HCDD**; collectively called **dioxins**) have been found to be teratogenic in laboratory animals, and to cause a skin condition in man. Although manufacturing methods have reduced the level of this contaminant to what is thought to be nontoxic, the final decision has not yet been made by regulatory agencies.

Sodium chlorate is still a widely used herbicide. Treated plants and clothing that have been contaminated are highly combustible and constitute real fire hazards. Additionally, many cases of chlorate poisoning of livestock have occurred both from the ingestion of treated plants and from accidental consumption of feed to which it was mistakenly added for salt. Cattle sometimes are attracted to sodium chlorate-treated foliage. Considerable quantities must be consumed before signs of toxicity appear. The minimum lethal dose of sodium chlorate is 1.1 gm/kg of body wt for cattle, 1.54 to 2.86 gm/kg for sheep and 5.06 gm/kg for poultry. Ingestion results in the conversion of hemoglobin to methemoglobin. The signs that result are due to methemoglobinemia. Treatment with methylene blue (℞ 633) must be repeated frequently because, unlike the nitrites, the chlorate ion is not inactivated in the conversion of hemoglobin to methemoglobin and is capable of producing an unlimited quantity of methemoglobin as long as it is present in the body. The IV administration of isotonic salt solution in large quantities may hasten the elimination of the chlorate ion.

Arsenicals: Some of the inorganic arsenicals (sodium arsenite and arsenite trioxide) still are used as herbicides, although the high incidence of livestock losses that frequently follow their use for this purpose has made them somewhat unpopular. Cattle sometimes readily consume toxic quantities of treated foliage. Deer often are attracted to trees poisoned with arsenite and apparently lick the chemical from the trees. The highly soluble arsenicals sometimes are concentrated in pools after a rain has washed them from recently treated plants. Animals that consume this water frequently develop arsenic poisoning (q.v., p. 966). The organic arsenicals and arsenic acid are frequently used as desiccants or defoliants on cotton. Feeding of cotton gin trash so treated has caused toxicity in cattle and sheep.

Organic arsenical herbicides (cacodylic acid and derivatives, MSMA, DMSA) produce signs and lesions resembling, in general, those found in inorganic arsenical poisoning. Toxic single oral doses for cattle and sheep range from 22 to 55 mg/kg. Poisoning may be expected from much smaller doses consumed on successive days.

Chlorobenzoic Acids: 2,3,6-TBA (Trysben), **chloramben** (3-amino, 2,5-dichlorobenzoic acid), **dicamba** (Banvel D): These herbicides are toxic to cattle and sheep in single oral doses in the range of 220 to 440 mg/kg of body wt. Such dosages can be obtained by these animals only through carelessness in handling and storage. The signs and lesions follow the pattern described for hormone type herbicides (*see* p. 988).

Phenylurea Compounds: Diuron (Karmex), **linuron** (Lorox), **monuron** (Telvar), **fenuron** (Dybar): For cattle and sheep these herbicides are toxic in single oral doses of 220 to 440 mg/kg of body wt. Such dosages can be obtained only through carelessness in handling and storage. Signs and lesions follow the pattern described for hormone type herbicides (*see* p. 988).

Triazine Compounds: Atrazine (Aatrex, Atratol, Gesaprim, Primatol A), **Propazin** (Gesamil, Primatol P), **simazine** (Gesatop, Primatol S), **prometone** (Primatol, Gesafram), and **Prometryne** (Caparol, Primatol, Gesagard, Lambast). These compounds are toxic to sheep and cattle in single oral doses ranging from 22 to 220 mg/kg of body wt. Cumulative action is not remarkable. The signs and lesions follow the pattern described for the hormone type herbicides (*see* p. 988).

Amide Compounds: Diphenamid (Dymid, Enide), **CDAA** (Randox): Diphenamid is much less toxic than CDAA, the toxic oral doses for cattle and sheep being in the range of 440 mg/kg and 22 mg/kg of body wt, respectively. The signs and lesions follow the pattern described for hormone type herbicides (*see* p. 988).

Thiocarbamate Compounds: Diallate (Avadex), **triallate** (Avadex B W, Far-go), **dichlormate** (Rowmate), **EPTC** (Eptam, Knoxweed), **vernolate** (Vernam), **chlorpropham, barban, CDEC, pebulate:** The toxic oral doses of these compounds for cattle and sheep are in the range of 220 to 440 mg/kg of body wt, quantities unlikely to be available except through spillage or careless handling. Signs and lesions are as for the hormone type herbicides (*see* p. 988). Hair loss may be seen in animals for some time after ingestion.

Dipyridyl Compounds: Diquat, paraquat: Used as herbicides and desiccants at rather low rate (2 oz/acre [150 gm/ha]), these compounds act rapidly, are inactivated on soil contact and decompose in light rapidly. They are extremely toxic on ingestion and extremely hazardous to people. Diquat has caused cataracts as well as being teratogenic. Paraquat has a biphasic toxic action on ingestion: primary kidney and liver involvement followed, after 1 to 2 weeks by irreversible pulmonary fibrosis. Signs of poisoning include evidence of pain, gastroenteritis, extreme depression, icterus and finally respiratory difficulty and failure. There is no known antidote. Deaths have occurred in man as a result of drinking from contaminated containers.

Methyluracil Compounds: Bromacil (Hyvan X), **isocil** (Hyvar Isocil): These cause very mild toxicity at levels of 50 mg/kg in sheep, 250 mg/kg in cattle, and 500 mg/kg in poultry when given for 8 to 10 daily doses. Signs include bloat, incoordination, depression, and anorexia. The normal application rate of 5 lb/acre (5.6 kg/ha) could be hazardous, especially for sheep, but no field cases of toxicity have been reported.

Phthalmic Acid Derivatives: Dimoseb, naptalam. Naptalam is moderately toxic at 25 mg/kg for 8 to 10 daily doses for cattle and sheep, and 2 daily doses in chickens; there is a hazard of poisoning at recommended application levels in range chickens. Signs are similar to those for the hormone type herbicides (*see* p. 988).

Dinitroaniline Compounds: Nitralin (Planavin), **trifluralin** (Treflan). The toxicity of nitralin is about 250 to 500 mg/kg daily for several successive days. This would not be encountered except through carelessness. Signs are diarrhea, anorexia, nervousness and lack of gain.

Miscellaneous Herbicides: Bandane (Polychlorodicyclopentadiene) is used on brush at 30 to 40 lb/acre (34 to 45 kg/ha); 100 mg/kg for 8 to 10 days has been shown to be toxic, causing anorexia, muscle tremors, hyperexcitability, incoordination and prostration.

Picloram (Tordon) is used on noncrop areas at 25 lb/acre (28 kg/ha); 8 or 9 daily doses of 250 to 500 mg/kg in sheep and cattle, respectively, have caused death. Signs are weakness, depression, and anorexia. It is eliminated in feces rather quickly with the herbicidal action still effective.

Glyphosate (Roundup) is used as a herbicide and desiccant on small grains. No toxicity is seen at recommended doses. Laying hens given oral doses at 25 mg/kg may produce soft-shelled eggs.

POISONING BY RODENTICIDES

A large group of poisons have been used against rodent pests. Farm animals, pets and wildlife often gain access to these poisons via the baits or the destroyed pests, or by malicious intent. This discussion covers only the rodenticides that are in most common use. Strychnine poisoning is discussed separately (*see* p. 970).

Red squill produces convulsions that alternate with paralysis, and is a rather potent emetic. Since the rat is incapable of vomiting, red squill is more toxic to that species than to most others. However, swine, dogs and cats occasionally have been poisoned despite the unpalatability of the squill for these species. The chief signs are vomiting, depression, weakness, ataxia, paresis that may progress to posterior or generalized paralysis, bradycardia, cardiac arrhythmias, dyspnea, cyanosis and sometimes cutaneous erythema. Vomiting does not always occur in swine and complete paralysis seldom develops in dogs. The clinical course seldom exceeds 24 to 36 hours. Death occurs suddenly as a result of ventricular fibrillation.

Treatment consists of complete isolation to prevent undue exertion that might result in cardiac embarrassment. Emetics and gastric lavage should be used if vomiting has not occurred. Saline cathartics may aid in elimination of unabsorbed glycoside. Atropine sulfate (℞ 511) administered subcut. at 6- to 8-hour intervals may prevent cardiac arrest. Phenytoin at 16 mg/lb (35 mg/kg), t.i.d. should be given to dogs to suppress arrhythmias.

Phosphorus, in its white (or yellow) form, was once used widely in preparations employed in the extermination of rodents and rabbits. These preparations were, and to a lesser extent still are, a hazard to domestic animals. The onset of signs of poisoning is sudden. The early signs include vomiting, severe diarrhea, which often is bloody, marked signs of abdominal distress and a peculiar garlic-like odor to the breath. On the third or fourth day of illness, the animal may appear to recover, but additional signs due largely to acute liver damage, develop. They include hemorrhage, severe abdominal pain and generalized icterus. The patient rapidly becomes prostrate and dies in convulsions. Postmortem findings include severe gastroenteritis, a fatty liver, multiple hemorrhages, black tarry blood that fails to clot, and the cadaver may be phosphorescent.

To be successful, treatment must be instituted early. The judicious use of emetics may be beneficial if vomiting has not already emptied the stomach. A 1% solution of copper sulfate is an effective emetic, and also forms a copper phosphide complex that is not absorbed. Gastric and gastrointestinal lavage using a 0.01 to 0.1% solution of potassium permanganate or a 1% solution of copper sulfate should be used in an attempt to oxidize the toxic allotrope. Gastric lavage should be followed by a saline cathartic. Any form of fat in the diet must be avoided for at least 3 to 4 days because fats favor the absorption of phosphorus. The administration of 100 to 200 ml of mineral oil has been recommended, however, since it dissolves phosphorus and prevents its absorption. No treatment has been successful after signs of acute liver damage have appeared.

Thallium sulfate is now infrequently used as a rodenticide. It is toxic to all species to which it has been fed. Mature animals are more susceptible than young ones. The signs of poisoning include vomiting, anorexia, excessive salivation, abdominal distress, severe diarrhea, ulcerative stomatitis, dyspnea, weakness, blindness, hyperesthesia, convulsions and loss of hair or wool after clinical recovery. Thallium will accumulate in the body, and repeated ingestion of small doses may lead to hair loss and further toxicity. The most prominent necropsy findings are those of marked ulcerative gastroenteritis and cutaneous erythema.

Treatment of acute thallium poisoning comprises the use of emetics, gastric lavage with a 1% solution of sodium iodide, and IV administration of a 10% solution of sodium iodide (℞ 636). Diphenylthiocarbazone (℞ 629) is antidotal. Symptomatic treatment of the diarrhea and convulsions is indicated with particular attention to fluid and electrolyte balance.

ANTU (α-naphthylthiourea): All animals tested have been susceptible to ANTU poisoning but most cases have occurred in dogs and swine. There is a marked variation in susceptibility with age, older animals being most susceptible. Animals with an empty stomach readily vomit after ingestion of ANTU and seldom are poisoned, while those with a full or partially filled stomach usually absorb fatal quantities of the chemical before vomiting occurs. The onset of signs is sudden and usually characterized by vomiting. Progressive weakness rapidly develops. Affected animals become ataxic, later exhibit a propensity to sit and finally remain recumbent. There may be vomiting, salivation and restlessness. Marked signs characteristic of pulmonary edema—dyspnea, dullness and flatness on percussion and moist rales—rapidly appear, and coughing is common. The pulse rate is rapid but weak; heart sounds are faint. The temperature gradually becomes subnormal. Diarrhea develops late in the course of the disease. Patients gradually become comatose and die from hypoxia. The course is rapid, many poisoned animals dying within an hour, the majority within 2 to 4 hours. Animals that survive 12 hours may recover.

The lesions are suggestive. The most striking finding is edema of the lungs with hydrothorax. Hyperemia of the tracheal mucosa, moderate to acute gastroenteritis, marked hyperemia of the kidneys and a pale mottled liver are found in most cases. A 10% solution of sodium thiosulfate, IV, has been reported to be beneficial. Positive-pressure oxygen therapy may help to relieve the pulmonary edema.

Sodium fluoroacetate (1080): This colorless, odorless, tasteless, water-soluble chemical has been found to be highly toxic (0.1 to 8 mg/kg) to all animals to which it has been fed. Fluoroacetate is not toxic in itself, but it is metabolized to fluorocitrate, which blocks the tricarboxylic acid cycle—a mechanism necessary for energy production by cells. It produces its effects by 2 general mechanisms: (1) overstimulation of the CNS resulting in death in convulsions, and (2) alteration of cardiac function that results in myocardial depression, cardiac arrhythmias, ventricular fibrillation and circulatory collapse. The CNS stimulation is the main reaction in dogs, while the cardiac effect is predominant in the horse, sheep and chicken. Swine, however, appear to be about equally affected by both.

The onset is rapid and occurs between 15 minutes and several hours after ingestion of the chemical, depending on the dose. Most species exhibit an initial period of nervousness and restlessness. This is followed in all species, except the dog and pig, by marked depression and weakness. Patients rapidly become prostrate, the pulse is weak and 2 to 3 times the normal rate. Death occurs as a result of cardiac failure. Usually, dogs and swine rapidly develop tetanic convulsions. Many exhibit evidence of severe pain. The clinical syndrome displayed is reminiscent of strychnine poisoning in these species. Vomiting is prominent in swine. The course is rapid, affected animals dying between 15 minutes and several hours after signs have appeared. Few animals that develop marked signs recover. The most common necropsy finding is the presence of subepicardial hemorrhages on a heart that has stopped in diastole. The blood is usually dark and tarry in appearance.

Treatment consists of administering emetics and gastric lavage. Barbiturates have been used with some success in mild cases; however, they must be used with caution since they may depress the respiratory center even more. Glyceryl monoacetate (monacetin) serves as a competitive antagonist of fluoroacetate. The recommended dose is 0.25 ml/lb (0.55 ml/kg), IM every half hour for several hours. This compound also may be administered IV in 5 parts of sterile isotonic saline solution. The use of this class of rodenticides has been severely restricted in the U.S.A. Compound 1080 has been banned for use on all federal land. A black dye must be mixed with 1080 for identification. Only certified, insured exterminators can purchase it. One further hazard is that any animal that consumes a rat killed by 1080 will be similarly poisoned—a biologic chain reaction.

Sodium fluoroacetamide (1081) causes similar signs and requires the same treatment.

Warfarin, pindone and **diphacinone** have potent antiprothrombin activity and are potentially dangerous to all classes of mammals and birds. Intoxications in domestic animals have been largely the result either of contamination of feed with warfarin concentrates or with malicious use of the chemical. Swine have been poisoned by feed mixed in equipment used immediately beforehand to prepare rodent bait. The clinical signs and treatment are as for sweet clover poisoning (q.v., p. 1017).

The anticoagulant rodenticides can cause poisoning by massive single doses or by repeated low doses: dogs—single dose of 50 mg/kg, or 5 mg/kg for 10 days; swine—a single dose of 3 mg/kg, or 0.05 mg/kg for 7 days. The half-life of warfarin in canine plasma is 15 hours.

Castrix (Crimidine) is a convulsant rodenticide antagonizing pyridoxine. Toxicity in dogs is low, but chronic ingestion of low doses leads to convulsions. Convulsions can be controlled by barbiturates.

Vacor is a rodenticide whose toxicity in most domestic animals is about 300 mg/kg body wt. The toxicity to cats is, however, 100 to 200 mg/kg. Clinical signs are restricted to extreme CNS depression.

Experimentally, large doses of nicotinamide are said to antagonize the action.

Zinc phosphide is employed as a rodenticide in baits; it has been used extensively around farms and barns because rats tend to die in the open; an esthetic advantage. The toxic dose is about 40 mg/kg, and onset is rapid in animals with a full stomach. The chief signs are anorexia, depression, dyspnea and vomiting with gastrointestinal pain. Convulsions may suggest strychnine poisoning, and death is due to respiratory arrest. Signs which are less frequently seen include visceral congestion and pulmonary edema. Treatment must include supportive therapy, calcium gluconate, and 0.17 M sodium lactate to reduce acidosis.

α-**Chloralose** is a compound used as an anesthetic and rodenticide by acting on the CNS. Its toxicity is very low—about 400 to 600 mg/kg—and signs of toxicity are mild ataxia followed by hyperexcitability. Some affected cats may become quite aggressive. These signs are followed by salivation, ataxia, dyspnea, hypothermia and prostration. Treatment is supportive with artificial ventilation, maintenance of normal body temperature and evacuation.

Norbormide is a selective rodenticide, being toxic to the Norwegian rat at 5.3 mg/kg and to other animals at extremely high levels, of more than 1 gm/kg. There have been no reported instances of poisoning in species other than rodents.

TOXICITY OF ORGANIC INSECTICIDES AND ACARICIDES

There has been criticism from many quarters of certain of the pesticides to be discussed in this section. There are changes proposed in State and Federal legislation, changes expected as the result of executive interpretation, changes as one ecologic interest challenges another. For these reasons, it is important that every user of pesticides make a particular effort to always read and follow current label directions—not just once, but each and every time a new container is purchased. (*See also* PROTECTION OF PERSONS HANDLING INSECTICIDES, p. 1009 and GENERAL PRECAUTIONS, p. 1009.)

The day-to-day and month-to-month changes that will occur will be the result primarily of pressure from environmentalists, consumers and others, rather than toxicologists concerned with the safety of livestock and other domestic animals, since the safety of these compounds for these animals has been rather carefully established in the past. It is of utmost importance that changing recommendations and regulations be treated with respect and full compliance. Prosecution of individuals, including veterinarians, has already occurred and will continue, for failure to follow label directions or to heed label warnings and for failure to warn the animal owner of the precautions to be taken.

Poisoning by the organic insecticides and acaricides may be caused by their direct application to animals, by the ingestion of the compounds on feed or forage treated for the control of plant parasites, or by accidental exposure. It is not within the scope of this section to cover all materials currently used as insecticides or acaricides. For this reason, discussion is limited to those organic compounds known to be most frequently hazardous as toxicants to livestock or as residues in animal products.

An ideal insecticide or acaricide should be efficacious without the risk of injury to livestock or the person making the application and without leaving residues in the tissues, eggs or milk. While many compounds meet some of these requirements, few of those presently available satisfy all of them.

Under present regulations, labels must carry warnings against use of many compounds on certain animals or under certain circumstances. These warnings may be concerned with acute or chronic toxicity or with the avoidance of residues in meat, milk or other animal products. In either case it is imperative that label instructions be followed to the letter.

PETROLEUM PRODUCTS

Petroleum fractions have been used as insecticides and acaricides for many years, either alone or as part of more-or-less complex formulations. Certain light mineral oils, kerosene and xylene may be applied to the skin in small quantities without harmful effects other than perhaps transitory erythema or discomfort. In general, such materials should not be used on cattle in excess of 60 gm per adult. When larger quantities are used, severe reactions may occur, such as drying, cracking or blistering of the skin, inappetence, depression, dyspnea, salivation and, occasionally, death. Xylene irritates the skin of cattle, and in sheep, excessive amounts produce generalized signs, including dizziness, trembling and narcosis. The toxic effects of xylene are observed within a few minutes of exposure and may last for several hours, depending upon the degree of exposure. The effects of oils and petroleum fractions are observed within the first few days after application and persist for several days or weeks. Through failure to recognize their toxic effects, many cases of poisoning or injury following the use of these substances have been wrongly attributed to the insecticide dissolved in them.

Treatment of poisoning or damage due to petroleum products should be directed to the removal of the material from the skin with the aid of soap or detergents and copious quantities of water. Further treatment is dependent upon the clinical signs.

SOLVENTS AND EMULSIFIERS

Solvents and emulsifiers are required in most liquid preparations of insecticides. These compounds may or may not be toxic; usually they are of very low toxicity, but like the petroleum products (which many are), they must be given consideration as possible causes of poisoning. In direct treatment there must be excellent emulsification, with an average droplet size of approximately 5 μ (preferably smaller), or excessive deposits will be made on the animals treated. Treatment should be as for the petroleum products.

PURITY OF PRODUCT

In all syntheses of chemicals, the reactions rarely yield 100% of the product of interest. In any synthesis, be it a natural crop or man-made, there will be present, in variable proportions, related compounds which may have different biologic effects from the compound sought. A prime example of this is to be found with TDE (Rhothane, DDD). The p,p′-isomer is an effective insecticide of low toxicity for most mammals. The o,p-isomer causes necrosis of the adrenal glands of human and dog and is employed to treat certain adrenal malfunctions. There is evidence that p,p′-DDT and o,p-DDT have a similar relationship.

Final purity may often rest with the consumer. Storage of products under extremes of temperatures may lead to deterioration as may the holding of partially emptied containers for unusually long periods. It cannot be overemphasized that storing any chemical in anything but the original container is hazardous. Some consumers continue to mix their own combinations, often to the disadvantage of the animals treated.

INSECTICIDES DERIVED FROM PLANTS

Most of the insecticides derived from plants have traditionally been considered safe for use on animals. Derris (rotenone) and pyrethrum are examples of such materials. Nicotine in the form of **nicotine sulfate** (Black-leaf 40) is an exception. Unless it is carefully used, poisoning may result. Animals poisoned by nicotine sulfate show tremors, incoordination, nausea and disturbed respiration, and finally become comatose and die.

Necropsy lesions of nicotine poisoning include pale mucous membranes, dark blood, hemorrhages on the heart and in the lungs, and congestion of the brain. Treatment of nicotine poisoning consists of removing the material by washing or by gastric lavage, applying artificial respiration, and providing the usual measures for cardiac arrest and shock. Mildly affected animals recover rapidly and spontaneously.

SULFUR AND LIME-SULFUR

Sulfur and lime-sulfur are 2 of the oldest insecticides. Elemental sulfur is practically devoid of toxicity, although poisoning has occurred occasionally when very high proportions were mixed in the feed of cattle. Specific toxic dosages are not known, but probably exceed 4 gm/kg of body wt. Lime-sulfur, which is a complex of sulfides, may cause irritation, discomfort, or blistering, but rarely causes death. Treatment consists of removing the residual material and applying bland protective ointments plus any supportive measures that may be indicated.

CHLORINATED HYDROCARBON COMPOUNDS

Those most commonly used (or that may have been used) on animals and in their environment are DDT, TDE (Rhothane), methoxychlor, lindane, benzene hexachloride (BHC), chlordane, toxaphene, dieldrin, aldrin and heptachlor.

Acute Toxic Doses

DDT poisoning of cattle, sheep, goats, hogs, horses and dogs is not observed, except under the most unusual circumstances. Poisoning of poultry and cats occurs occasionally. Cattle tolerate applications of sprays containing as much as 8% DDT. Sheep, goats, hogs and horses are not harmed by sprays or dips containing 1.5% of DDT, even when applied every 4 days for 4 applications. Dogs tolerate 1% dips and sprays. Cats have been reported to be highly susceptible to DDT, although exact toxic doses have not been presented. Chickens have been poisoned by 1% dips of DDT.

When administered orally, DDT is definitely toxic to cattle, sheep and goats in doses of 500 mg/kg of body wt. The minimum acute toxicity level is 250 mg/kg. Single doses of 100 mg/kg are tolerated by sheep, goats, cattle and horses. Horses have been given as much as 240 mg/kg without producing clinical signs.

When applied as a 0.5% spray to lactating cows, an average of 0.5 ppm appears in the milk with a peak of about 1.5 ppm 2 days after spraying. DDT appears in the milk of cows occupying barns sprayed with DDT unless precautions are taken to prevent contamination of the feed and contact between the animals and the treated walls and stanchions. DDT is not recommended for use on animals producing milk for human consumption.

DDT is stored in the fat of cattle that are sprayed with it or are consuming it in treated or contaminated feeds. A single spraying with 0.5% DDT produces a residue in the fat of cattle of about 11 ppm. Additional spraying at 2- or 3-week intervals gradually increases the residue. Six applications of DDT at 3-week intervals have produced a residue of 35 ppm in the fat of cattle, while 31 applications at 2-week intervals produced from 80 to 100 ppm. After the cessation of treatment, an interval of at least 24 weeks is required for the elimination from the fat tissue of a residue of 35 ppm. Cattle fed a diet containing 10 ppm of DDT for 28 days have shown a residue of 7 ppm in the fat. Sheep so fed had a residue of 3 ppm. DDT is no longer approved for use on livestock, and any residue is violative in many countries.

DDD or **TDE** (Rhothane) is chemically related to DDT and it is somewhat less toxic. Residues in the tissues and the amounts excreted in milk are also similar. Statements relating to DDT apply in general to this compound.

Methoxychlor is one of the safest available chlorinated hydrocarbon insecticides. Young dairy calves tolerate 264 mg/kg of body wt; 500 mg/kg is mildly toxic. While 1 gm/kg produces rather severe poisoning in young calves, sheep are not affected. One dog was given 990 mg/kg daily for 30 days without showing signs. The extent of absorption and storage of methoxychlor is less than with DDT or DDD (TDE), but the duration of storage is about the same. About 0.4 ppm of methoxychlor may be found in milk one day after spraying a cow with a 0.5% spray. Because of this excretion, sprays of methoxychlor are no longer recommended for use on animals producing milk for human consumption. Six applications of a 0.5% spray at 3-week intervals will produce a residue in the fat of cattle of 2.4 ppm. Cattle and sheep store essentially no methoxychlor when it is fed to them at the rate of 25 ppm in the total diet for 112 days. The established tolerance for methoxychlor in fat will not be exceeded, provided it is used only as recommended.

Benzene hexachloride (**BHC**, hexachlorocyclohexane) is a very useful insecticide for large animals and for dogs, but is highly toxic to cats in the concentrations necessary for parasite control. Only the gamma isomer of this compound is insecticidal. Unfortunately, the same isomer accounts for its acute toxicity. **Lindane** contains 99% or more of the gamma isomer. Because isomers other than the gamma are stored excessively and for long periods in body tissues, it is best that lindane be used in preference to the technical grade of BHC, which contains several isomers.

Cattle in good condition tolerated 0.2% lindane applications, but in stressed, emaciated cattle poisoning has resulted from spraying or dipping in 0.075% material. Horses and hogs appear to tolerate 0.2 to 0.5% sprays, thereby leaving an adequate margin of safety for these species. Ordinarily, sheep and goats tolerate 0.5% applications. Emaciation and lactation are known to increase the susceptibility of animals to poisoning by lindane; therefore, such animals should be treated with extreme caution. Very young calves are poisoned by a single oral dose of lindane at 4.4 mg/kg of body wt. Mild signs appear in sheep given 22 mg/kg and death occurs at 100 mg/kg. Adult cattle have been given 13 mg/kg without producing signs. BHC is stored in the fat of the body and excreted in the milk.

While all the isomers behave in this manner, lindane is eliminated rapidly, while the other isomers are excreted more slowly. Cattle sprayed or dipped in 0.075% lindane showed 23 ppm in their fat. This residue declined to zero over a period of 12 weeks. Chickens are susceptible to lindane poisoning to about the same extent as young calves, 0.05% dips producing about 10% mortality.

Chlordane: Livestock become exposed only through consumption of treated plants or through carelessness and accidents. Very young calves have been killed by doses of 44 mg/kg, and the minimum toxic dose for cattle is about 88 mg/kg. Cattle fed chlordane as 25 ppm of their diet for 56 days showed 19 ppm in their fat at the end of the feeding. Emulsions and suspensions have been used safely on dogs at concentrations up to 0.25%, provided freshly diluted materials were used. In dry powders, it has been safely used in concentrations up to 5% on dogs. No injury resulted to pigeons, Leghorn cockerels and pullets that had been subjected for 30 to 60 days to vapors emanating from chlordane-treated surfaces.

Toxaphene can be used with reasonable safety if recommendations are followed, but can produce poisoning when applied or ingested in excessive quantities. Dogs and cats are particularly susceptible to toxaphene poisoning and it should never be used on these animals. Young calves have been poisoned by 1% toxaphene sprays, while all other farm animals except poultry can withstand 1.0% or more as sprays or dips. Chickens have been poisoned by dipping in 0.1% emulsions and turkeys have been poisoned by spraying with 0.5% material. Toxaphene is primarily an acute toxicant and does not persist unduly in the tissues. Adult cattle have been mildly intoxicated by 4%, and definitely harmed by 8% sprays. Poisoning of adult cattle has resulted from dipping in emulsions that contained only 0.5% of toxaphene, an amount ordinarily safe, because the emulsions had begun breaking down, allowing the fine droplets to coalesce. The large droplets readily adhere to the hair of cattle and the resultant dosage becomes equivalent to that obtained by spray treatments of much higher concentration. Toxaphene is lethal to young calves at 8.8 mg/kg but not at 4.4 mg/kg. The minimum toxic dose for cattle is about 33 mg/kg, and for sheep between 22 and 33 mg/kg. Spraying Hereford cattle 12 times at 2-week intervals with 0.5% toxaphene produced a maximum residue of 8 ppm in the fat. Cattle fed 10 ppm of toxaphene in the diet for 30 days had no detectable toxaphene tissue residues, while steers fed 100 ppm for 112 days stored only 40 ppm in their fat. This amount was eliminated in 2 months after the feeding of toxaphene had been suspended.

Dieldrin has not been recommended for use on livestock in the U.S.A., with the exception of sheep, because of the residues that appear in meat and milk. In sheep, the material has given outstanding results in controlling the sheep ked when used as a 1.0 to 1.5%

dust. While residues limit its application, dieldrin is actually an insecticide of moderate toxicity. Young dairy calves are poisoned by oral doses of 8.8 mg/kg but tolerate 4.4 mg/kg, while adult cattle tolerate 8.8 mg/kg and are poisoned by 22 mg/kg. Pigs tolerate 22 mg/kg and are poisoned by 44 mg/kg. Horses are poisoned by 22 mg/kg. Because of its high effectiveness against insect pests on crops and pasture and consequent low dosage per acre, dieldrin is not likely to produce poisoning of livestock grazing the treated areas. Diets containing 25 ppm of dieldrin have been fed to cattle and sheep for periods of 16 weeks without producing any harmful effect other than a residue in their fat. Residues in animal fat are slow to disappear. Considerable judgment must be exercised in the marketing of animals grazing treated areas or consuming products from previously treated areas as no edible tissue residue is allowable in the U.S.A.

Aldrin is a potent insecticide and a near relative of dieldrin. It is of the same order of toxicity and the statements pertaining to dieldrin may be considered to apply in general to aldrin. It is not recommended for use on livestock because of its tendency to produce considerable tissue residue. The animal body converts aldrin to dieldrin and stores the material as dieldrin. Specific analyses for aldrin will, therefore, usually yield negative results, while dieldrin analyses reflect the true level of storage.

Heptachlor has not been recommended for use on livestock in the U.S.A. but since it is very effective against certain plant-feeding insects, it is encountered from time to time in areas grazed by livestock. Heptachlor is tolerated by young dairy calves in doses as high as 13 mg/kg body wt but is toxic to them at 22 mg/kg. Sheep tolerate 22 mg/kg but are poisoned by 40 mg/kg. Diets containing 60 ppm of heptachlor have been fed to cattle for 16 weeks without producing any harmful effect other than the residues in the fat tissues. Heptachlor must, therefore, be considered as another chlorinated hydrocarbon of moderate toxicity. It is converted by animals and stored in the body fat as heptachlor epoxide. For this reason, a specific analysis performed for heptachlor will usually yield negative results, while the epoxide method will reveal storage.

Clinical Findings: The chlorinated hydrocarbon insecticides are general stimulants to the CNS. They produce a great variety of signs, most of which are neuromuscular manifestations. The affected animal generally is first noted to be more alert. Fasciculation of the muscles is then observed, the process commencing in the facial region and extending backward until all the body musculature is involved. In poisoning by DDT, DDD and methoxychlor, progressive involvement leads to trembling or shivering movements that are followed by convulsions and death. With the other chlorinated hydrocarbons, the muscular twitchings are followed by convulsions, usually without the intermediate trembling. Convulsions may be clonic, tonic, or both and may last from only a few seconds to several hours or may be brief and frequent. Abnormal postures, such as touching the sternum to the ground while maintaining the standard position with the hind limbs, or keeping the head down between the forelegs, are often seen. Some animals stand with their heads pressed against a wall or fence. Many animals exhibit almost continual chewing movements. Occasionally, an affected animal becomes belligerent and will attack other animals or moving objects. There usually is a copious flow of thick saliva and incontinence of urine. Vocalizations of various sorts also are common. During the convulsive states, high fevers may occur due to intense muscular activity. Some affected animals show none of these active signs, but are depressed, almost oblivious to their surroundings and do not eat or drink. Such animals may live several days longer than those showing the more violent manifestations. In certain cases, there is an alternation of clinical signs, the animal first being extremely excited and then severely depressed. The severity of the signs observed at a given time is not a sure prognostic index. Some animals have only a single convulsion and die, while others suffer innumerable convulsions but subsequently recover. The signs of poisoning by these insecticides are highly suggestive, but are not sufficiently definitive to be diagnostic. Encephalitis or meningitis often present signs similar to those observed in insecticide poisoning.

Signs of acute intoxication by chlordane in birds are nervous chirping, collapse on hocks or side, excitability and mucous exudates in the nasal passages. Signs of subacute and chronic intoxication are molting, dehydration and cyanosis of the comb, loss of body weight and cessation of egg production. Molting and cyanosis of the comb are nonspecific signs.

Lesions: If death has occurred suddenly, there may be nothing more than cyanosis. More definite lesions occur as the duration of the intoxication increases. There is usually congestion of various organs, particularly the lungs, liver and kidneys, plus a blanched appearance of all organs if the body temperature was high before death. The heart generally is in systole, and there are usually many hemorrhages of varying size on the epicardium. In some cases, the appearance of the heart and lungs suggests a peracute pneumonia, and, if the animal was affected for more than a few hours, there may be edema of the lungs. The trachea and bronchi may contain a blood-tinged froth. Cerebrospinal-fluid volume is excessive in many cases, and the brain and spinal cord frequently are congested and edematous.

Treatment: There are no known specific antidotes for the chlorinated hydrocarbon insecticides. When exposure has been by spraying, dipping or dusting, a thorough bathing, using detergents (if possible, otherwise soap) and copious quantities of water is recommended. If the material was taken internally, gastric lavage is indicated together with saline purgatives. The use of oils for this purpose is contraindicated because they may increase, rather than decrease, absorption.

Regardless of the manner of exposure, the signs exhibited by the animal should be controlled. When these are of the excitatory type, the use of barbiturates or chloral hydrate is indicated. All disturbing elements of the environment should be reduced or removed. If the animal shows marked depression, anorexia and dehydration, therapy should be directed toward supplying appropriate nourishment and fluids by the use of IV injections and, if necessary, introduction of food and water through a stomach tube. Residues of insecticides remaining in the exposed animal may be reduced by treatments of activated charcoal slurry or providing charcoal in feed. Feeding 5 gm of phenobarbital per day may accelerate residue removal.

ORGANOPHOSPHORUS COMPOUNDS

A large number of organophosphorus compounds have been developed for plant and animal protection. They vary greatly in toxic effect, and each has its own characteristics in regard to tissue storage and excretion in milk. In general, however, this family of compounds offers a distinct advantage by producing little or no tissue residues. Experimentally, several organophosphorus compounds have shown delayed neurotoxicity, but field cases have been rare.

Recently several organophosphorus compounds have been prepared by microencapsulation, thus releasing the active compound slowly and increasing the duration of effectiveness. Preliminary work has shown that the toxicity is reduced by a factor of 5 in mature cattle but not in calves. Only the microencapsulated form of methyl parathion has been registered at the time of this writing, but several others are being prepared. Users of these compounds should be aware that the toxic properties are still present.

Tetraethyl pyrophosphate (TEPP) probably is one of the most acutely toxic of all insecticides. Although it is not used on animals, they may occasionally be exposed to it accidentally. One herd of 29 cattle ranging in age from calves to adults were accidentally sprayed with 0.33% TEPP emulsion; all were dead within 40 minutes.

Parathion, a widely used material for control of plant pests, is approximately one-half as toxic as TEPP. It has been used as a dip and spray on cattle in some countries, but not in the U.S.A. The majority of the cases of human poisoning (occupational) by insecticides thus far reported have been attributed to parathion or its degradation products. As a spray, it produces definite signs of poisoning in young calves at a 0.02% concentration and occasional transitory signs at 0.01%. Orally, parathion is toxic to sheep at 22 mg/kg of body wt, but not at 11 mg/kg. Young dairy calves are poisoned by 0.44 mg/kg while 44 mg/kg is required to poison older cattle. Parathion is used extensively in the control of mosquitoes and insects in the orchard and on truck crops. Normally, because so little is used per acre treated, it presents no particular hazard to livestock. Because of its potency, particular care should be taken to prevent accidental exposures to the compound. Parathion is not stored in animal tissues in appreciable amounts.

EPN is related to parathion, but is approximately one-half as toxic when externally applied. When given orally, it is of approximately equal toxicity. The oral LD_{50} in rats is 7 mg/kg, while the dermal LD_{50} is 22 mg/kg. The dog is not poisoned at doses greater than 100 mg/kg.

Malathion is one of the safest organophosphorus compounds and is roughly equivalent to toxaphene, 0.5% sprays not being toxic to young calves while 1% sprays are. Adult cattle tolerate 2% sprays. Given orally, malathion is toxic at 100 mg/kg but not at 55 mg/kg of body wt. Young calves tolerate 11 mg/kg, but are poisoned by 22 mg/kg. Malathion appears in the milk of dairy cattle.

Ronnel (fenchlorfos) produces mild signs of poisoning in cattle at 132 mg/kg of body wt, but severe signs do not appear until the dose is increased to about 440 mg/kg. The minimum toxic dose in sheep is 400 mg/kg. The oral LD_{50} in rats is 906 mg/kg. Concentrations as high as 2.5% in sprays have failed to produce poisoning of cattle, very young dairy calves or sheep. Poisoning by ronnel usually occurs in 2 stages: The animal first becomes rather weak and, although moving about normally, may be very placid. Diarrhea also may appear at this time, the feces often being flecked with blood, Later, salivation and dyspnea appear if the dose is high. At the lower dosages, the salivation and dyspnea will probably not be seen. Blood cholinesterase activity declines slowly over a period of 5 to 7 days. Ronnel produces residues in meat and milk, therefore strict adherence to label restrictions is essential. The residues may be removed by giving the animal activated charcoal for several days.

Coumaphos is used against cattle grubs (*Hypoderma* spp.), *Dermatobia hominis* and a number of other ectoparasites and for treatment of premises. The maximum concentration that may be safely used on adult cattle, horses and hogs is 0.5%. Young calves and all ages of sheep and goats must not be sprayed with concentrations higher than 0.25%. For them, the drug may be lethal at 0.5% concentrations. Adult cattle may show mild signs at 1.0% concentrations.

Diazinon: When sprayed, young calves appear to tolerate 0.05%, but are poisoned by 0.1% concentrations. Adult cattle may be sprayed repeatedly at weekly intervals with 0.1% concentrations without inducing poisoning. Orally, diazinon appears to be tolerated by young calves at 0.44 mg/kg of body wt but poisoning results at 0.88 mg/kg. Adult cattle tolerate 8.8 mg/kg orally, but are poisoned by 22 mg/kg. Sheep tolerate 17.6 mg/kg, but are poisoned by 26 mg/kg.

Trichlorfon: As a spray, the material is tolerated by adult cattle at a 1.0% concentration. When administered orally, this compound is tolerated by young dairy calves at 4.4 mg/kg of body wt, but it produces poisoning at 8.8 mg/kg. In adult cattle, 44 mg/kg appears to be tolerated, while 88 mg/kg produces poisoning. Sheep and horses are poisoned by 88 mg/kg, but appear to tolerate 44 mg/kg. Dogs were unaffected by the feeding of 1,000 ppm of trichlorfon for 4 months. Trichlorfon is metabolized very rapidly.

Ciodrin is of rather low toxicity; however Brahman cattle are markedly more susceptible to poisoning than are the European breeds. Cattle (except as above), sheep, goats and pigs all tolerate sprays containing ciodrin at 0.5% levels or higher. The toxic dose appears to be in the 2% range except for Brahmans where 0.144% to 0.3% may be toxic.

Dichlorvos is rapidly metabolized and excreted; it has many uses on both plants and animals. Residues in meat and milk are not a problem if label directions are followed. Dichlorvos is of moderate toxicity. The minimum toxic dose is 10 mg/kg in young calves, 25 mg/kg in horses, and sheep, and the LD_{50} in rats is 25 mg/kg, orally. A 1% dust was not toxic to cattle. "Flea collars" that contain this compound may cause skin reactions in some pets.

Dioxathion is a mixture of cis- and trans-isomers (70%) and reaction products (30%). It is used for both plant and animal protection. It is rapidly metabolized and is not likely to produce residues in meat greater than the 1 ppm official tolerance. Concentrations of 0.15% or less are generally employed on animals. The minimum toxic dose in calves is 5 mg/kg, orally, while the oral LD_{50} in rats is 19 mg/kg. Sprays of 0.5% have not been toxic in cattle or sheep, and sprays of 0.25% nontoxic in goats or swine. Orally, dioxathion has killed young calves at 8.8 mg/kg and produced intoxication at 4.4 mg/kg.

Ruelene is active both as a systemic and contact insecticide in livestock, has some anthelmintic activity, and is of rather low toxicity. Dairy calves have been poisoned by oral doses of 44 mg/kg and above, while adult cattle required 88 mg/kg for the same effect. Sheep have shown moderate intoxication by 176 mg/kg while Angora goats were about twice as sensitive. Pigs have been poisoned by 11 mg/kg and horses by 44 mg/kg. As a topical spray most livestock tolerate concentrations of 2%.

Carbophenothion: Dairy calves under 2 weeks of age sprayed with water-based formulations showed poisoning at 0.05% and higher concentrations. Adult cattle have been poisoned by concentrations of 1.0% and higher. Sheep and goats have been poisoned by oral doses of 22 mg/kg and higher but not at 8 mg/kg. The LD_{50} for rats is about 31 mg/kg; a daily dosage of 2.2 mg/kg for 90 days produced poisoning. Dogs tolerated a diet containing 32 ppm for 90 days.

Supona: Adult cattle were poisoned by sprays containing 0.5% and above, while young calves were poisoned only when the concentration was raised to 2%. The minimum oral toxic dose appears to be about 22 mg/kg for all ages of cattle.

Dimethoate: When administered orally, the minimum toxic dose for young dairy calves was about 48 mg/kg, while 22 mg/kg was a lethal dose for cattle one year of age. Daily doses of 10 mg/kg for 5 days in adult cattle lowered blood cholinesterase activity to 20% of normal but did not produce signs of poisoning. Horses have been poisoned by oral doses of 60 to 80 mg/kg. When applied topically, sprays of 1% concentration have been tolerated by calves, cattle and adult sheep.

Phorate (Thimet): The minimum toxic dose found in calves was 0.25 mg/kg, 0.75 mg/kg in sheep, and 1.0 mg/kg in cattle. The oral LD_{50} in rats is 1 mg/kg.

Disulfoton (dithiodemeton, Di-Syston): The maximum nontoxic oral dose is 0.88 mg/kg for young calves, for cattle and goats 2.2 mg/kg and for sheep 4.8 mg/kg. Several occurrences of intoxication have shown that cattle are very susceptible to this compound or its toxic metabolites when sprayed on forage crops.

Oxydemetonmethyl: The maximum nontoxic oral dose was 0.88 mg/kg for young calves, 2.2 mg/kg for cattle and 4.8 mg/kg for sheep and goats.

Azinphosmethyl: The maximum nontoxic oral dose for calves was 0.44 mg/kg, for cattle and goats 2.2 mg/kg, and for sheep 4.8 mg/kg.

Temophos (Abate, Bithion): The oral LD_{50} seen in rats is 1 gm/kg body wt while the dermal LD_{50} is greater than 4 gm/kg.

Chlorpyrifos (Dursban): The LD_{50} found in goats was 500 mg/kg orally while the rat had an LD_{50} of 97 mg/kg.

Demeton (Systox): The LD_{50} dose in goats was 8 mg/kg orally while the rat showed an LD_{50} of 2 mg/kg orally and 8 mg/kg on dermal application.

Famophos (famphur): The maximum nontoxic dose found in calves was 10 mg/kg, and 50 mg/kg in cattle, sheep and horses. This compound is effective against warbles in cattle, but care must be taken to follow directions as to time limits on application; if larvae are killed while migrating on the body, especially throat areas, there may be a reaction to the killed larvae.

Fenthion: The minimum toxic dose found on oral administration to cattle was 25 mg/kg; 50 mg/kg orally killed sheep.

Methyl parathion: The single, oral dose LD_{50} in rats is 9 mg/kg compared to 3 mg/kg for ethyl parathion. This compound is being microencapsulated by one manufacturer, and the lethal dose in cattle has thus been increased from 0.5% spray to a 2% spray as preliminary testing has shown a 5-fold decrease in toxicity.

Mevinphos (Phosdrin): The LD_{50} in rats is 3 mg/kg, whether given orally or topically.

Naled (Dibrom): The oral LD_{50} in rats is 430 mg/kg.

Phosmet (Prolate): The minimum oral toxic dose in cattle and calves is 25 mg/kg and 50 mg/kg in sheep. The LD_{50} in rats is 147 mg/kg, orally.

Tetrachlorvinphos (stirofos): The oral LD_{50} in rats is 4 gm/kg, while the minimum toxic dose found in swine was 100 mg/kg.

Clinical Findings: The organophosphorus compounds have in common a widely variable ability to inhibit cholinesterase activity. For some compounds, this appears to be the primary mechanism of poisoning, while for others, the inhibition is secondary. Not all of the actions of these materials are understood. When cholinesterase inhibition is the primary mechanism of intoxication, the clinical syndrome is associated with cholinergic signs such as mild-to-profuse salivation, dyspnea, signs of abdominal pain, ataxia, diarrhea and, occasionally, convulsions. When given in small, repeated doses, these compounds may progressively lower blood cholinesterase activity until no activity can be detected, yet no signs appear. In other cases, when the activity is lowered to 20% or less of normal, signs are noted. Sometimes poisoning may appear while the blood activity is rather high. In this respect, it must be remembered that signs are observed when nerve cholinesterase is inhibited and that the enzyme in the blood reflects only in a general way, the levels in the nerve tissues. Onset of signs after exposure may be within 5 or 6 minutes or may be delayed for 2 days or more. The course of intoxication is influenced principally by the dosage. Malathion, trichlorfon, parathion and TEPP produce poisoning of short duration, followed by death or full recovery within 24 hours. Ronnel and coumaphos produce their effects over a much longer period, in extreme cases signs of intoxication may be seen for as long as 30 days. In acute poisoning death appears to be immediately preceded by paralysis of the respiratory center.

Lesions: In most cases of acute poisoning with organophosphorus compounds the necropsy findings are essentially negative. In the more prolonged cases, there may be visceral changes usually associated with anoxia. Diagnosis of organophosphorus poisoning cannot be based solely upon necropsy lesions. Blood and tissue cholinesterase levels may not fluctuate proportionately; therefore, determination of blood cholinesterase levels is not an accurate index of the presence or degree of poisoning.

Treatment: Organophosphorus insecticide poisoning can usually be treated successfully with atropine sulfate, using the following amounts as average initial doses: cattle—30 mg/100 lb (0.66 mg/kg) of body wt, sheep—50 mg/100 lb (1.1 mg/kg), horses—6.5 mg/100 lb

(0.15 mg/kg), dogs—2 to 4 mg total. One-fourth to ⅓ of the dose should be given slowly, IV, the remainder subcut. or IM. It is important that atropinization be reached and maintained over several hours. The dosage may be repeated, judging time and amount by the response of the patient.

An improved treatment combines atropine with 2-PAM (pralidoxime chloride) (℞ 635); the latter encourages the regeneration of cholinesterase.

Treatment for removal of the poison from the animal, as suggested for the chlorinated hydrocarbons (p. 1002) should also be given. Rest and quiet surroundings are indicated. Artificial respiration or the administration of oxygen is advantageous. Phenothiazine-derived tranquilizers should be avoided. Succinylcholine should not be used for at least one week following the administration or exposure to use of any of the organophosphorus compounds.

CARBAMATE INSECTICIDES

Carbaryl (Sevin): The oral LD_{50} in rats is 307 mg/kg and greater than 500 mg/kg, dermally. A 2% spray is nontoxic to calves while 4% is nontoxic to cattle.

Carbofuran (Furadan): The oral LD_{50} in the rat is 8 mg/kg. The minimum toxic dose in cattle and sheep is 4.5 mg/kg, becoming lethal at 18 and 9 mg/kg, respectively. The LD_{50} in the dog is 19 mg/kg, orally. Swine have been poisoned after drinking water contaminated by this compound.

Methomyl (Lannate): The oral LD_{50} in rats is 17 mg/kg. Cattle have been reported to be poisoned after consumption of forage inadvertently sprayed by this compound.

Propoxur (Baygon): The oral LD_{50} in rats is 95 mg/kg. In goats, the LD_{50} was found to be greater than 800 mg/kg orally.

Clinical Findings and Treatment: The carbamate insecticides act similarly to the organophosphorus (OP) compounds in that they inhibit cholinesterase at nerve junctions. The inhibition is by a different mechanism, however, and the inhibiting bond is much less durable. Frequently, the inhibition cannot be seen in the laboratory because of this reversibility. Treatment of carbamate poisoning is similar to that of the OP compounds in that atropine sulfate injections readily reverse the effects of inhibition. Pralidoxime, or 2-PAM, is contraindicated in carbamate poisoning, at least for carbaryl poisoning, as it may increase the bonding and inhibition of cholinesterase. Signs and lesions are similar to those of the OP poisonings (*see* p. 1007).

CHEMICAL ANALYSIS IN DIAGNOSIS

Chemical analyses are of little value in establishing a diagnosis of poisoning by organic insecticides; most chlorinated hydrocarbon insecticides leave an easily detectable residue even when the health of the animal is unimpaired, while others, particularly the organic phosphorus compounds, may not leave detectable residues even when the true cause of death. The analytic methods available for these compounds are rather specialized and expensive. In all cases it is essential to confirm the identity and quantity of each suspected compound by at least 2 different types of analysis, particularly if there is a possibility of litigation. The validity of chemical analysis is highly dependent upon the care exercised by the collector of the tissues to avoid contamination with the compound from the skin or the environment.

PROTECTION OF PERSONS HANDLING INSECTICIDES

Absorption of insecticides occurs in man as it does in animals. Each exposure, no matter how brief or small, results in some of the compound being absorbed and perhaps stored. Repeated short exposures may eventually result in intoxication. Every precaution should be taken to minimize exposure. This may include the use of rubber gloves, respirators, rain gear or frequent changes of clothing, with bathing at each change. Respirators must have filters approved for the type of insecticide being used; ordinary dust filters will not protect the operator from phosphorus fumes. Such measures are generally sufficient to guard against intoxication. Overexposure to chlorinated hydrocarbon insecticides is difficult to measure except by the occurrence of signs of poisoning.

The cholinesterase-inhibiting property of the organophosphorus compounds may be used to indicate degree of exposure if frequent determinations of the activity of the blood enzyme are made. Serum esterase is usually inhibited first and, in the absence of declining erythrocyte activity indicates a recent exposure of only moderate degree. Depression of the erythrocytic-enzyme activity indicates a very severe acute exposure or a chronic exposure over a long period. It is important to remember that normal cholinesterase activity values vary from individual to individual and that a determination of activity has significance only when it can be compared with the normal value for that particular individual.

GENERAL PRECAUTIONS

Organic pesticides may have deleterious effects upon fish and wildlife as well as upon domesticated species. In no event should amounts greater than those specifically recommended be used, and maximum precautions must be taken to prevent drift or drainage to adjoining fields, pastures, ponds, streams or other premises outside the area in which the treatment is essential.

PESTICIDE POISONING IN DOGS AND CATS

Dogs and cats are exposed to many potentially toxic materials that can lead to poisoning. The ingestion of pesticides is a major hazard. Cats, although potentially exposed to the same poisons as dogs, are less frequently affected, possibly because of their selective eating habits. However, when poisonings do occur, signs observed are comparable to those in dogs.

Metaldehyde and N-methyl carbamates have supplanted arsenic, strychnine, and phosphorus as the major causes of poisonings in small animals. Anticoagulants, organophosphorus compounds and chlorinated hydrocarbons are also significant problems. A variety of other pesticides are also involved to a much lesser extent. Due to the recent reformulation of snail baits so that the inert ingredients are no longer attractive to most dogs, there has been a dramatic decrease in the number of metaldehyde poisonings (q.v., p. 981); however, a significant number of these cases still occur. Some of these are misdiagnosed as strychnine poisoning (q.v., p. 970) due to the similarity of signs.

In the rural and suburban areas, organophosphorus compounds are frequently a major cause of poisoning. Many crops are treated with them and dermal contact alone can lead to poisoning.

The N-methyl carbamates (esters of N-methyl carbamic acid) are widely used in home and garden types of insecticides as well as some snail baits and are a major cause of dog and cat poisonings. When ingested, the cholinergic signs can be dramatic but respond well to prompt treatment with sufficient amounts of atropine.

Although some of the older scientific literature suggests that oximes are contraindicated for carbamate treatment, recent experimental animal studies suggest that they are only contraindicated for treatment of poisoning by carbaryl (Sevin). If an animal is showing severe cholinergic signs and there is no information as to whether an organophosphorus compound or a carbamate was involved, oximes such as 2-PAM (℞ 635) should be considered for supportive treatment.

Cats and dogs are occasionally poisoned by feeding on animals or rodents that have died from pesticide exposure. Most flea collars contain organophosphorus compounds or carbamates and do not normally cause problems. However, young or debilitated dogs or cats may develop signs of cholinesterase inhibition or dermatitis. Solvents may contribute to pesticide poisonings or by themselves may cause the toxic effects. Whenever a pesticide exposure is suspected, the pesticide container should be obtained, as the toxic ingredients are given on the label, and treatment information for man is required on the labels of the more toxic pesticides.

(*See also* the table of contents of the TOXICOLOGY section, p. 964, and the INDEX for more general discussions of most of the poisons listed below.)

Some pesticides and solvents commonly involved in dog and cat poisoning are listed below with their signs and suggested treatment.

ANTICOAGULANTS

COUMARIN TYPES (Warfarin, Coumafuryl)

Clinical Findings: Hemorrhage; sudden death with no previous warning. In subacute cases, anemia, weakness, pale mucous membranes; dyspnea; moist rales; bloody feces; scleral, conjunctival and intraocular hemorrhage; staggering, ataxia, blood-tinged froth around mouth and nose and CNS signs may appear if hemorrhage is in the brain or spinal cord.

Treatment: In severe cases treatment should be initiated promptly, and include one or more of: sedation or light anesthesia to prevent trauma; oxygen therapy; citrated whole blood (9 ml/lb [20 ml/kg]) IV; thoracocentesis to remove blood, if present; vitamin K_1 (0.25 to 1 mg/lb [0.55 to 2.0 mg/kg]) given IV in dextrose solution. The animal should be kept warm and free from physical trauma for at least 24 hours. Oral vitamin K for 4 to 6 days is indicated.

1,3 INDANDIONE TYPES (Diphacinone/diphenadione, pindone)

These tend to be more toxic than the coumarins. The signs are similar to those of coumarin poisoning plus signs of cardiopulmonary and neurologic damage. Treatment is the same as for coumarins.

ARSENICALS

Clinical Findings: In general, organic arsenicals are less toxic than the inorganics. **Acute:** Intense abdominal pain, staggering, extreme weakness, trembling, salivation, vomiting, diarrhea, fast, feeble pulse, normal to subnormal temperature, collapse and death. **Subacute:** Anorexia, depression, watery diarrhea, increased urination followed by anuria, partial paralysis of hind limbs, stupor, subnormal temperature and eventual death.

Treatment: Acute: Treatment must be administered early: give emetics or gastric lavage only if signs are not yet present; if signs are present, give dimercaprol at the rate of 3 mg/lb (6 mg/kg) body wt IM every 4 hours for first 2 days then twice a day for the next 10 days. **Subacute:** Supportive therapy is indicated for additional signs such as dehydration and uremia.

N-METHYL CARBAMATES

Clinical Findings: These include: hypersalivation, gastrointestinal hypermotility, abdominal cramping, vomiting, diarrhea, sweating, dyspnea, cyanosis, miosis, muscle fasciculation (in extreme cases, tetany followed by weakness and paralysis) and convulsive seizures. Death is usually a result of hypoxia due to bronchoconstriction.

Treatment: Atropine sulfate, approximately 2 mg for an average dog. 2-PAM (℞ 635) and other oximes are also useful in addition to atropine treatment, however 2-PAM is contraindicated for treatment of carbaryl poisoning.

METALDEHYDE

Clinical Findings: Muscle weakness, frothing at the mouth, hypersalivation, incoordination, tachycardia, loss of consciousness, cyanosis and often convulsions are seen. Death is due usually to respiratory failure.

Treatment: Emetics, gastric lavage, ventilatory support for respiratory failure, glucose or calcium gluconate for treatment of possible liver damage are indicated. It is often necessary to anesthetize the animal to control convulsions.

CHLORINATED HYDROCARBONS
(Organochlorines)

Clinical Findings: These consist of apprehension, hypersensitivity and spasms of the eyelids and front quarters progressing to the hind quarters, and may be continuous to intermittent. Clonic-tonic seizures, loss of coordination, circling and abnormal posturing may also be seen and the animal may become comatose.

Treatment: Convulsions should be controlled with anesthetics such as chloral hydrate or pentobarbital. If exposure was oral, gastric lavage and saline cathartic should be administered. Diazepam may be successful in controlling violent neuromuscular activity.

ORGANOPHOSPHORUS COMPOUNDS

Clinical Findings: Sialosis; gastrointestinal hypermotility, tenesmus, vomiting, diarrhea; sweating, dyspnea; cyanosis; miosis; muscle fasciculation (in extreme cases, tetany, followed by weakness and paralysis); and convulsive seizures may all be seen. Death is usually a result of hypoxia due to bronchoconstriction.

Treatment: Atropine sulfate (0.25 mg/lb [0.5 mg/kg]), every 4 hr. 2-PAM (℞ 635) is useful to reactivate cholinesterase. Atropine therapy alone will not abolish the skeletal muscular manifestations of poisoning.

PHOSPHORUS

Clinical Findings: The chief signs are abdominal irritation and vomiting; the vomitus may be luminous in the dark and have a garlic-like odor. The animal may appear to recover for a few hours to a few days only to relapse into vomiting, abdominal pain accompanied by icterus, nervous signs, convulsions, coma, and death from severe hepatic and renal degeneration.

Treatment: Gastric lavage should be followed by oral administration of 0.1 to 0.2% potassium permanganate, or 0.2% copper sulfate. Cardiac stimulants and 5% glucose IV may be indicated. Avoid contact with gastric washings containing phosphorus as it can burn the skin and eyes.

STRYCHNINE

Clinical Findings: Signs appear 10 minutes to 2 hours after ingestion; they include apprehension, nervousness, tenseness and stiffness. Violent tetanic spasms may be spontaneous or the result of any external stimulus. Intermittent periods of relaxation may appear but become less and less frequent. Cyanosis, exhaustion, hypoxia and death follow. If not treated the entire syndrome may proceed from onset to death in less than 2 hours. When treated, the strychnine should be metabolized within 24 hours.

Treatment: Apomorphine (0.03 mg/lb [0.07 mg/kg], subcut.) is the emetic of choice for the dog if the animal is not convulsing. Xylazine (0.2 mg/lb [0.44 mg/kg], IM) is an effective, safe emetic for cats. Pentobarbital is indicated for short-term control of seizures; inhalation anesthetic or administration of methocarbamol for longer control; gastric lavage (using potassium permanganate solution, then activated charcoal), and forced diuresis with mannitol should follow. Positive pressure ventilation may be necessary, and the animal should be kept warm and in a quiet area.

VACOR

Clinical Findings: Vomiting, gastric pain, chills, nervousness and weakness are the chief signs. A few animals progress to a state of shock.

Treatment: Apomorphine (0.035 mg/lb [0.077 mg/kg], subcut.) should be used to empty the stomach if ingestion has been recent; also gastric lavage if a few hours have elapsed since ingestion. Nicotinamide is a useful antidote if given within one hour after ingestion. Symptomatic treatment may be useful for other developments.

ZINC PHOSPHIDE

Clinical Findings: The signs may be similar to those of strychnine poisoning. The onset is rapid with repeated vomiting as an early sign, and animals with signs rarely survive 24 to 48 hours. Signs include anorexia, lethargy, wheezing, vomiting, and abdominal pain; the vomitus often contains dark blood. Ataxia, weakness, recumbency and terminal hypoxia follow. The odor of phosphine (similar to acetylene) is detectable on the breath and vomitus. If an animal survives for 3 days the prognosis is favorable.

Treatment: Gastric lavage with sodium bicarbonate is followed by symptomatic and preventive treatment for acidosis and liver damage.

SOLVENTS

Acetone
Gastroenteric irritation, narcosis, kidney and liver damage are the main signs. Treatment consists of gastric lavage, oxygen, and a low-fat diet. Additional supportive treatment may be given as the signs dictate.

Isopropyl Alcohol
The signs are: gastroenteric pain, cramps, vomiting, diarrhea, CNS depression (dizziness, stupor, coma, death from respiratory paralysis). The liver and kidneys are reversibly affected. Dehydration and pneumonia may occur. Treatment consists of administration of emetics, gastric lavage, mild CNS stimulants, oxygen and artificial respiration.

Methanol
Nausea, vomiting, gastric pain, reflex hyperexcitability, opisthotonos, convulsions, fixed pupils and acute peripheral neuritis are the typical signs. Toxic effects are due in part to the alcohol itself and in part to formic acid produced by its oxidation. Treatment should include emetics (apomorphine) followed by gastric lavage with 4% sodium bicarbonate, administration of saline laxative, oxygen therapy, sodium bicarbonate solution IV and analgesics, although the prognosis is poor. Intensive and prolonged alkalinization is the mainstay of treatment. Ethyl alcohol retards the oxidation of methanol and may be given as an adjunct to alkali therapy.

Petroleum Derivatives (light mineral oils, xylene, kerosene)

Clinical Findings: Skin: Erythema, drying, cracking, blistering. **Systemic:** Inappetence, depression, dyspnea, vomiting, diarrhea, salivation, dizziness, coma (sometimes convulsions), trembling, narcosis, death. Effects of xylene are noticed within minutes and may last for hours. Signs of exposure to other solvents may appear after a few days or last for several weeks.

Treatment: Skin: Remove solvent from skin with copious quantities of water, soap or detergent. Thereafter, treat clinical signs symptomatically. **Systemic:** Treatment should be based on clinical signs. Gastric lavage, and laxative may be beneficial for ingestion incidents. There is no effective treatment for lipid-pneumonia induced by aspiration.

BRACKEN FERN POISONING

Bracken fern (*Pteridium aquilinum, Pteris aquilina*) is widely distributed in North America and in many other parts of the world. Ingestion of the plant produces a cumulative type of poisoning which requires 1 to 3 months to develop, depending on the quantity consumed, time of year, condition of the animal and other factors. It is sometimes difficult to convince farmers that the plant is poisonous because the disease can appear 2 or more weeks after removal of livestock from the fern-infested area. Most cases develop in the summer and early fall, following periods of drought. Even when present as a contaminant in hay, the plant is toxic and cases have been observed in stable-fed animals. Both the leaves and rhizomes contain the toxic principles, their concentrations varying with the seasons. The disease occurs in horses, cattle, sheep and possibly in swine.

In Australia the fern *Cheilanthes seiberi* (mulga or rock fern) is highly toxic to cattle and induces the same signs as bracken fern poisoning. Another syndrome resulting from many months of low-level consumption of *Pteridium* or *Cheilanthes* spp. is called **bovine enzootic hematuria.**

Etiology: Two toxic principles are involved: a thiaminase, which inactivates thiamin and is apparently not toxic to cattle and only partially so to sheep, and the so-called aplastic-anemia or radiomimetic factor, which depresses bone marrow function in cattle. Thiamin or other B-complex vitamins are ineffective in treating cattle.

In the rat and horse, bracken fern poisoning is manifested as a thiamin deficiency. In an affected horse, thiamin decreases from an average normal of 8.5 mcg/100 ml of blood to a low of 2.8 mcg and increases to 11.5 mcg during thiamin therapy. At the same time, the pyruvic acid content of the blood increases from a normal of about 2.0 mg/100 ml to a high of 8.5 mg with a decrease to about 2.0 mg upon treatment. This response is evident in 2 days.

Clinical Findings: Affected **horses** exhibit anorexia, incoordination, circumduction of the limbs and a crouching stance with arched neck and feet planted wide apart. When the signs are severe, tachycardia is present as contrasted to bradycardia at the onset. The animal dies in a clonic spasm with typical opisthotonos. In most cases, the rectal temperature is normal, but in some instances it reaches 104°F (40°C).

Affected **cattle** present 2 different syndromes described as the enteric and laryngitic types. The enteric type is the commonest and is marked by the passage of large clots of blood in the feces due to hemorrhage in the abomasum and intestines. The cecum and colon are often filled with clots of blood. The animals are depressed, anorectic, pyretic (106 to 110°F [41 to 43°C]), weak, and have pale mucous membranes with petechiae. There is often bleeding from the body orifices. The blood frequently fails to clot normally and, during the season when tabanid flies are abundant, the skin of affected cattle is marked by numerous streaks of blood where these insects have fed. Poisoned cattle often try to hide and may be aggressive when efforts are made to drive them. The laryngitic type is most frequent in younger animals and is marked by edematous swelling of the throat region, which may interfere with breathing. The signs of the enteric type of disease are also observed with this syndrome.

The physiologic processes in the bone marrow, and possibly elsewhere, are greatly affected as shown by the reduction of leukocytes and blood platelets. Once developed, this condition is not reversed by any currently used nutritional factor. The carcinogenic factor becomes evident in long-term and low-level feeding of bracken to cattle, resulting in endemic hematuria associated with bladder tumors. Blindness caused by progressive degeneration of the neuroepithelium of the retina was seen in sheep grazing bracken in Yorkshire ("bright blindness").

Diagnosis: The widespread hemorrhages are an important diagnostic aid in cattle, although the above signs easily can be confused with several infectious diseases and other poisonings marked by hematologic changes. Chief among these are leptospirosis, anaplasmosis, bacillary hemoglobinuria and *Crotalaria,* sweet clover or warfarin poisoning.

The morbidity in affected herds varies from 5 to 10% and occasionally is higher. Animals which develop acute signs seldom recover. The onset is sudden and death may occur in 12 to 72 hours, although chronically affected animals may linger for 4 to 10 days.

Prophylaxis: Bracken and other poisonous plants are usually grazed for the want of more suitable food. The disease has been prevented in cattle and horses by an alternative grazing plan whereby they are allowed on a bracken-contaminated pasture for 3 weeks and then are removed for 3 weeks. The fern growth is retarded by close grazing or trampling and the stand in a pasture can gradually be brought below dangerous levels by this alternative grazing system. Weed killers developed to date, or burning of pastures, are not effective in the control of bracken.

Treatment: In **horses**, thiamin usually is given subcut. at a dose of 100 mg in the morning and afternoon of the first day of treatment and 100 mg daily for 7 days thereafter. In extreme cases, 200 mg of thiamin has been administered for 14 days before the animals completely recovered.

In acutely affected **cattle**, the mortality rate is usually above 90%. Treatment with DL-batyl alcohol (℞ 630, 631) and antibiotics has been used with equivocal results. The herd should be removed from bracken-contaminated pasture. A feed high in protein and energy is indicated. If animals are anemic, blood transfusions (2 to 4 L) from a donor not grazing bracken may help prevent the development of acute signs. Injections of antibiotics will assist in combating secondary infection resulting from the leukopenia.

SWEET CLOVER POISONING

An insidious hemorrhagic disease occurring in animals that consume toxic quantities of spoiled sweet clover hay or silage. (*See also* table, p. 1020.)

Etiology: During the process of spoiling, the harmless natural coumarins in sweet clover are converted to dicoumarol (bishydroxycoumarin). When toxic hay or silage is consumed by animals, hypoprothrombinemia results, presumably because dicoumarol combines with the proenzyme to prevent formation of the active enzyme required for the synthesis of prothrombin. It probably also interferes with synthesis of Factor VII, and other coagulation factors (*see* HEMOPHILIA AND OTHER HEMOSTATIC DISORDERS IN DOMESTIC ANIMALS, p. 38). The toxic agent passes through the placenta in pregnant animals and newborn animals may become affected immediately after birth. All species of animals studied have been shown to be susceptible, but instances of poisoning have involved mainly cattle and, to a very limited extent, sheep, swine and horses.

Clinical Findings: All clinical signs are referable to the hemorrhages which result from faulty blood coagulation. The time of appearance of clinical disease after consumption of toxic sweet clover varies greatly and depends to a large extent on the dicoumarol content of the particular specimen of sweet clover fed and the age of the animals. If the dicoumarol content of the ration is low or variable, animals may consume it for months before signs of disease appear.

Initial signs of disease may be stiffness and lameness, due to bleeding into the muscles and articulations. Hematomas, epistaxis or gastrointestinal bleeding may be observed. Death sometimes occurs suddenly with little preliminary evidence of disease and is caused by spontaneous massive hemorrhage or bleeding after injury, surgery or parturition. Neonatal deaths may occur, rarely without signs in the dam.

Lesions: Hemorrhage is the characteristic necropsy finding; large extravasations of blood are commonly found in subcut. and connective tissue sites.

Diagnosis: This requires a history of continuous consumption of sweet clover hay or silage over relatively long periods, compatible signs and lesions, and markedly prolonged blood clotting time or demonstration of reduced prothrombin content of the plasma. Most other diseases with hemorrhagic manifestations, such as blackleg, pasteurellosis, bracken fern poisoning and aplastic anemia, can be readily differentiated on the basis of clinical, pathologic and hematologic findings. This is the only commonly acquired disease, except purpura hemorrhagica, a common occurrence only in the horse, in which such large hemorrhages occur.

Congenital or inherited diseases affecting various coagulation factors or blood platelets such as Hemophilia A may be characterized by large hemorrhages.

Prophylaxis: Cultivars of sweet clover that are low in coumarin content, and hence safe to feed, have been developed. If one of these is not available, the only certain way to prevent the disease is to avoid feeding sweet clover hay or silage. Although well-cured sweet clover in good condition is not dangerous, the absence of visible spoilage is insufficient evidence of safety. There is no chemical test for dicoumarol that can be quickly performed. Suspected feed may be fed to rabbits; a shorter feeding period is required to produce fatal hemorrhage, and determination, at intervals, of prothrombin time in the rabbits further reduces the test period. However, some rabbits are refractory to dicoumarin, requiring large doses before the coagulation mechanism is affected, thus making negative tests suspect.

Treatment: Immediate correction of the hypoprothrombinemia as well as the anemia can be accomplished to a degree by the IV administration of 2 to 4 liters of whole blood per 1,000 lb (450 kg) body wt (from an animal that has not been fed sweet clover). This procedure should be employed in all animals with marked signs, and repeated if necessary. In addition, parenteral administration of synthetic vitamin K_3 (menadione), repeated if necessary, will permit increased prothrombin production. All severely affected animals should receive this drug until their blood clotting time returns to normal. Either the administration of synthetic vitamin K or a blood transfusion is sufficient to correct mild cases of intoxication if feeding of the toxic hay is stopped. Vitamin K_1 (phytonadione) is more effective than vitamin K_3 but is usually precluded from use by cost.

SORGHUM POISONING OF HORSES

A condition seen sporadically in horses grazing sorghum, mostly hybrid strains. The unidentified toxic principle causes degeneration of axones and demyelination in the lateral and ventral funiculi of the spinal cord. Neuromuscular disturbances result in more or less incoordination of the gait, paralysis of the bladder and accumulation in the bladder of a characteristic yellowish to brownish, granular material. The bladder wall becomes edematous, inflamed and covered with fibrin and the sediment. The latter material, which has a strong odor of urine, often covers the hocks causing alopecia. A characteristic ataxic swaying gait develops early. Flaccid paralysis may result.

The toxic principle has not been identified but there is speculation that the axonal degeneration and demyelination might be the result of several sublethal doses of hydrocyanic acid or a derivative from the sorghum. *See also* CYANIDE POISONING, p. 971. Treatment is removal from the sorghum. Recovery is rare.

Quercus POISONING

(Poisoning by oak buds or acorns)

Cattle are poisoned in the fall by acorns and in the spring by oak buds if they consume too much of these gallotannin-containing materials in their diet. The primary lesion is severe kidney damage. Signs include loss of weight, rough hair coat, poor appetite, thin nasal discharge that may become red-tinged, polydypsia, polyuria and constipation followed by diarrhea that may contain mucus and blood. Edema may be noted subcut., in the body cavities and around the kidneys, ureters and vulva. Hemorrhagic abomasitis and petechia or ecchymoses on the edematous kidneys may be observed.

Preventing access to acorns or oak buds is necessary. Additional animals may become affected after removal from the source. Specific treatment is unknown. Partial protection can be provided cows on oak-containing pastures by supplying 4 lb (2 kg) daily (2 lb/head in a creep for calves) of a mixture of: cottonseed meal, 1,080 lb; dehydrated alfalfa meal, 600 lb; vegetable oil, 120 lb; and calcium hydroxide, 200 lb. Oak-bud poisoning may be prevented by removing cattle from the affected range during spring until the leaves reach maturity.

POISONOUS PLANTS OF TEMPERATE

Dangerous Season	Scientific Name	Common Name	Habitat and Distribution	Affected Animals
SPRING	*Hymenoxys* spp.	Bitterweed, Rubberweed, Pingue	Roadways, lakebeds, flooded areas, overgrazed range; southwest.	Sheep, also cattle
	Nolina texana	Sacahuista, Beargrass	Open areas on rolling hills and slopes; southwest.	Sheep, cattle and goats
	Cicuta spp.	Water hemlock	Open, moist-to-wet situations; throughout.	All
(also seeds in fall)	*Delphinium* spp.	Larkspurs	Either cultivated or wild. Usually in open foothills or meadows and among aspen; mostly western.	All grazing animals, mostly cattle
	Phytolacca americana	Pokeweed, Poke	Recent clearings, pastures, waste areas; eastern.	Cattle, swine
(and occasionally fall)	*Xanthium* spp.	Cocklebur	Fields, waste places, exposed shores of ponds or rivers; throughout.	All animals, more common in swine
	Peganum harmala	African rue	Arid to semiarid ranges; southwest.	Cattle and sheep
	Sarcobatus vermiculatus	Greasewood	Alkaline or saline bottom soils, not in higher mountains; western.	Sheep and rarely cattle
	Veratrum spp.	False hellebore	Low, moist woods and pastures, and high mountain valleys; throughout.	Cattle, sheep and fowl

NORTH AMERICA

Important Characteristics	Toxic Principle and Effects	Remarks and Treatment
Much-branched annual or perennial up to 2-ft high. Yellow flower head. Leaves divided into narrow glandular segments.	Sesquiterpene lactone (hymenovin) — depression, loss of appetite, abdominal pain, green nasal discharge, salivation, prostration.	Fresh or dry. Remove from pasture. Avoid overgrazing. Cumulative.
Perennial with many clustered, long narrowed leaves. Stem mostly underground. Several flower stems with many small white flowers in clusters.	Toxin in buds, flowers and fruit. Photosensitization. Anorexia, icterus, prostration.	Remove animals from range during blooming season. (*See* PHOTOSENSITIZATION, p. 530.)
White flower, umbels. Veins of leaflets ending at notches. Stems hollow except at nodes. Tuberous roots from chambered rootstock.	A higher alcohol—excessive salivation, violent convulsions, dilation of pupils, diaphragm contractions, pain.	Roots and young shoots. Death usually rapid. Use sedatives to control spasm and heart action. Intestinal evacuation followed by astringents may help.
Annual or perennial herbs. Flowers each with one spur, in racemes. Perennial with tuberous roots. Leave palmately lobed or divided.	Alkaloid delphinine and others—straddled stance, repeated falling, nausea, rapid pulse and respiration, constipation, bloating.	Young plants and seeds. Use Rx 507.
Tall, glabrous, green, red-purplish perennial herbs. Berries black-purple, staining, in drooping racemes.	More than one—vomiting, spasms, respiratory paralysis, ulcerative gastritis.	Roots most poisonous. 10 ml nikethamide (cattle). Tannic acid is helpful.
Coarse annual herb. Fruit one solid mass, 2 beaked, with 2 cavities, armed with hooked spines.	Hydroquinone — anorexia, depression, incoordination, twitching, paralysis, spasms of limb and neck, blindness in cattle.	Spring seedlings or old plants in silage. Milk, vegetable oil and fats may be beneficial; depressants.
Much-branched, leafy, perennial, bright green, succulent herb; leaves divided; flowers white, single.	Alkaloids—weakness of hind limbs, listlessness, subserous edema and hemorrhage of small intestine.	Unpalatable. Eaten only under drought conditions.
Large deciduous shrub with spiny stems; fleshy, alternate, round in cross-section. Flowers inconspicuous.	Oxalates—kidney lesions, weakness, depression, prostration, coma, death.	Poisoning occurs only on steady diet of greasewood leaves. Provide other forage.
Erect herbs; leafy-throughout, leaves large and plaited. Flowers small and white or greenish.	Sterolid alkaloids—salivation, prostration, depressed heart action, dyspnea; "Monkey-face" in lambs.	Remove animals from range. Provide other forage. Respiratory and heart stimulants.

POISONOUS PLANTS OF TEMPERATE

Dangerous Season	Scientific Name	Common Name	Habitat and Distribution	Affected Animals
	Tetradymia spp.	Horsebrush	Arid foothills and higher desert and sagebrush ranges; dense stands along trails; western.	Sheep
	Zygadenus spp.	Death camas	Foothill grazing lands, occasionally boggy grasslands; low, open woods; throughout.	Sheep, cattle and horses
SPRING and SUMMER	*Aesculus* spp.	Buckeyes	Woods and thickets; Eastern U.S.A. and California.	All grazing animals
	Amianthium muscae-toxicum	Fly poison, Stagger-grass, Crow poison	Open woods, fields, and acid bogs; eastern.	All grazing animals
	Lantana spp.	Lantana	Ornamentals and wild in lower Coastal Plain of Southeast, and southern California.	All grazing animals
	Quercus spp.	Oaks	In most deciduous woods; throughout.	All grazing animals
SUMMER and FALL	*Prosopis glandulosa (juliflora)*	Mesquite	Dry ranges, washes, draws; southwest.	Cattle
	Centaurea solstitialis	Yellow star thistle	Waste areas, roadsides, pastures; mostly western.	Horses

NORTH AMERICA (*Continued*)

Important Characteristics	Toxic Principle and Effects	Remarks and Treatment
Shrubs with yellow flowers in spring, not later. Leaves spiny, silvery white, early deciduous.	Resinous substances — weakness, "bighead" photosensitization; liver injury, death	Cumulative. Remove animals from range and light. Antihistaminics. (*See* PHOTOSENSITIZATION, p. 530.)
Perennial bulbous, unbranched herbs with basal flat grasslike leaves; flowers greenish, yellow or pink, in racemes or panicles. No onion odor.	Steroid alkaloids of the veratrum group—salivation, vomiting, staggering or prostration, coma and death. Abortion or congenital defects.	Hay with dried camas is poisonous. 2 to 3 subcut. injections of 2 mg atropine sulfate and 8 mg picrotoxin in 5 ml of water per 100 lb (45 kg) body wt.
Trees or shrubs. Leaves opposite and palmately compound. Seeds large, glossy brown, with large white scar.	Glycoside, aesculin and possibly others—depression, incoordination, twitching, paralysis, inflammation of mucous membranes.	Young shoots and seeds. Especially poisonous. Use stimulants and purgatives.
Bulbous perennial herb. Leaves basal, linear. White flowers in a compact raceme, the pedicels subtended by short, brownish bracts.	Alkaloid, of the veratrum group—salivation, vomiting, rapid and irregular respiration, weakness, death by respiratory failure.	No practical treatment. Especially dangerous for animals new to pasture. Keep animals well fed.
Shrubs. Young stems 4-angled. Leaves opposite. Flowers in flat-topped clusters, yellow, pink, orange, or red. Berries black.	Lantadene A, a polycyclic triterpenoid—erythema, pruritus, edematous suffusions and usually sloughing of skin, gastroenteritis, bloody watery feces.	Remove plants from pasture. Keep animals out of light sources after eating plant.
Mostly deciduous trees, rarely shrubs, with 2 to 4 leaves clustered at tips of all twigs.	Tannic acid — anorexia, constipation, dry muzzle, black pelleted feces followed by diarrhea with blood and mucus, frequent urination, thin rapid pulse.	Leaves, sprouts, acorns. Remove animals from oak source. Treat symptomatically. (*See* Quercus poisoning, p. 1019.)
Deciduous shrub or small tree with smooth or furrowed gray bark, paired spines; leaves divided. Legume pod long, constricted between seeds.	Malnutrition, excessive salivation, stasis and impaction of rumen; sublingual or submaxillary edema, loss of weight.	Believed that high-sucrose content of beans alters bacterial flora to extent that cellulose cannot be digested, and B-vitamins synthesized. Change pasture.
Annual weed. Leaves densely covered with cottony hair. Terminal spreading cluster of bright yellow flowers with spines below. Branches winged.	Involuntary chewing movements, twitching of lips, flicking of tongue. Mouth commonly held open. Unable to eat. Eventual death from starvation or thirst.	Force food far back into mouth. Change pasture.

POISONOUS PLANTS OF TEMPERATE

Dangerous Season	Scientific Name	Common Name	Habitat and Distribution	Affected Animals
	Oxytenia acerosa	Copper-weed	Arid, alkaline soils in foothills, and sage-brush plains; south-western.	Cattle, also sheep
	Eupatorium rugosum	White snakeroot	Woods, cleared areas, waste places, usually the more moist and richer soils; eastern.	Cattle and sheep
	Solanum spp.	Nightshades, Jerusalem Cherry, Potato, Horse nettle, Buffalo bur	Fence rows, waste areas, grain and hay fields; throughout.	All
	Apocynum spp.	Dogbanes	Open woods, roadsides, fields; throughout.	All
FALL OF WINTER	*Hapalopappus heterophyllus*	Rayless goldenrod, Burroweed	Dry plains, grasslands, open woodlands and along irrigation canals; southwestern.	Cattle, sheep and horses
	Halogeton glomeratus	Halogeton	Deserts, overgrazed areas, winter ranges, alkaline soils; western.	Sheep and rarely cattle
	Sophora secundiflora	Mescal bean	Hills and canyons, limestone soils; south-western Texas into Mexico.	Cattle, also sheep and goats
	Notholaena sinuata var. *cochisensis*	Jimmy fern, Cloak fern	Dry rocky slopes and crevices, chiefly lime-stone areas; southwest.	Sheep, goats and cattle

NORTH AMERICA (*Continued*)

Important Characteristics	Toxic Principle and Effects	Remarks and Treatment
Tall, perennial herb with narrow leaflets; flowers in many heads resembling goldenrod.	Green or dry. Weakness, stupor, loss of appetite, coma, death without struggling.	Supplement diet, or change pasture.
Perennial herb; leaves 3-nerved, taper-pointed, opposite; flowers small, white, many.	An alcohol, tremetol—trembling, depression, vomiting, labored respiration, coma, death. Acetone odor.	"Milk sickness." "Trembles." Cathartics and stimulants may help. Discard milk.
Fruits small, when ripe yellow, red, or black; structurally like tomatoes; clustered on stalk arising from stem between leaves.	Glycoalkaloids — weakness, trembling, dyspnea, nausea, constipation or diarrhea, death.	Leaves, shoots and berries may be poisonous. In cattle repeated doses of 2 to 3 mg carbachol or of injection of 15 mg strychnine may be useful. Pilocarpine usually helpful.
Erect, perennial herbs with milky juice, branched above. Leaves opposite. Flowers small, cream, in erect clusters. Seeds silky-hairy, from long, slender pods.	Resin and glycosides, mainly cymarin. Sweating, cold extremities, dilated pupils, sore and discolored mouth, death.	Green plants or dried in hay. Keep animals away, and plants out of hay. Tannic acid, atropine.
Bushy perennial 2 to 4 ft (~1 m) tall, with many yellow flower heads. Leaves alternate, linear, sticky.	An alcohol, tremetol—trembling, depression, vomiting, labored respiration, coma, death. Acetone odor.	"Milk sickness." Keep animals away by fencing. Discard milk.
Annual herb. Leaves fleshy, round in cross-section, tip with stiff hair. Axillary flowers inconspicuous. Fruits bracted and conspicuous.	Oxalates — dyspnea followed by rapid death.	Alfalfa hay or dicalcium phosphate, fed free-choice when added to 3 parts salt, is effective preventive in sheep. Avoid dense growths of weeds.
Evergreen shrub or small tree. Leaves alternate, divided and leathery; flowers violet-blue, fragrant; seeds large and bright red with hard seed coat, in legume pod.	Alkaloid sophorine—trembling, stiff gait, falling after exercise; recumbent for few minutes. then arise alert and fall again if exercised.	Not cumulative. Provide supplemental feed.
Evergreen, perennial, erect fern with divided leaves, folding when dry. Leaflets about as wide as long, scaly on back.	After exercise by walking, will have arched back, stilted movement of hind legs, and usually increased respiration. Continued walking induces violent trembling and death if not allowed to rest.	Avoid driving during danger period. Provide ample watering, placed to avoid long walks. Allow rest if poisoning occurs.

POISONOUS PLANTS OF TEMPERATE

Dangerous Season	Scientific Name	Common Name	Habitat and Distribution	Affected Animals
	Glottidium vesicarium, Sesbania spp.	Bladder pod, Rattlebox, Sesbane, Coffee bean	Mostly open low ground, abandoned cultivated fields; Southeastern Coastal Plain.	All
	Daubentonia punicea	Rattlebox, Purple sesbane	Cultivated and escaped in waste places; Southeastern Coastal Plain.	All
FALL, WINTER and SPRING	*Melia azedarach*	Chinaberry	Fence rows, brush, waste places; southeast.	Swine and sheep; others less susceptible
ALL SEASONS	*Baccharis* spp.	Silverling, Baccharis, Yerba-de-pasmo	Open areas, often moist; eastern and southwestern.	All grazing cattle
	Pteridium aquilinum	Bracken fern	Dry poor soil, open woods, sandy ridges.	All grazing animals
	Prunus spp.	Chokecherries, Wild cherries, Peaches	Waste areas, fence rows, woods, orchards, prairies, dry slopes; mostly eastern.	All grazing animals
	Acacia berlandieri	Guajillo	Semiarid range lands; southwestern Texas into Mexico.	Sheep, also goats
(especially spring)	*Agave lecheguilla*	Lechuguilla	Low limestone hills, dry valleys and canyons; southwest.	Sheep and goats, rarely cattle
	Asclepias spp.	Milkweeds	Dry areas, usually waste places, roadsides, streambeds.	All

NORTH AMERICA (*Continued*)

Important Characteristics	Toxic Principle and Effects	Remarks and Treatment
Tall annual. Legume pods flat, tapered at both ends, 2-seeded. Leaves pinnate-divided. Flowers yellow.	Saponins — intense inflammation of gastrointestinal tract, yellowish diarrhea, frequent urination, shallow and accelerated respiration, death.	Seeds poisonous. Remove plants from pasture. Keep animals off pasture after seed pods form.
Shrub. Flowers orange. Legume pods longitudinally four-winged.	A saponin—rapid pulse, weak respiration, diarrhea, death.	Seeds poisonous. Keep seeds from animals. Use saline purgative followed by stimulants and soft food.
Tree. Leaves 2 to 3 pinnate; fruit cream or yellow with a furrowed globose stone, persisting on tree through winter.	Nausea, constipation, excitement, or depression, often weakened heart action and death.	Fruit most poisonous. Use stimulants and cathartics followed by easily digestible diet.
Shrubs; numerous small, whitish flowers; leaves resin-dotted, and persistent southward.	Glucosidal saponin having digitaloidal properties—paralysis and death soon after ingestion. Depression, weakness, trembling, prostration.	Most dangerous during new growth in spring or root sprouts in fall, or after cutting.
Leaves firm, leathery, thrice pinnate.	(*See* BRACKEN FERN POISONING, p. 1015.)	
Large shrubs or trees. Flowers white or pink. Cherries or peaches. Crushed twigs with strong odor.	Prussic acid—slobbering, increased respiration rate, dyspnea, rapid weak pulse, convulsions, rapid death.	Wilted leaves, bark. (*See* CYANIDE POISONING, p. 971.)
Deciduous shrub or small tree; leaf divided; flowers white to yellowish in dense heads; fruit a legume with margins thickened.	Amine, N-methyl β-phenylethylamine—after eating for 6 to 9 months, may have locomotor ataxia called "limber leg." Mortality as high as 50% in extreme drought.	Dominates vegetation in some areas. Valuable to sheep industry due to high nutritive value and dominance. Supplement during drought.
Perennial stemless, with thick fleshy tapered leaves having sharply serrated margins. Flowering infrequently with tall terminal panicle.	A photodynamic agent; also a saponin that is hepatonephrotoxic—photosensitization, generalized icterus, listlessness, progressive weakness, coma, death.	Remove animals from range and provide shade. (*See* PHOTOSENSITIZATION, p. 1530.)
Perennial herbs with milky sap; seeds very silky-hairy from elongated pods.	Resinoid and others—loss of control, spasms, bloating, pulse rapid and weak, rapid breathing, coma, death.	Entire plant. Mainly due to drought or overgrazing. Fluids and nutrients; a cathartic may be helpful.

POISONOUS PLANTS OF TEMPERATE

Dangerous Season	Scientific Name	Common Name	Habitat and Distribution	Affected Animals
	Astragalus spp., *Oxytropis* spp.	Locoweeds, Poison vetch, Milk vetch	Nearly all habitats; mostly western.	All
	Drymaria pachyphylla	Inkweed, Drymary	Heavy alkaline clay soil in low areas or dry overgrazed pastures; southwest.	Cattle, sheep; also goats
	Gutierrezia (Xanthocethalum) microcephala	Broomweed, Snakeweed, Slinkweed, Turpentine weed	Widespread over dry range and desert; overgrazed lands; western.	Cattle, sheep, goats and swine
	Psilostrophe spp.	Paper-flowers	Open range lands and pastures; southwest.	Sheep
	Senecio spp.	Groundsel, Senecio	Grassland areas; mostly western.	Cattle, horses and sheep
(especially dry season)	*Triglochin* spp.	Arrowgrass	Salt marshes, wet alkaline soils, lake shores.	Sheep and cattle
	Hypericum perforatum	St.-John's-wort, Goatweed, Klamath weed	Dry soil, roadsides, pastures, ranges; throughout.	Sheep, cattle, horses and goats
	Agrostemma githago	Corn cockle	Weed, grain fields and waste areas; throughout.	All
(spring and fall)	*Dugaldia (Helenium) hoopesii*	Orange sneezeweed	Moist slopes and well-drained mountain meadows; western.	Sheep, also cattle

NORTH AMERICA (*Continued*)

Important Characteristics	Toxic Principle and Effects	Remarks and Treatment
Perennial stemmed or stemless herbs. Leaves with many small leaflets. Flowers like garden peas, in racemes.	Selenium or "locoine" in different species. Weakness, trembling, ataxia, or paralysis.	Cumulative. (*See* SELENIUM POISONING, p. 979 as one type.)
Much-branched, succulent, prostrate annual with opposite leaves and small white flowers.	Diarrhea, lack of appetite, arched back, coma, death.	Dangerous during drought, after rain, or at night. Avoid overstocking to improve range.
Much-branched, perennial, resinous shrub, with many yellow-flowered heads.	Saponin. Loss of appetite, listlessness, hematuria in severe cases. Abortion with retained placenta in cattle.	Supplement diet.
Perennial composite with erect, woolly stems branching from base. Many small heads of yellow flowers.	Sluggishness, stumbling, coughing, vomiting, depression, death.	About 2 weeks of grazing before signs appear. Pasture rotation, or placing animals on other feed.
Perennial or annual herbs; heads of yellow flowers with whorl of bracts below.	Alkaloids—aimless walking, slight staggering, staring expression, and running into fences or other objects. Hepatic cirrhosis, edema of visceral peritoneum and distension of gallbladder.	Cumulative, fresh or dry. Supplemental feeding. Treat signs. (*See* SENECIO POISONING, p. 1048.)
Grass-like, except leaves are thick; heads of fruits globular on erect raceme. Flowers inconspicuous.	Prussic acid in leaves—abnormal breathing, trembling, and jerking, convulsions. Rapid poisoning.	(*See* CYANIDE POISONING, p. 971.)
Perennial herb or woody below; leaves opposite, dotted; flowers many, yellow, with many stamens.	Primary photosensitizer; skin lesions in white skin, itching, blindness, convulsions, death.	Fresh or dry. Remove animals from infested areas. (*See* PHOTOSENSITIZATION, p. 530.)
Green winter annual with silky white hairs, opposite leaves, purple flowers, black seeds.	Sapogenin, githagenin—irritation of mucosa, vomiting, vertigo, diarrhea, rapid breathing, coma.	Toxin in seeds. Avoid grain screenings containing seed. Give oils, demulcents, cardiac stimulants.
Perennial herb with orange sunflower-like heads or yellow flowers. Leaves alternate.	Sesquiterpene lactone (hymenovin)—salivation, "spewing sickness," vomiting, weakness.	Cumulative. Cathartics may help. Avoid dense areas of weed.

POISONOUS PLANTS OF TEMPERATE

Dangerous Season	Scientific Name	Common Name	Habitat and Distribution	Affected Animals
	Helenium microcephalum	Smallhead sneezeweed	Moist ground; southern.	Cattle, sheep, and goats
	Lupinus spp.	Lupines, Bluebonnet	Dry to moist soils, roadsides, fields, and mountains; throughout, but poisoning mostly western.	Sheep, also cattle, goats, horses and swine
	Conium maculatum	Poison hemlock	Roadside ditches, damp waste areas; throughout.	All
	Crotalaria spp.	Crotalaria, Rattlebox	Fields and roadsides; Eastern and Central States.	All
	Datura stramonium	Jimson weed, Thorn apple	Fields, barn lots, trampled pastures, and waste places on rich bottom soils; throughout.	All
	Gelsemium sempervirens	Yellow jessamine	Open woods, thickets; southeastern.	All
(especially winter and spring)	*Kalmia* spp.	Laurel, Ivybush, Lambkill	Rich moist woods, meadows; or acid bogs; eastern and northwestern.	All, often sheep

NORTH AMERICA (*Continued*)

Important Characteristics	Toxic Principle and Effects	Remarks and Treatment
Annual, erect herb, simple-stemmed below, bushy above. Stem winged. Narrow leaves throughout. Flowers in small heads, disk pale red-brown, rays yellow.	Sesquiterpene lactone (helenalin)—dullness, weakness, trembling, "spewing sickness," salivation.	Cumulative. Remove from pasture. Cathartics may help.
Perennials; leaves simple or palmately divided; flowers blue, white, red, or yellow in terminal raceme.	Alkaloids D-lupanine, sparteine and others—nervousness, convulsions or coma.	Fresh or dry. Eating of pods with seeds frequent cause of poisoning. Not cumulative. (*See* MYCOTOXIC LUPINOSIS, p. 1037.)
Purple-spotted hollow stem; leaves resemble parsley, parsnip odor when crushed; tap root; flowers white, in umbels.	Alkaloid coniine and others—loss of appetite, salivation, feeble pulse, paralysis, trembling, coma.	Vegetative parts, later the seeds most poisonous. Give stimulants, tannic acid.
Annual or perennial legume with yellow flowers in racemes; pods inflated; bracts at base of pedicels of flowers and fruits persistent; leaves simple or divided.	Alkaloid monocrotaline—diarrhea, abnormally light or dark comb in fowl, Diarrhea, stupor alternating with apparent improvement, walking in circles in horse and mule. Bloody feces, anorexia, weakness in others. In all death.	Cumulative, fresh or dry. All parts, especially seeds, poisonous. Seeds often found in combined corn. No treatment known. Keep plant from fields and hay.
Leaves wavy; flower large (4 in.), white, tubular; fruit a spiny pod, 2 in. (5 cm) long.	Alkaloids atropine, hyoscyamine and hyoscine—nausea, vertigo, thirst, dilated pupils, convulsions, death.	All parts, mainly in hay or silage. Rapid death. KI or tannic acid per os; cardiac and respiratory stimulants. Physostigmine, pilocarpine and arecoline are antidotes.
Climbing or trailing vines with evergreen, entire, opposite leaves; yellow tubular flowers, very fragrant.	Alkaloids gelsemine and seminine — weakness, convulsions, rigid extremities, lowered respiration and temperature, death; "limp-neck" in fowl.	Use relaxing agents, sedatives; repeat as required.
Woody shrub with evergreen glossy leaves; flowers pink to rose, showy.	Andromedotoxin—salivation, nasal discharge, emesis, paralysis, coma, death.	Laxatives, demulcents, nerve stimulants.

POISONOUS PLANTS OF TEMPERATE

Dangerous Season	Scientific Name	Common Name	Habitat and Distribution	Affected Animals
	Nerium oleander	Oleander	Common ornamental in southern regions.	All
(especially winter and spring)	*Prunus caroliniana*	Laurel cherry, Cherry laurel	Woods, fence rows and often escaped from cultivation; southern regions.	All grazing animals
	Ricinus communis	Castor bean	Cultivated in southern regions.	All
	Sorghum vulgare	Sorghum, Sudan grass, Kafir, Durra, Milo, Broomcorn, Schrock, etc.	Forage crops, and escapes; throughout.	All
	Sorghum halepense	Johnson grass	Weed of open fields and waste places in south; scattered north to New York and Iowa.	All grazing animals
(especially winter)	*Pinus ponderosa*	Western yellow pine	Coniferous forests of Rocky Mountains at moderate elevations; western.	Cattle
	Brassica, Raphanus, Descurainia spp.	Mustards, Crucifers, Cress	Fields, roadsides; throughout.	Cattle, horses, swine

ENZOOTIC CALCINOSIS

(Enteque seco, Espichamento, Espichacao, Manchester wasting disease, Naalehu disease)

A disease complex of ruminants and horses, caused by plant poisoning or mineral imbalances and characterized by extensive calcification of soft tissues. The prevalence of the disease in cattle varies widely, from 10% to as high as 50%, in areas of Argentina, Papua-New Guinea, Jamaica, Hawaii and Bavaria. It is said to affect

NORTH AMERICA (*Continued*)

Important Characteristics	Toxic Principle and Effects	Remarks and Treatment
Evergreen shrub or tree, leaves whorled and prominently finely pinnately veined beneath. Flowers showy, white to deep pink.	Cardiac glucosides—nausea, depression, increased pulse rate, mydriasis, bloody diarrhea. Later weak and irregular heart beat, death.	Fresh, clipped or dried leaves most dangerous.
Leaves evergreen, shiny, leathery. Broken twigs with strong cherry bark odor. Fruit black.	Prussic acid—slobbering, increased respiration rate, dyspnea, rapid weak pulse, convulsions, rapid death.	Wilted parts most poisonous. (*See* CYANIDE POISONING, p. 971.)
Large palmately lobed leaves; seeds resembling engorged ticks, usually 3 in somewhat spiny pod.	Ricin, irritant blood poison — nausea, vomiting, diarrhea, thirst, cessation of rumination, death.	Seeds and "press cakes" most dangerous. Gastric lavage, warmth, sedation.
Coarse grasses with terminal flower cluster. Some to 8 ft (2.5 m) tall.	Prussic acid—slobbering, increased respiration rate, dyspnea, rapid weak pulse, convulsions, rapid death.	Dark green, short (2 ft (60 cm) second growth or stunted by dry weather most dangerous. (*See* CYANIDE POISONING, p. 971.)
Coarse grass with large rhizomes and white midvein on leaf. Topped by large, open panicle.	Prussic acid—slobbering, increased respiration rate, dyspnea, rapid weak pulse, convulsions, rapid death.	Dark green second growth or stunted by dry weather most dangerous. (*See* CYANIDE POISONING, p. 971.)
Tree, 150 to 180 ft (45 to 55 m); leaves in groups of 3 yellowish green, 7 to 11 in. (17 to 27 cm) long; bark platy, reddish orange.	Toxin in leaves; browsing cattle predisposed to abortion.	Needles. Remove from western yellow pine stands in later stages of gestation.
Annual herbaceous weeds with terminal clusters of yellowish flowers and slender elongated seed pods.	Mustard oils (isothiocyanates. Abortion, weakness, paralysis of heart and lungs.	Mainly seeds, and leaves and stems in quantity, fresh or in hay. Do not cut with hay.

17% of the sheep at Mattewara (India). Incidence elsewhere is less well documented; in many areas it is rare or nonexistent.

Etiology: Known causes fall into 2 categories: plant poisonings and mineral imbalances in the soil, the first being probably the more important. *Cestrum diurnum* (wild jasmine, day-blooming jessamine, king-of-the-day), *Trisetum flavescens* (golden oats or yellow oat grass), and *Solanum malacoxylon* (*glaucophyllum*) contain 1,25-dihydroxycholecalciferol glycoside or a substance that mimics its calcinogenic action. No concrete evidence incriminating other plants is available.

The imbalance of minerals in certain soils in Hawaii, India, Austria and possibly elsewhere has been thought to be the main etiologic factor; dietary mineral imbalance may contribute to the calcification chiefly associated with plant poisoning. Excessive phosphate or calcium, absolute or conditioned magnesium deficiency, and deficiency of potassium and nitrogen have all been incriminated or suspected.

Osteopetrosis of bulls following prolonged excessive calcium intake is a similar condition. The calcification of the cardiovascular system associated with aging and such cachectic diseases as tuberculosis is not identical.

Clinical Findings: The disease is progressive and chronic, extending over weeks or months. The earliest signs are stiffened and painful gait most pronounced when the animal gets up after prolonged rest. Forelimbs are particularly affected and some animals even walk or graze on their knees. When standing, the forelimbs bow forward as the joints cannot be extended completely. The animal shifts weight to the forepart of the hooves, or alternatively to each forelimb thus easing stress on the knee joint, which is thickened and painful. The distal joints become abnormally straight. When affected animals are forced to walk, their gait is awkward, stiff and slow, the steps short, and after only short distances breathing becomes shallow and diaphragmatic, the nostrils are flared, and the head and neck are extended. Varying degrees of heart murmur are detectable, usually as a double or blurred second sound; these are exaggerated after exercise. Pulse rate is increased after slight exercise. Jugular pulse is prominent in some cases.

As the disease progresses, the animal loses weight and becomes weak and listless. The coat becomes shaggy, lusterless and faded, particularly in cattle. There is wasting of muscles, a prominent skeleton, tucked up abdomen, kyphosis and raised tailhead. Ovarian function is impaired. Appetite is usually unimpaired but sometimes becomes depraved.

Osteopetrosis is observed in calcinosis due to *Trisetum flavescens* and *Cestrum diurnum* toxicities in Bavarian cattle and Florida horses, respectively. Severely affected horses stand with forelimbs somewhat abducted and luxated caudally at the shoulder joints. The flexor tendons, particularly the suspensory ligaments, are painful. Fetlock joints are overextended to varying degrees.

Lesions: Gross lesions are degeneration and calcification of soft tissues, emaciation, and presence of varying amounts of excess fluid in thoracic and abdominal cavities and pericardial sac. The cardiovascular system is the first to be involved, followed by lung, kidney and tendons. The heart and aorta show the most marked effects. The left auricle and ventricle are more affected than the right ones. In extreme cases, calcified foci are seen on valves and chordae tendinae. White, elevated plaques of irregular size and shape are seen on the luminal surface; in advanced cases, these occur throughout the length of the aorta and its main branches. Mineral deposits occur on the pleura, the surface and edges of the diaphragmatic and apical lobes of lungs, in the renal artery and pelvis of kidney, the ligaments and tendons, particularly of the forelimbs. Capsular thickening and irregular erosions of articular surface of cartilage and joints especially of the knee and hock occur.

The basic microscopic lesion is necrosis and calcification of connective tissue followed by cellular proliferation in the affected area.

Biochemical Alterations: These appear to vary from area to area: frequently serum calcium and inorganic phosphorus are both elevated but depending on the area one or both may be in the normal range. Hypomagnesemia may also be present in some areas.

Diagnosis: The disease is usually diagnosed from the history, signs and lesions but may be difficult at early stages. X-ray examination and electrocardiography may be helpful.

Control: Removal of the causal factor(s) is essential, but when the disease is associated with the soil mineral-content the control may present difficulty. Change of pasture, forage and environment may bring about clinical improvement and even diminish the soft-tissue mineral deposits.

BLISTER BEETLE (CANTHARIDIN) POISONING OF HORSES

There are many species of beetles containing cantharidin. The 3-striped blister beetles (*Epicauta* spp.) swarm in alfalfa hay when the hay is drying in the windrow and are baled with the hay. When fed to horses the highly irritant cantharidin causes severe pain associated with gastroenteritis, nephritis and cystitis. A frequent history is that the animal was normal when fed at night and found dead the next morning with signs of a violent struggle. The diagnosis is made by finding the beetles in the hay rack or hay. The condition has been reported in the South and Southwestern U.S.A. Laboratory analysis can confirm cantharidin in the stomach content or urine of affected horses. Treatment is symptomatic but not often successful.

MYCOTOXICOSES

(Fungal or Mold toxicoses)

Acute or chronic intoxications due to the ingestion of feed contaminated with toxins produced during growth of various saprophytic or phytopathogenic fungi or molds. The toxins may be produced on hay, cereals, pastures or fodder, or may be present in constituents used in the manufacture of meals or pelleted animal diets. Some animal diets, especially those containing grains or nuts, may contain several toxigenic species of molds, which may produce a number of mycotoxins having different toxic or pharmacologic properties. Under these circumstances, clinical effects and lesions found in disease outbreaks may not conform to the usual descriptions of outbreaks or to experimental findings in animals dosed with mycotoxins isolated from pure mold cultures.

Treatment of mycotoxicoses is ineffective but some animals recover if the source of toxin is removed; others are stunted or die. Since toxigenic molds are ubiquitous the aim should be to prevent damage to, and mold spoilage of, cereals, peanuts (groundnuts) and fodder by correct harvesting and proper storage. High relative humidity is a growth requirement for all molds but temperature requirements vary considerably.

Mycotoxic diseases that occur throughout the world are summarized in the table on pages 1038 to 1041.

AFLATOXICOSIS

This disease, recognized in many parts of the world, is caused by toxigenic strains of *Aspergillus flavus* and *A. parasiticus*. Aflatoxins are produced on peanuts, soy beans, corn (maize) and other cereals in the field or during storage as seeds, processed meals and cakes when moisture content and temperatures are sufficiently high for mold growth.

Aflatoxins likely have been partly responsible for other previously recognized mycotoxic diseases such as Moldy Corn Toxicosis, Poultry Hemorrhagic Syndrome and "Aspergillus Toxicosis."

Epidemiology: The disease affects growing poultry, especially ducklings and turkey poults. Young swine, pregnant sows, calves and dogs are highly susceptible. Adult cattle, sheep and goats are also susceptible when fed toxic diets over longer periods. The toxin is excreted in the milk. Experimentally, all species of animals tested have shown some degree of susceptibility to aflatoxins. Their potent carcinogenic effects upon the liver have been demonstrated in several species.

Clinical Findings: In all animals the first signs in an outbreak are inappetence, reduced growth rate or loss of condition. Other signs are rarely seen until about 7 to 14 days before death. Icterus, apathy and hemorrhagic enteritis may be evident.

Lesions: In all species, in acute cases, the liver shows severe fatty degeneration, is friable and may show small hemorrhages under the capsule. Icterus is often present. The kidneys are enlarged and may also show small hemorrhages. In chronic cases the liver is mottled and firm due to cirrhosis. In cattle, swine, sheep and dogs, a hemorrhagic enteritis with ulceration may also be present.

Diagnosis: The history of the outbreak, the necropsy findings and the histologic examination of liver tissue should establish the diagnosis. Aflatoxicosis may be confused with phosphorus poisoning (q.v., p. 991) in dogs, and with *Senecio* poisoning (q.v., p. 1048) and mycotoxic lupinosis (*see* below) in cattle and sheep.

If available, samples of the feed should be forwarded for laboratory examination. Testing for toxicity of extracts by dosing ducklings will also give positive evidence within 7 days.

MOLDY CORN TOXICOSIS

A hemorrhagic disease observed in swine, cattle and dogs that have consumed diets containing moldy corn (maize). Several molds may be implicated: *Penicillium rubrum* and *Aspergillus flavus*, isolated from toxic moldy corn, have been shown experimentally to produce lesions and signs similar to those observed in field toxicoses. More recent investigations have implicated *Fusarium* spp. in the etiology of outbreaks, in particular *F. tricinctum*, and the toxic trichothecene metabolites (most notably the T2 toxin) that are known to be produced on unharvested corn and in cereals stored at low temperatures. This toxicosis has been observed in late summer and fall in the Southeastern U.S.A. Mortality ranged from 5 to 55% in affected herds.

Gross icterus and tissue hemorrhages are the most constant findings at necropsy. In acute cases, massive hemorrhages are observed in most tissues. In chronic cases, extensive icterus and cachexia are the predominant gross findings. Acute signs occur within 8 to 12 hours after the ingestion of toxic corn or may extend over a period of 1 to 3 days. They may include depression, incoordination, anorexia and icterus. Chronically affected animals show general depression, anorexia and cachexia.

As in aflatoxicosis, early diagnosis of moldy corn poisoning may be difficult. There is no treatment.

MYCOTOXIC LUPINOSIS

Lupines (*Lupinus* spp.) cause 2 distinct forms of poisoning in domestic animals, viz. lupine poisoning and lupinosis. The former is a nervous syndrome caused by alkaloids present in bitter lupines. Lupinosis is an icteric disease caused by a mycotoxin of as yet

FUNGI AND MOLDS TOXIC TO DOMESTIC ANIMALS

Disease	Fungi or Molds	Toxins (where known)	Countries where reported	Contaminated Toxic Foodstuff	Animals Affected	Signs and Lesions
Aflatoxicosis	*Aspergillus flavus, A. parasiticus*	Aflatoxins	Widespread	Moldy peanuts, Soybean, Cottonseed, Rice, Sorghum, Corn, other cereals	All poultry, Swine, Cattle, Sheep, Dogs	(*See* AFLATOXICOSIS, p. 1036 and POULTRY MYCOTOXICOSIS, p. 1115.)
Aspergillus clavatus tremors	*A. clavatus*	Unknown	South Africa	Sorghum beer residue	Cattle	Hypersensitivity, incoordination, severe generalized muscular tremors, progressive paresis and paralysis. Necrosis of large motor neurones in CNS.
Diplodiosis	*Diplodia zeae*	Unknown	Southern Africa	Moldy corn	Cattle	CNS hypersensitivity followed by paresis. Recovery usual on removal from source.
Ergot	*Claviceps purpurea*	Ergot alkaloids	Widespread	Seedheads of many grasses	Cattle, Horses	(SEE ERGOTISM, p. 1045.)
	C. paspali	Nonalkaloidal ergot tremorgens	Widespread	Seedheads of paspalum grasses	Cattle, Horses, Sheep	(*See* PASPALUM STAGGERS, p. 1044.)
Facial eczema (Pithomycotoxicosis)	*Pithomyces chartarum (Sporidesmium bakeri)*	Sporidesmins	New Zealand, Australia, South Africa, probably U.S.A.	Toxic spores on pasture	Sheep, Cattle	(*See* FACIAL ECZEMA, p. 532.)

Fusariotoxicosis	*Fusarium tricinctum*, *F. roseum*, *F. culmorum*, *F. equiseti*, *F. scirpi* and other fusaria	T2 Toxin, Diacetoxyscirpenol and other Tricothecenes	U.S.A., U.S.S.R., Australia, Canada	Overwintered cereal crops, Growing maize, Tall fescue grass	Cattle, Horses, Swine, Poultry	Loss of appetite and milk production, diarrhea and staggers, recovery upon removal from crops. (Possibly also associated with FESCUE LAMENESS, p. 1043.)
Fusarium estrogenism and vulvovaginitis	*Fusarium roseum* (=*F. graminearum*) Sexual stage: *Gibberella zeae*	Zearalenone (estrogen)	Widespread	Moldy corn and pelleted feeds, Standing corn, Corn silage	Swine, Cattle, Sheep, Poultry	Vulvovaginitis in swine, estrogenism in cattle and sheep, reduced egg production in poultry. (*See Fusarium* ESTROGENISM, p. 1042.)
Leucoencephalomalacia	*Fusarium moniliforme*	Not known	Egypt, U.S.A., South Africa, Greece	Moldy corn	Horses	Dependent on degree and specific site of brain lesion.
Mold nephrosis	*Penicillium viridicatum*, *P. citrinum*, *Aspergillus ochraceus* and others	Ochratoxin, Citrinin?	Denmark, probably North America	Moldy barley, corn, wheat	Swine, Poultry	Perirenal edema, enlarged pale kidneys with cortical cysts, tubular degeneration and fibrosis.
Moldy corn toxicosis	Probably *Fusarium* spp., *Penicillium rubrum*, *P. purpurogenum*	Probably T2 Toxin and/or Rubratoxins	Widespread	Moldy corn	Horses, Swine, Cattle, Poultry	(*See* MOLDY CORN TOXICOSIS, p. 1037.)
Mushroom poisoning	(a) *Amanita verna*, (b) *A. muscaria*	(a) Amanitins, (b) Muscarine	U.S.A.	Eaten from pastures	Cattle	(a) Severe inflammation of intestinal tract. In severe cases, convulsions and death. (b) Parasympathomimetic stimulation.

FUNGI AND MOLDS TOXIC TO DOMESTIC ANIMALS (*continued*)

Disease	Fungi or Molds	Toxins (where known)	Countries where reported	Contaminated Toxic Foodstuff	Animals Affected	Signs and Lesions
Mycotoxic lupinosis (as distinct from lupine alkaloid poisoning)	*Phomopsis leptostromiformis*	Not known	Widespread	Moldy seed, pods, stubble and haulm of several *Lupinus* spp. affected by *Phomopsis* stem blight	Sheep, occasionally cattle and horses	Lassitude, inappetence, stupor, icterus, marked liver injury—usually fatal termination.
Myrothecio-toxicosis (Dendrodochiotoxicosis)	*Myrothecium verrucaria, M. roridum*	Verrucarins, Roridins	U.S.S.R.	Moldy rye stubble, straw	Sheep, Cattle, Horses	Acute: diarrhea, respiratory distress, hemorrhagic gastroenterocolitis, death. Chronic: ulcerations of intestinal tract, unthriftiness, gradual recovery.
Poultry hemorrhagic syndrome	Probably *Aspergillus flavus, A. clavatus, Penicillium purpurogenum, Alternaria* sp.	Probably Aflatoxins and Rubratoxins	U.S.A.	Toxic grain and meal	Growing chickens	Depression, anorexia, no gain in weight, death. Widespread internal hemorrhages, sometimes aplastic anemia. (*See* MYCOTIC DISEASES [POULTRY], p. 1114.)
Slobbers	*Rhizoctonia leguminicola*	Alkaloid, Slaframine	U.S.A.	Blackpatch-diseased legumes (notably red clover) eaten as forage or hay	Sheep, Cattle	Salivation, bloat, diarrhea, sometimes death—recovery usual when removed from clover.

Stachybotryotoxicosis	*Stachybotrys atra (alternans)*	Satratoxin (Trichothecenes)	U.S.S.R.	Toxic pastures or roughage, other contaminated feed	Horses, Cattle, Sheep, Swine	Stomatitis and ulceration, anorexia, leukopenia. (Horses may also show incoordination and blindness.) Extensive hemorrhages in many organs, inflammation and necrosis in the gut.
Sweet clover poisoning	*Penicillium* spp., *Mucor* spp., *Aspergillus* spp.	Dicumarol	North America	Sweet clover (*Melilotus* spp.)	Cattle, Horses, Sheep, Swine	(*See* SWEET CLOVER POISONING, p. 1017.)
Tremorgen-staggers syndrome	*Penicillium crustosum, P. puberulum, P. verruculosum, Aspergillus flavus, A. fumigatus* and others	Penitrems, Verruculogen, Paxilline, Fumitremorgens	U.S.A., Australia, New Zealand, Europe, South Africa	Moldy commercial feed, grass, litter, soil	Horses, Cattle, Sheep, Poultry, Dogs	Tremors, incoordination, ataxia, collapse, convulsive spasms. (*See* RYEGRASS STAGGERS, p. 1046.)
Vomiting and feed refusal in swine	*Fusarium roseum* (=*F. graminearum*) Sexual stage: *Gibberella zeae;* other fusaria	Same factor in both, Vomitoxin (Trichothecene)	U.S.A., U.S.S.R., Korea	Scabbed barley	Swine, Dogs	Vomiting and diarrhea. Recovery when diet is changed. Feed refusal when toxin is present in higher concentration.

undetermined structure and has been reported from Europe, Australia, New Zealand and South Africa. Sheep, cattle and occasionally horses are affected when they graze infested lupine material especially after rain when saprophytic growth has occurred.

The causal fungus is *Phomopsis leptostromiformis*, a phytopathogen causing *Phomopsis* stem-blight especially in white and yellow lupines, blue varieties being very resistant. It produces sunken linear stem lesions containing black stromatic masses, and also affects the pods and seeds. It is also a saprophyte and under favorable moisture and temperature conditions grows well on dead lupine material, e.g. haulm, pods and stubble. It can also be grown artificially on other substrates, e.g. corn.

The fungus produces a potent hepatotoxin and the syndrome may be confused with aflatoxicosis. In acute poisoning, lethargy, anorexia and ruminal stasis are the first signs encountered after a latent period of 2 to 3 days and this is followed by intense icterus and constipation. At necropsy the characteristic finding is a severe fatty degeneration of the liver. In more chronic cases varying degrees of cirrhosis are encountered, and in sheep almost complete cirrhosis may be seen, producing a "boxing glove" liver the size of a man's fist.

The diagnosis is confirmed by histopathologic examination of liver tissue and by the identification of the causal fungus on lupine material. Mycotoxic lupinosis can be avoided by growing lupine varieties (e.g. blue lupines) that are resistant to *Phomopsis* blight.

Fusarium ESTROGENISM
(Including Vulvovaginitis in swine)

Fusarium roseum (*graminearum*) produces at least 2 types of toxic metabolites: an emetic principle and a feed-refusal factor that have been shown to be the same compound (vomitoxin, a trichothecene mycotoxin) and zearalenone or F2 toxin. The latter is a potent estrogen that causes vulvovaginitis in swine, and the syndrome is produced when moldy corn infested with certain strains of this fungus, or even pelleted feed from such corn, is fed. (Zearalenone is one of a group of compounds known by the more general name of resorcylic acid lactones. As with many compounds, the toxicity is dose related; the RALs are useful as anabolic agents.) *Fusarium roseum* (*graminearum*) has been identified as a predominant advanced-decay mold, so it is unlikely that zearalenone is produced in significant quantity in the field before harvest.

The condition cannot be distinguished from excessive estrogen administration and the signs encountered are especially evident in young gilts. Conspicuous tumefaction of the vulva (with occasional prolapse of the vagina and rectum) and enlargement of the mammary glands due to ductular proliferation are the most obvious signs. There is hypertrophy of the uterus and a decrease in size of the ovaries.

Abortion and fetal resorption may be encountered and reproductive performance may be influenced. In young boars, arrest in the development of the genitalia may be seen. The condition can usually be rectified by removing the contaminated feed.

The corresponding disease has also occurred in sheep fed ensiled corn. Abortions, premature live births, prostration, paraplegia and a few deaths occurred in the ewe flock. A high content of zearalenone was shown in the corn silage and estrogenic effects were produced in rats when extracts were injected.

Similarly, dairy heifers feedlot-fed whole corn ensiled at the green stage showed weight loss, vaginal discharge, nymphomania, uterine hypertrophy with endometrial hyperplasia, mammary development, failure to conceive or early loss of conceptus, all overt signs of severe hyperestrogenism. Losses in terms of reproduction and subsequent productivity were severe.

FESCUE LAMENESS

(Fescue foot)

A condition, resembling ergot poisoning, caused by a toxic substance in tall fescue (*Festuca arundinacea*). It commences with lameness in one or both hind feet and may progress to necrosis of the distal part of the affected limb. The tail and ears also may be affected.

Etiology: The cause of fescue lameness is a toxic substance of tall fescue grass, which has actions similar to those produced by sclerotia of *Claviceps purpurea*, but which is not localized in the seed heads. Tall fescue is a coarse, rank growing grass that thrives in moist places and is used in Australia and New Zealand for stabilizing the banks of watercourses. In the Southeastern U.S.A. it is an important pasture grass.

Reliable reports of occurrence of fescue lameness have come from Kentucky, Tennessee, Florida, California, Colorado and Missouri as well as from New Zealand, Australia and Italy. "Alta" and "Kentucky 31" strains of tall fescue may, under some conditions, cause lameness.

Ergot poisoning (q.v., p. 1045) probably is not the cause of fescue foot. Ergot toxicosis is most prevalent in the latter part of summer when the seed heads of grasses mature. Fescue foot, on the other hand, can occur at any time of the year, but the incidence is highest in winter. Typical fescue foot has been produced in cattle by feeding dried grass free of seed heads and ergot. In recent years several toxic fungi including *Fusarium tricinctum* have been suspected of causing the disease, but none have so far been proven to do so.

Clinical Findings: In cattle, the first signs develop within 10 to 14 days of grazing on tall fescue grass. There is local heat, swelling, severe pain and lameness of one or more feet. Usually, one hind foot is affected first. With continued feeding on fescue, an indented line appears at some point, usually between the hock and the claws. Dry gangrene affects the distal part, which eventually may be sloughed. Low environmental temperature is thought to contribute to the lesions. At necropsy, there are no lesions other than those associated with the swelling or dry gangrene.

Although lesions similar to those of fescue foot have occasionally been reported in sheep, no authenticated outbreak of fescue foot has been recorded in any species other than cattle.

Control: Removal to other feed will result in recovery if the lesions have not progressed to dry gangrene, and the animals are kept warm. Risk of fescue lameness is reduced by maintaining legumes in the sward since tall fescue has proved to be one of the least palatable of our cultivated or wild grasses and, therefore, will not be consumed in large amounts when other forage is available. Most reports indicate an increased incidence of fescue lameness as the age of the stand increases. This may be due to an increased fungal infestation. Severe droughts may be followed by an increased number of cases of fescue foot. Tall fescue tends to survive protracted droughts more successfully than other commonly grown forage plants.

PASPALUM STAGGERS

An incoordination of animals resulting from eating paspalum grasses. The life history of this fungus is similar to that of *C. purpurea* (*see* ERGOTISM, p. 1045). The yellow-gray sclerotia, which mature in the seed heads in the autumn, are round and 2 to 4 mm in diameter. Ingestion of sclerotia causes nervous signs in cattle most commonly, but horses and sheep also are susceptible. Guinea pigs can be affected by experimental feeding. The toxicity is ascribed to a group of nonalkaloidal tremorgens chemically related to other tremorgenic mycotoxins such as penitrem A. Toxicity increases as the sclerotia mature.

A sufficiently large single dose will cause signs that persist for several days. Animals display continuous trembling of the large muscle groups. If they attempt to move, their action is jerky and limb movements are incoordinated. If they attempt to run, they fall over in awkward attitudes. Condition is lost after prolonged exposure and complete paralysis can occur. The time of onset of signs depends on the degree of the infection of seed heads and the grazing habits of the animals. Experimentally, early signs appear in cattle after about 100 gm of sclerotia per day have been administered for more than 2 days. Young sclerotia may be more toxic than mature ones.

Recovery follows removal of the animals to feed not contaminated with sclerotia of *C. paspali*. Topping of the pasture to remove affected seed heads has been effective in controlling this condition.

ERGOTISM

A disease of cattle and other farm animals resulting from the continued ingestion of sclerotia of the parasitic fungus *Claviceps purpurea* that replaces the grain or seed of rye and other small grains or forage plants, such as the bromes, bluegrasses and ryegrasses. The sclerotia may contain varying quantities of ergot alkaloids of which the levorotatory alkaloids, ergotamine and ergonovine (ergometrine), are pharmacologically most important.

Etiology: Ergot causes vasoconstriction by direct action on the muscles of the arterioles, and repeated dosages injure the vascular endothelium. These actions result initially in reduced blood flow and eventually complete stasis with terminal necrosis of the extremities due to thrombosis. A cold environment predisposes the extremities to gangrenous ergotism. In addition, ergot has a potent oxytocic action and also causes stimulation of the CNS, followed by depression.

Clinical Findings: Cattle may be affected by eating ergotized hay or grain or occasionally by grazing seeded pastures that are infected with ergot. Lameness is the first sign and may appear 2 to 6 weeks or longer after initial ingestion, the length of time depending on the concentration of alkaloids in the ergot and the quantity of ergot in the feed. Hind limbs are affected before forelimbs, but again the extent of involvement of a limb and the number of limbs affected depends on the daily intake of ergot. A high body temperature and increased pulse and respiration rates accompany the lameness.

Associated with the lameness are swelling and tenderness of the fetlock joint and pastern. Within about a week, sensation is lost in the affected part, an indented line appears at the limit of normal tissue and dry gangrene affects the distal part. Eventually, one or both claws or any part of the limb up to the hock or knee may be sloughed. In a similar way, the tip of the tail or ears may become necrotic and be sloughed. Exposed skin areas, such as teats and udder, appear unusually pale or anemic.

Lesions: The only constant lesions at necropsy are in the skin and subcut. parts of the extremities. The skin is normal to the indented line, but beyond it is cyanotic and hardened in advanced cases.

Subcut. hemorrhage and some edema occur proximal to the necrotic area.

Sheep given the alkaloid experimentally had ulceration in the mouth and gastroenteritis; the legs were not affected. A **convulsive syndrome in sheep** has been associated with the ingestion of ergot.

A syndrome of **agalactia in sows,** characterized by complete absence of hypertrophy of mammary glands in the preparturient period and subsequent starvation of the piglets, has followed the ingestion of ergot-infested grain. Piglets from such sows are often weak at birth.

Control: Control of ergotism consists of an immediate change to an ergot-free diet. Under pasture feeding conditions, frequent grazing or topping of pastures prone to ergot infection during the summer months to allow few or no flowering heads to develop should control the disease. Grain with any sign of ergot infection should not be fed to pregnant or lactating sows even if the degree of infection is low (i.e. less than 0.6% infected grain).

PERENNIAL RYEGRASS STAGGERS

A seasonal neurotoxic condition, characterized by tremors, incoordination and sometimes collapse, affecting sheep, cattle or horses during summer and fall. It is strongly associated with short grazing of perennial ryegrass (*Lolium perenne*) dominant pastures, particularly those containing abundant dead ryegrass litter. Severe outbreaks occur in dry seasons, usually a few days after rainfall. The disease, which occurs in North America, Australia and Europe, can cause serious disruptions to animal and pasture management.

Etiology: The cause is unknown, but mycotoxic tremorgens such as peritrems, verruculogen, fumitremorgens and paxilline, known products of several *Penicillium* and *Aspergillus* spp., have been strongly implicated. Experimental dosage of sheep and cattle with mold cultures containing tremorgens produces a disorder closely resembling the field disease. A multiple etiology, based on a spectrum of tremorgenic molds in soil and litter, seems likely.

Sclerotia of *Claviceps purpurea*, often coincidentally present on ryegrass, do not contain neurotoxic tremorgens. Cobalt supplementation gives protection from "phalaris staggers" but not from ryegrass staggers. Clinically, ryegrass staggers is indistinguishable from "paspalum staggers" (q.v., p. 1044), a disease mainly affecting cattle and produced by tremorgens, not alkaloids, in the sclerotia of *Claviceps paspali*.

Clinical Findings: Signs develop gradually over a few days. In undisturbed sheep and cattle, approached quietly, fine tremors and head nodding may be the first signs. Excessive noise and fright or sudden exercise may elicit more severe signs, such as marked tremors of head and limbs, jerky movements, marked incoordination and even collapse. Locomotion occurs in stiff bounding movements as the legs become rigidly extended. The animal may fall in lateral recumbency with opisthotonos, nystagmus, stiffly extended limbs and fasciculation of muscle groups. The attack quickly subsides, the animal sits with a dazed appearance and within minutes will regain its feet and rejoin the flock or herd. If again forced to run the episode will be repeated. Both cattle and sheep avoid rapid movements and stand and graze with hind legs abducted to maintain balance. Horses often walk with a reeling gait.

Generally, animals recover completely when pasture toxicity falls or when given alternative feed. Within flocks and herds individual susceptibility varies greatly; some are affected in most summers yet others are never affected. Morbidity may reach 80% but mortality is low and death is usually accidental. No constant gross or microscopic lesions are found at necropsy. The muscle dystrophy and cerebellar Purkinje-cell degeneration observed in some cases are regarded as lesions secondary to the incoordination and convulsive episodes.

Control: Since movement and handling of animals exacerbates signs, individual treatment is generally impractical. Recovery is spontaneous if animals are allowed to migrate (not driven) onto nontoxic pastures or crops. Injections of diazepam or mephenesin may reduce severe muscular spasms.

High stocking rates and overgrazing of ryegrass dominant pastures should be avoided during the dangerous season. Experimentally, good seasonal control has been achieved by prior injections of compounds known to stimulate liver mixed-function oxidase enzymes, which inactivate the tremorgens. Carcass residues preclude the use of these compounds but alternative stimulants may prove acceptable.

ANNUAL RYEGRASS STAGGERS

This disease occurs in Australia in sheep and cattle grazing annual (Wimmera) ryegrass (*Lolium rigidum*) pastures.

Etiology: The neurotoxicity is associated with seedhead galls which result from a primary infestation by a nematode (*Anguina lolii*) and subsequent infection of the gall with a bacterium (*Corynebacterium* sp.). The bacterial galls are toxic but not the nematode galls. A similar disease has been reported from Oregon when hay of *Festuca* *rubra* var. *commutata* (Chewing's fescue) with *Corynebacterium*-infected seedhead galls proved toxic to cattle and horses.

Clinical Findings: Signs are closely similar to those of perennial ryegrass staggers (q.v., p. 1046). However mortality in animals affected with annual ryegrass staggers is often 40 to 50%.

Control: No treatment is known. Topping of overgrown pastures and grazing management aimed at restricting seed formation is recommended.

Senecio POISONING

(Pyrrolizidine alkaloidosis, Seneciosis, Ragwort, Ragweed poisoning)

A chronic and infrequently acute poisoning caused by many toxic plants found most commonly in the genera *Senecio, Crotalaria* and *Heliotropium* but also in *Amsinckia, Echium, Cynoglossum* and *Trichodesma*. These plants grow mainly in temperate climates, but some (e.g. *Crotalaria*) require tropical or subtropical climates. Their distribution is worldwide and it is likely that their toxic effects are unique. The plants most commonly responsible are ragwort (*S. jacobaea*), woolly groundsel (*S. ridellii, S. longilobus*) and seeds of yellow tarweed (*A. intermedia*).

The toxic factors common to these plants are a number of pyrrolizidine alkaloids that affect mainly the liver. Cattle, horses and swine are the species most susceptible to intoxication. Sheep are much less susceptible. It is claimed that in sheep rumen liquor the alkaloids are reduced to the corresponding (nontoxic) 1-methylene pyrrolizidine derivatives. The organism responsible for this reduction has been isolated and characterized as a new species, *Peptococcus heliotrinreductans*. However, an alternative explanation advanced is that the marked species difference is due to differences in hepatic alkaloid metabolism rather than to rumen effects. Individual susceptibility varies greatly within species and may be influenced by sex, age and diet. Young growing animals are most susceptible because the alkaloids have a marked antimitotic effect on liver cells.

Under normal conditions these plants are unpalatable and are avoided by grazing animals. During drought conditions the growing plants may be eaten. Animals are also poisoned by eating the plant material in hay or silage. Seeds from *Crotalaria, Amsinckia* and *Heliotropium*, which have been harvested with grain, have been responsible for the disease in horses, cattle, swine and poultry.

Clinical Findings: The clinical signs and the pathologic effects are similar in all animal species affected regardless of the species of plant responsible or the toxic pyrrolizidine alkaloids it contains. The acute form of the disease, characterized by sudden death from acute hemorrhagic liver necrosis and visceral hemorrhages, is rare. The effects upon the liver of repeated low intake of toxic plants are cumulative and progressive; clinical signs may not be seen for several weeks (often after consumption of the plant has ceased). In *Heliotropium* spp. poisoning severe losses are produced in sheep only after the plants have been grazed for a second season.

In horses and cattle, some of the following signs are seen: loss of condition, anorexia, dullness and constipation or diarrhea. Tenesmus and passing of bloodstained feces may be followed by rectal prolapse, especially in cattle. Ascites and icterus may be present and cattle sometimes show intermittent photosensitization. Some animals may become progressively weaker and rarely move while others wander aimlessly with an awkward gait, either stumbling against or actively pushing headlong into fences or other structures. Still others may become frenzied and dangerously aggressive. Pica may be observed in some individuals. Death may occur suddenly or following prolonged recumbency with hepatic coma and high blood-ammonia levels.

Lesions: In acute cases the liver may be enlarged, hemorrhagic and icteric. In chronic cases the liver is atrophied, fibrous, misshapen, and usually pale with a glistening surface due to fibrous thickening of the capsule. Other livers are markedly icteric. The gallbladder is often edematous and grossly distended with thick mucoid bile. Edema of segments of the bowel, mesentery and associated lymph nodes is common and much ascitic fluid may be found in the abdominal cavity. In some cases numerous small hemorrhages are present in the abdominal serous membranes.

Characteristic histologic changes are found in the liver. Irreversible enlargement of individual hepatocytes (megalocytosis) is unique, and is conspicuous in the horse and sheep, but less pronounced in cattle. In cattle, marked perivenous fibrosis of sublobular veins is usually present, but this is not a consistent finding in the horse and sheep. In all species there are marked increases in connective tissue both within and around the lobules.

Diagnosis and Treatment: A diagnosis based on a history of the outbreak, clinical signs and gross necropsy findings can usually be confirmed by histologic examination of liver tissue obtained by biopsy or at necropsy.

Further intake of toxic plant material must be prevented. Animals showing clinical signs rarely recover and lesions present in asymptomatic animals may progress and result in further losses over several months. Since high-protein intake may prove harmful, diets with a high-carbohydrate ratio are indicated. Intravenous administration of methionine in 10% dextrose solution is claimed to be of value in treating horses.

The diminished ability of the liver to regenerate after pyrrolizidine alkaloid poisoning suggests that a guarded prognosis should always be given. Factors in preventing further outbreaks should be stressed.

Control: Sheep are commonly used for grazing control of *Senecio jacobaea, Heliotropium europaeum* and *Echium plantagineum,* though the practice carries risks unless sheep destined for early slaughter are used. Biological control of plants with predator moths and butterflies is being attempted and has met with limited success. Measures that enhance destruction of the alkaloids in the rumen of sheep have also shown some promise.

ALGAL POISONING

A usually acute and highly fatal condition caused by drinking water containing high concentrations of toxic blue-green algae. Fatalities and severe illness of livestock, pets, wild animals and people have been associated with algal blooms in the northern half of the U.S.A., Texas, Canada, Russia, Argentina, Australia and South Africa.

Poisoning usually does not occur unless there is a dense bloom of toxic algae. The factors leading to such blooms include warm, sunny weather, ample nutrients (especially nitrates), and a gentle prevailing wind that drifts and collects the algae against the shore where it produces a blue-green scum. Such conditions commonly occur during the summer months in drainage ponds and lakes used for watering livestock.

Etiology: More recent research has discounted the earlier beliefs regarding the alkaloidal nature of the toxic principle and incriminated a 7-amino acid cyclic polypeptide, which rapidly produced toxic signs. Strains of *Microcystis aeruginosa* (*toxica*), *M. flos-aquae, Aphanizomenon flos-aquae* and *Anabaena flos-aquae* are most commonly responsible for algal intoxication, although certain bacteria associated with the algae may also produce toxins, which are less potent.

Clinical Findings: Toxic signs usually appear within 15 to 45 min. after ingestion of the poisonous material. Death may occur in less than 24 hours and often within 1 or 2 hours after ingestion of the toxin. The most commonly reported sequence of events is rapid prostration, convulsions and death. Abdominal pain, muscular tremors, dyspnea, cyanosis and excessive salivation are common; less common are severe gastrointestinal manifestations which include diarrhea, bloody feces and icterus. Photosensitization frequently occurs in animals that survive for several days.

Control: Removal of animals from the affected water supply is essential. Algal growth may be suppressed with copper sulfate or other algicide treatment, but this does not remove the toxin already present in the water. If no other water supply is available, animals should be allowed to drink only from the shore kept clearest by the prevailing wind.

Animals dying from algal poisoning must not be used for food as the toxic principle is stable and consistently produces toxic symptoms in the consumer.

Treatment: Following removal from the contaminated water supply, affected animals should be placed in a protected area out of direct sunlight. Ample quantities of water and good quality feed should be made available. Administration of activated charcoal slurry and a laxative dose of heavy mineral oil has proven useful in removing toxins from the gastrointestinal tract. (CAUTION: Affected animals are usually very weak, and heroic procedures should not be employed.)

One to 2 oz (30 to 60 mg) of sodium thiosulfate in solution given IV or orally twice a day seems to be of benefit, even though the pharmacologic principle has not been identified. In surviving animals, a long recuperative period is to be expected.

SNAKE BITE

Venomous snakes fall into 2 classes: the elapine snakes, which include the cobra, mamba and coral snake, and the viperine snakes, which comprise 2 families—the true vipers, e.g. puff adder, Russell's viper and common European adder; and the pit vipers, e.g. rattlesnakes, cottonmouth moccasin and fer-de-lance. Elapine snakes have short fangs and tend to hang on and "chew" their victims. Their venom is mainly neurotoxic and kills by paralyzing the respiratory center; in cases of recovery there are seldom any subsequent ill-effects. Viperine snakes have long, hinged fangs; they strike once and then withdraw. Their venom is mainly hemotoxic, causing pronounced local damage; subsequent necrosis may lead to the loss of a limb even if the victim recovers. However, all snake venoms contain both neurotoxic and hemotoxic factors.

The active principles of venom include hyaluronidase, cholinesterase, proteolytic enzymes, phosphatases and neurotoxins. The latter have been shown to be basic polypeptides.

The severity of the bite of any species of snake is extremely variable, depending chiefly upon the amount of venom injected. The expulsion of venom from the glands is a voluntary action on the part of the snake, and is entirely under the reptile's control. In numerous cases the bite of a venomous snake entails no envenomation at all. Other factors that affect the outcome of a bite are the toxicity of the venom, the location of the bite, the size and species of the victim and its age and general condition of health. Experimental work suggests that the order of decreasing sensitivity is horse, sheep, ox, goat, dog, pig and cat.

Since the lethal dose of a poison is based upon the quantity of poison introduced per unit of body weight, horses and cattle seldom die as a direct result of snake bite, but lack of medical attention may result in serious secondary damage. Fatalities in horses and cattle have resulted from bites on the muzzle, head or neck.

Undoubtedly, the death rate from snake bite in all parts of the world is higher in dogs than in any other domestic animals. Due to the relatively small weight of the dog in proportion to the amount of venom injected, and to the fact that most bites occur on the head or neck, the bite of even a small snake is frequently fatal.

Clinical Findings and Diagnosis: The presence of hair may obscure the typical fang marks, though a close examination should reveal the point of entry of the venom. Venoms from viperine snakes may produce prolonged intense pain, muscular weakness, impaired vision, nausea, paralysis, edema, shock, cyanosis, hemolytic anemia, necrosis of tissue and bleeding tendencies. The venom of the rattlesnake causes an almost immediate reaction in the form of extensive swelling around the wound. When horses and cattle are bitten about the head, their lips, face and submaxillary region become grossly swollen, which results in pronounced dyspnea. Sloughing of the skin in the region of the wound may follow a bite. If a limb has been struck, the swelling usually causes lameness. In the case of an elapine snake bite the pain and local swelling may be absent, but the systemic signs are more pronounced.

Shock, in all its classical elements, accompanies all severe snake bites. Body temperature is frequently lowered. Lassitude and somnolence usually ensue. If a dog has been exercising violently, as is frequently the case, and if the venom is deposited in a highly vascular area, death commonly occurs in a matter of 5 to 10 minutes. Severe bacterial infections are sometimes sequelae to snake bites.

Treatment: The aims are: (1) to prevent or delay the absorption of venom into the general circulation, (2) to neutralize any absorbed venom with the most appropriate antivenin, (3) to counter the local and general effects of the venom with supportive measures, especially the maintenance of cardiorespiratory function. Speed is essential. As exercise increases the rate of absorption of the venom, the patient should be carried to the veterinarian, or kept quiet and still until his arrival. Should there by any delay in obtaining expert help, the following first aid treatment may be useful in the case of a bite by a viperine snake. It would be of little value in the case of an elapine bite. The animal should be placed at rest and the hair clipped from the wound. If the bite is on a limb, a wide tourniquet should be placed 2 in. (5 cm) above the site of the bite. The tourniquet must arrest venous and lymphatic flow, but not arterial circulation. It should be released every 15 minutes for a period of 1 or 2 minutes. After injection of antivenin, the tourniquet should be discarded.

In the case of a bite from a dangerous snake, such as a rattlesnake, the fang wounds should be enlarged with lineal incisions paralleling the blood supply. Suction should be applied to the incisions for at least 30 minutes. Ordinarily rubber suction cups have been shown to remove significant quantities of venom from FRESH VENOM SITES in 15 minutes. Oral suction should never be employed.

Early injection of polyvalent antivenin is most desirable; in fact, it is the only lifesaving measure in cases of bites from dangerous snakes, and for this reason is indicated in all cases of poisonous snake bites regardless of the interval between bite and institution of treatment. It has proved beneficial when administered for head bites of horses as late as 24 hours after the bite. The life of the animal will be endangered if (1) antivenin is withheld when there is clear evidence of envenomation; (2) the wrong antivenin is administered, as when the snake has been mistakenly identified; (3) an inadequate quantity of the appropriate antivenin is given; (4) the dose of antivenin is not repeated when the signs of envenomation persist.

The smaller the animal, the more antivenin is required. The initial dose for dogs may be as high as 100 ml; 1 to 5 ampules (15 ml each) should be administered to an average-sized dog, depending upon the kind and size of the snake and the condition of the victim. All antivenin should be given IV, but the subcut. or IP route is preferred for first-aid use in the field. A minimum of 3 vials of antivenin should be administered at once except in the case of a small snake such as the European adder, where a single vial will probably be enough. For a cow, 50 ml of antivenin may suffice. It is advisable to administer additional doses at 1- to 3-hour intervals as the patient's condition warrants.

Corticosteroids exert a beneficial effect on the shock that invariably accompanies snake bite. They also prolong survival time and help minimize tissue destruction. Broad-spectrum antibiotics should be administered. Infusions of isotonic saline and dextrose solutions, in addition to blood transfusions, are beneficial. Incision wounds should be kept open and draining until the animal shows marked improvement. An analgesic such as meperidine may be given if pain is severe. Permanganate should never be employed. Tetanus antitoxin should be given in prophylactic doses.

As a last resort, in the case of a bite by a dangerous viper or pit viper, if no antivenin is available, the area surrounding the bite may be excised.

Anaphylaxis is always a possibility after the administration of heterologous serum. As all antivenins are prepared by hyperimmunizing horses with appropriate venom, they are heterologous for all species other than the horse. The risk of foreign serum reaction may be minimized by giving the antivenin under the cover of epinephrine 1:1000, 0.5 to 1.0 ml subcut.

Contrary to former opinion, the use of excessive heat or cold is contraindicated in the treatment of the lesion. Since antihistamines have been shown to potentiate the effect of snake venom, their use is contraindicated. Certain cobras are capable of "spitting" their venom at the eyes of their victim from a distance of several feet, causing severe pain and often temporary blindness. Treatment consists of washing the eye with water or diluted serum.

PART III
POULTRY

COLIBACILLOSIS
(*Escherichia coli* infections)

A few of the many serotypes of *E. coli* can cause infection in poultry. Even though *E. coli* is part of the intestinal flora of all animals, only a small number of serotypes isolated from birds can cause disease in mammals. *E. coli* is a frequent cause of disease in birds although predisposing factors are usually involved. Among the more commonly observed lesions are: yolk sac infection, pericarditis, respiratory tract infections, peritonitis, salpingitis and less commonly joint infections, acute septicemia and panophthalmitis. Diagnosis is by isolation of *E. coli* from typical lesions.

Losses can be reduced by use of only clean and disinfected hatching eggs, hatchery sanitation and by the elimination of respiratory tract agents particularly *Mycoplasma* spp. In acute cases the nitrofurans, streptomycin, tetracyclines, gentamicin or sulfaquinoxaline are at times effective.

ERYSIPELOTHRIX INFECTION

An acute or subacute septicemic disease of turkeys, particularly males, caused by *Erysipelothrix rhusiopathiae* (*insidiosa*) and characterized by multiple diffuse hemorrhages in the large muscle masses and under the serous surfaces of the visceral organs. Outbreaks have also occurred in ducks and, occasionally, in geese and domestic chickens.

Etiology: In the acute septicemic infection of poultry, *E. rhusiopathiae* can be found in almost any part of the body including the blood. Contaminated soil probably is the source of infection and the organism probably enters the body through skin lesions. Uncooked fish meal or meat scraps in the feed are suspected as occasional sources of infection. In an outbreak the affected birds provide ample infective material for other members of the flock.

Clinical Findings: The disease usually appears in the fall and affects growing birds on range. Toms are more often affected than hens because of greater transmission during fighting. Affected birds lose their appetite, become listless and develop a greenish yellow diarrhea. They may show dyspnea and a nasal discharge. A red-purple swelling of the caruncle is highly suggestive but not pathognomonic.

In untreated flocks, the mortality may reach 40%. The most characteristic lesions are diffuse hemorrhages in the abdominal, pectoral and femoral muscles as well as in the fascial sheaths. Subserous hemorrhages in viscera are also common. The liver and spleen are usually congested and enlarged and may present hemorrhagic infarcts. There may be a catarrhal exudate in the intestines.

Diagnosis: A tentative diagnosis made on the basis of lesions and clinical signs should be confirmed by isolation and identification of *E. rhusiopathiae*. A gram-stained smear from a lesion may enable an experienced diagnostician to recognize the organism by its size, shape, and usual occurrence in a paired "V" arrangement.

Prophylaxis: Bacterins prepared from immunogenic strains of *E. rhusiopathiae* are widely used and are usually adequate under field exposure. Occasionally, vegetative endocarditis and myocarditis develops from chronic local infection in vaccinated birds.

Treatment: All birds in affected flocks should be treated with procaine penicillin, at 5,000 u/lb (11,000 u/kg) of body wt by subcut. or IM injection, and simultaneously injected with *E. rhusiopathiae* bacterin. Birds with clinical disease should be separated from the flock and inoculated IM with an additional 11,000 u/kg of potassium penicillin. Penicillin alone will suppress infection for only 4 to 7 days.

INFECTIOUS CORYZA

An acute disease of chickens, characterized by nasal discharge, sneezing and swelling or edema of the face. Less frequently there is a lower respiratory tract infection causing rales and difficult breathing.

Etiology and Epidemiology: *Haemophilus gallinarum*, the causative agent, is a hemophilic, gram-negative, pleomorphic, nonmotile bacterium. There are several serotypes with at least 3 distinct immunotypes. In recent years, the disease has been reported only from California to Florida in the U.S.A.; it occurs in many countries, especially those with temperate climates. Commercial poultry farms practicing the all-in, all-out procedure with essentially one age of chicken on a given premises have practically eradicated the disease.

Uncomplicated infectious coryza is characterized by rapid onset, the nasal discharge appearing on the first or second day following artificial inoculation. Under field conditions the disease may run a longer course, up to several months, depending on the presence of other complicating diseases such as mycoplasmosis.

The mortality may be negligible, but adverse effects on body weight and egg production may be severe. Secondary infections are common, resulting in a more chronic course. Chickens that recover may be carriers and are the commonest source of new outbreaks. Transmission takes place by airborne infective droplets and by contamination of drinking water and equipment.

Clinical Findings: In its mildest form, the only sign is a serous nasal discharge, with little or no systemic effect. In the more severe form, there is edema of the face that may extend (especially in males) to the intermandibular space and wattles. In chronic cases where other infectious agents are involved, sinuses become distended with a yellow caseous exudate. Other signs may be conjunctivitis, tracheitis, bronchitis and airsacculitis.

Diagnosis: The most reliable diagnostic procedure is the reproduction of the typical disease by contact or intranasal inoculation and demonstration of *H. gallinarum*. A history of a nasal discharge that quickly affects a large percentage of the chickens is good presumptive evidence. Swelling of the face and wattles must be differentiated from fowl cholera. Other diseases that must be considered are mycoplasmosis, laryngotracheitis, Newcastle disease and vitamin A deficiency.

Control and Treatment: In endemic areas, all replacements should be made with day-old chicks unless the bird source is known to be free of infectious respiratory diseases. Survivors of an outbreak should be completely and permanently separated from all other chickens either by segregation in a separate house or removal from the premises.

Early treatment is important, therefore water medication is to be recommended immediately until medicated feed is available. Erythromycin (℞ 37) is usually beneficial. Various sulfonamides (e.g. ℞ 93, 104, 261) have been used successfully but must not be used in layers. In more severe outbreaks, although treatment may result in improvement, the disease may recur when medication is discontinued.

Preventive medication may be combined with a vaccination program using a bacterin where started pullets are to be reared or housed on infected premises. A federally licensed bacterin (℞ 132) is available and some states have an approved bacterin.

LISTERIOSIS

This infection in birds occurs most frequently as a septicemia, but localized encephalitis similar to that seen in ruminants (q.v., p. 357) has been reported in chickens and turkeys, and encephalitis combined with septicemia has been observed in young geese. Chickens, geese, ducks and canaries appear to be the most commonly affected birds.

Etiology and Epidemiology: *Listeria monocytogenes* is widely distributed among avian species. Since it has been isolated from apparently normal birds and from birds dying from causes other than uncomplicated listeriosis, it is possible that birds may play an important role in the spread or perpetuation of the disease, not only in birds but also in mammals (including man). There is evidence that the bacterium may survive for at least 4 years in a chicken flock without manifestation of active disease. Further evidence incriminating birds as carriers is the frequent occurrence of relatively high agglutinating-antibody titers against *L. monocytogenes* in apparently normal birds and the common association of *L. monocytogenes* with other diseases.

Conjunctivitis due to *L. monocytogenes* in people employed in poultry-processing plants has been traced to the handling of apparently normal, but infected, chickens. There is strong circumstantial evidence that other forms of listeric infection, particularly listeric abortion in women, may result from contact with infected or carrier birds.

Clinical Findings and Diagnosis: Young birds appear to be more susceptible. In listeric septicemia among domestic birds, outbreaks are sporadic and mortality in the individual flock may vary within wide limits. Adult birds usually die suddenly with few clinical signs, while young birds waste slowly before death. At necropsy in uncomplicated listeric infection, the most striking lesions may be either massive necrosis of the myocardium with pericarditis and an increased amount of pericardial fluid, or focal hepatic necrosis, or both. The gram-positive *L. monocytogenes* may be found in the myocardial fibrils, and within or adjacent to the hepatic cells. There may be generalized edema, splenomegaly, peritonitis, enteritis and salpingitis. These lesions may be absent when listeric infection is associated with other disorders. The bacterium is most easily cultivated from the blood or from the affected organs. In some instances it may be necessary to refrigerate the tissue to be cultured before the bacterium can be isolated.

In listeric encephalitis, the signs are marked torticollis, a tendency to walk in circles and coarse tremors of the skeletal muscles. No gross lesions have been reported from this form of the disease, and *L. monocytogenes* can be isolated only from the brain.

Control: Recommended control includes rigid sanitation and culling and isolation of affected birds. The present widespread use of poultry feeds containing antibiotics may be an effective prophylactic measure against listeric infection.

AVIAN MYCOPLASMOSIS

Several *Mycoplasma* spp. have been isolated from avian hosts. Only 3 of these fastidious microbial species (*M. gallisepticum, M. meleagridis* and *M. synoviae*) have been demonstrated to be important pathogens of poultry. Each has significantly distinctive epidemiologic and pathologic characteristics.

MYCOPLASMA GALLISEPTICUM INFECTION (MG)

(PPLO infection, Chronic respiratory disease, CRD, Infectious sinusitis of turkeys)

MG infection in chickens is commonly designated as chronic respiratory disease (CRD) and has been identified in all major chicken- and turkey-producing areas of the world. It is very frequently complicated by other infections of both bacterial and viral etiology. In turkeys, MG infection is called infectious sinusitis.

Etiology and Incidence: The causative agent, *Mycoplasma gallisepticum*, can be isolated and propagated in embryonated chicken eggs and in a variety of specialized artificial media. Due to the activity of both the chicken and turkey industry in control and eradication procedures, most primary breeder flocks are free of the infection.

Clinical Findings: Spread both within and between pens is by aerosol transmission and may be rapid or slow depending on the virulence of the mycoplasma or other complicating respiratory infections or vaccinations. Most flocks are infected through egg transmission and such progeny commonly carry the infection in a latent form for weeks or months before clinical signs become evident. Clinical disease is often precipitated by stresses such as crowding, onset of egg production, live-virus vaccines, or field infection with a respiratory virus.

Affected chickens show varying degrees of respiratory distress; in uncomplicated cases there may be no obvious signs. Mortality is significant only if there are complicating infections. Feed conversion, rate of lay, hatchability, and chick and poult quality are adversely affected. Turkeys are likely to develop severe sinusitis.

Clinical recovery of the flock occurs after several weeks or months, but the infection remains and egg transmission can be expected to continue, though with decreasing frequency, for the remainder of life.

Lesions: Uncomplicated MG infections in chickens result in relatively mild sinusitis, tracheitis and airsacculitis. In broilers, in particular, *Escherichia coli* infections (q.v., p. 1058) are often concurrent and result in severe air-sac thickening and turbidity, with exudative accumulations together with fibrinopurulent pericarditis and perihepatitis. Localization in synovial tissues sometimes occurs. Turkeys develop severe mucopurulent sinusitis, and varying degrees of tracheitis and airsacculitis.

Diagnosis: Agglutination reactions with MG antigen are most commonly used for diagnosis. Occasional cross-agglutination from *M. synoviae* antibodies occurs. Isolation from affected tissues can be accomplished in MG-free embryos or chicks or in appropriate artificial media. Isolates must be identified as several different *Mycoplasma* spp. are found in birds. Intercurrent infections with Newcastle disease, infectious bronchitis, influenza, adenoviruses and other respiratory pathogens offer the major problems of differential diagnosis.

Treatment and Control: Since in the field many cases of MG infection are complicated with other pathogenic bacteria, the treatment to be effective must also attack the secondary invader. Most strains of MG are susceptible to a number of antibiotics such as chlortetracycline, erythromycin, magnamycin, oxytetracycline, spiramycin, streptomycin and tylosin.

The usual treatment in severe cases is an injectable antibiotic, followed by feed or water treatments for 5 to 7 days. In milder infections feed or water administration is usually sufficient.

Eradication of MG from both chicken and turkey breeding stock is well advanced in the U.S.A. and several other countries. Control has been based on identifying isolated groups of breeders that are uninfected as indicated by agglutination tests; also, by treating hatching eggs, usually with tylosin or by egg heating, to destroy the infecting organism. Progeny are hatched and maintained in isolation from infected stock and tested periodically.

MYCOPLASMA MELEAGRIDIS INFECTION (MM)

A widespread egg-transmitted infectious disease of turkeys in which the primary lesion in the progeny is airsacculitis. The organism commonly found in the respiratory and reproductive tracts is a specific pathogen for turkeys.

Etiology and Incidence: *Mycoplasma meleagridis* was recognized as a major pathogen of turkeys following the widespread elimination of *M. gallisepticum* from breeding stock. Infection is currently present in commercial flocks but some bloodlines have eradicated it.

Epidemiology: The primary source of infection is through egg transmission. However among adult turkeys transmission of *M. meleagridis* is unique, being related to genital contact. Early infections usually become quiescent by sexual maturity. The phallus and adjacent tissues of the tom retain infection and contaminate semen, which serves as a vehicle for infecting the vagina of the hen. Hens may retain infection in the bursa of Fabricius, which serves as a source of infection of the reproductive tract following rupture of the cloacal-vaginal occluding membrane at puberty. Such infections ascend the reproductive system and may reach the surface of the ovary. The high rate of egg transmission of *M. meleagridis* that results from infection of the reproductive tract of the hen is not true transovarian infection but rather infection incorporated during the formation of the egg following ovulation. Transmission also occurs between birds in young flocks with active infections of the respiratory tract. Hatchery transmission is also possible.

Clinical Findings: Egg infection appears to reduce hatchability, poult quality and growth rates. In stressful conditions poult mortality may be considerable during the first few weeks. It has been suggested that infections of the periarticular tissues of the hock joints and of the cervical vertebrae as well as adjacent bone during early rapid growth may produce major bone deformities resulting in crooked necks and hocks. Rales may develop in flocks at 3 to 8 weeks of age and persist for several weeks without significant mortality or serious interference with growth.

Lesions: Poults have airsacculitis with thickening, turbidity, and sometimes marked caseous exudative accumulations. Respiratory signs are seldom evident in the young bird. Tracheitis and airsacculitis may develop and produce clinical signs after a few weeks. Lesions often recede with advancing age but may be present at slaughter and cause considerable condemnation.

Treatment and Control: Dipping hatching eggs in, or injecting them with, tylosin is effective in reducing the incidence of egg transmission. Primary breeder flocks free of MM have recently been produced. Procedural precautions to minimize contamination during semen collection and artificial insemination help prevent infecting the female genital tract. Several serologic tests have been used experimentally to detect infection. Such tests are dependable during periods of active infection but often fail to show a reaction when the pathogen is quiescent.

INFECTIOUS SYNOVITIS
(Infectious arthritis)

An infectious disease of poultry, characterized by inflammation of the synovial membranes. It occurs most frequently in chickens 4 to 10 weeks of age, and has been found in turkeys. The condition has also been called enlarged hock condition. It has been reported from all of the important poultry-growing areas in the U.S.A., as well as from Canada and Great Britain.

Etiology: The causative agent, *Mycoplasma synoviae*, has fastidious growth requirements. The incubation period following artificial infection varies from 5 to 10 days; the disease usually is clearly evident in 7 days. Older birds are usually more resistant. Transmission occurs through the egg. The infection frequently remains latent until the start of egg production with the organism present in the respiratory tract and no clinical signs of infection.

Clinical Findings and Lesions: Although the disease has been reported in older birds, those between 4 to 8 weeks of age are more commonly affected. The first sign is lameness and swelling of the hock and other joints. Green droppings are also a frequent early feature. In field outbreaks, although mortality may be very low, the disease produces up to 30% of cull and crippled birds. Airsacculitis occurs when the organism is present with stress such as from Newcastle disease, infectious bronchitis or improper ventilation. The liver is enlarged and sometimes discolored green. The spleen is enlarged and the kidneys are enlarged and pale. These lesions are particularly characteristic early in the disease and are less apparent as the disease progresses. A yellow, viscid exudate is present in almost all synovial structures; it is most commonly observed in the keel, bursa, hock and wing joints. It is also seen in the mandibular, costal and digital articulations. In chronic cases, this exudate may become inspissated and orange in color.

Diagnosis: A presumptive diagnosis can be based on the lesions and clinical signs described above. The disease must be differentiated from viral arthritis and bacterial infections. There may be cross reactions in serum plate agglutination with *Mycoplasma gallisepticum* but the hemagglutination—inhibition test is specific.

Treatment and Control: Serologic testing and isolation similar to those of the *M. gallisepticum* program have resulted in eradication of the infection in most primary breeder flocks of chickens. Serologic testing in turkey flocks is not as effective. The administration of chlortetracycline or oxytetracycline in the feed at 0.022% is beneficial. The IM injection of 200 mg streptomycin per bird very early in the course of the disease is quite effective in operations where individual birds can be treated and withholding times can be met. The condition has been prevented experimentally by the administration of one of the tetracycline antibiotics at 0.011% in the feed and field use indicates similar results under natural conditions. Medication of breeder flocks is not effective in preventing egg transmission.

NECROTIC DERMATITIS

(Clostridial dermatomyositis, Gangrenous dermatitis, Gangrenous cellulitis)

An infectious disease of chickens characterized by sudden onset, a sharp increase in mortality and gangrenous necrosis of the skin over the thighs and breast. This disease occurs sporadically in growing chickens from 4 to 16 weeks of age and affects both broilers and layer replacement stock.

Etiology: *Clostridium septicum* is the most commonly isolated pathogen but other clostridia, notably *Cl. perfringens*, Type A, and *Cl. novyi* (*oedematiens*) have been reported. Other bacteria almost always accompany the clostridia in culture, particularly staphylococci and *Escherichia coli*. Recent research has established that immunosuppression induced by the virus of infectious bursal disease (IBD, q.v., p. 1102) in young chicks predisposes them to necrotic dermatitis. In addition, numerous environmental factors appear to be involved. These include: skin trauma from surgical procedures, mechanical devices or cannibalism, heavily contaminated, moist, built-up litter and devitalization of the skin as occurs in staphylococcal infections and in selenium deficiency. The disease has been produced by subcut. or IM inoculation of *Cl. septicum* in conjunction with a chemical irritant (calcium chloride). Inoculated chickens develop gangrenous necrosis of the skin and underlying musculature and death frequently occurs within 12 to 48 hours.

Clinical Findings: The first sign is usually a sudden drastic increase in mortality in the affected flock; overall mortality ranges from 10 to 60%. Affected chickens die within 8 to 24 hours after showing signs of extreme depression, lameness and prostration. Externally, there are patches of red-to-black gangrenous skin over the breast or thighs and frequently feather loss or sloughing of the epidermis is noted. Palpation of the affected areas often reveals crepitation owing to gas bubbles in the subcutis and musculature. At necropsy, there is accumulation of bubbly serosanguineous fluid in the subcutis and the underlying musculature has a cooked appearance. The liver and spleen are enlarged and may contain large areas of necrotic infarcts. The kidneys are usually swollen and the lungs congested and edematous. Atrophy of the bursa of Fabricius may be a frequent finding in chickens that were exposed to infectious bursal disease (IBD) virus in the first few weeks after hatching.

Diagnosis: Histopathologic demonstration of gas gangrene and numerous large filamentous bacilli in the skin, musculature and liver, and isolation of the causative clostridia, coupled with the history and clinical findings will differentiate this condition from exudative diathesis (selenium deficiency), staphylococcal infection and other diseases involving the skin.

Control: Usually this disease can be prevented by maintaining proper litter condition, minimizing mechanical injury and controlling cannibalism through effective debeaking or other procedures. The predisposing effects of early infection with IBD virus may be avoided by assuring a substantial maternal antibody level in day-old chicks. The causative organisms are sensitive to a wide variety of antibiotics *in vitro*. Administration of oxytetracycline or chlortetracycline at 0.02% in the feed has produced a rapid decline of mortality in field outbreaks.

NECROTIC ENTERITIS

An acute enterotoxemic disease of young chickens characterized by sudden onset, explosive mortality and confluent necrosis of the mucosa of the small intestine, and affecting primarily broiler chickens from 2 to 12 weeks old. The disease has been reported from the U.S.A., Canada and several other countries throughout the world.

Etiology: Recent evidence indicates that toxins elaborated by *Clostridium perfringens*, Types A and C, play an important role in inducing the lesions of necrotic enteritis. The marked intestinal clostridial proliferation and toxin production leading to enterotoxemia are likely to occur only when the lumenal environment is drastically altered. This may be brought about by variations in: 1) the intestinal substrate—rapid change in quality or quantity of ingesta may promote clostridial growth; 2) intestinal motility—depressed motility may enhance both clostridial multiplication and toxin absorption; and 3) viability of the intestinal mucosa—damage by more aggressive pathogens (e.g. *Salmonella* spp., coccidia) or toxins may promote clostridial colonization and invasiveness. Necrotic enteritis has been reproduced consistently only by infusing numerous clostridial cells and preformed toxin directly into the duodenum.

Clinical Findings and Lesions: Infected chickens are extremely depressed and may have diarrhea. The disease progresses rapidly, and death occurs within an hour or two. The disease persists in a flock for 5 to 10 days. Flock mortality varies from 2 to 50%. Necropsy reveals extreme dehydration and darkening of the breast muscle. The liver is usually swollen and congested, but necrosis is rare. The small intestine is ballooned and friable and contains foul-smelling brown fluid. The mucosa is covered with a brownish diphtheritic membrane.

Diagnosis: Lesions produced by *Eimeria brunetti* can be similar to those in necrotic enteritis, but uncomplicated coccidiosis is seldom as acute or severe clinically. Ulcerative enteritis can resemble necrotic enteritis clinically, but the intestinal lesions are usually focal and are located in the ileum, ceca and rectum. Large numbers of gram-positive bacilli observed in a stained smear of a mucosal scraping may assist in differentiation. The microscopic pathology consists of a coagulative necrosis of one-third to one-half the thickness of the mucosa, with accompanying masses of long filamentous bacteria in the fibronecrotic debris. *Cl. perfringens,* types A or C, can be isolated from liver and intestine by routine anaerobic culture.

Treatment and Control: Strict sanitation and efforts to prevent coccidiosis, salmonellosis and other intestinal infections minimize the risk of necrotic enteritis. Drastic changes in feed should be avoided, and feed and water should be monitored for contaminants that alter intestinal motility or devitalize intestinal mucosa.

Bacitracin is the drug of choice for preventing and treating necrotic enteritis. Preventive levels range from 0.05 to 0.1% in the feed, while 0.02 to 0.05% is therapeutic. Penicillin, erythromycin and the tetracyclines at 0.02% in the feed have also been effective.

OMPHALITIS

(Navel ill, "Mushy chick" disease)

A specific condition characterized by infected, unhealed navels in chicks, poults and other young fowl.

Etiology: This noncontagious disease is associated with excessive humidity and marked contamination of the incubator. The navels fail to close. Opportunist bacteria (coliforms, staphylococci, *Pseudomonas* and *Proteus*) are often recovered. Proteolytic anaerobes are prevalent in outbreaks. Losses may be increased by chilling or overheating during shipment.

Clinical Findings: The affected chicks or poults usually appear normal until a few hours before death. Depression, drooping of the head and huddling near the source of heat usually are the only signs. The navel is found inflamed and a scab may be present. The yolk sac is not absorbed and is often highly congested or broken, with extensive peritonitis. Edema of the sternal subcutis may occur. Mortality often begins with hatching and continues to the 10th to 14th day of age, with losses to 15% in chickens or 50% in turkeys. Persistent unabsorbed, infected yolks often produce stunted chicks or poults.

Prophylaxis: Careful control of temperature, humidity and sanitation in the incubator will prevent the disease. Only clean, uncracked eggs should be set. If eggs are washed, a sanitizing detergent must be used according to directions. Time, temperature and frequent changes of water are equally as critical as the concentration of sanitizer in both wash and rinse water. The rinse should be warmer than the wash water but not over 140°F (60°C).

The incubator should be thoroughly cleaned and fumigated between hatches and prior to the start of the hatching season. Fumigation must be carried out with closed vents at high temperature and humidity. Thirty ml of formalin (40% formaldehyde) and 15 gm of potassium permanganate should be used per 20 cu ft, or paraformaldehyde in a heating device should be used in strength recommended by the manufacturer. Contamination of the machines may readily occur following fumigation unless care is taken to clean and disinfect the exterior of the machines and the rooms in which they are located.

There is no specific treatment.

FOWL CHOLERA

A contagious, widely distributed disease that affects domesticated and wild birds. It usually occurs as a septicemia with sudden onset and high morbidity and mortality, but chronic and asymptomatic infections also occur.

Etiology: *Pasteurella multocida*, the causal agent, is a small, gram-negative, nonmotile rod which may exhibit pleomorphism after repeated subculture. In freshly isolated cultures or in tissues, organisms have a bipolar appearance when stained with Wright's stain. Although this organism may infect a wide variety of animals, strains isolated from nonavian hosts generally do not produce fowl cholera. Strains that cause fowl cholera represent a number of immunotypes that complicate prevention of the disease by the use of bacterins. The organism is susceptible to ordinary disinfectants, sunlight, drying and heat. Turkeys and waterfowl are more susceptible to the disease than chickens, and older chickens are more susceptible than young chickens.

Clinical Findings and Lesions: These vary greatly depending upon the course of the disease. In acute cases, dead birds may be the first indication of disease. Fever, depression, anorexia, mucus discharge from the mouth, ruffled feathers, diarrhea and increased respiratory rate are usually seen. Many of the lesions of acute cholera are related to vascular disturbances. Hyperemia is especially evident in the vessels of the abdominal viscera. Petechial and ecchymotic hemorrhages are common, particularly in subepicardial and subserosal locations. Increased amounts of peritoneal and pericardial fluids are frequently observed. Livers usually contain multiple small necrotic foci and may be swollen. Pneumonia is particularly common in turkeys.

The signs and lesions of chronic fowl cholera are generally related to localized infections. Sternal bursas, wattles, joints and footpads are often swollen because of accumulated fibrinosuppurative exudate. Exudative conjunctivitis and pharyngitis may occur. Torticollis may result from infections involving the meninges, middle ear or cranial bones.

Diagnosis: A presumptive diagnosis may be based on the observation of characteristic signs, gram-negative organisms in blood smears and lesions; a more conclusive diagnosis should include isolation and identification of *P. multocida.*

Prophylaxis: Good management practices are essential in preventing the disease. Polyvalent bacterins are widely used and are generally effective. A live vaccine which is administered in drinking water is available for use only in turkeys. It is generally effective and can produce immunity against different immunotypes of *P. multocida.*

Treatment: Drug therapy in the field is often handicapped by cold, damp weather, which favors the disease and reduces water consumption. Since the appetite is usually poor in sick birds, the drug intake may be below effective levels. Sulfaquinoxaline sodium (℞ 107) in feed or water usually controls mortality as do sulfamethazine (℞ 104) sulfadimethoxine (℞ 93) and sodium sulfamerazine (℞ 97). (Use sulfas with caution in breeders.) High levels of tetracycline antibiotics in the feed (0.04%) or parenterally may be useful. Penicillin administered IM is often effective in cases of sulfa-resistant infections.

Pasteurella anatipestifer INFECTION

(New duck disease, Infectious serositis)

A contagious disease caused by *Pasteurella anatipestifer*, which primarily affects young ducks, but may also affect other waterfowl, turkeys, chickens and pheasants. Usually it occurs in ducks 2 to 7 weeks of age.

Affected ducks often have ocular and nasal discharges, mild coughing and sneezing, tremor of the head and neck, and incoordination. Widely distributed fibrinous exudate is the most characteristic lesion. The exudate is most evident in the pericardial cavity and over the surface of the liver. Fibrinous airsacculitis is common and infection of the CNS can result in fibrinous meningitis. Spleens and livers may be swollen. Pneumonia may occur.

Diagnosis should be based on signs, lesions and isolation of the causative organism, since other diseases, particularly *Escherichia coli* infection (q.v., p. 1058), may produce similar lesions. Chocolate agar medium is recommended for isolation, with incubation at 37°C in a candle jar. Biochemical characteristics can be used to differentiate this organism from other bacteria which cause important diseases of ducks, particularly *E. coli* and *Pasteurella multocida* infections.

Careful management practices are important for prevention of infection. The use of bacterins combined with oral vaccine of low virulence gives better protection than bacterins alone. A combination of penicillin and streptomycin or sulfaquinoxaline (℞ 108) can be used for treatment.

AVIAN CHLAMYDIOSIS
(Psittacosis, Ornithosis)

An acute or chronic disease of wild and domestic birds, characterized by respiratory and systemic infection, transmissible to other animals and man. The disease is commonly called psittacosis in psittacine birds (parrots, budgerigars, etc.), ornithosis in other birds (turkeys, pigeons, etc.) and psittacosis or ornithosis in man depending upon the type of bird from which it is contracted.

Etiology and Occurrence: The cause is any avian strain of *Chlamydia psittaci*, an extremely fastidious organism that requires living cells in which to multiply. Other closely related mammalian strains produce an assortment of disorders in domestic animals including polyarthritis, reproduction problems, pneumonitis and enteritis. All chlamydial strains contain identical group-specific antigens but may differ in the antigenic specificity of their cell-wall antigens.

The disease occurs worldwide, being particularly important in colonially nesting species, in domestic poultry (turkeys, pigeons, ducks) and in caged birds passing through dealers' collecting houses.

Epidemiology: Aerosols and dusts from respiratory discharges or digestive dejecta are infective. Nestlings in colonies or breeding farms become infected and may become carriers if they survive. Such carriers, under environmental stress, may have a recurrence and transmit the infection. Chlamydial strains of unusually high virulence that cause high mortality have been found in gulls, egrets and turkeys. Strains of less virulence are usually found in psittacine birds, pigeons, ducks and chickens. All strains appear to be infectious to man.

Clinical Findings: Nasal discharge, diarrhea, dullness, weakness, inappetence and loss of weight are often seen.

Lesions: Air sacculitis, pericarditis, perihepatitis and peritonitis with serofibrinous exudate and hepatosplenomegaly are common findings in acutely affected birds. Chronic infections, seen frequently in psittacine and columbidan species, may be characterized only by an enlarged spleen or an enlarged, discolored liver or both.

Diagnosis: A tentative diagnosis may be made by detection of intracytoplasmic groups of chlamydiae in impression smears of diseased organs stained by the Gimenez, Giemsa or Machiavello method. Confirmation should be made by a laboratory competent to isolate and identify chlamydiae. Freshly collected liver, spleen, kidney and lungs should be shipped frozen. Attempts to isolate the chlamydiae from cloacal excretions may also be made if it is necessary to preserve the life of a valuable bird. Serologic tests, particularly complement fixation and agar gel precipitin, are of value.

Thyroid enlargement (from iodine deficiency), or *Sternostoma* mites are often causes of respiratory difficulty in pet birds. Swollen spleen and severe respiratory distress may result from hemosporidial infections (*Plasmodium, Leucytozoon, Haemoproteus*). Aspergillosis is common in birds. Influenza and mycoplasmosis produce respiratory signs and lesions. Chickens may have air-sac disease. Fowl cholera (q.v., p. 1069) may produce similar lesions in turkeys.

Prophylaxis and Treatment: Chlamydiosis is relatively rare in food birds. Why the outbreaks are sporadic is not clear. Preventive measures, such as screening houses against wild bird entry, are justified, but drug prophylaxis, in the absence of cases in the area, is unwarranted. Effective vaccines are not available.

Pet birds should come from breeding establishments free of the infection. If the infection status is not known, chlortetracycline (CTC) impregnated seed should be fed to the birds to reduce the possibility of infection during transport and during stays in pet stores. On tentative diagnosis, treatment with CTC should be initiated. Poultry flocks should be given 0.02% CTC in mash feed. In confirmed cases treatment should be continued for a minimum of 3 weeks. Such treatment will usually stop losses and allow the birds to be marketed without danger to processing plant workers or consumers. Birds should be marketed immediately after an appropriate drug withdrawal period and under no circumstances should they be retained for future production.

Smaller psittacines and other seed eaters can be effectively treated with hulled millet seeds impregnated with 0.05% CTC, whereas larger psittacines will require a 0.5%-level in pellets or mashes. Fruit and nectar eaters can be treated by adding oral CTC powder to nectar at a level of 0.05%. Birds with confirmed disease should be treated for 45 days.

Public Health Significance: The disease in man usually follows heavy exposure to infective aerosols or dusts. This most commonly occurs at dressing plants when large numbers of infected birds are processed, in breeding aviaries where large numbers of infected birds are held in close confinement and in pet-bird situations where continued close proximity to a single infected bird may effect transmission. Some individuals are more susceptible than others.

A simple preventive measure for the veterinarian examining dead birds is the use of a detergent disinfectant to wet the feathers. This also drowns lice and mites, helps prevent spread of other infective agents, and keeps feathers from floating in the air or sticking to the hands. Other protective measures to use while examining live birds include: dust masks, plastic face shields, fan-exhausted examining hoods or glove boxes.

Outbreaks should be reported to public health and regulatory officials.

THE SALMONELLOSES

Infections caused by *Salmonella* spp. may be divided into those caused by: (1) two species highly host-adapted to the chicken and turkey (*Salmonella pullorum* and *S. gallinarum*—now listed in Bergey's Manual as a single species), and (2) the remaining nonhost-adapted species comprising some 1,700 species. The latter group (paratyphoid) may infect and be transmitted among almost all animals. (*See also* SALMONELLOSIS, p. 299.) They have major public health significance because of possible infection of man from contamination of food.

A quite similar group of pathogens, important in turkeys, which are commonly called paracolons, and by many are regarded as salmonellae, are grouped as *Arizona hinshawii*.

PULLORUM DISEASE

Infections by *S. pullorum* usually cause high mortality in young chickens and turkeys and occasionally in adult chickens. The disease in other avian species usually occurs only if these are maintained in close contact with infected chickens or turkeys. Infections in mammals are rare. Once common, the disease now has been eradicated from most commercial stock.

Transmission is chiefly by direct egg transmission, but may also occur by direct or indirect contact. Egg- or hatchery-transmitted infection usually results in mortality during the first few days of life and continues to 2 to 3 weeks of age. Affected birds huddle near a source of heat, do not eat, appear sleepy and show whitish fecal pasting around the vent. Survivors frequently become asymptomatic carriers with localized infection of the ovary. Some of the eggs laid by such hens hatch and produce infected progeny.

Lesions: Lesions in young birds usually include unabsorbed yolk-sacs, focal necrosis of the liver and spleen, and grayish nodules in the lungs, heart and gizzard muscle. Firm cheesy material in the ceca and raised plaques in the mucosa of the lower intestine are sometimes seen. Occasionally synovitis is prominent. Adult carriers sometimes have no gross lesions but usually they have pericarditis, peritonitis or distorted ovarian follicles with coagulated contents. Acute infections in mature chickens produce lesions that are indistinguishable from those of fowl typhoid (q.v., below).

Diagnosis: Lesions may be highly suggestive, but diagnosis should be confirmed by isolation and identification of *S. pullorum*. It is readily isolated by direct plating on most nonselective solid aerobic media. Infections in mature birds can be identified by serologic tests followed by necropsy and culturing for confirmation.

Treatment and Control: Several sulfonamides, antibiotics and other antibacterials are effective in reducing mortality but none eliminate the infection from a flock. Furazolidone at a level of 0.022% in the feed is one of the most effective treatments. Control is based on a regular testing program of breeding stock to assure freedom from infection. Chickens are tested by a tube-agglutination or whole-blood method. The latter method is not dependable for testing turkeys, and either a tube-agglutination or serum-plate test is used. Variant or polyvalent antigens are sometimes necessary.

FOWL TYPHOID

The causal agent, *S. gallinarum*, is very similar to *S. pullorum*, and many workers consider them as one. Infection is now chiefly confined, in the U.S.A. and Canada, to a few areas. Although *S. gallinarum* is egg-transmitted and produces lesions in chicks and poults similar to those produced by *S. pullorum*, it has a much greater tendency to be spread among growing or mature flocks. Mortality at all ages is usually high.

Lesions in the older bird consist of dehydration, swollen, friable and often bile-stained liver with or without necrotic foci, enlarged spleen and kidneys, anemia and enteritis. Diagnosis is accomplished by isolation and identification of the causal agent by standard bacteriologic methods.

Treatment and control are the same as for pullorum disease (q.v., p. 1074) except that a rough strain of S. *gallinarum* (9R) is useful in controlling mortality. It is usually most effective if administered at 9 to 10 weeks of age before natural exposure occurs. The standard serologic tests for pullorum disease are equally effective in detecting fowl typhoid.

PARATYPHOID INFECTION

Paratyphoid infections may be caused by any one of the many nonhost-adapted salmonellae. Frequently several species infect a bird or flock concurrently. *S. typhimurium* is most common, but the prevalence of other species varies widely by geographic location and strain of bird. In the U.S.A., most infections are produced by 10 to 20 species. Probably all birds are susceptible, and infections are common in all species of domesticated birds. Usually the incidence in infected young flocks is high, but declines to a low percentage by maturity. Efforts to control paratyphoid infections in domestic poultry are chiefly stimulated by public health considerations.

Clinical Findings: Infections are often substantially subclinical. Mortality is chiefly confined to the first few weeks of age, and is higher in ducks and turkeys than in chickens. Some species or strains are more pathogenic than others. The stress of shipping, delayed feeding, chilling or overheating increases mortality. Clinical signs are not distinctive. Depression, poor growth, weakness, diarrhea and dehydration may occur. Lesions may include an enlarged liver with or without areas of focal necrosis, unabsorbed yolk sac with coagulation, and cecal cores. Occasionally infections localize in the eye or synovial tissues.

Diagnosis: Isolation and identification of the causal agent is essential. Direct culture from liver and yolk sac onto almost any standard type of aerobic media is adequate for isolation. Either a selenite or tetrathionate enrichment broth, transferred in 24 to 48 hours to brilliant green agar, may be used to isolate the organism from intestinal or environmental samples.

Treatment and Control: Several antibacterial agents are of value in preventing mortality; none is capable of eliminating flock infection. Furazolidone at 0.022% in the feed is commonly used. Turkeys, in particular, are commonly injected with one or more antibiotics after hatching.

Control methods have not been developed to the point of dependability. Strict sanitation in all hatching processes is helpful in preventing transmission between successive lots of birds in a house. Early fumigation of hatching eggs is recommended to prevent penetration by salmonellae on the shell surface. Washing should be done only if conditions are strictly controlled. No method has been devised to destroy the pathogens in the egg as a result of true egg transmission, although apparently such infection is relatively rare. The heat of pelleting is reasonably effective in destroying salmonellae in feed ingredients. Maintenance of poultry in confinement and exclusion of all pets, wild birds and rodents help prevent introduction of infection. The water source should be free of contamination. Early colonizing of the gut with selected normal microflora results in significant resistance to subsequent exposure.

Several methods of determining the salmonella status of breeding flocks have been devised. Periodic cultural examination of environmental samples from litter, dust and water, and culturing samples of hatchery debris and cull chicks can be reasonably accurate for detecting infection. Serologic tests are not highly dependable but have been of value in detecting *S. typhimurium* infection in turkey flocks.

ARIZONA INFECTION

(Paracolon infection)

An acute or chronic egg-transmitted infection, chiefly of turkeys, by any of the serotypes of *Arizona hinshawii* (*Paracolobactrum arizonae*). The classification of this organism has been a matter of discussion and by some it is considered to be a *Salmonella* sp.

Etiology and Incidence: More than 100 serotypes have been identified from a variety of birds, mammals and reptiles. Two serotypes, 7:1,7,8 and 7:1,2,6, account for most isolates from turkeys; foodborne infections of man occur occasionally, but usually are produced by other serotypes. One or more *Arizona* serotypes are present in a large percentage of turkey flocks. Reptiles captured in the vicinity of turkeys are frequently infected and are thought to act as a reservoir of infection. Clinical infections in other birds and mammals are relatively rare.

Clinical Findings: Neither signs nor lesions are distinctive. Mortality is usually confined to the first 3 to 4 weeks of age. Poults are unthrifty, and in some flocks a considerable percentage develop eye opacity and blindness.

Lesions: Yolk sacs are slowly absorbed and livers may be enlarged and mottled. Some flocks are extensively infected without developing appreciable mortality. Infection usually persists in a flock. Some birds develop peritonitis, salpingitis, or local ovarian infections, but infections of the intestinal tract are more common.

Diagnosis: A diagnosis must be based on isolation and identification of the organism. The same culture methods as those used for paratyphoids are satisfactory. Environmental samples may also be used for detecting infection. Egg transmission levels are often high so cultural examination of dead embryos, egg shells and cull poults may be used to identify infected breeding stock.

Treatment and Control: A variety of drugs are used to minimize mortality in poults. Streptomycin, spectinomycin or other antibiotics are commonly injected at the hatchery. Furazolidone at 0.011 to 0.022% in the feed is also often used during the first few weeks. Early fumigation of hatching eggs and rigorous hatchery sanitation are aids to reducing transmission.

SPIROCHETOSIS

An acute or chronic, febrile, bacterial disease of birds, characterized by listlessness and leg weakness. *Borrelia anserina*, the causal organism, is thin (0.4 μ), actively motile, and of variable length (6 to 30 μ). It may be culvitated in complex culture media containing serum, in chicken embryos, or in chicks. The disease occurs in many parts of the world, generally in tropical or temperate regions, being rarely found in the Southwestern U.S.A. It affects gallinaceous birds, waterfowl, and a wide variety of other birds. The disease is transmissible through droppings or other moist materials containing the organism, or indirectly through blood-sucking arthropods, notably *Argas persicus*.

Clinical Findings: Affected birds are droopy, weak in the legs, feverish, thirsty and have a yellow-green diarrhea with increased urates. Incoordination or complete paralysis may be seen. The most characteristic lesion is a swollen spleen with ecchymotic hemorrhages. The heart may be enlarged and pale, and the liver is usually enlarged and congested, with many small foci. There is catarrhal enteritis, with large amounts of yellow-green urates in the posterior gut.

Diagnosis: Darkfield microscopic examination of a thin wet smear of the blood reveals actively motile spirochetes, usually in great numbers. At crisis, late in the disease, agglutinins appear that clump the spirochetes in large round masses. Later still, they may be very scarce. Since it is possible to mistake filamentous protoplasmic extrusions from erythrocytes or motile haemosporidial microgametes for spirochetes, stained smears must be examined with care. Clumped organisms resemble smudged leukocytes, and it is easy to miss the occasional spirochete in late stages. Even at early stages, infection can be detected with the agar gel precipitin test employing infective blood and ox bile solubilized antigen.

Treatment and Control: Penicillin, streptomycin and tetracyclines have been effective. Bacterins are widely used but tend to be type specific and at times an autogenous bacterin may be required. Screening of houses and insecticide applications help reduce the level of exposure by vectors.

STAPHYLOCOCCOSIS

Staphylococcus aureus is a common skin inhabitant of all animals. In birds, infections of yolk sac, joints and wounds are common manifestations. Infection is uncommon except where predisposing factors are present such as: fecal contamination of eggs, injury to joints or contamination of wounds. Diagnosis is by microbiologic identification of the agent.

Large doses of novobiocin, penicillin, streptomycin or tetracyclines are sometimes effective as treatments.

STREPTOCOCCOSIS

Various *Streptococcus* spp. uncommonly affect many avian species. *Str. zooepidemicus*, which also affects domestic mammals, produces an acute septicemic infection, often with peritonitis, in mature chickens. *Str. faecalis* is part of the intestinal flora of all animals; in young birds it is a cause of egg-transmitted yolk-sac infection or of emaciation and can result in severe losses. In mature birds it is a cause of bacterial endocarditis. Diagnosis is by identification of the causative organism.

Erythromycin or tetracyclines or nitrofurazone in the feed (0.02%) may be of value against acute infections.

TUBERCULOSIS

A slow-spreading, usually chronic, granulomatous bacterial infection of birds, usually mature, characterized by gradual weight loss.

Etiology and Occurrence: *Mycobacterium avium* is the usual cause, although *M. tuberculosis* (*hominis*) or *M. bovis* may also infect birds, especially parrots. *M. avium* is very resistant, surviving in the soil for as long as 4 years, in 5% phenol up to 24 hours, in 3% hydrochloric acid for 2 hours or more, and in 4% sodium hydroxide for 30 min or more. The disease occurs worldwide, most commonly in small barnyard flocks with birds of several years running together, and in zoos; it is rarely found in large commercial flocks. Wild birds, such as starlings and raptors, have been found infected.

Infected birds excrete the organism in their feces. Cadavers and offal may infect predators and cannibalistic flockmates. Rabbits, swine and mink are readily infected. Cattle may be sensitized to tuberculin and johnin. Man is highly resistant but has been infected in a few instances.

Clinical Findings: Usually there are no signs until the disease has progressed to where the bird is thin and sluggish. Lameness may be observed. Granulomatous nodules of varying size are found in many parts of the body. In chickens, these are usually in the liver, spleen, bone marrow and intestine. Raptors usually have liver and spleen lesions, without intestinal involvement. Large pultaceous lesions may be found in body cavities. Bone marrow nodules and small mesenteric nodules may be found. Lesions are not calcified.

Diagnosis: The finding of acid-fast bacteria, usually present in large numbers, in impression smears from lesions permits a diagnosis. Live birds may be tested with avian and mammalian tuberculins, or serologically. False reactions due to exposure to other mycobacteria may occur.

Treatment and Control: Treatment is uneconomic in commercial poultry. It is probably inadvisable, and in some countries is illegal, even in valuable individuals, because of the possible danger to human health. In any case isoniazid is less effective against *M. avium*, and said to be toxic to birds. Streptomycin may also be toxic in the levels required to be effective.

In commercial poultry flocks, relatively rapid turnover of populations, together with improved general sanitation, has largely eliminated the once common infection. Infected poultry should be destroyed. If housed, the house should be thoroughly cleaned and disinfected. Dirt-floored houses should have several inches of the floor removed and replaced with dirt from a place where poultry have not ranged. All openings should be screened against wild birds. It is best not to reuse ranges where tuberculous poultry have been. The incidence of avian tuberculosis in zoos may be reduced by a regular program of tuberculin testing of new birds in quarantine and of all birds once a year.

ULCERATIVE ENTERITIS

(Quail disease)

An acute or chronic infection, primarily of the lower intestine, which is particularly severe in quail but also occurs in chickens, turkeys, pheasants, grouse, pigeons and probably other species.

Etiology: The etiologic agent, *Clostridium colinum*, is a gram-positive bacillus with subterminal spores. Bobwhite quail are highly susceptible whereas other species of birds are quite resistant; in chickens ulcerative enteritis often follows outbreaks of coccidiosis, infectious bursal disease and inclusion body hepatitis (q.v., pp. 1128, 1102 and 1104).

Clinical Findings: Susceptible quail may suffer an explosive disease with virtually 100% mortality in a few days. In other species, clinical signs are usually less dramatic; mortality is 10% or much lower during the clinical course of 2 to 3 weeks or more. Affected birds may die without obvious signs or weight loss. Infected quail discharge characteristic droppings streaked with urates and with a watery ring. Chronically affected birds are listless, anorectic and humped up, with the neck retracted and eyes partially closed. Recovered birds are resistant to reinfection but may act as carriers.

Lesions: The primary lesions are in the ceca and intestine. Acute lesions are punctate hemorrhages in the wall of the lower intestine accompanied by enteritis. Chronic lesions appear as necrotic ulcers in the mucosa surrounded by an inflammatory zone or as large ulcers with yellow diphtheritic membranes having depressed centers and raised edges. Perforating ulcers may result in local or diffuse peritonitis. Hepatic changes appear as yellow foci or irregularly shaped yellow areas in the parenchyma. The spleen may be enlarged and hemorrhagic.

Diagnosis: Although histomoniasis (q.v., p. 1134) and the hemorrhagic syndrome (q.v., p. 1104) may superficially resemble ulcerative enteritis, coccidiosis (q.v., p. 1128) causes the greatest problem of differential diagnosis. Often both infections occur simultaneously. The spore-forming rods can be demonstrated in Gram's stains of blood, liver and spleen from septicemic specimens. Histopathologic lesions of the affected intestine show severe tissue destruction and massive invasion by these bacteria. The organism can be isolated from infected livers and spleens by the inoculation of an enriched media such as blood-glucose-yeast agar and incubation under strict anaerobic conditions. Isolation can also be accomplished by injecting liver and spleen suspensions into the yolk-sac of 5-day-old chicken embryos. Heating the inoculum at 158°F (70°C) for 10 minutes prior to inoculation helps assure freedom from contaminating bacteria.

Prophylaxis and Treatment: *Cl. colinum* apparently is a frequent and highly resistant environmental contaminant. It is particularly useful to maintain quail on clean ground or on porches with wire or slat floors. Ground that has been contaminated with the organism should not be used for quail for at least 2 years. As recovered birds may act as carriers, they should be isolated from young stock.

The drugs of choice are bacitracin or streptomycin. Streptomycin is given (prophylactically or therapeutically) in the drinking water (℞ 74) or in the feed at 0.006%. Bacitracin is used in the feed at 0.005 to 0.01% or in the drinking water at the same rate as streptomycin. The tetracyclines (℞ 28, 60) and furazolidone at 0.02% in the feed are also effective.

Birds exposed to natural infection without treatment develop some immunity, but medicated flocks often have little resistance against reinfection. Therefore, contaminated litter should be removed and it may be necessary to continue or repeat treatment periodically.

AVIAN VIBRIONIC HEPATITIS

(Avian infectious hepatitis)

A contagious bacterial disease of chickens characterized by low mortality, high morbidity and a chronic course. It has been diagnosed in North and South America and in Europe. Turkey poults have been infected by IM inoculation.

Etiology: The cause is a gram-negative, motile, microaerophilic *Vibrio* sp., which appears as short comma forms, S-shaped forms and long spirals, and can be isolated from bile or liver on 10% blood agar under reduced oxygen tension. The inoculation of the yolk sac of 6-day-old chick embryos is excellent for isolating and propagating vibrio. Embryos die in 4 days and vibrios can be demonstrated in stained yolk smears or by culture of the yolk on blood agar. *Vibrio* isolates vary in their biochemical, serologic, and pathogenic properties.

Clinical Findings: Vibrionic hepatitis is insidious in onset. Usually only a few birds in a flock appear affected at any one time but occasionally the disease is acute, with sudden deaths. In subacutely affected pullet flocks, egg production lags, while in older flocks, egg production may decrease as much as 35% over extended periods. Severely affected birds lose weight, have shriveled, dry and scaly combs, are listless and roost or stand apart from the rest of the flock. Birds less severely affected may appear normal, but their egg-production pattern is intermittent.

Lesions: Older chickens exhibit variable hemorrhagic and necrotic changes in the liver. Some livers have many small hemorrhages, with occasional bubble-like hematocysts under the capsule. Severe hemorrhage sometimes ruptures the capsule, releasing blood into the body cavity. Other livers have a few pinhead-sized grayish-white necrotic foci, or are enlarged and mahogany-brown, or may be firm and friable with irregular asterisk- or cauliflower-shaped necrotic areas up to 1 cm in diameter. Other signs may include a bile-stained liver, ascites and hydropericardium, enlarged and pale kidneys, and catarrhal enteritis. In young chickens, the heart lesions are more severe and consistent than in mature birds.

The histologic changes in the liver range from early fatty metamorphosis and vascular changes to lymphocytic and heterophilic infiltration of the portal triad and focal necrosis of the parenchyma. Inflammatory cells may infiltrate the liver capsule and the kidneys may have focal accumulations of heterophils and lymphocytes. Blood examinations indicate an increase in the heterophil, thrombocyte and total leukocyte counts and a decrease in the hemoglobin content, packed cell volume, and erythrocyte and lymphocyte counts.

Diagnosis: A presumptive diagnosis of hepatitis can be made from a typical history of low egg production, an increased number of culls and characteristic lesions. A rapid technique for confirming diagnosis is the examination of bile with phase-contrast microscopy. *Vibrio* also can be isolated from the bile or liver using the technique described under etiology; typical vibrio forms appear in a stained smear or in a wet-mount with phase-contrast microscopy.

Other bacterial infections such as fowl cholera, pullorum and typhoid may produce liver lesions similar to vibrionic hepatitis.

Treatment: Dihydrostreptomycin sulfate (25 mg/lb [55 mg/kg] of body wt, one injection IM) or furazolidone (0.02% in mash on an all-mash diet for 14 days and 0.01% for a further 14 days) gives good control, if given early in an outbreak. Since exposure apparently leads to little immunity; reinfection sometimes occurs. As most strains of *Vibrio* have been found highly susceptible to erythromycin in sensitivity tests, this drug may be of value in treating infected flocks.

ACUTE RESPIRATORY DISEASE OF TURKEYS

(Turkey coryza)

An acute upper respiratory disease of turkey poults that occurs worldwide but sporadically.

Etiology: Although the cause is unknown, signs of the disease can be transmitted to susceptible poults by contact with sick ones suggesting involvement of an infectious agent. Nonspecific stresses on the recipient poults enhance transmission. The causal agent appears to be highly resistant to disinfection and remains on infected premises for long periods of time.

Clinical Findings and Lesions: In the absence of secondary microbiologic invaders, lesions of acute respiratory disease are limited to the upper respiratory tract. The most characteristic lesions are mucoid rhinotracheitis accompanied by structural collapse of the trachea. Rarely, fibronecrotic tracheitis occurs and a diphtheritic membrane forms. A mild splenomegaly is common. Secondary microorganisms can lead to severe airsacculitis and pericarditis in a few poults.

Signs occur in poults from 7 days to 20 weeks of age, the first sign being mild sneezing. Many poults lose their voices. There is a mucoid discharge from the eyes and the orbital opening becomes almond shaped. The signs progress into a severe rhinitis with sneezing, moist rales, depression and severe dyspnea. The peak death rate occurs from 7 to 14 days after the onset of signs and the mortality is markedly enhanced by secondary stresses, e.g. vaccination, dust or ammonia. Commonly, mortality is approximately 25%, but this may reach 70%. Signs are enhanced by weather extremes and may persist for 6 to 10 weeks.

Diagnosis: Diagnosis is based upon the clinical signs of the disease, the inability to isolate any etiologic agent and the histopathologic changes in the upper respiratory tract. Nasal turbinates and tracheas exhibit hypertrophy of mucous glands with excess mucus production. The tracheal mucosa is devoid of cilia and exhibits progressive squamous metaplasia.

Prevention and Treatment: No preventive measures or treatment are known; management practices to reduce stress are recommended.

AVIAN ENCEPHALOMYELITIS (AE)

(Epidemic tremor)

A viral disease marked by ataxia and tremor of head, neck and limbs, which occurs worldwide in chickens, pheasants, Japanese quail and turkeys. Ducklings, pigeons and guinea fowl are susceptible to artifical inoculation.

Etiology: The causative picornavirus can be grown in chicken embryos from nonimmune hens. It is transmitted through eggs laid by infected hens up to a month later.

Clinical Findings: Signs, sometimes present at hatching or delayed until several weeks of age, commonly appear at 7 to 10 days of age. The chief signs are unsteadiness, sitting on hocks, paresis and even complete inability to move. Muscular tremors are best seen after exercising the bird; holding the bird on its back in the cupped hand helps in detection. About 5% of the flock may be affected, although much higher morbidity and mortality may occur. The disease in adult birds is inapparent, except for a transient drop in egg production. The disease in turkeys is often milder than in chickens.

Lesions: No gross lesions of the nervous system are seen. Lymphocytic accumulations in the gizzard muscle may be visible as grayish areas. Lens opacities may occur weeks after infection. Infected embryos have poorly developed voluntary muscles. Microscopic lesions are lymphocytic foci in the pancreas, liver, gizzard, proventriculus, and CNS (perivascular cuffing), along with neuronal degeneration, endothelial hyperplasia and gliosis.

Diagnosis: AE must be differentiated from avian encephalomacia (vitamin E deficiency), rickets, vitamin B_1 or vitamin B_2 deficiency, Newcastle disease, equine encephalomyelitis, Marek's disease and encephalitis caused by bacteria, fungi (e.g. aspergillosis) or mycoplasma. Diagnosis is based on history, signs and histologic study of brain, spinal cord, proventriculus, gizzard and pancreas. Virus isolation in AE-antibody-free eggs is sometimes necessary to confirm the diagnosis. Serologic testing may be helpful. Microscopic lesions are sparse and difficult to find in infected adults.

Prophylaxis and Treatment: Immunization of breeder pullets between 10 and 15 weeks of age with a commercial vaccine is advised. Vaccination should be repeated at time of molt if flocks are to be held for a second laying year. Vaccination of table-egg flocks is sometimes advisable. Affected chicks and poults are ordinarily destroyed as few recover.

AVIAN INFLUENZA
(Including Fowl Plague)

A viral disease of domestic and wild birds characterized by the full range of responses from almost no signs of disease to very high mortality. The incubation period is also highly variable from a few hours to a few days.

Etiology, Epidemiology and Distribution: The causal orthomyxoviruses are type A influenza viruses. There are 9 known serologically distinct subtypes based on surface hemagglutinins, each with virulent and avirulent members. The viruses grow readily in embryonating chicken eggs and agglutinate erythrocytes. The specific inhibition of this hemagglutination is the basis for the important HI serologic test for influenza antibodies. The viruses have a worldwide distribution and are frequently recovered from clinically normal sea birds, migrating waterfowl and imported pet birds. While domestic turkeys are commonly infected in much of the U.S.A., chickens have rarely been involved.

Clinical Findings: Respiratory signs are commonest but disease signs range from only a slight decrease in egg production or fertility to a highly fatal fulminating infection. In severely affected hosts, cyanosis and edema of the head, comb and wattle with blood-stained oral and nasal discharges are common. Sinusitis is not uncommon in ducks, quail and turkeys.

Lesions: The location and severity of gross lesions are also highly variable and may consist of hemorrhages, transudation and necrosis in the respiratory, digestive and urogenital systems.

Diagnosis: Isolation of the virus in embryonating chicken eggs results in allantoic fluid that will agglutinate erythrocytes. The hemagglutination will not be inhibited by Newcastle disease antiserum. A crude antigen prepared by grinding the chorioallantoic membrane of infected embryos will give positive results with a gel-precipitation test using known positive influenza A antiserum. In its severe forms, the disease resembles acute fowl cholera and viscerotropic Newcastle disease. In milder forms, it may be confused with other respiratory diseases.

Prophylaxis and Treatment: The use of viable and nonviable vaccines is complicated by the 9 antigenically distinct hemagglutinin subtypes that may be responsible for the disease. The other major viral surface antigen, neuraminidase, is not as important in influenza immunity as the hemagglutinin (but is useful for identification). Treatment of affected flocks with broad-spectrum antibiotics to control secondary bacterial invaders, and increased house temperatures may help reduce mortality. Suspected outbreaks should be reported to regulatory authorities.

THE TRANSMISSIBLE AVIAN NEOPLASMS

(The Avian Leukosis Complex)

The complex consists of 3 groups of transmissible neoplastic diseases which may cause great losses among commercial poultry. The **leukosis-sarcoma group** mainly affects the hemopoietic system and is caused by C-type oncornaviruses, which contain ribonucleic acid (RNA). It includes lymphoid leukosis, erythroblastosis, myelocytomatosis and several other etiologically related conditions, including sarcoma, nephroblastoma, endothelioma and osteopetrosis. **Marek's disease**, like lymphoid leukosis, is a lymphoproliferative disease. In its "classical" manifestation it predominantly affects the nervous system. It is caused by a deoxyribonucleic acid (DNA) virus infection. In the acute form of Marek's disease, however, the viscera are more extensively involved. **Reticuloendotheliosis** primarily causes a tumorous enlargement of the liver and spleen with occasional necrobiotic foci. In the chronic forms there may be nerve enlargement and derangement of feather follicle function. It is caused by an oncornavirus immunologically and biologically distinct from those of the leukosis-sarcoma group.

The provisional classification of the avian leukosis complex is based on pathologic and etiologic differences among the disease groups. It differs from earlier classifications by dissociating the lymphoid lesions occurring in lymphoid leukosis from those occurring in Marek's disease. The term "visceral lymphomatosis" of previous classifications referred to the visceral lesions of both lymphoid leukosis and Marek's disease; to avoid confusion this term will not be used (except to note its use as a synonym for lymphoid leukosis, q.v., p. 1088).

The disease complex is a serious economic problem in domestic chickens, and sporadic occurrences have been recorded in other avian species. The economically important members of the complex are Marek's disease and lymphoid leukosis. The other forms usually occur sporadically, although rare flock outbreaks of myelocytomas, osteopetrosis, sarcomas, erythroleukosis and reticuloendotheliosis have been described.

Diagnosis: Differentiation of the entities in the leukosis-sarcoma classification of the avian leukosis complex can often be made by gross inspection of lesions. In uncertain cases, histologic sections of tissues, bone marrow and blood smears are needed for definitive diagnosis.

Differential diagnosis between lymphoid leukosis, Marek's disease and reticuloendotheliosis requires skill and experience because of their similar appearance and the lack of routine diagnostic tests.

Nonneoplastic disease characterized by the development of tumor-like inflammatory granulomas, such as tuberculosis and pullorum disease, must be differentiated from the neoplastic diseases in which discrete tumors develop. Inflammatory nodules can be differentiated from neoplasms by tissue distribution, color, consistency, texture and association with other inflammatory and degenerative lesions. In questionable cases, tissue smears or sections will reveal the presence of definitive microscopic characteristics such as bacteria, fungi and especially the cell type since secondary infection of a neoplasm may occur.

The neural involvement of Marek's disease must be differentiated from other diseases of the nervous system, such as Newcastle disease, encephalomyelitis, encephalomalacia and riboflavin deficiency.

Control: *See* p. 1093.

TABULAR COMPARISON OF LESIONS AND SIGNS

Feature	Lymphoid Leukosis	Marek's Disease
Age	Over 16 weeks	Any age after 3 weeks, most common from 12 to 24 weeks
Paralysis	Rare	Characteristic
Enlargement of peripheral or autonomic nerves and ganglia	Rare (if ever)	Common
Bursa of Fabricius	Nodular tumors are common	Atrophy or diffuse involvement
Neoplasia of ocular and feather follicular tissue	Rare	Common
Characteristic cells	Lymphoblastic tumors	Infiltrating pleomorphic lymphocytes

THE LEUKOSES

Etiology: Lymphoid, erythroid and myeloid leukosis, myelocytomatosis, the related soft-tissue neoplasms, and osteopetrosis are caused by closely related RNA-containing oncornaviruses most of which are able to produce more than one type of neoplasm. The viruses all have a common group-specific antigen, which can be demonstrated by the complement-fixation test for avian leukosis viruses (COFAL test). The group can be divided into at least 4 subgroups on the basis of host genotype range, interference and major antigenic properties. Virus neutralization is type-specific and if cross-reactions occur, they do so only between viruses of the same subgroup.

The leukosis viruses have the ability to act as "resistance-inducing factors" (RIF) that interfere with the neoplastic transformation of cell cultures of genetically susceptible chick-embryo fibroblasts by Rous sarcoma virus. This property is the basis of the RIF test for detecting leukosis viruses. A leukosis virus will only interfere with a sarcoma virus belonging to the same subgroup.

Certain sarcoma viruses are defective. Cells infected by them become morphologically transformed but do not produce infectious virus. When such nonproducer (NP) cells are super-infected with a leukosis virus the cellular genome is activated and infectious sarcoma virus is produced in addition to the helper leukosis virus. The phenomenon is the basis of the NP activation test.

Phenotypic mixing occurs readily among avian tumor viruses. There is an interaction between genetically different but related viruses infecting the same cell. This results in progeny virus with a protein coat of both parental types with a genome of only one parent and is the basis of the phenotypic mixing (PM) test for leukosis viruses. Leukosis-sarcoma virus may also phenotypically mix with reticuloendotheliosis virus and vesicular stomatitis virus.

The COFAL, PM and NP activation tests are group-specific, the RIF test is subgroup-specific and the neutralization test is type-specific. The tests are useful for detecting the presence of infection in a flock and for identifying viral types.

LYMPHOID LEUKOSIS

(Visceral lymphomatosis, Big-liver disease)

A contagious malignancy of lymphoid cells caused by an oncornavirus-induced neoplastic transformation of lymphocytes within the follicles of the bursa of Fabricius. Metastases of malignant lymphocytes subsequently occur to cause diffuse or focal involvement of the liver, spleen and other organs. The disease affects birds 4 months of age or older.

Transmission: The virus is widespread in poultry operations and is excreted in the feces and saliva of both diseased and carrier birds. Birds are most susceptible to contact infection during the hatching and brooding periods. Chicks from immune hens have maternal antibodies that provide a temporary passive immunity to contact infection during the first few weeks of life. In the absence of maternal antibodies, exposed birds develop specific antibodies that may or may not eliminate the virus. Some of the infected birds develop lesions of leukosis and others become asymptomatic carriers. Hens that continue to carry the virus pass the infection to some of their offspring through the egg. The infected embryos become immunologically tolerant to the virus, which results in a persistent viremia, a lack of antibody production and a lack of lesions after hatching, but they may develop lesions sometime after 3 months of age. Tolerant adult hens transmit the virus to all of their offspring in contrast to nonviremic carrier hens, which only transmit the virus intermittently. Infected birds of both sexes may transmit the infection horizontally by contact, but the male has no known role in vertical transmission to the embryo.

Clinical Findings: There are no characteristic signs; affected birds may be in good or poor condition, the comb is often pale and shrunken and an enlarged liver may be palpable.

Lesions: The initial lesions are focal tumors of the bursa of Fabricius, which may progress to cause massive enlargement of the whole organ. The neoplastic cells metastasize to other organs such as the spleen, kidneys, bone marrow, gonads and especially the liver. Gross lesions may vary from large single or sparsely scattered discrete gray-white nodular lymphomas to diffusely disseminated miliary foci of tumor cells. Often the lesion is manifested as a uniform enlargement and grayish discoloration of the affected organ. The initial metastatic lesion is comprised of a microscopic extravascular focus of homogeneous lymphoblasts. The microscopic foci subsequently enlarge and coalesce to form the grossly apparent lesions. Occasionally a concomitant leukemia develops.

Diagnosis: *See* p. 1086.

Control: *See* p. 1093.

ERYTHROID LEUKOSIS
(Erythroblastosis)

A blood dyscrasia characterized by neoplastic proliferation of immature erythroid cells. Intravascular accumulations of tumor cells cause enlargement of the liver and the spleen.

Erythroid leukosis occurs sporadically in the field, usually in birds 6 months of age or older. A specific viral etiology is supported by isolation of strains of virus from natural infections that are able to induce erythroid leukosis in young chicks within 2 weeks after exposure. Some strains of lymphoid leukosis virus also appear to be able to induce erythroid leukosis under appropriate conditions.

Clinical Findings: Birds become listless, cyanotic and die suddenly in the acute proliferative form of the disease. Chronically affected birds may survive several months during which signs of anemia (pallor or a yellowish discoloration of unfeathered parts), emaciation and diarrhea may develop.

Lesions: The characteristic gross lesions in fresh specimens are a diffuse bright cherry-red discoloration and enlargement of the liver, spleen and kidneys. The carcass is pale, and petechial hemorrhages may be apparent in various tissues. The marrow is hyperplastic and has a "currant-jelly" consistency. The dyscrasia is produced by the release of neoplastic basophilic erythroblasts from the bone marrow into the peripheral blood. The primitive cells accumulate in the sinusoids of the liver, spleen and other organs and they characteristically predominate in blood smears.

A chronic, anemic form of erythroid leukosis occurs in which excessive proliferation of erythroblasts and organ enlargement do not occur. In such cases the liver contains small groups of erythroblasts with foci of lymphoid and granulocytic reactive hyperplasia.

Diagnosis: Tissue sections, and blood and bone marrow smears contain characteristic neoplastic immature erythroid cells.

Control: *See* p. 1093.

Myeloid Leukosis
(Myeloblastosis, Granuloblastosis)

Essentially an extravascular growth of malignant granulocytes and a concomitant striking granulocytic leukemia. It usually occurs sporadically in mature birds. A specific viral etiology is supported by the existence of virus strains that predominantly produce myeloid leukosis, and the inability of lymphoid leukosis viruses to produce the disease.

Clinical Findings: These are similar to those associated with erythroid leukosis (*see* above).

Lesions: The liver, spleen and kidneys are diffusely enlarged. The liver may have a granular appearance and is discolored grayish yellow. The marrow is hyperplastic and pale. Leukemia results when neoplastic immature granulocytes pass from the bone marrow into the general circulation. These cells invade extravascular sites of the liver, spleen and other organs where they continue to proliferate.

Diagnosis: Tissue sections, and blood and bone marrow smears contain a predominance of neoplastic myeloblasts and myelocytes.

Control: *See* p. 1093.

Myelocytomatosis
(Knothead, Chloroma)

A viral disease characterized by myelocytic tumors of the skull, ribs and long bones. It occurs sporadically in immature birds.

Clinical Findings: Occasionally, birds have protuberances of the skull that may be hard, soft, or have a very thin layer of brittle bone overlaying the tumor.

Lesions: Soft, yellowish white tumors develop on the cranium, long bones and the pleural surface of the thoracic cage. Occasionally, muscular invasion, visceral metastasis, or a concomitant leukemia occurs. The tumors and leukemic cells are proliferating myelocytes with characteristic eosinophilic granules.

Diagnosis: The presence of neoplastic heterophils in smears or sections of tumors is diagnostic.

Control: *See* p. 1093.

Osteopetrosis
(Osteopetrotic lymphomatosis, Marble bone, Thick-leg disease)

Osteopetrosis is regarded as a dysplastic skeletal disease rather than a neoplastic disease. It is included in the avian leukosis complex because of its high frequency in transmission experiments with some strains of leukosis virus. It occurs sporadically in the field in birds of all ages, more often in males than in females. Virus strains have been isolated that usually produce the lesions of osteopetrosis alone, but it appears that the disease is also produced by some strains of lymphoid leukosis virus.

Clinical Findings: Most bones of the skeleton can be affected, but the most pronounced changes occur in the long bones. Enlargement of the metatarsus is obvious and thickening of other bones is evident on palpation. The affected bones are warm and skeletal involvement is usually bilateral.

Lesions: The dysplasia principally involves the diaphyses of the long bones. Abnormal bone is formed by hyperplastic activity of subperiosteal and endosteal osteoblasts that produces a thickened bony cortex and results in obliteration of the marrow cavity. Osteopetrosis may be accompanied by the lesions of lymphoid leukosis or may occur alone in which case splenic atrophy usually occurs.

Diagnosis: Bilateral skeletal dysplasia is characteristic of the disease.

Control: *See* p. 1093.

MAREK'S DISEASE

(Fowl paralysis, Neurolymphomatosis gallinarum, Acute leukosis)

A highly infectious disease of poultry, characterized by gross enlargements of the nerves and tumors of the visceral organs, skin and muscle produced by infiltration and proliferation of pleomorphic lymphoid cells. Atrophy of the follicles and interfollicular infiltration of the bursa of Fabricius may also occur.

Etiology and Epidemiology: Marek's disease is caused by a DNA virus belonging to the cell-associated or B-group of herpesviruses. The virus produces characteristic syncytial cytopathic effects in cell cultures of chicken kidney and duck embryo fibroblasts. Nuclei of such cultured cells, and the nuclei of cells of infected feather follicular epithelium, develop eosinophilic Cowdry Type A inclusion bodies which are outlined by a halo of marginated nuclear chromatin. Antigens are produced in the cell cultures and in the feather follicles, which will react with serum from infected birds in the agar gel precipitation and fluorescent antibody tests.

Transmission of the virus through the egg is not important. Infectious cell-free virus is not present in large quantities in the blood, visceral organs or tumors. The virus matures to its infectious form in the feather follicular epithelium and is disseminated in the dander from infected chickens. The virus spreads readily over long distances and infection of new hosts is thought to occur primarily by inhaled aerosols of infectious dander. Nearly all flocks of chickens are infected by the time they reach sexual maturity. Clinical disease, however, is an exceptional sequela to virus infection. Most birds develop antibodies that are passed to offspring as a form of temporary passive protection. The occurrence of disease depends on the genetic resistance of the chicken, the age at which the bird becomes infected, the dose of virus received and the pathogenicity of the virus strain.

Clinical Findings: Most commonly, the disease occurs in 12- to 24-week-old birds. Exceptional cases have occurred as early as 3 weeks and as late as 18 months of age. Birds classically develop lameness or paralysis of the legs, wings, neck, eyelids or other parts of the body. Occasionally, dyspnea, dilatation of the crop, diarrhea and emaciation occur. Young birds affected by the acute form may only show signs of anorexia and depression. Neoplastic lesions of the viscera, skin and muscle are the predominant lesions in such birds. When the eyes are involved, the iris is discolored gray and the pupillary margin becomes irregular. Light accommodation is eventually lost and blindness results.

Lesions: Birds commonly have enlargements of one or more of the peripheral or autonomic nerves. The brachial, sciatic, celiac and vagus nerves are most frequently involved. The thickened nerves lack striations and are grayish and edematous. Lymphomas are frequent in the ovary, but may also develop in the testis, liver, lung, skin, muscle, kidney, proventriculus and other organs. Lesions of the viscera (acute leukosis) are most common in young chickens. In sexually mature chickens, visceral lesions may appear very similar to those of lymphoid leukosis. The bursa of Fabricius usually undergoes atrophy in Marek's disease, but occasionally it is diffusely involved in the neoplastic process.

Microscopically, the nerve infiltrations and lymphomas are a mixture of large, medium and small lymphocytes. In some nerves the lesion appears as an edematous inflammation. The involved iris is infiltrated by the pleomorphic lymphocytes, which can also be found in some optic nerves and eye muscles.

Diagnosis: *See* p. 1086.

Control: *See* p. 1093.

RETICULOENDOTHELIOSIS

An infectious neoplasm of the lymphoreticular cells, affecting several avian species and resulting in enlargement of the liver, spleen and at times peripheral nerves.

Etiology and Epidemiology: Infection with the oncornavirus, type C, occurs sporadically in domestic chickens, ducks and geese and is more prevalent in turkeys and wild water fowl. The virus is transmitted horizontally and congenital transmission has been suggested. Pathogenicity varies widely with different isolated strains. Of some confusion as well as economic importance was a disease caused by Marek's disease vaccine contaminated with reticuloendotheliosis virus, as well as its natural presence in turkey blood used as a vaccine for Marek's disease. In some countries significant mortality among turkeys with tumorous enlargements has been attributed to reticuloendotheliosis virus.

Clinical Findings: The disease develops in 1 to 4 weeks after experimental infection and occurs naturally in chickens as early as 8 weeks and in turkeys up to 18 weeks of age. Signs include retarded growth, anemia, abnormal feathers, leg paralysis, emaciation and general weakness. Lesions are either proliferative or necrobiotic. Liver and spleen may be enlarged with pinpoint to large focal or even diffuse involvement. Other viscera may also be tumorous and one or more of the peripheral nerves may be enlarged. There may be atrophy of the thymus, bursa of Fabricius and less often the spleen.

Histologic changes are characterized by the infiltration and proliferation of large vesicular lymphoreticular cells in the various tissues. Some lesions have a moderate to heavy proportion of smaller lymphoid elements and nerve lesions contain mostly the latter elements and plasma cells.

Diagnosis: A tentative diagnosis may be based on typical gross and microscopic lesions but a definitive diagnosis requires the demonstration of the causative virus or its antibody. This virus, unlike those of lymphoid leukosis and Marek's disease, is not ubiquitous and its presence has considerable diagnostic value. Virus may be isolated in susceptible cell cultures and identified by specific antiserum using immunofluorescence or neutralization tests. Specific antibody in serum or egg yolk from exposed birds may be detected by the indirect immunofluorescence or virus neutralization tests.

CONTROL OF THE TRANSMISSIBLE AVIAN NEOPLASMS

There is no known treatment for any of these diseases. Currently, a vaccine is available to aid the control of Marek's disease only. Control of all members of the complex is based on hygienic rearing techniques and breeding for resistance.

Hygienic control is based on preventing the introduction of disease by careless caretakers, infected embryos or chicks, and prevention of contact infection between infected and uninfected stock.

The RNA viruses of the leukosis-sarcoma group of diseases are perpetuated by vertical transmission through the egg in contrast to the DNA virus of Marek's disease. Eggs or chicks from different strains or hatcheries, therefore, should not be hatched or brooded together because a congenitally infected chick can contaminate others with RNA viruses. Moreover, chicks in immunologic balance with other diseases endemic in their parent flock may not have resistance to the endemic diseases of another flock. Hens that are not shedding RNA leukosis viruses must be identified to obtain clean eggs. A minimum of 9 eggs comprising 3 pools, albumen samples, or vaginal-cloacal swabs must be tested from each hen by the COFAL, NP or PM tests before it can be regarded as a noncarrier. Chicks from such sources must then be raised in hygienic isolation to prevent exposure to oncogenic viruses as well as other pathogens.

Premises should be thoroughly cleaned and disinfected before the introduction of new stock. All-in, all-out brooding should be practiced for any one location. Effectiveness of disinfection depends on the thoroughness of technique. Insect control must be practiced to avoid mechanical carriers of virus. Birds should be maintained in isolation away from sources of Marek's disease, including aerosols of dust and dander, for the first 3 months of life. During this time they are extremely susceptible to the disease and a filtered, positive-pressure air supply within the house is necessary to insure the benefits of absolute isolation procedures.

Genetic composition influences the response of birds to the viruses that cause neoplasms. Available evidence indicates that selection for resistance to one group of diseases is unlikely to result in resistance to the others. At the cellular sites, genetic resistance appears to be specific for each subgroup of virus. In contrast, suppression of tumor growth implies a broader type of resistance. Response to virus exposure is used as the final criterion for selection regardless of the method used to identify genetic resistance including sib-, progeny- and line-testing, or longevity.

Live-virus vaccines have been developed to control Marek's disease. While the mechanism of protection is incompletely understood, it is evident that the development of lesions is prevented. Birds are vaccinated at one day of age because of the constant danger of exposure to ubiquitous virulent strains of virus if vaccination is delayed. Conscientious attention to manufacturer's recommendations for vaccine use is imperative for adequate protection. In the U.S.A., a cell-culture propagated turkey herpesvirus is used, usually given subcut. or IM at one day of age. Elsewhere a cell-culture propagated Marek's disease herpesvirus originating in chickens is utilized; this may be either a naturally occurring mild strain, or an attenuated virulent strain. Natural control of Marek's disease may occur in some field flocks when only wild strains of mild Marek's virus are present, or the mild virus infection occurs before the introduction of a virulent strain.

CORONAVIRAL ENTERITIS OF TURKEYS

(Bluecomb, Transmissible enteritis)

An acute, highly infectious disease of turkeys characterized by sudden onset, marked depression, anorexia, diarrhea and weight loss. Mortality may be high, particularly in young poults, but loss of condition in growing and adult birds may be more important economically.

Etiology and Epidemiology: The causative agent is a coronavirus, but the disease as seen in the field is complicated by secondary bacterial activity. Bluecomb spreads by direct or indirect contact with infected birds or premises. Droppings of infected birds are especially rich in virus, and recovered birds may continue to shed virus for months. Environmental factors do not appear to influence the occurrence; however, the stress of adverse environment may be a contributing factor to the severity of the disease.

Clinical Findings: A short incubation period, often 48 to 72 hours, is followed by general depression, anorexia and diarrhea in the flock. Young poults appear cold, chirp constantly and seek heat. Feed and water consumption drop markedly, and poults lose weight rapidly. Morbidity and mortality may approach 100% in uncontrolled outbreaks. Young birds have few lesions other than those associated with the intestinal tract. Intestines usually are distended and lack muscle tone. Contents are watery and gaseous (foamy).

Morbidity and mortality are variable in growing and adult turkeys. Profuse diarrhea, with droppings containing mucoid threads or casts, is common. Dehydration and weight loss are pronounced, and birds in recovery may require several weeks to regain lost weight. Cyanosis of the head is common. Birds in lay experience a severe drop in production.

Lesions in older birds are more extensive than in young poults. The body musculature is dehydrated. Petechial hemorrhages may be seen on the viscera. Kidneys commonly are swollen and contain an excess of urates. Severe catarrhal enteritis is usually seen, and mucoid casts may be present. The pancreas may present multiple chalky white areas. The crop may be distended and contain sour-smelling contents.

Diagnosis: Although clinical findings and lesions are highly suggestive, definitive diagnosis requires the use of laboratory techniques. Among these are: demonstration of coronaviral antigen in the intestines of affected birds by direct fluorescent-antibody techniques, reproduction of the disease in young poults with bacteria-free intestinal filtrates, and negative findings for common bacterial and protozoan infections. Disorders of young poults that may produce similar signs include hexamitiasis (q.v., p. 1133), salmonellosis (q.v., p. 1073), inanition and water deprivation. In older birds, septicemias such as fowl cholera (q.v., p. 1069) and erysipelas (q.v., p. 1058) may cause diagnostic confusion.

Prophylaxis and Treatment: Management and sanitation practices to minimize introduction of infection should be employed. Depopulation of problem premises followed by cleaning and disinfection of buildings and equipment is an effective method of breaking the cycle of infection. Such farms should be left vacant for at least 30 days before repopulation.

Commercial biologics are not available. "Controlled" exposure programs have been used with variable success on some problem farms, but such procedures are not recommended except in unusual circumstances.

The course of clinical outbreaks of disease may be altered by good nursing care and the judicious use of antibiotics and other drugs. Affected birds in the brooder house should be given supplemental heat and birds on range should be protected from adverse environmental conditions. Antibiotics and drugs are used to combat secondary bacterial infections and dehydration. The selection of an antibiotic is often empiric at best, but tetracyclines, neomycin, streptomycin, penicillin and bacitracin are among those that have been used with variable success. Antibiotics may be added to the drinking water in combination with calf milk-replacer and electrolyte, e.g. 25 lb (11.4 kg) calf milk-replacer, 450 gm of potassium chloride and 100 gm of antibiotic to 100 gal (380 L) of water. Birds should be medicated for a period of 7 to 10 days. During and after treatment birds should be observed closely for secondary intestinal mycosis, a common sequela of the use of antibiotic therapy.

EASTERN ENCEPHALITIS IN PHEASANTS

An acute viral disease of pheasants, characterized by neurologic signs, high morbidity and often high mortality. The disease is responsible for serious economic loss to producers unless adequate control measures are taken. The infective agent is the virus of the Eastern type of encephalitis (q.v., p. 288). Infection is normally transmitted by mosquitoes, but once established in a flock, transmission is facilitated by the birds pecking at one another. Serologic and other data clearly indicate that many other species of birds carry an inapparent infection. The virus has been isolated from mice, rats, foxes, dogs and other mammals.

Clinical Findings and Diagnosis: The lesions are typical of the viral encephalitides. Signs include inappetence, staggering and paralysis. Recovered birds may be blind, have unilateral or bilateral paralysis of various muscle groups and have difficulty in holding the head up. The morbidity may reach 90% and, in some outbreaks, the mortality in individual pens has been as high as 90%. While birds in some pens are affected, those in adjacent pens may show no signs. Diagnosis may be confirmed by inoculation of guinea pigs or mice, or by chick-embryo tissue culture methods. Prophylaxis may be accomplished in some instances by effective control of the mosquito population and by husbandry practices designed to reduce injuries from pecking, e.g. debeaking of the birds at regular intervals and the provision of adequate space for exercise. Preventive vaccination reduces mortality to less than 5%. It is recommended in endemic areas, particularly in flocks with a history of previous outbreaks. A dose is 1/10 the equine dose of either an Eastern or Bivalent Eastern and Western vaccine injected into the pectoral muscles, preferably at 5 to 6 weeks of age, or when the birds are released from brooder houses. Efforts should be made to have most birds vaccinated by the first week in July, since in Northeastern U.S.A. outbreaks usually commence some 2 weeks later.

FOWL POX

A relatively slow-spreading viral infection of chickens and turkeys characterized by the formation of nodules in the skin progressing to heavy scab formation, and of diphtheritic membranes in the upper digestive and respiratory tracts. The disease is worldwide.

Etiology and Epidemiology: Fowl pox virus, a large DNA virus, is highly resistant and may survive for years in dried scabs. Although in some characteristics the virus from turkeys differs from that of chickens, the differences are not significant and they may be considered together. The virus is present in large quantities in the lesions and is usually transmitted to pen mates through abrasions of the skin. A number of mosquitoes including *Aedes aegypti*, *A. vexans*, *Culex pipiens* and *Stegomyia faciata* may serve as vectors. Demonstrated capability of transmitting infection for at least 39 days suggests that mosquitoes serve as more than mechanical carriers. Transmission within flocks is rapid when mosquitoes are plentiful. Apparently some carriers remain following clinical recovery and reactivation may be caused by stress, such as moulting.

Clinical Findings: Lesions are prominent in some birds causing a significant decrease in flock performance. Cutaneous lesions usually occur only on the unfeathered parts of the head of the chicken and head and upper neck of the turkey; generalized skin infection occurs in some flocks. Lesions in chicks are usually limited to feet and legs. The lesion is initially a raised, blanched, nodular area that enlarges, becomes yellowish, and progresses to a heavy, dark scab. Multiple lesions usually develop which often coalesce. Lesions in various stages of development can often be found on the same bird. Localization around the nostrils may cause nasal discharge. Lesions on the eyelids may result in lacrimation, closing of the lids, large caseous exudative accumulations in the conjunctival sac and sometimes eventual loss of the eye if secondary infections occur.

Lesions may also occur in the buccal mucosa or in the esophagus, larynx and trachea (wet pox or fowl diphtheria). Occasionally lesions occur almost exclusively in one or more of these sites. Caseous patches firmly adherent to the mucosa of the larynx and mouth develop. Tracheal lesions, which may be diffuse and progress to a heavy, brown pseudomembrane, may cause death by suffocation.

Often the course of the disease in a flock is protracted due to slow spread of the lesions. Extensive infection in a flock results in a slowly developing decline in egg production with some loss of fertility. Cutaneous infections alone ordinarily cause little mortality and these flocks generally return to normal production upon recovery.

Diagnosis: Cutaneous infections usually produce characteristic lesions. When only small lesions are present, it is often difficult to distinguish the disease from the abrasions caused by fighting. A few isolates have been found that produce few or no inclusion bodies but appropriately stained sections or scrapings of affected areas usually reveal characteristic intracytoplasmic inclusion bodies which are diagnostic. Isolation may be accomplished by inoculation of the chorioallantoic membrane of embryonating eggs. The disease is readily reproduced by applying suspensions of lesions to scarified skin or denuded feather follicles laryngeal and tracheal lesions from infectious laryngotracheitis (q.v., p. 1103).

Prophylaxis and Treatment: In areas where pox is prevalent, vaccination of chickens and turkeys with live-embryo-propagated virus is practiced. The most widely used vaccines are attenuated fowlpox virus and pigeon pox virus isolates with high immunizing ability and low pathogenicity. In high-risk areas, vaccination should be done in the first few weeks of life; revaccination at 12 to 20 weeks is often sufficient. Because the infection spreads slowly, vaccination is often useful in limiting spread in affected pens if administered when less than 20% of the birds have lesions.

Vaccinated birds should be examined one week later for swelling and scab formation at the vaccination point. Lack of such a reaction indicates impotent vaccine, previously existing immunity, or improper vaccination. Revaccination is indicated, possibly with another serial lot of vaccine.

Birds in which caseous deposits interfere with breathing may be helped by removal of the material and swabbing the site with tincture of iodine.

Pox in Other Avian Species

Infections with pox virus have been recorded from a large variety of avian species. Some isolates are primarily infectious for only the homologous host species, whereas others are infectious for one or more additional species. Immunity is also unpredictable with other avian pox infections. Classification is usually based on host pathogenicity studies. Canary pox is usually severe with mortality sometimes approaching 100%. Cutaneous lesions may develop as well as systemic infection with cytoplasmic inclusion bodies in the salivary glands, liver, pancreas and other organs of epithelial origin. No effective vaccine is available in the U.S.A. for canaries.

HEMORRHAGIC ENTERITIS OF TURKEYS

An acute, infectious disease usually occurring in turkeys over 4 weeks of age and characterized by sudden death with the voiding of blood from the vent. It is important in many areas where intensified turkey growing is practiced.

Etiology and Transmission: Hemorrhagic enteritis (HE) is thought to be caused by an adenovirus but attempts at isolating, propagating and purifying the causal agent have, to date, met with limited success. The agent is highly transmissible via the intestinal contents, or feces, and is quite resistant to the influence of certain environmental conditions; hence it may persist for extended periods of time on contaminated farms and transmission from flock to flock occurs easily.

Clinical Findings: In affected poults, signs of the disease develop rapidly. Some appear depressed and recover quickly while others die suddenly from frank intestinal hemorrhage. These birds are usually anemic, have feed in the crop and have not lost weight. The infection spreads rapidly through the flock and losses vary from none, in a clinically inapparent infection, to as high as 60% in field outbreaks.

Lesions: The intestines are dark, distended and usually filled with blood and sloughed epithelial tissues. Spleens are enlarged and mottled. Occasionally the livers will possess hemorrhages and areas of necrosis. The lungs are usually congested.

Diagnosis: Often the diagnosis of HE can be made from the history, signs and lesions. Recovered birds will have neutralizing and precipitating antibodies. Additional confirmation of the presence of HE can be made by experimental inoculation of susceptible poults with intestinal contents from clinically affected birds.

Prevention and Control: Experimental avirulent HE vaccines have been prepared from infective spleen tissue, on farms and in areas where HE is endemic. They have been effective when administered in the drinking water. Convalescent antiserum obtained from healthy flocks may be injected at the first signs of HE and will assist in reducing losses in field outbreaks.

INFECTIOUS BRONCHITIS

An acute, rapidly spreading, viral respiratory infection of chickens, characterized by rales, coughing and sneezing, without the accompaniment or subsequent development of nervous signs.

Etiology and Incidence: Infectious bronchitis is caused by a virus that, so far as is known, infects only chickens. It is widespread in the U.S.A. and Canada and has been reported from other parts of the world. The virus is resistant to the action of antibiotics and can be cultivated readily in 9- to 11-day-old chick embryos. Embryonic mortality is variable. Six days after injection into the allantoic sac, living embryos should be examined for stunting or tight curling of the embryo or urate deposits in the mesonephros. Similar embryonic changes have been observed with the B_1 strain of Newcastle disease virus.

Epidemiology: Recovered birds are immune and do not remain carriers. The virus can be spread by droplet infection through the air or by contamination of feed sacks, equipment, clothing and shoes of caretakers. In the Northeastern U.S.A., the virus does not persist on premises more than 4 weeks after signs have ceased. Although bronchitis virus has been isolated from eggs laid by fowls in the acute stages of the disease, chicks that hatch from such eggs are not infected. Parentally conferred immunity protects the chick for a short period.

Clinical Findings: Coughing and rattling are manifest from 18 to 48 hours after exposure. Slight nasal discharge is seen occasionally in young chicks only. There is occasional facial swelling. Wet eyes are commonly seen. Spread to other birds in the same pen takes place in

24 to 48 hours and usually all susceptible birds on a farm become infected within a short time. The morbidity is practically 100%, although the severity of the signs may vary considerably. Respiratory signs cease in 2 or 3 weeks.

Mortality is highest in very young chicks and may reach 60%, but is negligible in birds older than 5 or 6 weeks. Feed consumption and egg production in laying fowls drop sharply. A decrease of 20 to 50% in egg production, with many misshapen, thin- or soft-shelled eggs of poor internal quality is not uncommon. Frequently, egg quality is impaired permanently.

Mortality may be reduced in young chicks by providing good environmental conditions. In older growing chickens, the prognosis is excellent and recovery is uneventful. However, laying birds may never reach their former egg-production level even months after recovery from the respiratory infection. Such flocks should be marketed.

Diagnosis: The isolation of the virus in chick embryos, with the production of embryonic lesions, is the most certain procedure. A history of an acute, rapidly spreading, respiratory disease, which is not Newcastle disease (negative to the hemagglutination-inhibition test) with typical changes in the eggs of producing birds, is good presumptive evidence. Serum neutralization tests (3 weeks after onset or later) will yield significant antibody titers. After recovery, birds are refractory to challenge with virulent bronchitis virus.

Postmortem examination reveals a catarrhal tracheitis, bronchitis and, occasionally, slight thickening and clouding of the air-sac membranes. In fatal cases, caseous plugs may be found in primary and secondary bronchi. Ova in producing birds are flaccid. Yolks and eggs with shells are often found in the abdominal cavity.

Control: No medication is available that will alter or shorten the course of the disease. Increasing the temperature in the room and under the hover by 5 to 10°F (3 to 4°C) may lower mortality. Food consumption should be stimulated by all possible means.

Immunization may be carried out by the use of live-virus vaccines, which produce relatively mild respiratory signs. These vaccines are usually given in the drinking water, or as a dust or spray. Such products should be used according to the manufacturer's specific recommendations.

Infectious bronchitis variant strains: At least 10 serologic variant strains are recognized. Although they share antigenic components with the previously recognized standard strain (Massachusetts) they pose problems in immunization and diagnosis. Standard vaccines may not afford complete protection against some of these variants, which has led to the use of a variant-strain vaccine in certain localized areas where infectious bronchitis outbreaks in broilers has become a significant problem. Outbreaks of infectious bronchitis with mortality due to nephritis have been associated with several of these variant strains in Australia and the U.S.A.

INFECTIOUS BURSAL DISEASE (IBD)

(Gumboro disease; Infectious avian nephrosis)

An acute, highly contagious viral disease of young chickens occurring worldwide and characterized by edema and swelling of the cloacal bursa, necrosis of lymphoid elements, vent picking, prostration and mortality. IBD has been confused with a nephritis or nephrosis syndrome caused by aberrant or variant strains of infectious bronchitis virus.

Etiology and Transmission: The causal virus (IBDV) has been isolated from the cloacal bursa, kidneys, spleen, thymus, liver, intestinal tract, lungs and blood. Organ suspensions, infective feces and embryo-propagated virus have reproduced the disease. Probably transferred by fomites, IBDV is difficult to eradicate from premises.

IBDV may be isolated in 8- to 11-day-old "clean" chicken embryos with inocula from birds in the early stages of disease. The chorioallantoic membrane is more sensitive to inoculation than is the allantoic sac. Embryo deaths generally occur within 3 to 7 days with virus titers of 10^2 to 10^6. In early transfers of IBDV, embryo tissue suspension should be employed; for subsequent adaptation to embryos, allantoic fluids can be used. IBDV is neutralized only by specific IBD antiserum. IBDV strains adapted to avian cell-culture systems produce a cytopathic effect; these cell cultures may be used in serologic tests. All isolates appear to be antigenically similar with no relationship to infectious bronchitis strains, including those that are nephropathic.

Clinical Findings: After an incubation period of 3 or 4 days, onset is sudden in birds 3- to 6-weeks old, causing severe prostration, dehydration, incoordination, diarrhea and straining, soiled vent feathers, vent picking and inflammation. The disease has been diagnosed in younger and older birds. Light breeds appear to be affected more severely than are meat-type chickens. Losses range to more than 20%. The recovery period often is less than a week, delaying broiler weight gains 3 to 5 days. Maternally conferred antibodies may persist as long as 5 to 6 weeks, altering the clinical pattern. Recovered birds have high resistance.

Serologic surveys reveal significant flock exposure to IBDV without clinical signs; clinical IBD thus may be exceptional.

In the early stages the bursa is swollen, appears gelatinous and occasionally is hemorrhagic. The kidneys may be swollen and show degenerative changes. Muscle congestion occurs often, IM hemorrhages occasionally.

Immunosuppression: Early IBDV infection can suppress the bird's immune system. Effects on the cloacal bursa, spleen and thymus may reduce the immune response to vaccination against Newcastle disease, infectious bronchitis, Marek's disease and, perhaps, other diseases. Intercurrent infections from other viruses (e.g. adenoviruses) and bacteria may precipitate necrotic dermatitis, inclusion body hepatitis or other syndromes. IBDV increases susceptibility to coccidiosis.

Control: There is no treatment. Depopulation and rigorous disinfection of contaminated farms have achieved limited success for IBDV is persistent and resists hostile environment. Unknown reservoirs of infection may exist. IBD vaccines, of chick-embryo or cell-culture origin, can be administered by eye drop, drinking water or subcut. routes at 1 to 7 days of age. The immune response at an early age can be altered materially by maternally derived antibodies; thus the active immunity stimulated may vary.

Chicks in broiler flocks (and in some commercial layer operations) should carry high levels of parental immunity to provide protection during early brooding, minimizing bursal damage from IBDV infection with supervening immunosuppression or subsequent infection or both. Breeder flocks can be vaccinated during the growing period and revaccinated, if necessary, during the laying year by drinking water or, preferably, the subcut. route. Immune status can be determined by virus-serum neutralization, embryo challenge or the agar gel-precipitin test.

INFECTIOUS LARYNGOTRACHEITIS

An acute, highly contagious respiratory disease of chickens and pheasants characterized by severe dyspnea, coughing and rales; or subacute disease with lacrimation, tracheitis, conjunctivitis and mild rales.

Etiology: The disease is caused by a virus and has been reported from most of the intensive poultry-rearing sections of the U.S.A. and many other countries.

Clinical Findings: In the acute form, gasping, coughing, rattling and extension of the neck during inspiration are seen from 6 to 12 days after natural exposure. Reduced productivity is a varying factor in laying flocks. Affected birds lose their appetite and become inactive. The mouth and beak may be bloodstained from the tracheal exudate. Mortality varies but may reach 50% in adults. Signs usually subside after about 2 weeks, although some birds may cough for a month.

The subacute form has a low mortality, a more protracted course, and is characterized by milder respiratory signs, lacrimation and conjunctival edema.

A small percentage of recovered birds remain carriers and may serve as sources of infection. Infection also may be spread by mechanical transfer.

Diagnosis: The presence of the clinical signs indicated above, and finding blood, mucus and yellow caseous exudate in the trachea or a hollow caseous cast in the trachea or, in the subacute form, punctiform hemorrhagic areas in trachea and larynx, and conjunctivitis with lacrimation permit a presumptive diagnosis. In uncomplicated cases, the air sacs are not involved. A conclusive diagnosis may be made by (1) demonstrating intranuclear inclusion bodies in the tracheal epithelium early in the course of the disease; (2) isolation and identification of the specific virus in chick embryos, tissue culture, or chickens; (3) intraorbital sinus or vent inoculation of known immune and susceptible birds. Neutralization of virus is less dependable but has been used. Microscopically, a desquamative necrotizing tracheitis is characteristic.

Prophylaxis and Treatment: Some relief from the effects of the disease is obtained by keeping the birds quiet, lowering the dust level and using mild expectorants, being careful that the latter do not contaminate feed or water. Vaccination should be practiced in endemic areas or farms where a specific diagnosis is made. Immediate vaccination of adults in the face of an outbreak will shorten the course of the disease. Vaccination is currently being done with modified strains of lower virulence applied by drop to the eye (conjunctiva). The use of so-called virulent strains applied by brush or drop method to the vent mucosa is now limited to California. Broiler flocks in some areas must be vaccinated when young, but protection is not likely to be solid when done under 4 weeks of age. Some vaccine producers recommend revaccination when birds are to be held to maturity.

HEMORRHAGIC ANEMIA SYNDROME

(Inclusion body hepatitis)

A disease of young chickens characterized by jaundice, anemia and depression. It has been known for many years but it is only recently that different aspects of the syndrome have been described and the conclusion reached that the disease is infectious.

Etiology: Several strains and serotypes of avian adenoviruses are the causative agents. Frequently, the disease is accentuated if immunosuppression has resulted from prior infection with infectious bursal disease (IBD, q.v., p. 1102). Concurrent administration of sulfonamides, particularly sulfaquinoxaline, appears to enhance the severity of the disease.

Clinical Findings: Generally affected flocks consist of young birds, broilers or pullets, reared on the floor. The disease has been diagnosed infrequently in mature birds. Individual chickens will show various degrees of depression, jaundice and pale comb and wattles. Hemorrhage in various tissues is an inconstant finding but may be seen in the subcut. tissue and muscle when it does occur. Hemorrhage into the anterior chamber of the eye is seen infrequently. Losses are variable; none may occur in clinically inapparent infections but they can be as high as 25% over a 2-week period. Secondary bacterial infections may alter the course of the disease and result in complications, e.g. necrotic dermatitis (q.v., p. 1066).

Lesions: The pathologic findings are variable depending on whether immunosuppression has taken place from IBD allowing a more complete expression of the adenovirus infection. The carcass may be icteric. Characteristically, petechial and ecchymotic hemorrhages in the various organs and tissues accompany an aplasia of the bone marrow. Livers are swollen and mottled with stellate subcapsular hemorrhages and necrotic foci in some birds. The presence of Cowdry Type A intranuclear inclusion bodies in the hepatic cells is pathognomonic. Hemoglobin values are low in severely affected birds. A regressed cloacal bursa is often present and probably is the result of IBD.

Diagnosis: The typical signs and lesions will usually suffice; however, in the early stages of the disease, the virus can be isolated in the yolk sac of specific pathogen free embryos or, alternatively, in an avian kidney cell-culture system.

Treatment and Prevention: Treatment is of little or no value and the disease will be self-limiting. Secondary bacterial infections may be treated with antibiotics but sulfonamides should be avoided. Contaminated poultry houses and equipment must be cleaned thoroughly and disinfected. Iodine-containing and sodium hypochlorite disinfectants are indicated sanitizers.

Chicks should originate from parent flocks that are immune to IBD to reduce the chances of immunosuppression from that disease. Such progeny are much more resistant to the clinical effects from both IBD virus and challenge from a potentially pathogenic strain of adenovirus. If the chicks are also carrying maternally derived adenovirus antibodies to the offending serotype on the farm, the effects of the disease may be minimized. Avian adenovirus vaccines are not available commercially.

It is often difficult to prevent the syndrome from occurring in spite of implementing the foregoing measures. The disease is diagnosed infrequently in chickens raised on wire floors compared with those maintained on litter particularly litter re-used from brood to brood. Good cleaning and disinfection practices are helpful in prevention especially when coupled with isolation procedures.

MARBLE SPLEEN DISEASE OF PHEASANTS

This disease is caused by a virus that apparently is antigenically similar to the virus that causes hemorrhagic enteritis of turkeys (q.v., p. 1099). It is thought to be an adenovirus but characterization is incomplete. Marble spleen disease (MSD) of pheasants is sometimes called **lung edema**, but the primary lesions are seen in the spleen. MSD is found in all ages of pheasants. Depression is noted and the death loss is variable. In some cases, however, sudden death occurs with no premonitory signs.

An enlarged, mottled spleen is generally present giving a marbling effect. Histologically, necrosis of the splenic lymphoid cells and hyperplasia of the white pulp is common. Basophilic intranuclear inclusion bodies are often present in the reticuloendothelial cells. Infective spleen tissue may be used as an antigen in the agar gel-precipitin test with specific antiserum to confirm a diagnosis of MSD. However, typical gross splenic lesions are generally diagnostic in the absence of known bacterial pathogens. How to control and prevent MSD is unclear at this time, although methods similar to those used in hemorrhagic enteritis in turkeys may be efficacious.

NEWCASTLE DISEASE

(Avian pneumoencephalitis)

An acute, rapidly spreading viral disease of domestic poultry and other birds in which the respiratory signs (coughing, sneezing, rales) are often accompanied or followed by nervous manifestations and, with infections with some strains, by diarrhea and swelling of the head.

Etiology and Occurrence: The causal agent is a hemagglutinative paramyxovirus, with strains whose pathogenicity for chickens vary from very low to very high. The respiratory-nervous isolates common in the U.S.A., even those that are highly pathogenic, produce no distinctive gross lesion while the viscerotropic isolates of the old world often do. Virus isolates kill 9-day-old chicken embryos in 2 to 6 days. The disease occurs worldwide in a variety of domestic and wild birds, and sometimes as an induced conjunctivitis in man.

Epidemiology: Virus is shed during the incubative stages throughout the clinical stage and for a varying but limited period during convalescence. Virus is present in exhaled air, in respiratory discharges, in feces, in eggs layed during clinical disease and in all parts of the carcass during acute infection and at death. Chickens are readily infected by aerosols and by ingesting water or food contaminated with the virus. While the primary source of virus is the chicken, other domestic birds and certain wild birds are susceptible and may spread the virus. Parrots, mynahs and such caged birds as pittas that moved in commercial channels were the principal source of infection during the 1970-72 pandemic (U.S.A.) of the virulent viscerotropic form of Newcastle disease.

Clinical Findings: Signs are respiratory or nervous or both in the most widespread forms of the disease. In the peracute disease of the old world, viscerotropic signs predominate. Disease appears almost simultaneously throughout the flock 2 to 15 days after exposure, the average being about 5 days. Respiratory signs are gasping and coughing. Nervous signs, which may accompany, but usually follow the respiratory signs, are: drooping wings, dragging legs, twisting of head and neck, circling, walking backward (particularly after drinking water), and complete paralysis. Clonic spasms are seen in moribund birds. Depression and inappetence are seen.

Viscerotropic signs include watery and greenish diarrhea and swelling of the tissues around the eyes and in the neck. Laying flocks may have partial or complete cessation of production and fail to recover. Eggs abnormal in color, shape, or surface, and with watery albumen are produced. Mortality depends on the virulence of the virus strain, the environmental conditions, and the condition of the flock. In general, mortality is higher in very young flocks (but 100% mortality may occur in adult flocks).

Lesions: Lesions are highly variable, reflecting the variation in tropism and pathogenicity of the virus. Petechiae of the serous membranes may be seen, and (with old-world strains) hemorrhages of the proventricular mucosa and hemorrhages of the intestinal serosa with accompanying branny, necrotic areas on the mucosal surface. Congestion and mucoid exudates may be seen in the respiratory tract, with opacity and thickening of the air sacs.

Diagnosis: Tentative diagnosis of a rapidly spreading, respiratory-nervous disease may be confirmed by isolation of the hemagglutinating virus, identified by inhibition with known Newcastle disease antiserum. Paired serum samples showing a rise in HI antibodies also serve to identify the disease.

Prophylaxis and Treatment: Live virus vaccines are widely used to prevent disease losses. Lentogenic strains, chiefly B1 and LaSota in the western world, are administered in drinking water or in spray or dust. Sometimes administration is by nose or eye drops. Healthy chicks are vaccinated as early as the fourth or even the first day of life. However, delay until the second or third week avoids partial blockage of the active immune response by maternal antibody. Mycoplasma and some other bacteria, if present, may be potentiated by mass vaccination methods. Failure to follow instructions (e.g. use of sprays in windy houses or use of chemically treated water to dilute the virus) may result in incomplete or no protection.

When other infections are present in the flock and where required by law, killed vaccines should be used. Vaccines with oil adjuvants give the longest protection. Whether killed vaccines, lentogenic mass vaccines, or wing-web or IM-injected mesogenic strains are used, some scheme of repeated vaccination is required to protect chickens throughout life. The frequency of revaccination is largely dependent upon the risk of exposure and the virulence of the field virus.

Disease control officials in the U.S.A. and some other countries use importation restrictions and eradication methods to prevent the establishment of the highly virulent, viscerotropic form of the disease. Other countries depend upon vaccination. Proper administration of a high-titered vaccine is essential for induction of a good immune response.

QUAIL BRONCHITIS

An infectious, contagious disease of bobwhite quail observed in the wild and captivity. It is a serious respiratory disease on certain farms where the birds are pen-reared and particularly when birds of different ages are maintained on the same premises. It apparently occurs worldwide.

Etiology: Quail bronchitis (QB) is caused by an adenovirus, generally regarded as avian serotype 1. The virus can be isolated readily in embryonated chicken eggs and avian cell cultures from the respiratory tissues of affected birds. It is highly transmissible and may persist on contaminated, densely populated farms. However, the disease is often self limiting.

Clinical Findings: The disease is characterized in quail chicks by a sudden onset of sneezing, coughing and rales, which spread rapidly through the flock. Lacrimation and conjunctivitis are seen frequently. The death loss ranges from 10 to 100% in birds under 8 weeks of age but with a progressive increase in age, it is generally lower.

Lesions: Mild tracheitis with excess mucus, mild airsacculitis, conjunctivitis, and inflammation of the nasal turbinates and infraorbital sinuses may be found.

Treatment and Control: Treatment is ineffective. Isolation of affected groups of the birds and attempts to prevent transmission to other groups is recommended since the virus can be transported with ease by physical or mechanical means. Effective cleaning and disinfection are especially helpful if the farm is depopulated prior to introducing newly hatched chicks. Young chicks should always be kept well-isolated from older birds since the latter may be carriers of QB virus. Survivors develop a significant antibody level for several months.

VIRAL ARTHRITIS

(Infectious tenosynovitis)

A sporadic disease, primarily of broiler chickens, affecting the tendons of the legs, generally seen as a bilateral swelling in the metatarsal area and the tendon bundle above the hock. Rupture of the gastrocnemius tendon is common.

Etiology and Incidence: Viral arthritis is caused by otherwise unidentified reoviruses. The viruses are ubiquitous in poultry and are found primarily in the digestive and respiratory tracts. Some serotypes become viremic and multiply in the tendon sheaths and tendons. Although the disease is seen primarily in the meat-type bird, it is occasionally seen in egg-type birds, but not in turkeys. The incidence is related to the weight of the bird and is more prevalent in males than in females. The disease is found wherever commercial broilers are raised.

Epidemiology: The disease is egg transmitted and is of short duration except where lateral transmission in a flock is prolonged. The respiratory and digestive infections in adult birds are also of short duration; however, the virus survives in the tendon sheaths and tendons for extended periods. Spread takes place through aerosols, fomites, contaminated equipment and by mechanical means. The virus is resistant to heat and acids.

Clinical Findings: An acute fulminating infection is occasionally seen in young chicks and embryos with cardio-, hepato- and splenomegaly with necrotic foci. The disease usually occurs in 4- to 8-week-old broilers as bilateral swelling of the shank and tendon bundle above the hock. The birds walk with a stilted gait, which is worsened when unilateral or bilateral rupture of the gastrocnemius tendon occurs.

In severely affected flocks many cull birds are seen around the feeders and waterers. Mortality ranges from 2 to 10% and morbidity from 5 to 50%. Severely affected birds rarely recover but less severely affected birds recover in 4 to 6 weeks. The infection is inapparent in many birds.

Diagnosis: A presumptive diagnosis can be made on the basis of bilateral swelling of the shank and tendon bundle above the hock. Virus isolation is made by cultivation in primary kidney, liver or lung cells or in the yolk sac of 5- to 7-day-old embryonating chicken eggs. The agar gel-precipitin (AGP) test is usually positive and a high percentage of birds are positive early in the infection. Virus neutralization tests are used to detect the specific virus serotype.

Prophylaxis: A commercial vaccine is available. Vaccination of dams passes parental antibody to the chick to prevent early infection and should reduce or prevent egg transmission. Since egg transmission is the principal means of spread, it is desirable to have breeder flocks immune to the infection. Such a program should be concerned with the serotypes present in the flock. Adult birds are resistant to the clinical disease if exposed by a natural route. There is no effective treatment.

DUCK PLAGUE

(Duck viral enteritis)

An acute, highly contagious herpesvirus infection of ducks, geese and swans of all ages, characterized by sudden death, high mortality and hemorrhages and necrosis in internal organs. It has been reported in domestic and wild waterfowl of Europe, Asia and North America, resulting in serious economic losses in the duck industries and a massive die off of wild waterfowl in the Mississippi flyway.

Etiology: The causal herpesvirus is nonhemagglutinating and nonhemadsorbing and produces intranuclear inclusion bodies in infected tissues and tissue cultures. All strains are antigenically similar but some vary in virulence. Field experience indicates the absence of egg transmission. Infection can be transmitted by parenteral or oral administration of infected tissues. Recovered birds may remain carriers.

Clinical Findings: The incubation period is 3 to 7 days. Sudden high and persistent mortality is often the first sign of the disease; mature ducks die in good flesh. Dead males may evidence prolapse of the penis. In laying flocks, a sharp drop in egg production may occur. Photophobia, inappetence, extreme thirst, droopiness, ataxia, nasal discharges, soiled vents and a watery or bloody diarrhea may be seen. Ducklings evidence dehydration, loss of weight, blue beaks and a blood-stained vent.

Lesions: These are tissue hemorrhage, free blood in the body cavities, destruction of lymphoid tissues and degenerative changes in the parenchymatous organs. Petechial and ecchymotic hemorrhages are found on the heart, liver, pancreas, mesentery and other organs. In the digestive tract, specific enanthematous lesions can be observed. These are macular mucosal hemorrhages that progress to yellowish-white encrusted plaques that can be found on the longitudinal mucosal folds of the esophagus, at the esophageal-proventricular junction, the surface of the intestinal annular lymphoid bands and in the cloaca. In young ducks, hemorrhages, and degenerative changes may be found in the thymus and bursa. Ruptured yolk and free blood may be found in the abdominal cavity of laying ducks.

Diagnosis: A presumptive diagnosis may be based upon the history and pathognomonic lesions. Isolation of the virus on the chorioallantoic membrane of susceptible embryonating duck eggs or in duck embryo fibroblastic tissue culture and the neutralization of the virus with specific antiserum confirms the diagnosis. The disease must be reported to the appropriate regulatory agency.

Prophylaxis and Treatment: Strict isolation of susceptible ducks is required. Contact with wild, free-flying waterfowl, or the introduction of infected waterfowl, must be avoided. Once the disease is introduced, control and eradication can be effected by depopulation, sanitation and disinfection of infected premises. A chick-embryo-adapted, modified live virus vaccine is effective in preventing losses and has been approved for use in domestic flocks.

DUCK VIRAL HEPATITIS (DVH)

An acute, highly contagious, viral disease of young waterfowl, particularly domestic ducklings, characterized by a short incubation period, sudden onset, high mortality and the development of rather characteristic liver lesions. It is of economic importance in all duck-raising areas of the world. Limited outbreaks occur in mallard ducklings and goslings.

Etiology: The causal picornavirus, readily propagated in chick and duck embryos, does not produce hemagglutination. Field experience indicates that egg transmission does not occur. Experimentally, infection can be transmitted by parenteral or oral administration of infected tissues. Variant viruses exist that are more difficult to isolate and replicate.

Clinical Findings: The incubation period is from 18 to 48 hours. Affected ducklings become lethargic, paddle spasmodically with their feet and die within a few minutes with typical opisthotonos. Although adult ducks may become infected, clinical evidence of the disease has not been seen in ducks over 7 weeks of age. Mortality may be as high as 95%. Practically all deaths occur within a week after the onset of the disease.

Lesions: The liver is pale red, slightly enlarged and covered with hemorrhagic foci up to 1 cm in diameter. The spleen is slightly enlarged and darker than normal. Kidneys may be swollen and renal blood vessels injected.

Diagnosis: A presumptive diagnosis may be based on the history and pathognomonic lesions. Virus isolation or serum neutralization tests may be used for positive identification. Variant virus forms will not be neutralized by DVH antisera.

Prophylaxis and Treatment: Prophylaxis can be achieved by strict isolation, particularly during the first 5 weeks of age. Immunization of breeder ducks with modified live virus vaccine using both type 1 and type 2 virus provides parental immunity that effectively prevents the high losses in ducklings. Antibody therapy (antiserum or yolk given IM) at the time of initial loss is the only effective flock treatment.

VIRAL HEPATITIS OF GEESE (GVH)

An acute disease of goslings and Muscovy ducklings (*Cairina moschata*). Peking ducklings are refractory. Both wild and domesticated geese are susceptible. Experimentally the incubation period is from 4 to 7 days; in natural infections most deaths occur between the 9th and 14th day of life. The disease is widespread throughout the world but has not been reported from Canada and the U.S.A.

Etiology: GVH is caused by a parvovirus (goose parvovirus type 1). It contains DNA, is 25 to 27 nm in diameter and highly resistant. The virus propagates in goose and Muscovy duck embryos and tissue cultures of these embryos. Egg transmission occurs. Most infections occur in the hatcher and in infected pens.

Clinical Findings: In young goslings, depending on their maternal antibody level, mortality varies from 7 to 100% in a flock. The birds lose their appetites, huddle together, and have polydipsia. Some have conjunctivitis, nasal discharge and fibrinous pseudomembranes on the tongue. Later they refuse food and water and die within a few days. Some birds have a more chronic disease; these lose their feathers, exhibit reddened skin and remain stunted after recovery. There is a strong age resistance and the disease has not been seen in geese over 4 weeks of age.

Lesions: At necropsy the most characteristic changes are seen in the swollen and occasionally firm liver, which sometimes has small pinpoint hemorrhages. Generally there is hydropericardium and ascites. The thyroid is enlarged. No lesions are seen in the lungs, kidneys and gut, which is important for differential diagnosis.

Diagnosis: The diagnosis may be based on the pathognomonic lesions of hepatomegaly, ascites and loss of feathers. Virus isolation on tissue cultures or goose embryos is confirmatory. The immunofluorescence test is practicable, using impression smears from the adrenal gland and the thyroid where virus concentrations are high.

Similar losses in geese are seen in **hemorrhagic nephritis and enteritis** of geese. This viral disease is peracute, there is no age resistance and no loss of feathers.

Prophylaxis: Convalescent serum or hyperimmune goose serum inoculated subcut. (1 ml/bird) shortly after hatching is an effective method of control. Immunizing breeder geese to increase their humoral antibody level is also useful. The virus is rapidly attenuated by passing in goose fibroblast cultures. A 40th passage can serve as a vaccine. A double vaccination with 3- to 6-week intervals should be terminated 3 weeks before the laying season starts. The virus has low immunogenic capacity and should be injected with adjuvant. The vaccination procedure must be repeated twice yearly to protect the goslings during the entire season.

VIRAL HEPATITIS OF TURKEYS

An acute, highly contagious, frequently subclinical infection of turkeys which produces hepatic and pancreatic lesions.

Etiology and Incidence: The causal adenovirus is isolated without difficulty from the liver or other tissues of poults, but is isolated less consistently from older birds. It grows readily in the yolk sac of 5- to 7-day-old chick or turkey embryos and in chick kidney cell cultures. It is thermostable, ether-, phenol- and creolin-resistant, and is susceptible to a high, but not low pH. The infection is widespread and common in some areas. Mortality has been reported only in poults.

Clinical Findings: Usually the disease is subclinical and becomes apparent only when the birds are stressed. Morbidity and mortality vary according to the severity of stress. In poults under 6 weeks morbidity may reach 100% and mortality 10 to 15%. Breeder flocks may suffer from decreased production, fertility and hatchability.

Lesions: In the liver, foci of necrosis range from 1 to 3 mm in diameter and may be confluent, as may hemorrhage or congestion that may nearly obscure the degenerative changes. Occasionally, the liver is bile-stained. The liver lesions resemble those of blackhead, but the absence of cecal lesions in hepatitis helps to differentiate the 2 diseases. Basophilic intranuclear inclusion bodies are seen rarely in the hepatocytes. The pancreas frequently exhibits relatively large, circular gray areas of degeneration.

In the subclinical form, the lesions are less extensive and hepatic hemorrhage or congestion is seldom prominent. Affected tissues return to normal in 3 to 4 weeks.

Paratyphoid and paracolon infections produce necrotic areas in the liver that may be confused with those of viral hepatitis. These and other bacterial and mycotic infections must be differentiated by appropriate culturing techniques. Granulomas may be identified grossly or histologically. Blackhead usually produces concurrent cecal lesions unless modified by medication. In the latter case, histopathologic examination or demonstration of the respective etiologic agents is necessary.

Prophylaxis and Therapy: There is no known treatment. Secondary bacterial invasion does not appear to be important, but if it does occur it should be treated on the basis of specific etiology. Although recovered birds possess demonstrable resistance to reinfection, no circulating antibodies have been found. Sanitation may be of value in preventing dissemination of the agent.

MYCOTIC DISEASES

ASPERGILLOSIS

(Brooder pneumonia, Mycotic pneumonia, Pneumomycosis)

A disease, usually of the respiratory system, of chickens and turkeys and less frequently of ducklings, pigeons, canaries, geese and many other wild birds. In chickens and turkeys, the disease may be endemic on some farms, whereas, in wild birds, it appears to be sporadic, frequently affecting only an individual bird.

Etiology: *Aspergillus fumigatus* is a cause of the disease. However, several other species of *Aspergillus*, as well as other genera, e.g. *Penicillium*, may be incriminated.

Clinical Findings: Dyspnea, hyperpnea, somnolence and other signs of nervous system involvement, inappetence, emaciation and increased thirst may be observed. The encephalitic form appears most commonly in turkeys.

Lesions: In young chicks or poults up to 6 weeks of age, the lungs are most frequently involved. Pulmonary lesions are characterized by cream-colored plaques from a few millimeters up to several centimeters in diameter. Such lesions may also be found in the syrinx, air sacs, and systemically, in the liver, intestines and occasionally the brain. An ocular form of the disease has been observed in chickens and turkeys in which large plaques may be expressed from the medial canthus.

Diagnosis: The fungus can be demonstrated by cultural methods or by microscopic examination of fresh preparations. One of the plaques teased apart and placed on a Petri dish of suitable fungus media usually results in a pure culture of the organism. Histopathologic examination using a special fungus stain, reveals granulomas containing mycelia. Confirmation of pathogenicity of the isolate is accomplished by injecting it into the air sacs of susceptible 3-week-old chicks.

Differential diagnosis from infectious bronchitis, Newcastle disease and laryngotracheitis is important. Aspergillosis is usually seen in birds 7 to 40 days old.

Prophylaxis and Treatment: The avoidance of moldy litter or feed serves to prevent outbreaks. Treatment of affected individuals is considered useless. The organism is frequently found in wet hay or sawdust litter. Often infection will clear up in young birds if the flock is culled, the house thoroughly cleaned and fresh litter from a different source used. All moldy litter should be removed and burned. The pen should be sprayed with 1% copper sulfate and all equipment cleaned and disinfected. Hamycin (20 mg/ml in drinking water), nystatin, amphotericin B, crystal violet and brilliant green, all have shown some fungistatic activity against *Aspergillus* sp.

MYCOTOXICOSIS

(Turkey X disease, Aflatoxicosis)

Disease caused by ingestion of alfatoxin, which is produced by *Aspergillus flavus* or *A. parasitcus* growing on the feed—groundnut (peanut) meal, cereals, etc. *See also* pp. 1038 *et seq.*

Clinical Findings: Depression, inappetence and reduced growth rate, together with loss of condition and mortality, are common. Turkey poults and ducklings are particularly susceptible and pheasant chicks are to a lesser degree. Ataxia, convulsions and opisthotonos are common signs.

Lesions: There may be a membranous glomerulonephritis and hyaline droplet nephrosis, and some degree of ascites and visceral edema may be apparent. The liver is pale and mottled with widespread necrosis. Excessive bile production is common. A marked catarrhal enteritis, especially in the duodenum, is characteristic. Diagnosis can be confirmed by histopathologic examination of the bile duct in which hyperplasia is common. The hepatic cells are enlarged with some necrotic foci.

Control: No specific treatment is known. The ingredients of the diet should be examined for the presence of peanut meal. *A. flavus* may be isolated but without further tests it is not confirmatory of the disease. Biologic assays for the toxin are available in which ducklings or poults are used. Chemical methods, using fluorescent techniques and chromatographic tests, are available. 8-Hydroxyquinoline, at 500 ppm in the mash, has been suggested as an antimycotic to prevent the growth of *A. flavus* in the feed. The successful use of thiabendazole (45 mg/lb [100 mg/kg] of grain) for this purpose has also been reported.

THRUSH
(Candidiasis, Moniliasis, Sour crop)

A mycotic disease of the digestive tract of chickens and turkeys caused by *Candida* (*Monilia, Oidium*) *albicans*. Lesions are most frequently found in the crop and consist of a thickened mucosa and whitish, raised, circular ulcer formations. The mouth and esophagus may show these same lesions. Hemorrhagic spots, necrotic debris and pseudomembranes are not uncommon. Depression and emaciation may be the only clinical signs. An accurate diagnosis may be established by demonstrating tissue invasion histologically and by culture of the offending organism. Young chicks and poults are most susceptible to infection.

No satisfactory treatment is known. All sick birds should be removed from the flock and a program of disinfection carried out. Copper sulfate at a dilution of 1:2,000 in the drinking water has been recommended. Nystatin at the level of 50 mg/lb (110 mg/kg) fed in the diet has shown significant protection against moniliasis.

ECTOPARASITISM

LICE

Biology: Chickens are infested with at least 7 species of biting lice but no sucking lice. They live on bits of skin, feathers, etc., but consume blood if it is available. The entire life cycle is usually completed on the body of the original host. Man can harbor chicken lice but only as a temporary carrier.

The common lice of chickens are the chicken body louse *Menacanthus stramineus* (on the skin), the shaft louse *Menopon gallinae* (on feather shafts), the chicken head louse *Cuclotogaster hetero-*

graphus (mainly on the head and neck) and the wing louse *Lipeurus caponis* (mainly on the wing feathers, rather inactive). Less commonly found on chickens are the fluff louse *Goniocotes gallinae* (very small, in the fluff), the brown chicken louse *Goniodes dissimilis* (brownish, on feathers, southern in distribution) and the large chicken louse *Goniodes gigas* (bluish gray, very large and strongly marked).

Turkeys, geese and ducks sometimes harbor chicken lice when raised with chickens, but, more commonly, turkeys are infested with the large turkey louse *Chelopistes meleagridis* and the slender turkey louse *Oxylipeurus polytrapezius*. Geese and ducks are infested with *Anatoecus dentatus*, whereas only ducks are infested with *Anaticola crassicornis* and *Trinoton querquedulae* (*luridum*). *Anaticola anseris*, which also occurs in ducks, and *Trinoton anserinum* are encountered on geese and swans. Ducks and geese seldom are heavily infested with lice.

Other domesticated and cage birds are infested with species of Mallophaga, which are usually specific for each host.

Clinical Findings: The irritation by the lice causes reduced egg production and rate of weight gains. Examination of birds particularly around the vent and under the wings, but also elsewhere, will reveal eggs on the feathers or moving lice on the skin or feathers.

Control: Lice and other ectoparasites of poultry must be considered as any other infectious disease; isolation from all possible means of contamination must be maintained.

Birds are seldom treated individually but a thorough dusting with sodium fluoride, if done twice about 10 days apart, is effective for most lice. Malathion (℞ 297) is effective, or the roost can be painted with nicotine sulfate (℞ 305). Where the birds or the litter or both have to be treated, a 4% dust of malathion or a 0.5% dust of coumaphos can be used. These 2 products may also be used as a spray.

THE FOWL TICK

(*Argas persicus*)

Biology: The fowl tick occurs worldwide in tropical and subtropical countries and is the vector of *Borrelia anserina* (spirochetosis). The tick is active in poultry houses throughout the year whenever temperatures are high enough. The adults and nymphs rarely are seen feeding on the birds, as they attack at night and hide in cracks and crevices during the day. The larvae may be found on the birds, as they frequently remain attached for as long as 2 days in taking their first blood meal. After feeding, the larvae molt into the nymph stage. Nymphs may feed and molt many times before reaching the adult stage. The adults feed repeatedly, with the females laying 50 to 100 eggs after each feeding. In warm weather, the eggs may hatch in 10 days, but cool weather prolongs the incubation period as much as 3 months or longer.

Clinical Findings: The fowl tick produces anemia and toxemia, with the anemia being of greater importance. Affected birds lose weight, appear anemic, are depressed and their egg production decreases. Red spots can be seen on the skin where the ticks have fed. Since the ticks are nocturnal, the birds may show some uneasiness when roosting. Death losses are rare, but production may be seriously depressed.

Control: The fowl tick is difficult to eradicate because the adults and nymphs are usually not on the birds in the daytime. Therefore the first efforts to control this pest must be isolation to prevent infestation, well-constructed housing to reduce hiding places, plus cleanliness in the poultry house.

Malathion (℞ 297) affords good control if applied at least 1 gal./1,000 sq ft (1 L/23 sq m) of surface. Malathion does not produce residues in the tissues of birds maintained in close contact with the treated areas and may be used where poultry houses cannot be depopulated.

For areas and buildings from which the birds can be removed, sprays or paints containing 0.5% lindane (℞ 295—use one-half strength), chlordane (℞ 273) or toxaphene (℞ 335) applied at a rate of at least 1 gal./1,000 sq ft (1 L/23 sq m) of surface, should effect control. Since these materials may appear as residues in the flesh and eggs of birds that come in contact with them, treated areas must be kept empty for periods specified by the manufacturer.

THE RED MITE

(*Dermanyssus gallinae:* Roost mite, Nocturnal mite)

Biology: This mite attacks chickens, pigeons, canaries and various wild birds. It is less than 1-mm long and gray until it engorges with blood and becomes red. These common pests are nocturnal feeders and during the day hide in the cracks and crevices of the chicken house where they lay their eggs. They propagate very rapidly during the warm months and more slowly in cold weather. The life cycle may be completed in as little as a week. Transmission is accomplished by contact or through the use of infested equipment. A house may remain infested for 6 months after birds are removed.

Clinical Findings: In laying flocks, egg production is lowered. Young birds become emaciated and death occasionally results. Birds may be uneasy on the perches at night. Examination of birds at this time, or of roosts during the day, particularly cracks and where roost poles touch supports, will disclose grayish accumulations. The mites can produce a serious anemia, and may transmit diseases such as spirochetosis and fowl pox. Severe irritation of the skin is common.

Control: Sanitation and isolation so that birds do not become infested must be stressed. Carbolineum or creosote diluted with equal parts of kerosene applied to roosts and supports and nests once a year when the pens are empty will prevent infection. The recommendations given for the use of malathion, coumaphos and nicotine sulfate for the control of lice (see p. 1118) will also control the red mite.

FEATHER MITES

(*Ornithonyssus sylviarum:* Northern fowl mite)
(*Ornithonyssus bursa:* Tropical fowl mite)

Biology: Feather mites are common on chickens, robins, swallows and sparrows throughout the U.S.A. and Canada. Slightly smaller than the red mite, they differ from it in that they occur continuously on the birds and the surroundings both day and night. They are quick to crawl onto a person handling birds.

Clinical Findings: Infestation commonly leads to lowered egg production and emaciation, and can be severe enough to cause death. Examination of the birds reveals the mites, which are often only recognized because the small dust-like particles move. They are voracious blood suckers and may produce scabs.

Control: Feather mites are extremely difficult to control. The following treatments are recommended: (1) nicotine sulfate (℞ 305) as a roost paint; (2) a 0.25% wettable powder spray of coumaphos used at the rate of 1 gal. (4 L) per 100 birds directly on the birds (Do not contaminate feed or water or use in conjunction with other organic phosphates. Do not use within 10 days of vaccination or other stress influences.); (3) 4% malathion dust or 2% spray application to the roosts, droppings, nests and over litter.

THE SCALY LEG MITE

(*Knemidocoptes mutans*)

This small mite usually tunnels into the epithelium under the scales of the legs, and the resulting irritation and exudation cause the legs to become thickened, encrusted and unsightly. It also may attack the comb and wattles. Under modern systems of sanitation it is not common. If possible the first cases should be culled. The roosts and nests should be painted with carbolineum. The legs may be dipped in 1 part of kerosene plus 2 parts of raw linseed oil.

THE DEPLUMING MITE

(*Knemidocoptes laevis* var. *gallinae:* Body mange mite)

This microscopic mite of chickens, pheasants, pigeons and geese causes intense irritation at the base of the feathers. The wing and tail feathers are usually lost. To control this mite, isolate affected birds and treat with an ointment of caraway oil and petrolatum (℞ 272) or dip in 1 gal. (4 L) water plus 2 oz (60 gm) wettable sulfur and 1 oz (30 gm) of soap.

THE SUBCUTANEOUS MITE

(*Laminosioptes cysticola*)

The subcut. mite is a small parasite that is most often diagnosed by observation of white-to-yellowish caseocalcareous nodules about 1 to 3 mm in diameter in the subcutis, perhaps a reaction of the bird's tissue to enclose a foreign body after death of the mite. Careful examination of the skin and subcutis of birds under the dissecting microscope may more frequently reveal the mite. No attempts are made to control this parasite except to destroy the bird.

THE AIR-SAC MITE

(*Cytodites nudus*)

The air-sac mite occurs in bronchi, lungs, air sacs and bone cavities of several species of birds. Opinions vary as to the amount of damage done to the host. It will be recognized as whitish dots on the surface of the air sacs. The recommendation for control has been to destroy the affected birds.

CHIGGERS

(*Trombicula alfreddugesi:* Red bugs, Harvest mites)

These small larval mites are parasitic on chickens, turkeys, man and wild animals. Chiggers are prevalent in the Southern U.S.A., particularly on heavy soil. They breed on the ground in waste areas, such as fence rows. Young birds may be severely affected, become emaciated, droopy and die. A vesicle or abscess may form at the point of attachment of the chigger.

Control is partly accomplished by keeping the grass on the range cut short. Dusting the range with about 50 lb (22.5 kg) of sulfur, 40 lb (18 kg) of 1% malation, ⅓ gal. (1.3 L) of 45% chlordane, or ½ gal. (2 L) of toxaphene per acre will control chiggers. One part of sulfur to 5 parts of petrolatum may be applied to the skin lesions.

BEDBUGS

(*Cimex lectularius*)

These reddish-brown, oval, flattened, wingless insects are about 6 mm in length. They are bloodsucking parasites and can subsist on the blood of wild and domestic animals and man. They can live without food for at least a year. Bedbugs have been known to become troublesome in old henhouses and in poultry-fattening cages. They may cause considerable trouble in pigeon lofts. The life cycle takes about 4 to 6 weeks. Control is best accomplished by thorough cleaning of the houses and reducing hiding places such as cracks, to which these insects retire during the day. Usually, spraying with malathion or with carbolineum or creosote oil diluted with kerosene, after removing birds from premises, is quite a satisfactory control measure. Most methods of control for mites are equally effective for bedbugs.

MOSQUITOES

Perhaps the most common mosquito in the Southern U.S.A., and in the same latitude around the world, is *Culex pipiens quinquefasciatus*. This mosquito feeds readily on poultry. Swarms of this and other species feeding on chickens have been known to be responsible for a marked drop in egg production and even death. Several viral diseases of birds are transmitted by them. The usual control measures are employed, such as oily preparations on nearby pools and other breeding places, and spraying of the walls and ceilings of evacuated chicken houses with 1% malathion water emulsion every 5 to 7 days.

FLIES AND GNATS

The **pigeon fly** (*Pseudolynchia canariensis*) is a small, flat, brownish fly which causes most trouble in pigeon lofts. The flies suck blood, move rapidly through the birds' feathers and may cause heavy losses in squabs. Most prevalent in the Southern U.S.A., it is the transmitter of *Haemoproteus columbae*, which causes pigeon malaria. The pigeon loft especially should be thoroughly cleaned every 20 days. Squabs can be dusted with pyrethrum powder. Derris powder (℞ 322) also is effective as a dust.

Black flies (members of the family Simuliidae), known as buffalo gnats or turkey gnats, are bloodsuckers and transmit *Leucocytozoon* disease (q.v., p. 1135). These small flies are less than 6 mm in length and breed in well-oxygenated water. They are commonest in the north temperate zones, but may occur in the South. They often attack in swarms and can cause anemia and death of birds. Control is exceedingly difficult since these flies breed in streams or shallow shores of some lakes. The range may be treated with a 1% DDT dust (where lawful) and all poultry houses should be screened.

FLEAS

The **sticktight flea** (*Echidnophaga gallinacea*) is commonest in the Southern U.S.A. After mating, the female burrows into the skin, causing ulcers on the birds. The eggs hatch and the larvae drop to the ground where they feed, and the life cycle is complete in 60 days. Other birds and mammals may become infested.

The "western" hen flea (*Ceratophyllus niger*) seems to be confined to the Pacific coast area. This flea actually breeds in the droppings and only feeds on birds occasionally.

The "European" chick flea (*C. gallinae*) is widespread in the U.S.A. It breeds in the nests and litter, and only goes on the birds to suck blood. It is known to attack many other birds besides chickens.

Control is accomplished by cleaning the houses and dusting the birds and treating the infected premise with malathion (℞ 298).

DIGESTIVE TRACT HELMINTHIASIS

Etiology: Some 60 species of worms occur in poultry in the U.S.A., while many additional species are found elsewhere in the world. Injury to the host results from direct destruction of tissues, with the amount of destruction proportional to the number of worms present. Damage is best measured in terms of reduced weight gains and egg production. Small farm flocks reared on range or in back yard pens may have large numbers of worms. Next most common are parasite problems in floor reared layers or broilers. With all-in, all-out and confinement reared management of broilers, only 2 or 3 species of parasites have survived to produce flock problems.

Of the 3 major classes of helminths, nematodes most commonly produce flock problems and are more pathogenic than trematodes or cestodes. With confinement rearing, the latter 2 groups have largely lost contact with the intermediate hosts necessary to complete their life cycles. Trematodes often require habitats near water, close to small intermediate hosts. With cestodes (*Choanotaenia infundibulum* and *Raillietina cesticillus*), only contact with houseflies and beetles without poultry houses continues to produce infections.

Clinical Findings: The signs are: general unthriftiness, retarded growth, inactive "colorless" birds with depressed appetite in an environment where sanitation has broken down. Specific lesions have not been associated with every parasite. There may be nodules, irritations, minute hemorrhages where worms are attached, and ulceration when fine-bodied worms invade the submucosa. Larval worms may do more damage than adults. Occasionally, *Ascaridia galli* worms migrate from the cloaca into the oviduct and become encapsulated within hens' eggs. Although the infection is harmless, concerned consumers may involve public health officials in attempts to trace the source. The problem can be prevented by careful candling of eggs or worm prevention measures.

Diagnosis: Since pathogenicity varies greatly with species, accurate identification will make all recommendations including flock prognosis, management changes, prevention and treatment more meaningful. Individual worms must be recovered and examined for identification. The digestive tract is opened, scraped, and the contents of each section put into a separate container of water. A good light source is essential; many worms are not actively motile. The esophagus and crop are removed in one piece and the inner surfaces stretched taut to expose capillarids "sewn" into the mucous membrane. The outer and inner surfaces of the proventriculus are examined for female *Tetrameres*. The gizzard lining must be removed to find gizzard worms. The ceca are split separately to find cecal worms; the cecal contents and scrapings are examined closely for the capillarids, which are thin and without movement. Scoleces of tapeworms may be located and recovered for species identification by floating the entire worm free under water; an incision deep into the mucosa under the attachment point is made with a sharp scalpel to free the scolex.

Prevention and Control: Most helminth parasite problems respond more readily to changes in management programs than to treatment regimens. Recommendations require consideration of economic benefits, the life cycle of the parasite and the method of infection, particularly if an intermediate host is involved. Sanitation in terms of moisture control is important; wet spots around drinkers or from leaky roofs should be avoided. A thorough inspection of the premises after diagnosis may locate the source of the infection.

Treatment: Flock treatment may be helped more by interrupting the life cycle than by removing adult worms from infected birds. This is particularly true of *Ascaridia galli* where more damage is done by the larval nematodes than the adults. With broilers, good control has been effected by regularly treating each successive flock with piperazine in the water between the fourth and the sixth week. The number of eggs in the litter may be sufficiently reduced to eliminate flock infection after treatment of 2 or 3 successive growouts. A similar approach using phenothiazine has been successful in eliminating *Heterakis gallinarum* and associated histomoniasis in broilers in Australia.

With layers, hygromycin B administered in the feed at 8.8 ppm has successfully reduced the population of *Capillaria*, *Heterakis* and *Ascaridia* if continued for at least 2 to 3 months. Coumaphos administered in the feed at 30 to 40 ppm has proved effective in controlling capillarias.

Tapeworms in chickens and turkeys may be removed by compounds containing proper levels of butynorate (℞ 355).

COMMON HELMINTHS IN THE DIGESTIVE TRACT OF CHICKENS AND TURKEYS

Parasite	Bird Host	Intermediate Host or Life Cycle	Organ Infected	Pathogenicity	Control
Nematodes					
Ascaridia galli	Chicken	Direct	Jejunum	Moderate migrates into hen's eggs	Management change. Piperazine, hygromycin B, coumaphos, butynorate.
Ascaridia dissimilis	Turkey	Direct	Jejunum	Moderate	
Ascaridia columbae	Pigeon	Direct	Jejunum	Moderate	
Capillaria obsignata	Chicken, turkey	None, direct	Small intestine, cecum	Moderate to severe	Hygromycin B, coumaphos.
Capillaria annulata	Chicken, turkey	Earthworms	Esophagus, crop	Moderate	
Capillaria caudinflata	Chicken, turkey	Earthworms	Small intestine, cecum	Moderate to severe	
Cheilospirura hamulosa	Chicken, turkey, quail	Grasshoppers, beetles	Gizzard	Moderate to severe	Management change.
Dispharynx nasuta	Chicken, turkey, pigeons	Sowbugs	Proventriculus	Moderate to severe	Management change.
Heterakis gallinarum	Chicken, turkey	Direct cycle, earthworm transport	Cecum	Very mild, transmits histomoniasis	Hygromycin B, phenothiaz.ne, coumaphos, butynorate.
Tetrameres americana	Chicken, turkey	Grasshoppers, cockroach	Proventriculus	Moderate	Management change.

Trematodes					
Echinostoma revolutum	Turkeys, geese, pigeons, 12 or- orders of birds	Snails, fish	Cloaca, lower intestine	Mild	Management change.
Prosthogonimus macrorchis	Chickens, wild birds	Snails, dragon flies	Oviduct, cloaca	Mild	Management change.
Cestodes					
Choanotaenia infundibulum	Chicken	House flies	Upper intestine	Moderate	Management change.
Davainea proglottina	Chicken	Slugs, snails	Duodenum	Severe	Management change. Butynorate.
Metroliasthes lucida	Turkey	Grasshoppers	Intestine	Unknown	Management change.
Raillietina cesticillus	Chicken	Beetles	Duodenum, jejunum	Mild	Management change.
Raillietina tetragona	Chicken	Ants	Lower intestine	Severe	Management change. Butynorate.
Raillietina echinobothrida	Chicken	Ants	Lower intestine	Severe, nodules	Management change. Butynorate.

FLUKE INFECTIONS IN POULTRY

Although trematodes continue to be of importance in some production systems, and as parasites of certain wild birds, they are of diminished importance where modern poultry production methods are used.

***Prosthogonimus macrorchis* Infection:** This pyriform fluke (about 7 mm by 5 mm) develops to maturity in the bursa of Fabricius except in those birds, such as chicken, turkey and pheasant, which do not have a functional bursa; in these it develops in the oviduct. Birds become infected by eating mature or immature dragonflies (secondary host) bearing the metacercariae. Development to adults requires about 14 days. The primary host is a snail.

In ducks and other birds with a functional bursa, only light infections are found, and no clinical signs are observed. In gallinaceous birds, where the parasites develop in the oviduct, heavy infections may occur. Such birds go off feed, become droopy, lose weight and lay fewer eggs. The eggs are soft-shelled and, in extreme cases, egg laying ceases. A calcareous discharge, presumably from uterine glands, soils the cloacal feathers. The lesions range from mild inflammation of the oviduct to distension and even rupture of the oviduct with exudate and egg material. Death may occur.

Since the fluke eggs appear in the bird's droppings only periodically, fecal examination is diagnostically unreliable. Necropsy may disclose flukes in the oviduct.

Infection can be prevented by keeping birds away from aquatic situations where they can feed on dragonflies. Carbon tetrachloride (1 to 5 ml, orally) has been used in treatment; however, it is extremely toxic to birds, especially chickens. Treatment on a total flock basis is impractical.

***Collyriclum faba* Infection:** This parasite is found in subcut. cysts in turkeys, chickens and other birds. The life cycle is unknown; probably it involves snails and insects such as dragonflies or mayflies. The cysts, about 4 to 6 mm in diameter, and usually containing 2 adults, may occur anywhere on the body, but most are found near the vent. Young birds may have locomotor difficulty and poor appetite; heavy infection may be fatal. The cysts ooze exudate, attract flies, and may become infected with bacteria. The worms can be removed surgically. Prevention is by keeping birds away from aquatic insects.

GAPEWORM INFECTION

The gapeworm, *Syngamus trachea*, inhabits the trachea and lungs of many domestic and various wild birds. Infection may occur directly by ingestion of infective eggs or larvae; however, severe field infection is associated with the ingestion of transport hosts, such as earthworms, snails, slugs and arthropods such as flies. Many gapeworm larvae may encyst and survive within a single invertebrate for years. Range infection is favored by seasonal climatic abundance of specific invertebrate hosts, e.g. great numbers of earthworms brought to the surface by spring rains. Although gapeworms are not a problem in confinement-reared poultry they are in game-farm pens and serious economic losses occur in range-reared chickens, pheasants, turkeys and peacocks. *Cyathostoma bronchialis* is the causative agent of the disease in geese and ducks.

Clinical Findings: Young birds suffer most. Sudden death and verminous pneumonia characterize early outbreaks. Signs of gasping, choking, shaking of the head, inanition, emaciation and suffocation may follow. Necropsy reveals adult gapeworms obstructing the lumina of the trachea, bronchi and lungs. Respiratory inflammation may be present. The blood-red female gapeworm is usually found attached to a much smaller, paler male whose head becomes permanently embedded deep in the host tissue. The joined pair have a "Y"-shaped, or forked appearance. The female worm may become detached from the male and feed freely within the lumen, or be coughed up and discharged from the body.

Prophylaxis and Treatment: To prevent wild birds from introducing infection, pens should be isolated by overhead and lateral screening. After infection occurs, pens should be "rested" and preferably rotated with crops; however, poultry and game birds should not be placed on newly plowed fields. Earthworm populations can be reduced prior to introduction of range-reared birds by soil treatments such as Shell D-D, ethylene dibromide, rotenone and chlordane. Various molluscacides, such as copper sulfate or pentachlorophenate, will destroy slugs and snails.

Administration of thiabendazole at 0.1% in the feed continuously for 10 days to 2 weeks is highly effective in eliminating gapeworms, and 0.05% feed medication when given continuously for 4 days or longer helps prevent and control infections. Tetramisole has been reported as effective at 1.6 mg/lb (3.6 mg/kg) for 3 consecutive days in the drinking water. Poultry treated while larvae are migrating in the body will develop immunity to gapeworms even though therapy may abort infection.

MANSON'S EYEWORM INFESTATION

Manson's eyeworm, *Oxyspirura mansoni*, is a slender nematode, 12 to 18 mm in length, occurring beneath the nictitating membrane of chickens and other fowl in tropical and subtropical regions. The parasite causes various degrees of inflammation, lacrimation, corneal opacity, and disturbed vision. Worm eggs deposited in the eye reach the pharynx via the nasolacrimal duct, are swallowed, passed in the feces and ingested by the Surinam cockroach, *Pycnoscelus surinamensis*. Larvae reach the infective stage in the roach. When infested intermediate hosts are eaten, liberated larvae migrate up the esophagus to the mouth, thence through the nasolacrimal duct to the eye, where the cycle is completed. Strict sanitary measures including the use of approved insecticides on roach-infested premises provide efficient control. Surgical removal of the nictitating membrane is reported to be a useful prophylactic measure. As a treatment, the eye is anesthetized with a local anesthetic and the worms in the lacrimal sac are exposed by lifting the membrane. One or two drops of a 5% cresol solution placed in the lacrimal sac kills the worms instantly. The eye should be irrigated with pure water immediately to wash out the debris and excess solution. The eyes show improvement within 48 to 72 hours after treatment, and gradually become clear if the destructive process caused by the parasite is not too far advanced.

AVIAN COCCIDIOSIS

A parasitic disease caused by one or more species of coccidia. Found in a wide variety of avian hosts, these protozoan organisms are host-specific, each species usually occurring in a single host species. Because some hosts support several species of coccidia there are as many types of coccidiosis as there are coccidial species. Except for renal coccidiosis in geese, all coccidia of domestic fowl parasitize the digestive tract.

Etiology: The life cycle of the genus *Eimeria*, responsible for most infections of poultry, is summarized under MAMMALIAN COCCIDIOSIS (q.v., p. 458). Coccidia are almost universally present in poultry-raising operations, but clinical disease occurs only after ingestion of relatively large numbers of sporulated oocysts by a susceptible host. Both clinically infected and recovered birds shed oocysts in droppings, which serve as means of contaminating feed, dust, water, litter and soil. Oocysts may also be transmitted by mechanical carriers such as equipment, clothing, insects and other animals. Newly passed oocysts are not infective until sporulated. Sporulation under optimum conditions (70 to 90°F [21 to 32°C] plus moisture and oxygen) varies from 1 to 2 days for the various species. The prepatent period varies from 4 to 7 days. Sporulated oocysts may survive for long periods depending upon environmental conditions such as pH, temperature and moisture. Oocysts are resistant to most disinfectants.

Pathogenicity of coccidia varies among strains of the species and by genetic susceptibility of the host. Markedly pathogenic species invade the mucosa, tunica propria and sometimes the submucosa; less pathogenic strains produce more superficial lesions. Acquired immunity of a portion of the flock from earlier subclinical infection can greatly moderate the disease. Flock management techniques are often designed to allow development of immunity without clinical disease by controlling infection. Birds are susceptible at all ages but disease is less frequent in older birds because of immunity from earlier exposure.

Clinical Findings: Chickens: In *E. tenella* infection, involvement of the ceca rather than the small intestine is a distinguishing characteristic. Clinically, the infection can be recognized by the accumulation of blood in the ceca and bloody droppings. Cecal cores, which are accumulations of clotted blood, tissue debris and oocysts, may be found in birds that are past the acute stage of the disease.

E. necatrix produces major lesions in the anterior or midportion of the small intestine recognizable by small white spots usually intermingled with rounded, bright- or dull-red spots of various sizes. The white spots are pathognomonic for this species if clumps of large schizonts can be demonstrated microscopically. In severe cases, the intestinal wall is thickened, the involved area is dilated to 2 or 2½ times the normal diameter, and there may be blood in the lumen. Fluid loss may result in marked dehydration; crops are often concurrently distended with water. While the damage is in the small intestine, the sexual phase of the life cycle is completed in the ceca; thus *E. necatrix* oocysts are found in the ceca. Oocysts of all other species develop in the area of major lesions.

E. acervulina and *E. mivati* infections, characterized by numerous gray or whitish transverse patches in the upper half of the small intestine, are not easily distinguished on gross examination. The clinical course in a flock is usually protracted. Poor growth and the development of culls are often observed with a low mortality. *E. maxima* causes dilatation and thickening of the small intestine, which may contain a grayish, brown, or slightly pink mucous exudate. The oocysts are large.

E. brunetti occurs in the lower small intestine, rectum, ceca and cloaca. In moderate infections, there is a catarrhal enteritis and thickening of the intestinal wall. A severe infection may cause an extensive coagulation necrosis and sloughing of the mucosa throughout the entire intestine. Oocysts are sometimes difficult to demonstrate.

Three other species (*E. hagani*, *E. mitis*, and *E. praecox*) that parasitize the upper half of the intestine are regarded as pathogenic but of less economic importance than the 6 species mentioned above.

Signs of coccidiosis are highly variable in flocks and range from decreased growth rate to a high percentage of visibly sick birds, severe diarrhea, and high mortality. Usually there is decreased feed and water consumption. Weight loss, the development of culls, decreased egg production in hens, and increased mortality are observed in clinical infections. Survivors of severe infections recover in 10 to 14 days but may require more time to return to normal production. The degree of acquired immunity of the host population prior to the development of clinical disease may influence the clinical severity and course of a flock infection.

Turkeys: Only 3 of the 7 coccidia of turkeys (*Eimeria adenoeides, E. gallopavonis* and *E. meleagrimitis*) are considered to be pathogenic. *E. dispersa, E. innocua, E. meleagridis* and *E. subrotunda* are said to be relatively nonpathogenic. Oocyst sporulation occurs in 1 to 2 days; the prepatent period varies from 4 to 6 days.

E. adenoeides and *E. gallopavonis* infect the lower ileum, ceca and rectum. The developmental stages are found in the epithelial cells of the villi and crypts. The affected portion of the intestine may be dilated and have a thickened wall. Thick creamy material, or caseous casts containing enormous numbers of oocysts are found. *E. meleagrimitis* chiefly infects the upper small intestine. The lamina propria or deeper tissues may be parasitized and result in a necrotic enteritis.

The common signs seen in infected flocks include reduced feed consumption, rapid weight loss, droopiness, ruffled feathers and severe diarrhea. Mortality is variable but may be very high. Bloody droppings do not occur, but wet droppings containing mucus are common. Clinical infections are seldom observed beyond the age of 8 weeks.

Ducks: A large number of specific coccidia have been reported in both wild and domestic ducks but there is a question of the validity of some of the descriptions. The following have been reported in the domestic duck: *Eimeria battahki, E. danailovi, E. saitamae, Wenyonella anatis, W. philiplevinei* and *Tyzzeria perniciosa. T. perniciosa* is known to be a pathogen; members of the *Eimeria* species have also been described as pathogenic while the other coccidia of domestic ducks are considered relatively nonpathogenic. A variety of coccidia have been reported from wild ducks.

Infrequent but dramatic outbreaks occur in ducklings between 2 and 5 weeks old. Morbidity and mortality may be high. *T. perniciosa* produces ballooning of the entire small intestine with mucohemorrhagic material that later becomes caseous. Other species apparently produce hemorrhagic enteritis with an anatomic distribution characteristic of the species.

Geese: The most striking coccidial infection of geese is that produced by *Eimeria truncata*, in which the kidneys are enlarged and studded with poorly circumscribed yellowish white streaks and spots. The tubules are dilated with masses of oocysts and urates. Mortality may be very high. At least 5 other species of *Eimeria* have been described as parasitizing the intestine of geese.

Diagnosis: The presence of coccidial infections is usually readily established by the demonstration of oocysts in feces or in intestinal scrapings. Responsible diagnosis of coccidiosis as a clinical problem in poultry sometimes demands a high order of skill as the observation of oocysts has little relationship to current or impending clinical disease. Knowledge of flock appearance, morbidity, mortality, feed intake, characteristic odor, and growth rate or rate of lay are often of critical importance for diagnosis. Necropsy of several representative specimens is advisable. Classical lesions of *E. tenella* and *E. necatrix* may be diagnostic. Familiarity with the lesions, area parasitized by different species, and the size, shape and location of oocysts allows a reasonably accurate differentiation of the coccidial species in most instances. Mixed coccidial infections are common.

A diagnosis of coccidiosis is warranted if oocysts, merozoites or schizonts are demonstrated mciroscopically and if lesions and flock history are compatible with the diagnosis. The frequency of subclinical coccidial infections in some individuals in a population demands care in eliminating other possible flock disorders.

Control: Complete prevention of infection cannot be expected by practical methods of management. Maintaining poultry at all times on wire floors to separate birds from droppings is usually adequate to prevent all but minor infections; only rarely is clinical coccidiosis observed under such circumstances. Other methods of control are designed to allow development of immunity from infection, or to minimize infection usually by use of drugs if no immunity is necessary. As chickens may experience serious problems from coccidiosis throughout life, methods to control the disease in this species will be discussed in detail.

Immunity: A species-specific immunity develops, the degree of which is largely dependent upon the extent of parasitism that occurs following exposure. Repeated infection with small numbers of oocysts produces greater immunity than from the same numbers given at one time, and is less damaging to the host.

"Vaccines" in the form of standardized doses of sporulated oocysts of the various coccidial species are available. The "vaccine" is administered in the drinking water during the first 14 days of age. As the "vaccine" serves only to introduce infection, the litter must be managed to allow oocyst sporulation; spraying the litter may be necessary to keep it moist but not wet.

Drug use when immunity needed: A great variety of anticoccidial drugs are available for use in preventing clinical infections. Ideally, the environmental conditions interacting with the suppressing effect of the drug should allow sufficient infection to produce a gradual development of immunity without clinical disease. Failures occur either by overly suppressing infection, which results in little or no immunity, or by inadequate suppression and the development of clinical infection. Different drugs are highly variable in degree of immunity suppression.

Drug use when no immunity needed: No immunity is necessary in chickens reared for meat production or in floor-reared layers to be moved to cages. Under these circumstances exposure and infection should be minimized. Litter should be dry to minimize oocyst sporulation, and highly effective anticoccidial drugs at relatively high levels may be used continuously to minimize infection. Drug withdrawal is only necessary (as required by the specific drug used) to avoid residues in meat or eggs.

Anticoccidial drugs: A variety of drugs are available for prevention and treatment of coccidiosis in chickens, and a smaller number for use with turkeys. These include aklomide, aklomide with sulfanitran, amprolium, amprolium with ethopabate, arprinocid, buquinolate, butynorate, butynorate with sulfanitran and dinsed, chlortetracycline, clopidol, decoquinate, furazolidone, lasalocid sodium, monensin, nicarbazin, nitrofurazone, nitromide with sulfanitran, robenidine hydrochloride, sulfadimethoxine with ormetoprim, sulfaquinoxaline and zoalene. All are provided by the manufacturer in premixes with detailed instructions for prophylactic use. Drugs are most effective in prevention since most of the damage occurs before signs become apparent and treatment may be initiated too late to benefit all the birds in a flock.

Drugs that show efficacy even if started late in the cycle, such as the sulfonamides, are preferred for treatment. Of the drugs effective prophylactically only a few are also effective therapeutically. Water medication is generally preferred over feed medication for treating infected flocks. Therapeutic drugs include: amprolium, chlortetracycline, furazolidone, nitromide with sulfanitran, pyrimethamine with sulfaquinoxaline, and sulfaquinoxaline. Increased levels of vitamins A and K or antibiotic drugs are sometimes used extemporaneously in the ration to improve the rate of recovery.

Proper drug levels depend upon authorized governmental approvals and various management considerations. For prevention, relatively low levels may be used continuously while higher levels may be used over short periods of time for treatment. Recommended dosage varies with the species of coccidia involved. Higher levels may be used if a high level of exposure is anticipated. Lower levels may be used if development of immunity is desired. Mild infections of intestinal species which would otherwise be classed as subclinical may cause depigmentation. *All manufacturer's warnings should be carefully observed.*

Continuous use of anticoccidial drugs may result in selection and survival of drug-resistant strains of coccidia. Fortunately there is little cross resistance among strains resistant to anticoccidials with different modes of action. Change of drug may be beneficial in areas where resistance problems have been established. However, little benefit may be expected from frequent changing of drugs.

HEXAMITIASIS

An acute, catarrhal enteritis of turkeys, pheasants, quail, chukar partridges and peafowl, now rare in North America. The highest mortality occurs in 1- to 9-week-old birds. Natural infection has not been observed in chickens. Pigeons are susceptible to another species of *Hexamita*.

Etiology: The causative protozoan parasite, *Hexamita meleagridis*, is spindle-shaped, averages 8 μ long by 3 μ wide and has 6 anterior and 2 posterior flagella. It has not yet been cultured in artificial media. It is transmitted directly by ingestion of infected feces. Many survivors become carriers and hexamitae are shed in the droppings.

Clinical Findings and Lesions: The unspecific signs include watery diarrhea, dry unkempt feathers, listlessness and rapid weight loss although the birds continue to eat. They may die in convulsions. Bulbous dilatations of the small intestine, especially of the duodenum and upper jejunum, filled with water contents are characteristic. The crypts of Lieberkuhn contain myriads of hexamitae, which attach themselves to the epithelial cells by their posterior flagella.

Diagnosis: Diagnosis depends on finding hexamitae upon microscopic examination of scrapings of the duodenal and jejunal mucosa. Hexamitae move with a rapid, darting motion (contrast the jerky motion of trichomonads). In order to avoid contamination of the instruments with other cecal protozoa, the duodenum should be opened first. Hexamitae may be demonstrated in the poults that have been dead for several hours if the scrapings are placed in a drop of warm (104°F, 40°C) isotonic saline solution on the slide. A few hexamitae in birds more than 10 weeks old do not justify a diagnosis of hexamitiasis.

Prophylaxis and Treatment: Because many birds remain carriers, breeder turkeys and poults should, if possible, be raised on separate premises; preferably with separate attendants. Wire platforms should be used under feeders and waterers. Pheasants and quail may be carriers and sometimes bring the infection to turkeys.

Furazolidone (℞ 346), oxytetracycline (℞ 60) or chlortetracycline (℞ 28) are used to prevent and treat hexamitiasis. Treatment does not substitute for adequate sanitation and management programs.

HISTOMONIASIS

(Infectious enterohepatitis, Blackhead)

A protozoan disease affecting turkeys, chickens, peafowl, ruffed grouse and quail. Turkeys of all ages are susceptible, but greatest mortality occurs in birds under 12 weeks old.

Etiology: Histomoniasis is probably the result of dual etiology, one being the protozoan *Histomonas meleagridis* and the other any one or more of a group of common bacterial inhabitants of the intestinal tract of chickens and turkeys. The protozoan does not seem capable of producing the disease in the absence of bacteria. As a rule both the liver and ceca of infected birds are involved. In the lumen of the ceca, *H. meleagridis* has one flagellum and tends to rotate in a counterclockwise direction. (A nonpathogenic species has 4 flagella.) In the tissues of both the ceca and liver, it assumes an ameboid form but recently electron microscope studies have shown an axostyle relating it more closely to trichomonads than the amebae.

This disease has traditionally been thought of as affecting turkeys, while doing little damage to chickens. This is not entirely true. The disease in chickens has an early cecal involvement. Mild liver lesions occur occasionally. Mortality is low but morbidity can be high in young chickens, especially those of broiler age. Tissue responses to infection may be gone in 4 weeks but the bird may be a carrier for another 6 weeks.

H. meleagridis may sometimes be transmitted directly by ingestion of infected feces, but it is more often transmitted by ingestion of the embryonated eggs of the cecal worm, *Heterakis gallinarum*, which can harbor *H. meleagridis*. A large percentage of chickens harbor this worm which, in itself, is not pathogenic. Its eggs are resistant and may remain viable in the soil for months or even years. Studies have shown that 3 species of earthworms can harbor *Heterakis* larvae containing *H. meleagridis* and that they are infective to both chickens and turkeys.

Clinical Findings: Signs are apparent 7 to 12 days after infection. These include: listlessness, drooping wings, unkempt feathers and sulfur colored droppings. The head may be cyanotic, hence the name "blackhead." Young birds have a more acute type of the disease and die within a few days after signs appear. Older birds may be sick for some time and become very emaciated before death.

Lesions: The primary lesions are in the ceca, which exhibit marked inflammatory changes and ulcerations causing a thickening of the cell wall. Occasionally these ulcers erode the cecal wall, causing a peritonitis and involvement of other organs. The ceca contain a yellowish-green caseous exudate or, in later stages, a dry cheesy core. The liver lesions are circular, yellowish green and characteristically depressed. In the turkey, they may be up to 4 cm in diameter.

The lesions in the liver and ceca are pathognomonic. However, the liver lesions must be differentiated from those of tuberculosis, leukosis, avian trichomoniasis and mycosis, which are raised and grayish or gray-yellow. In some cases, especially in chickens, histopathologic examination is very helpful. Histomonads are intercellular, although the parasites may be so closely packed between cells as to appear intracellular. The nuclei are much smaller than those of the host cells, and the cytoplasm less vacuolated. Scrapings from the liver lesions or from the ceca may be placed in isotonic saline solution for direct microscopic examination. It is important in such examinations to differentiate *Histomonas* from other cecal flagellates and from *Blastocystis.*

Prophylaxis and Treatment: Strict sanitation is indicated. The use of large wire platforms for feeders and waterers reduces the danger of infection. As healthy chickens often carry infected cecal worms, the practice of ranging chickens with turkeys should be avoided. Grouse and quail also may be carriers capable of bringing the infection to the turkey yards. Since *H. gallinarum* ova can survive in soil for many months, turkeys should not be put on ground contaminated during the past 12 to 24 months. A rotation system, in which the turkeys are moved every 3 to 5 weeks, helps to reduce the chances of infection.

The following drugs have been found to be effective in control: ronidazole (℞ 360); nitarsone (℞ 351); furazolidone (℞ 346); carbarsone (℞ 342); dimetridazole (℞ 343). Phenothiazine and tobacco dust are used to remove cecal worms, but have no direct effect on *Histomonas* itself.

LEUCOCYTOZOON DISEASE

A disease of birds, caused by protozoan parasites similar to those that cause malaria. The parasites invade various tissues as well as the blood cells. Many species have been described from different kinds of birds. Acute outbreaks of the disease have been reported in chickens, geese, turkeys and ducks.

Etiology: Several species of the parasites have been described from various wild and domestic birds, but few are known to cause serious disease. Those recorded from domestic birds are: *Leucocytozoon simondi (anseris)* from ducks and geese, *L. neavei* from guinea fowl, *L. smithi* from turkeys, and *L. sabrazesi*, *L. caulleryi* and *L. andrewsi* from chickens. Wild birds may be responsible in certain areas for initiating the infection in domesticated species each year.

Chronic infections may persist in birds from one year to the next with certain ornithophilous black-flies (Simuliidae) and biting midges (*Culicoides* spp.) serving as vectors and infecting healthy birds. (*L. caulleryi* is the only one transmitted by *Culicoides* spp.)

Black flies (q.v., p. 1121) deposit their eggs on rocks, vegetation, logs or other objects, in or near the edge of rapidly flowing streams, or occasionally in shallow lake margins. Adult flies emerge in late spring and early summer and fly or are carried by winds for some distance from the streams in which they develop but are more numerous close to their breeding places. Biting midges breed in wet ground.

Clinical Findings: Acute disease occurs when there is a high parasitemia; otherwise, the infection is subacute or chronic. The disease has a relatively sudden onset with anemia, leukocytosis, splenomegaly and hypertrophy of the liver commencing about one week after infection. Fatalities usually occur within a week after infection has appeared in the blood. Birds with heavy infections show lack of appetite, dullness, loss of equilibrium, lameness and weakness. Chickens with acute infections with *L. caulleryi* are anemic; some vomit and die from hemorrhage; some excrete green feces. Retarded growth and lowered egg production occur in those surviving. Death may be due to severe anemia, to pathologic changes in the liver and brain resulting therefrom, and to respiratory embarrassment caused by the presence of large numbers of gametocytes in the lung capillaries.

Outbreaks of the disease occur during the late spring and summer when black flies and biting midges are present. Low-grade chronic infections may be found in birds at other times. Highest mortality (up to 100% in ducks) has been reported in young birds, especially in operations where new stock is continually introduced. The disease in ducks is characterized by sudden onset and mortality usually of up to 35%. Death due to *L. caulleryi* is reported in 10 to 80% of infected older chickens.

Diagnosis: Laboratory diagnosis is based on an examination of thin blood films that have been stained with Wright's or Giemsa stain to reveal the sexual stages of the parasite in the peripheral blood cells. Red blood cells as well as lymphocytes may be invaded. The degree of alteration in the host cell varies with the species of parasite. The typical elongated cells, with attenuated ends, are observed in ducks, geese and turkeys, and in chickens affected with one species. Two other species in chickens occur in round cells only; *L. caulleryi* is often free from the host cell.

Control: Pyrimethamine, 0.00005% in the diet, sulfadimethoxine, 0.0025%, or sulfaquinoxaline, 0.005% in the diet or drinking water continuously, prevents infection with *L. caulleryi*. No satisfactory treatment is presently available for other species.

A method of preventing the disease in young turkeys is to dispose of all adults several weeks before the young birds are exposed to black flies. This method fails in areas where wild turkeys are also carrying the parasite. Tightly screening the houses is effective, but is practical only on a limited scale. Keeping ducks and turkeys inside may give some protection as black flies seldom feed inside buildings. Chickens cannot be protected this way as biting midges will feed inside buildings.

The large-scale rearing of ducks in areas where ornithophilous black flies are prevalent is to be avoided. It is difficult to eradicate the biting midges from paddy fields and swampy areas where they breed.

BLOOD SPOROZOA OF BIRDS

Aside from *Leucocytozoon*, birds may be infected with other malarial parasites belonging to the genera *Haemoproteus* and *Plasmodium*. Physical signs are similar to those observed in infections with *Leucocytozoon* (q.v., p. 1135). Diagnosis is made by examination of stained, thin blood smears and demonstration of the causative organisms in the red blood cells. During the acute stages of the disease, the liver and spleen are enlarged and dark.

Haemoproteus is common in pigeons, doves, quail, ducks and many species of wild song birds. It has been reported on a few occasions from turkeys. Fatalities have been observed among pigeons, doves and quail. The parasites are transmitted by bloodsucking flies of the genus *Lynchia*. In ducks, the vector is a *Culicoides*.

Plasmodium gallinaceum has not been observed in domestic poultry in North America, although it occurs in other parts of the world. *P. durae* has been reported as a severe pathogen in turkeys in East Africa. An unidentified *Plasmodium* has been reported in chickens in Wisconsin. Turkeys, but not chickens, are experimentally susceptible to *P. circumflexum* isolated from wild Canadian geese. A number of other species occur in a variety of wild birds, but chickens and turkeys are not susceptible to these species.

TOXOPLASMOSIS

The etiology and general characteristics of toxoplasmosis are discussed under the heading on p. 466. In chickens, clinical signs include anorexia, emaciation, paleness and shrinking of the comb, whitish feces, and sometimes diarrhea, incoordination and ataxia. Some birds walk in circles, and exhibit torticollis, muscular spasms, paralysis and blindness. The course may be rapid or protracted, lasting 2 to 3 weeks, and is often fatal. In turkeys and geese, infections are mild and may be undetected. Characteristically, there are lesions of the CNS, such as necrosis of the midbrain and optical chiasma and defects of the retina accompanied by a pericarditis, myocarditis, necrotic hepatitis, and ulceration of the proventriculus and intestines. The pericardial sac is distended and contains reddish serous fluid; subpericardial nodules may be present.

Since the Sabin-Feldman dye test is negative or only slightly positive, the diagnosis is confirmed by histologic examination and isolation trials. Treatment has not been established, but a sulfonamide-pyrimethamine combination (q.v., p. 468) may be of use.

TRICHOMONIASIS

A disease of domestic fowl, pigeons, doves and hawks, characterized, in most cases, by caseous accumulations in the throat, usually accompanied by loss of weight. It has been termed "canker," "roup" and, in hawks, "frounce." Falconers have known the disease for many centuries.

Etiology: The causative organism is a flagellated protozoan, *Trichomonas gallinae*, which lives in the head sinuses, mouth, throat, esophagus and other organs of birds. It is more prevalent among domestic pigeons and wild doves than among chickens or turkeys, although severe outbreaks have been reported among domestic fowl. Some strains are highly fatal in pigeons and doves. Hawks, which may become diseased after eating infected birds, commonly show liver lesions, with or without throat involvement. Parent pigeons and doves transmit the infection to their offspring in contaminated pigeon milk. Contaminated water is probably the most important source of infection for chickens and turkeys.

Clinical Findings: The course of the disease is rapid. The first lesions appear as small, yellowish areas on the oral mucosa. They grow rapidly in size and coalesce to form masses which frequently completely block the esophageal passage, and may prevent the bird from closing its mouth. Much fluid may accumulate in the mouth. There is a rapid weight loss and the bird becomes weak and listless. Death usually ensues within 8 to 10 days. Eye involvement is evidenced by a watery discharge and, in more advanced stages, the production of exudate about the eyes may finally result in blindness. In chronic infections, the bird appears healthy, although trichomonads usually can be demonstrated in scrapings from the mucous membranes of the throat.

Lesions: On necropsy, the bird may be riddled with caseous necrotic foci. The mouth and esophagus are a mass of necrotic material which may extend into the skull and sometimes through the surrounding tissues of the neck to involve the skin. In the esophagus and crop, the lesions may take the form of yellow, rounded, raised areas, with a central conical caseous spur, often referred to as "yellow buttons." The crop may be covered by a yellowish diphtheritic membrane which may extend to the glandular stomach. There is no involvement of the gizzard or intestine.

Lesions of internal organs are most frequent in the liver. They may vary from a few small areas of yellow necrosis to almost complete replacement of liver tissue by caseous necrotic debris. Adhesions and involvement of other internal organs appear to be contact extensions of the huge liver lesions.

Diagnosis: The lesions of *T. gallinae* infection are quite characteristic, but not pathognomonic; those of pox and other infections can be quite similar. Diagnosis should be confirmed by laboratory demonstration of the causative trichomonad. This is accomplished readily by microscopic examination of a smear containing mucus or fluid from the throat. The organisms can be cultured easily on a variety of artificial media; 0.2% Loeffler's dried blood serum in Ringer's solution or in saline-bicarbonate solution, or a 2% solution of pigeon serum in isotonic salt solution may be employed. Good growth is obtained at 37°C. Antibiotics may be used to reduce bacterial contamination.

Control: Because *T. gallinae* infection in pigeons is so readily transmitted from parent to offspring in the normal feeding process, chronically infected birds should be removed at once. In pigeons, recovery from infection with a less virulent strain of *T. gallinae* appears to be accompanied by some protection against subsequent attack from a more virulent strain. Metronidazole when given orally at 60 mg/kg of body wt has prevented mortality. Dimetridazole given orally at 50 mg/kg of body wt or in the drinking water (0.05% for 5 to 6 days) has suppressed the disease.

BOTULISM

(Limberneck, Western duck sickness)

A type of intoxication due to ingestion of food materials containing toxins of *Clostridium botulinum.*

Etiology: Type A and Type C toxins of *Cl. botulinum* are the commonest causes of botulism in poultry and wildfowl. This organism occurs commonly in the soil and may contaminate foodstuffs. In order to produce botulism, the organism must have multiplied and formed its toxin in the food before it is ingested. The principal causes are improperly sterilized, home-canned vegetables and occasionally other home-canned foods, improperly processed and spoiling foods of animal origin, such as sausages and hams, and decomposing carcasses and the fly maggots living in them.

"Western duck sickness" or "alkali disease" occurs in the Western U.S.A. and Canada, and kills millions of wild waterfowl in certain years. It occurs around lakes or marshes where flooding has occurred and where there is relatively shallow water containing decaying vegetation. Anaerobiosis results in such cases, killing the invertebrates that live there. *Cl. botulinum* multiplies in their bodies and forms toxins. Waterfowl become affected when they feed in these areas.

Clinical Findings and Diagnosis: No characteristic lesions can be seen. There may be a slight enteritis and an enlarged spleen. The toxin affects the nervous system causing a flaccid paralysis, which is well described by the common name, "limberneck." In addition, the feathers are characteristically loose and come out easily. Death usually is due to respiratory paralysis.

A presumptive diagnosis of botulism can be made from the physical appearance and a history of eating spoiled food, carcassses, or maggots. A positive diagnosis can be made only by injection of a filtrate from the suspected feed or the intestinal contents of affected birds into 2 sets of mice or guinea pigs, of which one set receives simultaneously injections of bivalent Type A and Type C botulinum antitoxin. Isolation of *Cl. botulinum* from the feed or intestine is valueless since it may occur in them normally.

Control: Chickens should not be fed spoiled foods that are considered unfit for human consumption. Carcasses should be picked up from chicken yards and buried deeply or burned. Laxatives, such as Epsom salts (℞ 502) are of value in treating exposed birds that have not shown signs of the disease. No feed should be given, but fresh water should be supplied. *Cl. botulinum* antitoxin (℞ 128) may be of some value. It has been used successfully in treating wild waterfowl with signs of western duck sickness, but relatively few birds can be handled in this way.

Much greater success has been obtained by herding ducks away from affected areas with pyrotechnics, airplanes or boats, by draining such areas and by distributing feed for the birds elsewhere.

DISORDERS OF THE REPRODUCTIVE SYSTEM

Ruptured Egg Yolks: A sporadic condition causing death in laying hens, in which the yolk-filled ova rupture into the abdominal cavity. It is common in flighty pullets. Yolk material covers the viscera and often results in peritonitis. Rupture may be accompanied by severe hemorrhage, but whether this or the escape of yolk into the abdominal cavity is the cause of death is unknown. The condition is frequently associated with chronic *Pasteurella multocida* or acute *Escherichia coli* infection.

Internal Laying: An aberration in which the fully formed egg comes to lie in the abdominal cavity. Such eggs act as foreign bodies and may become surrounded by inflammatory tissue resembling a tumor. No control or treatment is known.

Prolapse of the Oviduct ("Blowouts"): A displacement of the oviduct characterized by a large mass protruding from the vent. The following factors may be involved: sex hormone imbalance, hereditary predisposition, laying at too early an age, laying eggs of an unusually large size, and starting production when overly fat.

If the condition is observed early, affected birds should be removed from the flock, the prolapsed part washed and replaced by gentle pressure. If the tissues are swollen, dirty and injured, the bird should be destroyed. The condition invites cannibalism.

Salpingitis (Oviductitis): An inflammation of the oviduct characterized by distension of this structure with a foul-smelling exudate. A great variety of bacteria may cause salpingitis, but enteric species are commonest. The infection arises in some cases as a result of invasion from the intestinal tract. In young growing pullets, it is often associated with mycoplasmosis or infectious bronchitis. At necropsy, a severe peritonitis is usually found. The oviduct is enlarged and filled with white or yellow, thick, tenacious exudate. In cases of longer standing, the exudate may be firm, caseous or inspissated. The disease accounts for much of the mortality in laying flocks. Since so many different organisms seem involved, bacteriologic examination is of little value. Treatment is not practical and the affected bird should be destroyed.

DISORDERS OF THE SKELETAL SYSTEM

This discussion is of disorders of genetic or unknown etiology. Disorders due to specific infectious diseases are discussed earlier in this section (part III) while those due to nutritional deficiencies are discussed in part V (p. 1263 *et seq.*). (*See also* OSTEOPETROSIS, p. 1090.)

Spondylolisthesis (Kinky Back): A developmental anomaly of the spinal column of broiler chickens. The sixth thoracic vertebra twists in a longitudinal plane with downward angulation of the anterior end. Compression of the spinal cord at the junction of the sixth and seventh vertebrae causes posterior paralysis. A few birds affected with clinical spondylolisthesis are found in many broiler flocks between 3 and 6 weeks of age, and an incidence of 1% has been reported in some flocks. Many broiler chickens are affected with subclinical spondylolisthesis in which twisting of the sixth vertebra occurs without cord compression. Affected birds sit in a typical position with the weight on their hocks and tail and their feet off the ground. If disturbed the only movement they are capable of making is to struggle backwards on their hocks. Some fall on their sides and usually are incapable of righting themselves. A high rate of growth during the first week of life increases the incidence. It is thought that staphylococci may be the primary cause of this condition; in any case they cause stress and make it worse. There is some evidence that genotype is important in the development of spondylolisthesis. Clinically affected birds should be culled.

Twisted Leg: An outward or inward bending and twisting of the leg of chickens and turkeys. The deformity is generally unilateral and the main deformation occurs in the distal tibiotarsal and to a lesser extent in the proximal tarsometatarsal bone. In some cases the gastrocnemius tendon is displaced laterally. A few affected birds are found in most broiler chicken and turkey flocks; in some flocks an increased incidence may be encountered. The etiology is poorly understood. The incidence of the deformity has been shown experimentally to be influenced by genotype and brooding conditions. The incidence is increased when broiler chickens are raised in batteries. Affected birds should be culled.

Twisted leg superficially appears similar to **perosis (chondrodystrophy, q.v., p. 1424)**. In perosis shortening of long bones due to degenerative changes in growth plates occurs prior to deformation of the leg. Perosis is commonly due to a deficiency of manganese or one of several B-vitamins and is rare in poultry fed commercial rations.

Rotated Tibia: A rotation of the shaft of the tibiotarsus which results in the metatarsus pointing laterally. The hock joint is normal with neither displacement of the gastrocnemius tendon nor bending of the distal tibiotarsal bone. The lesion is unilateral and the affected leg is often abducted giving a "spraddle legged" posture. This leg deformity primarily affects young turkeys from 2 to 14 weeks of age and an incidence in some flocks of 15% has been reported. The etiology is obscure. Affected birds should be culled.

Tibial Dyschondroplasia: A persistent mass of hypertrophic cartilage in the proximal end of the tibiotarsal bone in growing broiler chickens and turkeys. In many birds the abnormal cartilage is restricted to the posterior medial portion of the proximal tibiotarsal bone, and birds are clinically normal. An incidence of 10 to 30% of birds with subclinical dyschondroplasia is common in many flocks. In more severe cases the abnormal cartilage occupies the whole metaphysis of the proximal tibiotarsal bone and also develops in the proximal tarsometatarsal bone. Birds with these more severe lesions may be lame with bowing of the affected bones. In some instances fractures have occurred below the abnormal cartilage. The incidence of tibial dyschondroplasia is affected by the genotype and the acid-base balance of the diet.

Crooked Toes: A common developmental anomaly in both young growing turkeys and chickens affecting a few birds in most flocks. Toes are bent either laterally or medially in a horizontal plane. Careful examination reveals twisting of the phalanges. This condition must be differentiated from curled toes due to a riboflavin deficiency in which the toes are curled downwards and the primary lesion is in the nervous system. Crooked toes impairs the mobility of the bird and probably reduces production efficiency. The cause is not understood but the incidence can be increased by infrared brooding and wire floors.

DEGENERATIVE MYOPATHY OF TURKEYS

(Green muscle disease)

A condition involving degeneration, necrosis and fibrosis of the deep pectoral (supracoracoideus) muscle. The highest reported incidence in any one flock is 25%. The defect is found principally in turkeys of breeding age, and only to a very limited extent in birds under 24 weeks old. Clinically, the disease causes little or no problem. The primary loss is from downgrading and condemnation of carcasses at processing. This condition should not be confused with the muscular dystrophy of birds that bilaterally affects the pectoral and wing muscles.

The myopathy may occur unilaterally or bilaterally and primarily affects the middle one-third of the muscle, often the middle and posterior two-thirds, and rarely involves the anterior one-third. In advanced cases the defect is grossly apparent by a depression of the breast on the affected side or sides. Early in the disease, the affected muscle may be greenish, hemorrhagic and edematous. Ultimately, there is liquefaction and absorption of necrotic tissue leaving a fibrotic atrophic portion of muscle. The lesion is felt to be caused by ischemia possibly due to insufficient vascular supply of the large-breasted birds or to pathologic changes of the vasculature limiting blood supply to the muscle.

The condition is a heritable characteristic of polygenic nature, variable in expressivity and penetrance. Experimental selective breeding for the trait has decreased the age of onset and increased the incidence. A similar myopathy has been observed in broiler breeder-type chickens, which supports the belief that the defect is a result of selection for breast development. Research to identify genetic carriers by serum enzyme tests has been inconclusive. Nutritional studies have ruled out the involvement of selenium, vitamin E, and methionine in the condition. Experimental results suggest that certain types of stress factors increases expression of the defect.

THE TURKEY LEG EDEMA SYNDROME

A condition of unknown cause in slaughter age turkeys. It is characterized by edema in the subcut. tissues of the leg and the inguinal space, accompanied by a disseminated focal myopathy.

First reported in 1967, it has occurred sporadically throughout the U.S.A. since that time, primarily in heavy toms, but sometimes also in heavy hen turkeys. It occurs throughout the slaughter season but is more frequent in August through October. Rarely diagnosed ante mortem, it is detectable by palpation. About 5% of all flocks are affected; incidence within flocks varies from 2 to 70%.

The condition is often unilateral. The defeathered skin over the area of the edema shows no evidence of trauma, but does appear blanched and is "slick" to the touch. The edema fluid contains a variable number of gas bubbles, and may be amber, red or greenish or may be manifested by an accumulation of yellowish inflammatory exudate. Microscopic evidence of muscle degeneration is also variable. The lesion usually appears as an abnormal segment separating normal appearing muscle tissue.

Although the cause remains obscure, reduction of transportation trauma is said to reduce losses.

ROUND HEART DISEASE (RH)

A disease affecting poultry, primarily turkeys, characterized by sudden death due to cardiac arrest. It has been described in pigs.

Incidence: In commercial flocks the incidence of the disease varies from 3 to 28% with an average mortality of 1 to 5%. Field reports suggest a higher incidence during the early brooding season of February to April, and higher mortality in severely affected flocks. Most deaths occur when the poults are 2 to 4 weeks old.

Clinical Findings and Diagnosis: The affected poult appears unthrifty and droopy, has ruffled feathers and is dyspneic. Necropsy usually reveals cardiomegaly with marked hypertrophy of the right ventricle, flaccidness of myocardium, ascites and pulmonary edema. Electrocardiographic recordings and assays of total serum protein and trypsin inhibition capacity (TIC) may be used for identification of RH poultry. The average TIC of unaffected poults has been reported as 1.086 ± 0.126 compared with 0.698 ± 0.081 in RH poults. Hypoproteinemia is pronounced with total serum protein values approximately 50% of that seen in normal poults.

Etiology: Various factors have been suggested as causative agents: hereditary predisposition, management practices such as the introduction of toxic materials with an affinity for cardiac muscle, serum protein deficiencies (e.g. α_1-antitrypsin), viruses and dietary deficiencies of trace materials (e.g. copper and selenium). The pathogenesis of the disease may involve the interaction of genetics with management practices and environmental factors.

Treatment and Prevention: In the absence of specific treatment, supportive therapy is recommended. This includes: (1) changing the feed to remove possibility of toxic contaminants, (2) lowering the level of dietary salt to 0.2 to 0.3% in corn-soybean diets, (3) curtailing activity of poults by reducing the amount of light, (4) checking brooder temperatures to prevent chilling of poults, (5) maintaining dry litter, and (6) improving ventilation in confined areas. Daily administration of immunosuppressive doses of cortisone (℞ 138) has been employed to reduce mortality in RH poults during the first 10 days after hatching. Poults that recover usually regain lost weight, but tend to be hypotensive.

Preventive measures are limited to the practice of good management. It is known that therapeutic doses of the feed additive, furazolidone, are extremely toxic to the young turkey poult resulting in a syndrome similar, if not identical, to spontaneous RH disease. Decrease in reported incidence of RH disease may be due to increased avoidance of toxic levels of this nitrofuran in the diet.

DISSECTING ANEURYSM IN TURKEYS

(Aortic rupture, Internal hemorrhage)

A fatal disease of turkeys, and less frequently of chickens, characterized by massive hemorrhage resulting from rupture of aneurysms formed in various parts of the blood vascular system by blood being forced between the coats of the arterial wall. The frequency with which the posterior aorta is affected has given rise to the term "aortic rupture."

The disease has been reported in the U.S.A., Canada and Great Britain. The largest and most rapidly growing male turkeys, between 8 and 24 weeks of age, in the best-managed flocks, are most often affected. The disease also occurs in females, but the incidence is lower. It is seldom observed in poorly managed flocks. The disease has been observed in most breeds of turkeys raised in the U.S.A. Dissecting aneurysms also occur in chickens, but the incidence is extremely low.

Etiology: The exact cause is still unknown. Three factors probably must be present before fatal dissecting aneurysms will occur: The birds must be fed and managed in such a way that they are growing rapidly, there is some evidence that the birds must have a genetic susceptibility, and there must be a prolonged lipemia during the period of rapid growth. The lipemia may result from a high dietary intake of fat or the effects of hormonal factors, such as high levels of estrogens. Although β-aminopropionitrile, the toxic agent in *Lathyrus odoratus*, is capable of producing dissecting aneurysms in turkeys, there is no evidence that the nitriles are responsible for the occurrence of dissecting aneurysms under natural conditions.

Clinical Findings: Affected birds are found dead with no premonitory signs of disease. Occasionally, a caretaker will observe an apparently healthy bird die within a few minutes. The incidence is usually less than 1%, but may rise to 10%. Formerly, when male turkeys were implanted with stilbestrol, the incidence was as high as 20%.

Lesions: Necropsy reveals markedly anemic cadavers with large quantities of clotted blood in the peritoneal cavity or pericardial sac. Occasionally, massive hemorrhage into the lungs, kidneys and leg muscles occurs. The rupture in the wall of the posterior aorta at about the position of the testes, or in the atrium, can readily be located by carefully washing away the clot. Ruptures in smaller blood vessels are more difficult to locate.

Histologic examination reveals that the aortic rupture is caused by an intramedial hemorrhage of the dissecting type. In almost every instance, there is either intimal thickening or a large, fibrous plaque in the region of the rupture. Staining for fats reveals that there is a marked accumulation of lipids in the thickened intima and in the fibrous plaques.

Treatment: There is no known treatment; coagulants and vitamin K are useless, since there is no defect in the clotting mechanism.

Losses sometimes may be reduced during the critical period between 16 and 20 weeks of age by limiting feed intake. High-fat diets should not be fed during this period. There is some evidence that continuous, low-level feeding of reserpine after 4 weeks of age reduces losses from this disease (0.0001% in the ration for not more than 5 days or 0.00002% continuously).

POISONINGS

See also the general section on TOXICOLOGY, p. 964 *et seq.* Generally birds are less susceptible to poisoning than are mammals. A point of some significance, however is the possibility of residues of toxic substances in eggs or poultry meat. Label recommendations regarding withdrawal times for all potentially toxic substances should be scrupulously followed.

Inorganic Sources

Carbon monoxide: This poisoning commonly arises from exhaust fumes when chicks are being transported by truck or from anthracite or oil heaters. The mortality may be high unless fresh air is provided immediately. At necropsy, the beak is cyanotic and a characteristic bright pink color is noted throughout the viscera, particularly the lungs. Diagnosis can be confirmed by a spectroscopic analysis of the blood.

Arsenic: Rat poisons, Paris green, lead arsenate and other arsenicals are common sources of poisonings in birds. Chickens are quite tolerant to arsenic and, unless large amounts are consumed, few deaths occur. Poisoned birds become restless and show spasmodic jerking of the neck. There may be a depraved appetite and loss of equilibrium. Large doses cause submucous inflammation of the crop and gizzard and a catarrhal enteritis. Severe kidney degeneration may be noted.

Copper: Copper sulfate in single doses above 1.0 gm is fatal. The signs are a watery diarrhea and listlessness. A catarrhal gastroenteritis accompanied by a greenish seromucous exudate throughout the intestinal tract is found at necropsy.

Lead: Lead poisoning usually is caused by paint or orchard-spray material. Amounts of 7.2 mg of metallic lead per pound of body weight are lethal. Clinical signs are depression, loss of appetite, emaciation, thirst and muscular weakness. Greenish droppings are commonly observed within 36 hours. As poisoning progresses, the wings may be extended downward. Young birds may die within 36 hours after ingesting lead. Diagnosis of acute lead poisoning may be made from the history and necropsy findings of a greenish brown gizzard mucosa, enteritis and degeneration of the liver and kidney. Chronic poisoning produces emaciation, and atrophy of the liver and heart. The pericardium is distended with fluid and the gall-bladder is thickened and enlarged. Urate deposits are usually found in the kidneys. Ingestion of lead shot often occurs in wild waterfowl on heavily gunned feeding grounds. The retention of only a few lead pellets in the gizzard can kill a duck.

Mercury: Poisoning occurs from mercurial disinfectants and fungicides, including mercurous chloride (calomel) and bichloride of mercury (corrosive sublimate). Clinical signs are progressive muscular weakness and incoordination. Diarrhea may occur, depending on the amount of chemical ingested. In some cases, the caustic action of the chemical produces gray areas in the mouth and esophagus, which usually ulcerate if the bird lives for more than 24 hours. Catarrhal inflammation of the proventriculus and intestines occurs in some birds. If a large amount of mercury is ingested, extensive hemorrhage may occur in these organs. The kidneys are pale and studded with small white foci. The liver shows fatty degeneration.

Selenium: The ingestion of feeds containing more than 5 ppm of selenium decreases the hatchability of eggs because of deformities of the embryos, which are unable to emerge from the shell because of beak anomalies. Eyes may be missing and feet and wings may be deformed or underdeveloped.

Selenium in a concentration of 10 ppm, as in seleniferous grains in the laying ration, usually reduces hatchability of fertile eggs to zero. Mature birds seem to tolerate more selenium in their feed than swine, cattle or horses, without exhibiting signs of poisoning other than poor hatchability of the eggs. Starting rations containing 8 ppm selenium have reduced the growth rate of chicks, but 4 ppm had no noticeable effect on growth rate. The feeding of rations containing as little as 2.5 ppm to poultry has resulted in meat and eggs containing concentrations of selenium in excess of the suggested tolerance limit in foods.

Sodium arsenite and some of the organic arsenicals, when administered to laying hens with selenium, have given some improvement in hatchability.

Salt: The addition of 0.5% salt (NaCl) to the ration of chickens and turkeys is recommended, but amounts in excess of 2% are usually considered dangerous. Rations for chicks have contained as much as 8% without injurious effect, but rations containing 4% were harmful to poults and levels of 6 to 8% have resulted in mortality. The addition of 2% sodium chloride to the feed, or 4 parts per thousand in the water, will depress growth in young ducks and lower the fertility and hatchability of the eggs in breeding stock.

Salt levels high enough to produce salt poisoning may be reached when salty protein concentrates are added to rations already fortified with salt or when the salt is poorly incorporated in the feed. Sporadic poisoning has also been reported from the accidental ingestion of rock salt or salt provided for other livestock. Necropsy findings are not diagnostic. Enteritis and ascites are common findings. Watery droppings and wet litter can often be suggestive of a high-salt intake.

Boric acid: This is quite toxic for birds, resulting in depression, diarrhea and progressive weakness. Necropsy findings include severe crop thickening, gastroenteritis and degenerative kidney changes.

Organic Sources

Various organic chemicals, especially those used to treat seed grain, are dangerous.

Thiram: This substance, used to treat seed corn, is toxic to chicks at 40 ppm and goslings at 150 ppm, causing leg deformities and loss of weight. Turkey poults tolerate up to 200 ppm.

EDB (ethylene dibromide): Certain grains treated with fumigants containing this chemical are toxic to laying hens. Egg weights are significantly reduced with as little as 0.5 mg of EDB per bird daily.

BAPN (β-aminopropionitrile): This substance is toxic for turkeys. In diets containing *Lathyrus odoratus* seeds, BAPN at 0.06% produced massive internal hemorrhage, particularly of the aorta in turkeys. BAPN at 0.03 and 0.06% of the diet of laying hens produced soft-shelled and malformed eggs and egg production and hatchability were significantly reduced.

DDT (dichlorodiphenyl-trichloroethane): This chemical, once much used for fly and insect control, is toxic to birds if consumed at levels about 0.03% of the diet. The clinical signs are dyspnea, tremor, convulsions and prostration. Death may occur. There are no significant lesions found at necropsy.

Crotalaria: Many species of *Crotalaria* seeds are toxic to chickens. Concentrations above 0.05% in the feed produce signs of toxicosis. There is a marked reduction in weight gain at 0.2 and 0.3% will cause death in 18 days. Lesions consist of ascites, swelling or atrophy of the liver and hemorrhages. Resistance to the toxin increases with age.

Common vetch: The seed of the common vetch, *Vicia sativa* will cause high mortality when fed at levels of 30 to 40% of the rations.

Nicotine: The usual source of poisoning from nicotine is "Black Leaf 40", which contains 40% nicotine sulfate. Amounts of 0.5 to 1 ml are fatal. This solution is used for the control of external parasites by painting it on the roosts. It is volatile at high temperatures. Affected birds show uneasiness, wing paralysis, dilated pupils and often vomit. Ecchymoses in the heart and lungs are seen at necropsy.

Toxic Fat: A crystalline halogen has been identified as the "toxic fat" factor in some feed, which produces hydropericardium and ascites in young chickens. In young pullets it reduces growth, retards sexual development and increases mortality. Hatchability is lowered. Turkeys and ducks are less susceptible than chickens. The signs of intoxication include ruffled feathers, droopiness and labored breathing. Lesions include ascites and hydropericardium, necrosis of liver, subepicardial hemorrhage and bile duct hyperplasia. Although the amount of toxin varies in feeds from different sources, 0.25 to 5% fed for 35 to 150 days produced typical lesions.

Carbolineum: Fumes resulting from this chlorinated coal-tar poultry house spray produce burns of the face, wattles and feet, together with gasping, ascites, and acute swelling and degeneration of the liver.

Gossypol: Cottonseed meal contains appreciable amounts of gossypol, which produces severe cardiac edema resulting in dyspnea, weakness and anorexia.

Polychlorinated biphenyl: PCB residues have recently been reported in chicken and turkey meat in excess of the 5 ppm permitted in edible tissue, and in egg products in excess of the permitted 0.5 ppm. The product has been traced to such sources as heat-exchange fluid and plastic wrappers from bakery goods that have been ground and included in poultry feed. Presently, spectrographic methods have been developed to clearly distinguish between PCBs and chlorinated pesticides such as DDD and DDT. PCBs depress egg production and markedly reduce hatchability. PCBs are found in the fatty tissue of the birds. Up to 40 ppm in tissue does not produce changes that are evident in birds by gross necropsy.

Autointoxication

Self-poisoning due to the retention of the waste products of metabolism or the absorption of products of decomposition including bacterial toxins that occur within the intestine. Signs include cyanosis, sluggishness and diarrhea. Congestion of the muscles and viscera with kidney congestion, swelling and blockage may be noted. A catarrhal enteritis is usually present. Antibiotics (e.g. chlortetracycline, oxytetracycline) given at 0.01% in the mash may be helpful together with a laxative (℞ 503).

MISCELLANEOUS CONDITIONS AFFECTING POULTRY

BREAST BLISTERS

A large abscess, usually found on the carinal apex of the sternum, containing a clear or blood-tinged fluid or thick, white-to-yellow pus. The condition in market chickens and turkeys causes serious financial loss when birds are sold. The etiology is obscure, but direct trauma and heritable predisposition suggest themselves. In birds raised on wire or contacting sharp-edged troughs, injuries may occur as early as 6 weeks of age. Staphylococci are commonly recovered from these lesions. Heavy turkeys raised on wire, or older roosting birds are also occasionally affected. Frequently the condition is not noticed until the birds are marketed.

Provided the blisters have not reached an advanced stage, the fluid can be drained surgically and flushed with a 1:10,000 solution of potassium permanganate. To be economically successful, this treatment must be carried out at least one month prior to marketing. Simple breast blisters should be differentiated from infectious synovitis (q.v., p. 1064), which usually affects other synovial structures.

BUMBLEFOOT

(Abscess of the foot pads)

A sporadic local infection of the feet of chickens and turkeys characterized by enlargement and lameness in one or both feet. The condition usually appears after an injury to the food pad. Various bacteria may be present, but staphylococci are most commonly found. A fowl cholera organism (*Pasteurella*) of low virulence and *Mycobacterium avium* have also been reported. The condition is commoner in the heavy breeds. Lameness is associated with a localized bulbous swelling of the foot pad. A superficial wound may or may not be present. In advanced cases, the entire leg may be involved. Although the condition may be obvious, it should be differentiated from infectious synovitis (q.v., p. 1064). The latter disease occurs usually in birds up to 12 weeks of age, whereas bumblefoot is more prevalent in older, heavier birds.

The incidence may be reduced by removal of high roosts and other objects which allow birds to jump from high places to concrete floors. Equipment should not have sharp projections or protruding nails as these may injure the feet. If treatment is elected, the hard core or pus in the swelling should be evacuated, bleeding controlled, and the resulting cavity thoroughly cleaned and painted with tincture of iodine, or packed with ammoniated mercurial ointment. Sulfathiazole ointment has also proved satisfactory.

GOUT

(Acute toxic nephritis)

A condition of low incidence, cause unknown, usually found in adult hens, characterized by the presence of urates in the viscera or joints. Two types of the disease occur, visceral and articular. Vitamin A deficiency and high-protein diets have both been suggested as of etiologic significance, but there is little evidence to support these views. Affected birds become dull and listless, and eventually die. The condition must be distinguished from thallium poisoning. At necropsy, the visceral type shows a white, flakelike, material (uric acid crystals) covering all abdominal organs. This material may also be present in the pericardial sac. In the articular type, which is uncommon, the joints may be enlarged and swollen. When opened, these joints exude a thick, white, tenacious fluid, composed almost entirely of synovia and uric acid crystals.

No specific treatment or control is known, but ample fresh water is indicated.

KERATOCONJUNCTIVITIS

A condition of chickens, ducklings and turkeys characterized by a severe conjunctivitis, keratitis and ulceration of the cornea, commonly leading to blindness in one or both eyes. The morbidity in turkeys may reach 40% and in chickens it may approach 100%. The condition should be differentiated from a clouding of the lens that is frequently found in avian encephalomyelitis (q.v., p. 1063) and sometimes Newcastle disease (q.v., p. 1106). Pox, fowl cholera, *Pseudomonas* spp. and other bacterial organisms are specific causes. The condition, however, is generally associated with a high atmospheric concentration of ammonia which arises from the litter under circumstances of poor ventilation and unsanitary surroundings. It can usually be controlled by changing to fresh, dry litter and improving the ventilation. Supplementing the ration with vitamin A may be helpful. Affected birds should be isolated, if possible, and treated individually with antibiotic eye ointments and vitamin A concentrates. If feed and water are convenient so blind birds can locate them, recovery will usually occur.

PENDULOUS CROP

(Crop bound, Sour crop, Impacted crop, Sagging crop)

A disease of both chickens and turkeys characterized by a greatly enlarged, dependent crop which becomes distended with food. The cause is unknown, but hereditary factors, impaction due to coarse, long-fibered food, or paralysis of the crop may be of etiologic importance. No treatment is completely satisfactory. Flooding the crop with isotonic salt solution or mineral oil through a dose syringe, to loosen the mass, may effect a cure. In valuable birds, surgical removal of the contents and reduction of the crop size is reasonably successful.

CANNIBALISM

A vice of chickens, turkeys and game birds reared in captivity, characterized by varying degrees of tissue loss from picking of the vent, tail, toe, head, wing, nose, back, snood and caruncle (listed in order of occurrence).

Etiology: Predisposing causes include: overcrowding, excessive light and temperature, insufficient or improperly placed feeder or drinking space, nutritional imbalances including mineral deficiencies, feeding only pelleted or concentrated feed, feeding high caloric diets heavy in corn or low fiber grains, insufficient secluded nests, injuries (e.g. freezing of comb or wattles or infection of ear lobes), blood present at the vent when birds lay large eggs, lack of canvas saddles to protect the backs of breeder hens from treading by tom turkeys in mating pens.

Types of Cannibalism: Feather pulling, wing and tail picking are most frequently seen in young birds. Head picking is generally noted in older birds in cages. Toe and vent picking are usually seen in young domestic or game birds, but vent picking can be serious in adult laying birds. Nose and tail picking are often observed in overcrowded quail 2-to-7 weeks of age. Back injury and picking with resultant discoloration occur more often in turkeys. Snood and caruncle injury and hemorrhage may often be noted in tom turkeys following fighting.

Prophylaxis and Treatment: Prevention is aided by ideal husbandry practices. Debeaking (removing the upper, or upper and lower, portion of the beak by electric cautery) is the commonest method of control. It may be done at day one or at any time in the life of the bird. Careless debeaking can cause permanent damage and prevent adequate feed consumption, likewise birds debeaked in high egg production will not eat properly and will often go out of production. Turkeys may also have a small ring placed in the upper beak to prevent cannibalism.

ARTIFICIAL INSEMINATION IN POULTRY

Low fertility in the turkey, caused by deficient mating resulting from large, heavily muscled birds or reduced sex drive, is a serious and costly problem in the production of hatching eggs. AI is widely used to overcome this problem. In chickens, the practice has not found wide application, but is routinely used in special breeding work.

Chicken and turkey semen is collected by stimulating the male to protrude its copulatory organ by massaging the underside of the abdomen and the back over the testes. This is followed quickly by pushing the tail forward with one hand and, at the same time, using the thumb and forefinger of the same hand to "milk" semen from the ducts of this organ. Ejaculation is more rapid in the chicken than in the turkey. The semen is usually collected with an aspirator. The volume of semen averages about 0.20 to 0.25 ml in the turkey, with a spermatozoon concentration of 6 to 10 million or more per cubic millimeter. In the chicken, semen volume is 2 or 3 times, and the spermatozoon concentration approximately one-half, that in the turkey.

Chicken and turkey semen cannot yet be stored for longer than about an hour without considerable loss of fertilizing capacity. Similarly, semen from either of these species is not normally diluted before being used for insemination. However, freshly collected turkey semen diluted 1:1 with 1.024% saline, having a freezing point depression of −0.65°C, gives as good fertility as undiluted semen when used immediately. This applies early in the season but fertility decreases rapidly later in the season. Further dilution tends to reduce drastically the fertilizing capacity of the semen. Several commercial semen diluents or extenders are available.

For insemination, pressure is applied to the abdomen around the vent. This causes the cloaca to evert and the oviduct to protrude so that a syringe or the plastic straw on the insemination gun can be inserted about an inch into the oviduct and the correct amount of semen delivered. Due to the high sperm concentration of turkey semen, 0.025 ml of undiluted pooled semen gives optimum fertility. However, amounts as small as 0.01 ml have also been shown to give excellent results. For maximum fertility, turkeys must be inseminated at regular intervals of 10 to 14 days. In the chicken, due to the lower spermatozoon concentration and shorter duration of fertility, 0.1 ml of undiluted pooled semen, at intervals of 5 to 7 days, is required to maintain fertility at a high level.

PART IV
FUR, LABORATORY AND ZOO ANIMALS

FUR-ANIMAL MANAGEMENT

MINK

The ranch should be located on well-drained soil, well away from urban areas. There are no practical means of reducing the odor of a mink farm. A guard fence around the ranch aids in preventing the escape of mink from the ranch, and keeping out stray dogs or skunks.

Mink are housed individually in wire mesh pens raised above the ground. A nest box with a hole for entry is attached outside or placed within the pen. Soft marsh hay free from awns, or fine wood-wool makes suitable nest material. Nest boxes should be cleaned and nest material replaced as required, especially before a female whelps, and during cold weather.

Sheds may be used throughout the year, provided lighting is adequate to supply the usual daylight hours and there is plenty of air circulation in the warmer months. Artificial lights in the sheds must be used with caution as they may influence the breeding season.

Mink are fed by placing a day's ration of a meat-cereal-water mixture on top of the wire. Most ranchers place food on pans inside the run for small kits which cannot reach the food on top of the pen. Mink require an ample supply of fresh water. Watering cups fastened to the outside of the pen with a lip protruding inside are commonly used. Automatic watering systems with individual nipples are used in sheds, until the temperature drops to freezing. Cold storage facilities are necessary to freeze and store the meat portion of the ration. A day's supply of meat and meat by-products is thawed, cereal is added and the combined ration is mixed with water to a consistency that will remain on the wire of the pen without dropping through. Ready-mixed feeds are available in some areas. This may be delivered daily, ready to feed, or may be in frozen blocks, which are kept in cold storage and thawed as required. Dry pelleted diets are used on some ranches for part of the year.

Mink are normally pelted in November or December. Several methods of killing are used, depending on the preference of the rancher. Cervical dislocation is commonly used. Magnesium sulfate, nicotine sulfate, ether or strychnine may be injected into the heart.

Ranchers usually keep one male for each 5 female breeders. March is the mating season. Mink are much more active at this time, and a clucking sound is characteristic, but there are no external signs of estrus. After a male is placed in a female's pen, mating should occur within an hour. If fighting ensues they should be separated. Ovulation is induced by coitus. Females may ovulate 2 or 3 times and 2 matings are usual to ensure a high conception rate but there should be an interval of 6 to 8 days between matings. Ova from 2 ovulations have been known to contribute to the same litter. There is delayed implantation of the fertilized ova, so the apparent gestation period varies from 40 to 75 days.

Mink have one litter a year of 1 to 12 kits (average 4). Most litters are born during the last week in April and the first 2 weeks in May. Kits are blind, hairless and weigh about 10 gm when born, but grow rapidly throughout the summer to reach a weight of about 800 gm (females) or 1,600 gm (males) by October. Kits are weaned at about 6 to 8 weeks of age, and may be separated shortly thereafter into singles, twos or threes. Adult mink are extremely agile, strong and vicious. Handling requires the use of special leather gloves or squeeze cages.

CHINCHILLA

The chinchilla is a small rodent with large, almost hairless ears, prominent tactile hairs protruding from the upper lip, and well-developed hind limbs. The fur, which is very soft and normally grayish, is produced in tufts of several strands from each hair follicle. The female, weighing about 1.5 lb (0.68 kg) is slightly larger than the male. The color and marking of both sexes are the same. There are now 3 recognized species, the Peruvian, *Chinchilla chinchilla chinchilla*, the Bolivian, *C. boliviana* (both formerly *C. brevicaudata*), and the Chilean, *C. villidera* (formerly *C. laniger*). The differences are minor, the former 2 species being slightly larger and darker.

Although chinchillas originated from the Andes mountains of South America, they can be raised almost anywhere in temperate zones. Ranchers with a smaller number of animals may keep them in dry and well-ventilated basements. If a special building is planned for chinchilla raising, it should be situated so that its length runs north and south, to allow the animals access to a maximum of sunlight.

Pens are usually constructed of wire mesh for easy cleaning and adequate circulation of air. A nest box may be used. Water is usually supplied from bottles or by an automatic system. A pan or box containing a mixture of Fuller's earth and white sand should be placed in the pen each day, to provide a dust bath. A hayrack and a self-feeder for pellets should be included as part of the equipment for each pen. Exercise wheels are not necessary, but a small block of wood should be provided on which the chinchilla may satisfy its urge to chew.

The pens must be cleaned regularly; the interval is dependent on the type of pen. Most mild disinfectants can be used. Cresol compounds should be avoided since they may cause a severe inflammation of the feet. Water bottles should be cleaned, disinfected and rinsed thoroughly at frequent intervals.

The breeding unit should have an area designated for the storage of hay and pellets. Some feed rooms have a solid bale-sized bin for hay. Metal refuse cans may be used to store pellets. Rodents, dogs and other animals must be kept away from feeds that the chinchillas are to consume.

Chinchillas may breed when they are 7 to 9 months old. Either pair-mating, or the controlled access of one male to a battery of 4 or 5 pens each containing a female, may be used. Mating often occurs at night and may be preceded by a fight. One of the best indications of a successful breeding is the finding of a "stopper" or plug-like structure in the bottom of the pen. This structure is formed in the vagina and is expelled at the time of breeding, but it may not be found because frequently it is consumed by one of the chinchillas. The gestation period varies with the species; for *C. villidera*, the average is 111 days, while for the other 2 it is 128 days. If the female has conceived, the mammary glands will enlarge soon after the 60th day. A litter consists of 1 to 4 young, the average being 2. The female comes in estrus within a few hours of parturition. The male is sometimes left in the pen during littering so that a mating may take place shortly thereafter, although the female may be aggressive at this time. A second estrus occurs within about 28 days.

Newborn chinchillas are furred and active at birth but should not be subjected to drafts. Heat (e.g. a small electric light bulb) should be provided in the nest box, especially in cold, damp weather. The young should be kept under observation for the first few days, to be certain that they are being nourished adequately. If the female is weak or the young are orphaned, a lactating guinea pig may be substituted for the mother. Dry fortified cereal such as that used for babies makes a satisfactory supplement for young chinchillas. Litters of more than 3 kits often require hand-feeding, although extra kits can usually be transferred to another female littering at the same time with only 1 kit. Unusual noises in the nest box indicate that the young chinchillas' teeth are so sharp that the dam will not allow them to nurse; such teeth can be filed with a small emery board. The young are weaned at about 60 days.

Tattoo marks are made in the ears so that individual animals can be identified. The pelt becomes prime from December to February, depending on local climatic conditions. The most convenient way to handle chinchillas is by grasping them gently at the base of the tail. If they become excited, the hair comes out in patches. Chinchillas may bite, but they are not considered vicious.

DISEASES OF MINK

DISEASES OF VIRAL ETIOLOGY

Aleutian Disease
(Plasmacytosis)

A slow virus infection of mink, characterized by poor reproduction, gradual weight loss, oral and gastrointestinal bleeding, uremia, renal failure and high mortality. Aleutian color phases (blue mink) are most susceptible. The cause is a parvovirus. Transmission occurs *in utero* or by direct and indirect contact with infected mink.

Following infection, mink frequently respond with marked increases in immunoglobulin levels detectable by the iodine agglutination test (℞ 658) and specific antiviral antibody demonstrable by counterimmunoelectrophoresis. Glomerulonephritis and arteritis result from tissue deposition of circulating immune complexes. Gross pathologic changes include enlargement of the spleen, kidney changes varying from swelling and petechiation to atrophy and pitting, and enlargement of mesenteric lymph nodes. Histopathologically, the most characteristic findings include proliferation of plasma cells in the kidneys, liver, spleen, lymph nodes and bone marrow; bile duct proliferation in the liver; hyaline changes in renal glomeruli and tubules; and fibrinoid arteritis.

Control of the disease is possible by first screening the herd with the iodine agglutination test followed by testing for specific antibody with counterimmunoelectrophoresis. All mink testing positive are considered to be carriers. Mink that are to be kept for breeding stock are tested in late fall (before selection of breeding stock and pelting) and in January or February (before breeding). New introductions to the herd should be tested. Because there is no vaccination or effective treatment, all positive reactors should be pelted.

The virus is present in the saliva, urine, feces and blood of infected animals. Pens should be cleaned with 2% sodium hydroxide. Care should be taken to disinfect equipment after handling, vaccinating, or testing mink on infected farms.

Distemper

Mink of all ages are susceptible to canine distemper. The incubation period varies from 9 to 14 days. The virus may be recovered from infected mink 5 days before the appearance of clinical signs.

Mink that have apparently recovered may continue to shed the virus for several weeks.

Transmission may be direct (through contact or aerosol) or indirect (the virus may persist for a day or more in the environment). The first signs are usually a nasal and ocular exudate followed by hyperemia, swelling, wrinkling, thickening and crustiness of the skin on the face, feet and ventral abdominal wall, neurologic signs (convulsions and "screaming fits") or a combination of these.

At necropsy, organs usually appear to be normal, but histopathologic examination may reveal eosinophilic intracytoplasmic or intranuclear inclusions in epithelial cells of the urinary bladder, kidney, bile ducts, intestine, lung or trachea. Similar inclusions may be seen in mink with Aleutian disease, but distemper inclusions are negative with the periodic acid-Schiff stain.

Treatment is not recommended; all mink showing signs of distemper should be destroyed. All apparently normal mink should be vaccinated prophylactically at 10 to 11 weeks of age (10 days after weaning) and breeding stock should be vaccinated annually, in January or February. Aerosol vaccines may be advantageous, since handling subclinically infected mink is avoided and thus the possibility of transmission of distemper or other diseases by handling the mink or by using contaminated needles, syringes or other equipment, is minimized.

MINK VIRAL ENTERITIS

A highly contagious, feline-panleukopenia-like disease of mink, caused by a virus related but not identical to that of feline panleukopenia. All ages are susceptible, but the disease is most common in kits. Transmission usually occurs by the fecal-oral route, and the incubation period varies from 4 to 8 days. Clinical signs include anorexia, depression and the passage of pale, mucoid, unformed feces, often containing blood and intestinal casts. Characteristic gross pathologic findings are flaccid dilation and marked hyperemia of the small intestine, with liquid, fetid content, but these changes are not present in all affected mink. Histopathologic examination usually reveals severe enteritis, with hydropic degeneration of epithelial cells in the intestinal mucosa; these cells may contain inclusion bodies similar to those of feline panleukopenia.

All mink showing signs of viral enteritis should be destroyed, and all clinically normal mink should be vaccinated with a formalized tissue culture vaccine as soon as the diagnosis is made. A modified live virus vaccine is available in Canada. After an outbreak, breeders should be revaccinated in January or February, and annual vaccination of kits is recommended in endemic areas. Although the viruses of mink and feline enteritis are cross-immunogenic, they do not appear to be cross-infective under natural conditions.

AUJESZKY'S DISEASE
(Pseudorabies)

Aujeszky's disease is occasionally reported in mink fed contaminated pork products. Mortality may be high, and clinical signs are referable to the CNS (tonic and clonic convulsions, excitement alternating with depression and, in some cases, self-mutilation). The diagnosis is confirmed by inoculation of brain tissue from suspect mink into rabbits. Since contaminated pork is usually the source of infection, suspect pork should be cooked before it is fed to mink.

TRANSMISSIBLE MINK ENCEPHALOPATHY
(Mink scrapie)

This scrapie-like disease has caused high mortality in adult mink. The incubation period in experimental infections is 8 months or longer, and clinical signs are similar to those of scrapie (hyperirritability, ataxia, compulsive biting, somnolence, coma and death). Histopathologic findings in brains of affected mink are similar to those of scrapie in sheep. Although mink have been experimentally infected by intracerebral inoculation of brain material from scrapie-infected sheep, and by the feeding of tissues from infected mink, the means of natural transmission is unknown. Control measures cannot be suggested, therefore, except to suggest exclusion of sheep by-products from the ration in endemic areas.

BACTERIAL DISEASES

BOTULISM

Botulism occasionally causes heavy losses in unvaccinated mink consuming food containing botulinus (Type C) toxin. Usually, many mink are found dead within 24 hours of exposure to the toxin, while others show varying degrees of paralysis and dyspnea. Postmortem findings are nonspecific and are related to death from respiratory paralysis.

Toxic feed should be removed, and stored feed or ingredients examined for the presence of toxin. Antitoxin therapy is of questionable benefit, and recovered mink are not immune to further challenge. Annual vaccination of kits and breeders with botulism (Type C) toxoid is recommended to prevent outbreaks. Mink are usually vaccinated subcut. with a combined virus enteritis-botulism vaccine. This may be administered at the same time as distemper vaccine, but must be injected at a different site, since the formalin from this vaccine may inactivate the modified live virus distemper vaccine.

Hemorrhagic Pneumonia

This pneumonia, caused by *Pseudomonas aeruginosa*, may result in serious losses. Mink of all ages are affected, particularly in the warm, humid days of the fall. Mink are usually found dead with no prodromal signs. A thin, bloody nasal exudate may be observed at the time of death. One or more lobes of the lung are consolidated, the others may be hemorrhagic. Immediate administration of sulfathiazole (1 oz/150 lb [410 mg/kg] of wet mixed feed) and an equivalent quantity of sodium bicarbonate for 7 days as a herd treatment is recommended. This regimen may have to be repeated. The mink should have ample water. *Pseudomonas* bacterins have been used successfully.

Tuberculosis

Mink, particularly Aleutian types, are susceptible to infection with avian, bovine and human tubercle bacilli. Infection is usually food-borne, and the disease may become endemic on some ranches. Clinical signs include weight loss, and in some cases, abdominal distension. At necropsy, the mink is severely emaciated and has an enlarged spleen and lymph nodes; in many cases, there is miliary involvement of the lungs, liver and other organs. The diagnosis is confirmed on the basis of acid-fast stains of smears of affected tissues. Treatment of affected mink is ineffective and impractical, and control consists of culling visibly affected mink, and using meat products from inspected processing plants for feed. Tuberculin tests are generally ineffective in detecting infected mink.

Urinary Infections and Urolithiasis

Urinary tract infections cause serious losses in female mink in late spring (during pregnancy and lactation) and in male mink in late summer and autumn (during the rapid-growth and furring period). Several predisposing factors have been suggested, including avitaminosis-A, diethylstilbestrol toxicity, and contamination of food, cages or nest boxes by pathogenic bacteria.

Affected mink usually die without showing clinical signs. Gross postmortem findings include acute hemorrhagic cystitis or pyelonephritis or both, usually associated with urinary calculi (magnesium ammonium phosphate) in the bladder or kidneys. A variety of organisms, including staphylococci, coliforms and *Proteus*, are commonly isolated.

In severe outbreaks, bacteriologic culture and sensitivity tests should be done to determine the causative organism, and the treatment of choice added to the feed. Where a continual problem exists, feed grade (75%) phosphoric acid may be added to the feed (0.8 lb/100 lb [8 gm/kg] of wet mixed feed) from March to October, to educe the pH of the urine, since magnesium ammonium phosphate alculi are soluble in solutions of pH 6.0 or less.

Miscellaneous Bacterial Diseases

Various diseases, including septicemia, pneumonia, pleuritis, abcesses, cellulitis and enteritis occur sporadically on mink ranches, ut occasionally they may become herd problems. Many bacteria ave been isolated from these diseases, including *Proteus*, *Klebsilla*, coliforms, streptococci, staphylococci and salmonellae.

Antibacterial sensitivity tests should be done to determine the reatment of choice in individual mink, or the herd if several mink re involved. Drugs may be administered orally or parenterally and many mink are to be treated drugs should be added to the feed. Dosage can be estimated on the basis of body weight—female mink veigh 1½ lb (680 gm), and males from 4 to 4½ lb (1.8 to 2.1 kg). Dosage levels recommended for cats should be used and adjusted or weight. However, some sulfonamides, such as sulfaquinoxaline r sulfamethazine, and streptomycin are not recommended for mink.

Whenever possible, the source of infection should be determined nd eliminated. For example, enteritis is often caused by spoiled eed, and abscesses by injury from wire or splintered wood in the ens, awns in hay or straw used for bedding, or spicules of bone in ne feed. Outbreaks of tularemia, anthrax, brucellosis and clostridial nfections have been caused by the feeding of contaminated feed, ften containing tissue of animals that have died or are carriers of nese infections. Careful selection of feed ingredients, and disinfecon of equipment and pens are very important in the prevention nd control of many infections of mink.

NUTRITIONAL DISEASES

Steatitis (yellow fat disease) is common in young, rapidly growing nink as a result of excessive rancid unsaturated fatty acids in the iet. Affected mink may be found dead, or they may exhibit slight ocomotor disturbances followed by death. Necropsy findings inlude yellow, edematous internal or subcut. fat that contains an acidst pigment. Control consists of removal of the source of the rancid its, and proper storage of feed. Stabilized vitamin E may be administered in the feed (15 mg/mink) for 2 weeks, and affected kits hould be injected parenterally with 10 to 20 mg for several days.

Chastek paralysis (thiamin deficiency) results from feeding cerain raw fish containing thiaminase. These include whitefish, freshvater smelt, carp, goldfish, creek chub, fathead minnow, buckeye hiner, sucker, channel catfish, bullhead and minnow, white bass, auger pike, burbot and saltwater herring. Affected mink gradually ose their appetite and weight, and die after terminal convulsions nd paralysis. Thiaminase-containing fish should be cooked, or fed aw only on alternate days. Affected mink may be injected IP with 1 mg/lb (2 mg/kg) of body wt of thiamin hydrochloride, and adequate thiamin (brewer's yeast) should be present in the ration.

Because of the rapid growth of mink kits, **rickets** is common where rations are deficient in vitamin D, calcium or phosphorus. Affected kits usually crawl unsteadily in a frog-like posture, have rubbery bones, and are smaller than normal. The diet should be supplemented as required, and severely affected kits may be treated on an individual basis.

Nursing sickness occurs in lactating female mink. Affected females become thin and weak, stop eating and wander about aimlessly, ignoring their kits and sometimes carrying food in thei mouths without eating it. Death occurs within a few days of onset o clinical signs. Gross postmortem lesions are nonspecific, but include lipidosis of liver and kidney, and dehydration. Kits from affected females must be weaned or fostered as soon as possible and affected females should be tempted to eat with liver, freshl killed sparrows, etc. To control this condition, kits should be encouraged to start eating solid food as early as possible by placing trays containing soft feed in the pen. Salt may be added (0.5% c ration) if it is not already present in the commercial cereal, and plenty of fresh water and feed should be available to nursing females at all times.

Cotton underfur usually indicates **anemia in mink**, and may be caused by certain fish (Pacific hake, coalfish, whiting) which inter fere with iron retention in the mink. This condition can be pre vented by cooking the offending fish, or by feeding it on alternate days.

Gray underfur occurs when high levels of turkey offal or uncooked eggs are fed to young mink. Avidin, a factor present in eggs inactivates biotin, a vitamin required for pigmentation. Affected mink may be injected with 1 mg biotin twice weekly for 4 weeks and turkey offal should be cooked or biotin added to the ration.

POISONINGS

Lead poisoning is common in mink that have ingested lead-containing paints from wire or other equipment. Affected mink gradually lose weight and die within 1 or 2 months. Dicalcium phosphate or calcium gluconate and vitamin D should be added to the ration on affected ranches.

Insecticides other than pyrethrum, piperonyl butoxide and rote none may be highly toxic to mink. The above insecticides should not be used on mink under 8 weeks of age, or where these mink can contact them (e.g. nest boxes). Other insecticides should be avoided whenever possible.

Wood preservatives (chlorinated phenols, cresols) cause mortality of kits in the first 3 weeks of life, and occasionally, in older mink

They should not be used where mink can chew on treated wood (pens or nest boxes).

Diethylstilbestrol-containing products cause reproductive failure and a high incidence of urinary tract infections in mink, and care should be taken not to include them in the ration. Similarly, **thyroids and parathyroids** included in meat trimmings may result in reproductive failure if present at high levels.

Chlorinated hydrocarbons and **polychlorinated biphenyls** (PCB) contained in the ration have caused reproductive failure in mink.

DMNA: The addition of sodium nitrite as a preservative to stale herring meal results in the formation of dimethylnitrosamine (DMNA), which is very hepatotoxic in mink, causing hepatic degeneration, ascites and extensive internal hemorrhage.

Sulfaquinoxaline upsets normal blood-clotting mechanisms of mink and causes extensive internal hemorrhage resulting in serious losses. **Streptomycin** is very toxic to mink and the use of this antibiotic should be avoided whenever possible.

MISCELLANEOUS DISEASES

Fur-clipping and **tail-biting** are common vices of mink, and may be related to abnormal behavior patterns of captivity. Fur-clipping decreases the value of the pelt, and tail-biting frequently results in fatal hemorrhage. There is no effective treatment, but it may be advisable to avoid using affected mink for breeding purposes.

Urinary incontinence (wet-belly disease) is a nonfatal condition usually affecting male mink in the late summer and autumn, characterized by dribbling of urine and staining of the pelt around the urinary orifice. Since affected areas of the pelt must be discarded, the condition is of economic importance. Although the cause of this condition is unknown, recent work suggests that the feeding of high levels of fresh raw chicken waste or fish may be a cause, and that cooking these ingredients may prevent the disease.

Starvation and **chilling** are common causes of death in mink fed inadequate fat or too little feed during the winter and early spring. Affected mink are very thin, and may run until they collapse and die, or they may be found dead in their cages. Such deaths are commonest after a sudden decrease in environmental temperature, especially in the early spring. Postmortem examination reveals emaciation and an absence of body fat, in some cases accompanied by lipidosis and gastric ulceration. This disease must be differentiated from plasmacytosis and other chronic diseases on the basis of gross postmortem and histopathologic examination.

Gray diarrhea in mink resembles chronic pancreatitis in dogs, and is characterized by a ravenous appetite and the passage of large amounts of gray, fetid feces. Affected mink appear to die of starvation. No pancreatic abnormalities, viruses, bacteria or parasites have been demonstrated as possible causes. Treatment is of questionable value.

Pregnancy disease occurs in female mink in late pregnancy, and is characterized by death of affected mink with extensive placental hemorrhage. The cause of this condition is unknown, but fresh feed, fresh water and good bedding in nest boxes may be effective in preventing the disease.

Gastric ulcers and hepatic and renal **lipidosis** are common in mink, and are usually associated with other diseases or with a period of inappetence.

Hereditary diseases (hydrocephalus, hairlessness, "screw neck," "bobbed tails," Ehlers-Danlos syndrome, hemivertebra) are occasionally seen in mink and must be controlled by pelting of the sire, dam and litter mates of the affected mink.

Coccidiosis occasionally occurs and may cause losses. Coccidiostats, such as monensin or lasalocid, are effective in inhibiting coccidial multiplication.

Flesh-fly infestation: Flies of the genus *Wohlfahrtia* are the most important external parasites of mink. The only satisfactory measure of control is to use 5% ronnel dust in the nest boxes beginning a few days prior to the occurrence of the flies in an area. One heaping teaspoonful is placed in the nesting hay of each nest box. It should not be used for kits less than 3 days old. Treatment may be repeated once after a 14-day interval. (*See CUTEREBRA* INFESTATION OF SMALL ANIMALS, p. 775.)

DISEASES OF CHINCHILLAS

Many diseases of chinchillas are herd problems and are diagnosed on the basis of postmortem examination. Because several diseases may produce identical or similar pathologic lesions, they must be differentiated on the basis of bacteriologic culture. Clinical signs may be vague, nonspecific or nonexistent, although certain conditions such as dermatomycosis and malocclusion can be detected in the living animal.

Treatment is usually administered on a herd basis by medication of the drinking water or feed. If chinchillas appear reluctant to drink medicated water, sugar may be added in small amounts until water intake is normal. Individual treatment by oral or IM routes is traumatic and impractical, except in clinically ill individuals. Often treatment must be repeated several times at weekly intervals to control disease outbreaks. No more than one treatment should be administered at a time; when more than one disease co-exists, each disease should be treated individually (e.g. first listeriosis, then pseudomoniasis, then giardiasis).

Whenever possible, antibacterial treatments should be selected on the basis of bacteriologic culture and sensitivity. Certain antibiotics such as penicillin, streptomycin and lincomycin may cause severe inappetence and impaction if administered orally. Broad-spectrum antibiotics may seriously upset the intestinal microflora if administered for prolonged periods, therefore 3- to 5-day treatments, repeated at weekly intervals if necessary, should be used. Since secondary disease outbreaks are common in chinchillas, all animals dying during an outbreak should be examined to determine the need for continuing or changing treatment.

Many diseases of chinchillas are transmissible to man, and chinchilla owners should be made aware of this.

Pseudomonas aeruginosa is an important pathogen of chinchillas, causing wound infections, conjunctivitis, otitis, pneumonia, enteritis, metritis or septicemia. Focal typhlocolitis is a characteristic postmortem finding, but diagnosis must be confirmed by bacteriologic culture. Bacterins are the treatment of choice and can be prepared by the practitioner or diagnostic laboratory. Supplementary chlorination of the drinking water is recommended during outbreaks.

Chinchillas are very susceptible to infections caused by ***Listeria monocytogenes.*** Affected animals often exhibit anorexia, posterior paralysis, other neurotropic signs and coma, although in many cases they succumb without showing clinical signs of disease. Mortality is high, and losses may continue for long periods in spite of treatment. Focal hepatic necrosis is the most common postmortem finding, but direct smears and bacteriologic culture are required to establish the diagnosis. Water-soluble chloramphenicol in the drinking water is the treatment of choice, and may have to be repeated several times. Treatment is given for 3 consecutive days at weekly intervals until losses cease.

Salmonellae occasionally cause outbreaks in chinchilla herds and must be differentiated from listeriosis on the basis of bacteriologic culture. **Streptococci** and **staphylocci** may cause conjunctivitis, pneumonia, metritis and death in chinchillas. ***Yersinia (Pasteurella) pseudotuberculosis*** infections may resemble listeriosis in many respects. ***Pasteurella multocida*** and ***P. haemolytica*** cause pneumonia or sudden death, and usually are readily detectable on bacteriologic culture or blood or tissue smears. Choice of treatment depends on culture and on antibiotic sensitivity tests. **Proteus** spp. are often isolated from metritis, and occasionally from conjunctivitis, otitis and enteritis, but, except in metritis, are of questionable pathogenic significance. Several other bacterial species are occasionally isolated from chinchillas, but are not considered to be important pathogens in this host.

Toxoplasma gondii has caused serious outbreaks in chinchilla herds. Clinical signs are nonspecific. Necropsy findings may include straw-colored fluid in the body cavities, pulmonary congestion, splenomegaly and enlargement of lymph nodes. Isolation of *Toxoplasma* by inoculation of tissue suspensions into susceptible laboratory animals and careful histopathologic examination of affected chinchillas must be done to establish the diagnosis. Sulfonamides (℞ 89) administered to the herd for 10 to 14 days may be effective in controlling outbreaks. Since cats are potential sources of *Toxoplasma* oocysts, they should be excluded from the animal house and care should be taken to avoid exposing chinchillas to feed or bedding materials contaminated by cats.

Giardia cysts and trophozoites are seen frequently in large numbers on intestinal scrapings and smears from chinchillas that have died after a period of intermittent watery diarrhea, impaction, or without clinical signs. Mortality may be high in such outbreaks, and often no other cause of death can be found. Fresh, unrefrigerated carcasses must be examined soon after death. Occasionally trophozoites or cysts can be seen in the feces of living chinchillas. Giardiasis often is secondary to other diseases, therefore bacteriologic culture should be done to eliminate this possibility. Treatment is done on a herd basis (℞ 357) and may have to be repeated if losses continue. Long-term therapy with thiabendazole may be useful.

Trichomonads are occasionally seen on intestinal smears of dead chinchillas, but are of questionable pathogenicity in this host.

Trichophyton mentagrophytes is the commonest cause of **ringworm** in chinchillas. Affected individuals usually have loss of hair and reddening in lightly furred areas (nose, around eye, at base of tail) but direct microscopic examination of plucked hairs and skin scrapings or culture on Sabouraud's agar are required to confirm the diagnosis. Ringworm should not be confused with fur-chewing, which is characterized by large patches of clipped fur. Topical ringworm treatments are of questionable value. Affected animals should be isolated and treated with griseofulvin (℞ 365). If several chinchillas are affected, herd treatment should be considered.

Fur-chewing is a common vice of chinchillas characterized by clipping of the fur on the flanks and other parts, leaving patches of short fur. Numerous causes have been proposed, but the condition probably is an abnormal behavior pattern precipitated by confinement, boredom or nervousness. The herd incidence, which may be high, has been reduced in some cases by the elimination of affected animals from the breeding herd, decreasing the environmental humidity and temperature and supplying good-quality hay free-choice to the animals.

Malocclusion is a common dental deformity of chinchillas, characterized by overgrowth and angularity of molar and incisor teeth. Affected animals are usually over a year of age, lose weight rapidly and salivate profusely (slobbers). Death results from starvation or secondary diseases. Examination of the mouth with an otoscope reveals overgrown, angular teeth. Since the condition is thought to be hereditary (caused by a recessive gene), and because it recurs after surgical correction, euthanasia of affected chinchillas should be recommended.

Metritis is a common cause of infertility in chinchillas and is characterized by a white or creamy discharge seen upon opening the vagina. Bacteriologic culture and sensitivity tests are required to determine the treatment of choice. After the infection has been controlled, estrogenic compounds may be injected to re-establish estrus in affected females. The value of hormone treatments in sterile chinchillas is questionable, however, since many of these do not conceive in spite of induced estrus.

Intestinal impaction, intussusception and **rectal prolapse** are seen commonly in chinchillas and often are secondary to pseudomoniasis, listeriosis or other infections. Impaction is characterized by the passage of small hard droppings that decrease in numbers until none is passed. Sometimes it can be relieved by oral administration of 0.5 to 2 ml of equal parts of mineral oil and milk of magnesia b.i.d., until the droppings are normal. Subcut. fluids may be administered to offset dehydration. Rectal prolapse or intussusception or both are associated with diarrhea or impaction. These conditions usually recur after surgical corrections, thus a poor prognosis should be given in affected animals. In all cases, the initial cause of these conditions must be determined to rule out the possibility of concurrent bacterial or parasitic infection.

Surgical procedures are occasionally required in chinchillas (e.g. cesarean, rectal prolapse) although the prognosis for life or reproductive capacity following surgery often does not make such procedures economically attractive. Ether, halothane or methoxyfluorane can be used as inhalation anesthetics, but chloroform is toxic to chinchillas and other rodents. Pentobarbital sodium (35 mg/kg) or thiopental sodium (40 mg/kg) can be administered IP for surgical anesthesia.

RABBIT MANAGEMENT

The housing required for rabbits raised outdoors is dependent on the climate and should be located on nearly level, well-drained soil. Shade should be provided over a portion of the hutch. All-wire construction will allow for ventilation and light. Hutches should be 2½-ft deep and 3-ft long (75 × 100 cm) for medium breeds. Hutch height should be 18 in. (50 cm). Giant breeds should have hutches 2 ft (60 cm) longer. Hutches should be constructed of 1×1 in. (2.5 × 2.5 cm) or 1×2 in. (2.5 × 5 cm) welded wire for the top and sides and 0.5 × 1 in. (1.3 × 2.5 cm) welded wire for the floors. Wood should be avoided as it will be chewed and soaked with urine. Welded wire hutches require no wooden bracing members. In northern regions, the sides and back of the hutch should be sheathed to prevent drafts, whereas in warmer climates only a roof is required. The hutches should be fenced for protection from dogs.

The hutch should be equipped with feed hoppers for pellets, water containers and nest boxes. The hoppers should be constructed so as to prevent contamination. Automatic watering systems are used on large farms. Water bottles are preferable to crocks for small operations. The nest box should be so constructed that it can easily be removed from the hutch for cleaning and disinfecting between litters. It should be of a size sufficient to prevent crowding, but small enough to keep the young warm. Welded wire nest boxes with corrugated cardboard liners are excellent. Straw or wood shavings make good bedding in either warm or cold weather.

More than 35 million pounds (15.9×10^6 kg) of domestic rabbit meat (liveweight) is consumed annually in North America. Large and increasing numbers of rabbits are used in research and teaching. For this purpose, many rabbits are raised indoors in relatively controlled environments.

The selection of breeding stock is dependent upon the purposes of the growers. The wool breeds include the English and French Angora. Among those bred for meat are the White New Zealand, Red New Zealand, Californian and Champagne D'Argente. The white breeds, the White New Zealand and the Californian, are the most popular as they produce a white pelt. Of the more than 30 rabbit breeds recognized in America, most laboratory usage is of the White New Zealand.

Rabbits are sexually mature from 5 months for the medium breeds, to 6 to 9 months for the giant breeds. The small breeds, such as the Polish and the Dutch, mature at about 4½ months. Rabbits do not have a regular estrous cycle. The receptiveness of the doe, which is an induced ovulator, is established by excitement or close proximity to other rabbits. A ratio of 10 does to one buck is considered to be maximum, with 4 or 5 matings per week for the buck occasionally employed, and 2 to 3 matings a week with continuous use. The breeding program should be carried on throughout the year. The gestation period is 31 to 32 days. The pregnant doe will make her own nest in the nest box 3 or 4 days before parturition (kindling). The does should be left as quiet as possible during this period. The young may be examined on the second or third day. Considering a nursing period of 8 weeks, one doe can produce 4 litters a year if breeding failures do not occur. By rebreeding the doe when the young are 6 weeks old, 5 litters per year are obtained in many commercial rabbitries. Accelerated programs with creep feeding practices produce as many as 8 litters annually. A false pregnancy may occur as a result of infertile mating or one female riding another. These females cannot conceive for 17 days (the period of false pregnancy). If the doe has conceived, the fetuses can be palpated about the 12th day after breeding.

Rabbits may be carried by grasping the loose skin over the withers with one hand and placing the other under the rump to support the weight from beneath. If they are not held properly and securely, fractures or luxations of thoracic and lumbar vertebrae may follow struggling; also the claws on the rear limbs may severely scratch the unprotected arms of handlers. Some breeders tattoo their animals for identification purposes. The right ear is reserved for registration marks applied by American Rabbit Breeders Association registrars.

The sex of the rabbit may be determined when the rabbit is a day old; however, it usually is done at weaning time. By depressing the external genitalia, the mucous membrane can be exposed. In the male, the mucous membrane protrudes and forms a circle, whereas, in the female, it will extend and form a slit. Castration has no advantage for meat-type rabbits, as the growth for males and females is about the same until after market age. Angora rabbits raised longer than 6 months are sometimes castrated. The technique is similar to that of castrating cats, although it should be noted that the testes in the scrotum are lateral-to-anterior to the penis, as in marsupials, and unlike most other placental mammals.

When they are unobserved, usually in the early morning or at night, rabbits re-ingest part of their feces by contorting themselves so that the mouth touches the anus. They feed only on the soft matter than has passed through the tract but once. This trait of rabbits, which is normal and not a sign of nutritional deficiency, is often called pseudorumination. This coprophagy serves an important nutritional function by supplying the animal with intestinally synthesized B-vitamins, particularly thiamin. Stability of the normal intestinal microflora may depend on normal coprophagy; wire-mesh cage or hutch flooring does not prevent coprophagy.

Feeding rabbits (q.v., p. 1357) has been greatly aided by commercially available pelleted diets, most of which are nutritionally adequate.

DISEASES OF RABBITS

Although most techniques suitable for dogs and cats may be applied to rabbits for physical examination and restraint, general anesthesia of rabbits with barbiturates is often accompanied by significant mortality. Inhalation agents such as halothane are safer to use. Use of such preanesthetic agents as chlorpromazine hydrochloride (25 mg/kg), diazepam and propiopromazine (5 mg/kg) or fentanyl and droperidol allays apprehension, may reduce the dosage of general anesthetic by 50%, and often prolongs anesthesia. Ketamine (35 mg/kg) and xylazine (5 mg/kg), given together, result in adequate general anesthesia.

VIRAL DISEASES

With the exception of rabbit pox, and a herpesvirus infection (Virus III), viral diseases in rabbits are restricted to the infectious fibromas and papillomatosis. The former are tumors composed of connective tissue and consist largely of fibroblasts and their products. They are located under, rather than in the skin, in which respect they differ from the papillomas. There are 2 known types of infectious fibrotic tumors that occur under natural conditions, the tumor of infectious myxomatosis and the Shope fibroma. Both are viral and restricted to rabbits, the former to domesticated species only, in the U.S.A., and the Shope fibroma to the cottontail.

Infectious Myxomatosis

A fatal disease of the domestic rabbit, Angoras, Belgian hares, Flemish Giants and the European wild rabbit. The cottontail and jack rabbit are quite resistant, as are man, dog and other animal species tested. The virus causing the disease is transmitted by mosquitoes, biting flies and direct contact.

In the U.S.A., myxomatosis is restricted largely to the coastal area of California and Oregon, where epidemics occur every 8 to 10 years during the months of May to August, which correspond to the height of the mosquito season. These areas represent the geographic distribution of the California brush rabbit (*Sylvilagus bachmani*), the reservoir of the infection. In the rabbitries involved, losses range from 25 to 90%. During intervening years, only sporadic outbreaks occur. Rabbits of all ages are susceptible, although young up to the age of a month appear more resistant than adult animals.

The first characteristic sign is conjunctivitis that rapidly becomes more marked and is accompanied by a milky discharge from the inflamed eyes. The animal is listless, anorectic and the temperature frequently reaches 108°F (42°C). In acute outbreaks, some animals may die within 48 hours after showing signs. Those that survive become progressively depressed, develop a rough coat, and the eyelids, nose, lips and ears become edematous, giving a swollen appearance to the head. The vent becomes inflamed and edematous, and in the male, swelling of the scrotum occurs. A characteristic sign at this stage is drooping of the edematous ears. A purulent nasal discharge invariably appears, breathing becomes labored and the animal goes into a coma just before death, which usually occurs within 1 to 2 weeks after the appearance of clinical signs. Occasionally, an animal will linger on for several weeks before death ensues. In these cases, fibrotic nodules appear on the nose, ears and forefeet. Animals inoculated experimentally with laboratory strains of the virus invariably develop small nodules at the point of injection after several days and these are followed by development of similar nodules on other parts of the body, particularly the ears.

No characteristic lesions are found at necropsy. The spleen is occasionally enlarged and black. The seasonal incidence of the disease, the clinical appearance of infected animals and the high mortality are all of diagnostic significance.

A live vaccine prepared from an attenuated myxomatosis virus has been shown to protect both field- and laboratory-infected animals.

The Shope Fibroma

The Shope fibroma occurs under natural conditions in the cottontail only, although domestic species of rabbits can be infected by inoculation of virus-containing material. The disease is a threat to commercial rabbits where it is endemic in wild rabbits and where husbandry practices allow contact with arthropod vectors. Were it to occur, the chief diagnostic problem would be infectious myxomatosis, q.v., p. 1176.

Papillomatosis

Benign tumors occasionally seen in domestic rabbits. They consist of small, grayish white, pedunculated nodules on the under surface of the tongue or the floor of the mouth. Individuals are not treated, but the balance of the herd may be vaccinated with an autogenous vaccine: To a 10% suspension of papilloma tissue in isotonic salt solution, 0.4% formaldehyde solution is added and allowed to stand at 41°F (5°C) for a week. Then it is cultured and, if bacteriologically sterile, inoculated subcut. in 0.5-ml quantities at 7-day intervals for 3 weeks. This virus (Papova virus) is distinct from the Shope papilloma virus (which is also distinct from the Shope fibroma virus) seen in wild rabbits, and reported in domestic rabbits in Southern California. Skin tumors caused by the Shope papilloma virus never occur in the mouth.

Rabbit Pox

An acute, generalized disease of laboratory rabbits, characterized by pyrexia, nasal and conjunctival discharge and skin rash. The mortality varies, but is always high. Only 6 outbreaks have been reported in the U.S.A. since 1930 and the disease apparently has not been recognized in wild rabbits. The causative virus is closely related to vaccinia virus and some outbreaks may have been caused by a virulent strain of vaccinia. The virus may be isolated and identified by methods appropriate to vaccinia (*see* POX DISEASES, p. 242). Spread of this disease through a rabbitry or an animal house is very rapid, but rabbits that have been inoculated with smallpox vaccine (vaccinia virus) are immune.

BACTERIAL AND FUNGUS DISEASES

Pasteurellosis

A highly contagious disease, common in domestic rabbits, transmitted either by direct or indirect contact. Apparently rabbits develop little immunity following infection. Some animals are healthy carriers and probably perpetuate the disease in the rabbitry. An indirect fluorescent-antibody test for use on nasal swabs has been found effective in identifying carriers, which may constitute up to 90% of apparently healthy rabbits in conventional colonies. *Pasteurella multocida* infections may be manifested as any of the following: snuffles, pneumonia, otitis media (q.v., p. 233), conjunctivitis, abscesses, genital infections or septicemia.

Snuffles or nasal catarrh: An acute, subacute or chronic inflammation of the mucous membranes of the air passages and lungs. The signs are a thin or purulent exudate from the nose and eyes. The fur on the inside of the front legs just above the paws will be matted and caked with dried exudate from the rabbits pawing at their noses. Infected animals usually sneeze and cough. Snuffles, in general, occurs when the resistance of the rabbit is low or at kindling time. Those animals that recover may become carriers. *Bordetella bronchiseptica* may play a role in some cases also. Pneumonia (q.v., p. 1179) can ensue.

Abscesses caused by *Pasteurella* may be found in any part of the body or head. Rabbits of all ages are susceptible. When bucks are penned together, their fight wounds frequently develop into abscesses. In most instances, it is advisable to eliminate rather than to treat the affected rabbit. The condition may terminate in septicemia and death within 48 hours. Necropsy reveals bronchial congestion, tracheitis, splenomegaly and subcut. hemorrhages.

A troublesome **genital infection** is often caused by *Pasteurella* but several other organisms also may be involved. It is manifested by an acute or subacute inflammation of the reproductive tract. This condition most frequently is found in adults, more often in does than bucks. If the condition is bilateral, the does often become sterile, but if only one horn of the uterus is infected, a normal litter may develop in the other. In the female, a pyometra is produced, of which the vaginal discharge of a thick, yellowish gray pus may be the only sign noted. The buck may exhibit a discharge of pus from the penis, but usually an orchitis is noted. Chronic infection of the prostate and seminal vesicles is most likely and since venereal transmission may ensue it is best to eliminate the animal. The infected hutch and its equipment should be thoroughly disinfected. For a valuable breeder, antibiotics (℞ 27, 60) may be used in combating the infection; however a poor prognosis should be given.

Yersiniosis
(Pseudotuberculosis)

Nodules resembling the tubercles of tuberculosis, and caused by *Yersinia* (*Pasteurella*) *pseudotuberculosis*, may be observed in the parenchyma of the liver, lungs, spleen and the intestinal wall. There is evidence that suggests the organisms enter the host through contaminated food or water. This is a chronic debilitating disease and the signs are lassitude, anorexia, emaciation and dyspnea. Since man is susceptible, these rabbits should be destroyed, and not marketed. The contaminated hutches should be cleaned and disinfected with a strong hot lye solution.

Listeriosis

A sporadic septicemic disease characterized by sudden deaths, abortions or both. Poor husbandry and stress may be important factors in initiating the disease. Clinical signs are variable and nonspecific including anorexia, depression and weight loss. In contrast to the disease in cattle and sheep, listeriosis seldom affects the CNS in rabbits but spreads to the liver, spleen and gravid uterus via the blood. At necropsy the liver consistently contains multiple pinpoint gray-white foci. Antemortem diagnosis is rarely made and therefore treatment is seldom attempted.

Staphylococcosis

Staphylococcus aureus infection occurs commonly in domestic and wild rabbits and is manifest as a fatal septicemia or suppurative inflammation involving almost any organ or tissue, often skin. Rabbits may be infected but show little or no clinical disease unless resistance is decreased, e.g. by skin wounds. Abscesses develop in chronic infections. In acute speticemia there is usually fever, depression and anorexia terminating in death. Time permitting, sensitivity testing should precede antibiotic treatment.

Mastitis
(Blue Breasts)

Mastitis occurs occasionally in domestic rabbits. The cause is usually streptococci or staphylococci. The malady may spread through the rabbitry, rapidly attacking lactating does. The mammary glands become hot, reddened and swollen; later, the glands may become cyanotic, hence the common name. The doe will not eat, but may crave water. A temperature as high as 105°F (40.5°C), or higher, is often noted. The condition may be treated by the parenteral injection of penicillin (℞ 63). Treatment of does where the inflammation is extensive is not advocated and euthanasia of both does and young is recommended; handraising infant rabbits is difficult.

Pneumonia

Pneumonia is not uncommon in domestic rabbits. It may occur in adult animals or may infect the young while they are in the nest box. Frequently, it is a secondary and complicating factor in the enteritis complex. The cause is bacterial with *Pasteurella* accounting for the greatest number of cases. Other bacteria involved may be *Klebsiella pneumoniae*, *Bordetella bronchiseptica* and pneumococci. Drafty, damp, unsanitary hutches and inadequate bedding are predisposing causes. The animals usually succumb within 4 days after the first signs have been noted. Affected rabbits are off feed with elevated temperature (104°F [40°C]), dyspnea, diarrhea and lassitude. Necropsy reveals a bronchopneumonia, pleuritis or pericardial petechial hemorrhages. Treatment consists of oxytetracycline (℞ 50), chlortetracycline (℞ 27) or penicillin (℞ 63). Combinations of penicillin and streptomycin (℞ 66) are also useful and effective for such mixed infections.

Conjunctivitis
(Weepy eye)

Mature bucks and young rabbits seem particularly susceptible. The cause is often *P. multocida* infection. Affected rabbits rub their eyes with their front feet. The exudate may vary in consistency and color. Any of the common ophthalmic ointments containing sulfonamides (℞ 411, 412), antibiotics (℞ 391) or antibiotics and a steroid (℞ 408) are satisfactory for treatment but recurrence is common. In cases of deep-seated infections, injections of penicillin (℞ 63) should be given. A conjunctivitis also accompanies rabbit pox (q.v., p. 1177) and myxomatosis (q.v., p. 1176).

Treponematosis
(Vent disease, Spirochetosis)

A specific venereal disease of domestic rabbits characterized by appearance of denuded or scab-covered areas about the external genitalia and caused by the spirochete *Treponema cuniculi*. It occurs in both sexes and is transmitted by coitus. It is not transmissible to other domestic animals or man. Small vesicles or ulcers are formed, which ultimately become covered with a heavy scab. These lesions usually are confined to the genital region, but in some cases the lips and eyelids may be involved. Infected animals should not be mated. Penicillin in daily doses of 50,000 units appears to be specific therapy. Lesions usually heal within 10 to 14 days and recovered animals can be bred without danger of transmitting the infection.

Necrobacillosis
(Schmorl's disease)

A sporadic disease characterized by necrosis, ulceration and abscess formation in the skin and subcut. tissue, usually on the face, head and neck. It is caused by *Fusobacterium necrophorum* (*Spherophorus necrophorus*). The organism is probably always present in the digestive tract and infection usually is associated with fecal contamination of skin wounds under unsanitary conditions. Clinical signs include swelling, necrosis and abscessation of the skin. The lesions are progressive and have a foul odor. Affected animals usually are removed to minimize contamination of cages and other rabbits. The lesions can be treated by opening and draining abscesses and applying iodine or a topical sulfonamide.

HUTCH BURN
(Vent disease, Urine burn)

Hutch burn is often confused with treponematosis. It affects the vent and external genitalia and is caused by wet and dirty hutch floors. Constant exposure to urine splashes and soiled corners chap the membranes of the vent and genital region, allowing the area to become secondarily infected. Brownish crusts cover the area and a bleeding and purulent exudate may be present. Keeping hutch floors clean and dry, and the application of antibiotic ointment to the lesions will hasten recovery.

SCABBY NOSE

Similar to hutch burn in many respects, this infection causes chapping and cracking of the skin on the nose and lips. Most cases are contracted from infected vents. When secondary infections develop, large brown scales are produced on the nose and lips. Cases of hutch burn should be dealt with first and those with scabby nose should be treated with an injection of 50,000 units of penicillin, repeated on the third day.

DIARRHEAS

Diarrhea is one of the most important causes of morbidity and mortality in domestic rabbits and usually is a complex problem rather than a simple disease entity. The disease has been referred to as **mucoid enteritis, mucoid enteropathy, enterotoxemia, scours or bloat.** Several known causes of diarrhea in the rabbit include salmonella, *Bacillus piliformis* (Tyzzer's disease), *E. coli* (colibacillosis), clostridia (enterotoxemia) and intestinal coccidiosis. This list is incomplete since there still is much to learn about diarrhea in the rabbit; the disease often occurs as a complex of mucoid enteropathy with one of the above infections.

The etiology of mucoid enteropathy is unknown although it can be classified as an enterotoxin-induced secretory diarrhea. The incidence is a function of age with most cases occurring in rabbits 7 to 10 weeks old, and occasional infections occur as early as 2 weeks or as late as 20 weeks of age. The disease runs an acute course up to 8 days. Clinical signs include anorexia, lassitude, subnormal temperature, rough hair coat and diarrhea with rapid weight loss. There may be polydipsia and the abdomen is bloated because of gas- and fluid-filled intestines. The perineum is stained with mucus and feces and at necropsy the colon often contains gelatinous mucoid material. Treatment is palliative, aimed at limiting secondary infections. Antibiotic supplements in the feed may reduce mortality due to mucoid enteropathy but generally will not prevent the disease or limit morbidity. Dimetridazole in the feed has been reported to be quite useful.

Tyzzer's disease, caused by *Bacillus piliformis*, has been recognized in recent years as a cause of severe diarrhea and death in some rabbit colonies. Outbreaks have affected mainly young rabbits 6 to 7 weeks old. The disease is characterized by profuse diarrhea, anorexia, dehydration, lassitude and death within 1 to 3 days. The lesions consist of necrotic enteritis along with focal necrosis in liver and heart. Infection occurs by ingestion and is associated with poor sanitation and stress. No treatment is known to be effective.

Ringworm
(Dermatophytosis)

An uncommon disease of domestic rabbits usually associated with poor husbandry. The lesions usually first appear on the head and may spread to any area of the skin. The affected areas are circular, raised, reddened and capped with white, bran-like, flaky material. The lesions may fluoresce under the Wood's lamp. The commonest cause is *Trichophyton mentagrophytes* var. *granulare*, which also affects man, guinea pigs, mice and rats. Because active cases are infectious for man and other animals, infected rabbits should be isolated and treated or killed. A degree of control can be obtained by continual application of powdered sulfur to all nest boxes prior to kindling or by use of topical agents such as those containing salicylic and benzoic esters of propylene glycol, aqueous solutions of sodium caprylate, and tinctures containing tannic, benzoic and salicylic acids. The drug of choice is griseofulvin at an individual dose of 12 mg/lb (25 mg/kg) body wt daily for 14 days or in the feed at 375 mg/lb (825 mg/kg) of feed (*see* RINGWORM IN DOGS AND CATS, p. 933).

Miscellaneous

Tuberculosis and tularemia are uncommon infections of the rabbit, now largely of historical interest. Other bacteria that may infect the rabbit but produce disease either poorly defined or of little importance include the genera *Salmonella*, *Proteus*, *Pseudomonas*, *Actinobacillus*, *Actinomyces*, *Brucella*, *Streptococcus*, *Diplococcus*, *Erysipelothrix* and *Leptospira*. Systemic mycotic infections are rare in rabbits although individual cases have been reported.

PARASITIC DISEASES

Coccidiosis

One of the commonest diseases of rabbits. Those animals that recover from this protozoan infection frequently become carriers.

There are 2 forms, hepatic coccidiosis, caused by *Eimeria stiedai*, and intestinal coccidiosis, the cause of which may be *E. magna*, *E. irresidua*, *E. media*, or *E. perforans*. So-called "nasal coccidiosis" is the result of the rabbits contaminating the mucous membrane of their nose while practicing coprophagy (*see* RABBIT MANAGEMENT, p. 1173).

Hepatic Coccidiosis: Severity of disease is dependent on the number of oocysts ingested. There may be an infection with no apparent signs or death may follow a short course. Young rabbits are most susceptible. Affected animals exhibit diarrhea, anorexia and a rough hair coat. Growing rabbits fail to make normal gains. The animals usually succumb within 30 days after a severe experimental exposure. At necropsy, in most cases, the lesions are easily recognized. Small, grayish white nodules or cysts are found throughout the parenchyma of the hepatic tissue. They may be sharply demarcated in the early cases, while in the later stages, they coalesce with other affected areas. The early lesions have a milky content, whereas older lesions may have a more cheese-like consistency. Microscopically, the nodules are composed of hypertrophied bile ducts. A large number of oocysts are seen. This form of coccidiosis is diagnosed from the gross and microscopic changes along with demonstration of the oocysts in the bile ducts.

Sulfaquinoxaline administered continuously in the drinking water (0.025% for 30 days) prevents the development of the clinical signs of hepatic coccidiosis in rabbits heavily exposed to *E. stiedai*. Sulfaquinoxaline may also be given in the feed at 0.025% for 20 days, or for 2 days out of every 8, until marketing. The rabbits acquire an immunity to subsequent infections. Lower concentrations of the drug are not satisfactory. The maximum prophylactic effect is obtained by 3 weeks of administration. A concentration of 0.10% of sulfaquinoxaline in the feed, or 0.05% in the feed and 0.04% in the drinking water, given continuously for 2 weeks, is recommended for therapeutic control of naturally occurring outbreaks. The drug should not be given within 10 days of slaughter of the rabbits for food. The above treatments will be of no avail unless a sanitary program is simultaneously instituted. The feed hoppers and water crocks should not become contaminated with feces. The hutches should be kept dry and the accumulated feces removed at frequent intervals. Sulfamethazine, sulfamerazine, or succinylsulfathiazole in the feed at 0.5% concentration have also been used during outbreaks.

Intestinal Coccidiosis: This form of the disease will occur in rabbits receiving the best of care, as well as in rabbits raised under unsanitary conditions. Inability to gain, anorexia and "pot belly" are prominent signs. The lesions are inconsistent: In early infections there are few changes, later, the intestine may be thickened and pale. All of the responsible coccidia develop in the small intestine. While losses due to liver coccidiosis may be held to a negligible level through a sanitary program, and will permit profitable production, the same program will not eliminate intestinal coccidiosis. It is important that any diseased rabbit be removed from the rabbitry and its feces examined for coccidia. Sulfaquinoxaline fed continuously for 2 weeks at 0.1% of the feed has been used for treatment.

Larval Tapeworm Infection

Rabbits are intermediate hosts for 2 tapeworms of the dog, *Taenia pisiformis* and *T. serialis*. The larval forms are found in the viscera of the rabbit. If the cysts develop under the skin, they can be surgically removed. The rabbit is also the intermediate host for the cat tapeworm, *T. taeniaeformis*. The larval stage, a segmented worm, is found in a white cyst in the liver. Dogs and cats should not be allowed near the rabbits' feed, water, bedding or feeding utensils as they may transmit tapeworm eggs in their feces, nor should dogs and cats eat the viscera of rabbits, as they may become infected and perpetuate the cycle.

Ear Mite Infestation

The ear mite, *Psoroptes cuniculi* is the commonest external parasite of rabbits. Head shaking and ear flapping, along with scratching at the ears with the hind feet are common signs. Torticollis and spasms of the eye muscles may be observed. Affected rabbits lose flesh, fail to produce and succumb to secondary infections. These infections frequently damage the inner ear and may reach the CNS. The mites irritate the lining of the ear, causing serum and thick crusts to accumulate. Under good restraint or even general anesthesia, the brown, crumbly exudate should be removed with cotton soaked in dilute hydrogen peroxide. After cleaning, the ears are swabbed with 1 part Canex (℞ 271) in 3 parts mineral or vegetable oil. The medication should be applied around the external ear and down the side of the head and neck as well. The application has to be repeated after 6 to 10 days. Additional treatments may be necessary. The hutches used by the affected rabbits must be carefully cleaned and disinfected. Incidence is much lower in wire than in solid cages.

Mange Mite Infestation

Not infrequently, rabbits are infected with either *Sarcoptes scabiei* or *Notoedres cati*. The rabbits scratch themselves almost continually. There is a loss of hair on the chin, nose, head, base of the ears and around the eyes. The condition is extremely contagious. It is difficult to eliminate the parasites on domestic rabbits. The owner should be advised to destroy the animals unless they are valuable breeders. They may be dipped in a lime-sulfur preparation, or Canex (℞ 271) may be rubbed into the lesions.

Nosematosis

Encephalitozoon (*Nosema*) *cuniculi* is a widespread protozoal infection of rabbits and occasionally of mice, guinea pigs, rats and dogs. It involves the brain and kidneys, mainly, but usually no clinical signs are produced. It is mildly contagious in a rabbitry or colony and is believed to be spread via urine or transplacentally. At necropsy, the lesions must be differentiated from those of *Toxoplasma gondii* (q.v., p. 466) by morphologic and staining criteria. It may be possible to eliminate carriers from a colony by examining brains of younger rabbits and then culling the dams of positive subjects. Toxoplasmosis, which is not as common in rabbits as nosematosis, may be diagnosed by available serologic methods, and serologic tests for *Encephalitozoon* are being developed.

Pinworms

Passalurus ambiguus, the rabbit pinworm, usually is not economically or medically important. If necessary, it can be controlled by phenothiazine in the feed (1 gm/50 gm of molasses-treated feed).

NONINFECTIOUS CONDITIONS

Moist Dermatitis (Wet Dewlap): Some rabbits have a heavy fold of skin on the ventral aspect of the neck. As the rabbit drinks, this skin may become wet and soggy ("**slobbers**") leading to inflammation of the area. Factors which may contribute to this condition include dental malocclusion and damp bedding. The hair may slip and the area may become infected or fly blown. To prevent the occurrence of wet dewlaps, the water receptacles should have small openings or be set on low, flat boards. The hair in the affected area must be clipped and an antiseptic dusting powder applied.

Cannibalism: Many times, young does will kill and consume their young. Although the exact causes are not known, cannibalism has been attributed to nervousness, lack of water or a poor ration. Does that are prone to kill their young should be culled. The young should not be examined too soon after kindling as this will excite the doe.

Wool-eating (Hairballs): In many instances, the stomach contents of rabbits contain small amounts of hair but impaction results only if a habit of wool-eating is formed. Rabbits may pull wool from the back of another rabbit or eat their own wool. It often is difficult to break this habit. Occasionally, wool balls will occlude the pyloric opening.

Heat Exhaustion: Rabbits are very sensitive to heat and hot, humid weather along with poorly ventilated hutches or transport in poorly ventilated vehicles may lead to death of many rabbits, particularly pregnant does. Affected rabbits lie on their sides and breathe rapidly. They should be immersed in a bucket of cool water. Hutches should be constructed so that they can be sprinkled in hot, humid weather. Free access to water and salt blocks should be provided. Where it is possible to control the environment, optimal criteria are: temperature 60 to 70°F (15.5 to 21°C), relative humidity 40 to 60%, with 10 to 20 air changes per hour. Wire cages are preferable to solid hutches.

Ketosis (Pregnancy Toxemia): A rare disorder that may result in death of does at kindling or a day or 2 before they are due to kindle. Predisposing factors include obesity and lack of exercise. The most significant finding at necropsy is fatty liver and kidneys. To prevent the condition, the daily intake of pellets of all pregnant does should be restricted prior to kindling.

Milkweed Poisoning: This type of poisoning is caused by feeding hay containing woolly pod milkweed, *Asclepias eriocarpa,* reported only from the Pacific Southwestern U.S.A. It sometimes is called "head down disease," inasmuch as the affected rabbits develop paralysis of the neck muscles and loss of coordination. If the animal has not consumed too much of the weed and the paralysis has not progressed too far, an attempt may be made to treat it. The head of the rabbit is held so that it can drink water and consume food. Leafy greens and carrots should be fed. Hay and bedding must be free of this weed in order to prevent the condition. The poisonous principle is a resinoid; consumption of approximately 0.25% of an animal's weight of green plant produces death. The use of rice straw or wood shavings for bedding will eliminate this hazard.

Dystocia: The gestation period of the rabbit rarely exceeds 32 days. If a pregnant doe is overdue and is straining or in distress, an injection of oxytocin (℞ 193) is generally effective, providing presentation, normally anterior or posterior, is acceptable.

Ulcerative Pododermatitis (Sore Hocks): This disease does not involve the hock but the metatarsal, and less commonly the metacarpal-phalangeal region. The cause is pressure on the skin from bearing the body weight on wire-floored cages with secondary infection of the necrotic skin. Several factors including accumulation of urine-soaked feces, excessive nervousness, posterior paralysis following spinal cord injury, and the type of wire may influence its development. Affected rabbits may otherwise appear healthy or suffer anorexia, weight loss and death. Treatment consists of using solid-bottom cages with clean, dry bedding and topical application of zinc or iodine ointment.

Dental Malocclusion: The incisors, premolars and molars of rabbits grow throughout life. Normal length is maintained by constant grinding of opposing teeth. Mandibular prognathism (malocclusion, brachygnathism) is probably the commonest inherited disease in the rabbit and leads to overgrowth of incisors with resultant difficulty in eating and drinking. Temporary correction can be effected by cutting, from time to time, the overgrown teeth. Occasionally, the cheek teeth overgrow, causing severe tongue or buccal lesions. The disorder can be selected against in the breeding program.

Congenital Malformations: There are many inherited defects that affect various organs in the rabbit. Some common malformations, the genetics of which are poorly known, include variation in the number of ribs (12 or 13 pairs), degree of sternebral ossification, craniofacial abnormalities, missing or misshapen gonads and ventral body wall defect. (*See also* DENTAL MALOCCLUSION, above.)

Muscular Dystrophy: Nutritional muscular dystrophy in the rabbit is an uncommon disease characterized by high neonatal mortality at 3 to 10 days of age with no prior signs. Occasional deaths occur in surviving young up to the age of 2 to 3 months. Breeding females undergo decreases in fertility. Gross lesions are absent; acute degenerative and inflammatory changes are present in sections of skeletal muscle. Dietary vitamin E deficiency is believed to be causal. Breeding females can be treated with oral DL-α-tocopherol acetate (25 to 60 mg orally 3 times weekly for 8 weeks) or by feeding a diet containing about 9.0 mg α-tocopherol per 100 mg of diet (*see also* MYOPATHIES AND RELATED CONDITIONS IN DOMESTIC ANIMALS, p. 590).

SPECIFIC-PATHOGEN-FREE (SPF) RABBITS

It is possible to obtain neonatal rabbits by hysterectomy and raise them behind an environmental barrier in the laboratory, to serve as a nucleus for an SPF colony. To be truly SPF, regular monitoring with reliable techniques must be carried out. Pasteurellosis, coccidiosis, ear mites and pinworms have been eliminated under such programs. General mortality from all causes can be drastically reduced.

In Britain, the 3 most frequently diagnosed rabbit diseases in conventional colonies are the diarrheas, coccidiosis and respiratory diseases. In North America, they are the diarrheas, pasteurellosis and genetic maladies such as mandibular prognathism.

DISEASES OF LABORATORY ANIMALS

This chapter deals with the more important diseases of those animals used in the largest numbers for research purposes: mice, rats, guinea pigs, hamsters, as well as various primate species and amphibians. Diseases of other domestic species that are also widely used research animals, such as dogs, cats, rabbits and chickens, are dealt with elsewhere in the MANUAL.

The guide for the Care and Use of Laboratory Animals: DHEW Pub. No. (NIH) 78-23 Revised 1978, is a primary reference for information on the basic principles and standards for the care and use of laboratory animals.

DISEASES OF MICE AND RATS

A disease prevention program is essential to exclude or limit infectious disease in mouse and rat colonies. Its elements should include: production and introduction of animals free of common pathogens, quarantine procedures, use of facilities designed to limit the introduction and spread of microbial pathogens, prophylactic or therapeutic intervention where appropriate, methods for isolation and use of principles of population epidemiology.

Bacterial Diseases

Murine respiratory mycoplasmosis (chronic respiratory disease) is a disease syndrome complex characterized by inflammation of the respiratory tract and middle ear. Signs include chattering and dyspnea in mice, and nasal discharge, snuffling, rales, dyspnea, head tilt, incoordination and circling in rats. Lesions include suppurative bronchitis and bronchopneumonia, mucopurulent rhinitis, and otitis media and interna. The primary etiologic agent is *Mycoplasma pulmonis;* however, *Pasteurella pneumotropica*, *Corynebacterium kutscheri*, *Bordetella bronchiseptica,* streptococci, pneumococci and viruses may act in concert with the primary agent. Diagnosis depends on lesions and isolation of the etiologic agent. The condition may be prevented by keeping a cesarean-derived colony behind a microbiologic barrier. Acute outbreaks of the disease may be controlled to a limited extent by oxytetracycline in the drinking water (℞ 55).

Tyzzer's Disease: This endemic disease is widespread in laboratory mice in Europe and Japan; outbreaks have been reported in a wide variety of laboratory animals in the U.S.A. The causative organism is a slender gram-negative rod, *Bacillus piliformis.* Stress or cortisone injections may precipitate epidemics in colonies where the organism is present. Signs are diarrhea, humped back, poor haircoat, or sudden deaths, especially in young animals. Lesions usually include focal necrosis of the liver and inflammation of the terminal ileum. Diagnosis depends on histologic demonstration of the bacilli in bundles within the hepatocytes surrounding the focally necrotic areas, and negative cultures for *Salmonella*, *Corynebacterium* or other pathogens. The organisms stain well with Giemsa stain. Outbreaks may be controlled by isolation of affected animals, strict hygienic procedures and oxytetracycline in the drinking water (℞ 55).

Salmonellosis (Paratyphoid): Organisms of the genus *Salmonella*, usually *S. typhimurium* or *S. enteriditis*, may cause enteritis and septicemia with focal necrosis of the liver or spleen in rats and mice. Antibiotics may ameliorate the acute infection (*see* SALMONELLOSIS, p. 299).

***Pseudomonas* Infection:** Pseudomonads are part of the normal intestinal flora, but may cause early deaths in stressed or X-irradiated mice. *P. aeruginosa* may also cause otitis media and interna in nonirradiated mice. Prevention and control are best accomplished by acidification (pH 2.5) or chlorination (10 to 16 ppm) of the drinking water.

***Pasteurella* Infection:** Pasteurellae may cause localized inflammatory lesions and septicemia in rats and mice. *P. pneumotropica* infection may be latent, but when host defenses are reduced, bronchopneumonia, conjunctivitis, metritis, cystitis, or dermatitis may occur. Oxytetracycline (℞ 55) has been used successfully in treating infections caused by this organism.

***Corynebacterium kutscheri* Infection (Pseudotuberculosis):** *C. kutscheri* (*murium*) is an opportunistic pathogen of rats and mice. Infection may be inapparent, or result in nasal and ocular discharge, dyspnea, arthritis, or skin abscesses. Lesions are variable, but usually include focal abscesses in organs with capillary nets, leg, liver, kidney, lung and lymph nodes, and occasionally purulent arthritis. Diagnosis depends on characteristic lesions and isolation of the organism or serology (agglutination). Treatment with penicillin (℞ 65) or tetracycline (℞ 55), may prevent clinically apparent disease but will not eliminate the carrier state.

***Citrobacter freundii* Infection:** This can cause marked mucosal hyperplasia, colitis, rectal prolapse and moderate mortality in mice. Experimentally, a 0.1% solution of sodium sulfamethazine as drinking water has been effective in reducing the incidence of colitis.

MISCELLANEOUS BACTERIAL INFECTIONS

Klebsiella pneumoniae may rarely cause bronchopneumonia, pleuritis, and abscesses in various organs of mice. *Streptococcus pneumoniae* is an important cause of acute bronchopneumonia, pleuritis, pericarditis, meningitis and splenic infarcts in rats. *Streptobacillus moniliformis*, a gram-negative, highly pleomorphic bacillus, may rarely cause arthritis, pericarditis, and focal necrosis of the liver and spleen. It also causes rat-bite fever or Haverhill fever in man. *Bordetella bronchiseptica* is a common inhabitant of the respiratory tract of rats and mice. Although its role as a primary pathogen in rats and mice is uncertain it has been identified as a primary cause of pneumonia. **Group A streptococcus** or **Type D enterococcus** may rarely cause clinical disease in mice. **Group A streptococcus** causes cervical lymphadenitis, fibrinopurulent pneumonia, pleuritis, pericarditis and peritonitis. **Type D enterococcus** causes focal enteritis and focal hepatic necrosis. Diagnosis of these infections depends on isolation of the organism. Therapy is governed by specific antibacterial sensitivity of the organisms.

Viral Diseases

Ectromelia (Mouse Pox) is a devastating disease of laboratory mice caused by "*Poxvirus muris.*" It may remain latent or cause low-grade endemic disease or violent epidemics. In the acute systemic form, there can be deaths with no lesions. In more chronic cases there may be facial swelling, conjunctivitis with a secondary rash, and ulcerating or scaly lesions of the head, tail or extremities. Occasionally, extremities become necrotic and slough. Other lesions include focal necrosis of the liver, spleen, pancreas and lymph nodes, and intestinal hemorrhage. Eosinophilic cytoplasmic inclusion bodies may be found in hepatocytes, pancreatic acinar cells or in swollen epidermal cells in areas of cutaneous inflammation. Diagnosis is based on characteristic lesions and serology (hemagglutination inhibition using vaccinia antigen, serum neutralization or indirect immunofluorescence). A single positive animal indicates that a colony is infected. Effective control is gained by vaccinating all susceptible animals every 6 months. A drop of vaccinia virus vaccine is placed near the base of the tail, and the skin is lightly scarified beneath the drop. A small papule occurs at the site of vaccination. Ectromelia-free colonies should be well isolated from wild and newly received rodents. Newly received mice should be isolated and observed for 2 to 3 weeks before they are introduced into the colony.

Diarrhea of Infant Mice: EDIM is characterized by high morbidity and diarrhea in mice 5 to 15 days of age. Death occurs late in the disease due to constipation or secondary bacteremia. Recovered animals may be stunted. Lesions include distension of the colon with light mustard-colored feces and vacuolation of epithelial cells at the tips of small intestinal villi. These vacuolated cells may contain small acidophilic intracytoplasmic inclusions. Diagnosis is based on characteristic clinical and pathologic findings. The disease can be controlled and eliminated from most colonies by using filter-top cages and culling infected mice.

Sendai Virus Infection: This usually remains subclinical in rats but can cause violent epidemics with high mortality in mice. The signs are due to pneumonia and include weight loss, dyspnea, chattering and increased mortality. Weanling and young mice usually are most affected. Diagnosis is based on characteristic histology of pneumonic lesions and serology on exposed or recovered animals. The disease is highly contagious and difficult to control. A vaccine has been developed to protect susceptible stocks.

Sialodacryoadenitis: The causal coronavirus causes severe self-limiting inflammation and necrosis of the salivary and lacrimal glands of rats. The infection is highly contagious and causes high morbidity but low mortality in susceptible colonies. Affected animals show exophthalmos, porphyrin pigment staining around the eyes, and swollen face and neck. Exophthalmos may cause corneal drying with severe secondary ocular lesions. The disease is self-limiting with most lesions resolving within 14 days.

Subclinical Viral Infections of Mice and Rats: A number of viruses can be isolated from clinically normal laboratory mice and rats. These viruses do not usually pose significant clinical disease problems in laboratory colonies. However, they may seriously disrupt research by directly affecting research results or causing disease in animals whose resistance has been diminished by experimental procedures. *See* TABLE (pp. 1192 and 1193).

PARASITIC DISEASES

Protozoa: At least 4 species of coccidia (*Eimeria* spp.) may infect the intestinal tract of laboratory rats, and 8 species may infect mice. In addition, one species (*Cryptosporidium muris*) occurs in the stomach. Diagnosis is based on identification of oocysts after fecal flotation, or by finding organisms in the epithelial cells of the intestinal tract. Renal coccidiosis due to *Klossiella muris* occurs in mice. Oocysts are passed in the urine. Coccidial infection of the intestine, stomach, or kidney rarely causes lesions or clinical signs.

Hexamita muris, a flagellated protozoan, may cause diarrhea, weight loss and sporadic deaths in mice. Lesions include duodenitis with crypts dilated by numerous hexamitae. Diagnosis is based on microscopic lesions and demonstration of organisms in saline mounts and fixed smears from duodenum. *Hepatozoon muris* occurs in the hepatic cells of rats and mice. *Pneumocystis carinii*, an organism of uncertain classification may be found in the lungs of rats; respiratory signs may result from stress or immunosuppression. This organism may be transmissible to human beings. *Toxoplasma gondii* is an intracellular parasite (q.v., p. 466) with a wide host range including rat, mouse and man. It may cause encephalitis, pneumonitis, or enterocolitis. Treatment of rats or mice with clinically apparent protozoan infections is not considered feasible.

SUBCLINICAL VIRAL INFECTIONS OF MICE AND RATS

Disease	Agent	Lesions	Diagnosis	Comments
Adenovirus Infection	Adenovirus	Focal necrosis: heart.	Serology: CF[1], SN[2]; intranuclear inclusions: heart, kidney, adrenal.	Stunting lethargy, death in suckling mice only.
K-Virus Infection	Papovavirus	Interstitial pneumonia with proliferation of endothelial cells.	Serology: HI[3], SN; intranuclear inclusions; endothelial cells.	Labored breathing and death in suckling mice.
Kilham Rat Virus	Parvovirus	Cerebellar necrosis in suckling rats.	Serology: HI	Hamsters more susceptible than rats. Contaminates tumors.
Lactic Dehydrogenase (LDH) Virus Infection	Unclassified RNA virus	None.	Elevation of plasma LDH.	Causes elevated plasma enzyme levels. Contaminates transplanted tumors.
Lymphocytic Choriomeningitis	Arenavirus	Lymphocytic choriomeningitis; necrosis: liver and lymphoid tissue.	Guinea pig or LCM-free mouse inoculation. Serology: I[4].	Clonic convulsions, transplacental infection. Transmissible to man.
Mammary Carcinoma	Bittner agent; RNA virus	Mammary adenocarcinomas, adenoacanthomas, carcinosarcomas.	Lesions.	Virus in milk of infected dam.
Minute Virus of Mice	Parvovirus	Encephalitis; choriomeningitis.	Serology: SN, HL.	Contaminates transplanted tumors. Also affects rats.
Theiler's Mouse Encephalomyelitis (GD-VII)	Picornaviruses	Necrosis: brain stem, spinal cord.	Serology: HI. Neonatal hamster inoculation.	Flaccid posterior paralysis, virus carried in intestine.
Mouse Hepatitis	RNA virus	Focal necrosis: liver, lymph nodes, brain.	Serology: CF. Mouse inoculation.	Hepatotropic and neurotropic viral stains; occ. jaundice & neurologic signs.

Mouse Pneumonitis (Nigg Virus Inf.)	*Chlamydia* sp. (*Miyagawanella*)	Interstitial and bronchopneumonia.	CF. Elementary bodies: bronchial epithelium.	Latent infection may be activated by intranasal instillations.
Mouse Thymic Agent Infection	Herpesvirus	Thymic necrosis.	Inoculation of newborn mice.	Affects newborn only.
Murine Leukemia	RNA viruses	Lymphocytic, granulocytic, or erythrocytic leukemia.	CO Mu L(5) and XC(6) tests.	Several viral strains cause several different types of tumors.
Pneumonia Virus of Mice Infection	RNA virus	Interstitial pneumonia; pulmonary edema.	Serology: HI, SN. Inoc. of PVM-free mice.	May affect rats also.
Polyoma Virus Infection	Papovavirus	Tumors in various sites.	Serology: HI, SN. Agglutinates RBC's *in vitro*.	Stunted growth and tumor development 1-6 months after inoculation.
Rat Coronavirus Infection	Coronavirus	Experimental pneumonia.	CF.	Naturally occurs in rats.
Reovirus Infection (Hepatoencephalomyelitis)	Reovirus Type 3	Necrosis: liver, myocardium, pancreas; neuronal degeneration; encephalitis.	Serology: CF, SN.	Jaundice, yellow feces, oily hair and skin, neurologic signs.
Salivary Gland Virus (Cytomegalovirus Infection	Herpesvirus	Intranuclear inclusions: salivary-duct epithelium.	Lesions.	Rats and mice have species specific infections.
Toolan H1 Infection	Parvovirus	Cerebellar lesions.	HI.	Naturally occurs in rats.

1. Complement Fixation; 2. Serum Neutralization; 3. Hemagglutination Inhibition; 4. Immunofluoroscence; 5. Complement Fixation for Murine Leukemia; 6. XC Cell Cytopathogenicity Test; 7. Indirect Immunofluorescence.

Blood Parasites: Several blood parasites have been reported in rats and mice. These include *Plasmodium berghei, P. vinckei, Trypanasoma lewisi, T. cruzi, Hepatozoon muris, Babesia muris,* and *Haemobartonella muris* (rats only). *Eperythrozoon coccoides* (mice only), now classified as a rickettsia, was formerly considered to be a protozoan. These organisms do not normally cause clinically apparent disease unless animals are splenectomized or severely stressed. Blood-sucking ectoparasites may transmit the disease.

Nematodes: *Heterakis spumosa* is found in the cecum and colon of rats and mice. No lesions have been reported. Diagnosis is based on identification of ova in the feces. *Nippostrongylus muris* occurs in the small intestine of rats and mice. Clinical signs include unthriftiness, diarrhea and dyspnea. Lesions include pneumonia and pulmonary hemorrhage due to larval migration through the lungs. Characteristic eggs are passed in the feces. *Gongylonema neoplasticum* occurs in the epithelium of the stomach, esophagus and tongue. There is little tissue reaction; infection does not produce neoplasms. The intermediate host is the cockroach. Embryonated eggs are passed in the feces. Adult *Trichinella spiralis* (q.v., p. 713) are found in the duodenum of rats and many other animals. The pinworms, *Aspiculuris tetraptera* and *Syphacia* spp., occur in the cecum and colon of rats and mice. Impaction by worms, colonic intussusception, or rectal prolapse may result. *Aspiculuris* eggs are passed in the feces; *Syphacia* eggs are deposited on the perianal region by the female worm. Diagnosis can be made by fecal flotation (*Aspiculuris*) and by the cellophane-tape method (*Syphacia*). Control is difficult because of reinfection due to the presence of eggs on fomites and in air currents. An effective treatment is trichlorfon plus atropine (Dyrex R, 2.5 gm/L of distilled water), in the drinking water for 2 weeks, combined with strict sanitation of equipment and facilities. *Capillaria hepatica* occurs in the liver parenchyma of mice and rats. Eggs cause yellow streaks and patches in liver due to the local chronic inflammatory response. Eggs are liberated only when the liver is eaten by some other animal. The eggs are then passed in the feces to develop on the ground to become infective. The nematode, *Trichosomoides crassicauda,* lives in bladder, kidney, pelvis and ureters of rats. Operculated eggs are passed in the urine. Larvae migrating through the lungs may cause focal granulomas.

The adult lungworm, *Angiostrongylus cantonensis,* occurs in the pulmonary artery of rats. The life cycle is complex and involves a snail or slug as an intermediate host and 2 moults within the brain of the definitive host. It has little pathologic significance for the rat but is transmissible to, and causes meningoencephalitis in man.

Acanthocephala: The thorny-headed worm, *Moniliformis monili-*

formis, inhabits the small intestine of rats, mice and other rodents. The thorn-like hooks on the head may cause enteritis, ulceration and occasionally intestinal perforation with subsequent peritonitis.

Cestodes: The dwarf tapeworm, *Hymenolepis nana*, occurs in the small intestine of rats and mice, and is transmissible to man. The life cycle may be either direct or indirect. The tapeworm, *Hymenolepis diminuta*, occurs in the anterior ileum of rats and mice. A flea, beetle or cockroach may act as an intermediate host. *Oochoristica ratti symmetrica* is a rare tapeworm of mice and is usually of little importance in laboratory mice. The treatment of choice for tapeworms is niclosamide (℞ 249). Rats and mice may also harbor the intermediate forms of *Taenia taeniaeformis* (*Cysticercus fasciolaris*) in the liver and *Taenia* (*Coenurus*) *serialis* in the connective tissue. The presence indicates probable fecal contamination of the food supply by the definitive host(s).

Ectoparasites: The mites, *Myobia muris-musculi* and *Radfordia affinis*, in mice may cause loss of hair, and scabby lesions over the head, neck and shoulders. Great variation in effect is seen in different host genetic strains. Breeding males seem to be most severely affected. *Myocoptes musculinus* and *Trichoecius* (*Myocoptes*) *romboutsi* may also cause hair loss and dermatitis. *Psorergates oettlei* (*simplex*) causes chronically inflamed epidermal cysts which are visible only on the inner surfaces of the skin. Mites affecting rats are *Ornithonyssus* (*Bdellonyssus*) *bacoti* and *Radfordia ensifera*, which cause dermatitis, and *Notoedres muris*, which causes vesicles, papules and wart-like projections on the ears, nose, tail, feet and external genitalia. Lice and superficial mites are most easily and consistently diagnosed by killing a suspect animal and observing it by parting the hairs and looking at the epidermal level with a magnifying glass or dissecting microscope. Migration may be hastened by placing the carcass or skin in the refrigerator, followed by examination of the carcass after removal to room temperature. The burrowing mite, *P. simplex*, may be diagnosed by examining for the subcut. pinpoint, white focal lesions.

Infestation of laboratory rats or mice with fleas such as *Xenopsylla cheopis*, *Nosopsyllus fasciatus*, or *Leptopsylla segnis* is uncommon. Infestation with lice, *Polyplax spinulosa* (rat) or *Polyplax serrata* (mouse), is more common than flea infestation and can cause loss of hair and pruritis in laboratory stocks or strains.

Ectoparasites can be eliminated only with cesarian derivation procedures. Clinical control may be achieved by placing 2 sq in. of resin strip containing dichlorvos on cage tops for 24- to 48-hour intervals every 2 weeks for 2 to 3 treatments. Restriction of air flow in the room or cage increases the effectiveness.

Mycotic Diseases

Ringworm (*see* RINGWORM IN GUINEA PIGS, p. 1198).

Histoplasmosis, coccidioidomycosis, sporotrichosis, cryptococcosis and phycomycosis do not usually pose significant problems in laboratory colonies, but they may seriously disrupt research because of an overwhelming effect on animals whose resistance has been diminished by radiation or immunosuppressive drugs.

Noninfectious Diseases

Fighting: Trauma due to fighting is often a significant cause of morbidity and mortality in male mice. Fighting usually occurs at night and results in bite and scratch wounds over the head, perineum and lumbosacral skin. Frequently, these lesions become septic. A high incidence of secondary amyloidosis has been reported in animals that have lesions stemming from fighting. Fighting can be prevented by separating males, or preferably, by grouping males at the time of weaning rather than later.

Chloroform Toxicity: Mature male mice of some inbred strains (C_3H, CBA, A, HR) are exquisitely sensitive to low levels of chloroform vapor in the air. A chloroform spill may result in the death of large numbers of mature males while immature males and females are unaffected. Lesions include necrosis of convoluted renal tubules. There is no practical treatment once signs have become apparent.

Ringtail is a condition of young rats and mice characterized by annular constriction and later edema, necrosis, and spontaneous amputation of the tail. The condition in rats can be experimentally produced by lowering the ambient relative humidity. The disease can be controlled by providing a relative humidity of at least 50%.

Nutritional Diseases

Highly standardized balanced rations for rats and mice are commercially available. Most manufacturers provide separate diets for maintenance, breeding and other specific purposes.

The rations should be stored properly and used promptly since nutritional quality falls during storage. Ideally rations for rats and mice should be fed within 90 days of the milling date. If colonies are fed fresh diets manufactured by a reputable company, the possibility of clinically apparent nutritional deficiency is remote. However, long-term *ad libitum* feeding of presently available stock diets to rats and mice can lead to obesity, increased prevalence or severity of certain age-associated lesions, and reduced longevity. The control of problems such as these is complex; but long-term restriction of caloric intake, reduced protein intake or both may be helpful.

Age-Associated Diseases

Rats and mice are used widely in aging research. Maximum longevity of many stocks and strains is 36 to 40 months, with a 50% survival time of about 30 months. Genetic and environmental factors influence longevity and the prevalence of age-associated diseases, and strain differences are known to occur. It is desirable to rear and maintain rats or mice that are intended for use in aging research under barrier conditions, to prevent exposure to infectious diseases. The principal age-associated non-neoplastic lesions of rats are chronic glomerulonephropathy, polyarteritis nodosa, myocardial degeneration and radiculoneuropathy. The most commonly occurring neoplasms in the rat are pituitary adenomas, pheochromocytomas of the adrenal gland, pancreatic islet cell tumors, testicular interstitial cell tumors, and leukemias. Mice are subject to comparable types of lesions as they age, with increasing prevalence or severity both in rats and mice after 12 months of age. The differentiation of spontaneous age-associated lesions and true lesions of aging is a major challenge in experimental gerontology. The use of diagnostic screening procedures in selecting old rats and mice for research may be helpful in culling animals bearing lesions that could add to the variability of research results, or in selecting for specific lesions of research interest.

DISEASES OF THE GUINEA PIG

Antibiotic Toxicity: Guinea pigs and hamsters are highly susceptible to the toxic effects of many of the commonly used antibiotics. It now appears that toxicity results from the overgrowth of *Clostridium difficile* or gram-negative overgrowth. This causes fatal enterocolitis, with diarrhea and death in 3 to 7 days. Antibiotics with an activity spectrum directed primarily against gram-positive organisms (e.g. penicillin, lincomycin, erythromycin, tylosin) should not be used in guinea pigs and hamsters. Broad-spectrum antibiotics should not be used orally because of their direct effect on the intestinal flora, but may be used parenterally with caution. Topical antibiotic ointments may also induce the syndrome if animals are allowed to ingest the ointment.

Metastatic calcification occurs most often in male guinea pigs over a year of age. Signs include slow weight gains, stiff joints and high mortality. At necropsy, calcium deposits are seen in the lung, liver, heart, aorta, stomach, colon, kidney, joints and skeletal muscles. There are conflicting reports concerning the etiology; however, most investigators agree that when animals are fed diets low in magnesium and potassium, the calcific lesions increase with the phosphorus content of the ration. It is believed that hyperphosphatemia results from the inability of the guinea pig to conserve fixed bases by excreting ammonia in the urine; thus, the low-base reserve impairs normal urinary excretion of phosphorus. The condition may be aggravated by increasing the vitamin D content of the ration beyond 6 IU/gm. The condition may be minimized or prevented by feeding diets that contain adequate magnesium (0.35%), a calcium:phosphorus ratio of 1.3 to 1.5:1, and not more than 6 IU of vitamin D per gram.

Scurvy: (Vitamin C Deficiency): Guinea pigs require a dietary supply of ascorbic acid (vitamin C) because they lack the enzymes necessary for conversion of L-gulonolactone to L-ascorbic acid. Signs of vitamin C deficiency are unsteady gait, painful locomotion, hemorrhage from gums, swelling of costochondral junctions and emaciation. Lesions include hemorrhages in the subcutis, and skeletal muscle around joints and on all serosal surfaces. Microscopically, there is disarray of cartilage columns and fibrosis of the marrow in areas of active osteogenesis. The condition may be prevented by providing 1 to 3 mg ascorbic acid per 100 gm body wt daily. Commercial guinea pig diets contain vitamin C which is stable for 3 months after milling. Marginal diets should be supplemented with greens or vegetables high in vitamin C.

Muscular Dystrophy: Guinea pigs are exquisitely sensitive to dietary deficiency of vitamin E. Signs are stiffness, lameness and refusal to move. Microscopic lesions include coagulative necrosis, inflammation and proliferation of sarcolemmal nuclei in skeletal muscle. Diets should contain 3 to 5 mg of vitamin E per 100 gm.

Pregnancy toxemia in guinea pigs is a metabolic disorder similar to that observed in sheep prior to parturition (q.v., p. 512). Predisposing factors are obesity and any stress that might induce temporary anorexia during the late stages of pregnancy. Clinical findings are anorexia, adipsia, muscle spasms, coma within 48 hours of onset, and death within 4 to 5 days unless the course is interrupted by parturition. Laboratory findings are aciduria, proteinuria and hyperlipemia. Microscopically, there is fatty degeneration of parenchymatous organs and hyperlipemia. Control may be achieved by prevention of obesity, avoidance of stress during late pregnancy and provision of a high-quality ration during pregnancy. Early treatment of affected animals with oral propylene glycol, IP calcium gluconate, or parenteral corticosteroids may be helpful although the prognosis remains poor.

Ringworm is a common mycotic infection in guinea pigs, usually caused by *Trychophyton mentagrophytes* or *Microsporum gypseum*. It causes characteristic, crusty, flaking lesions on the skin. Facial lesions are usually prominent. Diagnosis is based on characteristic lesions and cultural and microscopic identification of the causative organism. The disease is usually self-limiting if good husbandry and sanitation are maintained. Long-term feeding of griseofulvin (℞ 366) is effective. Isolated skin lesions may be treated effectively with tolnaftate cream (℞ 373). The disease is contagious to man.

Bacterial and Viral Diseases

Lymphadenitis: Inflammation and enlargement of the cervical lymph nodes is a common finding in guinea pigs. The causative organism is usually *Streptococcus zooepidemicus* although other bacteria may also cause the condition. The organisms may gain entry to the lymphatics from abrasions of the oral mucosa or from the upper respiratory tract. Clinical findings are large, often unilateral, swellings or abscesses in the ventral region of the neck. Microscopically, there is suppuration of the cervical lymph nodes. Diagnosis is based on clinical signs and isolation of the causative organism. The use of abrasive materials in feed or litter should be avoided. In addition, upper respiratory tract infections should be prevented and controlled. Affected animals should be culled since organisms from the draining abscesses may infect other animals in the colony. Antibiotic therapy is generally unrewarding because of antibiotic toxicity (q.v., p. 1197). It is reported that IM cephaloridine (℞ 13) is effective in controlling and eliminating the disease.

Pneumonia in the guinea pig may be viral or bacterial *Streptococcus zooepidemicus, S. pneumoniae, Klebsiella pneumoniae, Pasteurella pneumotropica, Bordetella bronchiseptica*). Clinical signs are those of respiratory distress. Diagnosis is based on signs, pneumonic lesions and isolation of the causative organism. Prevention and control depend on maintenance of good husbandry procedures and culling of affected animals. Treatment with antibiotics should be approached cautiously since most commonly used antibiotics are toxic for the guinea pig (q.v., p. 1197). Treatment with tetracycline orally (℞ 55) or parenterally (℞ 49), or chloramphenicol (℞ 25) may be helpful.

Salmonellosis in guinea pigs is similar to the disease in other animals (*see* p. 299).

Parasitic Diseases

Several protozoa (*Toxoplasma gondii, Eimeria caviae, Encephalitizoon* [*Nosema*] *cuniculi*), nematodes (*Paraspidodera uncinata*), and lice (*Gyropus ovalis, Gliricola porcelli*) may infect guinea pigs. (*See* p. 1194 et seq. for control and treatment of nematodes and ectoparasites.)

DISEASES OF THE HAMSTER

Bacterial Diseases

Hamsters are susceptible to infection by a number of common bacterial pathogens. These include streptococci, pneumococci, salmonellae, leptospires, staphylococci and pasteurellae.

Clinical signs and lesions are similar to those seen in other animals. Antibacterial therapy should be given with the utmost caution since hamsters are highly susceptible to the toxic effects of many antibiotics (*see* p. 1197).

Parasitic Diseases

Helminths: Many hamster colonies are infected by the tapeworm, *Hymenolepis nana*, and the pinworm, *Syphacia obvelata*. (*See* p. 1195 et seq. for lesions and therapy.)

External Parasites: Many external parasites, including *Notoedres*, *Sarcoptes*, and the tropical rat mite, *Ornithonyssus bacoti*, may infect hamsters. (*See* p. 1195 et seq. for lesions and therapy.) Two *Demodex* species, *D. criceti* and *D. aurati*, are commonly found on hamsters; alopecia over the back and hind quarters may result.

Nutritional Diseases

Hamsters are very sensitive to vitamin E deficiency which leads to skeletal muscular dystrophy. Balanced diets formulated specifically for hamsters are commercially available; however, hamsters also thrive on commercially available rat and mouse diets.

Other Disease Problems

Antibiotic Toxicity: (*see* p. 1197).

Proliferative Ileitis (wet tail, regional enteritis) is a specific, apparently infectious, disease syndrome of uncertain etiology. The disease is endemic in many laboratory and commercial colonies and may reach epidemic proportions. Clinical signs are diarrhea (wet tail), dehydration, anorexia and depression. Weanling animals are often affected. Lesions include ileitis or typhlitis or both, and colitis with marked hyperplasia of the ileal epithelium. This epithelial hyperplasia results in marked thickening and rigidity of the ileal wall with partial stenosis of the lumen. The condition may respond to oral therapy with neomycin sulfate (15 mg/animal/day in divided doses). After initial oral dosing, the drug may be administered in the drinking water for 4 to 5 days. Vigorous therapy for dehydration and acidosis is also usually necessary. It is advisable to isolate affected animals and maintain strict sanitation in contaminated rooms.

DISEASES OF PRIMATES

The primate species most widely used in research are *Macaca mulatta* (rhesus monkey), *M. fascicularis* (crab-eating monkey), *M. arctoides* (stump-tailed monkey), *M. nemestrina* (pig-tailed monkey), *Cercopithecus aethiops* (African green monkey), *Papio* spp. (baboon), *Saimiri sciureus* (squirrel monkey), *Aotus trivirgatus* (owl monkey), *Cebus* spp. (capuchin), *Ateles* spp. (spider monkey), and *Saguinus* and *Callithrix* spp. (tamarins, marmosets). There are increasing restrictions on the exportation or availability of primates from the countries of origin. A nationally coordinated program of domestic primate production has been established; and the need for primate conservation has been stressed (National Primate Plan, DHEW, NIH, 1977). Most primates for research still are imported. They may be carrying or be susceptible to numerous infectious diseases. They should be quarantined before use for 30 to 90 days, to permit adequate evaluation of their health status and adaptation to the laboratory environment.

Bacterial Diseases

Tuberculosis: All primates are susceptible to tuberculosis, although species differences exist. For example, rhesus monkeys (*Macaca mulatta*) are exquisitely sensitive, while crab-eating macaques (*Macaca fascicularis*) appear to be relatively resistant. Clinical signs are not a reliable indication of the extent of tuberculosis in the rhesus monkey. A vigorous appearing animal may have extensive miliary disease involving thoracic and abdominal organs; signs of debilitation may only appear shortly before death. A testing program is essential, and tuberculin tests on all newly received primates should be considered mandatory. The tests should be performed at the time of arrival and at 2-week intervals thereafter until at least 3 consecutive negative tests have been recorded for the entire group. After their release from quarantine, all primates should be skin-tested at least quarterly. The test consists of injecting Mammalian Tuberculin or Old Tuberculin (15 mg in 0.1 ml of water) intradermally in the upper eyelid or in the abdominal skin. The subject is examined at 24, 48 and 72 hours. A positive hypersensitivity reaction is marked by edema, induration or erythema, which may be subtle in some species such as the squirrel monkey (*Saimiri sciureus*). Roentgenographic examination of the chest may aid diagnosis of well-established cases, but the tuberculin skin test should be considered the primary diagnostic method for routine surveillance. All positive reactors should be destroyed. The presence of tuberculosis should then be confirmed by necropsy. Semi-annual skin tests or chest radiographs for personnel working in primate facilities should also be provided.

Isoniazid (INH) is an effective tuberculostat. It should not be administered during the quarantine period because it may suppress the skin test reaction, and thus prevent detection of positive reactors before the animals are released from quarantine. However, once animals are released, routine maintenance on isoniazid will effectively prevent development of tuberculosis. Despite a possible suppressing effect of isoniazid on the hypersensitivity reaction, skin testing should be performed regularly on all primates maintained on isoniazid. An effective daily dose of isoniazid is 5 to 10 mg/kg of body wt administered in a sugar cube or incorporated in the feed. There is no evidence that the continuous use of isoniazid will lead to the development of isoniazid-resistant mycobacteria.

Dysentery: The organisms most commonly associated with primate dysenteries are *Shigella*, *Salmonella*, and occasionally, *Escherichia coli*, *Pseudomonas aeruginosa* and *Aerobacter aerogenes*. Apparently healthy primates may be carriers of any of these organisms. Routine stool cultures for *Shigella* to identify carriers are of questionable value inasmuch as the identification, isolation and treatment of carrier animals has not been shown to prevent subsequent outbreaks of shigellosis in primate colonies.

Dysentery is a major problem in primates undergoing conditioning. Clinical signs include watery or mucoid blood-tinged feces, and rapid dehydration, emaciation and prostration. Rectal prolapse is an occasional sequela. The presence of helminths or protozoa may be a complicating factor. Mortality can be extremely high in acute outbreaks unless prompt treatment is instituted to restore and maintain normal fluid and electrolyte balance. The most common pathologic lesions at necropsy are hemorrhagic enteritis, enterocolitis, colonic ulcers or simply colitis.

Clinical signs and death are generally due to dehydration, hypokalemia and metabolic acidosis. Affected primates should be treated individually. A nasogastric tube can be passed readily in most primates; it is indispensable for direct therapy. Fluid mixtures containing electrolytes, antibacterial agents and protectives can be administered in this way (℞ 497). Hydration should be maintained with parenteral lactated Ringer's solution. Broad-spectrum antibiotics may also be given (℞ 10, 25, 49). The choice of antibiotics should be based on the specific antibiotic sensitivity pattern. If circumstances prevent individual therapy, mass treatment of a colony for shigellosis or salmonellosis can be accomplished by incorporating furazolidone in the food (℞ 117); however, this is less satisfactory than individual treatment.

Pneumonia: Upper respiratory disease and pneumonia of bacterial origin can cause widespread illness and mortality, particularly in newly imported primates. Causative agents include *Streptococcus pneumoniae*, *Klebsiella pneumoniae*, *Bordetella bronchiseptica*,

Haemophilus influenzae, and various species of streptococci, staphylococci and pasteurellae. Pneumonia may accompany or follow primary disease elsewhere; for example, pneumonia and dysentery often occur together. Clinical signs may include coughing, sneezing, dyspnea, mucoid or mucopurulent nasal discharge, lethargy, anorexia and unthriftiness. The principal lesions seen at necropsy are those of broncho- or lobar pneumonia.

Antibiotic therapy is generally helpful in treating primate pneumonias. Cultures from pharyngeal swabs are most useful in isolating the causative agent and determining the specific antibiotic sensitivity. Various penicillins, chloramphenicol, lincomycin, or cephalothin should be administered (℞ 15, 25, 44). Intensive nursing and other supportive therapy, such as fluid administration, may also aid recovery in selected cases.

Viral Diseases

Herpesvirus Infections: At least 7 herpesviruses have been isolated from primates. They exist as latent or subclinical infections in reservoir hosts; at least 3 have caused fatal infections when transmitted naturally to other hosts. *Herpesvirus simiae* (Herpesvirus B) is generally innocuous in *Macaca* spp. but in man it causes a highly fatal encephalitis and encephalomyelitis. Transmission may occur through a monkey bite or by contamination of a superficial wound with infected saliva; aerosol transmissions of the virus may also occur. Herpesvirus T causes mild herpetic lingual ulcers and stomatitis in squirrel monkeys (*Saimiri sciureus*); but fatal epidemics have followed natural transmission to owl monkeys (*Aotus trivirgatus*) and marmosets (*Saguinus*). *"Herpesvirus hominis"* occurs as a mild infection in man and certain primates, but owl monkeys are highly susceptible and may die of the infection. Similar fatalities have occurred in tree shrews (*Tupaia glis*). Manifestations of infection may include mucous membrane or skin ulcerations, conjunctivitis, meningitis, or encephalitis.

Hepatitis: Newly imported chimpanzees may carry and transmit to man the virus of infectious hepatitis. Elevated SGOT and SGPT values in chimpanzee sera are of diagnostic significance.

Inasmuch as vaccines are not available to protect primate colony personnel or the primates themselves against these virus infections, effort should be made to prevent exposure. This is best accomplished by careful training of personnel in the handling of primates; by use of protective clothing, face masks and gloves; by separating primates in species-specific rooms; and by strict attention to hygienic standards.

Miscellaneous Viral Diseases: Several other viruses produce clinical disease in primates. Rubeola (measles) infection can assume epidemic proportions. The virus causes a nonpruritic, exanthematous rash on the chest and lower portions of the body; it may also cause interstitial, giant-cell pneumonia, rhinitis and conjunctivitis. There is no specific treatment. The efficacy of human measles vaccine in protecting nonhuman primates against rubeola is unknown. Monkey pox may occur in primate colonies. It is characterized by a maculopapular rash and variolous pustules. Affected monkeys usually survive. After recovery, animals are immune to challenge with vaccinia virus.

PARASITIC DISEASES

Newly imported primates harbor numerous parasites. Some are commensal; others can be made self-limiting by strict sanitation and good husbandry. However, some parasites can cause serious diseases or debilitation and should be removed by specific treatment.

Helminths: *Oesophagostomum* may cause characteristic granulomatous nodules in the large bowel associated with development of the worms and with an immune reaction of the host. The nodules sometimes rupture and thus cause peritonitis. *Strongyloides* and *Trichostrongylus* are invasive; adults may cause enteritis and diarrhea; larvae may cause pulmonary lesions during migration. These helminths, as well as *Trichuris*, can be treated effectively with thiabendazole (100 mg/kg of body wt), administered orally at 2- to 4-week intervals. *Prosthenorchis* are filarid worms, common in Central and South American primates, that burrow into the mucosa of the ileocecal junction and sometimes perforate the bowel, or cause obstruction when present in large numbers. Cockroaches are intermediate hosts; their elimination, along with strict sanitation, is essential to freeing infected monkeys of these acanthocephalan worms. *Dipetalonema* and *Tetrapetalonema* occur in the peritoneal cavity. They may be present in large numbers without apparent harm to the host.

Protozoa: Primates may serve as hosts of various intestinal amobae. *Entamoeba histolytica* is the principal pathogenic form in nonhuman primates as it is in man. In a heavy infection it may cause severe enteritis and diarrhea, and cysts may be demonstrated in the feces in large numbers. Chloramphenicol (℞ 25), oxytetracycline (℞ 49) and furazolidone (℞ 117) have been used successfully to control amebiasis in conjunction with strict sanitary measures.

Blood parasites, such as *Plasmodium*, *Leishmania* and *Trypanosoma*, also are common. There is generally an equilibrium between the parasite and the natural host, but serious reactions may result from cross-infections. Transmission of simian malarias to man has occurred in areas where the appropriate mosquito vectors are present. The disease does not usually pose a clinical problem in primate colonies, but the presence of blood parasites may render infected primates unsatisfactory for some types of research; however, some primate species, such as owl monkeys, are excellent models for malaria research.

Naturally occurring toxoplasmosis (*T. gondii*) has been reported more frequently in Central and South American primates than in African or Asian primates. Clinical signs of infection tend to be nonspecific (lethargy, anorexia, diarrhea). Hepatic focal necrosis and fibrinous pneumonia with edema are common histologic findings. Toxoplasma can be demonstrated in blood smears in acute cases.

Arthropods: Pulmonary acariasis (*Pneumonyssus*) occurs commonly in wild-caught Asian and African primates, particularly rhesus monkeys and baboons. Infection is rare in laboratory-raised primates. The life cycle of *Pneumonyssus* is not well understood. Infections do not usually produce serious disease, although they may stimulate sneezing and coughing. Lesions include dilatation and focal chronic inflammation of terminal bronchioles. The gross lesions of mite infestation may occasionally be confused with tuberculous granulomas.

Mange mites (*Psorergates* spp., *Sarcoptes scabiei*) or sucking lice (*Pedicinus obtusus* [*longiceps*]) are seen occasionally and may produce dermatoses. Topical treatment of affected animals with pyrethrin-containing compounds is recommended (℞ 323). Use of more toxic parasiticides should be avoided because of the possibility of ingestion during grooming.

Mycotic Diseases

Microsporum and *Trichophyton* are known to affect primates. Topical treatment of ringworm with undecylenic acid ointment or tolnaftate (℞ 373), or oral administration of griseofulvin (℞ 366) is recommended. *Candida* are common saprophytes of the skin, alimentary tract and reproductive tract of primates, and act as facultative pathogens in debilitating conditions. Ulcers or white, raised plaques may be seen on the tongue or mouth; the fungus may also attack fingernails. Oral lesions must be differentiated from those of trauma, monkey pox, or herpesvirus infections. A topical cream containing chlordantoin (℞ 370) is effective in superficial infections. Oral nystatin (℞ 367) is effective for digestive tract candidiasis. Cutaneous streptothricosis caused by the actinomycete, *Dermatophilus congolensis*, has been reported in owl monkeys (*Aotus trivirgalus*). Papillomatous lesions are seen in the face and extremities. The infection is transmissible to man. Aspergillosis may occur in various primate species, and is usually a facultative pathogen. It is significant because it may be secondary to or predispose to tuberculosis.

Nutritional Diseases

All laboratory primates are susceptible to vitamin C deficiency. Vitamin-C-deficient animals usually succumb to infectious diseases before clinical signs of the deficiency appear. Commercial monkey diets contain vitamin C which is stable for 3 months after the diet is packaged. Supplemental sources are citrus fruits. Orally administered pediatric vitamin preparations containing ascorbic acid are readily accepted. Daily intake of approximately 4 mg of ascorbic acid per kilogram of body weight will prevent scurvy. Primates require vitamin D. Asian and African primates can utilize provitamin D_2 in plant materials to prevent rickets and osteomalacia. Central and South American primates cannot utilize this provitamin, but require provitamin D_3. Animal proteins and fish liver oils provide an adequate source of D_3; or as little as 1.25 IU/gm of diet can be added to the ration. In the absence of adequate D_3 New World primates may develop osteodystrophia fibrosa (q.v., p. 577).

Other Disease Problems

Acute gastric dilation is being recognized increasingly in primate colonies. The etiology is poorly understood; however, many cases occur following refeeding after experimental food deprivation. Clinical findings are similar to those seen in small animals (q.v., p. 134). The condition is often fatal and emergency treatment is necessary. The stomach must be evacuated and fluids replaced, in like volume, with Ringer's solution given parenterally. Shock and dehydration usually occur, and require prompt treatment. Periodic evacuation of the stomach may be necessary for several days until normal gastrointestinal function is restored. Metabolic alkalosis may result from continued loss of hydrochloric acid. Adequate sodium, chloride and potassium (Ringer's solution) must be provided parenterally.

DISEASES OF AMPHIBIANS

The most widely used amphibians are leopard frogs (*Rana pipiens*), bullfrogs (*Rana catesbiana*), African clawed toads (*Xenopus laevis*), marine toads (*Bufo marinus*), salamanders (*Ambystoma* spp.) and Mexican axolotls (*Seridon mexicanum*). The vast majority are caught wild for use in laboratories; relatively few breeding colonies exist. Malnutrition, parasitism, and certain bacterial and virus diseases are common. These problems have not been studied systematically from the perspective of veterinary medicine. Good husbandry and adequate feeding are key elements in managing amphibians intended for laboratory use. However, individual or mass treatment of diseased animals can be used selectively in overcoming certain disease states.

Bacterial Diseases

Most amphibians are carriers of *Aeromonas hydrophila*, a facultative pathogen that is the most common cause of the infection commonly called "red leg." Malnourished, newly received amphibians are particularly susceptible. Clinical signs may include lethargy;

emaciation; ulcerations of the skin, nose and toes; and characteristic cutaneous pinpoint hemorrhages of the legs and abdomen. Hemorrhages may also occur in skeletal muscles, tongue and nictitating membrane. In acute cases, these signs may be absent. Histologic evidence of systemic infection may include inflammatory or necrotic foci in the liver, spleen and other coelomic organs. Individual treatment with oxytetracycline (150 mg/kg of body wt, b.i.d.) or chloramphenicol (50 mg/kg of body wt, b.i.d.) is effective. The antibiotics should be administered in a small volume of distilled water (0.2 ml to a 30-gm frog) by stomach tube (No. 5 French) for at least 5 consecutive days. Treatment of groups of frogs can be attempted by placing them in holding tanks containing oxytetracycline in the water (1 mg/ml). Cutaneous absorption may not be adequate to provide therapeutic systemic levels; however, this procedure may help to control or limit the spread of infection.

Amphibian tuberculosis is generally less devastating than mammalian tuberculosis. It is seen most commonly in debilitated animals; healthy amphibians normally are resistant, even though *Mycobacterium* spp. are widely present in aquaria. The usual route of infection is by ingestion or by direct entry of mycobacteria through skin abrasions. Accidental infection from unsterile parenteral injections may also occur. Primary pulmonary tuberculosis is less common. Affected animals may exhibit typical tuberculous granulomas in the liver, kidney, spleen, lungs and other coelomic organs. Specific treatment is not feasible.

Viral Diseases

Renal adenocarcinomas (Lucké tumors) are relatively common in wild-caught *Rana pipiens* originating in the Northeastern and North-Central U.S.A. Few tumor-bearing frogs are seen in the summer; but the incidence may exceed 8% in the winter. The difference presumably is due to the effects of temperature on the causative agent, a herpes-type virus. Virus particles and inclusion bodies are seen only in tumors held in the cold. Metastasis of the tumor to liver, lungs and other organs is common; both the primary and metastatic tumors can become very large. There is no treatment, but the Lucké tumor is used for research on viral oncogenesis.

Parasitic Diseases

Helminth parasites, protozoa and ectoparasites are extremely common in wild-caught amphibians; but heavy parasite loads are often well tolerated. Inflammatory reactions to parasitism are often imperceptible. Laboratory-reared animals have a strikingly lower incidence of helminths than those collected in the field. The parasite loads of wild-caught amphibians can be reduced markedly by maintaining them under good conditions of husbandry and nutrition in the laboratory.

SOME PHYSIOLOGIC DATA

Species	Approx. Gestation Period* (days)	Approx. Litter Size	Age (Weight) when Mature	Total RBC ($\times 10^6/mm^3$)	Total WBC ($\times 10^3/mm^3$)	Average Body Temp. (C°)	Approximate Water Consumption** (per day)
Mice	19	6-10	6 wk (20-30 gm)	7-11	4-12	37	4-7 ml
Rats	21	6-14	3 mo (0.2-0.3 kg)	7-10	5-15	38	30 ml
Guinea Pigs	68	1-4	3-4 mo (0.4-0.5 kg)	5-7	7-14	39	0.15 L
Hamsters, golden	16	4-10	2 mo (0.1-0.2 kg)	6-7	7-10	38	0.1-0.2 L
Gerbils	25	2-9	3 mo (60-100 gm)	7-8	8-11	39	4.0 ml
Rabbits	30	4-12	5-6 mo (3-4 kg)	5-7	6-12	40	0.3-0.7 L
Squirrel Monkeys	170	1	3-5 yr (0.6-1.1 kg)	8.3	8.2	39	0.07-0.11 L
Rhesus Monkeys	165	1-2	3-5 yr (5-11 kg)	4-6	10-20	38	0.2-1.0 L
Chimpanzees	225	1	8-12 yr (40-50 kg)	4-6	6-14	37	0.6-1.5 L
Baboons	154-183	1	3-6 yr (11-30 kg)	4-5	5-9	39	0.3-0.5 L

* *See also* REPRODUCTIVE PHENOMENA, p. 794.
** Varies with no. of animals per cage, moisture in feed, temperature, etc.

Nutritional Diseases

Long-term laboratory maintenance of most amphibians requires live food. Rickets is one example of a nutritional deficiency that may occur in *Rana* spp. Live food such as crickets, sow bugs, meal worms, or flies should be fed. Coating of the insects with powdered multiple-vitamin preparations, including vitamin D, is one way to supplement a natural diet.

CARE OF CAGED BIRDS

HUSBANDRY, MANAGEMENT AND HOUSING

One of the characteristics of wild birds, including those in captivity, is that they show few signs of disease until the illness is severe. Thus many pet birds are critically ill before they are presented for veterinary care. Birds found on the floor of the cage, i.e. unable to perch, require immediate attention. Many birds that are completely off feed and near death will still come to the feed dish and go through the motions of feeding.

Temperature of the pet bird is between 105 and 106°F (41°C). The smaller birds have a high metabolic rate and a short digestive tract. Finches, canaries and parakeets should have 25 to 50 or more droppings a day; less than 25 indicates insufficient feed intake and that the bird is using body reserves for maintenance. For larger birds, color and character of the feces are more useful as indicators of general condition. Droppings should be well formed and comprise urates and feces in equal parts; imbalances in this ratio may indicate digestive or urinary system disorders. If the diet contains large amounts of salt (crackers), there is often an increased water content, which is transient. Newspaper, or preferably, a paper towelling floor covering should be changed daily as many diseases are transmitted as aerosols of feces, especially if these are allowed to dry.

Sandpaper perches do little for toenails and tend to cause calluses and corns on the feet. Branches from apple, maple or willow trees make excellent perches; they afford a choice of diameter for perching and the bark has some nutritional value and pecking at it can relieve boredom.

Caged birds should not be subjected to sudden variations of temperature. They seem especially susceptible to heat, particularly if accompanied by prolonged low humidity. If suddenly subjected to it, they may go into a premature molt. Healthy birds can withstand cold far better than excessive heat and it is essential that the cage be placed in the section of the room which has an even temperature and is well protected from drafts. Birds maintained in outdoor aviaries year-round, with adequate shelter for protection against severe winds and rains, often exhibit superior plumage.

Any newly purchased bird should be isolated from others in the home and allowed to adjust for several weeks before any training schedule is established. Birds may be allowed to fly freely about the house but there is danger of them flying into windows or mirrors or out through open doors or windows. It is usually preferable to reduce the ability to fly by clipping the first 6 or 7 primary feathers on each wing at the junction of primary and secondary feathers. This will allow the bird to glide normally if it attempts flight from a high object, and is much less likely to result in injury than is the clipping of one wing only. Alternatively one may trim all but the end (largest) 3 primary feathers on both sides; this prevents any sustained flight but gives the individual a somewhat better cosmetic appearance. Cage size ideally should be as great as possible but at least ample to permit extension of wings. Continually caged birds should have room for limited flight and exercise. Overcrowding can be a problem if a number of birds are placed in one cage. Cages containing several birds should have a number of feed and water cups as a more aggressive bird may prevent others from obtaining adequate feed and water. Sick or injured birds should be removed at once, especially if there is any bleeding as other birds will pick at the wound.

Hand trained birds may be given limited examinations on the hand or forearm but moving or examining birds usually require that the bird be caught and restrained. A suitable restraint is described below (*see* CLINICAL EXAMINATION, p. 1211).

Birds often develop vices if not distracted or relieved from boredom as with tug toys and pieces of rawhide. An item such as a cardboard cereal box placed in the cage may serve, as may a mirror; however, mirrors should not be used with birds in training. Such birds (in training) should also be isolated from other birds to encourage their relationship with the trainer. Training procedures are best carried out away from the cage, preferably in another room.

NUTRITION OF COMPANION BIRDS

Although important, nutrition of caged birds has received only limited study and feeding requirements are not nearly as well defined as for poultry. Companion birds originate from all parts of the world and frequently it is impossible to duplicate their native foods. To help make up for a lack of knowledge of specific requirements, a wide variety of foods should be offered.

Feed Mixture: Finches and Canaries—The smaller seeds are usually selected for finch mixes. The commercially available finch seed mix contains red, white and yellow millet and occasionally some oats. This mixture can usefully be combined with commercially available canary seed blends (which include anise, flax, lettuce, poppy, rape, saffron, sesame, watergrass, endive, caraway and carrot seeds) in equal proportions and offered in the same dish. Millet spray can also be added to the finch diet.

Budgerigars and Parrakeets: The basic ration for budgerigars is canary seed, red, white and yellow millet in equal parts with a proprietary seed mixture (sesame, ryegrass, millet, flax, oats, niger and watergrass seed). To each pound of this mixture ¼ pound of oat groats are added and these ingredients are mixed and fed together.

Cockatiels and Small Parrots: A mixture of ¾ pounds of small sunflower seeds and ¼ pound safflower seed is mixed in equal parts with the budgerigar diet.

Parrots and Cockatoos: A pound of commercial parrot mix (containing sunflower seed, red peppers, peanuts, wheat and pumpkin seed) is mixed with ¼ pound of safflower seed and ¼ pound of the budgerigar mix to make a basic diet for the parrots and cockatoos.

Soft Foods: Soft foods are fed to all birds and are used to balance the diet. These can be supplied with fruits and vegetables: carrots, apples, oranges, bananas, peas, beans, corn, chickweed, spinach, romaine, lettuce, Swiss chard, dandelion greens, etc., plus fresh grass. Whole wheat bread or toast with peanut butter or fruit jelly added can also be used as appetizers for reluctant birds. Egg yolks, hard-boiled eggs and scrambled eggs should also be offered. Canned dog or cat food, semi-moist or dry meals, and most all meats, cottage cheese and hard cheeses may also be offered. The larger birds may adapt to commercial monkey biscuits. The smaller birds will also eat these if they are finely crushed. It is imperative that soft foods be available when birds start nesting.

Other Supplements: All birds should be supplied with twigs from either apple, maple or willow trees. Birds will occasionally pick at a bone from chicken, turkey or beef. In addition, a vitamin and fatty acid supplement and gravel, the size depending on the size of the bird, should be routinely added. Lugol's solution should be added to the drinking water twice a week, the amount being 1 drop for a parrakeet or canary and increasing to 4 drops for a macaw. Corn on the cob can be added to most diets. In the home, small amounts of nearly everything from spaghetti to steak may be offered, but **caution:** all items should be fed in moderation; too much of any one item can create a dietary imbalance.

CLINICAL EXAMINATION AND RESTRAINT OF COMPANION BIRDS

Diagnosis is primarily made from history and clinical examination. Many of the routine ancillary diagnostic tests used in small animal practice are not directly applicable due to the small size of the patient and the lack of normal values, although some tests are being adapted for pet birds. An easy way to obtain a blood sample is to use a 26- or 27-gauge needle and the jugular vein. In some birds the right vein is larger.

History must include origin of the bird (private breeder or commercial importer), length of time in the client's possession, previous illnesses and considerable detail concerning eating habits and diet.

Clinical examination is performed in stages: observation in the cage, handling and systematic examination, and observation of behavior after being replaced in the cage. The general attitude and signs of disease may be observed while the patient is relatively undisturbed in the cage. General depression, puffed feathers, conjunctival inflammation, nasal exudate, dyspnea, soiled vent feathers, poor feather quality and other gross abnormalities are noted before closer examination is attempted.

Next, the bird is caught using an appropriately sized towel (the towel protects both bird and handler) or better, a protective glove. For all sizes of companion birds the key maneuver of restraint is for the handler to place thumb and forefinger under or on each side of the mandible and thus control the head movements. With larger birds, e.g. parrots, an assistant is useful to restrain the bird during examination. Small birds may be restrained in one hand of the examiner. Visual examination begins with the head: crown feathers are checked for general appearance; eyes are examined for conjunctival inflammation; infraorbital sinuses are gently palpated; the beak is examined for flaking or cracks, which may indicate nutritional deficiencies and for fractures, overgrowth, wry beak, atrophy, tumors or scissor bill; the mouth is gently forced open (by placing forceps between the mandible and the maxilla); to look for stomatitis, the commissures of the mouth are checked for granulation tissue or ulcerated fibroepithelial polyps; and the tongue, pharynx and nasal turbinates are examined for signs of inflammation. In many birds, especially yellow headed parrots, cockatiels and parrakeets, mature cataracts are found as are unilateral miotic pupils. Moving to the lower body, the crop is palpated to determine the extent of filling. The fingers are moved downward over the keel bone and breast musculature to determine general fleshing of the bird. (In the well-muscled bird, a finger placed on the keel bone edge should almost contact the muscle masses on both sides of the keel bone.) With practice the gizzard, lower digestive tract and portions of reproductive tract are palpable through the abdominal wall. The cloacal opening and surrounding regions should be examined for any fecal soiling and evidence of external parasites. Next the wings are examined for muscle bruising, broken feathers and external parasites. Finally the tail feathers and uropygial gland are examined by drawing the towel forward over the lower body. Abnormal dryness or dullness of the feathers may be caused by diseases of the uropygial gland. Throughout the examination, the original restraining hold under the mandible is maintained.

For the third stage of the examination, the bird is returned to the cage, released and observed for several minutes. Its recovery to a normal posture and attitude is an excellent measure of available energy reserve. The entire examination can be completed within 2 minutes; if more time is required the patient may breathe through the mouth with great effort after being released. In extreme cases it may lie on the bottom of the cage for several minutes before attempting to rise, which may cause both owner and veterinarian some concern.

Ancillary Diagnostic Tests: Several diagnostic tests are adaptable to companion birds: serologic techniques, fecal flotation, fecal cultures and radiography. A limited hemogram, including packed-cell volume, total protein, differential and total white blood cell count (WBC), can be obtained using a large bore capillary tube plus an additional drop of blood. (A successful way of obtaining a drop of blood is to cut a nail short, then, after obtaining the drop of blood, cauterize it with silver nitrate.) The capillary tube is centrifuged to determine packed-cell volume, and the plasma then is used to determine total protein. The drop of blood is smeared on a slide and a differential WBC is determined. Total WBC is estimated using the high-power field technique. Several high-power fields containing WBCs are counted but not differentiated. The error introduced is slight and not significant in clinical practice. An average of 2 per field is normal; 2 to 4 is indicative of moderate leukocytosis and 4 or more per field of severe leukocytosis.

Fecal flotation using the Fecalizer or similar technique is readily accomplished using standard containers and diluent volumes, and reveals coccidia and worm eggs (round, cecal, capillarid). Direct fecal smears are useful in detecting coccidia and other protozoa.

Fecal cultures are beneficial: A gram of feces is suspended in 5 ml. of nutrient broth. The broth is preincubated for several hours and a loopful is streaked onto blood agar and MacConkey plates. Interpretation is relatively simple. Moderate growth of gram-positive colonies on blood agar is expected. Heavy growth of hemolytic, gram-positive colonies on blood agar is considered abnormal and the bird is treated accordingly. Heavy growth of *Escherichia coli* bacteria on MacConkey's agar is abnormal. Moderate growth of coliforms on MacConkey's agar is acceptable, but the patient's general condition is monitored closely for disease signs.

Radiology is most commonly used to confirm suspected fractures. The contrast between skeleton and body mass is high. Techniques using high-speed screens and fast film are adequate.

INTRODUCTION TO DISEASES OF CAGED BIRDS

A sick bird, regardless of cause, will appear depressed and sit huddled with its feathers puffed out. Although other clinical signs will frequently indicate which systems are distressed, often the precise cause of the malady is unknown, and treatment must be symptomatic. Fortunately certain treatment procedures are beneficial for all sick birds regardless of the etiology. Confinement to a hospital cage is beneficial in any seriously ill bird. Such a cage can easily be devised by wrapping clear plastic wrap over the cage except for the door. This cage is then placed on a heating pad, a thermometer placed inside, and the heating pad set to maintain the temperature between 75 and 80°F (27 to 29°C). Hospitalization in such a cage insures confinement and rest and increases water consumption (which is often a route of medication). Attempts to insure adequate nutrition for all sick birds are beneficial. Avian metabolism is high and recovery from disease is dependent upon adequate nutrition.

Respiratory Disease: Respiratory disease is common in companion birds. The clinical signs include dyspnea, mouth gaping, wheezing, and nasal and ocular discharge. The severity and duration of respiratory distress varies widely. Mild upper respiratory disease is often detected during routine physical examination. Chronic air sac infections are usually presented after the bird has been depressed for some time.

Mild **upper respiratory disease** is usually characterized by conjunctivitis, often with nasal discharge. Such signs may be an indication of systemic respiratory disease or the inflammation may be localized in the upper respiratory system. Localized inflammation can be caused by physical insults (e.g. temperature changes, dust) or by various bacterial infections. Streptococci, staphylococci, pasteurellae and occasional coliform bacteria are recovered from exudates.

Treatment of localized upper respiratory disease should include both local and systemic antibiotic medication. Chloramphenicol in the drinking water (12 drops of 100 mg/ml solution per 30 ml water) is usually adequate systemic medication. If higher levels are needed, chloramphenicol solution may be placed directly in the birds mouth twice daily (2 drops for a parrakeet, 0.1 ml for cockatiels, and up to 0.5 ml for parrots using 100 mg/ml solution). Alternatively 1% tetracycline solution may be administered similarly. Small animal ophthalmic ointments containing either antibiotics alone or antibiotic-steroid combinations may be used. Nasal decongestants intended for animal or human use may be administered by placing 1 or 2 drops in each nostril several times daily. Decongestants should not be used over an extended period of time.

Airsacculitis is the most serious and life threatening disease syndrome encountered in pet birds. Various infections of the relatively large air sacs commonly occur. Clinical signs include extreme depression, anorexia, dypsnea and rales detectable upon thoracic or abdominal auscultation. Upper respiratory disease signs may or may not be present. Causes include *Chlamydia, Mycoplasma, Escherichia coli, Klebsiella, Pasteurella,* Paramyxovirus (Newcastle disease virus), Orthomyxovirus (influenza virus), yeasts and *Aspergillus.* With such a wide range of infectious agents, microbiologic cultures and virus isolations should be attempted whenever possible.

Regardless of the original cause, most serious airsac infections are complicated. Chlamydial infections (q.v., p. 1071) are often encountered in pet-bird practice and may spread to both practitioner and owner. Such infections are most apt to occur in newly imported birds and thus should be considered when severe airsacculitis occurs in newly purchased or in groups of birds recently released from quarantine. Conversely chlamydial infections are unusual in birds that have been in the owner's possession for a number of years.

Prognosis should be guarded in even apparently mild airsac infections and radical treatment is indicated. Treatment includes high level antibiotic therapy combined with hospitalization and good nursing. Therapy is best initiated with a series of antibiotic injections and followed by oral antibiotics. For chlamydial, mycoplasmal and some bacterial infections, chloramphenicol (100 mg/ml) injections are administered IM (0.03 ml for parrakeets, 0.1 ml for cockatiels and up to 0.5 ml for parrots), followed by oral medication with chloramphenicol as described under upper respiratory diseases (q.v., p. 1214). If gram-negative bacteria, in particular, are suspected, gentamicin sulfate (50 mg/ml) injections should be administered (0.03 ml for parrakeets, 0.1 ml for cockatiels, and 0.5 ml for parrots). These injections must produce a beneficial response in 3 to 5 days or an alternative antibiotic should be used. An alternative is injections of tetracycline solution, 10 mg/ml (0.03 ml for parrakeets, 0.1 ml for cockatiels, and up to 0.5 ml for parrots). This injection series can be followed with tetracycline water medication as described above for upper respiratory disease.

When airsacculitis is caused by chronic fungal infections, treatment may be attempted with nystatin suspension or amphotericin B. (Amphotericin B is only effective IV as it is not absorbed orally. At 75 mg/kg in the first dose, followed with 0.5 mg/kg daily for 1 week, nystatin suspension [100,000 u/ml] is used at the rate of 1 ml for a parrot.)

Enteric Disease: Enteric diseases also are commonly seen in pet-bird practice. Clinical signs include generalized depression, anorexia, emaciation, abnormal feces, soiled feathers and visible lesions in the mouth, pharynx or cloaca. Duration of the disease can usually be estimated from the degree of emaciation present. Enteric diseases can be divided clinically into diseases of the upper and lower digestive system.

Diseases of the upper digestive system include inflammation of the mouth, pharynx, esophagus, crop and true stomach. Clinical signs indicative of upper digestive system distress are reluctance to eat and regurgitation. Visible examination of the mouth, pharynx and upper esophagus may facilitate diagnosis. Either diffuse or focal inflammation of the mouth and pharynx is commonly caused by gram-negative bacteria, especially *Pseudomonas* sp. Mild inflammation of the pharynx is often associated with upper respiratory disease and medicated as part of that syndrome (q.v., p. 1214). Avian pox (q.v., p. 1097) can cause both diffuse and focal inflammation of the mouth and pharynx in parrakeets, lovebirds and some parrots. When inflammations occur in the mouth or pharynx, the patient is reluctant to eat. Therapy must include a soft-food diet which can be ingested with minimal pain. Antibiotic medication is indicated in all inflammations of the mouth; the antibiotics should be placed directly into the mouth in an attempt to obtain a local as well as systemic effect. Chloramphenicol solutions may be used in mild inflammations at the dosage level as given for oral chloramphenicol medication in respiratory diseases (q.v., p. 1214). Medication should be continued until inflammatory tissues have healed. If inflammation is severe and abscesses to be expected, oral medication twice daily with gentamicin sulfate, 50 mg/ml (2 drops for parrakeets; 0.1 ml for cockatiels; 0.5 ml for parrots) may be beneficial.

Inflammations of the crop and true stomach usually cause regurgitation as their outstanding clinical sign. A variety of disease agents, including yeast, protozoa and certain metazoan parasites may cause inflammation of the crop wall. Direct smears may help to determine the cause, as capillarid eggs, yeast and protozoa may be visible. Accurate diagnosis is necessary for effective treatment. *Capillaria* infections of the crop may be treated by using levamisole soluble powder in the drinking water at the level of 2 gm/gal. (0.5 gm/L) for several days. Yeast infections of the crop wall may respond to twice daily oral medication with nystatin pediatric solution, 100,000 u/ml (again 2 drops for a parrakeet, 0.1 ml for a cockatiel and up to 0.5 ml for parrots). Protozoan infections of the crop usually respond readily to water medication with dimetridazole (0.05% in water for 7 to 10 days). In addition to infections, ingested toxic substances may severely irritate the crop wall. Such conditions must be treated symptomatically.

Inflammations of the true stomach are usually associated with the inflammations of the crop and indicated by violent regurgitation of ingesta. Since these are most often caused by ingestion of foreign substances, treatment is highly symptomatic. Oral medication with anticholinergic and coating products are beneficial. As with other species, these products (usually with kaolin base) may be given as often as needed.

Inflammation of the lower digestive tract is usually characterized by various degrees of diarrhea. Vent feathers are often stained with feces. Normal feces in most pet birds contain approximately equal parts of urates and fecal material. The fluid contained in a normal bowel movement should diffuse out on a newspaper to approximately the size of a dime (17 mm diameter). Larger circles of fluid diffusion indicate fluid loss from the bird. Most inflammations of the lower gut are caused by either bacteria or intestinal parasites. Several viruses also infect the gut (notably Newcastle disease); however, these diseases usually have other signs associated with them.

Intestinal parasitism in pet birds is commonly caused by round, capillarid and cecal worms. Roundworms respond to piperazine given at 4 times the dosage recommended for mammals. Thiabendazole medication (also given at 4 times the recommended dosage for mammals) is beneficial in removing cecal worms. Capillarids present a special problem. It is necessary to use levamisole at 2 gm/gal. (0.5 gm/L) of drinking water for several days.

The most commonly encountered inflammations of the lower digestive tract in pet birds are caused by a variety of bacteria. Birds in good flesh are usually in the early phases of this disease. Birds having diarrhea for a period of time may be severely emaciated, hence treatment must include improvement of diet (including forced feeding if necessary) as well as antibiotic medication. A broad-spectrum antibiotic such as chloramphenicol given either in the water or orally is indicated. Chloramphenicol dosages for both water and oral usage are included under treatment of respiratory diseases (q.v., p. 1214). Alternatively tetracyclines may be given by the same routes (these dosages are also included under treatment of upper respiratory diseases). Water medication with sulfa drugs often produces a beneficial response in diarrheic conditions when antibiotic medication has failed to do so. Any of the sulfa drugs can be used at approximately 2 to 4 times the dosage level recommended for mammals. Sulfadimethoxine (12 drops of 12.5% solution per ounce of drinking water) has proven beneficial.

Systemic Diseases: While a variety of bacteria, viruses and other infectious agents are capable of causing systemic disease in pet birds, **Newcastle disease** (ND) deserves special mention. Even though government regulatory agencies attempt to prevent entry of ND into the U.S.A. and several other countries, outbreaks occasionally occur, most often in quarantine facilities or aviaries with newly imported birds. ND virus affects respiratory, enteric and nervous systems. The most obvious signs are usually respiratory, although it may occur as an enteric disease syndrome; nervous system malfunctions are also possible. In summary, ND may cause nearly all of the clinical disease signs mentioned for pet birds.

When ND is suspected, diagnosis will usually be made by postmortem examination and virus isolation attempts. Hemagglutination inhibitory antibodies may be detected from serum samples but to determine whether antibody titers are the result of active infection or the consequence of previous infections requires serologic profiles. The disease is not treated. Affected birds are destroyed by government mandate and any suspicion of presence of the disease should be reported to appropriate regulatory officials. (*See also* NEWCASTLE DISEASE, p. 1106.)

THERAPY FOR BACTERIAL AND YEAST INFECTIONS IN CAGED BIRDS

Bacteria	Drug	Conc. (mg/ml)	Dose (Drops/oz Drinking Water)
Gram-Positive	Lincomycin	100	6
Gram-Positive	Tylosin	50	12
Gram-Positive	Erythromycin	200	3
Gram-Positive or Gram-Negative	Chloramphenicol	100	6
Gram-Negative	Ampicillin	200	2
Gram-Negative	Kanamycin	50	8
Gram-Negative	Spectinomycin	100	4
Yeast	Chlorhexidine	20	1 ml/qt (L) drinking water for not more than 5 consecutive days
Yeast	Nystatin (Mycostatin)	100,000 u/ml	0.25 ml/oz body wt b.i.d.

Disorders of the Feathers and Skin: Birds in normal molt will often be presented with the complaint of feather disorders because the bird is losing feathers and the feather coat is rough. Birds are often moved from one hemisphere to another, from a warm to a cold climate or vice versa, or to a location where there is increased daylight, and as any of these changes can initiate molting, molting in pet birds can occur at any time. It should be explained to the owner that this is a natural process. Owners of birds with excessively dry feathers may be advised to use an ounce of a good bath oil in 15 oz (450 ml) of water, sprayed from a spray bottle from a distance of 3 ft (1 m), in 2 or 3 "bursts" of spray.

A second commonly encountered complaint is that birds are losing feathers in localized or generalized areas of the body, particularly from the neck down. Spots on the wings or breast may be nearly devoid of feathers, while the remainder of the feather coat is in generally good condition. On close examination it is usually found that these birds are pulling or plucking their own feathers. While irritation and feather picking may be due to external parasites (lice and mites), it is usually a psychologic problem. Having no outlet for their activities, birds through boredom may turn to picking their own feathers. The key to the diagnosis of this problem is that the feathers on the head and neck are normal. This vice is best relieved by using toys or other devices to relieve boredom. A cardboard or plastic doughnut-shaped collar can be placed over the head so that self-inflicted trauma and the pulling of feathers can be controlled.

Several feather disorders of hormonal origin also occur. The most common is in the male canary that has gone through a molt and stopped singing. The molt can be almost completed, however, the bird still continues to molt very slightly. Careful examination reveals the presence of a few new feathers. This is associated with low testosterone levels. Feather growth and return to singing can usually be accomplished by a series of repositol testosterone injections (0.015 ml of 50 mg/ml IM every 3 to 4 weeks). Other hormonal problems may occur as inability to grow feathers and a completely bald bird. These birds also may respond to testosterone. If the bird is obese it may be hypothyroid. A 1-grain (65-mg) thyroid tablet crushed in the feed daily should provide a therapeutic intake of the drug.

Of the true dermatoses occurring in pet birds, fungal infections seem to be the commonest. Rather exotic fungal agents occasionally infect the larger pet birds as many of these birds originate in tropical and semitropical climates where fungal growth is abundant. These fungi may infect the feather follicle of both old and new feathers.

Treatment for such fungal infections is difficult. Mild infections may respond to a series of chlorhexidine baths. (Chlorhexidine at 1 ml/pt [2 ml/L] of water is placed in a common house plant sprayer and the bird is sprayed liberally twice daily.) Treatment of the more severe infections may be attempted using oral treatments with griseofulvin at approximately 4 times the mammalian dosage.

Diseases of the Urogenital System: Most of the urogenital disorders are either bacterial infections of the kidney and ureters, or the egg-bound female. Occasionally in birds presented with signs of listlessness and anorexia, close examination of droppings will reveal an abnormally high ratio of urates to fecal material. The amount of fluid in each dropping may be increased and the fluid spot on the dropping paper larger than expected. These are usually signs of disorders of the urinary system, although pancreatic disorders can occur and confuse the picture. (Diabetes has been diagnosed in companion birds.) Close examination may reveal tenderness along the lower back, or the bird may actually tend to pick at the feathers along the lower back. These are additional signs of urogenital tract infections.

Most infections of the urinary tract are caused by the gram-negative bacteria: *Escherichia coli*, *Salmonella* spp., *Klebsiella* sp. and *Citrobacter* sp. Vigorous treatment is necessary for even a moderate degree of success. A series of injections utilizing an antibiotic selected for gram-negative bacteria should be administered, e.g. gentamicin (50 mg/ml) injections (0.03 ml for parrakeets, 0.10 ml for cockatiels and up to 0.5 ml for larger parrots) daily for 3 to 5 days. A beneficial response during this time is essential as kidney diseases are usually acute and rapidly cause debilitation and death. The series may be followed by chloramphenicol water medication (as mentioned in the section on respiratory diseases, q.v., p. 1214). Once a beneficial response has been obtained, alternate treatments can include other antibiotics such as kanamycin and spectinomycin, which are directed specifically against the gram-negative bacteria. In kidney diseases, it is imperative that the birds be placed in a hospital cage where temperature is maintained and water consumption will be maximized. Maximum movement of water through the kidneys is of significant therapeutic benefit.

A condition known as **external and visceral gout**, in which urates are deposited in the joints or the serous membranes, usually appears clinically as swelling of the joints or as a distressed urinary system without visible pain in the kidney region. Gout is thought to be a metabolic disease in which high levels of proteins, purine and pyrimidines are improperly metabolized. Treatment consists of use of a hospital cage to increase water consumption and a water soluble antibiotic such as chloramphenicol to prevent secondary bacterial infections. Allopurinol may be administered for external gout; this will prevent extension of the disease, although it will not alleviate the condition already present. Alkaline drinking water may also be helpful (use a pinch of bicarbonate of soda in the drinking water daily).

Perhaps the most commonly encountered urogenital syndrome in companion bird medicine is the **egg-bound female.** The female will be found crouching on the floor of the cage trembling and apparently in pain. There is usually a history of egg laying. Depending on the amount of time in labor, the bird can be approaching or in shock. Gentle palpation of the abdomen may or may not reveal an egg in the abdominal cavity. Increasing the cage temperature to 85°F (30°C) will often result in the delivery of the egg. If this fails, the bird is turned on its back and a warm lubricant placed in the cloaca. The egg is propelled backward by constant and gentle pressure using the thumb and forefinger. A small amount of lubricant is applied to the egg as it comes into view. Care must be taken to prevent breaking the egg as this can cause a serious medical problem. A lubricated cotton applicator can be rotated around the egg while pressure is being applied. If necessary, episiotomy can be performed.

If the cloaca prolapses following severe straining, the protruding portion can be gently replaced and if necessary a purse string suture placed for 12 to 24 hours. The bird should be placed in a warm hospital cage until recovered. It should be isolated as other birds will peck at the inflamed tissues. Appropriate measures should be instituted to prevent shock by injecting steroids such as triamcinolone (2 mg/ml), 0.02 ml IM for a parrakeet.

CARE OF ZOO ANIMALS

The immediate surroundings and the management of captive wild animals have a direct and important bearing on their well-being. If animals are to be kept in zoological collections, then an attempt must be made to meet their physical, psychological, social, nutritional and medical requirements. The design of the enclosures to meet these requirements can themselves create management and medical problems. The natural looking exhibit with soil and vegetation makes adequate sanitation and parasite control difficult.

Management and Observation: The backbone of a complete medical program is a qualified and dedicated keeper staff who observe their animals for abnormalities such as anorexia, inactivity, abnormal feces and changes in behavior that may reflect early medical problems. Overzealous reporting of inconsequential observations is preferable to indifference. Since many exotic species instinctively mask overt outward signs of illness until the problem is well advanced, it is necessary to make keepers perceptive of what may seem to be trivial changes. Also, many animals associate the veterinarian's presence with past experiences, arousing responses that mask subtle changes observable by the keepers.

Environment: Except for tropical specimens, healthy captive mammals and birds do not require a great deal of heat. Reptiles require access to temperature gradients of up to 95°F (35°C), but must not be kept in direct sunlight on hot days for prolonged periods. A moderate temperature of 65 to 68°F (18 to 20°C) is adequate for most mammals and birds. Some species native to warmer climates adjust surprisingly well when allowed access to their outdoor cages during the winter months and often show improvement in the appearance of their pelage or plumage during the cold weather. Local experience regarding climatic needs for different species is valuable information. The fact that certain species can endure extremes of climate is no license to subject them to adverse conditions; proper shelters and close observation are always indicated. During cold weather, the floor of the sleeping quarters for mammals should be insulated, heated or covered with clean, dry bedding to prevent excess loss of body heat. It is necessary to provide adequate shelter and observe if it is being used. Some animals may not use the shelters and suffer cold injuries, such as frostbite of the ears, horns and hooves, or even die of exposure. Many times the dominant animals will use the shelter and keep subordinate animals in the cold. The energy requirements of animals subjected to colder environment is increased, requiring changes in diet.

Handling of Animals: The treatment of disease conditions in captive wild animals does not differ substantially from that of domestic species once the diagnosis is made, except in the method of restraint. Most undomesticated animals resent being handled and will usually fight manual restraint. Struggling with an animal to administer medical or surgical treatment may do more harm than can be offset by the treatment. It is, therefore, advantageous to conceal medication in food or drinking water whenever possible, eliminating anxiety for both animals and caretakers.

Restraint is indispensable, and the squeeze cage or chute is frequently used. While the dimensions and construction vary depending on the species to be handled, all operate on the principle of moving one wall to restrain the animal against the opposite wall of the cage. Useful procedures can be carried out on an unanesthetized animal so confined, e.g. limited physical examination, giving injections, obtaining blood samples, trimming ingrown claws or applying topical medication. Squeeze cages should ideally be designed as part of the animal's regular quarters. Whenever possible, patients should be enticed into the cage rather than forcibly compelled to enter it, or the cage should be constructed in a normal shifting area. Immobilizing drugs can be administered IV or IM with the aid of a squeeze cage.

Many zoos install small nest boxes or catch pens within the exhibit enclosure. Such retreats are equipped with doors that can be operated remotely and can be used to trap or catch animals. From these catch pens, the confined animal can readily be transferred to a squeeze cage, anesthetic chamber or into a shipping crate.

Smaller animals and birds may be caught and restrained in long-handled hoop nets. These nets must be sufficiently deep so that the animal may be dropped into a blind end of the net and the upper part twisted to prevent escape. The operator doing this work should wear protective gloves.

Drug Administration: A useful instrument for administering drugs to wild animals is a gun to propel a projectile syringe. Intramuscular injections as of antibiotics or immobilizing agents in volumes as large as 10 ml can be made accurately at a distance of approximately 60 yards (55 m). Practice with projectile darts is mandatory prior to their clinical use because expert marksmanship is essential; such weapons in the hands of a novice can be fatal. Other methods of injecting animals over a shorter distance include a syringe pole or a blow gun. Safe immobilization and anesthesia in wild animals are of special concern. Many procedures, routinely accomplished on domestic animals with minimal restraint, will require chemical immobilization of the zoo specimen for the welfare of both the patient and handler.

Dissociative anesthetics (phencyclidine and ketamine) are the commonest anesthetic agents for most small to medium sized mammals and birds. These are usually combined with a tranquilizer to speed induction, minimize excitement, increase muscle relaxation and provide a smoother anesthetic procedure. Etorphine (M99), alone or in combination with other agents (acepromazine, xylazine) has been extensively used for immobilization in ungulates, elephants and rhinoceroses. One advantage of etorphine is that a rapid-acting antagonist, diprenorphine (M50-50), can be given IV. Xylazine used alone can also provide adequate immobilization in some species of ungulates.

The factors affecting response to immobilizing drugs include age, sex, stage of reproductive cycle and general nutritional status. There are marked species as well as individual variations. The mental state of the patient prior to the drug administration is also important. An excited animal usually requires more drug and, once immobilized, has a higher tendency for hyperthermia and acidosis. The literature should be consulted for appropriate dosage information. Emergency resuscitative and supportive equipment and trained personnel should be at hand. Some immobilizing procedures and dosages may work well in a particular species in one collection but not in another collection.

When anesthesia must be maintained, inhalation anesthetics as halothane or metofane can be used. Nitrous oxide, in combination with halothane, is used unless the animal is a ruminant or has a large cecum.

Preventive medicine is primary to adequate zoological care; this includes quarantine procedures, routine parasitic examinations, routine physical examinations and testing, as well as specific vaccination programs. All newly acquired animals should be quarantined. Isolation quarters should be separate from the exhibit areas, serviced by separate caretakers, and so constructed that they can be easily cleaned and disinfected. Death losses of zoo animals are often greatest during initial acclimation, and care is therefore required in noting dietary intake, character of feces, signs of disease or any abnormal behavior. Adjusting animals to new feeds and feeding schedules is frequently difficult. Some specimens may require force-feeding.

Wild animals are vulnerable to a wide variety of endo- and ecto-parasitic infections, somewhat parallel to those found in domestic animals. The impact of these parasites on individual animals is variable, but is probably greatest at the time of the animal's shipment and arrival at the zoo. During this period of extreme stress, many normally commensal parasites, especially protozoa, appear to be capable of establishing pathogenic processes. Acute diarrhea may result from massive infections of *Trichomonas, Giardia* or *Balantidium.* Amebiasis is fairly common in primates and reptiles and may terminate in death.

Periodic examination of the skin and pelage and fecal specimens should be made during the quarantine procedure. For ecto- and endoparasites, an appropriate treatment regimen should be instituted. Parasites with indirect life cycles will less frequently impose a public health problem if the exhibit area is clean and free of intermediate hosts. If ectoparasites are found on newly received animals, proper spraying of the shipping crate and its contents is recommended before the crate leaves the quarantine area. Some zoos routinely use an organophosphate spray for such purposes.

Diagnostic tests should be routine. Tuberculosis is a potential threat in primates, especially Old World primates, and may spread rapidly if introduced into a colony. For this reason, no primates should be added to a collection without first having been found negative on 3 tuberculin tests at 2-week intervals. Testing of primates should be maintained on a biannual or annual basis. Tuberculosis is also a problem in exotic ungulates and TB testing should be a part of the preventive medical program. The keeper staff should also be tested periodically; such testing not only protects the staff but also protects the animals from infected personnel.

Vaccination of exotic Carnivora, which are susceptible to canine distemper, hepatitis and feline panleukopenia, is essential. The type of vaccine to use (modified live or killed) is still unresolved and continued study is needed. Other vaccines for feline upper respiratory disease are used in some collections, with good results.

Newly arriving specimens require caution and patience during uncrating and release since they are often frightened and fatigued. Ungulates have been fatally injured when released from shipping crates by running directly into barriers. Birds often try to fly through the glass cage fronts. Canvasses or colored plastic drop cloths suspended from the fences or cage walls or obscuring the glass windows with soap offer some measure of protection against such accidents by producing a visual barrier.

Though the new arrivals may appear famished, it is preferable to limit the quantity of food and especially water supplied at the first feeding. Later, the frequency and volume of feed can be increased.

More often, the newly arrived animal refuses to eat for the first few days. Such individuals must be pampered and fed their former diets, and only gradually weaned to the standard zoo diet for the species. Despite elaborate precautions, a number of new animals fail to adapt to a zoo environment and die, especially reptiles.

With larger numbers of birds or mammals, and especially when several species are housed in one exhibit or flight cage, it is recommended that several feeding and watering stations be established. Multiple feeding areas at appropriate elevations will help reduce injuries and death resulting from territorial invasions. If different types of feed are offered to mixed groups in one enclosure, it may be beneficial to feed these types of food separately. Multiple feeding stations may help reduce the size of individual territories.

All zoos should be conservation-minded and interested in animal reproduction. It is therefore important that the nature of the animal and its social behavior be understood. Species should be maintained alone, in pairs or in groups, depending upon their established social system and how social behavior is influenced during the breeding season. For example, in mixed species groups of Artiodactyla it is possible to establish estrous cycles by species and thus have only one male in the enclosure at a time. The other males can be rotated to coincide with the estrous periods of their species. Such measures often will reduce injuries. At parturition it is advisable to remove the males for several weeks to prevent attack on the postpartum females or their offspring.

Trimming beaks and nails of birds should be routine procedure. Pinioning of birds to prevent flight is readily accomplished by amputating one wing just distal to the radiocarpal joint or performing a tenectomy and fusing the radiocarpal joint. Other pinioning methods are also used and can be found in the literature. Pinioning of young birds is easier and more successful than the same procedure in adults. (*See also* p. 1210.)

Much can be learned about the diseases affecting zoo animals if a complete necropsy is made following all deaths. The prosector should constantly be aware of the variations in anatomy as such observations may aid in disease diagnosis and treatment.

Some Principles of Treatment: Bone fractures are repaired under general anesthesia. Since maintaining a splint on a wild animal is often difficult, rigid internal fixation is preferable whenever possible. When a cast is applied, freedom of movement and a minimum of discomfort to the patient must be assured as the cast must be left as applied for 3 to 4 weeks. Newer light-weight, strong and waterproof casting material is especially applicable in zoological medicine. Any fracture fixation should be rigid, strong, and require minimal postoperative care to obtain the best results.

Antibiotic therapy in exotic species has been empirical. Doses have been extrapolated from other mammals, but little consideration has been made for the different metabolic rates of the patients, such as snakes versus birds. Thus, the pharmacokinetics of drugs in the various species is important. When prescribing antibiotics and other drugs, these factors must be kept in mind if beneficial results are to be obtained.

Dentistry in zoo animals may present unique problems. The roots of canine teeth in monkeys and carnivores are more extensive than the exposed crown and it is not possible to remove such a tooth intact by simple traction and rotation; dislodging with a dental elevator is essential. A small electric drill or bone chisel may have to be used to remove a section of maxilla around the labial margin of the root. The incisor teeth of rodents, such as beavers, porcupines and capybaras, grow continually throughout life, and unless these animals are supplied with coarse feed or logs to gnaw on, their incisors will grow excessively long and interfere with their ability to feed. Periodontal disease in exotic species is treated by routine cleaning and providing adequate chewing substances to supplement the soft, prepared diets fed many animals.

CARE OF MARINE MAMMALS

The 3 principal groups of marine mammals are: the Cetaceans, the Pinnipeds and the Sirenians. Adventitious species such as the sea otter and the polar bear are not generally classed with the above but are considered under zoo animals in general. Sea otters are kept in captivity in very limited numbers at present.

The Cetaceans are made up of 2 groups, the toothed whales or Odontocetes, and the baleen whales, or Mysticetes. The Mysticetes are not discussed here as few if any are kept in captivity. The Odontocetes, on the other hand, are represented by a number of small species, which readily adapt to captivity and display. The Sirenians, the only entirely herbivorous marine mammals, are kept in captivity at a few oceanariums. In the U.S.A., all marine mammals are protected under the Marine Mammal Protection Act of 1972 and the Endangered Species Act of 1973.

The Pinnipeds are subdivided into 3 groups: the true seals (Phocidae), the sea lions and fur seals (Otariidae) and the walruses (Obodenidae). Of these groups the animals that are kept in captivity are the harbor seal, harp seal, California sea lion, Stellar sea lion, elephant seal and walrus. Few fur seals are kept in captivity.

The Odontocetes usually kept for display or research purposes are the bottlenosed dolphin (*Tursiops truncatus*), the white-sided dolphin (*Lagenorynchus* spp.), the killer whale (*Orcinus* spp.), the pilot whale (*Globicephala* spp.), Risso's dolphin (*Grampus* spp.), and the false killer whale (*Pseudorca* spp.).

Restraint of marine mammals, as with all others, is necessary for some examinations and treatments. The presence of familiar and trusted attendants during such efforts can be of great help. Small cetaceans may be netted in the pool and hauled out onto sponge rubber mats where most will lie quietly. The tail may be dangerous but a large attendant can usually control this by sitting on the tail head. If necessary the mouth can be held closed by one attendant with a towel, or open by 2 attendants with towels.

At the other extreme, very large animals are best lowered onto sponge rubber matting by draining of their pools. A killer whale may be sufficiently restrained for most purposes if a stout nylon rope is looped over the tail and fastened to the pool edge.

Small seals may be restrained by having an experienced attendant sit on the back and hold the neck. Sea lions are more difficult, and can give severe bite wounds. Netting and manual restraint may suffice but specially designed in-pool squeeze cages are better.

Tranquilizers, sedatives and anesthetics should only be used by those experienced in administering them to wild species. It is not recommended unless specially designed equipment is available.

The cetaceans and pinnipeds are entirely marine with some exceptions in each group. The pinnipeds also are capable of "hauling out" for long periods. Many pinnipeds are kept in fresh water tanks with apparently few ill effects provided their diets are supplemented with sodium chloride. However, pinnipeds that are kept in simulated or actual sea water should have access to fresh water for drinking purposes. This may be done by providing a hose that "leaks" fresh water suspended over the pool. On the other hand, cetaceans, with 1 or 2 rare exceptions, cannot be kept in fresh water for long periods as after about 10 days their dermal epithelial cells start to balloon and slough, followed by secondary bacterial infection. They, and other marine mammals, need an aquatic environment with a minimum concentration of 2% sodium chloride. Mid-ocean water is about 3.5% sodium chloride and has a pH of around 8.

It is recommended that those animals having access to fresh water have their diet supplemented with sodium chloride at the rate of 3 gm/kg of food daily and their plasma electrolytes monitored (at least daily) until they have stabilized within normal limits. If these remain below normal the salt supplementation can be increased until homeostasis is achieved. It is also recommended that the animals *always* have access to fresh drinking water while on salt supplementation, as in some cases animals are penned during off-hours and cannot get to their pools.

The clinical signs of **hyponatremia** are anorexia and weakness and are sometimes seen in captive California sea lions, northern fur seals, Stellar sea lions and harp seals. Harbor seals seem to tolerate fresh water much better than harp seals. These animals are probably borderline Addisonian (adrenocortical atrophy) and only show clinical signs when another stress such as vitamin deficiencies or molting are superimposed. The same clinical syndrome would probably occur in small cetaceans kept long enough in fresh water, however the inimical effect of the water on their skin supersedes any noticeable electrolyte imbalance.

Standards and Regulations for Humane Handling, Care, Treatment and Transportation of Marine Mammals, (U.S. Fed. Reg. 43 #182, Sept. 19, 1978), have been proposed. It is anticipated that these will become available from the U.S. Superintendent of Documents.

SIRENIANS

There are no published reports on diseases found in this group of herbivorous marine animals. From personal communications, the dugongs have died from malnutrition, fecal impactions and gastric ulcers. All deaths of manatees in captivity have resulted from severe trauma or respiratory problems.

Animals of both genera that appear ill have been treated with all the drugs traditionally used on dolphins or extrapolated from similar clinical situation in dogs, but with equivocal results.

PINNIPEDS AND CETACEANS

Husbandry and Nutrition

The 2 most important aspects of keeping marine mammals in captivity are nutrition and management (housing, etc.). All marine mammals, including those that haul out, should be kept in water with at least 2% but less than 3% salt. The water temperature should range between 55 and 80°F depending on the species. Cetaceans usually frequent an environment close to their critical temperature. Cold water does not seem to affect pinnipeds noticeably, provided they have been acclimated to decreasing temperatures. All animals that haul out should be provided with shelter from the wind and shade (*see also* p. 1235). Where large fluctuations in both air and water temperatures occur, devices should be installed for both cooling and heating water and for protection from very cold air temperature, i.e. a canopy over the water so that animals do not inhale extremely cold air.

For nutrition, only good quality, unspoiled food should be fed. This should include as wide a variety of fish as are available. Those responsible for maintenance of health in captive marine mammals should be familiar with what constitutes good quality fish. High quality frozen fish is preferred as spoilage is controlled and fresh fish may transmit infective parasites. Such a diet should be supplemented with a multivitamin preparation at least 2 to 3 times a week.

Thiamin Deficiency: Many fresh-water and salt-water fishes contain thiaminase, an enzyme that results in thiamin deficiency in animals fed exclusively on a diet of such fish. Clinical signs are anorexia and neurologic manifestations. Treatment consists of injections of thiamin hydrochloride plus supplementing the diet with oral thiamin. The response is quite dramatic and complete. The oral preparation should be concealed in fish that contains no thiaminase (q.v., p. 1354) and fed at least ½ to 2 hours before the regular feeding. This gives sufficient time for the thiamin to be absorbed before risking inactivation by the other fish in the diet.

Bacterial Diseases

Erysipelas: The most serious infectious disease of captive cetaceans and pinnipeds is erysipelas. The organism, *Erysipelothrix rhusiopathiae (insidiosa)*, is the same as that which causes erysipelas in swine and other domestic species, (q.v., p. 348). The disease may be peracute, acute or chronic. Peracute disease is usually unaccompanied by signs; the animals die quickly, within a very few hours. The acute form is characterized by depression and inappetence; fever, though probably present, has not been recorded for obvious reasons. At necropsy, widespread petechiation may be seen. In chronic disease the typical rhomboid skin lesions are usually seen; these animals usually recover after treatment with penicillin or tetracyclines and good nursing. Arthritis has also been found in animals that have died after the manifestation of the more chronic form of the disease. The diagnosis of the disease must be made by culture and identification of the organism.

Primary vaccination of all animals should be with a bacterin followed in 6 months with a modified live vaccine. Annual revaccination is recommended. Some aquaria do not vaccinate their pinnipeds but all captive cetaceans should be immunized. The animals are usually vaccinated in the dorsal musculature anterior and lateral to the dorsal fin. (In some instances where the vaccine was administered posterior and lateral to the dorsal fin the ensuing reaction immobilized the animals for a number of days.) No more than 3 to 5 ml of the vaccine should be used at any one site.

Leptospirosis: An infectious disease of California sea lions and the northern fur seal caused by *Leptospira* spp., characterized by depression, reluctance to use the rear quarters and back, and extreme thirst and fever. In aquaria the disease usually afflicts subadult males (2 to 8 years). At necropsy a severe, diffuse, interstitial nephritis has been observed; some of the tubules appear almost occluded by the spirochetes. The gall bladder may contain inspissated black bile, but hepatitis may not be obvious although hyperplasia of Kupffer's cells, erythrophagocytosis and hemosiderosis have been noted. Gastritis has been seen in a few animals as well as an enteritis. With fluorescent antibody techniques the following species have been identified: *L. canicola*, *L. icterohemorrhagiae*, *L. autumnalis* and *L. pomona*.

It is believed that *Leptospira* spp. cause many abortions in the wild California sea lion population as well as in northern fur seals. This expression of the disease has not been reported in captive sea lions. However since rehabilitated strandlings are now being sent to all parts of the country, the possibility exists that a subclinically infected animal may be among them, thereby posing a threat to the resident animals. The newly bought animal should probably be examined serologically in order to determine its exposure to the disease.

Puddles of infected urine are believed to be the source of contact since these animals are gregarious and do come onto land to breed and give birth. Captive animals can be vaccinated or treated with a penicillin-streptomycin combination, or both. The organisms are infective for man and suitable precautions should be taken, especially during necropsies of aborted fetuses that appear to have died of a hemorrhagic septicemia.

Pneumonia is probably the chief cause of death in captive marine mammals. Most of the organisms cultured from terrestrial species with pneumonic conditions have also been incriminated in pneumonias in marine mammals. Viruses have been suspected but none has ever been isolated. Pneumonias secondary to lungworm infections (q.v., p.1233) are common. It is not known how critical the difference is between air and water temperature, but cold environmental air conditions have been suspected in some cases of unexplained pneumonias, especially in cetaceans. Since small cetaceans normally inhabit water near to their bodily critical temperatures, breathing cold air may predispose them to infections. Pinnipeds that have been acclimated to cooling temperatures are quite hardy. However sea lions have died of fulminant pneumonia when they have been moved from warm environments to outside aquaria in cold weather.

Clostridial myositis has been found in captive cetaceans (killer whale, pilot whale and bottlenosed dolphin). It is recommended that all marine mammals in facilities where the disease has occurred be vaccinated with a commercially available clostridial bacterin.

Viral Diseases

In wild pinnipeds, 2 viral diseases have been diagnosed. These are San Miguel sea lion virus (SMSLV) disease and seal pox. The only significance to the presence of SMSLV in pinnipeds is the potential hazard to the health of agricultural animals since the virus is almost identical to that of vesicular exanthema (q.v., p. 261).

Seal Pox: A viral disease that has been reported in harbor seals, California sea lions and South American sea lions. It is manifested as a proliferative epithelial lesion consisting of multiple cornified papillomas located in the area of the head and neck. The disease usually occurs in newly arrived animals or in a stable captive population after the introduction of a new animal. The agent is a typical poxvirus producing the same signs and lesions as in other species (q.v., p. 242 and 1097). It occurs primarily in young animals and is characterized by raised nodules. The often dramatic lesions do not produce any ill effect and are self-limiting.

Since most seal pox lesions regress spontaneously, it is usually enough to isolate the animal and treat any complicating problems. If single lesions persist they may be removed surgically. An autogenous vaccine may be prepared and used in cases with multiple persisting lesions. Finely ground wart material with 10 volumes of 50% glycerol-saline solution has been used. Two to 5 ml are injected subcut.; this is repeated in 10 to 14 days.

No viral diseases have been diagnosed in captive cetaceans. Many disorders such as pneumonitis, hepatitis and skin diseases have been suspected of having a viral etiology; however no viruses have been isolated. Antibodies against human influenza virus (after challenge) and poliomyelitis virus have been found in *Tursiops truncatus*. Scoliosis has been observed in some small cetaceans, but the relationship to the polio virus has not been established.

Fungus Diseases

Cutaneous streptotricosis (infection with *Dermatophilus congolensis*) has been reported in pinnipeds. It must be distinguished from seal pox (*see* above) or other dermal lesions. Diagnosis is based on demonstration of the organism through either special strains, histopathology or culture. Systemic fungicides have been used with equivocal results. Simultaneous lesions of streptotricosis and pox have been recorded in sea lions. Cutaneous streptotricosis is usually manifested as sharply delineated nodules which cover the entire body.

Many fungus diseases have been diagnosed in marine mammals. Unfortunately most are diagnosed at necropsy, and few are amenable to treatment even if diagnosed early. Attempts have been made with the latest antifungal drugs but with equivocal results. Perhaps the most distressing mycotic infection in cetaceans is **candidiasis.** This disease may occur spontaneously or as the result of prolonged and indiscriminate antibiotic therapy. The lesions are usually found around the body openings—the blowhole, recto-genitourinary openings and the mouth. At necropsy, the pathognomonic lesions of the esophagogastric area are found.

Aspergillosis has been found in the bottlenosed dolphin as has **cryptococcosis.** In both instances the pulmonary lesions were advanced and believed to be the cause of death. **Mycotic dermatitis** due to *Trichophyton* sp. has been reported in the dolphin.

Nocardiosis has been reported in the pilot whale, harbor porpoise, killer whale, the false killer whale, and the spinner dolphin. *Mucor* spp. and *Entomophthora* spp. have been found in the bottlenosed dolphin. **Blastomycosis** has been reported in the bottlenosed dolphin as has a single case of **actinomycosis. Cheloidal blastomycosis** (Lobo's disease) has been found in bottlenosed dolphins. It does not appear to bother the host significantly, but it is unsightly. This is a disease that has been reported only in man and the dolphin.

In all cases of cutaneous and systemic mycoses reviewed, there has been no definitive evidence of horizontal transmission. Rather, each case appears to have been secondary to stresses, such as transport, stranding, beaching, or the artificial conditions of captivity and confinement. There is some evidence of a geographic distribution for some of these fungi. Tentative diagnoses may be suspected from clinical signs and the presence of pulmonary nodules on radiography in respiratory cases. Thoracic radiographs may be effective diagnostic tools in cases of respiratory mycosis for cetaceans and pinnipeds weighing under 200 kg. Confirmatory diagnoses are possible only by culture and identification of the organisms, or by histopathological demonstration. Wet mounts in lactophenol and cotton blue may render an immediate diagnosis with some of the morphologically distinct fungi. Tissue smears may be cleared in warm 10% potassium hydroxide and examined.

In pinnipeds, *Nocardia* has been reported in the leopard seal. **Aspergillosis** has caused the death of a California sea lion. **Blastomycosis** has been found in a Stellar sea lion and **histoplasmosis** in a harp seal. **Coccidioidomycosis** has been found in the California sea lion. *Microsporum canis* has been the cause of dermatological lesions in a harbor seal. Although candidiasis is common in cetaceans it has not yet been reported in the pinnipeds. *Mucor* spp. has been found and believed to be the cause of death of a harp seal. Although the mycotic disorders of captive marine mammals are not considered to be contagious, every precaution should be taken during examination both ante and post mortem on these animals. The usual route of entry is through inhalation or by contact of injured skin or mucous membrane.

Topical application of medication on marine mammals is futile unless the animals are kept out of water for sufficient period of time for the medication to have an effect or be absorbed. This is not a problem with pinnipeds, and most smaller cetaceans can be kept out of water for at least 2 to 3 hours provided they are kept moist. This can be accomplished by spraying a fine mist over all areas of the body not being treated.

Parasites

One of the major problems with captive pinnipeds is the control of parasites. Starting with the head there are **nasal or lung mites** of both seals and sea lions. Unfortunately their life cycles have not been worked out and there is no known treatment although perhaps systemic parasiticides such as levamisole or one of its analogues may be effective. The lung mites probably contribute to excessive mucus secretion in the respiratory tract with subsequent rattling coughs that the host exhibits. Nasal mites seem to cause little discomfort.

Demodectic mange occurs in California sea lions. The lesions are usually found on the flippers and contact surfaces. They are nonpruritic and are characterized by alopecia, hyperkeratosis, scaling and excoriation. Diagnosis is made by repeated deep skin scrapings and identification of the mite. Secondary bacterial infection resulting in pyoderma occurs if the condition is allowed to become chronic. Treatment is the same as for the dog; it is not always successful. Until the predisposing factors are elucidated nothing is known about the control of the infection.

All species of pinnipeds have **lice**, both biting and sucking. Heavy infestations, especially by the sucking lice, can result in severe anemia. The lice can be seen grossly, and are readily transmitted. They share with other lice a high sensitivity to chlorinated hydrocarbons. The affected animal should be removed from the water, allowed to dry before being dusted, and kept away from water at least 12 hours. Treatment must be repeated in 10 to 12 days.

Animals in captivity often rid themselves of parasites providing no new sources of infection are introduced. Caution should be exercised if the newer insecticides are used as some of these species are extremely sensitive.

Lungworms are common in all pinnipeds. Sea lions are parasitized by *Parafilaroides decorus,* while true seals are usually parasitized by *Otostrongylus circumlitus. O. circumlitus* has also been found in the hearts of some true seals; however it does not produce a microfilaremia. The presence of lungworms can be determined by fecal or bronchial mucus examination. Anorexia, coughing and sometimes blood-flecked mucus are the first signs of pulmonary parasitism. Treatment consists of antibiotics for the concomitant pneumonia and an appropriate anthelmintic for the lungworms.

Lungworms, at least in sea lions, often remain hypobiotic for long periods until the animal becomes debilitated for other reasons, when they cause a clinically apparent infection. However, they are regarded as self-limiting so long as no new larvae are introduced through feeding of fresh fish that are the intermediate host of *P. decorus*. Prevention of reinfection is fairly easy when only frozen fish is fed. Under no circumstances should fresh fish be fed as they are intermediate hosts for not only lungworms but many other parasites as well.

Heartworms (*Dipetalonema spirocauda*) are a common finding in true seals at necropsy; however this worm does not affect sea lions. Sea lions, on the other hand, are universally infected with a subcut. nematode, *Dipetalonema odendhali*, as well as *Dirofilaria immitis* in endemic areas. *D. immitis* may affect the true seals. Diagnosis is made by identifying the microfilariae in the blood. Treatment is as for canine heartworm (q.v., p. 704). Unfortunately the mode of transmission of the heartworms of marine mammals is unknown except for *D. immitis*. *D. immitis* infection in sea lions in endemic areas has been successfully prevented with diethylcarbamazine (2.5 mg/kg of body wt, daily in the diet for as long as exposure to mosquitoes is possible). This drug is also effective as a larvicide in microfilariae-positive animals.

Members of all 3 groups of helminths are present in the digestive tracts of the pinnipeds. Of the **trematodes**, *Zalophotrema hepaticum* in the sea lion is the most important. Successful treatment with bithional (Lorothidol) has been reported. (The level reported was 20 mg/kg of body wt.) The **cestode** *Diphyllobothrium pacificum* is commonly found in sea lions. It is thought to cause intestinal obstruction during heavy infection. Niclosamide has been suggested as an effective treatment. Of the **nematodes**, members of the Anasakidae are the most pathogenic, causing blood loss and ulceration where they attach. Raw fish is most often incriminated as the source. **Hookworms** (*Uncinaria* spp.) are also found in pinnipeds; however only the fur seals seem to be severely affected. Newborn pups are infected via the colostrum. Benzimidazole anthelmintics such as thiabendazole have been found to be effective against some of these nematodes.

Coccidia (new species) have been found in harbor seals exhibiting severe diarrhea. They may be susceptible to anticoccidial drugs used in other species, e.g. amprolium. No other pinnipeds have been found to have these parasites.

MISCELLANEOUS DISEASES

Eye Problems: Corneal opacities occur quite frequently in captive pinnipeds, although they also occur in the wild population. Opacities and ulceration also occur in animals kept in both fresh and salt water. Treatment by moving animals that are kept in fresh water into salt water and vice versa has not yielded definitive results. Diets have been changed and supplemented with minerals and vitamins, with similar responses. A recent hypothesis is that it is a light-induced phenomenon, i.e. the effect of excessive light on the eye (intraocular as opposed to extraocular). Most institutions that have animals on display have brightly colored pools with both bright incident light and reflected light. The light intensity and aerial accommodation cause marked miosis to occur. Marked miosis in the pinnipeds causes the peripupillary vascular arcade to become markedly prominent and may even swell to the point of touching the inner surface of the cornea resulting in an ulcer. In cetaceans a comparable situation occurs when the iris operculum swells until the same result obtains.

It is recommended that animals that are kept in fresh water be moved into salt water (*see* p. 1227) and that they be placed into a pool with non-reflecting sides and bottom and perhaps also in an area with decreased light intensity. If this is not possible at least an effort should be made to provide some darkened or shaded area in which to escape from the light. Of course proper attention should be given to the diet and sanitation of the environment.

Ulcers: Ulcers of the first compartment of the cetacean stomach are a common necropsy finding. A number of reasons have been suggested for their formation: increased histamine content of spoiled fish, anxiety due to change of environment or personnel, training procedures that are too strenuous, parasites, introduction of new animals, etc. Diagnosis is not easy; radiography may be tried, gastroscopy with a fibroscope, or aspiration of contents for visualization of the host's red and white cells. Alleviation of pain by demulcents is indicated. However, the constant attention of familiar trainers to make the animals feel secure (companionship) cannot be overemphasized. The ulcers in cetaceans very seldom perforate. **Foreign bodies** have been found frequently in the first compartment of the cetacean stomach (*see* below); whether they are the cause or result of the ulceration is unknown. Acid from the second compartment does regurgitate into the first as a part of the digestive and maceration process. Whether fasting of the animals for a period of time would allow ulcers to heal is unknown.

In pinnipeds, on the other hand, gastric ulcers do perforate with resulting peritonitis and death. The causes are probably the same as for the cetaceans. Treatment consists of elimination of any known cause and good nursing with fluids and broad-spectrum antibiotics until the problem is resolved.

Trained marine mammals when well are very playful and have a tendency to swallow small objects. In cetaceans the opening to the second stomach compartment is quite small with the result that these swallowed foreign objects remain in the first compartment. They may be visualized by radiography, gastroscopy, or by manual palpation via the esophagus, or direct observation that "an object" has just been swallowed. If the object has no sharp points it may be regurgitated at a future time with no consequence; if irregular and sharp it must be removed, as death has resulted from nails perforating the gastric wall and causing a peritonitis.

Skin Problems: Pinnipeds have many skin problems in addition to the infectious diseases mentioned above. **Dermal abscesses** occur most commonly in young, debilitated animals, either as pustules or as grossly infected lesions. Many organisms have been cultured, although the gram positive ones seem to predominate. The lesions should be excised, drained and treated both systemically and locally. Appropriate antibiotics and antiseptics can be used successfully in conjunction with good hygienic principles.

Focal dermatitis is an infrequently encountered condition occurring in California sea lions. The entire skin surface is affected with slightly raised epidermal eruptions. The lesions are not pruritic and are self-limiting with an alopecic period before new hair growth. This disease is somewhat infectious and seasonal. A viral etiology is suspected. It has been claimed that long term broad-spectrum antibiotics are effective.

Gastroenteritis is perhaps commoner than suspected as totally aquatic animals normally pass soft stools and in water they are dispersed almost immediately. However dolphins with suspected pancreatic disorders may void foamy feces that float. Another frequent cause may be poor quality food fish. In most instances the problem can be easily corrected by vitamin supplementation, control of the quality of food fish and strict adherence to compatible environmental conditions.

California sea lions and Stellar sea lion pups secrete no intestinal dissacharidases, hence cannot tolerate sucrose, lactose, cellobiose and trehalose. The enteritis produced if these carbohydrates are fed is severe and fermentative and can be rapidly debilitating. Removal of the cause will correct the condition. Sea lions also have been reported to have died from enterotoxemia due to clostridial organisms; but the diagnosis is open to question.

Miscellaneous Conditions: Many different kinds of **tumors** have been found in captive and wild marine mammals. They are infrequent and of little consequence with perhaps the exception of malignant lymphoma in harbor seals, where horizontal transmission may occur in a closed population.

Osteomyelitis (pyogenic spondylitis) has been found in the spine of a dolphin believed to have died from a concomitant staphylococcal septicemia. The organisms were found in the osteomyelitic lesions. **Fibrous osteodystrophy** has been reported in the common dolphin. The cause of the condition could not be determined. Fractures and congenital abnormalities have been reported in dolphins, but are rare. Transport-associated **myopathy** has been suspected in a dolphin. Depression and immobility were seen about a day after transport. Creatine phosphokinase and lactic dehydrogenase activities were increased, the animal responded to corticosteroid and antibiotic therapy and recovered.

Many **traumatic lesions** (cuts, wounds from gunshots or propeller blades) are found on marine mammals. They should be cleaned, debrided and allowed to heal as an open wound. Antibiotics should be administered during the convalescent period.

Stranded juvenile pinnipeds are found frequently on coasts. It is not known in most cases whether these animals are abandoned, lost or injured. Whatever their source they must be fed, which in most instances, means they must be force fed. As they are usually newly weaned or about weaning age, they should be fed a diet resembling mother's milk as well as one containing some solid nutrients to introduce them to eating fish. The following diet has been used successfully.

Lactated Ringer's solution	120 ml
Predigested protein (protein hydrolysate 15 gr/oz)	25 ml
Similac[1]	60 ml
Whipping cream	240 ml
Thiamin (500 mg)	1 ml
Nutri-cal[2]	11.6 gm
Herring	550 gm

[1]Or Similac-Isomil, Ross Labs., Columbus, Ohio, 43216.
[2]Evsco Pharm., Buena, New Jersey, 08310.

The material is blended and fed via stomach tube. The mixture above will provide 3 feedings of 240 ml, each containing approximately 463 Kcal or, with 6 feedings, 2,780 Kcal/day.
On analysis the formula provides the following:

Protein	9.4%
Fat	18.5%
Moisture	70.0%
Carbohydrate (by difference)	1.3%
Ash	0.84%
Calcium	0.06%

It is known that sea lion milk contains no lactose and that the species lacks intestinal dissacharidases (*see* above). However, the above diet has not caused any noticeable problems in the juveniles in which it has been used.

VACCINATION OF EXOTIC MAMMALS

Rabies: Wild-caught animals, even when young, may have been exposed to rabies virus. A short observation period is inadequate as incubation may be prolonged. Because of the potential danger of rabies, the keeping of wild animals as pets should be discouraged. There are, of course, other excellent reasons for discouraging this practice.

Most exotic pets presumably are closely confined, minimizing danger of being exposed to rabies in free-living animals. Rabies vaccination of exotic pets should be undertaken with great caution; it must be emphasized that there is marked variation between species and among individuals in their response to vaccines. Clinical disease and death are common sequelae when modified live-virus vaccines, safe for domestic Canidae and Felidae, are used for wild animals in captivity.

If vaccination is considered necessary, only inactivated rabies virus vaccine should be used; inactivated nervous tissue vaccine, caprine or ovine origin, or inactivated tissue-culture vaccine (20% tissue suspension) is administered subcut., preferably in 2 sites at the rate of 5 ml for up to 25 lb (11 kg) of body wt and an additional 1 ml for each additional 5 lb (2.3 kg) of body wt up to a total of 15 ml. Young animals are vaccinated at 3 to 4 months of age. Vaccination must be repeated annually.

Distemper: All members of the Canidae, Procyonidae, Mustelidae and Hyaenidae, and some members of the Viverridae, are considered to be susceptible to distemper. There is some doubt about the susceptibility of the Ursidae. Distemper in exotic animals generally resembles that in the dog but may also cause the affected animal to lose its fear of man, thus resembling rabies.

Caution is advised in vaccinating wild-caught species, because of the danger that they may have been exposed to the virus, and thus may be incubating the disease. There is marked variation between species and individuals in their reaction to modified live-virus vaccines, therefore only inactivated virus vaccines should be used unless there is a precedent. Most of the information available is from the experience of zoo veterinarians and there are differences in reports of apparent safety and efficacy of immunizing products; therefore recommendations can be made only as a guide and with the reservations above. Annual revaccination is recommended.

Killed tissue vaccines: Inactivated canine-distemper virus vaccine: Young should be vaccinated shortly after weaning, 2 doses of 2 ml each at 14- to 21-day intervals. For larger adult animals, the initial dose should be doubled.

Modified live-virus vaccines: (*See* DISTEMPER IN MINK, p. 1163.) Mink distemper vaccine (chick-embryo or cell-culture origin) is given subcut. (1 to 2 ml, or according to the manufacturer's directions and size of the animal). Modified canine-distemper live-virus, chick-embryo or cell-culture origin is also given subcut. (2 ml or according to the manufacturer's directions and size of the animal). Live ferret attenuated vaccines are pathogenic for many species (e.g. mink, raccoon) and should not be used.

Panleukopenia: All Felidae, most of the Mustelidae and some of the Procyonidae and Viverridae are believed to be susceptible to panleukopenia (feline distemper) virus infection (*see* VIRUS ENTERITIS OF MINK, p. 1164). Caution should be exercised when undertaking prophylaxis, and inactivated virus vaccines are recommended (*see* DISTEMPER IN EXOTIC MAMMALS, above). Booster doses are recommended when animals are handled or moved, and also annually. Inactivated virus feline-distemper vaccine (mink- or feline-tissue origin): for small species, 1 ml (IM or subcut.); for large cats, 2 ml/10 lb body wt (maximum 40 ml), or 2 to 4 ml, and repeated at 10-day intervals for 2 to 4 times (depending on the size of the cat).

Infectious Hepatitis: Canidae are susceptible (the disease in foxes is called **encephalitis,** as the chief manifestations are nervous signs). A modified live-virus combination, canine distemper-hepatitis vaccine, has been used in cases where the use of a modified live-virus vaccine is advisable (*see* DISTEMPER). Annual booster doses are given.

Canine distemper-hepatitis vaccine (modified live virus, tissue culture origin or combined chick embryo-tissue culture origin) is given subcut., 2 ml, repeated in 14 days. Canine-hepatitis vaccine, modified live virus (porcine-tissue-culture origin), is given subcut., 2 ml.

Leptospirosis: When they are at risk, Canidae, Procyonidae and Mustelidae may be vaccinated with *Leptospira canicola-icterohaemorrhagiae* bacterin. Young are vaccinated at 6 to 8 weeks of age (4 ml subcut., repeated in 14 days). Booster doses are given every 6 months.

DISEASES OF REPTILES

Reptile diseases have causes similar to those in higher vertebrates. For ease of reference the diseases of snakes, lizards and chelonia are dealt with separately. Veterinarians, who already cope with much comparative medicine, should be able to adjust readily to diagnosing and treating reptiles.

SNAKES

Bacterial Diseases

Subcut. abscesses, necrotic stomatitis, infectious dermal ulceration and terminal septicemia are common. The major pathogenic bacteria are *Aeromonas* and *Pseudomonas*, both of which cause high mortalities, but *Proteus*, *Enterobacter*, *Escherichia*, *Streptococcus*, *Salmonella*, *Citrobacter* and *Serratia* are regularly recorded aerobic organisms. *Bacteroides* and *Clostridia* are the anaerobic organisms isolated. Often several organisms are isolated from the same lesion.

Subcutaneous Abscesses: The abscess material is usually inspissated and shells out after incision. The abscess cavity is cleaned under general anesthesia, swabbed with povidone-iodine and packed with a suitable antibiotic ointment. Culture and sensitivity determination of the organism is indicated.

Necrotic Stomatitis: This condition affects lizards and chelonians as well as snakes. In snakes there are 3 forms of infection of the mouth, pharynx and esophagus. All species of reptile become anorectic.

Necrotic stomatitis (**Mouth Rot**): In this form the gingival mucosa develops petechiation and ulcerates. A necrotic plaque forms, which may seal the mandibular arch to the maxilla. As the condition worsens, deeper structures become involved. Osteomyelitis of the mandibles and the maxillary and premaxillary bones is common in advanced cases.

Esophagitis in snakes causes ventral edema from the intramandibular space caudally. Confirmation is by examination of the esophagus by speculum, when necrotic plaques are seen.

Infected "ranula" in snakes causes head edema and is confirmed by seeing marked swelling of the mucous membrane at the back of the mouth.

Treatment of all 3 forms is carried out under general anesthesia and comprises debridement and a thorough but gentle cleansing with hydrogen peroxide or povidone-iodine. In severe cases antibiotics are given both topically and orally (or parenterally) according to bacterial sensitivity.

Subspectacle Abscess: Incorrectly called conjunctivitis, this infection occurs between the spectacle and the cornea. Under general anesthesia an incision is made around 1/3 to 1/2 of the spectacle to produce a flap, the pus is washed out and an antibiotic ointment is instilled before the spectacle flap is replaced.

Infectious Dermal Ulceration (Scale rot): The lesions are normally multiple, early lesions showing small subdermal hemorrhages before they "blister" and ulcerate. Infection is almost certainly blood borne and therefore a bacteremia is usually present. Lesions apparently improve after ecdysis but never heal spontaneously and untreated snakes invariably die. Treatment requires isolation of the causal organisms, which are frequently multiple; instigation of strict vivarium hygiene; and daily dressing of lesions with either an antiseptic such as povidone-iodine, or a topical medication containing polynoxylin or an antibiotic preparation to which the organisms are sensitive. To treat the bacteremia, the correct antibiotic(s) is given orally or parenterally. A snake with any form of scale lesion will refuse food (for as long as 11 months) and the owner must be instructed to force-feed it regularly to avoid starvation.

Septicemia: Snakes that are seen writhing and throwing their ventral scales upwards have either septicemia, meningitis or some other cause of acute pain, and prognosis is poor.

Protozoan Infections

Amebiasis due to *Entamoeba invadens* causes massive hemorrhagic enteritis and in reptile collections can assume epidemic proportions. Treatment is with metronidazole (160 mg/kg up to a maximum of 400 mg daily for 3 days) given by stomach tube.

Other intestinal flagellate infections in reptiles cause wet cloacal voidings and polydipsia. When freshly voided material is examined under the microscope (×100) the live flagellates can be seen in great numbers. Treatment is a single dose of metronidazole (160 mg/kg) as an aqueous suspension by stomach tube.

Environmental Diseases

The artificial habitats created to house and display captive reptiles contribute to many diseases. Bacterial, fungal, protozoan and viral diseases are frequently directly associated with either careless hygiene or neglect. Rostral abrasions occur in active reptiles that continually push, probe and rub their rostral shields in attempts to escape. Treatment is both by topical application of a suitable preparation to promote healing and providing a place for the reptile to hide. It is useful to paint a black strip 20-cm high along the bottom of the entire glass frontage; this strip represents a solid barrier and reptiles rarely attempt to penetrate it.

Bites and lacerations occur between reptiles in the same vivarium and from the poor management practice of placing live rodent prey in the vivarium (when the rat bites the reptile). The treatment of fresh lesions is to cleanse the wound prior to suturing it to obtain primary intention healing. Large open infected wounds and defects must be allowed to heal by granulation.

Crush injuries occur in snakes, lizards and crocodiles when tree trunks and improperly supported rocks topple over and trap the reptile. X-ray examination allows assessment of skeletal damage.

Severe thermal **burns** occur when reptiles are able to get too close to poorly regulated heating devices such as sun lamps, tubular heaters and exposed lamp bulbs. The affected area should be gently cleansed and the appropriate antiseptic, and if necessary antibiotic, dressings applied. Since healing in reptiles takes about 10 times as long as in mammals a second degree burn will not be healed for 9 to 12 weeks. Much fluid may be lost from thermal burns and adequate rehydration with Ringer's solution is important.

Bruising in any snake is a serious and often fatal condition. Many snakes with 5 or 6 bruises to the musculature will die in 10 days. Gentle handling is essential at all times.

Fungus Diseases

Little is known about mycotic diseases of reptiles but fungal hyphae are from time to time identified at biopsy or on histopathologic examination of granulomatous lesions. Hyphae can also be seen on direct wet-smear examination. Topical treatment of lesions with povidone-iodine is useful.

Viral Diseases

The following confirmed viral diseases are known. A virus kills fer-de-lance snakes within 12 days, the signs being loss of muscle tone with terminal excessive activity and pupillary dilatation. At necropsy the body cavity and the lungs are full of fluid and a bronchopneumonia is evident. An oncornavirus has been isolated from a large (117 gm) mesenteric mass in a snake that became progressively weaker. Another oncornavirus has been isolated from a subcut. mass in another snake. The arbovirus of western equine encephalitis has been isolated from 25 species of snake, 14 species of lizard and 12 species of chelonia in the U.S.A., but is not associated with disease in the reptiles.

Nutritional Diseases

Only recently have true nutritional diseases of snakes been recognized, and these are rare, showing themselves as abnormal calcification of the ribs and spinal column. Both reduced calcification and the production of osteophytes or exostoses can be identified radiographically. Successful treatment must await research.

Severe debility and inanition is an induced condition in which snakes refuse to eat. Initially body weight drops slowly but once the fat between the muscle fibers starts being used there is not only a dramatic weight loss but also muscle wasting. To prevent such a deterioration force-feeding should be instigated early while the gastric mucosa will still accept and digest the food. Offering a different type of food, raising the temperature in the vivarium and supportive therapy such as giving vitamins may all be useful. Fresh water must be available at all times.

Endoparasites

Both wild and captive snakes can be infected by intestinal **nematodes** and **cestodes. Trematode** infections also occur. Nematode eggs are easily seen on microscopic examination of fresh feces. Cestode segments are voided but are less commonly observed. Nematode infections may be treated with a suspension of thiabendazole 110 mg/kg, mebendazole 50 mg/kg, or levamisole 25 mg/kg of body wt. given by esophageal tube. Cestode infections are treated with a suspension of niclosamide 150 mg/kg by esophageal tube.

Ectoparasites

The mite *Ophionyssus natracis* and many other species affect snakes. Herpetologists usually become aware of these parasites after a slough. If the infested snake is placed in a small plastic vivarium and a piece of dichlorvos (Vapona) strip (¼ in./10 cu ft) is suspended therein for a maximum of 4 days, all mites on the snake will die. The dichlorvos is then placed in the infected vivarium for 21 days to kill all nymphs and larval forms that hatch out of eggs laid in the crevices. All wood and bark should be burned.

LIZARDS

There are about 3,000 species of lizards, or saurians (suborder Sauria, Order Squamata). They range from the large iguanas and Monitor lizards through chuckwallas, anoles and skinks to spiny tailed lizards like the uromastix and agamids to small species. Also there are legless lizards like the glass lizard and the slow worm, the wall-climbing geckoes and poisonous lizards.

The major differences between legless lizards and snakes are that lizards have eyelids, visible tympanic membranes and are able to regenerate their tails by autotomy after losing them.

Bacterial Diseases

The same major pathogenic bacteria that affect snakes cause diseases of lizards.

Subcutaneous Abscesses: These are extremely common in iguanas and may be multiple. It is possible to wash out a single abscess with an antiseptic solution (cetrimide 1%), but when multiple abscesses occur it is best to amputate part of the tail as the infection is blood borne. The organism should be cultured and sensitivity determined.

Necrotic Stomatitis: This is less common in lizards than in snakes but does occur as swelling of the lips. Incision and evacuation of the pus is possible. The cavity should be cleansed with an antiseptic and packed with an antibiotic ointment.

Deep-Seated Abscess: These can occur due to blood-borne infection and cause large encapsulated swellings of inspissated pus in almost any part of the body; between muscles of the legs is a common site. The lizard loses weight; muscle wasting and signs of inanition follow if the lizard is neglected. Treatment of all forms must be under general anesthesia with total enucleation of the abscess, swabbing the cavity with povidone-iodine and repeated packing with antibiotic ointment until healing is complete. Intracoelomic abscessation presents a less favorable prognosis. Antibiotics should not be given until the sensitivities of the organism(s) are known.

Protozoan Infections

The same protozoa that affect snakes occur in lizards but the conditions are less commonly encountered. Treatment is a single dose of metronidazole, 160 mg/kg of body wt, as an aqueous suspension by stomach tube.

Environmental Diseases

See the discussion of these conditions in snakes, p. 1241.

Fungus Diseases

Fungal hyphae are seen from time to time when lizard biopsy and necropsy material is examined. Mycotic disease is not as common as bacterial or viral disease.

Viral Diseases

A virus has been isolated from the erythrocytes of Australian geckoes. These geckoes get a progressive anemia and on a blood smear inclusion bodies are seen inside the red cells. The virus of western equine encephalitis has been isolated from 14 lizards. Many lizards develop skin papillomata and a virus is associated with these papillomas in green lizards. Recently a herpesvirus has been isolated from a series of clinically ill South American iguanas.

Nutritional Diseases

Nutritional osteodystrophy is an extremely common finding in iguanas and water dragons kept in captivity. On X-ray examination, extremely poor skeletal calcification, greenstick fractures and old unhealed fractures will be visible. Often these iguanas swallow pebbles and gravel, presumably in an attempt to obtain calcium, and on X-ray films these pebbles will be apparent in the intestinal tract.

Some of the skeletal changes are irreversible but attempts to correct the calcium to phosphorus ratio to 1:1 by adding additional soluble calcium such as calcium gluconate or powdered cuttle fish to the diet are indicated. Vitamin A and iodine, but not excessive vitamin D, should be added to the diet. The deposition of calcium on the aorta and major blood vessels must not be allowed to occur and should be looked for in subsequent X-ray examinations.

Ectoparasites

Many species of mite affect lizards although herpetologists may be unaware that their reptiles are affected. Mites cause a degree of anemia and skin irritation, particularly round the eyes and ears. Also they may transmit blood-borne diseases as well as bacteria, and may initiate subcut. abscesses. It is imperative that newly acquired lizards be quarantined and treated for mite infestation. For treatment *see* the discussion of this condition in snakes, p. 1243.

Endoparasites

If a helminth infection is present, worm eggs and occasionally larvae will be seen on microscopic examination of fresh feces. Thiabendazole (110 mg/kg) or mebendazole (50 mg/kg) administered by stomach tube is effective.

CHELONIANS

This group includes the land tortoises, fresh-water terrapins and salt-water turtles.

Bacterial Diseases

The most severe diseases are those caused by bacteria that multiply rapidly in water. *Pseudomonas* sp. and salmonellae are commonly encountered in the terrapins and turtles. Bacteria can invade not only the viscera but also affect the shell.

Terrapins and turtles also get **pneumonia** and when so affected have difficulty in swimming. If only one lung is affected the chelonian will swim with the affected side lower in the water. Tortoises are often affected with a **rhinitis** with a serous nasal discharge. Mild rhinitis can be treated by raising the environmental temperature and smearing a mentholated ointment (e.g. Vick's) on the mandibles so that the vapor loosens the secretions. The nasal sections should be submitted for bacteriologic culture and sensitivity, and appropriate antibiotic therapy should be instituted.

Stomatitis and Glossitis: This is a common condition of tortoises that come out of hibernation. The reptile refuses to eat and when the mouth is examined ulcers and plaques of necrotic material will be seen on the tongue and elsewhere. Treatment requires that the mouth be cleaned with povidone-iodine and the reptile force-fed.

Fungus Diseases

As in other reptiles, these diseases are rare. If they occur on the shell of the terrapin, treatment with malachite green at a 1:15,000 dilution for 10 to 30 seconds is recommended.

Viral Diseases

A virulent herpesvirus has been recently isolated from aquatic chelonians. The overt disease is peracute with the affected turtles dying within 24 hours after initial signs of lethargy.

Environmental Diseases

Dirty water in terrapin and turtle vivaria is the commonest cause of the spread of disease. Rotting, decaying food is worse than a build-up of excretory products. In order to avoid this it is advisable to remove these reptiles to a separate feeding tank and return them to their vivarium after they have eaten. This technique also safeguards smaller species from having toes and limbs bitten off in the feeding frenzy of larger reptiles, which bite indiscriminately at anything that moves at feeding time.

Carapace and Plastron Injuries

Carapace and plastron injuries to tortoises and terrapins occur by being run-over by a car wheel, being dropped, gnawed by dogs, burnt in bonfires or sliced by the rotating blades of grass mowers. Injuries to the bony dermal shell can be repaired in 3 stages under general anesthesia: Local soft tissue damage is treated first. The fractured fragments are then lifted and where possible the normal anatomy is re-established. Finally the defect is covered with fiberglass and epoxy resin patches, being careful not to get the epoxy resin between the bony fragments thus preventing bridging and bony union.

Nutritional Diseases

Nutritional osteodystrophy causes the shell to become soft and deformed; a common complaint from the owner of terrapins and turtles. This is due to an incorrect diet with a calcium to phosphorus ratio that may be as wide as 1:40. Treatment requires that the Ca:P ratio be made 1:1 by the addition of soluble calcium salts such as calcium gluconate or calcium lactate to the diet. Also a multivitamin preparation with some iodine may be useful.

Hypovitaminosis A is a frequent occurrence in young terrapins and turtles. The Harderian glands under the eyelids become hypertrophied and hyperkeratinized so that the eyelids cannot open. Without sight the reptiles do not eat. There is also disturbance to the reptile's fluid balance and edema occurs round the base of the limbs and renal damage is seen at necropsy. There is a dramatic response to the IM injection of 5,000 IU of vitamin A, providing treatment starts before gross ocular swelling, leg edema and renal lesions have occurred. The vitamin A injection should be repeated in 7 days and the diet corrected. If the reptile is blind, force-feeding is necessary.

FISH DISEASES

In developed countries the principal purpose of aquaculture has been to provide salmonid and centrarchid fishes for restocking sport fisheries. In developing countries it has served primarily as an extension of fish capture, in large ponds or rice paddies and has thus been extensive in nature. Intensive food-fish culture is now expanding rapidly throughout the world and many species of fresh-water and marine fishes are being grown. Additionally, intensive techniques are being applied to the culture of ornamental temperate and tropical species both in U.S.A. and Europe, and also in the third world where aquarium fish production is a significant foreign exchange earner. Pond culture of small fish for bait fishing is a significant industry in Southern U.S.A. Many millions of tons of shellfishes including oysters, clams, mussels, shrimps and crayfishes are cultured for the table, although the technology required for these species and their diseases in intensive culture are less well understood.

The relationship between any aquatic animal and its environment, and its response to changes in that environment are critical in deciding how suitable it will be for artificial culture. All aquatic animals are susceptible to microbial, neoplastic, parasitic and nutritional diseases, and also to conditions of a pathophysiologic nature related to their environmental circumstances. Once an understanding of the principal characteristics of the aquatic environment and the physiologic differences between fishes and higher vertebrates is achieved, clinical appraisal of fish diseases is remarkably similar to intensive poultry or pig medicine.

The vertebrate fishes are poikilotherms and thus are dependent on water temperature for the rate at which they can fulfill bodily functions ranging from protein synthesis to swimming or digestion. They are hyperosmotic compared to the environment in fresh water; hypo-osmotic in salt. Fish skin ulceration is thus extremely serious in terms of its effects on fluid balance and although small ulcers are rapidly epithelialized at all temperatures by migration of neighboring epithelial cells, large or infected ulcers can result in circulatory collapse. Fish have no lymph nodes or Kupffer's cells, their phagocytic tissue being in the atrium of the 2-chambered heart and in the hemopoietic tissue of the spleen and kidney.

The fish kidney, located retroperitoneally as a long strand of tissue against the backbone, is a mixed organ consisting of glomeruli (usually) and proximal and distal tubules embedded in a stroma of hemopoietic and phagocytic tissue. The excretory kidney of fish is only responsible for divalent ion excretion; nitrogenous and monovalent ion excretion (e.g. NaCl from water) is via the gills. Thus gill damage is extremely significant, affecting as it does both gaseous and nitrogenous exchange and conversely, extensive renal lesions are often only of chronic significance.

The aquatic environment, particularly in intensive culture, is the dominant factor in determining whether a disease occurs, and its ultimate outcome. Temperature, pH, dissolved oxygen concentration, concentration of nitrogenous products of fish metabolism and amount and nature of suspended solids are all important and most are interrelated, e.g. as temperature rises oxygen carrying capacity decreases; as pH rises so the shift from un-ionized to ionized and highly toxic ammonia increases.

Requirements and minimal survival levels for all of these factors vary greatly with individual fish species. In general the salmonids are the most demanding in terms of oxygen, etc. while cultured pond fishes can survive up to 30°C and 2 ppm oxygen. With few exceptions, epidemic disease in fish culture, or in aquaria can be related to handling trauma or to some deterioration in environmental conditions, even transitory. Because the rate of pathogen multiplication as well as the rate of fish metabolism is temperature dependent, the speed with which a clinical condition develops can vary by several days, and in assessing environmental effects it is important to remember that at low temperatures the initial insult may have been some days or even weeks previously.

One physical condition responsible for high levels of mortality in cultured and aquarium fish is "**gas bubble disease**" due to gaseous embolism, detectable as bubbles of gas in the eye, gill or skin and nervous behavior. This is due to the fish obtaining supersaturated oxygen or nitrogen that comes out of solution in the blood—akin to "diver's bends" in man. The condition is generally due to a leaky pump diaphragm or a long water supply pipe sucking in air and compressing it, but it can also occur in water drawn from river spillways.

Immunization is currently only marginally successful in fish culture, with suitable bacterins of proven efficacy existing only for a very few conditions. Since dosing of large numbers of fish parenterally is uneconomic, oral vaccination has been attempted with limited success. Vaccine baths used after fish have been exposed to a hyperosmotic solution are also advocated and appear to work although the precise method of bacterin absorption is unknown.

Although most drugs active in higher animals have similar efficacy in fish, and there are a number of bath treatments, often based on empirical experience, only a few have been approved by the FDA (U.S.A.) or Medicines Commission (U.K.) for use in fish intended as food.

BACTERIAL DISEASES

All fish pathogens generally require some form of environmental stress to induce their clinical manifestation but the degree of stress, whether environmental, handling or nutritional, depends on the particular host and its pathogen.

The commonest bacterial pathogens of fishes are gram-negative rods of the genera *Aeromonas, Pseudomonas* and *Vibrio.* Clinical signs in very young fish may be simply darkening and acute mortality. In older fishes the general features of an acute septicemia are found with, if the fish survives long enough, the development of deep necrotic ulcers.

Specific conditions caused by gram-negative rods are: **furunculosis**—a condition of salmonids caused by the obligate nonmotile pathogen *Aeromonas salmonicida.* It is a major cause of mortality in all ages of fish and usually produces the characteristic "furuncle," a deep necrotic lesion of the flank or dorsum which ulcerates to release lightly infectious reddish fluid. Variant strains of this organism are also responsible for **carp erythrodermatitis,** a shallow ulcerative condition of pond fish, which is again responsible for heavy mortality.

Sulfonamides (e.g. ℞ 97) and oxytetracycline (℞ 60) have been successful in controlling furunculosis, and chloramphenicol is particularly successful for carp erythrodermatitis; however the latter is not available for use in fish in most developed countries. Potentiated sulfonamides have of late become particularly valuable in all gram-negative infections and nitrofurazone (℞ 125) is also valuable.

A group of closely related, but motile, aeromonads known collectively as the *Aeromonas liquefaciens* group, which are facultative in any richly organic water, are responsible for **hemorrhagic septicemias** with red skin lesions at the base of fins and in internal organs in a wide range of cultured pondfishes, aquarium fishes, and to a lesser extent, salmonids. Species of *Pseudomonas,* particularly *P. fluorescens* and *P. putida* are responsible for a similar condition. Treatment for the hemorrhagic septicemias is essentially the same as for furunculosis, but environmental factors must also be considered.

Vibriosis caused by *Vibrio anguillarum,* a halophilic species otherwise very similar to *V. cholerae,* is the most serious disease of marine and brackish water species, especially if they are handled excessively in intensive culture. Lesions are similar to those of furunculosis, but there is a severe anemia in long-standing cases. Bacterins suitable for use in mass medication by bathing are now available but must not be used as a substitute for careful husbandry. Epidemics are usually treated with oxytetracycline (℞ 60) or potentiated sulfonamides (e.g. ℞ 114).

The enteric bacteria *Yersinia ruckeri* and *Edwardsiella tarda* are also responsible for mortalities of a more specific nature, the former being responsible for **enteric redmouth in trout,** where the entire head becomes reddened with subcut. hemorrhage. ***Edwardsiella* septicemia** is generally found in catfish and eels and is characterized by gas-filled malodorous bullae in the muscle. Again tetracyclines and sulfonamides have been used for treatment but often refractory cases occur.

Pseudotuberculosis of cultured yellowtail in Japan, caused by *Pasteurella piscicida* is successfully treated with sulfonamides. A disease of wild white perch in U.S. waters characterized by mass mortality, has been ascribed to the same microorganism.

Flexibacteria, formerly known as myxobacteria, or slime bacteria, long, gliding, gram-negative rods producing tenacious mucoid colonies, are linked with several conditions in cultured fishes. All are associated with an environmental insult. **Columnaris disease,** caused by *Flexibacter columnaris* is usually associated with sublethal temperature levels (>15°C) in salmonids and with skin trauma in the warm water species. Generally it takes the form of an external infection with grayish white plaques of tenacious bacteria overlaying a red-rimmed ulcer. Such ulcers extend on the skin or may involve the gills, when systemic spread, and death, are more rapid. Environmental manipulation to lower water temperature below 50°F (15°C), bathing in diquat, or antibiotic treatment with oxytetracycline (℞ 60) or nifurpirinol (℞ 120) are effective.

Peduncle disease or cold-water disease, caused by the flexibacter *Cytophaga psychrophila,* affects salmonids and marine species when environmental water conditions are less than suitable. Benzalkonium chloride as a bath (℞ 424), sulfisoxazole (℞ 113) and oxytetracycline (℞ 60) have given good results, and improvement of water conditions, particularly by decreasing the level of waste products and suspended solids as well as, where possible, raising water temperatures is useful.

Bacterial gill disease is initiated by environmental trauma, particularly high silt levels, or suspended food particles in young salmonids. A variety of myxobacteria may be involved and affected fish have distended opercula, and the bacteria in their gray mucoid suspension are readily observed in smears taken from the gill surface and examined as wet mounts under the microscope. The excessive mucus clogging the sites of gaseous interchange is the main reason for the hyperpnea and death, and treatment with detergent-bactericidal compounds such as benzalkonium chloride is valuable.

Gram-positive bacteria play little part in fish pathology except for one particularly significant pathogen, the unnamed agent of **bacte-**

rial kidney disease. Putatively placed among the Corynebacteriaceae this minute coccobacillus is a serious cause of mortality in all salmonid culture. It is both vertically and horizontally transmitted and produces a chronic granulomatous condition of the kidney and spleen and a cavernous caseation of the muscle. Since it is slow and progressive, affected fish are often moribund before any signs other than poor growth are observed. Terminally, lesions include exophthalmos and ulcers, or small hemorrhages on the flanks. Erythromycin and oxytetracycline have been used for control but with little success since they merely contain the infection until therapy ceases.

Mycobacteria and the weakly acid-fast *Nocardia asteroides* are responsible for **chronic granulomatous conditions** particularly of the liver, spleen and kidney. The mycobacteria in particular are zoonotic and can cause both **skin infections** and **allergic dermatitis** in aquarists handling affected fish. A wide range of other bacterial species have occasionally been associated with specific disease outbreaks and again therapy should comprise a judicious mixture of husbandry improvement and antibiotic or disinfectant therapy. One specific disease confined to fishes but widespread, particularly in aquarium or marine species, is **epitheliocystis**, caused by a chlamydial agent replicating within the epidermal cells of the gills or skin. The small vesicles arising from the distension of the host cell are readily seen in the low-power field of the microscope. Treatment is best aimed at osmotic lysis of the epithelial cysts, but mortalities are rarely high unless there is a heavy gill infection.

VIRAL DISEASES

Viruses of fishes are generally aquatic members of the same groups as those that affect higher vertebrates. They are cultured and typed in fish-cell lines at lower temperatures, and do not infect higher vertebrates. Because each virus disease has a relatively closely defined temperature range, variation in temperature may enable control although often it merely induces latency. Vaccines are not yet commercially available and avoidance of infection by closed stock policy or purchase of stock from known disease-free sources is essential.

Channel catfish virus disease is an acute, virulent herpesvirus infection of fry and fingerlings that often causes mortality in excess of 80% at water temperatures of 77°F (25°C) or more. There is evidence of vertical transmission (from parents to eggs). Victims show ascites, exophthalmia and hemorrhages in fins. Originally known only from the Southern U.S.A., the virus has been transported as far west as California and as far south as Central America. It is readily isolated in cell cultures from members of the freshwater catfish family. It induces syncytia and intranuclear inclusions. Serum neutralization is used for identification.

Herpesvirus disease of salmonids is a newly recognized viscerotropic infection of young rainbow trout and kokanee salmon in the U.S.A. It requires temperatures of 50°F (10°C) or less to develop and an incubation period of about a month to cause death. The virus produces anemia, exophthalmia and ascites; mortality is at least 50%. It is readily isolated in salmonid cell cultures at 50°F (10°C) or less, and produces syncytia and intranuclear inclusions. Identification is presumptive and based on cell culture changes.

Herpesvirus disease of turbot is a condition of wild and cultured turbot causing massive hypertrophy and fusion of epithelial cells of the skin and gills of young fish. Mortality is associated with heavy gill infections and poor water quality. Maintenance of high levels of oxygenation is essential in such respiratory distressed fish. Diagnosis is by examination of skin scrapings or histologic sections, when the characteristic fusion of giant cells can be observed.

Infectious hemopoietic necrosis is an acute rhabdovirus infection of salmonids that is vertically transmitted and, at temperatures of 54°F (12°C) or lower, produces high mortality in fry and fingerlings. Victims darken, show pale gills and exophthalmia, and shed thick fecal pseudocasts. Renal hemopoietic and excretory tissues are necrotic, as are pancreatic acinar cells and granular cells of the intestinal stratum compactum. The virus is readily grown in a variety of fish cells, if incubated at 59°F (15°C) or less. Identification is by the serum neutralization test. It is now known in North America and Japan.

Infectious pancreatic necrosis is an acute vertically transmitted disease that can produce high mortality in young trout or occur subclinically or chronically in other salmonids. Victims whirl about their long axis and may have a whitish exudate (but no food) in the stomach and intestine. Pancreatic acinar cells and intestinal mucosal cells show severe cytolytic necrosis. The disease is prevalent in North America, Europe and Japan. Most fish cell lines are susceptible and identification is by the serum neutralization, fluorescent antibody, or complement fixation test. The causal agent has RNA and is icosahedral; it probably represents an undescribed virus group.

Pike fry rhabdovirus disease is an acute hemorrhagic infection of young northern pike, thus far known only in Europe. Affected fry have pale gills, exophthalmia and hydrocephalus. Kidney tubules show degeneration and necrosis. The causal agent is readily isolated in a variety of cell cultures. Identification is by the serum neutralization test.

Spring viremia of carp is an acute, virulent, usually hemorrhagic rhabdovirus disease of cultured carp; it can cause death in the adults as well as in the young. Victims lose motor control, are ascitic—sometimes grossly so—and show petechiation of the skin and gills, and sometimes of the entire visceral mass. This is the most important viral disease of carp and is known only from Europe and Russia. The virus is readily isolated on common fish cell lines and identified by a serum neutralization test. It forms part of the carp-dropsy complex (*see* below). Prophylaxis against the secondary aeromonad infections, which are often responsible for ultimately high mortalities, is achieved by inoculation of susceptible fish with chloramphenicol (℞ 26) or oxytetracycline (℞ 60) just before the spring temperature rise is anticipated.

Viral hemorrhagic septicemia is an acute virulent rhabdovirus disease of rainbow trout of all ages, which is thus far confined to Europe. Typical outbreaks occur at water temperatures of 50°F (10°C) or less. Victims become very dark and show exophthalmos and severe anemia due to the petechial hemorrhages or more extensive hemorrhages that can develop anywhere but particularly within the abdomen and musculature. There is necrosis of liver and renal hemopoietic and excretory tissues. Cell culture isolations are made at 59°F (15°C) or less and identification is by a serum neutralization test.

Lymphocystis disease is a unique, typically chronic, viral infection of many marine and fresh water species; it results in the development of benign growths that are characteristically external and composed of enormously hypertrophied dermal fibroblasts. Feulgen-positive cytoplasmic inclusions and a hypertrophied, centrally located nucleus are pathognomonic. The causal agent is an icosahedral DNA virus about 300 nm in diameter of the same group; the iridoviruses, as African swine fever virus. Lymphocystic growths can be readily removed surgically from aquarium fish and ultimately a cell-mediated immunity appears to develop.

Viral erythrocytic necrosis is a recently recognized blood dyscrasia of salmon, herring, cod and other marine species. Erythrocytes show a cytoplasmic inclusion, karyorrhexis and icosahedral virions—presumably DNA. The impact on the host is uncertain, but presumably deleterious. The agent has not been isolated.

Carp pox, salmon pox, walleye epidermal hyperplasia, walleye sarcoma and **eel stomatopapilloma** are all conditions with which a virus is associated, but none of the agents have been isolated.

Eels in Japan and North America harbor an icosahedral virus, a rhabdovirus, and an orthomyxovirus-like agent. The effects of these agents on their host have yet to be determined.

The carp-dropsy complex: Ascites and exophthalmos are characteristic of many conditions of carps and goldfish. In cultured carp it is collectively called the carp-dropsy complex and fish exhibiting these characteristic features may be suffering from bacterial hemorrhagic septicemia (q.v., p. 1249), spring viremia (q.v., p. 1252), carp erythrodermatitis (q.v., p. 1249) or **carp swim-bladder disease.** The latter is a chronic condition of young fish characterized by progressive shrinkage of the swim bladder, which becomes filled with necrotic debris. Mortality increases over a period of 6 months. Antibiotic therapy has a marginal effect on mortality by reducing secondary infections but the cause is unknown.

PROTOZOAN DISEASES

The protozoan subphyla and genera most responsible for diseases of fishes are: Sarcomastigophora (*Amyloodinium, Costia* [*Ichthyobodo*], *Cryptobia, Hexamita, Oodinium* and *Trypanosoma*); Ciliophora (*Brooklynella, Chilodenella, Cryptocaryon, Ichthyophthirius, Trichodina, Trichodinella* and *Trichophrya*); Sporozoa (*Eimeria* and *Haemogregarina*); Cnidospora (*Ceratomyxa* and *Henneguya*), *Myxosoma* of the Myxosporida, and *Glugea, Nosema* and *Pleistophora* of the Microsporida).

All degrees of host-specificity exist, ranging from strict tissue- and species-specificity to no specificity at all. Ectoparasitic forms can be readily treated by adding drugs and chemicals to the water but environmental improvement is usually also necessary for continued control. Little information is available on the systemic treatment of the tissue-inhabiting forms.

Diagnosis is usually by preparation of gill or skin wet-mount preparations which are viewed under the low- or medium-power microscope lens.

The dinoflagellates *Amyloodinium* and *Oodinium* are responsible for velvet disease of aquarium fishes. *Amyloodinium* invades primarily the gills but in heavy infections may also attack the skin. *Oodinium* normally invades both the gills and skin. Transmission of both is by a motile, infective dinospore stage. Baths with low concentrations of copper sulfate (℞ 430) or copper acetate usually eliminate these protozoans.

Costia, Cryptobia and *Hexamita* are parasitic flagellates. *Costia*, an external parasite, is the most ubiquitous and troublesome, but can be controlled with dilute formalin (℞ 436) or a formalin-malachite green mixture (℞ 437). Repeated treatment may be required. The parasite feeds on the skin and gills and is transmitted directly. *Cryptobia* lives in the blood, and *Hexamita* in the intestinal tract. Both have been implicated in salmonid epidemics, but pose no major problems.

Brooklynella and *Chilodonella*, marine and freshwater forms respectively, are ectoparasitic ciliates, and *Brooklynella* can produce severe lesions on gills of marine fish kept in aquaria, *Chilodonella* can be a serious pathogen in fresh-water fishes. Dilute formalin (℞ 436), a formalin-malachite green mixture (℞ 437), or acetic acid (℞ 421) will usually remove these protozoa from the fish.

Trichodina and *Trichodinella* are also external ciliates which occasionally cause epidemics in cultured and aquarium fishes. They are controlled by applications of formalin (℞ 436) or formalin malachite green (℞ 437); but continuing problems with these and the other ectoparasitic protozoa is indicative of a primary water quality problem, which no amount of formalin will alleviate.

Two of the most ubiquitous pathogenic ciliates are *Ichthyophthirius* of fresh-water fishes and *Cryptocaryon* of marine fishes. *Ichthyophthirius* is a severe problem in aquarium culture and also causes epidemics in natural waters and particularly in cultured fish. *Cryptocaryon* has not caused epidemics in nature, but does so under aquarium conditions. Both of these ciliates invade the epidermis, causing white spots. They feed on host cells and produce irritation which causes the fish to flash and rub against the aquarium. Death is from loss of osmotic control associated with the skin damage of emergence of maturing trophozoites and physical trauma due to abrasion from scratching.

The miliary white spots containing the maturing trophozoites are pathognomonic. They emerge, settle upon the substrate, encyst and undergo multiple divisions within the cyst until an infective unit, the tomite, is formed. As many as 1,000 tomites are produced in a single cyst. Tomites are free-swimming but die if they do not make contact with a host within about 24 hours (the exact time depending on water temperature).

The free-swimming tomite is easily eliminated with formalin (℞ 436) or formalin-malachite green (℞ 437). Because bath treatments do not effectively reach trophozoites within the tissue, it is necessary to make several treatments. Infected fish in tanks should be treated daily until relief is obtained. In ponds, treatments should be made at 3- or 4-day intervals until the disease is controlled. *Ichthyophthirius* causes an estimated $1 million loss per year in the U.S.A. alone.

The *Haemogregarina* and *Eimeria* species of coccidia contain fish pathogens producing liver lesions, parasitic castration, occlusion of the air bladder, or even in the case of *Haemogregarina sachae*, a leech-vector transmitted lymphoma of cultured turbot characterized by high mortality and economic loss.

Ceratomyxa, *Henneguya*, and *Myxosoma* are histozoic myxosporidans that are serious pathogens of fish. *Ceratomyxa* destroy the musculature of anadromous and fresh-water salmonids and have been responsible for major losses of rainbow trout. *Myxosoma* parasitize many fish species. The most important species is *M. cerebralis*, the causal agent of whirling disease of salmonids. Whirling disease affects rainbow trout in their first year of life. The mode of transmission is unknown. After gaining entrance, the parasite localizes in cartilage and begins to erode it. The whirling behavior is caused by damage to the cartilage of the semicircular canals. The blacktail condition is caused by destruction of infected cartilage in the vertebral column adjacent to sympathetic nerves controlling caudal pigment cells. Since there is no effective treatment for infected fish, control involves thorough disinfection of all hatching and fish-rearing facilities and destruction of infected fish and, since maturation of the parasite requires habituation in earth ponds, the maintenance of young fish in fiberglass or concrete tanks until cartilages have ossified.

Henneguya, a myxosporidan parasite of warm-water fishes that has its greatest effect in catfish culture, produces cysts in the skin and gills. It has caused heavy mortalities of small fingerling catfish. As with other Myxosporida, there is no known effective treatment for infected fish. Prevention is aided by general disinfection.

The mode of infection of fish by microsporidans is unknown. These protozoa are obligate cytozoic parasites that reproduce within individual host cells, often inducing massive hypertrophy (xenomas). These can range in size from several microns (e.g. *Nosema hertwigi* in smelt) to nearly a centimeter (e.g. *Pleistophora cepedianae* in gizzard shad). Other important microsporidans of fish are *Pleistophora ovariae*, causing castration of bait fishes, and *P. salmonae* in gills of trout.

MYCOTIC DISEASES

The most frequent and troublesome fungal diseases of fishes reared by fish culturists and aquarists are caused by members of the genus *Saprolegnia*. Species of *Achyla*, *Aphanomyces*, *Branchiomyces*, *Ichthyophonus* and *Pythium* may also occur on, and in, fish and fish eggs.

Life cycles of fungi are complex, and those of many are unknown. The sex organs, which are sometimes needed for taxonomic differentiation, are produced only on special media. Transmission of *Saprolegnia* is by flagellated zoospores, which are produced within sporangia. *Saprolegnia* is known to be an occasional primary invader of fish and fish eggs but both it and other fungi are generally saprophytic opportunists that take advantage of necrotic tissue associated with physical injury or lesions induced by viruses, bacteria, or parasites. Treatment consists of the addition of malachite green (℞ 444) to the water. Copper sulfate (℞ 430) is helpful if water chemistry permits use of this compound.

Branchiomyces is known to invade the gills of warm-water fish in Europe, North America and other areas of the world. It causes necrosis of gill tissue. Control is effected by the destruction of infected fish, followed by pond disinfection with calcium oxide (℞ 427).

Ichthyophonus is a fungus that causes recurring epidemics in wild Atlantic herring, plaice, whiting, mackerel, and yellowtail flounder, the incidence of infection ranging from 2 to 80%. Infections have been found in hatchery-reared salmonids especially if fed on infected, wet trash fish, and in tropical freshwater fish in various parts of the world. The organism causes granuloma-like lesions of the heart, muscle, brain, liver and kidney. Control in farmed fish consists of elimination of contaminated raw-fish products in the feed.

PARASITIC HELMINTHS

Worm parasites are common in fish, and include representatives of all major groups of helminths. Most do not appear to injure the host seriously, unless they are exceptionally abundant. Many species of ectoparasitic monogenetic trematodes (e.g. *Gyrodactylus* and *Dactylogyrus* of fresh-water and brackish-water fish, and *Benedenia* and *Microcotyle* of marine fish) may multiply rapidly under favorable conditions. A few are viviparous, but most lay eggs. A ciliated larva (onchomiracidia) hatches from the egg and swims about seeking a suitable host. Contact with the fish host must be made within a definite time period. If contact with a fish is made, the parasite attaches to the skin or gills, sheds its ciliated epidermis and begins to grow at the expense of the host. Because they are obligate parasites and do not have an intermediate host, treatment with formalin (℞ 436) or Masoten (℞ 445) is usually effective. The marine forms (*Benedenia* and *Microcotyle*) can be controlled by immersing infected fish in fresh water for 1 to 5 minutes.

Internal flukes (digenetic trematodes) have complicated life cycles that involve 2 or more intermediate hosts. All life cycles require a molluscan host (usually a snail), a food organism or forage fish, and a predatory fish or a fish-eating animal.

Some digenetic trematodes occur as larval forms in fish tissues. These larvae (cercaria) emerge from the molluscan host, actively seek out and penetrate fish, and encyst in a specific site such as the eye lens, or gonad. Forms that encyst in the skin or muscle often induce a pigmented host-capsule and the larvae (metacercariae) are conspicuous as black or yellow spots. Fishermen refer to the cysts as "grubs." Heavy infections may affect the functioning of the organs involved, e.g. castration may be caused by infections in the gonads and blindness may follow eye infection. No treatment is known for infected fish. Control can sometimes be achieved by elimination or reduction of molluscan host populations, or increasing flow rates and reducing stocking densities to make host finding more difficult for the cercariae. Elimination of final host predators is often notably successful, especially with the eye-flukes.

Other digenetic flukes occur as adult worms in the digestive or urogenital systems of fish. Such helminths also require a primary molluscan host, but cercariae penetrate a food organism of the fish and encyst in its tissues. When these are consumed by the proper fish species, the larval worms mature in the intestinal tract and produce eggs. Flukes of this type are common in natural waters but are not known to cause significant problems in fish culture.

Tapeworms, nematodes, and spiny-headed worms (*Acanthocephala*) are also common parasites of fishes. Sexually mature adults are usually found in the gastrointestinal tract of fishes and fish-eating animals, while larval or immature worms may be found in tissues of fish that serve as food for predatory fishes or higher animals. A typical example is *Diphyllobothrium latum*, the broad fish tapeworm of man, whose larvae occur in the flesh of fish. There is no treatment for larval infections in fish tissues. Adult tapeworms may be removed by including tin dilaurate or di-n-butyl tin oxide (℞ 432), in the diet. No treatment has been defined for nematodes or spiny-headed worms but empirical clinical evidence suggests that the responses to anthelmintics by fish helminths are similar to those of higher animal parasites.

Leeches transmit blood parasites of fishes (e.g. *Trypanosoma*, *Cryptobia*, *Haemogregarina*), and may cause severe anemia if exceedingly numerous on fish in pond culture. Treatment consists of draining the pond and liming during the dry season.

PARASITIC COPEPODS

Copepods constitute another large group of parasites that attack the body and gills of fresh-water and salt-water fishes. All are highly specialized for a parasitic life; the bodies of some have become so greatly modified that they resemble worms more than crustaceans. When abundant on fish, they may cause serious injuries. The most serious are the anchor worm (*Lernaea*), the salmon louse (*Lepeophtheirus*) and the fish louse (*Argulus*). All are capable of serious damage by themselves but they also provide foci for invasion by opportunist bacteria and fungi. These parasites can usually be controlled by applying Masoten (℞ 445) but care must be taken to avoid residue problems. The salmon louse can usually be eliminated by exposure to fresh water.

NUTRITIONAL DISEASES

Although the food requirements of different species of fish vary from exclusively animal protein to exclusively plants, there is a remarkable similarity between them and indeed with higher animals of similar dietary requirement, in terms of protein, energy and vitamin requirements. Although satisfactory diets are available for most commercially cultured species the possibility of deficiency or toxic conditions is ever present. **Fat rancidity** is a particularly serious problem resulting in pale-colored liver, anemia and poor growth.

Avitaminoses produce lesions similar to those found in higher animals, for instance **deficiency of thiamin** (B_1) results in CNS lesions, **riboflavin deficiency** results in vascularization of the cornea and **α-tocopherol (E) deficiency** produces typical bland myopathy and deformity. Generally, group deficiency is multiple rather than related to one specific component and thus supplementation should be given with a vitamin B complex.

Toxic conditions associated with diet include **aflatoxicosis** or poisoning with toxins of the fungus *Aspergillus flavus*, which grows on various oil seeds. Rainbow trout are particularly susceptible to aflatoxicosis, which results in the induction of rapidly growing **hepatomas** and very high mortality. **Pansteatitis** due to unsuitable fish meals incorporated in a diet of low vitamin E status results in swim bladder thickening and infiltration of all fat tissues with inflammatory cells, causing heavy mortality in severe outbreaks. Polycellulose binders used to bind wet diets can be toxic to certain species, causing liver and kidney fibrosis, and dry diets can be a source of salt poisoning in marine cultured salmonids when the salinity of the holding area is high. Fresh water should be presented to such fish, or the diet should be dampened with fresh water.

NEOPLASTIC DISEASES

Neoplasia in fishes is similar to that in higher animals. The high incidence of reported **skin tumors** probably reflects their ease of observation rather than any higher incidence, but **papillomas** of viral, chemical, or unknown origin are widely recognized, particularly in Pacific flatfish.

One particular tumor, the **malignant melanoma of the guppy-swordtail cross**, has been shown to be genetically mediated and others such as the **pseudobranch tumor of cod** and **malignant lymphosarcoma of northern pike** may also have a genetic component. Goldfish are particularly liable to develop small hard skin tumors, particularly on the head—called variously **neurilemomas** or **fibromas**. They are of little significance but can be removed surgically.

MISCELLANEOUS NONINFECTIOUS DISEASES

Coloration anomalies and **yolk-sac anomalies** or deformities are common in cultured fish and may be of genetic or environmental origin. **Blue-sac disease**, for instance, a condition of larval rainbow trout, is believed to be associated with unsuitable hatchery water and **pseudoalbinism** in cultured flatfish with excessive light levels shortly after hatching.

Sunburn can occur in surface swimming fish or can be induced by feeding photodynamic drugs such as phenothiazine even in bottom dwellers although ultraviolet light penetrates poorly into water.

Nephrocalcinosis and **visceral granuloma** are conditions found particularly in salmonid culture, induced supposedly by high levels of carbon dioxide in the water producing a metabolic acidosis and urinary and tissue precipitation of calcium around which extensive granulomata develop.

Proliferative kidney disease is a condition presently restricted to Europe in which the hemopoietic tissue and fibrous tissue of the kidney proliferate in the presence of large blast-like cells of possible ameboid origin. The condition appears to be related to certain types of water supply, which should be avoided where possible.

Ulcerative dermal necrosis is a condition of the head of Atlantic salmon and sea trout as they enter fresh water. The large deep ulcers that develop on the head rapidly become secondarily infected and the mortality may be very high. No cause is recognized but the condition appears to be cyclic. It is only reported from Northern Europe and affected fish usually recover if secondary infection is kept down by painting the lesions with dilute malachite green (℞ 444).

DIAGNOSTIC LABORATORIES

The following is a partial listing of laboratories equipped to help with diagnosis of fish diseases in the U.S.A. Permission should be sought before material is submitted for diagnosis.

Southeastern Cooperative Fish Disease Laboratory
Auburn University
Department of Fisheries and Allied Aquacultures
Auburn, Alabama 36830

United States Fish and Wildlife Service
Fish Farming Experimental Station
Stuttgart, Arkansas 72160

Fish Disease Laboratory
California Department of Fish and Game
407 West Line Street
Bishop, California 93514

Fish Disease Unit
California Department of Fish and Game
Mojave River Hatchery
P.O. Box 938
Victorville, California 92392

Fish Disease Control Center
U.S. Fish and Wildlife Service
P.O. Box 917
Fort Morgan, Colorado 80701

National Aquarium
Commerce Building
U.S. Department of the Interior
U.S. Fish and Wildlife Service
Washington, D.C. 20230

North Georgia Diagnostic Assistance Laboratory
College of Veterinary Medicine
University of Georgia
Athens, Georgia 30602

Louisiana Wildlife and Fisheries Commission
P.O. Box 4004
District II
Monroe, Louisiana 71203

Department Inland Fisheries and Wildlife
8 Federal Street
Augusta, Maine 04330

National Fish Hatchery
East Street
Belchertown, Massachusetts 01007

Wolf Lake State Fish Hatchery
RR No. 1
Mattawan, Michigan 49071

Fish and Wildlife Pathology
Department of Natural Resources
390 Centennial Office Building
St. Paul, Minnesota 55155

Idaho Department of Fish and Game
Fish Disease Laboratory
Hagerman State Hatchery
Hagerman, Idaho 83332

Fisheries Research Laboratory
Southern Illinois University
Carbondale, Illinois 62901

State Conservation Commission
Big Spring Hatchery
Elkader, Iowa 52043

U.S. Fish and Wildlife Service
P.O. Box 4389
2531 N. West Street
Jackson, Mississippi 39216

United States Fish and Wildlife Service
Fish Cultural Development Center
Route 2
Box 333
Bozeman, Montana 59715

New York State Department of Environmental Conservation
Rome Fish Pathology Laboratory
8314 Fish Hatchery Road
Rome, New York 13440

The Department of Interior Fish and Wildlife
P.O. Box 158
Pisgah Forest, North Carolina 28768

Warm Water Hatchery Biology Center
National Fish Hatchery
Tishomingo, Oklahoma 73460

Oregon Department of Fish and Wildlife
Department of Microbiology
Nash Hall
Oregon State University
Corvallis, Oregon 97331

Benner Springs Fishery Research Station
Pennsylvania Fish Commission
P.O. Box 200-C
Bellefonte, Pennsylvania 16823

Marine Pathology Laboratory
University of Rhode Island
Kingston, Rhode Island 02881

Wildlife Park and Forestry
3305 West South Street
Rapid City, S.D. 57701

Eastern Fish Disease Laboratory
U.S. Fish and Wildlife Service
Leetown, Route No. 1, Box 17
Kearneysville, West Virginia

Fish Pathology Laboratory
Michigan Department of Natural Resources
P.O. Box 507
Grayling, Michigan 49738

New York Aquarium
N.Y. Zoological Society
Seaside Park, Coney Island
Brooklyn, New York 11224

Western Fish Disease Laboratory
Building 204 Naval Support Activity
Seattle, Washington 98115

Western Fish Nutrition Laboratory
Cook, Washington 98605

PART V
NUTRITION

DAIRY CATTLE NUTRITION

NUTRITIONAL REQUIREMENTS

The specific dietary needs of dairy cattle are greatly modified by rumen activity. For the first 3 to 5 weeks after birth, dairy calves have dietary requirements similar to those of swine and dogs and must obtain these nutrients from milk or a milk replacer. These include high-quality, easily digested feeds to supply available energy, essential amino acids and all of the vitamins and essential minerals. Soon after 1 month of age, as roughage and grain consumption increases, microorganisms in the rumen become increasingly active in synthesizing the essential amino acids and B-vitamins and in digesting cellulose. Mature dairy cattle, therefore, can thrive largely independently of a dietary supply of essential amino acids or high-quality protein and the B-vitamins. In common with other ruminants, they utilize coarse feeds, high in cellulose, which are less useful for nonherbivores such as man. Veal calves, which are fed solely a milk or milk-replacer diet and no dry feed, continue to exist as nonruminants, in terms of their nutritional requirements.

The daily nutrient requirements of dairy cattle published by the Committee on Animal Nutrition of the National Research Council in 1978 are summarized in TABLE 1 for growing cattle and TABLE 2 for lactating and pregnant cows. Specific requirements are shown for large breeds for total feed, energy, total protein, calcium, phosphorus and vitamins A and D. TABLE 3 summarizes the concentration of all the known nutrients in the diets recommended for different classes of dairy cattle. Where maximum tolerances are known, these are also included.

TABLE 1. DAILY NUTRIENT REQUIREMENTS OF GROWING DAIRY CATTLE AND MATURE BREEDING BULLS

Body Weight (kg)	Large Breed, Age (wk)[a]	Daily Gain (gm)	Feed DM (kg)	Feed Energy					Total Crude Protein (gm)	Minerals		Vitamins	
				NE_m (Mcal)	NE_g (Mcal)	ME (Mcal)	DE (Mcal)	TDN (kg)		Ca (gm)	P (gm)	A (1,000 IU)	D (IU)
Growing Dairy Heifer and Bull Calves Fed Only Milk													
42	1	400	0.63	1.25	0.70	2.93	3.31	0.75	148	8	5	1.8	280
50	3	500	0.76	1.40	0.90	3.61	4.01	0.91	180	9	6	2.1	330
Growing Dairy Heifer and Bull Calves Fed Only Milk													
50	3	500	1.45	1.45	0.96	4.82	5.42	1.23	198	10	6	2.1	330
75	10	700	2.10	1.96	1.37	6.71	7.67	1.72	318	15	8	3.2	495
Growing Dairy Heifers													
100	16	700	2.80	2.43	1.47	8.09	9.26	2.10	402	18	9	4.2	660
150	26	700	4.00	3.30	1.68	10.49	12.17	2.76	510	19	12	6.4	990
200	36	700	5.20	4.10	1.96	13.01	15.20	3.45	620	21	14	8.5	1320
300	57	700	7.20	5.55	2.38	17.07	20.11	4.56	771	24	18	12.7	1980
400	77	700	8.60	6.89	2.66	20.40	24.03	5.45	864	25	20	17.0	2640
500	98	600	9.50	8.14	2.52	22.26	26.28	5.96	903	27	21	21.2	3300
600	127	200	9.58	9.33	0.90	19.60	23.68	5.37	879	25	18	25.4	3960
Growing Dairy Bulls													
100	15	800	2.80	2.43	1.68	8.47	9.63	2.18	427	19	10	4.2	660
300	45	1000	7.40	5.69	2.95	18.67	21.78	4.94	862	27	20	12.7	1980
500	74	900	10.00	8.95	3.60	25.56	29.76	6.75	973	29	23	21.2	3300
700	117	500	11.40	11.53	2.25	26.94	31.75	7.20	998	30	23	29.7	4620

Growing Veal Calves Fed Only Milk

45	1.0	800	1.06	1.36	1.52	5.04	5.60	1.27	259	8	5	1.9	297
75	5.8	1050	1.48	1.96	2.10	7.05	7.83	1.78	334	15	9	3.2	495
150	15.4	1300	2.22	3.30	2.99	10.58	11.75	2.66	428	20	12	6.4	990

Maintenance of Mature Breeding Bulls

500	—	—	7.80	9.60	—	15.95	19.27	4.37	673	20	15	21	—
900	—	—	12.13	14.55	—	24.79	29.94	6.79	1017	31	23	38	—
1300	—	—	15.98	19.17	—	32.67	39.46	8.95	1316	41	31	55	—

[a] Age in weeks indicates probable age of animals when they reach the weight indicated.
NE_m, net energy for maintenance; NE_g, net energy for body gain; ME, metabolizable energy; DE, digestible energy.
(From *Nutrient Requirements of Dairy Cattle*, National Research Council, 1978.)

TABLE 2. DAILY NUTRIENT REQUIREMENTS OF LACTATING AND PREGNANT COWS

Body Weight (kg)	Feed Energy				Total Crude Protein (gm)	Calcium (gm)	Phosphorus (gm)	Vitamin A (1,000 IU)
	NE_1 (Mcal)	ME (Mcal)	DE (Mcal)	TDN (kg)				
Maintenance of Mature Lactating Cows[a]								
400	7.16	11.90	13.86	3.15	373	15	13	30
500	8.46	14.06	16.39	3.72	432	18	15	38
600	9.70	16.12	18.79	4.27	589	21	17	46
700	10.89	18.10	21.09	4.79	542	24	19	53
800	12.03	20.01	23.32	5.29	592	27	21	61
Maintenance Plus Last 2 Months of Gestation of Mature Dry Cows								
400	9.30	15.47	17.89	4.10	702	26	18	30
500	11.00	18.29	21.25	4.84	821	31	22	38
600	12.61	20.97	24.37	5.55	931	37	26	46
700	14.15	23.54	27.35	6.23	1035	42	30	53
800	15.64	26.02	30.24	6.89	1136	47	34	61
Milk Production—Nutrients Per Kg Milk of Different Fat Percentages								
(% Fat)								
3.0	0.64	1.07	1.24	0.282	72	2.40	1.65	
3.5	0.69	1.16	1.34	0.304	82	2.60	1.75	
4.0	0.74	1.24	1.44	0.326	87	2.70	1.80	
4.5	0.78	1.31	1.52	0.344	92	2.80	1.85	
5.0	0.83	1.39	1.61	0.365	98	2.90	1.90	

[a] To allow for growth of young lactating cows, increase the maintenance allowances for all nutrients except vitamin A by 20% during the first lactation and 10% during the second lactation.

NE_1, net energy for lactation; ME, metabolizable energy; DE, digestible energy.

(From *Nutrient Requirements of Dairy Cattle*, National Research Council, 1978.)

Water

Dairy cattle will suffer more quickly from an inadequate water intake than from a deficiency of any other nutrient. Milk production and feed intake will be depressed if they are not allowed all the water they wish. Cows will consume 3 to 5 lb of water for each lb of dry matter consumed and another 3 to 4 lb for each lb of milk produced. Thus, cows yielding 80 lb of milk may drink over 300 lb per day. On succulent feeds, water consumption is less. In winter, cows will drink more water if it is warmed slightly; in very warm weather, intake may be trebled.

Calves during the latter part of the milk feeding period, heifers and bulls should be offered water *ad libitum*. Water may have to be restricted to young calves to prevent excessive intake.

Energy

The principal use of feed by the body is as a source of energy. All organic nutrients, e.g. protein, carbohydrates and fats supply energy. Thus, the energy values of the organic components of a feedstuff are combined and expressed as total digestible nutrients (TDN), digestible energy (DE), metabolizable energy (ME) or net energy (net energy-maintenance, NE_m; net energy-gain, NE_g; net energy-lactation, NE_l). TDN and DE account for energy losses in the feces, ME from the feces, urine and combustible gases from the gut, and NE equals ME minus the heat increment or energy losses from the metabolism of feed nutrients. The latter connotation reflects a truer value of the feedstuffs for productive purposes and more accurately compares concentrates with roughages. For a quick field reference as to overall diet adequacy, TDN is still a useful statistic.

Insufficient intake of energy is a more frequent cause of retarded growth, delayed puberty or depressed milk production than probably any other nutritional deficiency. The energy requirements (Tables 1 to 3) serve primarily as guides. Lower intakes than suggested will reduce growth rates and decrease milk production. Larger intakes will increase growth rates and may increase production or fat deposition or both in lactating cows.

Under rigid experimental conditions, calves have been shown to require the essential fatty acids, but under usual feeding conditions, even when low-fat milk replacers are used, the deficiency does not occur. A specific dietary fat requirement for ruminating cattle does not appear to exist or is at least met by normal feedstuffs.

Protein

The total protein values in Tables 1 to 3 represent the approximate minimum requirements. However, it is important to recognize that when high-protein feeds are cheap, they can safely be used to

TABLE 3. RECOMMENDED NUTRIENT CONTENT OF RATIONS FOR DAIRY CATTLE

Nutrients (Concentration in the Feed Dry Matter)	Lactating Cow Rations				Nonlactating Cattle Rations					Maximum Concentrations (All Classes)
Cow Wt (kg)	Daily Milk Yields (kg)									
≤400	< 8	8–13	13–18	>18						
500	<11	11–17	17–23	>23						
600	<14	14–21	21–29	>29						
≥700	<18	18–26	26–35	>35	Dry Pregnant Cows	Mature Bulls	Growing Heifers and Bulls	Calf Starter Concentrate Mix	Calf Milk Replacer	
Ration No.	I	II	III	IV	V	VI	VII	VIII	IX	Max.
Crude Protein, %	13.0	14.0	15.0	16.0	11.0	8.5	12.0	16.0	22.0	—
Energy										
NE_l, Mcal/kg	1.42	1.52	1.62	1.72	1.35	—	—	—	—	—
NE_m, Mcal/kg	—	—	—	—	—	1.20	1.26	1.90	2.40	—
NE_g, Mcal/kg	—	—	—	—	—	—	0.60	1.20	1.55	—
ME, Mcal/kg	2.36	2.53	2.71	2.89	2.23	2.04	2.23	3.12	3.78	—
DE, Mcal/kg	2.78	2.95	3.13	3.31	2.65	2.47	2.65	3.53	4.19	—
TDN, %	63	67	71	75	60	56	60	80	95	—
Crude Fiber, %	17	17	17	17[a]	17	15	15	—	—	—
Acid Detergent Fiber, %	21	21	21	21	21	19	19	—	—	—
Ether Extract, %	2	2	2	2	2	2	2	2	10	—
Minerals[b]										
Calcium, %	0.43	0.48	0.54	0.60	0.37	0.24	0.40	0.60	0.70	—
Phosphorus, %	0.31	0.34	0.38	0.40	0.26	0.18	0.26	0.42	0.50	—
Magnesium, %[c]	0.20	0.20	0.20	0.20	0.16	0.16	0.16	0.07	0.07	—
Potassium, %	0.80	0.80	0.80	0.80	0.80	0.80	0.80	0.80	0.80	—
Sodium, %	0.18	0.18	0.18	0.18	0.10	0.10	0.10	0.10	0.10	—
Sodium chloride, %[d]	0.46	0.46	0.46	0.46	0.25	0.25	0.25	0.25	0.25	5
Sulfur, %[d]	0.20	0.20	0.20	0.20	0.17	0.11	0.16	0.21	0.29	0.35
Iron, ppm[d, e]	50	50	50	50	50	50	50	100	100	1,000
Cobalt, ppm	0.10	0.10	0.10	0.10	0.10	0.10	0.10	0.10	0.10	10
Copper, ppm[d, f]	10	10	10	10	10	10	10	10	10	80
Manganese, ppm[d]	40	40	40	40	40	40	40	40	40	1,000
Zinc, ppm[d, g]	40	40	40	40	40	40	40	40	40	500
Iodine, ppm[h]	0.50	0.50	0.50	0.50	0.50	0.25	0.25	0.25	0.25	50
Molybdenum, ppm[i, j]	—	—	—	—	—	—	—	—	—	6
Selenium, ppm	0.10	0.10	0.10	0.10	0.10	0.10	0.10	0.10	0.10	5
Fluorine, ppm[j]	—	—	—	—	—	—	—	—	—	30

Vitamins[k]										
Vit A, IU/kg	3,200	3,200	3,200	3,200	3,200	3,200	2,200	2,200	3,800	—
Vit D, IU/kg	300	300	300	300	300	300	300	300	300	—
Vit E, ppm	—	—	—	—	—	—	—	—	300	—

[a] It is difficult to formulate high-energy rations with a minimum of 17 percent crude fiber. However, fat percentage depression may occur when rations with less than 17 percent crude fiber or 21 percent ADF are fed to lactating cows.

[b] The mineral values presented in this table are intended as guidelines for use of professionals in ration formulation. Because of many factors affecting such values, they are not intended and should not be used as a legal or regulatory base.

[c] Under conditions conducive to grass tetany magnesium should be increased to 0.25 or higher.

[d] The maximum safe levels for many of the mineral elements are not well defined; estimates given here, especially for sulfur, sodium chloride, iron, copper, zinc, and manganese, are based on very limited data; safe levels may be substantially affected by specific feeding conditions.

[e] The maximum safe level of supplemental iron in some forms is materially lower than 1,000 ppm. As little as 400 ppm added iron as ferrous sulfate has reduced weight gains.

[f] High copper may increase the susceptibility of milk to oxidized flavor.

[g] Maximum safe level of zinc for mature dairy cattle is 1,000 ppm.

[h] If diet contains as much as 25 percent strongly goitrogenic feed on dry basis, iodine provided should be increased two times or more.

[i] If diet contains sufficient copper, dairy cattle tolerate substantially more than 6 ppm molybdenum.

[j] Maximum safe level of fluorine for growing heifers and bulls is lower than for other dairy cattle. Somewhat higher levels are tolerated when the fluorine is from less-available sources such as phosphates (see text). Minimium requirement for molybdenum and fluorine not yet established.

[k] The following minimum quantities of B-complex vitamins are suggested per unit of milk replacer: niacin, 2.6 ppm; pantothenic acid, 13 ppm; riboflavin, 6.5 ppm; pyridoxine, 6.5 ppm; thiamin, 6.5 ppm; folic acid, 0.5 ppm; biotin, 0.1 ppm; vitamin B_{12}, 0.07 ppm; choline, 0.26 percent. It appears that adequate amounts of these vitamins are furnished when calves have functional rumens (usually at 6 weeks of age) by a combination of rumen synthesis and natural feedstuffs.

NE_l, net energy for lactation; NE_m, net energy for maintenance; NE_g, net energy for body gain; ME, metabolizable energy; DE, digestible energy.

(From *Nutrient Requirements of Dairy Cattle,* National Research Council, 1978.)

furnish more than the amounts recommended. The requirements are expressed as crude protein (N × 6.25), although it is recognized that dairy cattle, except young calves, can also make use of nonprotein nitrogen sources such as urea and ammonium compounds. Bacteria in the rumen are able to convert the nonprotein nitrogen into true protein which is then digested by the host. When urea or ammonium salts are appreciably cheaper than protein-rich feeds or when protein supplements are not available, it is good nutritional practice to use nonprotein feeds to balance the ration of dairy cows and heifers. The exception may be the high-producing dairy cow. Urea can furnish one-fourth of the nitrogen in concentrate mixtures if care is taken to ensure that it is thoroughly mixed to prevent an excessive intake, which may prove toxic. Palatability may be a problem if over 2.0% of the total concentrate is urea, while levels of over 1.0% of the total diet dry-matter will be used inefficiently. Since rumen bacteria must adjust to urea, such feeds should be gradually introduced over a 3-week period. Dairy cattle thrive on protein from a single feed source. It is therefore unnecessary to use feeds from a wide variety of sources, since protein quality is relatively unimportant for ruminating dairy cattle. Balancing feed protein sources based on their degradability in the rumen may however be accepted in future as a means of increasing efficiency of protein utilization by high-producing cows.

Minerals

Dairy cattle need a dietary source of calcium, phosphorus, magnesium, sulfur, potassium, sodium, chlorine, iron, iodine, manganese, copper, cobalt, zinc and selenium. A few of the ones needing special attention in practical feeding are discussed below.

Salt (sodium chloride) is not supplied by ordinary feeds in amounts large enough to meet the needs of dairy cattle with the possible exception of good pasture. Allowing animals free access to salt is the most satisfactory way of meeting the requirement. Block salt licks are adequate. It is also desirable to add 1 to 1.5% of salt to concentrate mixtures for growing calves, young stock, milking cows and bulls. Milk furnishes adequate salt to young calves. Excessive salt is not harmful when adequate water is available. After periods of salt deprivation, it should be reintroduced gradually.

Calcium and phosphorus must be added to almost all dairy cattle diets except those receiving milk. The calcium and phosphorus contents of certain feeds and supplements are shown in TABLE 4. It will be observed that alfalfa and clover hays are rich in calcium but somewhat low in phosphorus. This is true for most legumes. Nonlegume forages are poor in calcium.

All concentrate feeds used for dairy cattle are relatively deficient in calcium. Wheat bran, distillers' solubles and cottonseed meal are

TABLE 4. SOME GOOD SOURCES OF CALCIUM AND PHOSPHORUS (AS FED)

Feed	Calcium %	Phosphorus %
Alfalfa hay	1.17	0.21
Clover hay	1.31	0.22
Dried skim milk	1.17	0.97
Dried whey	0.91	0.75
Wheat bran	0.11	1.17
Cottonseed meal	0.16	1.21
Distillers' solubles	0.35	1.37
Bone meal	29.0	13.2
Defluorinated rock phosphate	31.7	13.7
Dicalcium phosphate	22.7	18.0
Limestone	36.0	0.02

the common feeds richest in phosphorus, but they are low in calcium. Bone meal, defluorinated phosphates and dicalcium phosphate are the most common supplements of calcium and phosphorus. Limestone (feeding grade) is the cheapest single source of calcium. It is recognized that both the ratio of calcium to phosphorus and the presence of vitamin D affect calcium and phosphorus utilization. The NRC recommendations (TABLE 3) call for calcium:phosphorus ratios of about 1.4 to 1 for growth, maintenance and milk production. For growth, ratios up to 7 to 1 are not detrimental. Mature bulls receiving 3 to 5 times their requirement develop a high incidence of osteopetrosis, which markedly reduces their ability to walk and to mount. Milk fever has been reduced by reducing calcium intake to about 30 gm/day 2 weeks before calving and increasing it to 150 to 200 gm/day after calving. It is a useful and convenient practice to allow animals free access to steamed bone meal, dicalcium phosphate or defluorinated rock phosphate in a sheltered box mixed 50:50 with iodized salt. When necessary, other mineral elements may be added as well. A surer method to guarantee satisfactory intakes is to add the supplements to the concentrate ration as cattle will not balance their diets precisely. This is especially true for high-producing cows.

Iodine is required by the animal for the synthesis by the thyroid gland of iodothyroglobulin and the hormone thyroxine, by which the thyroid exercises a degree of control over the basal metabolic rate and the functions of growth, reproduction and lactation. In the newborn calf, simple goiter (q.v., p. 203) is evident when maternal intake is deficient. The iodine requirement is increased by the presence of goitrogenic substances in feeds, such as raw soybeans, linseed, certain clovers and cruciferous crops generally. Pasture plants vary greatly in their ability to take up iodine from the soil. The only feeds naturally rich in iodine are the salt-water fish meals and dried kelp, so that any deficiency is more readily treated with stabilized iodized salt containing 0.007% iodine or as a part of a trace mineral mixture in the concentrate. Lactating cows require more than nonlactating ones because about 10% of it is excreted into the milk.

Since the thyroid can store iodine, the daily requirement does not have to be met each day. Excessive quantities, however, fed over short periods will give rise to signs of iodism. Iodine deficiency, which occurs on deficient soils such as around the Great Lakes and westward to the Pacific Coast, is discussed under NUTRITIONAL DEFICIENCIES IN CATTLE AND SHEEP:**Iodine** (q.v., p. 1397).

Cobalt is required by ruminants for the normal ruminal metabolism. When the intake of cobalt is inadequate, the bacterial population in the rumen is altered and the synthesis of vitamin B_{12} is greatly lowered. The animal requires the vitamin at the cellular level.

In many areas, the soil and hence the forages are deficient in cobalt. Usually the legumes are richer than the grasses. Corn appears to have a low content, while linseed meal is a rich source. When the forage contains less than 0.07 ppm of cobalt (dry basis), signs of cobalt deficiency may occur in cattle. Effective supplementation of the ration of dairy cattle can be achieved by adding 2 gm of cobalt sulfate to each ton of concentrate mixture. Details of cobalt deficiency are given under NUTRITIONAL DEFICIENCIES IN CATTLE AND SHEEP:**Cobalt** (q.v., p. 1397).

Copper is required by the animal as a constituent or activator of certain enzyme systems concerned with hemoglobin synthesis, melanin production, hair growth and the functional integrity of bone and nervous tissues. Except in very general terms, it is not possible to set a uniform copper requirement for all areas because it is markedly influenced by the level of other dietary constituents, particularly molybdenum, inorganic sulfate and phosphorus. The levels of these minerals being normal, the daily requirement of copper for dairy cattle may be satisfied by forage that contains not less than 10 ppm (dry basis).

There are many areas in the U.S.A. where, either because of a low copper content of the herbage or the presence of complicating factors such as high molybdenum, the copper content of the ration must be supplemented to maintain normal health, growth, production and reproduction in dairy cattle (*see* NUTRITIONAL DEFICIENCIES IN CATTLE AND SHEEP:**Copper** (p. 1398).

Vitamins

Young calves up to 4 to 5 weeks of age should receive all of the known vitamins in their feed except niacin and ascorbic acid. Niacin is synthesized from dietary tryptophan and normal tissue synthesis of ascorbic acid is adequate.

As bacterial function develops in the rumen, the B-vitamins are synthesized in large amounts and need not be supplied in the diet thereafter. Milk, cereal grains and other feeds consumed by young calves contain sufficient of the B-vitamins to meet their needs before rumen synthesis begins. Milk replacers should probably contain all the added B-vitamins (TABLE 3). Thus supplying the B-vitamins is not an important practical problem in cattle.

Vitamins A, D and E: A deficiency of any of these vitamins is relatively rare for cattle receiving natural mixtures of high quality feeds. White muscle disease (muscular dystrophy) due to a deficiency of vitamin E or selenium is uncommon in dairy calves although not infrequent in beef calves and lambs in areas where the soil is low in selenium.

When cows are fed poor-quality, bleached roughage for long periods, they may show reproductive failure from vitamin A deficiency, or they may give milk low in vitamin A. The best assurance against vitamin A deficiency in dairy cattle is to provide abundant pasture in summer and high-quality, properly cured hay or silage in winter. When adequate good-quality forage is not available, vitamin A supplements may be desirable. Most commercial concentrates now contain about 200 IU of vitamin A per pound as insurance against deficiency.

All natural feeds except sun-cured hay have a low vitamin D content. Animals that are exposed to sunlight for as little as an hour a day synthesize ample vitamin D and do not require high levels in their feed. Vitamin D deficiency may be observed in young calves which are closely confined and do not consume sun-cured roughage. Whole milk and skim milk are always low in vitamin D. Concentrate mixtures are also naturally low in the vitamin. As little as 200 IU of vitamin D per pound of calf feed is an adequate amount. Feeding sun-cured hay *ad libitum* to young calves will prevent vitamin D deficiency. Under normal conditions, even wilted legume silage furnishes ample vitamin D for dairy calves and thus dairy animals receive enough vitamin D from ordinary roughages and from exposure to sunlight. Feeding 20,000,000 IU of vitamin D per cow per day 3 to 5 days before the expected calving date and continuing through the first day after calving (maximum feeding period 7 days) has markedly reduced the incidence of milk fever in milk fever-prone cows.

Vitamin E has been added to dairy concentrates to help preserve the flavor of milk. Vitamin K is synthesized in the rumen in ample quantities.

In spite of the widespread use of vitamins A, D and E in dairy concentrates, the appearance of a frank deficiency in the field when not included is unlikely. Injections of vitamins A, D and E at the time of drying off were of no value to cows fed normal diets. Milk replacers should be fortified with vitamins A, D and E.

FEEDING AND MANAGEMENT PRACTICES

Dairy cattle will require some concentrates until the age of 8 to 10 months, although forage will supply an increasing percentage of the ration after about 4 months. In addition, concentrates will be needed for cows producing milk and as a supplement to poor-quality unpalatable sparse forage.

In determining the amount and kind of concentrate mixture needed, it is essential to know what type of roughage is available; a concentrate can then be selected that will supply the amounts of additional nutrients needed at lowest cost. As an aid in formulating concentrate mixture, the nutrient requirements stated as amounts per kg of feed are shown in TABLE 3. Note: These data are for total feed including forage and concentrates.

The appropriate amounts of nutrients furnished by some of the common dairy cattle feeds are listed in TABLE 5. Hays and silages of the same species vary greatly in composition depending upon the stage of maturity at the time of cutting and curing and preservation methods. Thus, although the precise value of a hay or silage cannot be known without chemical analysis (or even a feeding experiment), its approximate value can be estimated from TABLE 5, and a concentrate mixture of appropriate composition can be made or purchased to balance the roughage available. In many states a forage testing service is available either through Cooperative Extension or local feed companies, which can give more precise information as to composition.

High-protein feeds, such as soybean meal, cottonseed meal, linseed meal and coconut meal usually are higher in price than the cereal grains. Therefore, it is generally good economy to use concentrate mixtures as low in protein as will supply an adequate amount of total protein. Simple mixtures are as effective as complex ones, although feed companies pass on significant economies by using by-product feeds in complex mixtures.

Palatability and nutrient content rather than the number of ingredients in a mixture largely determine the value of feeds for dairy cattle.

Calves should receive colostrum for at least the first 3 days and then milk at the rate of 10% of body weight during the first few weeks after birth. A milk replacer or fermented colostrum (2 to 1 with water) are also excellent liquid feeds. Mastitic or hospital milk is satisfactory as well. Calves usually can be weaned at 4 to 6 weeks of age or when they are regularly consuming 1 to 2 lb (0.5 to 1 kg) of starter daily. During the first week, starter containing at least 18% protein and hay should be placed before calves. The calf should be allowed all the starter it will eat up to a maximum of 5 lb (2.3 kg) a day. Calves do not like finely ground and dusty feeds. They will readily consume coarsely cracked or rolled grains or feeds in which the "fines" are pelleted. While often economical, hay is not required during the first 2 months. With a coarse starter, calves begin to ruminate within 2 weeks. If hay is fed, early-cut green, leafy, soft-stemmed material is the best kind for calves. They can be offered all the hay they will eat. After 4 to 6 months of age the calf starter can be replaced with a cheaper type of grower ration or regular milk cow ration containing 16% total protein. Hay crop or corn silage can be fed to young calves, although they will consume it more effectively after 4 months of age.

Heifers and young stock that are well-grown normally will not need concentrates after 8 months of age if fed fine quality forage. More rapid gain or improved condition if desired or needed, will result from the addition of 2 to 3 lb (1 to 1.5 kg) of concentrates. It is advisable to feed 5 to 6 lb (2 to 3 kg) daily if the forage is of poor quality or scanty.

Pregnant cows and heifers should receive as much attention just before calving as after parturition. Having them too fat will predispose them to ketosis. Having them in good condition, plus a high level of feeding after calving will tend to reduce ketosis. During most of the dry period cows in good condition fed good quality hay or pasture require no concentrates. All-corn silage (plus protein and calcium) often will result in too-fat cows at parturition. Two weeks before parturition, cows and heifers should be offered grain (alone, in a complete feed, or as a part of corn silage [50% corn grain]) up to 6 to 10 lb (3 to 4 kg) per day by calving time to adjust the rumen to grain. At calving a complete feed of 60% concentrate, 40% roughage (dry basis) can be offered immediately to meet the energy needs of early high production and to challenge the cow to produce to her potential. If grain is fed separately, an increase at the rate of 1.5 lb (0.7 kg) per day to a maximum of 30 to 36 lb (14 to 16 kg) will be fast enough to generate production but not so fast as to produce digestive upsets or inappetence. For poor eaters, greater intakes are possible if cows are fed concentrates more often, i.e. 3 times a day, and roughage several times in between. After the peak of lactation, the concentrate level should gradually be adjusted to that needed for the amount and fat percentage of the milk produced and the quality of the forage available and consumed. Suggested daily intakes of concentrates for cows of high and low testing breeds receiving good or poor roughage are shown in TABLE 6. Cows fed complete feeds should be grouped by age and production and offered rations ranging from 60% concentrate, 40% roughage (dry basis) for fresh cows to 20% concentrate, 80% roughage for the low producing group. Care should be taken that the total diet contain at least 17% of crude fiber (or 21% acid detergent fiber [ADF]) to protect against milk fat depression. Protein levels of concentrates that will meet the requirements for different forage qualities are: nonlegume, including all-corn silage 23%, mixed legume-nonlegume 16%, all-legume 12

TABLE 5. THE ESTIMATED NUTRIENT CONTENT OF SOME FEEDS FOR DAIRY AND BEEF CATTLE (DRY MATTER BASIS)[a]

Feed	DE	ME	NE_m	NE_g	NE_l	TDN	Total Protein	Crude Fiber	Ca	P	Vitamin A Value	Dry Matter
	Mcal/kg					%	%	%	%	%	1,000 IU/kg	%
Dried roughage												
Alfalfa hay												
good (early bloom)	2.56	2.13	1.24	0.59	1.30	58	17.2	31	1.25	.23	34	90
poor (mature)	2.29	1.87	1.11	0.36	1.15	52	13.5	37	1.17	.17	3	91
Lespedeza hay	2.20	1.78	1.07	0.28	1.10	50	14.5	30	1.19	.26	22	93
Other legume hays	2.60	2.18	1.26	0.62	1.32	59	14.9	30	1.49	.25	13	88
Grass hay												
early cut	2.73	2.31	1.33	0.73	1.40	62	10.0	32	.53	.26	21	88
late cut	2.24	1.82	1.09	0.32	1.13	51	6.0	35	.28	.18	11	88
Weathered range grass (undoubtedly poorer than late cut grass hay)												
Corn stover	2.60	2.18	1.26	0.62	1.32	59	5.9	34	.60	.09	2	87
Cottonseed hulk	1.68	1.24	0.86	0.00	0.81	38	4.3	50	.16	.73	0	90
Silages												
Corn silage	3.08	2.67	1.54	0.97	1.59	70	8.0	24	.27	.20	18	35
Sorghum silage	2.42	2.00	1.17	0.48	1.23	55	8.3	26	.32	.18	5	29
Grass silage	2.73	2.31	1.33	0.73	1.40	62	10.0	32	.53	.26	21	33
Legume silage	2.56	2.13	1.24	0.59	1.30	58	17.2	31	1.25	.23	34	33
Concentrates												
Beet pulp (dried)	3.44	3.02	1.79	1.19	1.79	78	8.0	22	.75	.11	0	91
Barley	3.65	3.24	1.96	1.31	1.91	83	13.9	6	.05	.37	0	89
Brewers grains (dried)	2.90	2.49	1.44	0.86	1.50	66	26.0	16	.29	.54	0	92
Citrus pulp (dried)	3.40	2.98	1.76	1.16	1.76	77	6.9	14	2.07	.13	0	90
Corn	3.35	3.11	1.86	1.24	1.84	80	10.0	2	.03	.31	1	89
Corn gluten feed	3.61	3.19	1.93	1.29	1.89	82	25.0	9	.33	.86	4	90
Cottonseed meal	3.30	2.89	1.69	1.11	1.72	75	44.8	13	.17	1.31	0	93
Distillers grains	3.88	3.47	2.16	1.42	2.03	88	29.8	10	.16	.79	2	92
Linseed meal	3.34	2.93	1.73	1.14	1.74	76	38.6	10	.43	.91	0	91
Milk, whole	5.73	5.16	3.61	2.01	—	130	25.8	—	.89	.72	15	12

Milo (sorghum)	3.52	3.10	1.86	1.24	1.84	80	11.7	2	.03	.33	0	88
Molasses, cane	3.17	2.76	1.60	1.03	1.64	72	4.3	—	1.19	.11	0	75
Oats	3.34	2.93	1.73	1.14	1.74	76	4.3	12	.17	.39	0	89
Soybean meal	3.56	3.15	1.89	1.26	1.86	81	54.0	3	.36	.75	0	89
Wheat	3.88	3.47	2.15	1.42	2.03	88	14.4	3	.05	.45	0	89
Wheatbran	3.08	2.67	1.53	0.96	1.59	70	18.0	11	.12	1.32	1	89

[d] To convert to an "as fed" basis, multiply the value by the factor $\frac{\text{Dry Matter}}{100}$.

DE, digestible energy; ME, metabolizable energy; NE_m, net energy maintenance; NE_g, net energy for body gain; NE_l, net energy for lactation.

(Adapted from *Nutrient Requirements of Dairy Cattle*, National Research Council, 1978.)

to 14%. Feed consultants and company representatives and Cooperative Extension personnel can assist in determining least-cost concentrate feeds to use in a local area. All dairymen should be encouraged to join some type of testing association as a means of evaluating their herd and its feeding and management program.

TABLE 6. POUNDS OF CONCENTRATES TO BE FED DAILY

Daily Milk Yield		Fat Percentage of the Milk			
		3.5%		5.0%	
		Excellent Roughage	Poor Roughage	Excellent Roughage	Poor Roughage
lb	kg	lb	lb	lb	lb
20	9	—	9.0	—	11.0
25	11.5	—	11.0	3.0	14.0
30	13.5	—	13.0	6.0	17.0
35	16	3.0	16.0	9.0	20.0
40	18	5.0	18.0	11.0	22.0
45	20.5	8.0	22.0	14.0	26.0
50	23	10.0	25.0	17.0	29.0
55	25.5	13.0	28.0	22.0	33.0
60	27.5	16.0	31.0	26.0	37.0
65	29.5	19.0	35.0	31.0	
70	32	24.0	38.0	35.0	
75	34	29.0			
80	36.5	33.0			
90	44				

Feed to maximum appetite

BEEF CATTLE NUTRITION

NUTRITIONAL REQUIREMENTS

Beef cattle production, whether on range, improved pasture or in the feedlot, is most economical when roughages are used effectively. Young growing grass or other pasture crops usually supply ample nutrients needed by beef cattle, and mature cattle can consume sufficient good quality mixed pasture for normal growth and maintenance. However, mature and weathered pasture or other crops harvested in such a fashion that excessive losses occur due to shattering, leaching or spoilage, may be so reduced in nutritive value (particularly protein, phosphorus and vitamin A) that they are suitable only as a maintenance ration for adult cattle. Such feeds must be supplemented if they are to be used for other than maintenance.

Furthermore, the major- and trace-mineral content of pasture and forage crops may be influenced by corresponding levels in the soil or by excess minerals reducing the availability of other minerals. Normally, supplemental minerals are supplied in a free-choice mineral mix. Certain nutrients are required by beef cattle in the daily ration. Others can be stored in the body in rather large amounts and a deficiency is improbable over short periods. When body stores are high (vitamin A, for example), dietary supplementation is not necessary until these stores become reduced.

The following dietary constituents are required for maintenance and successful growth, fattening and reproduction in beef cattle:

Water

Beef cattle must have an abundant supply of good water at least once daily. Range cows consume a minimum of 2.5 gal. of water in winter and up to 12 gal. per head in summer (1 gal. ~ 3.8 L). When salt is fed with a protein concentrate to control the protein intake, more water is needed to aid in excreting the excess salt. Breeding cows, yearlings, and 2-year-old steers need about 10 gal. of water daily and fattening calves will drink 6 to 8 gal. With fresh, succulent feeds, less water is required.

Energy

Beef cattle, with the exception of young calves, can meet their energy requirements for maintenance from roughage, provided they have the capacity to handle such feed and it is sufficiently palatable. A shortage of energy occurs on overstocked pastures, with inadequate feed allowance or during a drought. For performance above the maintenance level, additional energy from concentrates may be necessary, especially with fair or poor quality forages.

For maintenance, especially in cold weather, roughages of varying quality may have similar energy values. The heat released during the digestion and assimilation of feeds contributes to the maintenance of body temperature for wintering stock cattle where little productive energy is required. For fattening, reproduction and lactation, however, much productive energy is needed, thus the necessity of good-quality feeds.

The energy requirement for wintering mature pregnant beef cattle ranges from 130 to 180 Kcal digestible energy per 100 lb (45 kg) of body wt. For growing calves, lactating cows, or fattening cattle, the requirement is much greater.

Protein

Since protein quality is relatively unimportant, except in young animals, beef cattle can thrive on protein from a single feed source. Nevertheless, a certain amount of digestible protein in the daily ration is essential. Except for a deficiency of energy because of low feed intake, a protein deficiency is the most common factor limiting growth, milk production and reproductive performance. Protein deficiencies of long duration eventually depress appetite with consequent weight loss and unthriftiness even though ample energy is available.

Feeds vary greatly in protein digestibility. For example, the protein of common grains and most protein supplements is about 75 to 85% digestible, that of alfalfa hay about 70%, while that of grass hays usually varies from 35 to 50%. The protein of feeds such as weathered grass hay and cottonseed hulls is very poorly digested. Thus, total protein intake may be "adequate" but digestible protein insufficient to meet the animal's needs.

Lack of protein in the ration also affects adversely the microbial population in the rumen and this, in turn, reduces the digestibility of low-protein feeds. Much of the potential nutritive value of roughages (especially energy) may, therefore, be lost if protein levels are not adequate. There is very little storage of available protein in the body and thus it must be present in the daily ration for best results.

Digestible protein requirements vary with body weight, growth, fattening and reproduction. Growing beef calves require about as much digestible protein as mature, nonpregnant beef cows. Steers on a full feed of grain, making maximal gains, have a much higher requirement than cattle of the same age and weight that are making only moderate gains. The digestible protein requirement for maintenance of beef cattle is about 0.6 lb/1,000 lb (0.6 gm/kg) of body wt daily, and for rapid growth and fattening, it is nearly double this amount. Cows nursing calves need about twice as much digestible protein as dry cows.

Urea is commonly used in commercial protein supplements to supply one-third or more of the total nitrogen. It is well utilized at this level, provided the ration has ample phosphorus, trace minerals, sulfur and soluble carbohydrate (starches and sugars). The amount of crude protein (N × 6.25) supplied by nonprotein nitrogen must be stated on the feed tag. Toxicity is not a serious problem where urea is fed at the recommended levels and thoroughly mixed with the feed. The rapid ingestion of urea at levels above 20 gm/100 lb (45 kg) body wt may, however, lead to toxic effects. Several urea-molasses mixtures, which may contain nearly 10% urea, are now being self-fed beef cattle. Caution should be exercised when cattle are started on these supplements.

Minerals

Qualitatively, the mineral requirements of beef cattle are essentially the same as those of dairy cattle; quantitatively, however, they generally are much lower than for high-producing dairy cows. In practice, the minerals most likely to be deficient in beef cattle rations are sodium and chlorine (as salt), calcium and phosphorus. (*See* NUTRITIONAL DEFICIENCIES IN CATTLE AND SHEEP, p. 1393.) In the interior areas of the U.S.A., iodine may be deficient in rations for pregnant cows. Natural feeds usually contain adequate amounts of the other required mineral elements, i.e. potassium, magnesium, sulfur, iodine, iron, copper, cobalt, manganese, selenium and, probably, zinc. Under certain circumstances, however, feedstuffs may not provide adequate amounts of some essential minerals and it becomes necessary to supplement the diet. The actual method used is determined very largely by the type of husbandry. Under intensive systems of stocking, calcium, phosphorus, potassium and magnesium are best applied as fertilizer to the pasture, since, in addition to supplying the necessary minerals to the animal, this practice may well increase the total yield of forage. Copper and cobalt also may be added to the fertilizer mixture. Perhaps the most economical and widely used methods of supplementation in the U.S.A. are to add a calcium and phosphorus source to trace mineral salt, preferably in the loose form, or to purchase a commercial mineral supplement.

The salt (NaCl) requirements of beef cattle are not well established. Beef calves wintered on dry roughage and a small amount of protein supplement made slower and more expensive gains than others receiving salt. In contrast, fattening calves full-fed grain gained as rapidly and efficiently with no salt as others fed salt. Similar comparisons have not been made in the U.S.A. with grazing cattle, but, when salt is provided free-choice, cattle on pasture consume more salt than those in dry lot.

Range cattle usually consume 2.0 to 2.5 lb (1 kg) of salt per head per month when the feed is succulent and 1.0 to 1.5 lb per month with dryer feed. When salt is added to protein feeds to limit the protein intake, beef cows often obtain more than 1.0 lb a day over long periods without injury, if they have plenty of water.

In Australia and New Zealand, cattle grazing on good pasture are rarely fed salt and there is some question whether the amounts provided in the U.S.A. (where it is usually fed free choice) are really necessary.

Calcium is relatively high in most roughages, but low in cereal hays, corn silage, and sorghum grains and other concentrates. Legume hay is a richer source of calcium than grass hay or stray, but even nonlegume roughages will often supply sufficient for maintenance. When the roughage is produced on soil exceptionally low in calcium, or when cattle are full-fed grain with corn or sorghum silage or only a limited amount of nonlegume hay, a calcium deficiency may arise. Finishing rations are more likely to be deficient in calcium than growing rations. Since the beef cow produces less milk than the dairy cow and usually is consuming more roughage, a deficiency of calcium is unlikely. However, it is good husbandry to supply a free-choice mineral mix at all times. This may consist of two-thirds dicalcium phosphate and one-third iodized or trace mineral salt. In addition, iodized or trace-mineralized salt should be supplied free choice. A commercial mineral supplement can also be used in the total ration. A calcium:phosphorus ratio of about 2:1 in the total ration is thought to be most desirable, although it appears that wider ratios can be tolerated if the minimum requirement for each element is met and adequate vitamin D is available. Range cattle should be provided a mineral supplement that has more phosphorus than calcium.

Phosphorus is much more apt to be deficient in ordinary beef cattle rations, since it is often low in roughages. Many soils in the beef-producing areas of the world are low in available phosphorus. Further, when weathered native range grass is the only roughage, or when such feeds as cottonseed hulls, stover or cobs are fed, the phosphorus level may drop precariously low. When the phosphorus content of forages drops below 0.16%, maximum performance is not attained. For best digestibility of feeds, the mineral phosphorus level in the rations should be approximately 0.2%. Most protein feeds are relatively good sources of phosphorus; therefore, when such feeds are given in amounts necessary to supplement poor-quality roughage, adequate phosphorus intake is assured. However, a mineral mix offered free-choice is recommended. Steamed bone meal, dicalcium phosphate, defluorinated rock phosphate, monosodium phosphate, sodium tripolyphosphate and ammonium polyphosphate are good sources of phosphorus. Since most grains are good sources of phosphorus, fattening cattle usually obtain their requirement from the grain. A phosphorus intake of 2 to 3 gm/100 lb (44 to 66 mg/kg) body wt is considered ample for fattening cattle.

A deficiency of **cobalt** in beef cattle usually arises from a low level in the forage as a consequence of a soil deficiency. Such deficiencies are known in many parts of the world. With some of the other minerals, e.g. iodine, copper, and selenium, and possibly zinc, the explanation is not so clear. There may be a simple deficiency in the soil and, therefore, in the plant. Further, the level in the food may be reasonably high, but the animal is unable to utilize the particular element because of unusual amounts of other substances in the diet. Therefore, induced deficiencies develop, which fortunately can be overcome by suitable supplements. These conditions are described under NUTRITIONAL DEFICIENCIES IN CATTLE AND SHEEP, p. 1393.

VITAMINS

While cattle probably require all the known vitamins, a dietary source of vitamin B complex and vitamins C and K is not necessary, because, in all but the very young animal, the vitamin B complex and vitamin K are synthesized in the required amounts by the ruminal microflora, and vitamin C is synthesized in the tissues of all cattle. If, however, rumen function is impaired or the bacterial population is inhibited by starvation, shortage of protein, cobalt deficiency or excessive levels of antibiotics or medicaments, synthesis of these vitamins may not occur at a normal rate.

Vitamin A: Since most beef cattle are produced in range and semiarid regions and are fattened on large amounts of grain and limited quantities of roughage, a shortage of vitamin A is always a potential danger. Many stock cattle and pregnant cows are wintered on low-quality roughages low in carotene. With the exception of newly harvested yellow corn, grains and other concentrates are almost devoid of vitamin A precursors. Since cattle on green pastures have the ability to store large quantities of vitamin A and carotene in their bodies, the length of time elapsing before a deficiency becomes apparent varies considerably. Thus, depending on the amount of green feed obtained during the previous grazing season, weaner calves may have sufficient liver stores to last 80 to 140 days on low-carotene rations before showing evidence of deficiency, yearling cattle about 100 to 150 days and mature cattle about 6 to 8 months. Newborn calves have very small liver stores of vitamin A and, therefore, must depend on colostrum and milk to meet their needs. These sources may not be sufficient if the dam is fed a ration low in carotene during gestation and while nursing the calf. Therefore, severe deficiency signs may become apparent in the young suckling calf within 2 to 4 weeks of birth, while the dam appears normal.

It is sound practice to supply from 2 to 5 lb (1 to 2 kg) of early-cut good quality legume or grass hay, or 0.5 to 1.0 lb (.25 to .5 kg) of dehydrated alfalfa meal, in the daily ration of stocker cattle and pregnant cows as assurance against a vitamin A deficiency. Many commercial protein and mineral supplements may be economically fortified with dry, stabilized vitamin A. When certain trace minerals are added, vitamin A must be protected against destruction. Access to green pasture, even for short periods, is the ideal method of alleviating a deficiency. The daily requirement for beef cattle appears to be approximately 5 mg of carotene or 2,000 IU of vitamin A per 100 lb (45 kg) body wt. Lactating cows may require considerably more than this in order to maintain high vitamin A levels in the milk.

Vitamin A deficiency under feedlot conditions has caused considerable loss to cattle feeders, especially where high-concentrate and corn silage rations low in carotene have been fed. Destruction of carotene during hay storage or in the digestive tract, or the failure to convert carotene to vitamin A may all be involved in increasing the need for vitamin A supplementation of these cattle. Growing and finishing steers and heifers fed these rations for several months will require 1,000 IU of vitamin A per pound of air-dry ration. Commercial vitamin A supplements are not expensive and should be used when such rations are fed and any danger of a deficiency exists.

Vitamin D deficiency is comparatively rare in beef cattle, since they usually are outside in direct sunlight and fed sun-cured roughage and receive vitamin D in this manner. In northern latitudes, during long winters, or in purebred herds where show calves are kept in the barn or turned out only at night, a vitamin D deficiency is possible. Direct exposure to sunlight, feeding sun-cured roughage or supplementary vitamin D, 300 IU/100 lb (45 kg) of body wt, are considered adequate to protect against a deficiency.

The interrelationships of **vitamin E** and selenium in reproduction and in the etiology of various myopathies of calves are discussed under MYOPATHIES AND RELATED CONDITIONS IN DOMESTIC ANIMALS (p. 590).

FEEDING AND MANAGEMENT PRACTICES

Feeds for beef cattle vary widely in quality, palatability and essential nutrient content. The composition of some common feeds for beef cattle is shown in TABLE 5 (pp. 1280-1281). To be most effective, any supplement must be patterned to fit the kind and quality of roughage available. Under certain systems of management, beef cattle are wintered as economically as possible on low-quality roughages and thus may not receive the recommended nutrients for optimum performance. This may not be undesirable if no severe deficiency develops and the cattle can make up for poor winter gains on abundant summer pasture. However, where maximum performance is desired (cows nursing calves, rapid growth of calves, steers on full feed), an attempt should be made to meet or exceed the nutrient requirements as shown in TABLES 7 and 8.

Feeding and management practices for 3 systems of beef production are discussed separately.

THE BREEDING HERD

In most areas, a spring calving program is followed (February to May) depending on the available feed, growth of early spring pasture and prevailing climate. Fall calving is on the increase, particularly in the South, and wintering the lactating cow presents a much greater nutritional problem than wintering pregnant cows. Beef calves are commonly weaned at 6 to 8 months of age; their dams are bred again while on summer pasture. Heifers may be bred to drop their first calves as 2-year-olds (24 to 27 months of age) if good winter feeding is practiced to assure maximum development and prevent high death losses at parturition. Heifers should weigh at least 600 to 650 lb (275 to 300 kg) at breeding time and should be fed well thereafter to allow for continued growth, good milk production and early conception. It is a good practice to breed the heifers to calve 2 to 4 weeks ahead of the cow herd. They can receive more attention at calving and have a longer interval from calving to breeding, which will improve conception rate.

TABLE 7. NUTRIENT REQUIREMENTS OF GROWING AND FINISHING BEEF CATTLE.[1,2]
(NUTRIENT CONCENTRATION IN DIET DRY MATTER)

Weight kg	Daily gain kg	Min. dry matter consumption kg	Total protein %	Dig. protein %	NE_m Mcal/kg	NE_g Mcal/kg	ME Mcal/kg	TDN %	Ca %	P %
A. Steer calves and yearlings										
150	0.5	4.0	11.0	7.0	1.35	0.75	2.2	62	.35	.32
	0.7	3.9	12.6	8.5	1.60	1.00	2.5	70	.46	.36
	0.9	3.8	14.1	9.7	1.81	1.18	2.8	77	.61	.45
	1.1	3.7	15.6	11.1	2.07	1.37	3.1	86	.76	.54
250	0.7	5.8	10.7	6.7	1.56	0.95	2.5	70	.31	.28
	0.9	6.2	11.1	7.1	1.64	1.02	2.6	72	.35	.31
	1.1	6.0	12.1	8.0	1.81	1.18	2.8	77	.43	.35
	1.3	6.0	12.7	8.5	2.07	1.37	3.1	86	.50	.38
350	0.9	8.0	10.0	6.1	1.64	1.02	2.6	72	.25	.22
	1.1	8.0	10.4	6.5	1.81	1.18	2.8	80	.29	.25
	1.3	8.0	10.8	6.9	1.98	1.31	3.0	83	.32	.28
	1.4	8.2	10.9	7.0	2.07	1.37	3.1	86	.34	.29
450	1.0	10.3	9.3	5.5	1.64	1.02	2.6	72	.19	.19
	1.2	10.2	9.5	5.7	1.81	1.18	2.8	80	.23	.22
	1.3	9.3	10.4	6.3	2.07	1.31	3.1	86	.26	.25
	1.4	9.8	10.0	6.1	2.07	1.37	3.1	86	.26	.23

TABLE 7. NUTRIENT REQUIREMENTS OF GROWING AND FINISHING BEEF CATTLE.[1,2] (NUTRIENT CONCENTRATION IN DIET DRY MATTER) (continued)

Weight kg	Daily gain kg	Min. dry matter consumption kg	Total protein %	Dig. protein %	NE_m Mcal/kg	NE_g Mcal/kg	ME Mcal/kg	TDN %	Ca %	P %
B. Heifer calves and yearlings										
150	0.5	4.1	11.0	7.1	1.32	0.70	2.2	61	.34	.29
	0.7	4.0	12.4	8.2	1.56	0.95	2.5	69	.45	.35
	0.9	4.0	13.5	9.2	1.81	1.18	2.8	77	.57	.42
	1.1	4.0	15.0	10.5	2.07	1.37	3.1	86	.70	.50
250	0.5	6.5	9.5	5.7	1.24	0.60	2.1	58	.20	.20
	0.7	5.8	10.5	6.5	1.64	1.02	2.6	72	.29	.26
	0.9	5.9	11.1	7.1	1.81	1.18	2.8	77	.36	.29
	1.1	6.5	11.4	7.4	1.89	1.25	2.9	80	.38	.31
350	0.5	8.3	8.7	5.1	1.32	0.70	2.2	61	.18	.18
	0.7	7.9	9.2	5.4	1.56	0.95	2.5	69	.19	.19
	0.9	8.1	9.5	5.7	1.72	1.10	2.7	75	.21	.21
	1.1	8.3	9.9	6.0	1.89	1.25	2.9	80	.24	.23
450	0.2	8.7	8.5	4.7	1.17	0.50	2.0	55	.18	.18
	0.5	9.3	8.6	4.9	1.40	0.78	2.3	64	.18	.18
	0.8	9.1	9.0	5.3	1.72	1.10	2.7	75	.18	.18
	1.0	8.5	9.5	5.6	2.07	1.37	3.1	86	.22	.22

[1] Adapted from National Academy of Sciences, Publication 1137, *Nutrient Requirements of Beef Cattle,* 1976.
[2] The concentration of vitamin A in all diets for finishing steers and heifers is 2,200 IU/kg dry diet.
NE_m, net energy for maintenance; NE_g, net energy for body gain; ME, metabolizable energy.

TABLE 8. NUTRIENT REQUIREMENTS OF BEEF CATTLE BREEDING HERD.[1, 2]
(NUTRIENT CONCENTRATION IN DIET DRY MATTER)

Weight kg	Daily gain kg	Min. dry matter consumption kg	Total protein %	Dig. protein %	NE_m Mcal/kg	NE_g Mcal/kg	ME Mcal/kg	TDN %	Ca %	P %
A. Pregnant yearling heifers—Last third of pregnancy										
325	0.4	6.6	8.8	5.1	1.09	0.38	1.9	52	.23	.23
	0.8	9.4	9.0	5.3	1.24	0.60	2.1	58	.23	.21
375	0.4	7.2	8.7	5.0	1.09	0.38	1.9	52	.21	.21
	0.8	11.0	8.7	5.0	1.17	0.50	2.0	55	.20	.20
425	0.4	7.8	8.8	5.1	1.09	0.38	1.9	52	.20	.20
	0.8	12.1	8.7	5.0	1.17	0.50	2.0	55	.18	.18
B. Dry pregnant mature cows—Middle third of pregnancy										
350	—	5.5	5.9	2.8	1.09	—	1.9	52	.18	.18
450	—	6.7	5.9	2.8	1.09	—	1.9	52	.18	.18
550	—	7.7	5.9	2.8	1.09	—	1.9	52	.18	.18
650	—	8.8	5.9	2.8	1.09	—	1.9	52	.18	.18
C. Dry pregnant mature cows—Last third of pregnancy										
350	0.4	6.9	5.9	2.8	1.09	—	1.9	52	.18	.18
450	0.4	8.1	5.9	2.8	1.09	—	1.9	52	.18	.18
550	0.4	9.1	5.9	2.8	1.09	—	1.9	52	.18	.18
650	0.4	10.2	5.9	2.8	1.09	—	1.9	52	.18	.18
D. Cows nursing calves—Average milking ability[3]										
350	—	8.2	9.2	5.4	1.09	—	1.9	52	.29	.29
450	—	9.3	9.2	5.4	1.09	—	1.9	52	.28	.28
550	—	10.5	9.2	5.4	1.09	—	1.9	52	.27	.27
650	—	11.4	9.2	5.4	1.09	—	1.9	52	.25	.25

TABLE 8. NUTRIENT REQUIREMENTS OF BEEF CATTLE BREEDING HERD.[1, 2] (NUTRIENT CONCENTRATION IN DIET DRY MATTER) (continued)

Weight kg	Daily gain kg	Min. dry matter consumption kg	Total protein %	Dig. protein %	NE_m Mcal/kg	NE_g Mcal/kg	ME Mcal/kg	TDN %	Ca %	P %
E. Cows nursing calves—Superior milking ability[3]										
350	—	10.2	10.9	6.4	1.17	—	2.0	55	.44	.39
450	—	11.3	10.9	6.4	1.17	—	2.0	55	.40	.37
550	—	12.4	10.9	6.4	1.17	—	2.0	55	.37	.35
650	—	13.4	10.9	6.4	1.17	—	2.0	55	.35	.33
F. Bulls. growth and maintenance (moderate activity)										
300	1.0	8.8	10.2	6.3	1.40	0.78	2.3	64	.31	.26
500	0.7	12.1	8.8	5.1	1.32	0.70	2.2	61	.18	.18
700	0.3	12.9	8.5	4.8	1.17	0.50	2.0	55	.18	.18
900	—	11.4	8.5	4.8	1.17	—	2.0	55	.18	.18

[1] Adapted from National Academy of Sciences, Publication 1137, *Nutrient Requirements of Beef Cattle,* 1976.
[2] The concentration of vitamin A in all diets for pregnant heifers and cows is 2,800 IU/kg dry diet; for lactating cows and breeding bulls, 3,900 IU/kg.
[3] First 3 to 4 months postpartum.
NE_m, net energy for maintenance; NE_g, net energy for body gain; ME, metabolizable energy.

Older cows have greater body reserves and lower nutrient requirements than heifers; therefore, they can be wintered on poorer rations. They usually are fed all the hay, fodder, silage or dry grass they will consume. This roughage ration should provide a minimum of 5.9% total protein in the dry matter. If it does not, then 1.0 to 2.0 lb (.5 to 1 kg) of a 20 to 30% protein supplement or its equivalent should be fed daily. A mineral mix should be provided.

Mature beef cows may lose 150 lb (67 kg) or more of body weight from fall until after calving in the spring. This weight loss does not impair reproductive performance if spring and summer pastures are adequate. Under most profitable systems of management, a cow will maintain her weight from fall to fall. Lactation is a much more severe strain than gestation. Feeding beef cows more than is necessary for satisfactory production, such as frequently occurs in purebred herds, is unnecessary. Large accumulations of body fat may lead to low conception rates, difficult calving, a lower calf crop and a shorter life span.

Beef calves are castrated and dehorned before 3 months of age. At this time, they may be vaccinated for blackleg and malignant edema. Spaying heifers depresses gain and is seldom profitable. Often, a system of "creep-feeding" is practiced whereby suckling calves are allowed access to grain mixture in an enclosure or feeder. A typical creep-feed mixture contains 6 parts of corn, 3 parts of oats and 1 part of protein supplement. The mixture should preferably be ground as coarse as possible.

Most beef cows are pasture-bred, and in the better herds the bulls remain with the cows for a 2-month period. Bulls for pasture mating should be at least 15 months of age and well developed. Not more than 12 to 15 females should be mated to a yearling bull, while mature bulls can safely settle 30 to 35 cows. Where pastures are large, or the terrain is rough and mountainous, 1 bull per 15 to 20 cows may be necessary. Growing bull calves and yearlings should receive about 2 lb (1 kg) of protein supplement, 3 to 5 lb (1.5 to 2 kg) of grain and good-quality roughage. Mature bulls are commonly wintered in the same manner as the cow herd, with a greater feed allowance during the late winter. Highly fitted show bulls may have to be "let down" by gradual reduction in the ration and much exercise before they are suitable for pasture mating.

Stocker Cattle

It is common practice to winter calves or yearlings to make moderate gains, with faster and cheaper gains on summer pasture. Such cattle may be sold as feeders or fattened out in dry lot the following fall. The cost of winter gain on harvested feeds is invariably higher than summer gain on grass; hence, it is advisable to winter cattle so as to make the greatest possible gain on grass. In order to maintain good health, weanling calves should gain at least 1 lb (.5 kg) per day. Two pounds (1 kg) of grain plus 1 to 2 lb (.5 to 1 kg) of protein supplement are recommended, in addition to nonlegume roughage. If legume roughage is fed, no protein supplement will be needed. Other cattle, particularly if they enter the winter in fleshy condition, may do well to maintain their fall weight. A free-choice mineral mix and trace-mineralized salt should be supplied. Limited amounts of grain fed to older cattle on pasture during the late summer may increase their market value.

FATTENING CATTLE

This phase of beef production consists of full feeding grain and limited amounts of roughage until slaughter condition is attained. Older cattle may fatten on pasture alone, or with a few pounds of grain to improve market grade. Weanling calves are commonly shipped direct to the feed lot for a 120 to 150 day warm-up program followed by finishing rations for 100 to 150 days; yearlings require about 150 days and older steers from 100 to 125 days. Grain consumption of cattle on full feed is approximately 2.0 to 2.5 lb/100 lb (1 kg/45 kg) of body wt. Roughage consumption usually is limited to about one-fourth to one-third of the total grain intake after cattle are on full feed. Cattle self-fed mixed rations will consume about 3% of their body weight daily. For calves, about 1.5 to 2.0 lb (<1 kg) of 30 to 35% protein supplement are required daily for best gains and market grades where nonlegume roughage is fed.

The grain allowance for fattening cattle should be increased gradually. Feeding too much grain early in the period may lead to lactic acidosis, founder, severe scouring and cattle that go "off feed." About 4 to 6 weeks are required to get calves on a full feed of grain, while a shorter time is necessary for older cattle. Self-fed, mixed rations should contain at least 50% roughage as cattle are started on feed.

Corn or sorghum silage is a very palatable roughage for fattening cattle, and plain cattle of lower grade may be fattened principally on silage supplemented with protein. Alfalfa or grass silage is relatively high in protein, carotene and minerals, but is somewhat lacking in available energy. This is especially true when no grain or molasses is added as a preservative. Alfalfa hay is an excellent roughage, but may cause bloat in calves if fed as the only roughage. Grains for fattening cattle have about the same relative value as is indicated by their TDN content. Plant sources of protein are equal in value and can be replaced in part by feeding urea-containing commercial supplements. These supplements are also fortified with minerals, vitamins and feed additives. A small amount of molasses (1 lb [.5 kg] per head daily) may improve rations containing low-quality roughages, such as corn cobs, weathered hays or cottonseed hulls.

A number of nonfeed hormone or hormone-like supplements are ısed to increase gains in fattening cattle, either as feed supplements or as injectable implants. The use of these, e.g. diethylstilbestrol, eranol, progesterone-estradiol benzoate or testosterone propionate vith estradiol benzoate and certain antibiotics, commonly result in ppreciable improvement in rates of gain and feed efficiency, but he uncertainty of official regulations governing their use preclude he inclusion of specific recommendations here. Strict compliance vith the manufacturer's directions is the safest course.

The newest additive is monensin, which causes cattle to consume 10% less feed but gain at the same rate as cattle not fed monensin. mproved efficiency of feed conversion is brought about by increased production of propionic acid in the rumen.

The use of tranquilizers to reduce stress and weight loss during veaning or shipment has not proved consistently beneficial. Various means of processing rations, such as pelleting, flaking and high-noisture ensiling, have been shown to be beneficial, at least in ome situations.

Conditioning Feeder Cattle After Shipment

Research results from university experiment stations have confirmed the value of therapeutic oral dosages of a combination of hlortetracycline (CTC) and sulfamethazine (SMZ) for feeder cattle rom 14 to 21 days immediately following shipment. Both drugs, vhen fed in combination at a daily dose of 350 mg each for this eriod, will lower significantly the incidence of the shipping fever yndrome and also will result in more rapid regain of shrinkage uffered during shipping. Size of the animal as related to levels of CTC and SMZ is not critical. Some animals may not respond to this reatment and should be isolated for individual attention. The nutriional program which is recommended for such cattle is a full feed of nedium-quality roughage plus 1 to 2 lb (<1 kg) per head daily of a 2% protein supplement which derives at least two-thirds of its rotein from natural sources. The prescribed daily dose of CTC and MZ for one animal may thus be incorporated into each 1 to 2 lb (.5 1 kg) of the protein supplement.

SHEEP NUTRITION

The economical and efficient production of lamb and wool is ontingent on maximum production per ewe. Economical maintenance of breeding animals, a high percentage of the lamb crop veaned, continuous and rapid growth of lambs, heavy weaning eights and a heavy fleece weight are important to efficiency; all re based largely on adequate nutrition.

TABLE 9. DAILY NUTRIENT REQUIREMENTS OF SHEEP (100% DRY-MATTER BASIS)

Body Wt		Wt Gain or Loss		Dry Matter[1]			Nutrients per Animal										
				Per Animal		Percent	Energy: TDN	Energy: DE[2]	Energy: ME	Total Protein	DP[3]	gm DP per Mcal	Ca	P	Carotene	Vit A	Vit D
(kg)	(lb)	(gm)	(lb)	(kg)	(lb)	Live Wt	(kg)	(Mcal)	(Mcal)	(gm)	(gm)	DE	(gm)	(gm)	(mg)	(IU)	(IU)
EWES[4]—Maintenance																	
50	110	10	0.02	1.0	2.2	2.0	0.55	2.42	1.98	89	48	20	3.0	2.8	1.9	1275	278
60	132	10	0.02	1.1	2.4	1.8	0.61	2.68	2.20	98	53	20	3.1	2.9	2.2	1530	333
70	154	10	0.02	1.2	2.6	1.7	0.66	2.90	2.38	107	58	20	3.2	3.0	2.6	1785	388
80	170	10	0.02	1.3	2.9	1.6	0.72	3.17	2.60	116	63	20	3.3	3.1	3.0	2040	444
Nonlactating: first 15 weeks gestation																	
50	110	30	0.07	1.1	2.4	2.2	0.60	2.64	2.16	99	54	20	3.0	2.8	1.9	1275	278
60	132	30	0.07	1.3	2.9	2.1	0.72	3.17	2.60	117	64	20	3.1	2.9	2.2	1530	333
70	154	30	0.07	1.4	3.1	2.0	0.77	3.39	2.78	126	69	20	3.2	3.0	2.6	1785	388
80	176	30	0.07	1.5	3.3	1.9	0.82	3.61	2.96	135	74	20	3.3	3.1	3.0	2040	444
Last 6 weeks gestation or last 8 weeks lactation suckling singles[5]																	
50	110	175 (+45)	0.39	1.7	3.7	3.3	0.99	4.36	3.58	158	88	20	4.1	3.9	6.2	4250	278
60	132	180 (+45)	0.40	1.9	4.2	3.2	1.10	4.84	3.97	177	99	20	4.4	4.1	7.5	5100	333
70	154	185 (+45)	0.41	2.1	4.6	3.0	1.22	5.37	4.40	195	109	20	4.5	4.3	8.8	5950	383
80	176	190 (+45)	0.42	2.2	4.8	2.8	1.28	5.63	4.62	205	114	20	4.8	4.5	10.0	6800	444

***First 8 weeks lactation suckling singles or last 8 weeks lactation suckling twins*[6]**																
50	110	−25 (+80)	−0.06	2.1	4.6	4.2	1.36	5.98	4.90	218	130	22	10.9	7.8	6.2	4250	278
60	132	−25 (+80)	−0.06	2.3	5.1	3.9	1.50	6.60	5.41	239	143	22	11.5	8.2	7.5	5100	333
70	154	−25 (+80)	−0.06	2.5	5.5	3.6	1.63	7.17	5.88	260	155	22	12.0	8.6	8.8	5950	388
80	176	−25 (+80)	−0.06	2.6	5.7	3.2	1.69	7.44	6.10	270	161	22	12.6	9.0	10.0	6800	444
First 8 weeks lactation suckling twins																	
50	110	−60	−0.13	2.4	5.3	4.8	1.56	6.86	5.63	276	173	25	12.5	8.9	6.2	4250	278
60	132	−60	−0.13	2.6	5.7	4.3	1.69	7.44	6.10	299	187	25	13.0	9.4	7.5	5100	333
70	154	−60	−0.13	2.8	6.2	4.0	1.82	8.01	6.57	322	202	25	13.4	9.5	8.8	5950	388
80	176	−60	−0.13	3.0	6.6	3.7	1.95	8.58	7.04	345	216	25	14.4	10.2	10.0	6800	444
***Replacement lambs and yearlings*[7]**																	
30	66	180	0.40	1.3	2.9	4.3	0.81	3.56	2.92	130	75	21	5.9	3.3	1.9	1275	166
40	88	120	0.26	1.4	3.1	3.5	0.82	3.61	2.96	133	74	20	6.1	3.4	2.5	1700	222
50	110	80	0.18	1.5	3.3	3.0	0.83	3.65	2.99	133	73	20	6.3	3.5	3.1	2125	278
60	132	40	0.09	1.5	3.3	2.5	0.82	3.61	2.96	133	72	20	6.5	3.6	3.8	2550	333
***RAMS—Replacement lambs and yearlings*[7]**																	
40	88	250	0.55	1.8	4.0	4.5	1.17	5.15	4.22	184	108	21	6.3	3.5	2.5	1700	222
60	132	200	0.44	2.3	5.1	3.8	1.38	6.07	4.98	219	122	20	7.2	4.0	3.8	2550	333
80	176	150	0.33	2.8	6.2	3.5	1.54	6.78	5.56	249	134	20	7.9	4.4	5.0	3400	444
100	220	100	0.22	2.8	6.2	2.8	1.54	6.78	5.56	249	134	20	8.3	4.6	6.2	4250	555
120	265	50	0.11	2.6	5.7	2.2	1.43	6.29	5.16	231	125	20	8.5	4.7	7.5	5100	666
***LAMBS—Finishing*[8]**																	
30	66	200	0.44	1.3	2.9	4.3	0.83	3.65	2.99	143	87	24	4.8	3.0	1.1	765	166
35	77	220	0.48	1.4	3.1	4.0	0.94	4.14	3.39	154	94	23	4.8	3.0	1.3	892	194
40	88	250	0.55	1.6	3.5	4.0	1.12	4.92	4.04	176	107	22	5.0	3.1	1.5	1020	222
45	99	250	0.55	1.7	3.7	3.8	1.19	5.24	4.30	187	114	22	5.0	3.1	1.7	1148	250
50	110	220	0.48	1.8	4.0	3.6	1.26	5.54	4.54	198	121	22	5.0	3.1	1.9	1275	278
55	121	200	0.44	1.9	4.2	3.5	1.33	5.85	4.80	209	127	22	5.0	3.1	2.1	1402	305

(continued on next page)

TABLE 9. DAILY NUTRIENT REQUIREMENTS OF SHEEP (100% DRY-MATTER BASIS) (continued)

Body Wt		Wt Gain or Loss		Dry Matter[1]			Nutrients per Animal										
				Per Animal		Percent	Energy			Total Protein	DP[3]	gm DP per Mcal	Ca	P	Carotene	Vit A	Vit D
							TDN	DE[2]	ME								
(kg)	(lb)	(gm)	(lb)	(kg)	(lb)	Live Wt	(kg)	(Mcal)	(Mcal)	(gm)	(gm)	DE	(gm)	(gm)	(mg)	(IU)	(IU)
Early—Weaned[9]																	
10	22	250	0.55	0.6	1.3	6.0	0.44	1.92	1.58	96	69	36	2.4	1.6	1.6	850	67
20	44	275	0.60	1.0	2.2	5.0	0.74	3.21	2.63	160	115	36	3.6	2.4	2.4	1700	133
30	66	300	0.66	1.4	3.1	4.7	1.02	4.49	3.68	196	133	30	5.0	3.3	3.3	2550	200

[1] To convert dry matter to an as-fed feed basis, divide dry matter by percentage dry matter.

[2] 1 kg TDN = 4.4 Mcal DE (digestible energy). DE may be converted to ME (metabolizable energy) by multiplying by 82%.

[3] DP = digestible protein.

[4] Values are for ewes in moderate condition, not excessively fat or thin. Few fat ewes feed at next lower weight; for thin ewes feed at next highest weight. Once maintenance weight is established, such weight would follow through all production phases.

[5] Values in parentheses for ewes suckling singles last 8 weeks of lactation.

[6] Values in parentheses for ewes suckling twins last 8 weeks of lactation.

[7] Replacement lambs (ewe & ram) requirements start at time they are weaned.

[8] Maximum gains expected—if lambs are held for later market, they should be fed similar to replacement ewe lambs. Lambs capable of gaining faster than indicated need to be fed at higher level; self-feeding permits lambs to finish most rapidly.

[9] 40-kg early weaned lamb fed same as finishing lamb of equal weight.

(From *Nutrient Requirements of Sheep*, National Research Council, 1975.)

Definition of the nutritional requirements for maintenance, reproduction, growth, finishing and wool production of sheep is complicated because sheep are maintained under a wide variety of environmental conditions. Not only do farm and feedlot conditions differ markedly from those in range areas, but there is also considerable variation from farm to farm and from ranch to ranch.

NUTRITIONAL REQUIREMENTS

An adequate diet for sheep should include water and feeds containing energy (carbohydrates and fats), proteins, minerals and vitamins. TABLE 9 lists the daily nutrient requirements suggested by the National Research Council, 1975. These amounts generally are sufficient to promote optimum growth and production. There may be occasions, under field conditions of particular stress, when additional nutrients should be provided.

WATER

The usual recommendations are approximately 1 gal. (3.8 L) of water per day for ewes on dry feed in winter, 1½ gal. per day for ewes nursing lambs and approximately ½ gal. per day for fattening lambs.

In many range areas, water is the limiting nutrient and even when present may be unpotable because of dirt, filth or high-mineral content. For best production, range sheep should be watered once a day during warm weather. However, the cost of supplying water sometimes makes it advisable to water range sheep every other day. When soft snow is available, range sheep do not need additional water. If the snow is crusted with ice, the crust should be broken to allow access to the supply. When dry feeds such as alfalfa hay and pellets are fed, sheep may not obtain sufficient water from snow.

ENERGY

Because so much of the diet depends on grass and forage that is either sparse or of poor quality, the provision of adequate energy is important. Poor forage, even in abundance, may not provide sufficient available energy for maintenance production. The energy requirement of the ewe is greatest during the first 8 to 10 weeks of lactation. Since milk production declines after this period and the lambs are foraging themselves, the requirement of the ewe is reduced to a level equivalent to that of ewes one month before lambing. This is of considerable economic importance.

PROTEIN

Good quality forage and pasture generally will provide adequate protein for mature sheep. It should be emphasized, however, that sheep do not digest the protein of poor-quality, mature and weathered forage as efficiently as cattle and that there are instances when a protein supplement should be fed with mature grass, hay and winter range.

Sheep can convert nonprotein nitrogen, such as urea, ammonium phosphate, and biuret, into protein in the rumen. This source of nitrogen can provide most of the necessary supplemental nitrogen in high-energy diets, containing a nitrogen:sulfur ratio of 10:1. In lamb-finishing diets, the inclusion of alfalfa and implanting with hormones enhances nitrogen utilization.

MINERALS

Sheep require the major minerals: sodium, chlorine, calcium, phosphorus, magnesium, sulfur, and potassium; and the trace minerals: cobalt, copper, iodine, iron, manganese, molybdenum, zinc and selenium. Trace mineralized salt, commonly fed to sheep, contains 8 of these necessary minerals and provides an economical method of preventing deficiencies; these are: sodium, chlorine, iodine, manganese, cobalt, copper, iron and zinc. As of 1978 selenium has been approved by the FDA of the U.S.A. and presumably it will be allowable to add selenium to salt. Since sheep diets usually contain sufficient potassium, iron, magnesium, sulfur and manganese, no discussion of these minerals will be presented.

Salt: Except on certain alkali areas of the western range and along the seacoast where forage and soil are high in salt, sheep are provided with salt (sodium chloride). Sheepmen in the U.S.A. and Canada believe that sheep need salt to remain thrifty and make economical gains. However, salt supplements are rarely fed to sheep on good pasture in New Zealand and Australia. Mature sheep will consume 0.02 lb (10 gm) of salt daily and lambs one-half this amount. Range operators commonly provide from 0.5 to 0.75 lb (225 to 350 gm) of salt per ewe per month.

Calcium and Phosphorus: In plants, generally, the leafy parts are relatively high in calcium and low in phosphorus, whereas the reverse is true of the seeds. Legumes, in general have a higher calcium content than grasses. As grasses mature, phosphorus is transferred to the seed (grain). Furthermore, the phosphorus content of the plant is markedly influenced by the available phosphorus in the soil. Low-quality pasture devoid of legumes, and range plants tend, therefore, to be naturally low in phosphorus, a situation that is accentuated as the forage matures and the seeds fall, and by a deficiency of phosphorus in the soil, which is characteristic of much range country. Consequently sheep subsisting on mature, brown, summer forage and winter range sometimes develop a phosphorus deficiency (q.v., p. 1396). Sheep kept on such forages or fed low-quality hay with no grain should be provided with a phosphorus supplement.

Since most forages have a relatively high-calcium content, particularly if there is an admixture of legumes, natural feeds usually supply adequate amounts of this element. However, when corn silage or other feeds from the cereal grains are fed exclusively, each sheep should be fed ground limestone daily at the rate of 0.02 to 0.03 lb (10 to 15 gm).

Sheep seem to be able to tolerate wide ratios as long as they contain more calcium than phosphorus. On the other hand, an excess of phosphorus may be conducive to development of urinary calculi or osteodystrophy; a Ca:P ratio of 1.5:1 is appropriate for feedlot lambs. For pregnant ewes, the diet should contain not less than 0.18% of phosphorus and, for lactating ewes, not less than 0.27%. A content of 0.20 to 0.40% of calcium is considered adequate.

Iodine: Sometimes, either as a consequence of a low-available-iodine content of the soil or the presence in the food of goitrogenic substances, which interfere with the utilization of iodine by the thyroid, the iodine requirements of sheep are not met in the natural diet and iodine supplements must be fed. Regions naturally deficient in iodine are known throughout the Western U.S.A., in the Great Lakes area and in many other parts of the world. A deficiency of iodine (q.v., p. 203) can be prevented by feeding stabilized iodized salt to the pregnant ewe.

Cobalt: Sheep require about 0.1 ppm of cobalt in their total diet. Normally, legumes have a higher content than grasses. Since cobalt levels of the feedstuffs are seldom known, a good practice is to feed trace mineralized salt containing cobalt.

Copper: Pregnant ewes require approximately 5 mg of copper daily and this amount is provided, under normal conditions, when the forage contains not less than 5 ppm. However, the amount of copper in the diet necessary to prevent a copper deficiency (q.v., p. 1398) in the animal is influenced by the intake of other dietary constituents, notably molybdenum and inorganic sulfate. High intakes of molybdenum in the presence of adequate sulfate increases the requirement for copper. Since sheep are more susceptible than cattle to the toxic effects of copper, care must be taken to avoid copper toxicosis. Toxicity may be produced in lambs by continued feeding of diets with 20 to 30 ppm of copper. This is particularly true where the molybdenum and sulfate contents in the soil and feed are low.

Selenium: Selenium has been shown to be an essential mineral for sheep, and it is effective in at least partial control of nutritional muscular dystrophy (q.v., p. 594). Areas east of the Mississippi River and in the Northwestern U.S.A. appear to be low in selenium. It can be provided by IM injections or oral feeding. The dietary requirement is approximately 0.1 ppm. Levels above 7 to 10 ppm may be toxic.

Zinc: The requirement of growing lambs for zinc is approximately 30 ppm. The requirement for normal testicular development is somewhat higher. Since many feeds do not contain this much zinc the possibility of a deficiency is real. Furthermore, a high-calcium intake will increase the need for zinc.

VITAMINS

Sheep diets usually contain an ample supply of vitamins A, D and E. Under certain circumstances, however, supplements may have to be provided. The B-complex vitamins and vitamin K are synthesized by the rumen microorganisms and, under practical conditions, supplements are unnecessary. However, polioencephalomalacia (q.v., p. 666) sometimes occurs in sheep. This condition is apparently due to destruction of thiamin in the rumen, and animals respond to supplements. Vitamin C is synthesized in the tissues of sheep.

On diets rich in carotene, such as high-quality pasture or green hays, sheep have the ability to store large quantities of vitamin A in the liver, sufficient often to meet their requirements for 6 to 12 months. Daily supplies are unnecessary and deficiencies are rarely a problem. (*See* NUTRITIONAL DEFICIENCIES IN CATTLE AND SHEEP: **Vitamin A,** p. 1401.)

Vitamin D supplies are derived from sun-cured forage or by exposure of the skin to ultraviolet light. When the exposure of the skin to sunshine is reduced by prolonged cloudy weather or confinement rearing and when the vitamin D content of the diet is low, the amount supplied may be inadequate for the animal's needs. The requirement for vitamin D is increased when the amounts of either calcium or phosphorus in the diet are low or when the ratio between them is wide. Fast-growing young lambs kept in sheds away from intense sunlight or maintained on green feeds (high carotene) during the winter months (low irradiation) may suffer impaired bone formation and show other signs of vitamin D deficiency (q.v., p. 1402). Normally, sheep on pasture seldom need vitamin D supplementation because of exposure to the sun.

The major sources of **vitamin E** in the natural diet of sheep are green feeds and the germ of seeds. A deficiency of this vitamin, therefore, is uncommon in mature sheep. Vitamin E deficiency in young lambs may contribute to nutritional muscular dystrophy if selenium intake is low. (*See also* pp. 590 et seq.)

FEEDING FARM SHEEP

The nutrient requirements as outlined in TABLE 9, with the tables on feed composition (p. 1438 et seq.), can be used to calculate adequate rations for sheep. Using these data and the results of practical experience, suggestions for the feeding of sheep are outlined below.

Specialized Sheep Production: There has been much information compiled in recent years concerning larger sheep units under a confined system of management. Such innovations as early weaning or artificial rearing of lambs, slotted floors, accelerated lambing, synchronization of breeding and production testing are being used.

It is questionable if the extensive use of pasture for lambs in the Midwest and Eastern U.S.A. will expand.

Use of Forage: Good hay is a highly productive feed; poor hay, no matter how much is available, is suitable only for maintenance unless improved by some processing method. Hay quality is determined primarily by: (1) its botanic composition, e.g. a mixture of palatable grasses and legumes—brome, alfalfa or bluegrass and clover, (2) the stage of maturity when cut, e.g. the grass before heading and alfalfa before one-tenth bloom, (3) method and speed of harvesting as it affects loss of leaf, bleaching by sun and leaching by rain and (4) spoilage and loss during storage and feeding. In general, the same factors influence the quality of silage. Sheep make excellent use of high-quality roughage stored either as hay or low-moisture, grass-legume silage, or occasionally chopped green feed.

FEEDING EWES

The period from weaning to breeding of the ewe is critical if a high rate of twinning is desired. Ewes should not be allowed to become excessively fat but they should make a very slight daily gain from weaning to breeding. The rate of gain depends on the desired weight gain. If pasture production is inadequate, ewes may be confined and fed high-quality hay and, if necessary, a small amount of grain to make this desired weight increase. There is evidence that breeding on legume pastures, particularly red clover, tends to depress the size of the lamb crop. Mixed pasture 2 weeks before and during breeding is, therefore, preferred.

After mating, ewes can be maintained on pasture, thus allowing feed to be conserved, if necessary, for other times of the year. Good pasture for this period will put the ewes into the winter feeding period in good condition. One of the rations outlined in TABLE 10 may be used when pasture is unavailable.

During the last 6 to 8 weeks of pregnancy, intra-uterine growth of the lamb is rapid and, from a nutritional viewpoint, this is a critical period particularly for ewes carrying more than one fetus. Com-

TABLE 10. RATIONS FOR PREGNANT EWES UP TO 6 WEEKS BEFORE LAMBING

Feed	Ration No.			
	1	2	3	4
	lb	lb	lb	lb
Legume hay, such as alfalfa, clover, or lespedeza	3.0-4.5	1.5-2.0	—	—
Corn or sorghum silage	—	4.0-5.0	—	6.0-8.0
Legume grass, low-moisture (50%) silage	—	—	6.0-8.0	—
Cottonseed, soybean, linseed, or peanut meal 90%; limestone 10%	—	—	—	0.25

mencing 6 to 8 weeks before lambing, therefore, the plane of nutrition should be increased gradually and continued without interruption by the addition of supplements such as those described in TABLE 11. The amount offered will depend on the condition of the ewes. If ewes are in fair to good condition, 0.5 to 0.75 lb (225 to 350 gm) daily are usually sufficient. The roughage of the ration should provide all the protein required by ewes for most efficient feeding of the farm flock. If necessary, the ewes may be classified according to age and condition and divided into groups for differential treatment.

TABLE 11. GRAIN MIXTURE FOR PREGNANT EWES

Feed	Mixture No.			
	1	2	3	4
	%	%	%	%
Whole barley, corn or wheat	60	75	75	50
Whole oats	30	—	25	50
Beet pulp, dried	—	25	—	—
Wheat bran	10	—	—	—

Lactating Ewes: Succulent pasture furnishes adequate energy, protein, vitamins and minerals for ewes and lambs; no added grain is necessary. When pasture is not available or not used under confinement rearing, ewes should be fed one of the rations outlined for pregnant ewes in TABLE 10, and 1 to 15 lb (450 to 650 gm) of one of the grain mixtures in TABLE 11. Ewes should have access to trace-mineralized salt and dicalcium phosphate as previously discussed. Ewes with twin lambs should be separated from those with single lambs and fed more grain. Ewes nursing twin lambs produce 20 to 40% more milk than those with singles. Under confinement rearing or accelerated lambing, it is a common practice to wean lambs at 2 months of age. The ewe's milk production declines rapidly after this period and since the lambs are consuming feed from a creep it results in more efficient use of feed.

FEEDING LAMBS

At about 2 weeks of age, the lambs should have free access to a creep except if they are born on succulent pasture. If pasture is to be used later they should be creep-fed for 1 to 2 months until it is available. If it will not be available until the lambs are 3 or 4 months of age, they should be finished in dry lot. The grain should be ground coarse or rolled at first, but may be fed whole later. At first, small amounts are fed and the feed is kept clean and fresh. The amount is gradually raised until the lambs are on full feed.

Feeding lambs from birth to market in dry lot together with early weaning at 2 to 3 months of age is becoming increasingly popular throughout the U.S.A. A complete diet of hay, grain and supplement is ground, mixed, and either fed in this form or made into a 3/16- or 3/8-in. (5 or 10 mm) pellet. These lambs usually reach market weight in 3½ to 4 months. Some examples of creep ration used in dry-lot feeding are shown in TABLE 12.

TABLE 12. CREEP RATION FOR YOUNG SUCKLING AND EARLY-WEANED LAMBS

Feed	Mixture No.			
	1	2	3	4
	%	%	%	%
Alfalfa hay, leafy ground	25	30	40	—
Dehydrated alfalfa leaf meal	54.5	—	20	48
Corn, shelled	—	—	—	35
Corn or wheat	—	55	—	—
Oats or barley	—	—	20	—
Soybean, linseed or cottonseed meal	19	10	10	10
Molasses	—	3.5	8.5	5.5
Bone meal or dicalcium phosphate	1	1	1	1
Limestone	1	—	—	—
Trace mineralized salt	0.5	0.5	0.5	0.5
Antibiotic	—	—	0.002	0.002

Rearing Lambs on Milk Replacer: In today's intensified type of sheep production, lambs such as orphans, extras or those from poor-milking ewes should be raised on milk replacers. They should first receive colostrum, if not from a ewe then from a frozen supply from cows. Milk replacers designed specifically for lambs are available. They contain approximately 30% fat and 25% protein and a high level of antibiotic. It is advisable to inject lambs with vitamins A, D and E and a combination of penicillin and streptomycin.

Multiple nipple pails or containers are used and the milk should be offered cold after the first week. Cold milk replacer can be used by older lambs, which will nurse more often, and the milk will not sour as quickly. The lambs should be given water to drink in addition to the milk when a creep ration is offered to them at 9 to 10 days of age. They can be weaned from the milk abruptly at 4 to 5 weeks of age if consumption of creep feed is at a reasonable level.

FINISHING FEEDER LAMBS

Preconditioning before the lambs leave the producer's property should be encouraged. This would include starting on feed, vaccination, worming and, under some conditions, shearing. If this is not done, then the lambs should be rested for several days and fed dry, average-quality hay. Following this rest, the above-mentioned practices should be performed. Vaccination should be against enterotoxemia and possibly contagious ecthyma.

Feeding Method: There is no best method or diet for finishing lambs. They may be finished on alfalfa or wheat pasture with no grain. They may be started on pasture or crop aftermath and fed grain later. When fed in dry lot they are usually self-fed. These diets may be either completely pelleted, ground and mixed, a mixture of alfalfa pellets and grain or a high-concentrate type. Self-feeding means more efficient use of labor and this provides the opportunity to increase the size of operation. Self-feeding usually results in maximum feed intake and gain. Hand-feeding can be mechanized with an auger system or self-unloading wagon. It involves feeding at regular intervals so that the lambs clean up the feed before they are fed again. Feed consumption and gain can be controlled. Corn silage should be hand-fed.

Starting on Feed: Feeders who feed lambs the year-round or feed heavy lambs usually prefer to place the lambs on full feed as rapidly as possible. This means full feeding within 10 to 14 days. Lambs can safely be started on self-fed, ground or pelleted diets containing 60 to 70% hay. Within 2 weeks the hay may be reduced to 30 to 40% when the ration is not pelleted. Other roughages such as cottonseed hulls or silage can be used in a similar manner. Lambs can be started and finished on pelleted rations that contain less grain than needed for nonpelleted rations. Digestive disturbances are usually reduced also. Feed cost may be higher depending on processing charges.

Two practices are helpful in starting lambs on feed more rapidly and in feeding diets that may be entirely of a concentrate nature: these are vaccination against enterotoxemia and feeding tetracyclines at a level to supply 25 to 30 mg per lamb daily.

Feeds: Corn, sorghum or alfalfa silage can replace about half the hay with hand-feeding but finish and yield will be decreased to some extent. Rations which could be used in self-feeding are given in TABLE 13. Corn barley, milo or wheat, or a mixture of these grains are also satisfactory. If these grains are used, 0.5% salt and 0.5% bone meal or equivalent should be added to the grain. Pelleting of rations for fattening lambs is beneficial when low-grade roughages or high-roughage rations are used. Caution should be used when feeding large amounts of wheat; lambs not adapted to it are more apt to develop acute indigestion than if on grains such as corn, sorghum or barley.

Mineral supplements including salt should be offered separately whether or not they are included in the grain mixture. The hormone implants usually increase growth rate 10 to 15% and feed efficiency 8 to 10% but tend to decrease carcass quality.

TABLE 13. RECOMMENDED FORMULAS FOR FINISHING LAMBS*
(lb/ton or kg/metric ton)

	Starter 10-day period		High Roughage		High Concentrate	Corn Silage
	Loose	Pelleted	Loose	Pelleted		
Grain-corn, barley or milo**	500	200	780	400	1500	540
Alfalfa hay	1280	1700	1000	1400	200	
Molasses	100	100	100			
Oil-seed meal	100		100			100
Urea					45	
Beet pulp				200	200	
Silage						1350
Limestone	10				35	10
Trace mineralized salt	10		20	20	35	
Antibiotic	50 gm	20 gm	20 gm	10 gm	20 gm	10 gm
Vitamin A (IU/ton)						1,000,000

* Feeder lambs should have about 14% crude protein in rations (dry basis).
** Wheat can be substituted for other gains, but allow a period of time for adaptation.

FEEDING MATURE BREEDING RAMS

Mature breeding rams should be grazed on pasture when available, or fed rations 1, 2 or 3 outlined in TABLE 10. If rams are in a thrifty condition at breeding time and the ewes are on a good flushing pasture, it should not be necessary to grain-feed the ram while with the ewes. In warm climates rams should be shorn prior to mating and turned with the ewes at night only, if the daytime temperature is above 90°F (32°C).

FEEDING RANGE SHEEP

The condition of the sheep, the amount and kind of forage on the range and the climatic conditions will determine the kind and amount of supplement to feed. Supplements usually consist of high-protein pellets or cottonseed meal and salt, medium-protein pellets, low-protein pellets or corn, alfalfa hay and minerals.

When the diets of sheep on the western winter range are properly supplemented, the lamb crop can be increased 10 to 15% and wool production increased 400 to 500 grams per ewe. Each operator will need to determine if this increased production will more than cover cost of supplementation. One recommended practice is to feed about ¼ lb (100 gm) of high-protein (36%) supplement or 0.33 to 0.5 lb (150 to 225 gm) of medium-protein (24%) pellets about 3 weeks before the breeding season, during the breeding season, during extremely cold weather and for about 30 days before green feed starts in the spring (TABLE 12). In addition, small lambs, small yearling ewes, old ewes with poor teeth and thin ewes should be separated from the large band and fed one of the above supplements from about December 1 until shearing time. In many instances, the old ewes, lambs and yearlings from more than one band can be herded together in a special flock.

When sheep are unable to obtain a full ration of forage because of deep snow, 1 to 3 lb (500 to 1,500 gm) of alfalfa hay and 0.2 to 0.3 lb (90 to 150 gm) of a low-protein pellet mixture (TABLE 14) or corn should be fed. If alfalfa hay is not available 0.5 to 1 lb (225 to 450 gm) per head of a low-protein pellet mixture should be fed daily for emergency feeding periods.

Deficiencies of Range Forages: Deficiencies most apt to occur among range forages are protein, energy and phosphorus. These are most prevalent as the forages approach maturity or are dormant and they may appear singly or in combination. Range sheep often travel long distances and are exposed to cold weather. This results in a higher energy requirement. Protein supplements such as soybean or cottonseed meal increase digestibility and utilization of forage as well as providing needed protein and phosphorus. Most ranges used for winter grazing are considered adequate in carotene be-

TABLE 14. PATTERN FOR RANGE SUPPLEMENTS FOR SHEEP

Main Groups	Sub-groups	Feedstuff	Proportions of Individual Feeds			
			Suggested Maximum	Recommended Amount of Protein		
				high	medium	low
			%	%	%	%
Energy feeds	Grains	Barley	75		33.0	57.5
		Corn	60	5.0	10.0	15.0
		Wheat	60			
		Milo	60			
		Oats	15			
		Screenings No. 1	10			
	Mill feeds	Wheat mixed feed	10			
		Shorts	10			
		Molasses	15	5.0	5.0	10.0
		Beet pulp	10			10.0
Protein supplements	30–40% Protein feeds	Cottonseed meal	75	62.5	32.5	5.0
		Linseed meal	25			
		Soybean meal	75	10.0	10.0	
		Peanut meal	25			
	20–30% Protein feeds	Corn gluten feed	15			
		Corn distillers' dried grains	10			
		Wheat distillers' grains	10			
		Brewers' dried grains	5			
		Safflower meal	25			
		Cull beans	15			
Mineral supplements		Bone meal or defluorinated phosphate		4.0	3.0	2.0
		Dicalcium phosphate				
		Disodium phosphate				
		Monocalcium phosphate				
		Monosodium phosphate				
		Salt or trace mineralized salt		0.5	0.5	0.5
Vitamin supplements		Dehydrated alfalfa meal	20	12.5	6.0	
		Sun-cured alfalfa meal	20			
		Vitamin A and carotene concentrates				
Total				100.0	100.0	100.0
Suggested composition						
Total crude protein %				36.0	24.0	12.0
Phosphorus %				1.5	1.0	0.5
Carotene mg/kg				35.0	17.0	—
Rate of feeding, gm/day—ewes				115	150 to 255	90 to 450

cause most browse species, even in the dormant stage, furnish as much carotene as sun-cured alfalfa hay. However, when sheep are required to graze dry-grass ranges for periods longer than 6 months without intermittent periods of green feed, vitamin A supplements are recommended.

Mineral Mixtures: On the range, portable mineral boxes are convenient for sheep. Suggested mineral mixtures high in phosphorus are given in TABLE 15. One of these mineral mixtures should be fed free choice along with salt in a 2-compartment mineral box. Mixture 1 is used if there are no iodine or trace mineral deficiencies, Mixture 2 where an iodine deficiency exists and Mixture 3 if deficiencies of trace minerals are present.

TABLE 15. SUGGESTED MINERAL MIXTURES FOR SHEEP

Ingredient	Mixture No.		
	1	2	3
	%	%	%
Salt	50	—	—
Iodized salt	—	50	—
Trace mineralized salt	—	—	50
Bone meal or phosphorus supplement	50	50	50

Under winter range conditions, the amount of phosphorus supplement that should be added to range pellets will vary with the type of range forage available, the rate of feeding and the ingredients used in the pellets. It is suggested that 36, 24 and 12% protein pellets contain 1.5, 1.0 and 0.5% phosphorus, respectively. It is assumed that the 36% protein pellets will be fed at the rate of 115 gm per head daily, the 24% protein pellets at the rate of 150 to 225 gm and the 12% protein pellets at the rate of 90 to 225 gm together with alfalfa or clover hay.

SWINE NUTRITION

NUTRITIONAL REQUIREMENTS

Advanced technology contributes to the many phases of modern swine production. This is most evident in nutrition as formulation of diets becomes more precise and economical with synthetic nutrients, by-products and new feeds. The nutrient requirements for swine, given in the following tables, are from the report issued by the Committee on Animal Nutrition of the National Research Council (NRC), entitled *Nutrient Requirements of Swine*, revised in 1979. These requirements should be distinguished from therapeutic doses of many times the normal needs, which may be administered singly or over short periods to correct deficiencies. Factors such as stress conditions, availability of nutrients or variability in animals may dictate increased levels of some nutrients to optimize performance. Natural diets may contain more of some nutrients than the table recommends, but the effect is minimal except in extreme cases of imbalance. Ingredient concentration should be modified to prevent serious imbalances. Data on the composition of feedstuffs for swine are presented in TABLE 47, p. 1444.

The nutrients required by swine may be classified as water, energy (chiefly carbohydrates and fat), protein (amino acids), minerals and vitamins. In TABLES 16 and 17 nutrient requirement values are expressed per kilogram of total air-dry diet; those in TABLE 18 are expressed as daily needs. Certain antibiotics and chemotherapeutic agents are added to swine diets to increase the rate and efficiency of gain, but are not considered to be nutrients.

WATER

This constituent can be best supplied by allowing the pigs free and convenient access to it. The water allowances for full-fed pigs are given in TABLE 16. The water consumption in kilograms of growing-finishing pigs can be estimated fairly closely by multiplying by 2 the amount (in kilograms) of air-dry feed consumed. Yearling brood sows on experiment consumed about 1 gal. (3.8 L) of water daily during the winter gestation period. For maximum milk production, lactating sows should be given all the water they will consume.

TABLE 16. WATER ALLOWANCES FOR FULL-FED PIGS

WEIGHT OF PIG	WATER CONSUMPTION FREEWILL, DAILY PER PIG			
	Spring Pigs		Fall Pigs	
lb	lb	gal.	lb	gal.
50	5.5	0.60	4.5	0.56
100	9.0	1.12	7.5	0.94
150	10.0	1.25	9.0	1.12
200	9.0	1.12	9.6	1.20
300	6.0	0.75	6.0	0.75
400	5.2	0.65	5.2	0.65

(From Evvard, J. M., 1929. *Iowa Agricultural Experiment Station Research Bulletin* 118.)

ENERGY

The amount of feed consumed by growing pigs fed *ad libitum* is controlled principally by the energy content of the diet. If diets contain excessive amounts of fiber (exceeding 5 to 7%) without commensurate increases in fat, the rate and especially the efficiency of gain are adversely affected. Energy requirements of swine are expressed in terms of kilocalories (Kcal) either as digestible energy (DE) or metabolizable energy (ME). The ME values increasingly are finding favor for use by swine nutritionists as values for more and more feedstuffs are determined.

Feeding Levels

Daily feed intake estimates may be obtained from the figures in Table 17 for growing-finishing pigs. Such information is useful as a guide in projecting total feed requirements or prescribing medication via the feed.

The feeding levels set forth by the NRC provide a daily intake of 4.0 lb (1.8 kg) for pregnant gilts and sows. Sows and gilts need little more energy during pregnancy than is required for maintenance of body weight and good health. The diets upon which these recommendations are based would be classified as high-energy diets (corn-

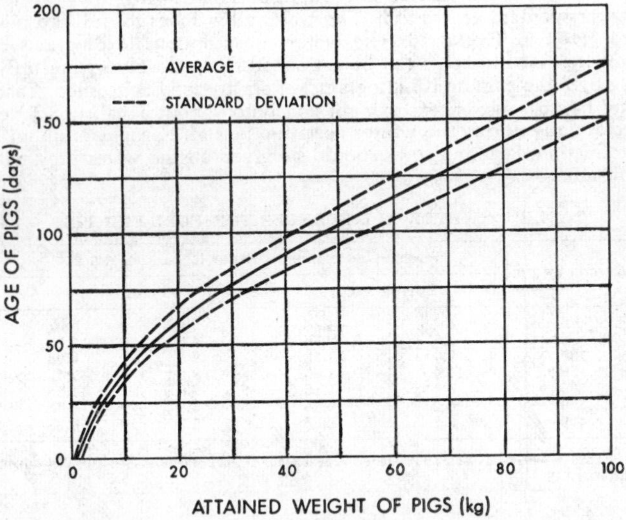

Figure 1: Weights, with standard deviations, that pigs are expected to attain at given ages under full-feeding conditions. The deviations around the mean tend to be skewed toward the right. (Figure from *Nutrient Requirements of Swine*, NRC, 1973)

soybean meal type) with no oats, alfalfa meal or other energy diluent. Voluntary intake by pregnant swine is difficult to control even with a high fiber or a high mineral level and invariably both excessive intake and weight gain occur.

A feeding method for pregnant gilts and sows receiving wide acceptance is that of feeding only one day out of 3, the total quantity of feed offered being the same (e.g. 5.4 kg every third day instead of 1.8 kg daily). The feed is spread out to allow opportunity for individuals to eat simultaneously. Sows may also be self fed a complete diet for a limited time (8 hr) every third day.

For feeding during lactation the NRC recommends 8.8 lb (4.0 kg), 10.5 lb (4.8 kg) and 12.1 lb (5.5 kg) of feed daily for sows producing 10.5, 13.2 and 16 lb (4.8, 6.0 and 7.3 kg) of milk daily, respectively. High-energy diets are usually fed during lactation. Many producers are restricting the feed offered to sows during the latter part of lactation (i.e. beyond 3 weeks) or are offering feed to sows based on the number of nursing pigs.

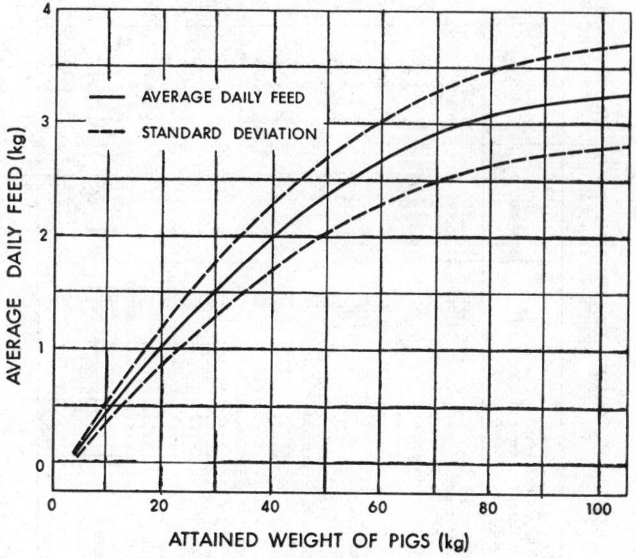

Figure 2: Expected daily feed intake (3,500 Kcal DE per kg of feed). (Figure from *Nutrient Requirements of Swine,* NRC, 1973)

TABLE 17. NUTRIENT REQUIREMENTS OF GROWING-FINISHING SWINE FED *AD LIBITUM*: PERCENT OR AMOUNT PER KILOGRAM OF DIET[a]

Liveweight (kg)		1-5[a]	5-10	10-20	20-35	35-60	60-100
Expected Daily Gain (gm)		200	300	500	600	700	800
Expected Efficiency (gm gain/kg feed)		800	600	500	400	350	270
Expected Efficiency (feed/gain)		1.25	1.67	2.00	2.50	2.86	3.75
Digestible energy[b]	Kcal	3,700	3,500	3,370	3,380	3,390	3,395
Metabolizable energy[b]	Kcal	3,600	3,400	3,160	3,175	3,190	3,195
Crude protein[c]	%	27	20	18	16	14	13
Indispensable amino acids							
Lysine	%	1.28	0.95	0.79	0.70	0.61	0.57
Arginine	%	0.33	0.25	0.23	0.20	0.18	0.16
Histidine	%	0.31	0.23	0.20	0.18	0.16	0.15
Isoleucine	%	0.85	0.63	0.56	0.50	0.44	0.41
Leucine	%	1.01	0.75	0.68	0.60	0.52	0.48
Methionine + cystine[d]	%	0.76	0.56	0.51	0.45	0.40	0.30
Phenylalanine + tyrosine[e]	%	1.18	0.88	0.79	0.70	0.61	0.57
Threonine	%	0.76	0.56	0.51	0.45	0.39	0.37
Tryptophan[f]	%	0.20	0.15	0.13	0.12	0.11	0.10
Valine	%	0.85	0.63	0.56	0.50	0.44	0.41
Mineral elements							
Calcium	%	0.90	0.80	0.65	0.60	0.55	0.50
Phosphorus[g]	%	0.70	0.60	0.55	0.50	0.45	0.40
Sodium	%	0.10	0.10	0.10	0.10	0.10	0.10
Chlorine	%	0.13	0.13	0.13	0.13	0.13	0.13
Potassium	%	0.30	0.26	0.26	0.23	0.20	0.17
Magnesium	%	0.04	0.04	0.04	0.04	0.04	0.04
Iron	mg	150	140	80	60	50	40
Zinc	mg	100	100	80	60	50	50
Manganese	mg	4.0	4.0	3.0	2.0	2.0	2.0
Copper	mg	6.0	6.0	5.0	4.0	3.0	3.0
Iodine	mg	0.14	0.14	0.14	0.14	0.14	0.14
Selenium	mg	0.15	0.15	0.15	0.15	0.15	0.10

Vitamins							
Vitamin A	IU	2,200	2,200	1,750	1,300	1,300	1,300
or β-carotene	mg	8.8	8.8	7.0	5.2	5.2	5.2
Vitamin D	IU	220	220	200	200	150	125
Vitamin E	IU	11	11	11	11	11	11
Vitamin K (menadione)	mg	2.0	2.0	2.0	2.0	2.0	2.0
Riboflavin	mg	3.0	3.0	3.0	2.6	2.2	2.2
Niacin[h]	mg	22	22	18	14	12	10
Pantothenic acid	mg	13	13	11	11	11	11
Vitamin B_{12}	μg	22	22	15	11	11	11
Choline[i]	mg	1,100	1,100	900	700	550	400
Thiamin	mg	1.3	1.3	1.1	1.1	1.1	1.1
Vitamin B_6	mg	1.5	1.5	1.5	1.1	1.1	1.1
Biotin	mg	0.10	0.10	0.10	0.10	0.10	0.10
Folacin	mg	0.60	0.60	0.60	0.60	0.60	0.60

[a] Requirements reflect the estimated levels of each nutrient needed for optimal performance when a fortified grain-soybean meal diet is fed, except that a substantial level of milk products should be included in the diet of the 1-5 kg pig. Concentrations are based upon amounts per unit of air-dry diet (i.e., 90 percent dry matter).

[b] These are not absolute requirements but are suggested energy levels derived from corn-soybean meal (44 percent crude protein) diets. When lower energy grains are fed, these energy levels will not be met, consequently, feed efficiency would be lowered.

[c] Approximate protein levels required to meet the need for indispensable amino acids when a fortified grain-soybean meal diet is fed to pigs weighing more than 5 kg.

[d] Methionine can fulfill the total requirement, cystine can meet at least 50 percent of the total requirement.

[e] Phenylalanine can fulfill the total requirement, tyrosine can meet at least 50 percent of the total requirement.

[f] It is assumed that usable tryptophan content of corn does not exceed 0.05 percent.

[g] At least 30 percent of the phosphorus requirement should be provided by inorganic and/or animal product sources.

[h] It is assumed that most of the niacin present in cereal grains and their by-products, is in bound form and thus unavailable to swine. The niacin contributed by these sources is not included in the requirement listed. In excess of its requirement for protein synthesis, tryptophan can be converted to niacin (50 mg tryptophan yields 1 mg niacin).

[i] In excess of its requirement for protein synthesis, methionine can spare dietary choline (4.3 mg methionine is equal in methylating capacity to 1 mg choline).

(From *Nutrient Requirements of Swine*, National Research Council, 1979.)

TABLE 18. NUTRIENT REQUIREMENTS OF BREEDING SWINE: PERCENT OR AMOUNT PER KILOGRAM OF DIET[a]

		Bred Gilts and Sows; Young and Adult Boars[b]	Lactating Gilts and Sows
Digestible energy	Kcal	3,400	3,395
Metabolizable energy	Kcal	3,200	3,195
Crude protein[c]	%	12	13
Indispensable amino acids			
Arginine	%	0	0.40
Histidine	%	0.15	0.25
Isoleucine	%	0.37	0.39
Leucine	%	0.42	0.70
Lysine	%	0.43	0.58
Methionine + cystine[d]	%	0.23	0.36
Phenylalanine + tyrosine[e]	%	0.52	0.85
Threonine	%	0.34	0.43
Tryptophan[f]	%	0.09	0.12
Valine	%	0.46	0.55
Mineral elements			
Calcium	%	0.75	0.75
Phosphorus[g]	%	0.60	0.50
Sodium	%	0.15	0.20
Chlorine	%	0.25	0.30
Potassium	%	0.20	0.20
Magnesium	%	0.04	0.04
Iron	mg	80	80
Zinc	mg	50	50
Manganese	mg	10	10
Copper	mg	5	5
Iodine	mg	0.14	0.14
Selenium	mg	0.15	0.15
Vitamins			
Vitamin A	IU	4,000	2,000
or β-carotene	mg	16	8
Vitamin D	IU	200	200
Vitamin E	IU	10	10
Vitamin K (menadione)	mg	2	2
Riboflavin	mg	3	3
Niacin[h]	mg	10	10
Pantothenic acid	mg	12	12
Vitamin B_{12}	μg	15	15
Choline	mg	1,250	1,250
Thiamin	mg	1	1
Vitamin B_6	mg	1	1
Biotin	mg	0.1	0.1
Folacin	mg	0.6	0.6

[a] Requirements reflect the estimated levels of each nutrient needed for optimal performance when a fortified grain-soybean meal diet is fed. Concentrations are based upon amounts per unit of air-dry feed (i.e., 90 percent dry matter).

[b] Requirements for boars of breeding age have not been established. It is suggested that the requirements will not differ significantly from that of bred gilts and sows.

[c] Approximately protein levels required to meet the need for indispensable amino acids when a fortified grain-soybean meal diet is fed. The true digestibilities of the amino acids were assumed to be 90 percent.

[d] Methionine can fulfill the total requirement; cystine can meet at least 50 percent of the total requirement.

[e] Phenylalanine can fulfill the total requirement; tyrosine can meet at least 50 percent of the total requirement.

Protein and Amino Acids

Amino acids normally incorporated into proteins long have been recognized to be essential for maintenance, growth, gestation and lactation of swine. Many amino acids are synthesized in the animal; however, some amino acids cannot be synthesized at a sufficiently rapid rate to permit normal growth and must be provided in the diet. The dietary amino acids indispensable for the growing pig are: arginine, histidine, isoleucine, leucine, lysine, methionine, phenylalanine, threonine, tryptophan and valine. The suggested feeding levels for crude protein in TABLE 17 are offered as guidelines for providing the required levels of amino acids when diets are based on corn and soybean meal. The essential amino acid requirements of swine are given in part in the tables. Further research is needed to clarify the amino acid requirements, particularly for boars.

The 3 amino acids of greatest practical importance are lysine, tryptophan and threonine. Corn, the basic grain in most swine diets, is markedly deficient in lysine and tryptophan. The other principal grains for swine, sorghum, barley and wheat, are low in lysine. The limiting amino acid in soybean meal is methionine, but sufficient is provided when soybean meal is combined with cereal grains into a complete diet containing the recommended level of protein. Milk protein is well balanced in essential amino acids, but usually is too expensive to be used in swine diets except for very young pigs. Corn and animal-protein (tankage, fish meal, meat meal, meat and bone meal) diets have proved inferior to corn-soybean meal diets, and have been improved significantly by additions of tryptophan or supplements that are good sources of tryptophan.

Minerals

The requirements for calcium, phosphorus, salt and other essential mineral elements are present in the tables.

Calcium and phosphorus, although used primarily in skeletal growth, play important metabolic roles in the body. Adequacy of these minerals are also essential to gestation and lactation; however, the quantitative needs are not increased greatly. The dietary requirements are stated by the NRC to be 0.6% calcium and 0.5% phosphorus for the growing pig and 0.5% calcium and 0.4% phosphorus for the finishing swine. These levels were established with more purified diets and although adequate for maximal growth (rate

---

[f] It is assumed that usable tryptophan content of corn does not exceed 0.05 percent.

[g] At least 30 percent of the phosphorus requirement should be provided by inorganic and/or animal product sources.

[h] It is assumed that most of the niacin present in cereal grains and their by-products is in bound form and thus unavailable to swine. The niacin contributed by these sources is not included in the requirement listed. In excess of its requirement for protein synthesis, trytophan can be converted to niacin (50 mg tryptophan yields 1 mg niacin).

(From *Nutrient Requirements of Swine*, National Research Council, 1979.)

of gain) they do not allow for maximal bone mineralization. The usual recommendation for such diets is the continued feeding of 0.5% phosphorus to market weight. Even higher levels of phosphorus (0.6%) may be required to maximize bone strength of growing boars. The use of feedstuffs such as tankage, meat meal, meat and bone meal and fish meal that are rich sources of calcium and phosphorus, may preclude the need of adding a phosphorus supplement. Calcium sources normally used in swine diets, limestone and oyster shell, have a high biologic availability. Steamed bone meal, defluorinated phosphate, soft phosphate or dicalcium phosphate may be used to increase both dietary calcium and phosphorus. There is some variation in the biologic availability of the phosphorus in these supplements.

Sodium chloride: The recommended salt allowance is 0.25% of the total diet. Animal and fish by-products as well as certain cereal by-products contribute appreciable amounts of salt.

Iodine is used by the thyroid gland to produce thyroxine, which affects cell activity and the rate of metabolism in the body. The iodine requirement of pregnant sows is approximately 0.44 mg/100 kg of body wt daily. Growing swine probably require somewhat less than this. Stabilized iodized salt containing 0.007% iodine, fed to meet the salt requirement, will meet the iodine needs of swine.

Iron and copper are necessary for hemoglobin formation and to prevent nutritional anemia. Fifteen milligrams of iron per pig daily for the first 3 weeks after birth will maintain normal levels of hemoglobin. The requirement for copper is listed by the NRC as 3 to 6 mg/kg total diet. It has been reported that pigs receiving 11 mg or more of copper per kilogram of body weight daily do not show copper deficiency signs.

Iron, which is severely deficient in milk, can be supplied orally to the suckling pig by mixing ferric ammonium citrate with water in a baby pig waterer or periodically dropping a mixture of iron sulfate and a carrier, such as corn, on the floor of the farrowing cage. Baby pig anemia (q.v., p. 23) can also be prevented with injectable iron compounds, which is the preferred method. Feeding iron and copper salts to pregnant or lactating sows or injecting iron dextran into these sows has not resulted in sufficient placental transfer or mammary uptake of these minerals to prevent anemia in baby pigs.

Cobalt is present in the vitamin B_{12} molecule and if the diet contains adequate vitamin B_{12} a growth response to added cobalt is unlikely.

Manganese is essential for normal reproduction and growth, but the quantitative requirement is unknown. It appears that 4 to 10 ppm in the diet is adequate for growth, gestation and lactation.

Potassium: When practical diets are fed, no deficiency is encountered because natural feedstuffs contain adequate amounts of potassium to meet the pig's needs.

Magnesium is a dietary essential for growing swine. The requirement has been established at 400 ppm (181 mg/lb) in the complete diet. Because of the content of this mineral in ordinary feedstuffs, a deficiency is unlikely under practical conditions. Magnesium oxide supplementation has been used to prevent cannibalism but controlled research does not support this practice.

Zinc is interrelated with calcium in swine nutrition. Supplemental zinc is recommended at the rate of 50 to 70 ppm (45 to 64 gm/ton) to prevent the occurrence of parakeratosis (q.v., p. 935). When diets contain excessive calcium (i.e., 1% or more) 100 ppm Zn is recommended.

Selenium: The selenium content of soils and ultimately crops is quite variable. Areas generally west of the Mississippi contain considerable amounts of selenium while soils east of the river tend to yield crops deficient in selenium. Under practical conditions 0.1 ppm selenium in the diet should meet the minimum requirements provided the diet is supplemented with vitamin E.

Vitamins

Requirements for vitamins are given in Tables 17 and 18.

Vitamin A: The use of stabilized vitamin A has become commonplace in manufactured feeds and in vitamin supplements or premixes. Concentrates containing natural vitamin A (fish oils for the most part) may be used to fortify diets, but both natural vitamin A and carotene, a precursor of vitamin A from plants, are rather easily destroyed in the presence of air, light, high temperatures, rancidity, and certain mineral elements. For these reasons less reliance is placed on natural feedstuffs as sources of vitamin A activity for swine. The NRC has set 1 mg of β-carotene equal to 500 IU of vitamin A for the pig. Green forage is an excellent source of carotene, as are high-quality legume hays. Dehydrated alfalfa meal is available as a standard feed ingredient and can be purchased with a guaranteed carotene content. Corn is not a reliable source.

Vitamin D: This antirachitic fat-soluble vitamin is necessary for proper bone growth and ossification. Vitamin D_2 (irradiated plant sterol) and vitamin D_3 (irradiated animal sterol) can be used by the pig to meet the vitamin D requirement. The requirements given in Tables 17 and 18 are 200 to 220 IU of vitamin per kilogram of diet for growing pigs weighing 20 kg and less, while the requirement for heavier swine is 125 IU/kg, when the diets contain recommended amounts of calcium and phosphorus. Vitamin D needs can be met by exposing pigs to direct sunlight for a short period each day. Sources of vitamin D include irradiated yeast, sun-cured hays, activated plant or animal sterols, fish oils and vitamin A and D concentrates.

Vitamin E (tocopherol) is required by swine of all ages. It is interrelated with selenium in nutrition of swine and is included at

11 to 22 IU/kg of a diet where selenium and vitamin E deficiencies have been reported. Vitamin E supplementation can only partially obviate a selenium deficiency. Green forage, legume hays and meals, cereal grains and especially the germ of cereal grains contain appreciable amounts of vitamin E. Vitamin E activity appears to be reduced in feedstuffs stored under high moisture conditions.

Vitamin K, the antihemorrhagic fat-soluble vitamin, is necessary to maintain normal blood clotting time. Hemorrhagic conditions have been reported in newborn as well as growing swine, perhaps indicating deficiencies of vitamin K in swine fed practical diets. It may be important to include supplemental vitamin K (2 mg/kg diet) as insurance in problem areas.

Thiamin: This water-soluble vitamin is not of practical importance in diets commonly fed to swine because grains and other feed ingredients supply ample amounts to meet the requirement of about 1.1 to 1.3 mg/kg of total diet.

Riboflavin: The requirement of breeding stock and of light-weight pigs is 2.6 to 3.0 mg of riboflavin per kilogram of diet. For 35 kg or heavier growing pigs, 2.2 mg/kg diet is required. Riboflavin is a constituent of several enzyme systems in the body. Swine diets are normally deficient in this vitamin and the crystalline form is added in premixes. Natural sources include green forage, milk by-products, brewer's yeast, legume meals and some fermentation and distillery by-products.

Niacin (nicotinic acid): The requirement for niacin is 22 mg/kg diet for the 10-kg pig, 14 to 18 mg/kg diet for the 20-kg pig and 10 mg for heavier pigs. Niacin is a component of co-enzymes concerned with utilization of carbohydrates. The pig can convert some tryptophan to niacin but this conversion is inefficient. Corn contains 9 to 10 mg of niacin per pound, but the niacin from corn and other cereal grains appears to be unavailable to swine. Swine diets are normally deficient in this vitamin and the crystalline form is added in premixes. Natural sources of niacin include fish and animal by-products, brewer's yeast, peanut meal and distillers' solubles.

Pantothenic acid: The requirement for pantothenic acid per kilogram of diet is 13 mg for 5- to 10-kg pigs, and 11 mg for pigs of other weights, and about 12 mg for breeding animals. Pantothenic acid is especially important in the female, since it is necessary for reproduction. Swine diets are normally deficient in this vitamin and the crystalline form is added in premixes. Natural sources of pantothenic acid include green forage, legume meals, milk products, brewer's yeast, fish solubles, wheat bran, peanut meal and rice polishings.

Pyridoxine (vitamin B_6): The requirement for pyridoxine is 1.5 mg/kg diet for 1- to 20-kg pigs and 1.1 mg/kg diet for heavier pigs. It is important in amino acid metabolism in the body and is present in plentiful quantities in the feed ingredients usually fed to swine.

Choline is essential for the normal functioning of the liver and kidneys. The pig can synthesize some choline from methionine in the diet. The requirement for choline is listed as 1,100 mg/kg of feed for 1- to 10-kg pigs and 900 mg/kg for 10- to 20-kg pigs but recent evidence indicates that the requirement is not greater than 330 mg/kg of feed. Corn-soy diets are not deficient in choline for starting, growing or finishing pigs. It has been shown that supplemental choline chloride at 440 to 770 mg/kg of feed will increase litter size in gilts and sows. Natural sources of choline include fish solubles, fish meal, soybean meal, liver meal, brewer's yeast, tankage and meat meal.

Vitamin B_{12}: The requirement for vitamin B_{12} is 22 mcg/kg diet for the 1- to 10-kg pig, 15 mcg/kg diet for the 10- to 20-kg pig and 11 mcg for heavier swine. A level of 15 mcg/kg diet is suggested for breeding stock. Vitamin B_{12} is needed by the young pig for growth and normal hemopoiesis. It is present in animal, marine and milk products, but the B_{12} potency of natural feed sources is quite variable. Swine diets are often deficient in this vitamin and the crystalline form is added in premixes.

Biotin, folic acid and ascorbic acid: Biotin and folic acid are essential for pig growth. Ascorbic acid apparently is synthesized by the pig at a rapid enough rate to meet its needs. There is no evidence to indicate the need to supplement practical swine diets with biotin, folic acid or ascorbic acid.

FEEDING AND MANAGEMENT PRACTICES

Swine Feeding Plan: A fundamental principle of economic pork production is the feeding of a diet in which the nutrient deficiencies of economically available cereal grains are corrected by supplementation. Dependable mineral and vitamin premixes to feed with cereal grains and soybean meal or complete manufactured supplements are available.

The consumption of creep-feed prior to 3 weeks of age is minimal. Litters nursing beyond this age should be self-fed a palatable starter diet until weaning. Supplemental feed is needed for optimum performance since milk production peaks at 3 to 4 weeks of age while the pig's demands are increasing rapidly.

Preparation and Feeding of Farm Grains: An improvement in gain and particularly feed efficiency can be expected from grinding grain. The older the pig the greater the response that can be expected from grinding. Grain should be reduced to a medium-fine particle size. Pelleting of diets may result in a small improvement in gain and especially feed efficiency. In general a greater benefit is obtained by pelleting diets containing higher levels of fiber.

Corn (maize) is the most widely used grain in North America for feeding pigs. It is high in metabolizable energy and relatively low in crude protein.

Oats: Because of the relatively low-energy content of oats they should not account for more than 20% of the cereal grain in the diet. On that basis finely ground oats can replace corn on a pound-for-pound basis.

Wheat contains 2 to 3% more protein than corn, but little or no increased substitutive value is gained since lysine content in wheat is only slightly greater than that of corn. The metabolizable energy values of wheat and corn are nearly identical. Wheat should be coarsely ground before feeding.

Barley: Ground or rolled barley has about 90% the feeding value of corn even though it usually contains 2 to 3% more protein than corn. Pelleting of diets containing high levels of barley results in improved swine performance over similar diets fed in mash form. Scabby barley should not be fed. Pelleted barley diets containing adequate amounts of all required nutrients are nearly equal to diets based on ground yellow corn and the necessary supplements.

Sorghum: This has become a significant energy source for swine in the Western and Southwestern parts of the U.S.A. The protein content will vary from 6 to 12% depending upon whether the crop is grown on irrigated or nonirrigated land and whether the soil was fertilized. In general, sorghum may be substituted for corn on an equal-weight basis in formulation procedures, being similar in metabolizable energy and lysine content.

Management of Sows and Litters: Preventing baby pig fatalities increases profits in the hog enterprise. About one-fourth of all pigs die before reaching weaning age. The following are management tips that will help reduce this loss: 1. The more vigorous a pig is at birth, the better are its chances of survival. To produce healthy pigs, the gestation diets need to be adequate in all nutrients. 2. The condition of the sow at farrowing and the need for using a laxative feed at farrowing is primarily a reflection of feeding during gestation. Constipation problems are minimal if the sow is limit-fed (1.8 kg/day) throughout gestation. After farrowing, the sow should be allowed to return to appetite as she chooses. 3. As the pigs are born, the navel should be dipped with tincture of iodine. The value of dipping the navel is lost once the cord dries. Needle teeth should be clipped, taking care not to injure the gums. The tails should be docked to preclude the possibility of tail biting at some subsequent time. 4. Care should be taken to see that each pig has nursed. If necessary the milk flow (or let-down) may be stimulated in some sows (℞ 193). If the sow is slow in coming to milk, weak pigs may gain from receiving artificial milk, but success depends on good management and sanitation. Greater returns may be gained by dividing pigs evenly among litters. Ear-notching pigs helps to identify the more productive litters at a future date. 5. An effective nutritional anemia-prevention program is essential to a successful swine production system (*see* p. 1318). 6. A palatable pig starter diet should be available from 2 weeks of age until time of weaning. 7. Boar pigs should be castrated at 2 weeks of age or earlier. 8. The use of some type of farrowing stall generally results in reduced baby pig mortality. The time of moving sow and litter to a nursing area (if this is part of the system) and the age of weaning vary with the physical facilities. Pigs are normally weaned between 3 and 5 weeks of age. With proper management and facilities pigs are often weaned in groups as they reach 12 to 15 lb starting at about 3 weeks of age. 9. Parasite control programs should be established for both external (q.v., p. 750) and internal parasites (q.v., p. 688).

Management of Growing Swine: The nutritional needs of growing-finishing pigs are best met by a program of full-feeding. Limited feeding will reduce the rate of gain but may improve feed efficiency and the carcass quality of finishing pigs. Proper design and adjustment of self feeders is necessary to prevent feed wastage.

TABLE 19 indicates space needs of growing swine. The management recommendations for growing pigs given herein are adapted from a report by the Nutrition Council of the American Feed Manufacturers Association. Recommendations for housing and space needs of swine are rapidly changing. It is currently recommended that growing-finishing swine be provided 4 sq ft of floor space from 50 to 125 lb, and 8 sq ft from 125 to 200 lb body wt, when the pigs are maintained on slatted or partially slatted floors. This assumes adequate ventilation. Where high summer temperatures are a problem, installation of sprays or fogging nozzles may be profitable.

TABLE 19. SPACE NEEDS OF GROWING-FINISHING SWINE

Items	Weaning to 75 lb	75 lb to 125 lb	125 lb to Market Size
Sleeping-space or shelter per pig, square feet			
Summer	4	5-6	8
Winter	4	5-6	8
Pigs per linear foot of self-feeder space (or per hole)			
On dry lot	4	3	3
On pasture	4-5	3-4	3-4
Percent of feeder space for protein supplement			
On dry lot	25	20	15
On pasture	20-25	15-20	10-15
For hand-feeding or hand-watering, running feet of trough per pig[1]	¾	1	1¼

[1] Access from one side.

One automatic watering cup should be provided for every 20 pigs (an automatic waterer with 2 openings is considered equivalent to 2 cups). Pigs varying widely in weight should not be raised together. Ordinarily, the range in weight should not exceed 20% above or below the average.

Growth Stimulants: Antibiotics and other chemotherapeutic agents are commonly added to swine diets to promote growth. Antibiotics in general have resulted in a larger and more consistent response than the arsenicals when added to growing-pig rations. The levels of antibiotics fed to various-age swine should be in accordance with the recommendations of the manufacturers. Efficacy and approval for feeding is based on prescribed levels. The following statements summarize the research results dealing with feed additives for growth promotion:

1. The inclusion of effective antibiotics in diets for growing swine tends to increase the rate of gain by about 10% on the average. This has been observed for both pasture and dry-lot feeding. 2. The average increase in feed efficiency due to chemotherapeutic feeding of growing pigs is approximately 5%. 3. The feed additives commonly used are penicillin (alone or in combination with streptomycin), chlortetracycline, oxytetracycline, bacitracin, tylosin, carbodox and virginiamycin. There are now legal restrictions on this use of some antibiotics. 4. For best results, the antibiotic should be left in the diet throughout the growing-finishing period. 5. It may help to reduce the number of runts and unthrifty pigs and cause such pigs to make more rapid and efficient gains. 6. It helps in preventing and controlling scours and certain forms of enteritis. (This advantage may be lost if resistant strains of enteritis-causing organisms develop.) 7. Results of several studies indicate that feeding antimicrobial agents at breeding time and at farrowing result in improved reproductive performance but not always. 8. There is considerable variability in the response from adding antibiotic to pig starters fed to suckling pigs. The inclusion of such agents in pig starters is recommended because of the possible value in controlling scours and overcoming the added stress imposed by weaning. 9. The feeding of antimicrobials to swine will not substitute for good management. Management includes practically all facets of production, but specifically, nutrition, genetics and environmental factors must be considered. An effective sanitation and disease-control program is absolutely essential in any successful swine operation.

HORSE NUTRITION

The feeding recommendations given below are drawn both from practical experience and scientific research. Horses are kept for a much longer time than most farm animals, and feeding programs must support the development of sound feet and legs which will sustain a long, useful and highly athletic life.

NUTRITIONAL REQUIREMENTS

Although horses obviously utilize hay and other roughage more efficiently than do other nonruminants, such as poultry or swine, the arrangement of the equine digestive tract limits this ability as compared with the ruminant. The site of fermentation in the horse is the cecum and large intestine, where large numbers of microorganisms digest hemicellulose and cellulose, utilize protein and nonprotein nitrogen and synthesize certain vitamins. Some of the products of fermentation such as volatile fatty acids and vitamins are absorbed and used. The microbial protein synthesized from nitrogen entering the cecum and colon undergoes only limited proteolysis, and the supply of essential amino acids from an unbalanced dietary nitrogen source is not satisfactorily balanced by microbial amino acids for optimum growth. The horse, therefore, is more dependent upon the quality of the diet than the ruminant.

Water

Water requirements depend largely upon environment, amount of work being performed, the nature of the feed and the physiologic status of the horse. Daily consumption may vary from 5 to 12 gal. (20 to 45 L). The working horse should be watered at least 3 to 4 times during the day. If the horse is hot, it should be cooled out first before being given unlimited access to water. If a horse is not being worked, it may be provided water *ad libitum*.

Energy

Energy requirements may be classified into those needed for maintenance, growth, pregnancy, lactation and work. Recent studies with light horses have resulted in prediction equations for estimating energy requirements. These equations permit the calculation of energy needs at any state of performance or production. Such estimates are provided in Tables 20 and 21. Individual differences of considerable magnitude exist in the need for energy, and some horses are "easy keepers," while others require prodigious amounts of feed. Thus, while these formulas provide a sound basis for estimating energy needs, the horseman should be aware of his responsibility to make a personal judgment of the energy needs of any individual horse.

Maintenance: To maintain body weight and support normal activity of the nonworking horse, digestible energy (DE) needs in Kcal/day equal 155 $W^{0.75}$, where W equals weight of the horse in kilograms.

$$\text{DE (Kcal/day)} = 155\ W_{kg}^{0.75}$$

WEIGHT CONVERSION TABLE

lb	kg	$kg^{0.75}$	lb	kg	$kg^{0.75}$
100	45.4	17.5	800	362.9	83.1
200	90.7	29.4	900	408.2	90.8
300	136.1	39.8	1000	453.6	98.3
400	181.4	49.4	1100	499.0	105.6
500	226.8	58.4	1200	544.3	112.7
600	272.2	67.0	1300	589.7	119.7
700	317.5	75.2	1400	635.0	126.5

Growth: The DE requirements for growth (to be added to that for maintenance) can be estimated from the following equation in which Y equals the Kcal DE/day/gm of gain and X equals the fraction of adult weight.

$$Y \text{ (Kcal DE/day/gm gain)} = 3.8 + 12.3X - 6.6X^2$$

Pregnancy: Maintenance energy intakes are adequate until the last 90 days of gestation when most of the tissue growth occurs. During this latter period, digestible energy requirements are 12% greater than for maintenance alone. Voluntary intake of roughage will decrease as the fetus gets larger, and it may be necessary to increase the energy density of the diet by using some concentrate.

Lactation: The National Research Council has estimated that 792 Kcal of DE/kg of milk produced per day should be added to maintenance needs to support lactation. Some data on average milk production of mares are shown below.

Months after foaling	Average Daily Milk Production (kg)		
	Draft horse	Light horse	Shetland pony
0 to 1	15.4	13.9	10.3
1 to 2	16.8	14.7	11.8
2 to 3	18.2	16.9	12.5
3 to 4	17.0	15.1	9.5
4 to 5	14.7	10.9	9.1

Work: Many factors such as type of work, condition and training of the horse, fatigue, environmental temperature and the skill of the rider or driver can influence the energy requirements of work. A guide to the amount of DE required above maintenance for various activities of light horses is shown below.

Activity	DE (Kcal/hr/kg body wt)
Walking	0.5
Slow trot, some cantering	5.0
Fast trot, cantering some jumping	12.5
Cantering, galloping, jumping	24.0
Strenuous effort, competitive racing	39.0

Protein and Amino Acids

Although some amino acid synthesis occurs in the cecum and large intestine, the entire amino acid needs of the growing, working or lactating horse cannot be met in this way. For this reason, the protein quality of the feeds used for horses is important. Weanlings require 0.6 to 0.7% lysine, and yearlings 0.4% lysine, in the diet. While other dietary amino acid requirements have not been established, the feed recommendations presented in Tables 20 to 22B contain an adequate distribution of those amino acids considered essential for the nonruminant.

Nitrogen needs expressed as crude or digestible protein are presented in Tables 20 and 21. The young growing horse has a considerably greater need for protein than the mature horse. Also, the protein requirements of growing horses of the heavier breeds are higher at the same body weight than those of the lighter breeds. Fetal growth during the last fourth of pregnancy increases protein requirements slightly, while lactation increases requirements still further. Work apparently does not increase the protein requirement, providing the increased energy requirements are met. If a horse is ridden or driven hard without being fed enough to meet the increased demands for energy, body fat and then muscle will be metabolized, resulting in a net nitrogen loss.

Minerals

Because the skeleton is of such fundamental importance to the performance of the horse, its mineral requirements deserve careful attention. However, excessive intakes of certain minerals may be as harmful as deficiencies. For this reason mineral supplements should be based on the consumption of the basic feeds in the diet. For example, if the horse is consuming mostly roughage with little grain, phosphorus is more likely to be in short supply than is calcium. However, if little roughage and much grain is being consumed, a shortage of calcium is more likely. The total mineral contribution and availability from all parts of the diet (roughage, grain, commercial products and supplements) must be considered in evaluating the mineral intake of the animal. Aside from actual feeding trials, no suitable test for availability of minerals now exists. Some caution is necessary in interpreting mineral requirements.

Calcium and phosphorus: *See* Tables 22A, 22B. The need during early growth is much greater than for maintenance of the mature animal. Work does not increase requirements as a percent of diet. The last fourth of pregnancy and lactation increase the need appreciably. Aged horses may require 30 to 50% more calcium and phosphorus than is required for maintenance of younger horses. However, excesses of dietary calcium will interfere with the utilization of magnesium, manganese, iron and probably zinc. The calcium:phosphorus ratio should be maintained at not less than 1:1. A desirable ratio is

TABLE 20. DAILY NUTRIENT REQUIREMENTS OF GROWING HORSES AND PONIES[1]

Age	Body Weight	Fraction of Adult Weight	Daily Gain	Daily Feed[2]	Daily Nutrients per Animal					
					Digestible Energy	Crude Protein	Digestible Protein	Ca	P	Vitamin A[3]
Mo	kg		gm	kg	Mcal	gm	gm	gm	gm	IU (thousands)
Growing ponies 200 kg adult weight										
3	60	0.30	700	2.50	8.17	410	380	18	11	2.4
6	95	0.48	500	3.15	8.81	470	310	19	14	3.8
12	140	0.70	200	3.20	8.14	350	200	12	9	5.5
18	170	0.35	100	3.45	8.25	320	170	11	7	6.0
24	185	0.92	50	3.45	8.25	300	150	10	7	5.5
Growing horses 400 kg adult weight										
3	125	0.31	1000	3.95	12.77	650	500	27	17	5.0
6	185	0.46	650	4.65	13.02	660	430	27	20	7.4
12	265	0.66	400	5.50	13.80	600	350	24	17	10.0
18	330	0.82	250	6.10	14.36	590	320	22	15	11.5
24	365	0.91	100	5.95	13.90	520	270	20	13	11.0
Growing horses 500 kg adult weight										
3	155	0.31	1200	4.65	15.18	750	540	33	20	6.2
6	230	0.46	800	5.55	15.60	790	520	34	25	9.2
12	325	0.65	550	6.65	16.82	760	450	31	22	12.0
18	400	0.80	350	7.20	17.16	710	390	28	19	14.0
24	450	0.90	150	7.35	16.57	630	330	25	17	13.0

Growing horses 600 kg adult weight

3	170	0.28	1400	5.15	16.71	840	780	36	23	6.8
6	265	0.44	850	6.05	16.92	860	570	37	27	10.6
12	385	0.64	600	7.50	18.85	900	500	35	25	14.0
18	475	0.79	350	8.15	19.06	750	430	32	22	13.5
24	540	0.90	200	8.20	19.27	740	390	31	20	13.0

[1] Adapted from *Nutrient Requirements of Horses*, National Research Council—National Academy of Sciences, Revised 1978.

[2] Ninety percent dry matter.

[3] One milligram of β-carotene equals 400 IU of vitamin A for the horse.

TABLE 21. DAILY NUTRIENT REQUIREMENTS OF MATURE HORSES AND PONIES[1]

Body Weight	Daily Feed[2]	Daily Nutrients per Animal						Daily Milk Production
		Digestible Energy	Crude Protein	Digestible Protein	Ca	P	Vitamin A[3]	
kg	kg	Mcal	gm	gm	gm	gm	IU (thousands)	kg
Mature Horses and Ponies, Maintenance								
200	4.15	8.24	320	140	9	6	5.0	—
400	7.00	13.86	540	240	18	11	10.0	—
500	8.30	16.39	630	290	23	14	12.5	—
600	9.45	18.79	730	330	27	17	15.0	—
Mature Horses and Ponies, Last 90 Days Gestation								
200	4.10	9.23	390	200	14	9	10.0	—
400	6.90	15.52	640	340	27	19	20.0	—
500	8.15	18.36	750	390	34	23	25.0	—
600	9.35	21.04	870	460	40	27	30.0	—
Mature Horses and Ponies, Lactating Mare, 1st 3 Months								
200	5.80	14.58	710	540	24	16	13.0	8
400	9.30	23.36	1120	680	40	27	22.0	12
500	11.20	28.27	1360	840	50	34	27.5	15
600	13.10	33.05	1600	990	60	40	33.0	18
Mature Horses and Ponies, Lactating Mare, 3 Months to Weaning								
200	5.55	12.99	600	340	20	13	11.0	6
400	8.60	20.20	910	510	33	22	18.0	8
500	10.40	24.31	1100	620	41	27	22.5	10
600	12.10	28.29	1290	730	49	30	27.0	12

[1] Adapted from *Nutrient Requirements of Horses,* National Research Council—National Academy of Sciences, Revised 1978.

[2] Ninety percent dry matter.

[3] One milligram of β-carotene equals 400 IU of vitamin A for the horse.

about 1.5:1 although, if adequate phosphorus is fed, foals will tolerate a ratio of 3:1 and mature horses a ratio of 6:1.

Sodium and chlorine: Salt requirements are markedly influenced by perspiration losses. Fifty to 60 gm of salt may be lost daily in the sweat and 35 gm in the urine of horses at moderate work. Supplemental salt may be provided at the rate of 1% of the grain ration plus extra salt *ad libitum* to replace the losses during hard work and hot weather. If more convenient, the entire salt needs may be provided *ad libitum;* salt poisoning is unlikely unless a salt-starved animal is suddenly exposed to an unlimited supply of salt, or water is not available.

Magnesium: The daily magnesium requirement for maintenance has been estimated at 3.6 to 5.9 mg/lb (8 to 13 mg/kg) of body wt. For the growing foal, magnesium at 0.37 to 0.57 gm/lb (0.85 to 1.25 gm/kg) of body wt gain must be added to the maintenance requirement. Outbreaks of tetany that respond to magnesium therapy have been reported from humid grassland areas. The addition of 5% magnesium oxide to the salt mixture has been protective.

Potassium: Foals require up to 1% potassium in a purified diet, while mature horses require about 0.4% potassium in a natural diet (27 mg/lb [60 mg/kg] of body wt). Since most roughages contain at least 1.5% potassium, a diet containing at least 35% roughage will provide sufficient potassium. Protein supplements are also high in this element.

Sulfur: It is doubtful that sulfur beyond that in methionine is a dietary essential. If the protein requirement is met, the sulfur intake of horses will usually be at least 0.15%—a level which is apparently adequate.

Iodine: Most iodized salts will provide the dietary iodine requirement which has been estimated to be 0.1 ppm. The iodine should be in a stable but available form. Pentacalcium orthoperiodate, calcium iodate, cuprous iodide, ethylenediamine dihydroiodide (EDDI) and stabilized potassium iodide are generally satisfactory. Iodine is poorly available from diiodosalicylic acid. Iodine toxicity has been noted in pregnant mares consuming as little as 40 mg of iodine per day. Goiter due to excess iodine was noted in both mares and their foals, and several cases were associated with use of large amounts of dried seaweed (kelp) in the diet.

Cobalt: The dietary requirement for cobalt is apparently less than 0.05 ppm. It is undoubtedly incorporated into cyanocobalamin (vitamin B_{12}) by the microorganisms in the cecum and colon. Absorption of the synthesized vitamin is probably sufficient to obviate any need for preformed vitamin B_{12}.

Copper: The dietary copper requirement for horses probably does not exceed 8 ppm. The presence of 5 to 25 ppm of molybdenum in forages has interfered with proper copper utilization.

Iron: The dietary maintenance requirement for iron is probably

TABLE 22A. REQUIRED NUTRIENT CONCENTRATIONS IN DIETS FOR HORSES AND PONIES[1, 2]

	Digestible Energy	Crude Protein	Digestible Protein	Ca	P	Vitamin A[3]	Example Diet Proportions: Hay Containing 2.0 Mcal DE/kg[4]		Hay Containing 1.8 Mcal DE/kg[5]	
	Mcal/kg	%	%	%	%	IU/kg	Concentrate[6]	Roughage	Concentrate	Roughage
Mature horses and ponies, maintenance	2.0	7.7	3.5	0.27	0.18	1,450	0	100	15B	85
Mares, last 90 days of gestation	2.25	10.0	4.9	0.45	0.30	3,000	25B	75	35A	65
Lactating mares, 1st 3 months	2.6	12.5	8.0	0.45	0.30	2,500	45A	55	55A	45
Lactating mares, 3 months to weaning	2.35	11.0	6.0	0.40	0.25	2,200	30B	70	40A	60
Stallions, breeding season	2.6	12.5	8.0	0.45	0.30	2,500	45A	55	55A	45
Creep feed	2.85	16.0	11.0	0.65	0.45	1,800	70A	30		
Foal (3 months of age)	3.2	16.5	13.5	0.70	0.45	1,800	75[10]	25	80[10]	20
Weanling (6 months of age)	2.8	14.5	9.5	0.60	0.45	1,800	65A	35	70A	30
Yearling (12 months of age)	2.55	12.0	7.0	0.50	0.35	1,800	45B	55	55A	45
Long yearling (18 months of age)	2.35	10.0	5.5	0.40	0.30	1,800	30B	70	40B	60

Two year old (light training)	2.6	9.0	5.0	0.40	0.30	1,800	50B	50	60B	40
Mature working horses (light work)[7]	2.25	7.7	4.5	0.27	0.18	1,450	25B	75	35B	65
(moderate work)[8]	2.6	7.7	4.5	0.27	0.18	1,450	50B	50	60B	40
(intense work)[9]	2.8	7.7	4.5	0.27	0.18	1,450	65B	35	70	30

[1] Ninety percent dry matter.
[2] Adapted from *Nutrient Requirements of Horses*, National Research Council—National Academy of Sciences, 1978.
[3] One milligram of β-carotene equals 400 IU of vitamin A for the horse.
[4] Good quality legume—grass hay.
[5] Grass hay.
[6] Concentrate containing 3.2 Mcal DE/kg. A or B refer to suitable concentrates (see Table 22B).
[7] Western pleasure, bridle path hack, equitation.
[8] Ranch work, roping, cutting, barrel racing, jumping.
[9] Race training, polo.
[10] Concentrate containing 3.6 Mcal DE/kg.

TABLE 22B. CONCENTRATES SATISFACTORY FOR USE WITH HAYS AS INDICATED IN TABLE 22A

Ingredient[1]	Formula A	Formula B
Corn[2] or sorghum grain, rolled or cracked	45	55
Oats[2], rolled or crimped	24	24
Soybean meal (44% CP)	20	10
Cane molasses[3]	8	8
Limestone (38% Ca)	0.5	0.5
Monodicalcium phosphate (18% Ca, 21% P)	1.5	1.5
Trace mineral salt[4]	1	1
	100	100
Analyses		
Digestible energy, Mcal/kg	3.2	3.2
Crude protein, %	16	12
Digestible protein, %	12	8.5
Calcium, %	0.60	0.58
Phosphorus, %	0.67	0.62

[1] Except for the cane molasses, all figures are on 90% dry matter basis.
[2] Barley may be used to replace the corn or sorghum *and* the oats, by using weights of barley equal to the combined weights of the grains replaced.
[3] Cane molasses is not an essential part of a concentrate mixture, but it minimizes separation of "fines" and reduces dustiness.
[4] Providing NaCl, Fe, Cu, Mn, Co, I, Zn plus Se (from sodium selenite) to provide 0.2 mg selenium/kg concentrate.

less than 40 ppm. For rapidly growing foals the requirement is estimated to be 50 ppm. Work with other species suggests that ferric oxide and ferrous carbonate are not effective iron supplements, and ferrous sulfate is the compound of choice.

Manganese: The amounts found in the usual forages are considered sufficient.

Zinc: Based on work with other species, the zinc requirement is estimated at 50 ppm of the ration. This mineral is relatively innocuous and intakes several times the requirement are considered safe.

Fluorine: Fluorine has been shown to retard dental caries in humans, but the effects of excessive ingestion are of much more concern in horse nutrition. Rock phosphates, when used as mineral supplements for horses, should contain no more than 0.1% fluorine. Fluorine intake should not exceed 50 ppm in the diet or 0.45 mg/lb (1 mg/kg) of body wt.

Molybdenum: Although an essential cofactor for xanthine oxidase activity, no quantitative requirement for the horse has been demonstrated. Excessive levels may interfere with copper utilization.

Selenium: The requirement for selenium is inversely related to the α-tocopherol content of the diet. The dietary requirement probably does not exceed 0.2 ppm, but there are regions of the world (including the lower Great Lakes states and part of New Zealand) where soils are deficient. In other areas (including parts of North and South Dakota) feeds may contain from 5 to 40 ppm of selenium, producing a characteristic toxicity (q.v., p. 979).

Supplementary minerals: Perhaps the most satisfactory method of providing supplementary calcium, phosphorus and salt for horses is to furnish trace mineral salt on one side of a double-compartment box and a mixture of one-third trace mineral salt and two-thirds dicalcium phosphate on the other. If relatively more phosphorus than calcium is desired, a mixture of mono- and dicalcium phosphate is appropriate. The mineral box should always be protected from rain.

VITAMINS

Carotene and vitamin A: The vitamin A requirement of the horse can be met by carotene, a precursor of vitamin A in plants, or by the vitamin itself. Fresh green forages and good-quality hays are excellent sources of carotene. However, because of instability to oxygen and light, the carotene content decreases with storage, and hays that are a year old or more may not furnish sufficient vitamin A activity to meet requirements. Dietary β-carotene is converted to vitamin A by horses so that 1 mg is equivalent to approximately 400 IU. Horses that have been consuming fresh green forage will usually have sufficient liver vitamin A stores to maintain adequate plasma vitamin A levels for 3 to 6 months. The National Research Council has estimated that the vitamin A requirements for maintenance, growth, pregnancy and lactation are 25, 40 and 50 IU/kg (11.3, 18.1 and 22.7 IU/lb) of body wt, respectively. These requirements expressed per kilogram of feed may be found in TABLE 22A. Prolonged feeding of excess vitamin A may cause bone fragility, hyperostosis and epithelial exfoliation.

Vitamin D: Grazing horses or horses that exercise regularly in sunlight and consume sun-cured hay normally will have their requirements for vitamin D met. However, if exposure to sunlight is restricted by confinement, hay may not always supply the requirement. Extrapolations from other species indicate that 6.6 IU of vitamin D per kg (3 IU/lb) of body wt should be sufficient. Vitamin D toxicity is characterized by general weakness, loss of body weight, calcification of the blood vessels, heart, other soft tissues, and bone abnormalities. Dietary excesses as small as 10 times the requirement may be toxic and will be aggravated by excessive calcium intake.

Vitamin E: No minimum requirement has been established. It seems quite likely that selenium concentration in the feed is related to the need for this vitamin. Based on work with sheep and cattle, evidence of vitamin E deficiency might be most likely to appear in the foal nursing a mare on dry winter pasture or given only low-quality hay unsupplemented with grain. Horses forced to exert severe physical effort are also likely to develop deficiency signs if they are fed low-vitamin E diets grown in low-selenium areas. If selenium intakes are 0.15 ppm of the diet, it is likely that 10 to 20 IU of vitamin E per kilogram (5 to 10 IU/lb) of diet would be adequate. (*See also* p. 1334.)

Vitamin K: This vitamin is synthesized by the microorganisms of the cecum and colon, probably in sufficient quantities to meet the normal requirements of the horse.

Ascorbic acid: Ascorbic acid is synthesized by the tissues of the horse, and this synthesis has been shown to be adequate for maintenance of mature horses.

Thiamin: Although thiamin is synthesized in the cecum and colon by bacterial action and about 25% of this may be absorbed, thiamin deficiency has been observed in horses fed poor-quality hay and grain. While not necessarily a minimum value, 25 mcg of thiamin per pound (55 mcg/kg) of body wt per day (about 1.4 mg/lb [3 mg/kg] diet) will maintain peak food consumption, normal gains and normal thiamin levels in skeletal muscle. Occasionally, horses are poisoned by consuming certain plants that contain thiaminases or antithiamins (*see* BRACKEN FERN POISONING, p. 1015).

Riboflavin: Under certain conditions, riboflavin may be required in the diet. Early reports implicated riboflavin deficiency in periodic ophthalmia, q.v., p. 226, but this relationship has not been substantiated. One report indicates that the riboflavin requirement may be met by supplying 20 mcg/lb (44 mcg/kg) of body wt per day.

Cyanocobalamin (vitamin B_{12}): Intestinal synthesis of this vitamin is probably adequate to meet ordinary body needs, provided sufficient cobalt is present in the diet. Absorption of vitamin B_{12} from the cecum has been established, and the feeding of a B_{12}-free diet had no effect on the normal hematology of adult horses. Parenteral injections of vitamin B_{12} into race horses has been shown to result in rapid and nearly complete excretion of the injected dose.

Niacin: This vitamin is probably synthesized in adequate quantities by the bacterial flora of the cecum and colon, and is synthesized in the tissues from tryptophan.

Pantothenic acid: Bacterial synthesis in the intestinal tract probably meets the requirements for this vitamin. Although not necessarily a minimum figure, Shetland ponies appeared healthy when provided with 18 mcg/lb (38 mcg/kg) of body wt daily; 0.9 mg/lb (2 mg/kg) of diet should be sufficient.

Folacin, biotin and vitamin B_6: All these vitamins are probably synthesized in adequate quantities in the intestine.

FEEDS AND FEEDING PRACTICE

The horse is an athlete and to produce top performance it must be properly nourished and appropriately trained. Proper nourishment implies more than a simple provision of essential nutrients. The master horseman not only provides the essential nutrients, but provides them in an appropriate form at the proper time. Horses do best when regularly fed and, because they have a relatively limited capacity for roughage at any one time, they may need to be fed frequently. For a hard-working horse in harness or under saddle, this may mean feeding 3 or more times a day. Under these circumstances, the principle of "feeding a little at a time and often" is a good one. A horse should not be worked on a loaded stomach and if 3 meals a day are offered, the daily roughage ration should be split between the morning and evening meals and should be offered at least 1 to 2 hours before work starts. The noon feeding should be light and 1 to 3 lb (0.5 to 1.5 kg) of grain should suffice. An alternative to this plan would be to feed one-fourth of the hay ration in the morning, a second fourth at noon and the remaining half at night.

Hot horses should be offered only small amounts of water until they are cooled out. This water should be clean and fresh.

Because horses are particularly sensitive to toxins found in spoiled feeds, all grains and roughages should be of good quality and free from mold. Likewise, dusty feeds should not be fed because of their tendency to initiate or aggravate respiratory problems.

Feeds

Pasture: The use of good pasture makes an ideal feeding program because it provides both nutrients and the opportunity to exercise. The pasture should be managed in such a way as to keep it free of weeds. Old, excessively mature growth should be clipped. A legume-grass mixture is ideal because it offers the advantages of good nutrient supply, a long grazing season and a long-lived stand. Alfalfa and smooth bromegrass make a good combination for many parts of the world, although many choices exist. Most grasses are improved by the presence of legumes.

Hay: The same species which make a good pasture usually make a good hay. Exceptions are low-growing plants, such as bluegrass and ladino clover. Legume-grass mixtures are generally high yielding and contain considerably more protein, minerals and vitamins than do grasses alone. However, they may be more difficult to cure in a humid climate, and moldy hay should be avoided.

Concentrates include the grains and by-product feeds high in energy or protein. In many instances it may be desirable to process them before feeding to improve nutrient availability and to increase their bulkiness (increase their volume per unit of weight). The bulkier concentrates are less apt to produce intestinal impaction and colic. Also the speed of digestion in the upper digestive tract is very important. Should any large volume of undigested grain reach the lower gut, the consequences can be serious. Excessive fermentation of such grain can result in founder.

Oats, perhaps the grain of choice, may be fed whole but rolling or crimping will increase its bulk 20 to 30% and will improve digestibility. Newly harvested oats may be dangerous due to the development of molds if their moisture content exceeds 14%.

Barley is a good grain for horses; it is higher in energy than oats but lower than corn. It may be fed as the only grain to horses that have a high energy need. It should be rolled or crimped.

Corn is a high-energy feed, useful for horses that are working hard or which are being fattened. It is low in bulk and more prone to produce colic than oats or barley if carelessly used. A good method of feeding is on the cob. This promotes salivation and the horse cannot bolt the grain. To maximize digestibility shelled corn may be cracked or rolled, but the moisture level should be low enough to avoid spoilage during storage.

Sorghum grain and **wheat** may be fed to horses with care to avoid colic. These grains should be cracked or rolled. **Wheat bran** is a bulky, mildly laxative feed that is well liked by horses. It is a good feed on idle days and may be substituted for part or all of the regular concentrate ration on those days when a hard-working horse is not under saddle or in harness.

Soybean meal is a palatable protein supplement with good amino acid balance for use with grains. It might be fed when pastures or hay are low in protein and are of poor quality or when protein requirements are greatest, such as during early growth or lactation. **Linseed meal** is also a very useful protein supplement. Its mucin content gives it a mildly laxative effect which may be helpful in certain feeding programs. The amino acid balance is not as good as that of soybean meal, being particularly low in lysine.

Cane molasses is frequently used to stimulate the appetite of poor eaters. It also minimizes separation of "fines" and reduces dustiness of concentrate mixtures. The sugar increases the desire for water.

Corn oil may occasionally be useful to improve the appearance of the hair coat when the diet is of poor quality and the intake of dietary essential fatty acids is low. Approximately 2 oz (60 ml) of corn oil per day, placed on the feed, is quite effective. It should be fresh and free of rancidity.

Limestone of a high grade (38% calcium) may be used as a supplementary source of calcium when this element alone is needed. Such a situation might prevail when poor-quality grass pasture or grass hay is the only roughage provided. Grains, being low in calcium, will not help much. When both supplementary calcium and phosphorus are needed, dicalcium phosphate, steamed bone meal, or defluorinated rock phosphate is recommended. Dicalcium phosphate is particularly good because it is low in cost per unit of phosphorus, odorless, the elements are quite available and there is no danger of anthrax. Monocalcium-dicalcium phosphate mixtures will supply relatively more phosphorus than calcium, when the need for supplemental phosphorus is greater than that for calcium. A supplement of both calcium and phosphorus might be needed when poor-quality grass pasture or grass hay is provided without grain. Grain containing appreciable phosphorus would tend to correct any deficiency of this element.

Salt (NaCl) should be provided in a block or in loose granular form *ad libitum*. It may be desirable to use a "trace mineralized" salt containing added iodine, iron, copper, cobalt, manganese, zinc and selenium. The need for these additional minerals will vary with the locality, but trace mineral salts are readily available and not costly. They may provide some nutritional insurance in areas where trace element deficiencies are a problem.

Succulent feeds: These feeds are high in water, are somewhat laxative and tend to stimulate the appetite. They should be introduced gradually when offered for the first time. Carrots are the safest and most satisfactory. A daily allowance of 1 to 3 lb (0.5 to 1.5 kg) is a desirable feeding rate. An artificial succulent feed can be made by soaking dried beet pulp in water sweetened with cane molasses. Well-preserved silage of good quality and free from mold affords a highly nutritious succulent forage during the winter months. As horses are much more susceptible to mold, botulism and digestive disturbances than are cattle and sheep, none but choice fresh silage should ever be fed. Various types of silages may be successfully used but corn silage and grass-legume silage are the most common. Mechanical silo unloaders may blend good and spoiled silage together and the spoilage may go undetected until digestive disturbances develop. Thus, the use of silage for horses is fraught with considerable danger.

Silage should not replace more than one-third to one-half of the roughage ration, considering that 6 lb (2 kg) of wet silage is approximately equivalent to 2 lb (1 kg) of hay. Thus, the silage allowance does not usually exceed 10 to 15 lb (4 to 7 kg) daily for a mature animal, although in some instances much larger amounts have been fed satisfactorily.

Rate of Feeding

Individual differences in the need for energy and nutrients make it difficult to generalize about the amount of feed to provide. The following rules of thumb will serve as guides and will usually satisfy the requirements. However, there is no substitute for observation and good judgment.

Horses at light work: Allow about 0.5 kg of concentrate and 1.25 to 1.5 kg of hay per 100 kg of body wt.

Horses at moderate work: Allow about 1 kg of concentrate and 1 to 1.25 kg of hay per 100 kg of body wt.

Horses at intense work: Allow about 1.25 to 1.5 kg of concentrate and 1 kg of hay per 100 kg of body wt.

The total allowance of concentrates and hay will fall within the range of 2 to 2.5 kg daily per 100 kg of body wt. No grain should be left from one feeding to the next and all edible forage should be cleaned up at the end of each day.

The need for grain while on pasture depends on pasture quality, but is more important for young than for mature horses. It is desirable to creep-feed nursing foals and they will frequently eat good-quality hay even when on pasture. They may be given free access to a concentrate mixture if accustomed to this regime gradually.

Suggested Rations

Example proportions of roughage and concentrate are present in Table 22A, with concentrate formulas in Table 22B. While these will generally meet the needs of the horses for which they were designed, many other choices exist. It is logical to use feeds that are locally available and in certain areas of the world several of the feeds suggested are not grown or are too high in price. Alternatives should be chosen on the basis of nutrient composition, palatability and general suitability for the horse.

Complete pelleted feeds, incorporating both concentrate and roughage, have been developed for horses. They have the advantage of uniform quality, complete control over nutrient intake, suitability for horses with bad teeth, less dustiness (which complicates respiratory problems), and reduced bulk for storage and transport. Because these feeds can be eaten so quickly, confined horses may exhibit increased boredom, and stable vices, such as wood-chewing, may be aggravated. This can be minimized by feeding some long hay. Damage to stable and fences can be reduced by treating wood with creosote or by covering or replacing wood with metal in vulnerable areas.

DOG NUTRITION

The dog, although classified as a carnivore, utilizes a wide variety of foodstuffs efficiently and can meet its nutritional requirements from a remarkable diversity of diets.

NUTRITIONAL REQUIREMENTS

Dogs regulate their food intake to meet their energy requirements, not to meet their requirements for any nutrient. The ideal way to provide a dog with its nutrient needs is to incorporate its exact daily nutrient requirements into precisely the amount of food consumed each day for energy. A series of tables listing the energy and nutrient requirements for average-sized dogs has been prepared by the Subcommittee on Canine Nutrition of the National Research Council. Modifications of several of these tables are used in this discussion (Tables 23, 24 and 25). For those interested in a more detailed account of the dog's nutritional requirements, the ɔulletin *Nutrient Requirements of Dogs*, published by the National Research Council, 2101 Constitution Ave., Washington, D.C., provides an excellent source of material.

PROTEIN

The dog's protein requirements usually are met by commercial dog foods having a minimum of 22 to 28% good quality protein, on a dry-matter basis. This protein should constitute approximately 20% of the diet's total calories. The ability of a protein to meet the dog's amino acid requirements depends on its ability to supply amino acids in the correct quantity and proportion. The higher the quality of protein fed, the lower the percentage of total protein needed in the diet. Soybean meal and corn, eggs, dairy products, muscle meats and the less tendinous organs are all satisfactory sources of amino acids for dogs.

The protein level needed for maintenance of dogs may be as low as 16%; at least 22% protein is required by the lactating bitch for maximum milk production.

TABLE 23. NUTRIENT REQUIREMENTS (AND SELECTED RECOMMENDED ALLOWANCES) OF DOGS (AMOUNTS PER KG OF BODY WT PER DAY)

Nutrient		Adult Maintenance	Growing Puppies
Protein	gm	4.8	9.6
Fat	gm	1.1	2.2
Linoleic acid	gm	0.22	0.44
Minerals			
Calcium	mg	242	484
Phosphorus	mg	198	396
Potassium	mg	132	264
Sodium chloride	mg	242	484
Magnesium	mg	8.8	17.6
Iron	mg	1.32	2.64
Copper	mg	0.16	0.32
Manganese	mg	0.11	0.22
Zinc	mg	2.2	4.4
Iodine	mg	0.034	0.068
Selenium	mcg	2.42	4.84
Vitamins			
Vitamin A	IU	110	220
Vitamin D	IU	11	22
Vitamin E	IU	1.1	2.2
Thiamin	mcg	22	44
Riboflavin	mcg	48	96
Pantothenic acid	mcg	220	440
Niacin	mcg	250	500
Pyridoxine	mcg	22	44
Folic acid	mcg	4.0	8.0
Biotin	mcg	2.2	4.4
Vitamin B_{12}	mcg	0.5	1.0
Choline	mg	26	52

Adapted from *Nutrient Requirements of Dogs*, National Research Council, 1974.

TABLE 24. NUTRIENT REQUIREMENTS (AND SELECTED RECOMMENDED ALLOWANCES) OF DOGS (PERCENTAGE OR AMOUNT PER KG OF FOOD)[a]

		Type of Diet			
		Dry Basis	Dry Type	Semi-moist	Canned or Wet
Moisture level (%)		0	10	25	75
Dry matter basis (%)		100	90	75	25
Nutrient		Requirement			
Protein	%	22	20	16.5	5.5
Fat	%	5.0	4.5	3.75	1.25
Linoleic acid	%	1.0	0.9	0.75	0.25
Minerals					
Calcium	%	1.1	1.0	0.8	0.3
Phosphorus	%	0.9	0.8	0.7	0.22
Potassium	%	0.6	0.5	0.45	0.2
Sodium chloride	%	1.1	1.0	0.8	0.3
Magnesium	%	0.040	0.036	0.030	0.010
Iron	mg	60	54	45	15
Copper	mg	7.3	6.5	5.5	1.8
Manganese	mg	5.0	4.5	3.8	1.2
Zinc[b]	mg	100	90	75	25
Iodine	mg	1.54	1.39	1.16	0.39
Selenium[c]	mg	0.11	0.10	0.08	0.03
Vitamins					
Vitamin A	IU	5,000[d]	4,500	3,750	1,250
Vitamin D	IU	500[e]	450	375	125
Vitamin E	IU	50[f]	45	37.5	12.5
Thiamin	mg	1.00	0.90	0.75	0.25
Riboflavin	mg	2.2	2.0	1.6	0.5
Pantothenic acid	mg	10.0	9.0	7.5	2.5
Niacin	mg	11.4	10.3	8.6	2.8
Pyridoxine	mg	1.0	0.9	0.75	0.25
Folic acid	mg	0.18	0.16	0.14	0.04
Biotin[c]	mg	0.10	0.09	0.075	0.025
Vitamin B_{12}[c]	mg	0.022	0.020	0.017	0.006
Choline	mg	1,200	1,100	900	300

[a] Based on diets with ME concentrations in the range of 3.5-4.0 Kcal/gm of dry matter. If energy density exceed this range, it may be necessary to increase nutrient concentrations proportionately.

[b] Zinc based on recent unreported data.

[c] Based on research in other species.

[d] This amount of vitamin A activity corresponds to 1.5 of all-*trans* retinol per kilogram of dry diet (One IU of vitamin A activity equals 0.3 mcg of all *trans* retinol).

[e] This amount of vitamin D activity corresponds to 12.5 mcg of cholecalciferol per kilogram of dry diet (One IU of vitamin D activity equals 0.025 mcg of cholecalciferol).

[f] This amount of vitamin E activity corresponds to 50 mg of DL-α-tocopheryl acetate per kilogram of dry diet (One IU of vitamin E activity equals 1 mg of DL-α-tocopheryl acetate).

Adapted from *Nutrient Requirements of Dogs,* National Research Council, 1974.

Carbohydrates

The dog utilizes carbohydrates with almost the same efficiency as man. Carbohydrates are economical sources of energy and help spare proteins from being used as energy. Carbohydrates can supply 60% of dietary calories with ample formula room for proteins, fats, minerals and vitamins. Raw starches are poorly digested and are cooked during processing of dog foods.

Lactose (milk sugar) is poorly digested by some dogs, which have low lactase production. Large quantities of cow's milk should not be given to either puppies or adult dogs since cow's milk contains more lactose than bitch's milk. Undigested lactose may ferment in the intestinal tract and produce diarrhea.

Fats

Dietary fat supplies concentrated energy, essential fatty acids, and palatability. While only 2% fat as corn oil (50% linoleic acid) is needed to provide the essential unsaturated fatty acids, fat levels of 6 to 8%, on a dry matter basis, may be added to diets to supply palatability. Dogs can tolerate rations containing up to 50% fat; however these diets are not economically feasible. High fat rations result in a proportionate reduction in total food intake, therefore all nutrients must be present in proper ratios to the metabolizable caloric content for a balanced diet.

The addition of corn oil and its high linoleic acid will help alleviate the dry, scaly coat condition produced by a previous dietary unsaturated fat deficiency; 1 ml/4 kg of body wt added to the daily diet will usually produce an improvement. Opened containers of food oil should be kept refrigerated to inhibit oxidative rancidity.

Fats added during the manufacture of dry dog foods are stabilized with antioxidants to retard rancidity since fats becoming rancid

TABLE 25. SUGGESTED CALORIC ALLOWANCES FOR MAINTENANCE AND DAILY FOOD INTAKES OF AVERAGE ADULT DOGS OF VARIOUS BODY WEIGHTS

Weight		Kcal ME per kg body wt	Daily Rations of Dog Food in Grams*		
(lb)	(kg)		Dry Type	Semi-moist	Canned
2	1	132	36	45	104
4.5	2	106	62	73	168
11	5	88	126	154	347
15	7	81	160	202	448
22	10	75	213	263	591
33	15	70	297	364	829
44	20	62	350	434	980
77	35	53	524	650	1465
110	50	48	678	840	1893

* Needs for growth may be estimated by multiplying adult requirements by appropriate multiples of maintenance as follows:

Weaning to 40% adult size-weight—2X maintenance; 40 to 80% adult size-weight—1.5X maintenance; 80% adult size-weight to maturity—1.2X maintenance.

Adapted from *Nutrient Requirements of Dogs,* National Research Council, 1974.

destroy fat-soluble vitamins, particularly vitamins A and E, and may precipitate deficiencies of these vitamins. This condition may sometimes be observed in show dogs to which an excess of polyunsaturated oils is fed in an effort to produce an attractive hair coat.

VITAMINS

Dogs require at least 13 vitamins. Although the precise requirements for some vitamins have not been determined, satisfactory levels for dogs have been confirmed by years of satisfactory formulation use and are presented in TABLES 23 and 24.

Ascorbic acid (Vitamin C) is synthesized by most dogs; perhaps one in each thousand dogs may benefit from ascorbic acid added to the daily diet; 100 mg ascorbic acid per 25 kg of body wt daily is adequate.

Adding vitamin supplements to complete and balanced commercial rations for healthy dogs is unnecessary. Some diseases may increase specific vitamin requirements and suggested prescribed supplementation may be useful. (*See* NUTRITIONAL DEFICIENCIES IN DOGS, p. 1415).

MINERALS

The dog requires a number of dietary minerals for health (TABLES 23 and 24). Most balanced commercial foods contain these minerals in ample amounts. The metabolism of many minerals is interrelated and they are best utilized when provided in the proper ratio to one another. Calcium and phosphorus, for example, are usually best utilized when provided in a ratio of 1.2:1 with normal levels of vitamin D. Supplemental calcium should not be added to adequate rations, particularly for growing dogs, since excessive amounts of ingested calcium increase the requirement for phosphorus, manganese, zinc and other nutrients. Excess absorbed calcium may be deposited in soft tissue and joints producing arterial plaques and arthritis, or concentrated in the urine where it may become a urolithic constituent.

DOG FOODS

Commercial dog foods can be found in 5 general types—dry, canned, semi-moist, treats and frozen—depending more on processing methods and water content than on ingredient and nutrient content. Since energy and nutrients are part of dry matter, dog food should be compared on a dry-matter basis. This can be done by eliminating the water mathematically (i.e. subtracting the percentage of moisture from 100%). To obtain the percent that each nutrient contributes to the total dry matter, the percentage of each nutrient is divided by the total dry-matter percentage.

Dry dog foods are available as biscuits, pellets and flakes or expanded chunks. The latter form has become the most popular, and provides about 80% of total dog nutrition. It is made by combining vegetable proteins, meat and meat by-products, cereal grains, fats and minerals; subjecting the mixture to heat and pressure, then forcing the resultant doughy mass through an extruder. The heat of processing converts starches into a more easily digestible form and destroys undesirable enzymes. Since heat also adversely affects heat-labile members of the B-complex vitamins and vitamin A, these are added at elevated levels in the basal ration or with fat sprayed on the surface after drying. Since dry foods usually contain less than 10% moisture, more nourishment is available from them, pound for pound than from any other type. They require no refrigeration and partially emptied containers can be returned to the shelf. Dry foods may become rancid or infested with insects or vermin with prolonged storage. The overall digestibility of most dry foods will average between 70 and 80% and they will contain between 1,500 and 1,600 Kcal/lb (3,300 to 3,500 Kcal/kg) of metabolizable energy.

Canned dog foods are available in "all meat," "meat," "dinners," or a flavored dog food. With the exception of 100% or "all meat" dog foods, all classes of canned food are usually complete and balanced.

"All meat" or "100% meat" dog foods contain the one ingredient plus added water, preservatives or condiments and the legally required "decharacterizing agents" (to render the food undesirable for human consumption). These cannot be complete foods since the vitamins and minerals necessary for a complete diet cannot be added according to definitions established by the Association of American Feed Control officials who monitor and regulate pet foods in each state. Few, if any, 100% meat or all meat products will be found on the market.

When an ingredient or combination of ingredients derived from animal, poultry, or fish constitutes 95% or more of the total weight of all ingredients in a pet food mixture, the name of that ingredient may be used as a basis for the product name, e.g. Beef For Dogs. Thus Beef For Dogs can be a complete and balanced product since the additional 5% of formula space can include the needed vitamins and minerals to produce a balanced food.

When an ingredient or combination of ingredients derived from animals, poultry, or fish constitutes at least 25% of the total weight of the food formula the name of the ingredient can constitute a part of the name in combination with a descriptive term such as "dinner" or "cakes." This means "fish cakes for cats" probably contains 25% fish.

Flavored pet foods need not contain any of the substance named in the title as long as the substance's flavor can be identified by the animal; e.g. "beef flavor" dog food may be expected to contain beef but the name assures only that it contains the flavor.

Generally, canned dog foods in these categories (except for 100% or all meat) contain a wide array of ingredients including vitamins and minerals and most are formulated to be complete and balanced. Canned pet foods usually contain about 76 to 78% water; stews, gravies, sauces, broth and milk replacers may contain more than the 78% permitted for canned foods. Digestibility of the total dry matter in canned foods usually exceeds that of dry foods because of the higher fat content on a dry matter basis and may average 75 to 85% digestibility and contain about 500 Kcal/lb or 1,100 Kcal/kg.

Semi-moist foods are designed anthropomorphically to provide a simulated meat appearance for the owner feeding the pet; they are available in patties, chunks and simulated hamburger shapes. Since semi-moist foods contain about 25 to 40% moisture they must rely on bacteriostats, fungistats, and humectants to aid in preservation. Soybean meal, meat and bone meal, and sucrose constitute the major ingredients with vitamins and minerals added. The processing destroys relatively few nutrients. Although semi-moist foods generally do not require refrigeration, once the package is opened they generally lose moisture rapidly. The digestibility of semi-moist foods usually ranges from 80 to 85% with about 1,300 to 1,500 Kcal/lb or 2,800 to 3,200 Kcal/kg. Most semi-moist foods are somewhere between dry and canned food in acceptability. Semi-moist foods in which the pH is controlled through acidulants generally produce an acid urine and are indicated when urolithic conditions prevail.

Treats can be fed extensively with this in mind. Most commercial treats are nutritionally complete and will not create an imbalance.

Frozen foods are available in small market areas and usually are combined dry food, ground meat, and water frozen into cake form primarily for show dogs. They must be kept frozen or spoilage occurs rapidly. Frozen food varies from 1,200 to 1,600 Kcal/lb or 2,600 to 3,500 Kcal/kg or even more if high fat meat is used. Most frozen foods are 85 to 90% digestible and highly palatable.

DRUGS AND CONTAMINATING SUBSTANCES IN DOG FOODS

Seldom will extraneous drugs, chemicals, or toxins be found in commercial pet foods. Pet foods use categories of ingredients approved by the U.S. Food and Drug Administration, and the better pet food plants adhere to good manufacturing practices designed to prevent contamination. Some extruded foods contain fewer bacteria per gram than pasteurized milk sold for human consumption.

The food storage area in the kennel or home should be cleaned periodically to discourage growth of mold and proliferation of mites, which may pass through the digestive tract and create confusion for the uninitiated parasitologic observer.

GENERAL CONSIDERATIONS IN FEEDING DOGS

When evaluating the nutritional problems of dogs consider: (1) The conditions under which the dog lives affect its need for nutri-ents. (2) The role the owner plays in dog nutrition is of as much practical importance as the dog's actual requirements. Owners may ndulge their animals with foods that subject them to careless and haphazard feeding practices. (3) The water content of the diet, which can produce suboptimal nutrient intake in some dogs and contribute to the consumption of poisonous house plants and dan-gerous toys.

Label guarantees and conventional chemical analyses are not very informative about the true value of a food. Protein, for example, s determined by analysis for nitrogen, which is multiplied by a constant and expressed as protein. (No information is given on the package or label regarding that protein's digestibility or biologic value.) Many commercial producers of dog foods maintain elaborate esearch facilities designed to help evaluate and improve their prod-ucts. During recent years many foods on the market have improved emarkably and supplementing their formulation may do more harm han good.

Whenever supplementation is necessary, it should always be cal-culated on a dry-matter basis. For example, the addition of 4 oz of corn oil to 1 lb (250 ml/kg) of canned food (which contains about 4 oz of dry matter) results in the addition of fat equal to the amount of dry matter. However, if 4 oz of corn oil are added to 1 lb of dry food which contains about 14.4 oz [430 gm] of dry matter) the fat added s only 27%. While both of these examples probably represent exces-ive fat additions, that amount added to dry food might be tolerated by the dog. The same amount, added to canned food, however, would lower the intake of protein, minerals and vitamins to the xtent that serious nutritional deficiencies could develop. Diets, marginal in one or more nutrients, having their fat level, hence their caloric density, increased, often produce a deficiency due to the decrease in the actual quantity of food eaten. Dogs that are fed mostly table scraps often have an excess of fat in their diet. TABLE 5 gives average caloric intakes needed to maintain dogs at various weights. Such a table only serves as a starting place, however. It is necessary to consider each dog individually and adjust each diet to he case at hand. A variety of things affect the dietary needs of a dog; hese are:

Stages of the life cycle: Growth requires about twice the intake of nutrients, per pound of body weight, that adult maintenance does. Gestation may require an increase in food intake during the last weeks. Lactation requires as much as 300% increase in energy hence food intake) by the third week of lactation for large litters.

Environment: Seasonal variations in environmental temperatures influence dietary intake, which varies inversely with the temperature. The winter energy requirement may be double the summer requirement. Dogs confined to small pens or apartments generally have lower energy needs than dogs permitted to exercise in large pens or yards.

Exercise: Hard-working dogs, such as hunting dogs, racing dogs, and herding dogs may have their energy requirement increased as much as 200 to 300% above maintenance. High-energy, concentrated rations are available for dogs with high-energy requirements. When increased energy is not provided the animal may continue to work for a time, but only at the expense of body reserves, resulting in weight loss and debilitation. While extensive exercise helps promote good muscular condition, it is not necessary for normal health. Dogs receiving limited exercise should be given a restricted diet to avoid undesirable gains in body weight.

Increased metabolism: Theoretically, hyperthyroidism, tissue injury and fever increase the basal metabolic rate and produce increased nutritional demands. It has been estimated that each 1°F (0.5°C) of fever increases the calorie demand by 7%, although dogs with elevated fever may not feel like consuming more.

Malnutrition and corrections of weight deficiency: Neglect, the lost dog, and convalescence following severe blood loss, debilitation or parasitism are some of the common circumstances that necessitate diets high in protein, calories and vitamins. Protein levels of 1 to 2 gm/lb (2 to 5 gm/kg) of body wt, a 50 to 70% increase in caloric intake above maintenance, and moistening the food to increase acceptability to exceed the dog's minimum daily requirement, are good principles to follow when feeding such animals. It is better to bring these patients along slowly for the first few days than to force gains too rapidly. Frequent daily feedings accompanied by extra attention may help to increase the total food intake.

Obesity and correction of excessive weight: Dogs receiving little exercise and those that are mature or approaching old age are often indulged by their owners. Because of the table "treats" such dogs often receive, they are fed poorly balanced diets, high in sugars and fats; commercial treats are usually nutritionally balanced. Discontinuation of all snacks and restriction of the amount of total food consumed to that amount which supplies only 60% of the calories needed to maintain the dog's normal body weight is indicated for obesity control. An adequate vitamin and mineral intake is important. It may be desirable to provide a high level of protein intake (i.e. 1 to 2 gm/lb [2 to 5 gm/kg] of body wt daily). Such animals usually are more content and have better bowel action if a fairly high level of fiber (e.g. 8% on a dry-matter basis) is included in their daily ration. The veterinarian's efforts to correct obesity are often undermined by lack of cooperation from owners, which may prove an insurmountable problem.

Disease: Many diseases respond favorably to dietary modification. Notable among these are chronic renal disease, congestive heart failure and gastrointestinal disorders. The primary objective in the dietary management of any disease should be to provide the dog with adequate nourishment while simultaneously compensating for metabolic or organic dysfunctions. (*See* FEEDING THE SICK DOG, p. 1389).

CAT NUTRITION

Nutritional Requirements: Like the dog, the cat is able to meet its nutritional needs from a wide variety of diets. Nutrient requirements are usually increased during growth, pregnancy, lactation and fever. TABLES 26 and 27 list some requirements and allowances: the National Research Council's bulletin, *Nutrient Requirements of Cats* (1978) is an excellent source for more details.

Protein: The cat has a high protein requirement. Healthy adult cats need at least 2.0 gm of protein having a biologic value of 100, per kilogram of body weight per day, about twice that needed by the dog. Optimal diets for cats should contain at least 25% of the calories from protein. This amounts to 30 to 40% of protein on a dry-weight basis. Growing kittens are more sensitive to the quantity and quality of dietary protein than adult cats. Protein suitable for cats must supply amino acids including taurine in the proper ratio and quantity. The more a protein is able to do this, the less of it is required to provide the cat's requirements. Animal proteins are, in general, more suitable for cats than plant proteins.

Fats: As much as 60% of the calories in a cat's diet can come from fat, but diets containing between 14 and 40% on a dry-matter basis have been used successfully. Diets containing the upper limits tend to produce obesity. If there is insufficient vitamin E in the diet, too much polyunsaturated fat may lead to steatitis. Whatever the level of fat in the diet, it should contain not less than 1% linoleic acid. Fat has an important effect on the palatability of a cat's diet, and a small addition may materially improve a diet's acceptability.

Carbohydrates: Although carbohydrates may not be essential in the cat's diet, they offer a less expensive calorie source than fat or protein. Starches must be cooked or they will be digested poorly. Except for an occasional case of lactose or sucrose sensitivity, most carbohydrates are well tolerated but will be poorly accepted unless incorporated into a diet properly formulated to appeal to the cat's palate.

TABLE 26. ESTIMATED DAILY FOOD ALLOWANCES OF CATS

Cat	Weight of Cat, kg	Dry Type (90% Dry Matter) ME 3.60 Kcal/gm		Semimoist (70% Dry Matter) ME 3.15 Kcal/gm		Canned (25% Dry Matter) ME 1.25 Kcal/gm	
		gm/kg body wt	gm/cat	gm/kg body wt	gm/cat	gm/kg body wt	gm/cat
Kitten							
10 weeks	0.4-1.0	70	28-70	80	32-80	200	80-200
20 weeks	1.2-2.0	36	43-72	42	50-84	104	125-208
30 weeks	1.5-2.7	28	42-76	32	48-86	80	120-216
40 weeks	2.2-3.8	22	48-84	26	57-99	64	141-243
Adult							
Inactive	2.2-4.5	20	44-90	22	48-99	56	123-252
Active	2.2-4.5	24	53-108	27	59-122	68	150-306
Gestation	2.5-4.0	28	70-112	32	80-128	80	200-320
Lactation	2.2-4.0	70	154-280	80	176-320	200	440-800

Adapted from *Nutrient Requirements of Cats*, National Research Council, 1978.

TABLE 27. RECOMMENDED NUTRIENT ALLOWANCES FOR CATS
(Percentage or amount per kilogram of diet, dry basis)

Nutrient		Amount	Nutrient		Amount
Protein	%	28	Vitamins		
Fat	%	9	Vitamin A	IU	10,000
Linoleic Acid	%	1	Vitamin D	IU	1,000
Minerals			Vitamin E	IU	80
Calcium	%	1	Thiamin	mg	5
Phosphorus	%	0.8	Riboflavin	mg	5
Potassium	%	0.3	Pantothenic Acid	mg	10
Sodium Chloride	%	0.5	Niacin	mg	45
Magnesium	%	0.05	Pyridoxine	mg	4
Iron	mg	100	Folic Acid	mg	1.0
Copper	mg	5	Biotin	mg	0.05
Manganese	mg	10	Vitamin B_{12}	mg	0.02
Zinc	mg	30	Choline	mg	2,000
Iodine	mg	1			
Selenium	mg	0.1			

Adapted from *Nutrient Requirements of Cats*, National Research Council, 1978.

Vitamins: Cats require about 12 dietary vitamins to maintain health: TABLE 27 presents the currently recommended vitamin allowances. Most commercial cat foods are fortified with vitamins, making supplementation unnecessary or possibly even dangerous.

Minerals: Since there have been practically no studies of the cat's mineral requirements, recommended dietary allowances for minerals listed in TABLE 27 have been derived from diets that have been used successfully. The ratio of one mineral to another is as important as its dietary level. Injudicious supplementation with one or more minerals is likely to do more harm than good.

Cat Foods: Commercial cat foods can be obtained in 3 different types: canned, dry and semi-moist. Like dog foods, cat foods should be reduced to a dry-matter basis for comparison (q.v., p. 1344). Many dog foods are not satisfactory for cats. Some cat foods are also unsatisfactory, e.g. a food derived from a single source may be nutritionally incomplete.

Canned cat foods are available as either ration-type or meat and meat by-product ("gourmet") foods. The latter may contain only a single ingredient, such as liver, shrimp or fish, and be with or without fortifying mineral and vitamin mixes. Others may contain the full range of animal by-products seen in dog foods. Canned cat foods contain from 72% (ration) to 78% (meat) water. They are probably among the most palatable foods available for the cat. Heat, used in processing, may destroy some of the vitamin potency in any canned food.

Dry cat foods are available as expanded pellets that may be molded into various shapes. The heat of processing can destroy some nutrients. Most dry cat foods contain between 7 and 9% water. One of the most essential husbandry practices for cats eating dry foods is maintaining a constant water supply by moistening the food. The acceptability of dry cat foods ranges from very high to very low.

Semi-moist cat foods are available in several shapes. Their advantages and disadvantages are similar to soft-moist foods for dogs. Soft-moist foods contain about 25% water and their nutrients are between 75 and 85% digestible by the cat. Their acceptability is variable, but some are so palatable that their feeding must be restricted or the cat will become obese.

Drugs and Contaminating Substances in Cat Foods: The ingredients used in manufacturing cat foods may become contaminated in many ways. The levels of many of these contaminating substances are restricted by law, but usually at levels considered hazardous for humans. Generally speaking, cats become intoxicated at much lower levels than either humans or dogs. Consequently, cats may react to foods containing "safe" levels of contaminants. In particular, such substances as estrogens, chlorinated hydrocarbons and those with phenyl and cresyl bases are likely to be injurious.

General Considerations in Feeding Cats: Healthy cats eat a variety of foods. Being occasional feeders by nature, they may eat only about once every 24 hours. If fed more often, or continuously, they often become highly selective in what they eat. While odor, consistency, taste and learned dietary habits will determine which food a cat selects, such things as noises, lights, food containers, the presence or absence of man or other animals, and disease will determine how much food the cat will eat. Cats dissatisfied with their diet are quite capable of starving themselves. Conditions requiring dietary modifications are:

Stages of the life cycle: Growth, pregnancy and lactation require greatly increased nutrient intakes. Because growing kittens and pregnant and lactating queens cannot, physically, consume enough at one feeding to meet their daily needs, they should be fed several times a day.

Environment: Seasonal variations in temperature may require a cat to eat more during winter months. This is especially true of cats that remain outdoors year-round or at night.

Alterations in optimal body weight: Cats may become either underweight or overweight. The diet must supply a balanced nutrient intake and a properly augmented or reduced energy intake given if either condition is to be corrected.

Disease: Numerous diseases may require dietary changes. Any time the diet is so deficient as to cause disease the diet must, obviously, be changed to an adequate one. Diseases unrelated to deficiency may produce a more subtle, but equally important, dietary need. Among these are parasitic diseases, renal diseases, pancreatic diseases, hepatic diseases, gastrointestinal diseases and most metabolic disorders. (*See* FEEDING THE SICK CAT, p. 1392, NUTRITIONAL DEFICIENCIES IN CATS, p. 1418, and UROLITHIASIS, p. 868).

FUR ANIMAL NUTRITION

MINK

Although he wants optimal growth, quality fur development and top reproduction-lactation performance of his mink, the mink rancher must consider feedstuff availability and cost as well as nutritional balance of the diet. Modern ranch diets are formulated with a combination of fortified cereal, liver, muscle meats (horsemeat, nutria, rabbits, whole poultry), cooked eggs, packing house by-products (lung, rumen, spleen), poultry by-products (heads, feet, entrails) and fish (whole or fillet scrap). The fortified cereal provides digestible carbohydrates, and is a carrier for vitamin concentrates and trace minerals.

The ingredient formula of the practical ranch diet will vary from region to region depending upon the availability and economics of various ingredients. However, the nutrient content within the final dietary mixture will be relatively similar throughout the industry. Ash levels, largely derived from bone, of 7 to 8% on a dry-matter basis, provide ample calcium and phosphorus for the mink. Protein levels should be consistent with the energy concentration of the diet, i.e. a good 10 percentage points above the level of fat present (e.g. minimum of 35% protein in a diet containing 25% fat measuring each on a dry-matter basis).

It is important to stress the proper preparation and storage of fresh and frozen products. Bacteria in the finished feed must be kept to a minimum if top performance is to be expected. Spoiled, off-odor feed products cannot be tolerated by the mink.

Proper nutritional balance in terms of protein, fat and minerals is essential for top performance and minimum feed cost per pelt produced, hence feed analyses during each phase of the year are important (low-energy diets can be very expensive in terms of feed volume while excessive-energy diets may result in deficient intakes of essential nutrients).

There should be ample water at all times and ample feed provision for the mink. Feed may be restricted in late February, March and early April to keep animals trim for breeding and whelping but throughout the rest of the year the amount fed should be determined by the appetite of the animal. Mink may consume (on the average) as much as 8 to 10 oz (250 to 300 gm) of wet-mixed feed daily in the period from weaning to pelting. In the critical months of May and June they may be fed 2 to 3 times daily to meet the high nutritional demands for lactation and fast early growth of the young. Twice daily feeding in July and August is common, while once a day feeding is practical during the fur production months of September to December.

A typical ranch diet would contain 20% fortified cereal, 80% of fresh or frozen meat or fish products and enough water to provide a hamburger-like consistency which will hold up when fed on the cage wire. Common diets contain about ⅓ dry matter (feed solids) when fed to the mink on wire netting.

Nutrient requirements for the mink are given in TABLE 28. Water must be made available at all times via water cups, troughs or automatic pressure nipples. Starter feed for the young kits (about 3 weeks of age) should be like porridge with a high water content, and should be offered on a board, in the cage.

The National Research Council (NRC) recommendation for the after-weaning protein requirement is 25% on a dry-matter basis, most practical diets provide 35 to 40% protein in combination with 20 to 25% fat and 25 to 35% carbohydrate. A lean, high-protein diet with emphasis on cooked eggs, liver and muscle meats is used for the breeding-reproduction period from January into early May. Higher energy levels may be used during the lactation-early growth period (May-June) with higher levels of protein added to the high caloric density diets. For the late growing period of July and August, good growth and minimum feed volume may be achieved with a diet containing 20% fortified cereal in combination with 25% fat and 35 to 37% protein on a dry-matter basis. For the fur production period (September-December), many ranchers use a "leaner" diet (20 to 22% fat on a dry-matter basis) and place a stronger emphasis on quality proteins like cooked eggs and muscle meats.

In recent years diets have been formulated from dry ingredients such as meat and fish meals, blood meals and cereals that can either be mixed with water and fed on the wire, or offered as pellets in special feeders.

In planning diets, consideration must be given to a number of factors in addition to nutritional content of the feedstuff. Ranchers must avoid products containing diethylstilbestrol residues and must be careful to exclude thyroid and parathyroid tissues from the mink's diet. Many freshwater fish such as carp, bullheads and smelt as well as ocean herring (but not freshwater herring) contain a thiaminase enzyme which destroys vitamin B_1 and causes Chastek paralysis in the mink (q.v., p. 1167). High levels of Pacific hake and Atlantic hake or whiting should not be used inasmuch as their formaldehyde content may inhibit iron absorption and lead to the development of

TABLE 28. NUTRIENT REQUIREMENTS FOR MINK
(In percentage of dietary dry matter, or amount per kilogram of dry matter fed)

Nutrient	Growth (Weaning to pelting)	Maintenance (Mature)	Pregnancy	Lactation
Energy (Kcal ME/kg dry diet)	5,300	4,250	5,300	*
Protein, %	25			
Vitamins				
Vitamin A, IU	3,500			
Vitamin E, mg	25			
Thiamin, mg	1.2	1.1		
Riboflavin, mg	1.5			
Pantothenic acid, mg	6.0			
Niacin, mg	20			
Pyridoxine, mg	1.1			
Folic acid, mg	0.5			
Minerals				
Salt (NaCl), %	0.5	0.5	0.5	0.5
Calcium, %	0.4	0.3	0.4	0.6
Phosphorus, %	0.4	0.3	0.4	0.6
Ca:P ratio	1:1 to 2:1	1:1 to 2:1	1:1 to 2:1	1:1 to 2:1

* Energy requirements for lactation increase sharply with (a) number of young produced and (b) growth of the young. The recommended level for growth may be taken as basal and increased according to the above criteria.
From *Nutrient Requirements for Mink and Foxes*, National Research Council, 1968.

"cotton fur." Eggs must be cooked to denature the avidin, which would inhibit biotin absorption and lead to achromotrichia and alopecia.

Fresh or frozen liver is an excellent dietary supplement for top reproduction-lactation performance of the mink and should be fed at a 5 to 10% level (preferably the latter) during the period from March 1st into early June.

Commercial, fortified cereal products are generally quite digestible for the mink if they contain high proportions of cooked or toasted cereal grains. Most raw grains except oat groats must be heated in some way prior to incorporation in the diet, as the starches present in raw grains are relatively indigestible.

The quality of fat used is important throughout the year. Unsaturated fat (fish oils or horse fat) can cause a disease known as "yellow fat disease" unless the diet contains high levels of vitamin E. High levels of fat in the fall fur production months may contribute to a problem known as "wet belly disease" (q.v., p. 1169), in which soiling of the inguinal region with urine may cause pelt damage. The use of a lean diet in September and higher levels of fortified cereal in late fall (late October and November) will minimize this problem.

Mineral supplementation of the diet is not required if the rancher is using a quality, fortified cereal product. Diets containing 35 to

40% of bone-in products provide more than ample calcium and phosphorus for the needs of the mink. Extra salt supplementation (0.5% NaCl) may be used in the period from May 15th to late June to prevent the dehydration problem known as nursing anemia.

With the use of a quality fortified cereal, there is no need for extra vitamin supplementation unless the rancher is using high levels of fish scrap or rancid fish or horesmeat; such diets require a higher level of vitamin E. If the rancher is making his own cereal formulation, he may use commercial vitamin supplements with vitamin concentrations in the diet similar to those recommended by the NRC Sub-Committee on Fur Animal Nutrition. Vitamin A must be provided as the vitamin and not as β-carotene, which is inefficiently utilized by the mink.

CHINCHILLA

In their native habitat, chinchillas live at high elevations in the South American Andes. The flora in this region consists of coarse grasses. The chinchilla, a herbivore, developed a highly efficient digestive system in order to survive in those regions. It is said to have the largest cecum of any animal in proportion to its size, and the whole gastrointestinal tract is long.

Diets low in fiber, and containing large amounts of grains, nuts, meals, succulent grasses and other easily digested carbohydrates may cause bloat, diarrhea, prolapse or other digestive disturbances.

Chinchillas are naturally nocturnal and usually feed early in the evening or during the night. They can be raised successfully on a diet consisting of a good grade of rabbit pellets and hay, which should be adjusted to just the quantity they will clean up in one 24-hour period—about 10 to 15 gm of pellets a day. It is believed that chinchillas require from 14 to 16% plant protein in their diet. Variations from this level may lead to difficulty.

The animals should have hay before them at all times to supply the large quantity of roughage they require. The more hay they consume in proportion to the amount of pellets, the better. Several different kinds are being fed: alfalfa, timothy, bean straw and orchard grass or prairie hay. Although the chinchillas prefer alfalfa, there have been no controlled experiments to show which is superior. All of the hays should be fed dry and must not be moldy. The alfalfa and timothy hay should be clean, bright-green and with pliable stems. Alfalfa hay is prone to absorb moisture and will mold rapidly at the temperatures of many chinchilla houses. Dietary changes in hay should be gradual. The hay should not have been sprayed with commercial insecticides, such as chlordane, since chinchillas can tolerate only small quantities of such chemicals.

Only weak, debilitated animals require supplementary feeding. Such feeding to the entire herd may result in obesity in many of the ɪnimals. Various supplements may be chosen, depending on the ɪnimal's needs. Wheat germ meal is a good source of vitamin E and ıs palatable to chinchillas. It must, however, be stored in a clean, dry place or it will become rancid. Raisins, apples and prunes may stimulate the appetite as well as serving as supplementary sources of B vitamins and trace minerals. Small quantities of succulent green feeds, such as dandelion leaves and lawn clippings may be ısed to supply carotene or vitamin A. They should always be fed with (not in place of) dry hay, and they should be clean and free of ɪnimal wastes. Salt spools containing trace minerals may be provided. Animal protein or pellets containing cod or other fish oils should not be fed.

RABBIT NUTRITION

The rabbit is a nonruminant herbivore with certain unique characteristics of its digestive system. It has a monogastric digestive ract with a large, active cecum that supports a large population of ecal microorganisms. They utilize much undigested, unabsorbed naterial, primarily cellulose, as a source of nutrients to produce heir own typical cells and a number of nutritionally important byproducts. When the rabbit recycles this material as it does by conuming the soft feces (coprophagy), the normal digestion and aborption processes make available bacterially synthesized nutrients uch as protein, B-vitamins and volatile fatty acids. Some previously ound minerals become available also.

Rabbits digest cellulose poorly but need a generous amount of iber in their diets to promote intestinal motility. Caged rabbits have higher incidence of enteritis problems on low fiber diets than on igh ones, as exercise is restricted.

For growth, rabbits are dependent upon adequate intake of esential amino acids, but these have not yet been well-defined. A lietary supply of the fat soluble vitamins A, D and E is necessary. Bacteria in the gut synthesize vitamin K. Good rabbit feeds will upply most B-vitamins. The amount needed will depend upon the erformance rate desired or economically necessary. Disease and tress increase the daily vitamin requirements. Vitamins A and E re more easily destroyed through oxidation than the other vitanins; thus feed preparation and storage must be carried out to ninimize losses. Rabbits voluntarily adjust their feed intake to meet heir energy needs when appropriate feed is available. Pelleted abbit feeds have largely supplanted home-grown feeds and provide good nutrition at reasonable cost. A summary of suggested requirenents is provided in TABLE 29. Fresh, clean water should always be vailable. When rabbits are fed hay (alfalfa or clover) and grain (corn, oats, barley), a salt block with added trace minerals should be provided.

TABLE 29. REQUIREMENTS OF SOME NUTRIENTS FOR RABBITS

	Protein					
	Total %	Digestible %	Fat %	Fiber %	Digestible Carbo-hydrates (NFE, %)	Total Digestible Nutrients %
Maintenance	12	9	1.5-2.0	14-20	40-45	50-60
Growth and Fattening	16	12	2.0-4.0	14-16	45-50	60-70
Pregnancy	15	11	2.0-3.0	14-16	45-50	55-65
Lactation (with litter of 7 or 8)	17	13	2.5-3.5	12-14	45-50	65-75

NFE = nitrogen-free extract.

EXOTIC AND ZOO ANIMAL NUTRITION

Captive wild animals are cared for today by many individuals in addition to the more traditional zoos and institutional organizations and accumulated experience has greatly increased the opportunities for success. Particular care must be exercised with newly captured animals, which are susceptible to fright and shock, and attention to some simple management practices can minimize losses. Such practices include avoiding overcrowding; separating males, especially in company of females; use of bedding material over slippery flooring and removal or covering of sharp, projecting objects. Use of appropriate tranquilizing drugs or ataractics can aid in the adaptation of wild animals. Extremely excitable animals usually respond to proper holding and exhibit areas that are quiet and initially provide limited visual and auditory stimuli.

Basic to the continuing care of wild animals is attention to their dietary needs. Wild animals require the same basic nutrients as their domestic counterparts: carbohydrates and fats as sources of energy, proteins, minerals and vitamins and it is the translation of these requirements into practical and acceptable rations that varies from species to species. Zoos have historically been successful in maintaining the health of large herbivores, as these animals adapt readily to a variety of roughages and grain supplements. In contrast captive carnivores (both birds and mammals), primates and reptiles have suffered gross nutritional abuse. The problems in feeding such species have been aggravated by the biochemical and microbiological instability of fresh diet ingredients, and may be reduced by ubstituting preserved feedstuffs (canned, dried or frozen) in nutri-onally adequate mixtures. In the past, inadequate and inappropri-te nutritional programs have been blamed for advanced nutritional isease, physical deformities and early mortalities in from 25 to 75% f exotic carnivorous species imported as pets or for zoological isplay.

Problems are encountered when feeding large groups or mixed roups of species in insuring that each animal is eating the desired mount of the proper diet. A method to evaluate proper nutrition is measure the individuals' weight gain and loss at selected inter-als. This is especially important in young and growing animals for e overall evaluation of a specific diet. This information should be btained when the animals are handled or restrained for various iagnostic or therapeutic procedures. When appropriate a complete ostmortem examination is important to evaluate the nutritional atus of an individual.

The following tables should be used as guidelines; their use hould be flexible and reflect new information as it becomes avail-ble.

More recently, numerous commercially prepared diets have been pecifically designed for exotic species (monkey pellets, marmoset iet, feline canned diet or sausage and carnivore sausages, pellets r moose, deer and other herbivores as well as rodents, parrot ellets, mynah bird pellets, and omnivore foods). Such specific repared diets and commercial diets developed for the domestic or boratory animal trade have virtually eliminated the excuse for idespread nutritional disease in exotic pets or zoological speci-ens formerly fed mixtures of fresh foods cafeteria style. Commer-ally available human milk substitutes, bitch's milk, queen's milk, ilk replacer, and whole cow's milk may be used as diets in suck-ngs of appropriate species.

Trace mineral salt blocks or spools (95% NaCl) should be made vailable *ad libitum* to all species of terrestrial and arboreal mam-als and psittacine birds. The block should be securely affixed to e outside of the cage of large primates to prevent them from using as a missile.

Good quality hay is the basic ingredient in diets for most her-ivores, including antelope, buffalo, deer, elephants, giraffes, hip-opotami, rhinoceri and zebras. Either legume, such as alfalfa, or rass hay may be used; the former is usually considerably higher in lcium and protein contents. It is important that such hay should e reasonably green and leafy and free from mold, dirt and other ontaminants, including toxic weeds. Approximately 2 kg of hay for very 100 kg of body weight is a guide to estimate hay intake. alatability of hay may be increased by spraying it with a solution of olasses in water. The molasses should be discontinued if animals ow signs of diarrhea.

TABLE 30. SUGGESTED DIETS FOR ZOO ANIMALS
MAMMALS

Animal	Prepared or Additional Feeds	Meat	Egg	Milk	Greens	Bread	Apple	Orange	Banana	Sweet Potato	Carrot	Oatmeal	Corn	Bone Meal	Meal Worms	Alfalfa Hay	Timothy Hay	Apricots, Grapes, Prunes, Raisins
Monotremes																		
Echidna		+	R	+														
Marsupials																		
Virginia Opossum	Dog meal, pellets or canned dog food		+	+	+	+	+		+									
Tasmanian Devil	Canned dog food, young mice																	
Wombat	Equine pellets, rabbit pellets																	
Phalanger	Canned dog food, monkey pellets				+	+	+	+	+	+	+							
Kangaroo and Wallaby	Equine pellets, rabbit pellets															+		
Tree Kangaroo	Equine pellets, rabbit pellets				+	+	+		+	B	+	+						+
Insectivores																		
Hedgehog	Canned dog food, earthworms		B	+											+			

Philippine Tree Shrew	Canned marmoset diet		B		+				+		+				+			
Mole	Canned marmoset diet		B	+			+								+			
Solenodon	Crushed fruits and carrots, canned marmoset diet		R	+			+	+	+		+				+			
Carnivores																		
Cats	Canned feline diet, feline or carnivore sausage																	
Hyena	Canned feline diet, feline or carnivore sausage																	
Ringtail or Cacomistle	Dog pellets, canned feline diet		R				+	+	+					+				
Raccoon, Kinkajou and Coatimundi	Canned or semimoist dog food, dog pellets		R			+	+	+	+		+							
Genet, Civet, Skunk	Dog pellets, canned feline food or feline sausage		R				+		+									
Fox, Wolf	Dog pellets, semimoist dog food																	
Fennec Fox	Dog pellets, semimoist dog food						+		+									
Badger	Dog pellets, semimoist dog food			+														
Otter	*																	

R = raw B = boiled
* *See* SPECIAL MIXTURES FOR MAMMALS, Table 31.

continued on next page

MAMMALS (*Continued*)

Animal	Prepared or Additional Feeds	Meat	Egg	Milk	Greens	Bread	Apple	Orange	Banana	Sweet Potato	Carrot	Oatmeal	Corn	Bone Meal	Meal Worms	Alfalfa Hay	Timothy Hay	Apricots, Grapes, Prunes, Raisins
Giant Panda	*																	
Lesser Panda	*																	
Bear	Dog pellets; fish, omnivore diets	+				+	+				+							
Sea Lion	Fish (mackerel, herring; butterfish)																	
Rodents Squirrel, Marmot, Prairie Dog	Rabbit pellets, laboratory animal pellets, nuts, oats, sunflower seed				+	+	+	+	+		+		+			+		
Palm Squirrel	Rabbit pellets, laboratory animal pellets, sunflower seed, chopped fruits, dog pellets				+								+					
Kangaroo Rat, Pack Rat ...	Chopped fruits, dog pellets, rabbit pellets laboratory animal pellets				+	+							+			+		

Jerboa	Oats, millet seed, monkey pellets, laboratory animal pellets				+		+		+							+		
Beaver	Twigs and willow branches, rabbit pellets, laboratory animal pellets				+	+	+			+	+		+					
Porcupine	Dog pellets, branches (evergreen for American porcupines), rabbit pellets, laboratory animal pellets				+	+	+				+		+			+		
Hutia-conga	Rabbit pellets, laboratory animal pellets				+	+	+	+	+		+	+						
Agouti	Laboratory animal pellets, monkey pellets, rabbit pellets				+	+	+	+	+	+	+		+			+		
Paca	Oats				+	+	+		+	+	+		+			+		
Capybara	Oats, rabbit pellets, monkey pellets, laboratory animal pellets				+	+	+		+		+		+			+		
Edentates																		
Anteater	*																	
Armadillo	Canned dog food; meat, eggs and milk, mixed	+	R	+														
Sloth	Leaves and twigs				+	+	+	+	+		+							
Aardvark	*																	

R = raw B = boiled
* *See* SPECIAL MIXTURES FOR MAMMALS, Table 31.

continued on next page

MAMMALS (*Continued*)

Animal	Prepared or Additional Feeds	Meat	Egg	Milk	Greens	Bread	Apple	Orange	Banana	Sweet Potato	Carrot	Oatmeal	Corn	Bone Meal	Meal Worms	Alfalfa Hay	Timothy Hay	Apricots, Grapes, Prunes, Raisins
Even-Toed Hoofed Animals																		
Antelope	Herbivore pellets or dairy conditioner (morning and evening feeding)															+	+	
Deer	Moose and deer pellets				+		+				+					+	+	
Camel	Herbivore pellets and dairy conditioner				+		+				+					+	+	
Llama, Alpaca, Vicuna	Herbivore pellets and dairy conditioner				+		+				+					+	+	
Giraffe	Oats, dairy conditioner				+	+	+		+		+					+		
Hippopotamus	Equine pellets, dairy conditioner (equal parts)				+	+	+				+					+	+	
Odd-Toed Hoofed Animals																		
Zebra, Ass	Equine pellets, herbivore pellets				+		+				+						+	
Rhinoceros	Equine pellets, dairy conditioner				+	+					+					+	+	

Tapir	Equine pellets, dairy conditioner				+	+	+	+	+		+					+		
Elephant	Equine pellets, dairy conditioner				+	+	+				+					+	+	
Hydrax	Rabbit pellets, barley				+	+	+				+					+		
Primates Lemur	Rabbit pellets, (moistened), leaves, berries and flowers, small stems				+		+	+	+									
Slow Loris, Galago	Monkey pellets (moistened)		B	+	+	+	+	+	+		+					+		+
Gibbon, Baboon, Woolly Monkey, Macaque, Colobus, Grivet, Spider Monkey, Squirrel Monkey, Capuchin, Mangabey	Monkey pellets, semi-moist dog food		B	+	+	+	+	+	+	B	+					+		+
Marmoset	Boiled egg, monkey pellets, canned marmoset diet, lizards			+	+		+	+	+		+				+			
Tarsier	Grasshoppers, chameleons (*Anolis*); young mice, canned marmoset diet			+														
Gorilla, Orangutan	*monkey pellets	+	B	+	+	+	+	+	+	B	+			+		+		+

R = raw B = boiled
* *See* SPECIAL MIXTURES FOR MAMMALS, Table 31.

continued on next page

BIRDS

Bird	Prepared or Additional Feeds	Greens	Apple	Banana	Orange	Sweet Potato	Bread	Scratch Feed*	Millet, Canary, Wild Grass Seeds	Mackerel	Smelts	Minnows	Herring	Soft Food Mixt. I*	Carnivorous Bird Diet	Soft Food Mixt. II*
Koel			+	+	+											+
Owl	Whole or small rodents occasionally														+	
Frogmouth	Whole mice														+	
Nighthawk	Must be hand-fed														+	+
Trogon, Quetzal	Quetzal food*		+	+	+											
Kingfisher	Mice										+	+			+	
Laughing Jackass	Mice														+	
Motmot, Hornbill	Mice		+	+	+										+	+
Barbet, Toucan	Mice, meal worms, insects		+	+	+										+	+
Cock of the Rock	Young mice		+	+	+											+
Manakin, Pitta, Old World Oriole	Canned dog food for Pittas		+	+	+											+

Crow, Magpie, Jay	Young mice														+	+
Bower Bird, Bird of Paradise	Insects, grapes, young mice		+	+	+											+
Babbling Thrush																+
Tyrant Flycatcher	Insects															+
Bulbul, Mockingbird, Thrasher, Thrush	Insects		+	+	+											+
Shrike															+	+
Starling, Mynah	Mynah bird pellets		+	+	+											+
Honey Eater	Liquid food*			+	+											+
Sugar Bird	Liquid food*			+	+											+
Warbler	Many insects															+
Finch, Waxbill, American Oriole, Blackbird	Soft Food Mixt. II for orioles; insects, thistle seed	+	+	+	+				+							
Tanager	Liquid food*	+	+	+	+											+
Grosbeak, Finch	Seeds including sunflower seeds	+							+							+
Ostrich, Rhea, Emu, Cassowary	Game bird pellets, chopped alfalfa, ratite pellets, laboratory animal pellets, young mice	+													+	
Tinamou	Game bird pellets	+							+							+

C = chopped B = boiled

* *See* SPECIAL MIXTURES FOR BIRDS, Table 32.

BIRDS (*Continued*)

Bird	Prepared or Additional Feeds	Greens	Apple	Banana	Orange	Sweet Potato	Bread	Scratch Feed*	Millet, Canary, Wild Grass Seeds	Mackerel	Smelts	Minnows	Herring	Soft Food Mixt. I*	Carnivorous Bird Diet	Soft Food Mixt. II*
Penguins Emperor, King	2 drops of saturated solution KI and one 000 capsule cod-liver oil every other day. Also butterfish									+						
Humboldt, Ringed, Galapagos, Fairy											+					
Loon, Grebe	Butterfish										+	+				
Pelican	Butterfish									+	+		+			
Cormorant, Snake Bird	Butterfish										+		+			
Heron, Bittern, Stork	Butterfish										+	+			+	
Ibis, Spoonbill	Kibbled dog biscuit, ground carrots										C				+	
Flamingo	Flamingo mix*															
Screamer	Game bird pellets	+						+								
Duck, Goose, Swan	Game bird pellets, duck pellets	+						+								

Secretary Bird, Vulture, Hawk	Rats, mice, rabbits														+	
Galliformes including Guan, Grouse, Quail, Pheasant, Peacock	Game bird pellets, ground peanuts for quail	+						+	+							
Crane, Rail	Game bird pellets	+						+				+	C		+	
Gallinule, Sun Bittern	Chopped boiled egg	+									C			+	+	
Pigeon, Dove	Pigeon pellets	+						+	+							
Fruit Pigeon	Grapes, pigeon pellets		+	+	+											+
Gull, Tern, Avocet, Stilt, Plover	Cut butterfish									C	+		C	+	+	
Parrot, Macaw, Cockatoo	Carrots, sunflower, hemp, canary seeds, large millet seeds, oats, peanuts, parrot pellets, pigeon pellets, monkey pellets	+	+	+	+											
Lory, Lorikeet	Liquid food*, canary seed, parrot pellets, pigeon pellets	+	+	+	+											
Parakeet	Millet, oats, pigeon pellets	+	+	+	+				+							
Touraco, Cuckoo	Canned dog food, whole mice for some Cuckoos		+	+	+											+

C = chopped B = boiled
* *See* SPECIAL MIXTURES FOR BIRDS, Table 32.

REPTILES

Animal	Prepared or Additional Feeds	Canned Dog Food (all meat)	Fish	Smelt	Egg	Bread	Lettuce	Carrots, grated	Greens, chopped	Tomatoes (canned)	Apple	Banana	Melon
Alligator	Insects for immature; whole rodents for adults		+										
Crocodile	Insects for immature; whole rodents for adults		+										
Caiman	Insects for immature; whole rodents for adults		+										
Turtle, Tortoise Snapping Turtles	Insects	+	+										
Alligator Snapper			+										
Mud Turtle	Earthworms	+	+										
Box Turtle		+	+			+	+			+	+	+	+
Giant Tortoise		+				+	+		+	+	+	+	+
Snakes	Mice, rats, guinea pigs, rabbits, toads, frogs, lizards												

King Cobra	Eats only other snakes in captivity, e.g., water snakes												
Lizards													
Iguana	Mice, dandelions	+			+		+	+	+		+	+	
Gecko	Live insects												
Basilisk Lizard	Live insects	+			+			+	+		+	+	
Monitor	Day-old chicks	+	+		+								
Skink	Tomatoes occasionally	+			+					+			
Chameleon	Flies, grasshoppers, spiders (must be alive)												
Salamander	Meal worms, earthworms	+											
Electric Eel				+									

Branches and small limbs from unsprayed willow, poplar, mulberry, maple, or eucalyptus should be made available daily to gnawing forms of mammals (capybara, beaver, porcupine and small rodents) to maintain proper occlusion of the ever-growing incisors. Such material may also be offered to all species of primates as a form of low calorie constructive occupation. Alfalfa hay may be offered if continuous access to branches is not possible. Dental problems can occur in carnivora that receive only the soft prepared diets. The diet should be supplemented with bones, e.g. oxtails, to help control dental disease and provide recreational chewing.

Some species of fish fed to exotic mammals, birds and reptiles (smelt, herring and minnows) have high tissue levels of thiaminase. The method of handling and storage of these fish can alter the

TABLE 31. SPECIAL MIXTURES FOR MAMMALS

Otter

Daily:
- 2 lb fish
- ½ lb raw meat
- ½ lb mixture of ground meat, dog or mink food and bone meal, with vitamin-mineral concentrate added (minimum 10 mg thiamin/lb of fish).

Lesser Panda

Morning:
- 1 cup Pablum
- ½ cup evaporated milk
- ½ tsp honey
- 1 raw egg
- Vitamin-mineral concentrate

Evening:
- Cut fresh fruits
- Fresh bamboo sprays

Giant Panda

Morning:
- Formula as for Lesser Panda, increased quantity.

Evening:
- 6 apples
- 6 carrots
- 4 bananas
- 2 loaves of bread
- Greens (green soybeans, cornstalks in season and fresh bamboo sprays)
- 1 qt dog biscuits

Anteater, Aardvark, Aardwolf

Mix together:
- 4 boiled eggs
- 8 oz ground meat
- 8 oz evaporated milk
- 16 oz water
- 2 oz Pablum or canned dog food
- 8 oz dog pellets
- Multivitamin-mineral concentrate

Mix in blender for best acceptability.

Gorillas, Orangutans (4 to 6 years of age)

Morning:
- 1 to 2 pints skim milk and cereal (whole grain)
- 1 orange, 1 banana and 1 apple
- 2 tsp multivitamin-mineral preparation
- 2 cups gelatin dessert

Noon:
- 1 to 2 pints skim milk
- ½ cup cottage cheese
- 1 banana, 1 apple, 1 boiled sweet potato, 1 orange

Evening:
- 4 oz canned or ground meat
- 4 slices bread
- 2 bananas
- 4 apples
- 3 oranges
- Greens
- Sugarcane
- 3 prunes or dried apricots
- 6 raw carrots
- 3 boiled sweet potatoes
- 1 hard boiled egg
- 1 to 2 pints skim milk

thiaminase level and nutritional value. Either they should be cooked before mixing with other diet ingredients, or diets containing such fish should be supplemented with thiamin at 10 mg/lb (20 mg/kg) of fish to prevent the appearance of clinical thiamin deficiency (q.v., p. 1167 and p. 1354).

A source of potable water should be available 24 hours per day. Accidental dehydration occurs often in winter when water sources freeze over and during the heat of late summer when higher intakes are required.

Recommended foodstuffs for preparing a dietary program for an exotic pet or zoological specimen are listed in TABLES 31 and 32.

It should be stressed that a complete prepared product should be supplemented with only minimal amounts (10 to 15% of the total diet) of fresh foods. To reverse this, i.e. to offer the prepared diet only as a supplement to a great mound of fresh food, will produce poor results.

TABLE 32. SPECIAL MIXTURES FOR BIRDS

Scratch Feed

Oats
Cracked Corn
Kafir
Wheat

Quetzal Food

2 tbsp zwieback crumbs
2 tbsp steamed brown rice
2 tbsp grated carrot
1 tbsp grated hard boiled egg
1 tbsp cottage cheese
1 tbsp Pablum
½ tbsp brewer's yeast
15 drops cod-liver oil
Mix well and make into marble-sized pellets. Also feed diced bananas, grapes, cherries and raisins.

Soft Food Mixture I:

Puppy meal
Grated carrot
Dried flies
Powdered shrimp
Finely ground cooked meat

Soft Food Mixture II

A. ¾ gal. puppy meal finely ground. Mix 1 oz cod-liver oil with the meal.
¼ gal. dried flies.
Mix with the above 6 lb diced bananas, ⅓ lb grated apple and ½ head finely chopped lettuce or escarole.
B. 5 grated hard boiled eggs
1 cup steamed brown rice
1 cup grated carrot
C. Ground scalded heart.
Place a small portion of each on each feeding dish.

Liquid Food

A.M.
2 tsp honey
1 tsp Pablum
1 tsp condensed milk
Beef extract
3 drops vitamin concentrate
Water (q.s. ad 8 oz)
P.M.
Water } Equal parts
Honey }

Flamingo Diet

2 lb mixed, precooked cereal
9 lb trout Chow no. 4
1 cup oyster shell flour
1 tbsp iodized salt
1¼ cup brewer's dried yeast
3 lb shrimp meal, dried
8 cups Super Caradee
4 cups laying mash
Mix well with 4 gal. water to soupy consistency. (1 day's ration for 25 birds)

POULTRY NUTRITION

NUTRIENT REQUIREMENTS

Poultry place high in their ability to convert feed into food, and this efficiency in feed conversion has been greatly increased in recent decades. The nutrient requirement figures in the seventh revision of *Nutrient Requirements of Poultry* published by the National Academy of Sciences (1977) are derived from experimentally determined levels found to be adequate for normal growth, health, productivity and quality of product. While the requirement figures should cover most populations, such factors as varying nutrient composition of feed ingredients and differing feed mixing and storage conditions may reduce nutrient levels to below those intended. Because of this and since such factors as high environmental temperature may increase nutrient needs, the feed formulator may wish to add "margins of safety" by increasing the levels suggested in TABLES 33 to 38, shown below. These requirements are in terms of percentages or units per kilogram of feed, which accords with customary practice.

ENERGY, PROTEIN AND AMINO ACIDS

The metabolizable energy (ME) requirement values are corrected to nitrogen equilibrium as most poultrymen and feed manufacturers express available energy for poultry diets on this basis. These values are apparent metabolizable energy (AME) values as they have not been corrected for metabolic fecal energy or endogenous urinary energy. Under practical conditions, where birds are consuming close to maximum intake levels, the correction for metabolic and endogenous energy is very small in relation to energy intake and hence AME values differ little from the true metabolizable energy (TME) values, which are corrected for these energy losses. Where feed intake is appreciably below normal, AME values can be significantly lower than TME values. Under practical conditions, TME values are 1.097 times the optimal AME value. Hence the TME requirement of a bird is also 1.097 times its AME requirement. It is difficult to establish energy requirements per unit of feed since birds adjust their feed intake in an attempt to satisfy energy needs. Protein requirements are usually stated in relation to the energy level of the diet. However, since environmental temperature can have a marked effect on the birds' requirement for energy, and dietary energy level influences the degree of fat deposition in a bird, the optimal calorie:protein ratio varies depending on a given situation. The calorie:protein ratio concept extends also to amino acids. Some of the amino acid requirement figures in TABLES 33 and 34 were established by direct experimentation while other values

TABLE 33. ENERGY, PROTEIN AND AMINO ACID REQUIREMENTS OF CHICKENS

	Broilers			Replacement Pullets (Egg or Meat Type)			Laying and Breeding Hens
	0-3 wk	3-6 wk	6-9 wk	0-6 wk	6-14 wk	14-20 wk	(Egg or Meat Type)
Metabolizable energy (Kcal/kg)	3,200	3,200	3,200	2,900	2,900	2,900	2,850
Protein (%)	23	20	18	18	15	12	15
Arginine (%)	1.4	1.2	1.0	1.0	0.83	0.67	0.8
Glycine and/or serine (%)	1.5	1.0	0.7	0.7	0.58	0.47	0.5
Histidine (%)	0.35	0.3	0.26	0.26	0.22	0.17	0.22
Isoleucine (%)	0.80	0.7	0.60	0.60	0.50	0.40	0.5
Leucine (%)	1.35	1.18	1.00	1.00	0.83	0.67	1.2
Lysine (%)	1.20	1.00	0.85	0.85	0.60	0.45	0.6
Methionine + Cystine (%)	0.93	0.72	0.60	0.60	0.50	0.40	0.50
Methionine (%)	0.50	0.38	0.32	0.32	0.27	0.21	0.27
Phenylalanine + Tyrosine (%)	1.34	1.17	1.0	1.0	0.83	0.67	0.8
Phenylalanine (%)	0.72	0.63	0.54	0.54	0.45	0.36	0.4
Threonine (%)	0.75	0.65	0.56	0.56	0.47	0.37	0.4
Tryptophan (%)	0.23	0.20	0.17	0.17	0.14	0.11	0.11
Valine (%)	0.82	0.72	0.62	0.62	0.52	0.41	0.5

TABLE 34. ENERGY, PROTEIN AND AMINO ACID REQUIREMENTS OF TURKEYS*

	Age (wk)						Breeders	
	Male 0-4 Female 0-4	4-8 4-8	8-12 8-11	12-16 11-14	16-20 14-17	20-24 17-20	Holding	Mature
Metabolizable energy (Kcal/kg)	2,800	2,900	3,000	3,100	3,200	3,300	2,900	2,900
Protein (%)	28	26	22	19	16.5	14	12	14
Arginine (%)	1.6	1.5	1.25	1.1	0.95	0.8	0.6	0.6
Glycine and/or serine (%)	1.0	0.9	0.8	0.7	0.6	0.5	0.4	0.5
Histidine (%)	0.58	0.54	0.46	0.39	0.35	0.29	0.25	0.3
Isoleucine (%)	1.1	1.0	0.85	0.75	0.65	0.55	0.45	0.5
Leucine (%)	1.9	1.75	1.5	1.3	1.1	0.95	0.5	0.5
Lysine (%)	1.7	1.6	1.35	1.0	0.8	0.65	0.5	0.6
Methionine + Cystine (%)	1.05	0.90	0.75	0.65	0.55	0.45	0.4	0.4
Methionine (%)	0.53	0.45	0.38	0.33	0.28	0.23	0.2	0.2
Phenylalanine + Tyrosine (%)	1.80	1.65	1.4	1.20	1.05	0.90	0.8	1.0
Phenylalanine (%)	1.00	0.9	0.8	0.7	0.60	0.50	0.4	0.55
Threonine (%)	1.00	0.93	0.79	0.68	0.59	0.50	0.4	0.45
Tryptophan (%)	0.26	0.24	0.2	0.18	0.15	0.13	0.10	0.13
Valine (%)	1.2	1.1	0.94	0.80	0.70	0.60	0.50	0.58

* Adapted from *Nutrient Requirements of Poultry*. National Research Council, Revised 1977.

were calculated, assuming the amino acid requirements to be proportional to protein requirements.

The amino acids shown in TABLE 33 are considered to be essential for poultry. While glycine can be synthesized by poultry there must be enough dietary serine present to provide for this need.

TABLE 35. VITAMIN, MINERAL AND LINOLEIC ACID REQUIREMENTS OF CHICKENS[1]
(In percentage or amount per kilogram of feed)

	Starting Chickens (0-8 wk)	Growing Chickens (8-10 wk)	Breeding Hens	Laying Hens
Vitamin A activity (IU)	1,500	1,500	4,000	4,000
Vitamin D (ICU)[2]	200	200	500	500
Vitamin E (IU)	10	5	5	10
Vitamin K_1 or equivalent activity (mg)	0.5	0.5	0.5	0.5
Thiamin (mg)	1.8	1.3	0.8	0.8
Riboflavin (mg)	3.6	1.8	2.2	3.8
Pantothenic acid (mg)	10	10	2.2	10
Niacin (mg)	27	11	10[3]	10[3]
Pyridoxine (mg)	3	3	3	4.5
Biotin (mg)	0.15	0.10	0.10	0.15
Choline (mg)[4]	1,300	500	500	500
Folacin, starch diet (mg)	0.55	0.25	0.25	0.35
Folacin, sugar diet	1.2	?	?	?
Vitamin B_{12} (mg)	0.009	0.003	0.003	0.003
Linoleic acid (%)	1.0	0.8	1.0	1.0
Calcium (%)	0.9	0.6	3.25	2.75
Phosphorus (%)[5]	0.7	0.4	0.5	0.5
Sodium (%)[6]	0.15	0.15	0.15	0.15
Potassium (%)	0.2	0.16	0.1	0.1
Manganese (mg)	55	25	25	33
Iodine (mg)	0.35	0.35	0.30	0.30
Magnesium (mg)	600	400	500	500
Iron (mg)	80	40	50	80
Copper (mg)	4	3	3	4
Zinc (mg)	40	35	50	65
Selenium (mg)	0.1	0.1	0.1	0.1
Chlorine (mg)	800	800	800	800

[1] These figures are estimates of requirements and include no margins for safety.

[2] See text, page 1380. These levels of vitamin D are satisfactory when levels of calcium and readily available phosphorus conform to this table.

[3] In diet that contains 0.15% of tryptophan.

[4] See text, page 1381.

[5] At least 0.4% of the total feed of starting chickens should be inorganic phosphorus. All the phosphorus of nonplant feed ingredients is considered to be inorganic. Approximately 30% of the phosphorus of plant products is non-phytin phosphorus and may be considered part of the inorganic phosphorus required. A portion of the phosphorus requirement of growing chickens and laying and breeding hens must also be supplied in inorganic form. For birds in these categories the requirement for inorganic phosphorus is lower and is not as well defined as for starting chickens.

[6] Equivalent to 0.37% of sodium chloride.

Adapted from *Nutrient Requirements of Poultry*, National Research Council, Revised 1977.

Cystine and tyrosine are considered essential even though they can be replaced by methionine and phenylalanine, respectively. There are 2 important relationships between individual amino acids and vitamins in practical feed formulation; methionine can spare choline as a methyl donor, and tryptophan can be used to synthesize niacin. These are practically important interrelationships since the 2 vitamins can be supplied in diets more economically than the 2 amino acids.

A number of feeding programs have been devised to restrict energy, protein and amino acid intakes of replacement pullets to

TABLE 36. VITAMIN, LINOLEIC ACID AND MINERAL REQUIREMENTS OF TURKEYS[1]
(In percentage or amount per kilogram of feed)

	Starting Poults (0-8 wk)	Growing Turkeys (8 wk - market)	Breeding Turkeys
Vitamin A activity (IU)	4,000	4,000	4,000
Vitamin D (ICU)[2]	900	900	900
Vitamin E (IU)	12	10	25
Vitamin K_1 or equivalent activity (mg)	1.0	0.8	1.0
Thiamine (mg)	2.0	2.0	2.0
Riboflavin (mg)	3.6	3.0	4.0
Pantothenic acid (mg)	11	9	16
Niacin (mg)	70	50	30
Pyridoxine (mg)	4.5	3.5	4.0
Biotin (mg)	0.2	0.1	0.15
Choline (mg)	1,900	1,100	1,000
Folacin (mg)	1.0	0.8	1.0
Vitamin B_{12} (mg)	0.003	0.003	0.003
Linoleic acid (%)	1.0	0.8	1.0
Calcium (%)	1.2	0.8	2.25
Phosphorus (%)[3]	0.8	0.7	0.70
Sodium (%)[4]	0.15	0.15	0.15
Potassium (%)	0.4	0.4	0.4
Manganese (mg)	55	25	35
Magnesium (mg)	500	500	500
Iron (mg)	60	40	60
Copper (mg)	6	4	6
Iodine (mg)	0.4	0.4	0.4
Zinc (mg)	75	40	65
Selenium (mg)	0.2	0.2	0.2
Chlorine (mg)	800	800	800

[1] These figures are estimates of requirements and include no margins for safety.

[2] See text, page 1380. These levels of vitamin D are satisfactory when levels of calcium and readily available phosphorus conform to this table.

[3] At least 0.4% of the total feed of starting chickens should be inorganic phosphorus. All the phosphorus of nonplant feed ingredients is considered to be inorganic. Approximately 30% of the phosphorus of plant products is non-phytin phosphorus and may be considered part of the inorganic phosphorus required. Presumably, a portion of the requirement of growing and breeding turkeys must also be furnished in inorganic form.

[4] Equivalent to 0.37% of sodium chloride.

Adapted from *Nutrient Requirements of Poultry,* National Research Council, Revised 1977.

TABLE 37. NUTRIENT REQUIREMENTS OF PHEASANTS AND QUAIL[1]
(In Percentage or Amount per Kilogram of Feed)

Nutrient	Pheasants		Bobwhite Quail		Japanese Quail	
	Starting	(6-20 wk) Growing	Starting and Growing	Breeding	Starting and Growing	Breeding
Metabolizable energy (Kcal/kg)	2,800	2,700	2,800	2,800	3,000	2,800
Protein (%)	30[2]	16	28[3]	24	24[4]	24
Lysine (%)	1.5	0.8	1.4	0.7	1.4	1.1
Methionine + cystine (%)	1.0	0.6	0.9	0.6	0.75	0.8
Glycine + serine (%)	1.8	1.0	1.6	0.9	1.7	0.9
Vitamin A (IU)	3,000	3,000	3,000	3,000	5,000	5,000
Vitamin D (ICU)	1,200	900	900	900	480	1,200
Riboflavin (mg)	3.5	2.6	3.8	4.0	4.0	4.0
Pantothenic acid (mg)	10	10	12.6	15	10	15
Niacin (mg)	60	40	31	20	40	20
Choline (mg)	1,500	1,000	1,500	1,000	2,000	1,500
Linoleic acid (%)	1.0	1.0	1.0	1.0	1.0	1.0
Calcium (%)	1.0	0.7	0.65	2.3	0.8	2.5
Chlorine (%)	0.11	0.11	0.11	0.15	0.15	0.15
Phosphorus (%)[5]	0.8	0.6	0.65	1.0	0.65	0.8
Sodium (%)	0.1	0.1	0.085	0.15	0.15	0.15
Iodine (mg)	0.3	0.3	0.30	0.30	0.30	0.30
Magnesium (mg)	600	400	600	400	150	500
Manganese (mg)	90	70	90	70	90	70
Zinc (mg)	60	50	50	50	25	50

[1] These figures are estimates of requirements and include no margins of safety. For nutrients not listed see requirements for turkeys as a guide.
[2] At energy level of 2,800 Kcal of metabolizable energy per kilogram of feed.
[3] May be reduced to 20% at 6 weeks of age.
[4] May be reduced to 20% at 3 weeks of age.
[5] At least 0.3% of the total feed should be inorganic phosphorus as defined in TABLES 35 and 36.
From *Nutrient Requirements of Poultry*, National Research Council, Revised 1977.

retard growth and to delay the onset of sexual maturity in order to obtain optimal results in the laying and breeding periods. These systems are particularly important for broiler-strain pullets. Restricted feed programs are also used to limit the energy intake of hens during the laying period. Not only does such a practice result in a saving in feed costs but also an enhancement in performance is noted, especially with broiler breeders.

VITAMINS

Vitamin requirements are presented in TABLES 35, 36, 37 and 38 in terms of milligrams per kilogram of diet except in the case of vitamins A, D and E, which are given given in International Units (IU) or International Chick Units (ICU).

One IU of vitamin A activity is equivalent to 0.6 mcg of β-carotene; 1 mg of β-carotene = 1,667 IU of vitamin A. In the chicken, as in the rat, 0.6 mcg of β-carotene is equivalent to one USP unit of vitamin A, except when the carotene intake provides vitamin A activity greatly in excess of the requirement. The vitamin A requirements recommended herein are based on the use of stabilized vitamin A preparations and are thus somewhat lower than previously recommended levels.

Requirements for vitamin D are expressed in ICU. Birds use vitamin D_3 from fish oils and irradiated animal sterol quite effectively, but vitamin D_2 from irradiated ergosterol is less efficacious

TABLE 38. NUTRIENT REQUIREMENTS OF DUCKS AND GEESE[1]
(In percentage or amount per kilogram of feed)

Nutrient	Ducks		Geese		
	Starting	Growing	Starting (0-6 wk)	Growing (after 6 wk)	Breeding
Metabolizable energy (Kcal/kg)	2,900	2,900	2,900	2,900	2,900
Protein (%)	16[2]	15	22	15	15
Lysine (%)	0.9	0.7	0.9	0.6	0.6
Methionine + cystine (%)	0.8	0.55	—	—	—
Vitamin A (IU)	4,000	4,000	1,500	1,500	4,000
Vitamin D (ICU)	220	500	200	200	200
Riboflavin (mg)	4	4	4	2.5	4
Pantothenic acid (mg)	11	10	—	—	—
Niacin (mg)	55	40	55	35	20
Pyridoxine (mg)	2.6	3	—	—	—
Calcium (%)	0.6	2.75	0.8	0.6	2.25
Phosphorus (%)	0.6	0.6	0.6	0.4	0.6
Sodium (%)	0.15	0.15	—	—	—
Manganese (mg)	40	25	—	—	—
Magnesium (mg)	500	500	—	—	—

[1] For nutrients not listed see requirements of chickens as a guide.
[2] Increasing protein level to 22% for the first 2 weeks will increase early growth.

for birds than for mammals. In recent years more active forms of vitamin D have been isolated and synthesized. These are 25-OH vitamin D_3, which is synthesized in the liver and 1,25-$(OH)_2D_3$ which is synthesized in the kidney. One ICU of vitamin D represents the vitamin D activity of 0.025 mcg of pure vitamin D_3.

One IU of **vitamin E** is equivalent to 1 mg of synthetic DL-α-tocopherol acetate The requirements of vitamin E will vary depending upon the type and level of fat in the diet, the level of selenium, the levels of trace minerals and the presence or absence of antioxidants other than vitamin E.

The growing chicken can use **betaine** as a methylating agent, but betaine cannot replace **choline** in preventing perosis. Betaine is widely distributed in practical feedstuffs and may be important as a sparer of choline. **Vitamin B_{12}** can also reduce the requirement of the chick for choline. The choline requirement values presented are applicable to diets containing the specific levels of vitamin B_{12}.

MINERALS

The calcium requirement of laying hens is difficult to define. Adding too much calcium to diets interferes with the utilization of several other minerals and fat, and tends to reduce the palatability of the diet and to cause roughening of the egg shells. The recommended level of 3.25% for laying birds is adequate for most conditions but hens subjected to high environmental temperature or high producing hens in the later stage of egg production may require slightly elevated levels.

UNIDENTIFIED NUTRIENTS

The chick is known to have a quantitative requirement for 39 nutrients, including metabolizable energy. There is evidence that there may still be some unidentified growth and hatchability factors which, under certain stress conditions are required for maximum performance.

ANTIBIOTICS

Antibiotics have been used in poultry feeds since 1950 as a means of increasing growth rate and improving feed efficiency. They are still effective for this purpose and are used at a level of 2 to 10 mg/kg of feed depending on the antibiotic used. However, in some countries regulations now restrict this usage for certain antibiotics, and care should be taken to comply.

FEED REQUIRED FOR GROWTH AND EGG PRODUCTION

Data on the amounts of feed required and time required to attain certain weights in pullets and turkeys are presented in TABLES 39 and 40. The values are typical for the breeds under consideration.

The figures in TABLES 39 and 40 are intended merely as a guide

TABLE 39. GROWTH RATE AND FEED INTAKE OF PULLETS*

Age in weeks	egg-strain pullets				meat-strain pullets			
	Average body wt		Feed consumed per bird to date		Average body wt		Feed consumed per bird to date	
	(kg)	(lb)	(kg)	(lb)	(kg)	(lb)	(kg)	(lb)
2	0.14	0.3	0.18	0.4	0.18	0.40	0.23	0.5
4	0.23	0.5	0.50	1.1	0.41	0.90	0.73	1.6
6	0.36	0.8	0.86	1.9	0.68	1.50	1.45	3.2
8	0.50	1.1	1.41	3.1	1.00	2.20	2.27	5.0
10	0.64	1.4	2.00	3.3	1.18	2.60	3.14	6.9
12	0.77	1.7	2.68	5.9	1.36	3.00	4.09	9.0
14	0.91	2.0	3.41	7.5	1.55	3.40	5.00	11.0
16	1.05	2.3	4.23	9.3	1.73	3.80	5.91	13.0
18	1.18	2.6	5.00	11.0	1.41	4.20	7.05	15.5
20	1.27	2.8	5.91	13.0	2.09	4.60	7.95	17.5
22	1.41	3.1	6.81	15.0	2.27	5.00	8.64	19.0

In order to obtain these weights and feed consumption, some type of nutrient restriction usually has to be employed.

* From *Poultry Nutrition Handbook*, Ontario Ministry of Agriculture and Food, 1978.

in estimating the amount of feed required for a particular purpose. Considerable variation from the figures presented may result from differences in the nutrient density of feed, the strain or breed used, the amount of feed wasted, and the environmental temperature.

FEEDING AND MANAGEMENT PRACTICES

Most of the diets used in feeding poultry are commercially mixed rather than home-mixed; in general they are prepared by feed manufacturing companies, most of which employ trained nutritionists. The formulation and mixing of poultry feeds is a highly technical job involving the use of an increasing amount of knowledge and experience in purchasing ingredients, the use of computers, experimental testing of formulas and laboratory control of ingredient quality. Improper mixing can result in vitamin and mineral deficiencies, lack of protection against disease or chemical or drug toxicity.

The physical form of the feed exerts an important bearing on the results to be expected. Most feeds for starting and growing birds are sold in the form of crumbles or pellets. The pelleting process involves treating the mash with steam and then passing the hot, moist mash through a suitably sized die under pressure. The pellets are then cooled quickly and dried by means of a forced air draft. The conditions used in pelleting have an important bearing on the nutritional quality of the pellets, or the crumbles that result from rolling the pellets.

METHODS OF FEEDING

"All-mash" rations, or so-called "complete" feeds are, in general, those that are to be used without supplementation with whole grain

As intimated above, "all-mash" may in fact be in the form of crumbles or pellets and not mash so that the designation "complete" feeds is perhaps more correct. For newly hatched or starting birds of any species, the use of a "complete" feed in crumble form is the program of choice regardless of other considerations. The use of "complete" feed programs for growing stock, and particularly for laying and breeding stock, is also highly recommended. Among the advantages of the complete-feed program over the "mash and grain" system are the simplicity of feeding, accuracy of medication, improved balance of dietary nutrients, and superior feed conversion efficiency.

Regardless of the system of feeding employed, the poultryman should follow the recommendations of the feed manufacturer with regard to the feeding of extra calcium, grit or whole grain. Plenty of fresh, clean water should be available at all times.

MANAGEMENT OF GROWING CHICKENS

Chicks are brooded in pens in which a portion has been fenced off with plastic and brought up to a comfortable temperature or are placed under heated brooders encircled with a chick guard to keep the birds near the source of heat. As the birds become older the pen or brooder temperature is dropped and the plastic curtain or chick guard is moved out until the birds finally have the run of the whole pen. Plenty of feeder and watering space should be available and should be well distributed in the pen.

TABLE 40. GROWTH RATE, FEED EFFICIENCY AND FEED CONSUMPTION OF LARGE WHITE TURKEYS*

Age (weeks)	Hens				Toms			
	Average weight per bird		Feed consumed per bird to date		Average weight per bird		Feed consumed per bird to date	
	(kg)	(lb)	(kg)	(lb)	(kg)	(lb)	(kg)	(lb)
2	0.21	0.48	0.28	0.61	0.28	0.62	0.35	0.78
4	0.65	1.42	0.95	2.09	0.75	1.65	1.06	2.34
6	1.45	3.20	2.32	5.12	1.68	3.70	2.66	5.85
8	2.32	5.11	4.13	9.10	2.82	6.30	4.90	10.79
10	3.36	7.40	6.59	14.50	4.20	9.25	7.70	16.93
12	4.24	9.32	9.28	20.41	5.45	12.00	11.29	24.84
14	5.14	11.30	12.38	27.23	6.82	15.00	15.41	33.90
16	5.82	12.81	15.72	34.59	8.14	17.90	20.01	44.03
18	6.45	14.20	19.30	42.46	9.45	20.80	25.34	55.74
20	7.09	15.60	22.76	50.08	10.77	23.70	31.24	84.78
22	7.45	16.40	26.46	58.22	12.27	27.00	38.54	68.73
24	7.95	17.50	29.67	65.28	13.45	29.60	45.72	100.60
26	—	—	—	—	14.55	32.00	53.09	116.80

In order to obtain these weights and feed consumption, some type of nutrient restriction usually has to be employed.

*From *Poultry Nutrition Handbook*, Ontario Ministry of Agriculture and Food, 1978.

At least 3 in. (7.5 cm) of suitable litter, spread to an even depth, is provided at the start. Litter must be free from mold; it should be able to absorb moisture without caking, be nontoxic and of large enough particle size to discourage its being eaten. Clean litter should be used for each brood. Chicks are started with 24 hours light, and thereafter given at least ½ hour of darkness each 24 hours to get them used to lights going out. Both length of day and intensity of light are important considerations. In general during rearing, length of day should never be decreased. Feeding systems are often combined with day-length control during rearing to influence the rate at which birds mature. Where light intensity cannot be controlled, pullets should be debeaked at 4 to 7 days of age. In controlled environment housing, with dim lights, this job may be delayed until later in the growing period.

Pullets should be treated for external and internal parasites as required. Vaccination can control many diseases and should be utilized for the problem diseases of the area (*see* the infectious diseases portion of the poultry section, p. 1055 *et seq.* for details).

MANAGEMENT OF LAYING CHICKENS

Most laying pullets are now housed in cages and they should be moved to these facilities at least a week before egg production commences. If breeders are to be moved from a growing to an adult house they should also be given at least a week to adjust to their new environment before the stress of egg production commences. Beaks should be retrimmed as necessary and culls removed at time of housing.

Feeders should be of the proper type, size and height for the stock and management system. Feeders that are too shallow, too narrow or lack a lip or flange on the upper edge may permit excessive wastage of feed.

Artificial Lights: Sufficient light should be used to provide an average 14- to 16-hour light period daily for both market egg and hatching egg layers. An intensity of at least one foot-candle of light at the feed trough (10.76 lux) should be provided; this is approximately equal to one 60-watt light bulb to each 100 sq ft (about 9 sq m), hanging 7 ft (2 m) above the birds. Production may be impaired if light intensity is reduced during the laying period. With cage systems of all types, more even illumination is achieved by using smaller wattage bulbs closer together rather than large bulbs suspended over the center of each aisle. With 2- or 3-tiered cages, the bulbs are suspended at a height 6 to 7 in. (15 cm) above the level of the top cage.

Record Keeping: To be successful in intensive poultry keeping,

TABLE 41. SPACE REQUIREMENTS FOR EGG-STRAIN BIRDS

CAGES

Age in Weeks	Floor Area per Bird		Straight Trough Feeder Space per Bird Not Less Than		Birds per Nipple	Birds per Cup	Trough Space per Bird	
	sq in.	sq cm	in.	cm			in.	cm
0-6	25	156	1.0	2.5	15	25	1.0	2.5
7-18	43	277	2.0	5.0	8	12	1.0	2.5
19 onward	60	388	3.0	7.5	8	12	2.0	5.0

LITTER AND SLATS

Age in Weeks	Floor Area—Litter Only or Combined With Slats		Straight Trough Feeder Space per Bird		Pans (15″ Dia.) per 100 Birds		Drinkers		
							Birds per Fount	Trough per Bird	
	Sq ft/bird	Birds/ Sq meter	in.	cm	Full Fed	Restricted		in.	cm
0-6	0.5	20	1.0	2.5	3	—	100	1.0	2.5
7-13	1.0	10	2.0	5.0	4	5	50	1.0	2.5
19 onward	1-1.5	7-10	3.0	7.5	4	—	30	2.0	5.0

records should be kept of everything that happens to the flock including such things as hatch date, regular body weights, quantity and type of feed given, mortality (so that amount of feed to be given can be accurately calculated), disease history, medications, vaccination dates, light program and pen temperatures.

Floor Space, Feeding and Watering Requirements: There is a trend to house egg-production and even broiler stock in cages right from the start. For broiler breeders, buildings with up to ⅔ slatted floor area have distinct advantages over all-litter types. For egg-strain pullets reared from day of age to end of egg-production cycle in cages, there is little chance of altering the feeding and watering space available, but periodic checks are necessary to ensure that feed and water are being continuously supplied. With the success of nipple- and cup-type waterers and the various types of automatic feeding arrangements it becomes more difficult to give specific recommendations for feeding and watering space. The poultryman must make the decisions as to proper floor space and feeding and watering requirements based on advice from equipment manufacturers, careful observation, and past experience as to profitability.

The space requirements for egg-strain and meat-strain birds set forth in TABLES 41 and 42 will serve as a useful guide.

TABLE 42. SPACE REQUIREMENTS FOR MEAT-STRAIN BIRDS

Age	Floor Space	Feeder Space*	Cups or Founts* (per 1,000 birds)
From Day 1	Heated area 5 sq ft (0.46 sq meter) of brooder per 100 chicks	10 trays per 1,000 (feed little and often)	8
From Week 1	1 sq ft per bird (10-11 birds per sq meter)	2 in. (5 cm) per bird	20
From Week 8	2 sq ft per bird (5-6 birds per sq meter)	4 in. (10 cm) per bird	30
Mated Adults	All litter: 3 sq ft per bird (3.6 birds per sq meter)	4 in. (10 cm) per bird	30 (60 in hot weather)
	½ to ⅔ slats: 2¼ sq ft per bird (4.3 birds per sq meter)		

* For feeder and drinking trough space, count both sides of the trough. Drinking trough space (all ages) is 1 in. (2.5 cm) per bird, except double this for adults in hot weather.

Pen Size: The smaller the pen population the better the average flock performance. The ideal flock size depends on several factors, including labor and cost and can only be determined by the individual poultryman.

NUTRITION OF SICK ANIMALS

The response of sick animals to certain rations or specific nutrints will depend on the nature and duration of the illness. Two asic aspects must be considered: (1) determining and eliminating he cause of the illness, and (2) supplying the necessary nutrients which will facilitate, as rapidly as possible, a return to health and fficient production. Nutrition of sick animals requires clinical wisom, knowledge of disease processes and applications of the prinliples of medicine and nutrition.

asic Considerations: In general, well-fed animals are more resistnt to bacterial and parasitic infections but are probably more suseptible to viral infections. Good nutrition is of value during the ecovery phase of any disease process, whether it be of viral, bacteal or toxic origin. Diseases that precipitate inappetence, vomiting, iarrhea and high fever cause the greatest depletion of nutrients om the body. Efforts should be directed to minimizing nutritional epletion. Feeds and nutrients that improve appetite and restore sses from the digestive tract are most important. Specific theraeutic diets should be considered in distinct entities such as a lowodium diet in cardiovascular disease, a low-fat diet in pancreatic isturbances and the use of lipotropic nutrients such as choline and ethionine in liver diseases. It is also important to understand the cause and effect" relationship characterizing nutritional therapy. ven though a nutrient markedly influences recovery from an illess, it may be erroneous to conclude that the original disturbance as due to a nutritional deficiency.

eneral Principles: Nutritional therapy consists of providing a noral ration modified to provide for the nutrients lost during the ourse of the disease, and if necessary, to increase its palatability.
The oral route is the method of choice for administering nutrients. there is complete anorexia, nutrients may be given in warm water y stomach tube. Parenteral therapy to provide immediate nourishent is indicated in prostrate animals. Depending on the nature of e illness some general principles to consider are:

Restoration of appetite: Because inappetence accompanies many lnesses, palatability assumes a particular importance. Ruminants ill often eat good-quality roughage, including green forage, when ey will not consume concentrate mixtures. Rations high in urea ot only tend to be unpalatable but may also be toxic in sick animals. lso in ruminants, factors required in rumen fermentation such as e mineral elements, especially cobalt, should be fed. Inoculation the rumen with cud material may be helpful in chronic disturnces of the rumen. Sweetening rations with a small amount of molasses will often induce feed consumption. Small amounts of fresh feed every few hours is better practice than a large amount at one feeding. Most feed not readily consumed should be removed before the next feeding as it may become stale and unpalatable. Housing sick animals in close proximity to animals eating normally will often encourage feed consumption. Parenterally administered glucose, protein hydrolysates, vitamin B_{12} and other vitamins aid in stimulating the appetite and supply immediate supportive treatment.

Readily available energy: This is especially important in animals in which digestion and metabolism are impaired or reduced. Energy is required to meet the normal requirements of body functions. During fever, requirements are estimated to be increased by 5 to 7% with each increase of 1°F (0.5°C) in body temperature. Low blood glucose values may produce serious neurologic disturbances. Administration of glucose aids the liver in detoxifying toxic products. Meeting energy requirements minimizes tissue nitrogen catabolism. In addition to parenteral glucose, to correct an acute weakness, a low-fiber, appetizing type of ration should be fed. In cold environments, body heat loss should be minimized by providing heated stabling or covering the animal with blankets.

Quality and quantity of protein: It may be important to supply an improved quality of protein for sick animals. This may be accomplished by feeding proteins of high biologic values such as milk or eggs. Vital tissue protein must be replaced, as well as proteins associated with other vital substances, such as enzymes and hormones, and those needed to form immune substances to resist infection. In most diseases, the quantity of protein may be increased 4 to 5% to replace the losses due to increased catabolism. High levels of protein are not indicated during impaired renal function because of the threat of accumulating nitrogenous end products in the blood.

Fat: Good-quality fat has merits in some therapeutic diets. In the monogastric animal it increases palatability, is a concentrated source of energy, and aids in the metabolism of the fat-soluble vitamins. It also supplies the essential fatty acids that may aid in correcting skin disturbances.

Fluids, Electrolytes and Minerals: Fluid and electrolyte imbalance are deterrents to organ function. Proper extra- and intracellular electrolyte composition must be maintained. During enteric disturbances, large volumes of water and electrolytes, especially sodium and potassium, may be excreted. Alkalosis or acidosis will dictate the choice of electrolyte solutions to be used in therapy. Caution should be exercised in potassium administration as indiscriminate use may be harmful. Fresh clean water should always be easily available. Anemia is present in many illnesses due to either increased loss of blood or deficient synthesis of hemoglobin. The diet of anemic animals should be carefully balanced, and the presence of adequate amounts of vitamins K and B_{12} and iron should be assured. *See also* DEHYDRATION—FLUID AND ELECTROLYTE IMBALANCE, p. 77.

Vitamins and unidentified growth factors: In sickness the requirement for vitamins and possibly for unidentified growth factors is increased. The depletion of water-soluble vitamins is relatively rapid, that of fat-soluble vitamins is much slower. In therapy, a 5- to 10-fold increase in the intake of water-soluble vitamins over the normal requirements is suggested. Vitamins A and E are indicated in chronic illness and during stress. Lesions of the gastrointestinal tract and liver may also interfere with the synthesis and metabolism of vitamins. Liver and milk are suggested as good sources of unidentified growth factors.

A balanced ration: In sick, as in normal animals, a balanced ration should be fed. The vitamins and minerals are required together with other substances in metabolizing the energy and protein portion of the diet. The use of a specific nutrient in the treatment of an illness may be only temporarily helpful. An effort should be made to supply all the nutrients in their proper proportions at the same time. Under field conditions this can sometimes be accomplished by substituting rations formulated for species having higher and more critical nutritional requirements. For example, weanling pigs recovering from an enteric infection might be fed a chick starter ration for a few days.

FEEDING SICK AND HOSPITALIZED DOGS

The best planned diet is useless unless eaten. Anorexia is a major problem in dogs hospitalized for medical reasons but, in general, animals recovering from surgery show normal appetite. If this is not the case, investigation should be undertaken to find the cause.

It is often difficult to tempt sick animals to eat anything, especially food to which they are unaccustomed. Individual persuasion, such as talking to and petting the dog, hand feeding, or even forced feeding may be necessary, at least initially. Attempts may be made to stimulate the appetite by giving warm food (i.e. heated to about 37°C but not beyond) or by offering several different types of food, e.g. milk pudding, beef gravy, chicken, fish, or perhaps raw or cooked red meat or liver. Variation in the water content of the food may also be helpful as some dogs have a marked preference for a certain consistency. (In general, dogs find wet textures more palatable than dry.) No sudden changes should be made as the appetite recovers. Uneaten food should not be left to become stale.

Hospitalized dogs should be fed familiar types of food (if not contraindicated by illness) by attendants who like dogs and will cater to them as occasion demands. The value of such care cannot be overstated. Vitamins (particularly of the B group) may help to improve appetite but, in general, other stimulants or medicaments (e.g. corticosteroids) should not be used primarily for this purpose. Infection and nutritional status influence each other. Nutrition influences resistance of the host to infection and its consequences, while infection affects the appetite and nutritional status of the host and often the dietary requirements as well.

The basic dietary requirements of healthy dogs (q.v., p. 1340) may have to be modified rather drastically in the face of altered physiology or disease. Some changes may be temporary (as the intake of lactating bitches) and some are relatively permanent (as in the diets for chronic diseases such as nephritis or diabetes). Many disease conditions respond well to diet modification. Often the diets needed are difficult to prepare, but commercial diets are available to fill the needs in most common maladies. The best of these dietary foods are more expensive than regular maintenance dog foods, but are effective and convenient. Where such foods are not suited to the particular patient the veterinarian must formulate a diet. By keeping in mind the basic nutritional requirements of normal dogs and using the following principles as guides, diets that enhance other therapeutic measures can be produced.

Parasitism: Demodectic mange may occur as a familial problem in certain strains of dogs on poor diet although it can also occur in healthy, well-fed animals. Hookworm infection is more likely to be a problem in thin, underfed dogs, even though the actual contents of the diet are satisfactory. Puppies fed high-energy, high-protein diets can often withstand massive roundworm infection. Any animal that is suffering from malnutrition is more susceptible to parasite infection or to the effects of an already present parasite burden.

Renal disease: One of the main functions of the kidney is the excretion of nitrogenous waste products. It is important during renal insuffficiencies to provide low, but adequate, quantities of dietary protein. The aim should be to keep the dog barely in nitrogen balance. This can be done by providing approximately 1.3 gm of high-quality protein per kg of body wt daily. Additional amounts will be needed in cases where urinary protein losses are high. Fats and carbohydrates should be increased to make up the normal caloric requirement and other ingredients supplied as in the normal diet. Patients can be kept on a high-sodium intake advantageously (by using sodium bicarbonate or bouillon cubes as supplements) and should be allowed liberal quantities of water. Many of these animals have polydipsia and polyuria, and water intake should not be restricted under any circumstances.

Gastrointestinal and digestive disease: Both inflammatory and functional disorders of the alimentary tract call for a diet that is nonstimulating (soft consistency, low residue). Eggs, dairy products, potatoes, chicken breasts, white bread and cooked rice are especially useful in such cases (but an excess of dairy products may cause diarrhea). Generally the best practice is to feed small amounts frequently. Constipation may be seen in older, overindulged house pets that have restricted opportunities for exercise. Such patients are often helped by feeding high-residue or bulky diets. Cooked oatmeal, bran and fibrous vegetables may be used to add bulk to the diet. It is important that adequate protein be supplied. An increased fluid intake may also be helpful.

Pancreatic disease can sometimes be managed by diet control alone. A diet high in protein and calcium but low in fat and starch is desirable. Supplemental enzyme and medium chain triglyceride therapy may be necessary.

Hepatic disease: What to feed the dog with liver disease is controversial: recent work suggests low-protein, moderate-fat diets. Probably more important than the level of either fat or protein is the assurance that adequate amounts of readily available carbohydrates are included in the diet of the dog with liver disease.

Diabetes mellitus: Diabetic patients can usually be maintained in satisfactory condition for several years when insulin and intelligent diet therapy are coordinated. Uniformity of day-to-day treatment is desirable in each case. A constant daily dose of insulin requires uniform exercise and a consistent dietary intake. A high-protein, high-fat diet with carbohydrates provided in nonconcentrated form is most desirable. After the quantity of protein and carbohydrates is established, the necessary calories are provided by adding fats. It is best to feed diabetic patients small amounts frequently in order to maintain a relatively stable blood glucose level.

Heart failure: Many older dogs develop congestive heart failure. Rest and diuresis are the prime requirements in these cases but restriction of the sodium intake is an important part of therapy, though unfortunately dogs find low-sodium diets unattractive. Rations should be prepared without the use of salt, baking soda or baking powder. Generally, muscle meat, freshwater fish, whole-grain cereals, rice and macaroni products, salt-free yeast bread, fresh or frozen vegetables and cooking oils or lard are desirable ingredients to use in low-sodium diets. Proprietary dog foods, regular bread, most processed foods and canned meats and vegetables are usually high in sodium because of added salt.

Food-induced allergy: (*See also* p. 7.) Some dogs may become allergic to almost any dietary protein but beef, milk and gluten are the commonest allergens. Unlike the situation in man, food-induced allergies are remarkably specific in dogs. It is essential to the diagnosis of dietary allergy to have the dog sign-free. This is most successfully accomplished in 1 of 3 ways: (1) by withholding all food for several days, (2) by feeding a special elimination diet, (3) by feeding a hypoallergenic diet. Nonallergenic diets may be foods not normally included in the dog's diet; these may include chicken, lamb and rice. Once sign-free, the dog should be fed one food at a time for 5 days. If signs do not recur, the food can be considered nonallergenic. The object is not to determine to what foods the dog is allergic, but to determine a sufficient number of foods to which the dog is not allergic to formulate an adequate diet. If a dog should develop a response to a food, withdraw that food and allow the dog to become sign-free again before proceeding further. Food-induced allergies are among the most difficult to handle because owners may "cheat" or dogs may accidentally eat foods to which they are allergic.

Surgery: Preoperative feeding is dictated by the surgical procedure scheduled. Generally, an empty gastrointestinal tract is desired, but excessive fasting, either before or after surgery, may be contraindicated since it may weaken the animal or deplete its glycogen reserves. The most successful pre- and postoperative diet is one that is known to be capable of supporting puppy growth.

FEEDING THE SICK CAT

Much feline illness involves the upper GI and respiratory tracts and anorexia is an early clinical sign that can rapidly lead to dehydration and emaciation, if not promptly countered.

Anorectic cats require water, electrolytes and B-vitamins. Patient intermittent oral force-feeding of sweetened fluids and gruels using a plastic hypodermic syringe is often successful. For the extremely ill and weak patient, it may be advisable and beneficial to pass a stomach tube via the nostril and feed a concentrated, high calorie, liquid food. This practice should not be continued any longer than needed, the cat being encouraged to eat on its own as soon as possible. Often just a little food in the stomach will revive the dormant appetite. Offering tuna, liver or kidney, or other special foods the cat is known to enjoy, often tempts the difficult cat to start eating.

Proper feeding can be an important factor in the therapy of several diseases of the cat. While there are but a few diets available commercially for specific diseases of the cat, many special diets can be formulated to meet the cat's needs. Even the commercial diets may need to have special foods or supplements added in small amounts to improve their acceptance by the sick cat.

Parasitism: Cats, like dogs, can withstand much greater burdens of both external and internal parasites when fed a diet containing adequate amounts of protein, energy, minerals and vitamins.

Renal disease: The cat's protein requirement is over twice that of the dog, but the by-products of protein metablism are excreted in the same manner, via the kidneys. During renal disease, therefore, protein must be restricted in the cat's diet, but not to the degree that it is for the dog, otherwise, hypoproteinemia results. The minimum that will keep a cat in positive protein balance is between 1.0 and 1.4 gm of high quality protein per lb (2.2 to 3 gm/kg) of body wt per day.

Gastrointestinal disease: Most cats with gastrointestinal disease can be fed in a manner similar to other monogastric animals with such a condition. One disease syndrome is worthy of note, however: chronic constipation caused by **megacolon** or **Hirschsprung's disease** should be managed, not with the bulk and roughage conventionally fed during ordinary constipation, but with highly digestible, low-residue foods. Since denervation is associated with the syndrome, the stimulatory effects of bulk and roughage are lost and such foods merely tend to further fill and stretch an already atonic colon and rectum.

Urolithiasis: While high-ash diets do not cause urolithiasis in cats, diets with restricted levels of magnesium may prevent the recurrence of urethral plugging. Since both urinary magnesium concentrations and urinary specific gravity seem to be factors, the following steps should help prevent recurrence of urethral plugging: 1) Restrict the diet to ingredients low in magnesium. Since about 70% of the magnesium in an animal's body is in its skeleton, foods containing whole fish, whole ground chicken or ground bone should be avoided. 2) Increase the cat's water intake. Since dry foods contain only about 10% water and semi-moist foods only about 25%, neither should be fed to cats prone to urolithiasis. Fresh waterishould be available to cats at all times. The addition of ¼ to ½ teaspoonful of table salt to the cat's food each day will often increase the water intake noticeably. Water containers should be washed daily, and supplied with cool (not cold) fresh water. (*See also* pp. 868 and 1349.)

NUTRITIONAL DEFICIENCIES IN CATTLE AND SHEEP

Nutritional deficiencies involving energy, protein, certain minerals, and vitamins A, D, E and K have been reported for ruminants under natural conditions. Experimentally, it has been possible to produce and study deficiencies of thiamin, riboflavin, biotin, choline and pantothenic acid in preruminant dairy calves, deficiencies that may never occur in the field.

A simple, uncomplicated deficiency, as observed in carefully controlled experiments is rarely if ever seen in the field. More likely, a deficiency of several nutrients contributes to the signs observed. Many of the signs of nutrient deficiencies are nonspecific and are often the total result of a low plane of nutrition. Further, the interactions of one nutrient with another and with other dietary constituents, in the development of deficiencies, are not usually clearly defined. This is well illustrated by the interrelationship of copper molybdenum and sulfate, of vitamin E and selenium, of zinc and calcium, and of iodine and the various goitrogens.

ENERGY

It is generally agreed that, given a balanced, high-energy ration, ruminants will consume feed until they satisfy some physiologic need for energy. In the strict sense most ruminants are energy deficient (for maximum performance) since they are not fed *ad libitum*, e.g. growing heifers, mature cattle or sheep on "satisfactory" pasture or stovers, and dry cows. Veal calves, cows in high production or fattening steers, on the other hand, are fed *ad libitum*. The commonest energy deficiency is due to the inappropriate allotment of feed with a resulting reduced production efficiency. Generally this is unintentional or thought to be "economical" or it may be forced on the feeder by drought, poor pastures or low quality, highly lignified, unpalatable forage.

A frank caloric deficiency is often subclinical in nature, resulting in lowered production, retarded growth, delayed puberty and lowered reproductive performance. In severe cases it is often complicated with other deficiencies particularly of vitamin A, protein and phosphorus. Appetite remains good. Young ruminants may be temporarily or permanently stunted and mature animals become thin and unthrifty. Milk production rapidly decreases in proportion to the deficiency and non-fat milk solids decrease. Pregnant animals will likely produce weak young and milk production will be inadequate to support the newborn. Surviving calves and lambs will often not do well and be unthrifty at weaning time if continually underfed.

Livestock in poor physical condition are most susceptible to the ravages of weather and parasites. They also are more likely to consume toxic plants if grazing poor pastures.

Research has shown that a slow growth rate until puberty will extend the lifespan of most species. Excessive feeding of potential breeding stock in early life produces unnecessarily fat animals which often have trouble conceiving and lactating later. It is better to allot enough energy to allow female dairy and beef cattle to reach the breeding stage at 12 to 15 months, the proper age for effective management. Even when cattle are underfed until 2½ years of age, they are still able to recover most of the loss in size and to produce normally when fed well, although their first production cycle is delayed. Under current livestock conditions in the U.S.A., dramatic underfeeding by design is not justified; growing animals should progress at a steady rate but not allowed to become too fat.

The energy requirement for maintenance is 25 to 100% greater when grazing than when stall fed.

PROTEIN

A deficiency of protein often goes hand in hand with an energy shortage and may be the first limiting factor in practical cattle and sheep feeding when these animals are on poor pasture. Nonlegume forages, especially roughages, if poorly fertilized with nitrogen, are often too low in protein for optimal performance. Legume forage is always ample in protein. Adequate amounts of protein (or nitrogen) are required, not only by the animal itself, but also by the rumen microflora whose composition and function may be markedly altered on a low-protein diet. Intake of low-protein feeds is depressed and growth is seriously retarded. Other signs may be similar to those encountered with insufficient energy. Weight gains and the condition of fattening cattle and sheep are reduced, milk production is lowered and, if severe or prolonged, the animals become thin and emaciated and blood protein is low. Weight losses may occur even though ample energy is available. In addition, with sheep, the growth of the wool fiber is restricted and "breaks" occur in the fleece.

Pregnant cows or ewes on a low-protein diet may lose considerable body weight and become thin and weak. Estrus may become irregular and conception delayed. Such females may have difficult parturition, be troubled with retained placenta, milk poorly and produce offspring that have poor chances of survival or, at best, are small and thin at weaning. Such unthrifty stock are susceptible to adverse weather, disease and parasites.

MINERALS

Sodium Chloride (Salt): Sodium chloride is an essential component of the acid-base mechanism in the body and is needed for the maintenance of proper osmotic relationships. Animals promptly adjust to low-salt diets by reducing sodium excretion in the urine. Continued deprivation results in an intense craving for salt in which animals chew and lick various objects such as wood, metal and dirt. Feed consumption declines, loss of body weight and a drop in milk production occurs. Feed efficiency is poor. As death approaches, milking cows shiver, show incoordination, weakness and cardiac arrhythmia.

The animal is able to judge its need for salt and a salt block or loose salt should be available throughout life. Following a salt deficiency it should be offered to the animal gradually. Salt intoxication is unlikely if adequate water is available.

Calcium: The bones and teeth contain about 99% of the body calcium in their structure and serve as a reserve of this element. The 1% remaining is found in the soft tissues and body fluids and is essential for proper nerve function, cardiac and other muscular activity and blood clotting. A dynamic equilibrium exists between these 2 pools.

A calcium deficiency in the young prevents normal bone growth and may lead to spontaneous fractures. General growth and development is retarded. Frank rickets (q.v., p. 580) may occur. If bone reserves are substantial in the adult, it requires a lengthy depletion period before bone mineral loss is sufficient to result in fragile bones. Under these conditions milk yield is depressed but not its calcium content. Blood calcium will be low only after an extended period of deficient intake. For positive diagnosis, the calcium content of the feed should be checked.

In practical feeding conditions, calcium deficiency is always suspected except where milk and legume forage are used extensively. Almost all concentrates and nonlegume forages including corn silage require calcium supplementation. Heavily lactating animals have the greatest need due to significant excretion in the milk. During early lactation, a high-producing cow will always be in negative calcium balance but will restore her reserves in late lactation if fed adequate levels. Young animals absorb calcium much more efficiently than older ones, hence there is a need to provide adequate levels throughout life. Animals heavily fed on concentrates with little forage will need supplemental calcium. Milk fever (q.v., p. 513) is characterized by a reduced blood calcium but is not due to a calcium deficiency.

Ground limestone, steamed bone meal and dicalcium phosphate are excellent sources of calcium. Addition of lime to fields may increase the potential of that field to grow legumes and hence provide more feed calcium.

Phosphorus: About 75% of the body phosphorus is present in the bones and teeth. The remaining 25% in the soft tissues are found in phosphoprotein, nucleoprotein, phospholipids, and hexose phosphate which are essential in organ structure, nutrient transport and energy utilization.

A deficiency of phosphorus in the young results in slow growth, poor appetite and unthriftiness, and has produced a knock-kneed condition in lambs. Energy utilization is reduced. In the adult, milk production declines, bones become fragile and feed intake is poor. The animals may become lame and stiff. Anestrus and low conception rates may occur. The phosphorus content of the milk does not decline. While a depraved appetite (chewing of wood, dirt, etc.) has long been recognized as often occurring with a phosphorus deficiency, this sign is not specific. Many animals engage in this vice on well-balanced diets.

In contrast to calcium, blood phosphorus declines rather quickly on a phosphorus-deficient diet. (Normal values are 4 to 6 mg/100 ml and 6 to 8 mg/100 ml for calves under 1 year of age.)

Forages produced on deficient, unfertilized soils may be marginal in phosphorus content and deficiencies occur when these roughages form the entire ration. Over much of North America, pasture and especially range forage have a low phosphorus content. Most of the winter range areas of the West are deficient in phosphorus, particularly those ranges characterized by a predominance of dry leached grass and shad scale. Use of phosphorus fertilizers markedly increases crop yields in these areas and may also raise the percentage of phosphorus in the forage. Fortunately, grains, protein supplements and by-product feeds usually are adequate in phosphorus and may supplement low-phosphorus roughages effectively.

Phosphorus deficiency can be corrected or prevented most easily by feeding phosphorus supplements, such as bone meal, dicalcium phosphate or defluorinated rock phosphate. Bone meal contains approximately 14% phosphorus, while dicalcium phosphate and defluorinated rock phosphate normally contain 18 and 14% phosphorus, respectively. Rock phosphates should contain less than 0.1% fluorine to avoid toxicity from this element. Colloidal clay phosphates (so-called "soft" phosphates) contain phosphorus in a relatively unavailable form and also may have a considerable fluoride content. Wheat bran, cottonseed meal, linseed meal and soybean meal are rich in phosphorus and their use in concentrate mixtures will insure adequate intakes. While the ratio of calcium to phosphorus may vary widely in natural feeds, ratios up to 7 to 1 are tolerated by growing calves, with requirement levels being about 1.4 to 1. A ratio of less than 1 is highly undesirable. Vitamin D is essential for the absorption and utilization of both calcium and phosphorus. In milk fever prone cows, low calcium intakes are recommended before parturition. (*See* DAIRY CATTLE NUTRITION, p. 1267.)

Iodine: About 80% of the body iodine is stored in the thyroid gland in the form of thyroglobulin, thyroxine and trace quantities of other iodinated amino acid derivatives including triiodothyronine. Iodine apparently exerts its total physiological role as a component of the thyroid hormones, which control cellular energy exchange, metabolic rate and tissue growth and development.

A simple iodine deficiency results in an enlargement of the thyroid gland or goiter (q.v., p. 203) with a reduction of thyroxine secretion. Pregnancy is the most critical period. Iodine deficiency occurs in areas in which soil and hence plant and water iodine is low such as around the Great Lakes and in the Northwest. Some plants such as cabbage, soybeans, and yellow turnips may promote goiter development because they contain substances (goitrogens) that inhibit thyroxine production. The goitrogenic effect of raw soybeans is only partially destroyed in processing.

Iodized salt is an effective source of iodine and is widely used. The iodine in the salt should be stabilized since weathering can reduce the content below the required level. The same is true for trace-mineralized salt. In both types of salt 0.007% iodine (0.01% KI) is usually added. Neither iodized nor trace-mineralized salt should be added to a concentrate supplement used to limit feed intake.

Cobalt: While cobalt is considered a dietary essential, the tissues actually require vitamin B_{12}, which contains cobalt and is synthesized by rumen microorganisms. Vitamin B_{12} will alleviate signs of a cobalt deficiency.

Cobalt deficiency develops very rapidly as little is stored. Deficient animals show a normocytic, normochromic anemia with a concomitant loss of appetite, retarded growth, general emaciation, rough hair coat and a loss of milk production. While herbage and liver analyses are helpful in diagnosing the deficiency, the proof positive is the prompt improvement in feed intake following the feeding of cobalt.

Natural forages containing less than 0.07 ppm of cobalt are usually considered deficient for sheep and cattle. Regions where, from time to time, these minima are not reached exist in Florida, Michigan, Wisconsin, New Hampshire and New York, in Western Canada, Scotland, South Africa, Australia and New Zealand.

Drenches of about 1.0 mg of cobalt, given twice a week, have corrected the deficiency syndrome in sheep. In cattle, feeding 5 to 15 mg of cobalt daily will cure cobalt deficiency and as little as 1 mg will prevent is occurrence. The inclusion of 15 to 30 gm of cobalt chloride or sulfate per 100 lb (45 kg) of salt is usually adequate to prevent deficiency in both cattle and sheep. The use of such trace-mineralized salt is the most common method of supplying cobalt to ruminants in the U.S.A. In New Zealand and in other intensively farmed areas, cobalt is applied to the soil annually at the rate of 5 oz (150 gm) of cobalt sulfate per acre, either as a spray or included in the phosphate fertilizer. A cobalt "bullet" (90% cobalt oxide baked hard in 10% clay) given orally dissolves slowly over many months in the rumen, and has been used with success as a preventive. This "bullet" is used quite extensively under some range conditions where other methods of oral administration are not practical. In about 5% of sheep, the bullet is regurgitated and lost, and in a further small percentage, it is covered with a deposit which prevents solution of the cobalt. Injections of cobalt are not effective since the site of B_{12} synthesis is the rumen. Extremely large doses of cobalt (300 times the requirement) may be toxic.

Copper and Molybdenum: Copper is involved at the functional level in the formation of the porphyrin nucleus of hemoglobin and in maintaining the function of bone osteoblasts. It is also essential in melanin production and in keratin (wool) formation. General signs of a deficiency include anemia, brittle or fragile bones, loss of hair or wool pigmentation and in sheep, poor wool growth characterized by a loss of crimp (steely wool).

Specifically in cattle, poor growth, anemia, bone fragility, diarrhea and a myocardial fibrosis occur. Ends of leg bones become enlarged and the hair loses its color. Milk production and body condition are poor, fertility is low and calves may show congenital rickets. With sheep, anemia and depressed growth are less common. Demyelination of certain tracts in the fetal and neonatal CNS results in incoordination which leads to immobilization, blindness and death. The disease is known as **swayback** or **enzootic ataxia.** Bone fragility may also occur.

In many cases, copper deficiency can be a simple deficiency of the element (primary). In other areas where excessive molybdenum and sulfate exists in the feed, these elements act to reduce copper solubility in the digestive tract and induce a copper deficiency (conditioned deficiency).

A normal level of sulfate in the diet counteracts the effects of molybdenum toxicity by increasing its rate of excretion. Higher sulfate levels, however, appear to enhance molybdenum intoxication with a detrimental effect on copper utilization. Frank cases of molybdenum toxicity occur on pastures containing an excess of the element, and are characterized by a profuse scouring; these can be alleviated by copper supplementation at levels of 0.25 gm of copper sulfate per 100 lb (45 kg) body wt daily.

The requirement for copper is about 5 ppm of the dry diet for sheep and 10 ppm for cattle. Adequate intakes can be met if feeds have this level or by providing 0.5% copper sulfate in a trace-mineralized salt. Toxic levels are about 10 times the minimum requirement and sheep are much more susceptible than cattle. Poultry litter used to supplement sheep rations may be a source of toxic levels of copper.

Iron: Normal hemoglobin formation requires iron as a component of the heme molecule. A microcytic normochromic anemia develops in calves on an iron-low diet (milk). Most feedstuffs contain adequate iron and a deficiency in adult cattle is not a problem. Young calves or lambs confined to a milk diet and prevented from consuming dry feed will develop anemia. Providing 30 ppm iron will prevent pathological anemia in milk- and milk replacer-fed calves. On normal feeding regimes where dry feeds are offered from birth, no special iron supplements are needed.

Magnesium: About 60% of the tissue magnesium is found in the bones where it is relatively difficult to mobilize. The normal calcium:magnesium ratio is about 55:1. A variable amount (15 to 50%) is bound to serum proteins. It plays a vital role as an activator of many enzyme systems involving energy exchange. It also is involved in maintaining normal nerve irritability and function. Signs of a magnesium deficiency are always accompanied by a low blood magnesium level (1.0 mg/100 ml) but not vice versa.

By feeding experimental rations deficient in magnesium or by giving whole milk as the only food for 8 to 10 months, magnesium deficiency has been produced in calves. (*See* HYPOMAGNESEMIC TETANY OF CALVES, p. 522.)

Throughout the world, adult lactating cows on early spring pasture that has been fertilized with nitrogen or potassium or both, during a cool spring may develop signs of "grass tetany" (q.v., p. 580). While this is clearly derived from a low-blood magnesium and animals respond to magnesium drench or infusion, it is not a simple case of a dietary magnesium deficiency. The etiology is complex and not well understood. Pastures fertilized to provide sward containing 0.25% magnesium will prevent the condition.

Sulfur: All ruminants require sulfur to synthesize the sulfur containing amino acids cystine and methionine. A sulfur deficiency results in poor growth and in sheep a marked impairment of wool growth. In cattle it results in reduced feed intake, lower digestability, slower gains and depressed milk production. If the diet is adequate in natural proteins, the sulfur intake will be satisfactory. If high levels of nonprotein nitrogen such as urea are used, sources of sulfur such as inorganic or organic sulfur should be added. Elemental sulfur is satisfactory but less well utilized. A NPN to sulfur ratio of 12:1 is recommended for cattle. This element is a cofactor of many enzymes and an integral part of others.

Manganese: Manganese has been less extensively studied in ruminants. In cattle a deficiency results in skeletal abnormalities, delayed estrus, reduced fertility, abortions and deformed young. The calves have deformed legs with "over-knuckling" and enlarged joints and grow poorly. Newborn calves often exhibit ataxia. Deficient dairy heifers are slower to exhibit estrus and conceive.

Most feeds are adequate in manganese precluding a need for supplementation. As corn grain is relatively low (5 ppm), beef cattle on high concentrate diets may need attention. A level of 40 ppm in the diet is adequate.

Zinc: Many enzymes that are distributed widely throughout the body contain zinc such as carbonic anhydrase, many dehydrogenases and alkaline phosphatase. It is probable that zinc is related intimately to the processes of cell division. Zinc deficiency signs have been produced experimentally with highly specialized diets. In lambs such a diet produced slipping of wool, swelling and lesions around the hooves and periorbital regions of the eyes, excessive salivation, anorexia, wool-eating, general listlessness and reduction of growth. Beef calves develop parakeratosis, and the mouth becomes inflamed. They are stiff in the joints and unthrifty in appearance. Dairy calves show alopecia, a general dermatitis of the neck and head, listlessness, reduced testicular growth and swollen feet. Wounds fail to heal properly. Calves can develop the deficiency in 3 weeks and adjust quickly to variations in the zinc content of the diet by altering the amount they absorb. The requirement is about 40 ppm. The toxic level is at least 10 to 30 times the requirement.

Selenium: Selenium has been shown to be an integral part of glutathione peroxidase, which functions to eliminate the effect of free radical damage resulting from fatty acid peroxidation. Its function is inextricably entwined with that of vitamin E. The predominant deficiency disease in ruminants is nutritional muscular dystrophy or white muscle disease (q.v., p. 594). Prevention and cure has been effected under field conditions by supplementation with either vitamin E or selenium. Retained placentas in cattle have been reduced with selenium treatment.

A deficiency of selenium is a geographic one, found in many parts of the world due to inadequate soil levels. New York, Ohio and the Pacific Northwest are examples. Striking responses to selenium therapy by lambs suffering unthriftiness have also been reported in New Zealand. Selenium therapy or prophylaxis is possible by injection of selenium compounds and recently approval (U.S.A.) has been given to incorporate it into the feed for ewes and ewes with lambs up to 8 weeks of age. It is permitted at a level in the total feed of 0.1 ppm or in the salt-mineral mixture at a level of 30 ppm.

A dietary level of 0.1 ppm is adequate for ruminants. Levels of 3 to 5 ppm are toxic and result in loss of appetite, loss of hair from the tail, sloughing of hoofs and eventual death. Some plants are selenium accumulators when grown on high selenium soils such as are found in parts of South Dakota, Wyoming and Utah.

VITAMINS

Vitamin A: This vitamin serves to maintain the integrity of all epithelial tissues including germinal epithelium. Thus a deficiency of vitamin A, besides reducing the efficiency of the epithelium *per se*, permits much of this tissue to be exposed to a secondary invasion of indigenous pathogens. Most signs of a deficiency can be traced to this signal function. Since vitamin A is related to epithelium and not metabolism, the requirements are generally related to body weight.

Tissue vitamin A may be derived from either provitamin A (carotene), a yellow pigment in plants that is converted in the intestinal wall to vitamin A, or from preformed vitamin A *per se*.

Carotene is destroyed when rougage is dried and bleached, hence a deficiency may occur in cattle and sheep under drought conditions or when they are fed old, weathered roughage for long periods. Carotene is abundant in growing pasture, silage and well-cured hay that has been stored less than 6 months. Grains (with the exception of yellow corn) and cereal by-products contain little or none of this provitamin.

Usually, the first signs of vitamin A deficiency are excessive lacrimation, thin or watery diarrhea, nasal discharge, coughing and pulmonary involvement. Night blindness may develop in the early stages; in fact, this sign has been used experimentally to establish minimum carotene requirements. Vitamin A levels in the blood decline to less than 8 to 10 mcg/100 ml of plasma in calves and below 12 to 15 mcg in yearlings and older cattle. Considerable individual variation, however, is often observed in plasma vitamin

A levels: carotene blood levels of cattle are consistently low in a deficiency and are indicative of insufficient carotene intake. Sheep have only traces of carotene in the blood even on high carotene intakes.

Calves and lambs have very low vitamin A blood levels at birth and depend on colostrum (a very rich source of vitamin A) to protect them against a deficiency until sufficient vitamin A or carotene from other sources can be obtained. Calves and lambs from dams with vitamin A deficiency may be born dead or so weak that they die within a few days; females may abort during the latter stage of pregnancy. Injury to the optic nerve as a result of stenosis of the optic foramen may occur in growing animals. Cerebrospinal fluid pressure is elevated and, as a result, staggering gait, muscular incoordination and convulsions ("fainting" of feedlot cattle) have been frequently reported. Anasarca is often observed in fattening cattle, and opacity and cloudiness of the cornea and xerophthalmia with subsequent infection and blindness may result.

Young bulls and rams may become sterile as a result of failure of spermatogenesis. Vitamin A-deficient mature bulls show muscular incoordination which makes them unable to mount. This occurs before spermatogenesis is altered.

While there is little difference in normal plasma carotene levels among the major beef breeds, there is considerable difference among dairy breeds because of the variations in their ability to metabolize carotene to vitamin A. Colored breeds have high carotene levels. The liver can store large quantities of vitamin A. Most animals off good pasture can live 200 days on their liver reserves.

With the exception of irreparable changes in the eye or bone tissues, signs of vitamin A deficiency can be corrected rapidly by high intakes in vitamin A. At this point, treatment should be by injection of preformed vitamin A. The requirement is about 2,000 IU/100 lb (45 kg) live wt. Up to 100 times this level is not detrimental as a curative dose. Changing to diets adequate in carotene or vitamin A is imperative. The rate of conversion of carotene to vitamin A by ruminants is considered to be 1 mg β-carotene equivalent to 400 IU of vitamin A. This is lower than in simple stomached animals. It also fluctuates widely and unpredictably. Therefore, many commercial feeds are now fortified with dry, stabilized vitamin A and supplements are used to fortify home-grown rations. Such a source of vitamin A may be more economical and dependable than carotene from natural feeds. The vitamin A requirement is 47 IU/kg of live wt. Single injections of 1 million IU of vitamin A apparently protects from a deficiency for 2 to 4 months.

Vitamin D: Calcium, phosphorus and vitamin D are closely related in metabolism. Vitamin D is essential for the adequate absorption of calcium and phosphorus. It is converted by the liver to 25-hydroxycholecalciferol which in turn is hydroxylated by the liver to

1,25-dihydroxycholecalciferol, which stimulates the synthesis of a calcium binding protein in the intestinal mucosa. Its effect on phosphorus absorption is by a different mechanism. Vitamin D is also necessary for the proper mineralization of the cartilaginous matrix that develops at the epiphyses. Poor mineralization results in cartilaginous overgrowth and disorganization leading to swollen leg joints and beaded ribs (rickets). Plasma calcium and phosphorus drop and serum phosphatase increases. An absolute or relative deficiency of calcium, phosphorus or vitamin D will result in rickets (q.v., p. 579). Vitamin D deficiency in adult cattle has not been well defined.

In practice, vitamin D deficiency is a possibility but not a probability even for the young. Milk is not especially rich in vitamin D but the calf or lamb can obtain adequate amounts by skin irradiation if exposed to the sunlight for 1 to 2 hours per day. Sun-cured forage is the best natural source of vitamin D. Even silages have sufficient dead leaves (thus sun-cured) to provide ample vitamin D to growing calves that are housed indoors. However, it is probably prudent to provide a vitamin D supplement to young calves in their milk replacer and starter until they are turned out or are consuming adequate forage, i.e. 6 to 8 weeks. Older ruminants should need no added vitamin D if consuming normal forages.

Vitamin E: Most natural feeds contain vitamin E, but oxidation rapidly destroys it so that old hay or ground grain may be poor sources. A deficiency of vitamin E or selenium is recognized as a common cause of muscular dystrophy (q.v., p. 591) in calves and lambs. Vitamin E does not seem to be associated with reproductive failures in ruminants and thus it is of practical importance only with the young. Milk replacers should be fortified. The interaction of vitamin E and selenium are discussed above.

Vitamin K: A deficiency is seen only in the presence of dicoumarin from moldy sweet clover. This results in the so-called "sweet clover disease" (q.v., p. 1017) in which the ruminant may die from hemorrhage following a minor injury, or even from apparently spontaneous bleeding. This vitamin is synthesized by rumen bacteria and is distributed widely in green, leafy forages.

B-complex vitamins: Deficiencies have not been observed in ruminants past 1 to 2 months of age except where they have been restricted to special diets. Rumen bacteria have the ability to synthesize all the B-complex vitamins if other factors necessary for their synthesis are present (for example, cobalt in B_{12} synthesis). Niacin (nicotinic acid) is also synthesized from tryptophan within the tissues of even young calves. This, together with that synthesized in the rumen, fully meets the needs of ruminants. Most of the other B-vitamins have been shown to be essential in the diet of very young calves before rumen function becomes established. However, milk and other natural feeds contain adequate amounts to meet the needs of young calves and lambs. Milk replacers should be fortified for insurance.

It must be borne in mind that the ruminant is dependent upon bacterial synthesis for B-complex vitamins and might actually undergo a shortage of these if it goes "off feed" for long periods. Further, low-protein diets of mineral-deficient feeds may depress the number of bacteria and the synthesis mechanisms of the rumen microflora. The practice of administering certain B-complex vitamins or yeast preparations to ruminants that have been "off feed" for a considerable period has been tried with apparent success in the field.

Vitamin C (ascorbic acid): Since it is synthesized in the tissues even of young ruminants, deficiencies of this vitamin do not occur and it is not required in the diet.

NUTRITIONAL DEFICIENCIES IN SWINE

The diagnosis of nutritional deficiencies by outward observation of signs in swine is difficult. Quite often, the clinical signs observed are due to a complex of poor management, infectious diseases and parasitism, as well as malnutrition. For most nutrient deficiencies, the signs are not specific. For example, poor appetite, reduced growth and unthriftiness are common to most nutrient deficiencies. A deficiency of a single nutrient may bring about inanition; the subsequent starvation may cause multiple deficiencies. Then, too, a nutritional deficiency may exist without the appearance of definite signs. In the field, the deficiency may be only slight or borderline, making the diagnosis difficult.

The diagnosis of a nutrient deficiency by observing the response to nutritional therapy is not always clear cut. The 1973 report by the Committee on Animal Nutrition of the National Research Council in the bulletin entitled *Nutrient Requirements of Swine* states:

"Some acute conditions that are produced in the laboratory by omitting an essential constituent from the diet can be dramatically reversed by supplying the missing constituent. It does not follow, however, that long-standing conditions can be made to recede in the same way. Many functional and anatomical lesions resulting from inadequate diets are irreversible."

A positive diagnosis of a nutritional deficiency should be made only after: (1) observance of several of the clinical signs expected and (2) a careful review of the dietary, disease and management history of the animals.

The usual clinical signs of dietary deficiencies are outlined in TABLE 43. A brief discussion of each along with related matters follows.

TABLE 43. SIGNS OF NUTRIENT DEFICIENCIES IN SWINE

Nutrient	Signs of Nutrient Deficiency	
	Clinical	Subclinical
Energy	Weakness, low body temperature, loss of weight, coma, and death	Hypoglycemia Loss of subcutaneous fat Elevated hematocrit and serum cholesterol Reduced blood glucose, calcium, and sodium
Protein: Amino acid	Impaired growth Unthriftiness Reduced resistance to bacterial infection	Kwashiorkor-like signs in baby pigs, including reduced serum protein and serum albumin, anemia, gross edema, and increased lipid liver concentration
Fat: Linoleic acid	Scaly dermatitis may appear	Small gallbladder Elevated triene/tetraene in tissue lipids
Vitamin A	Incoordination Lordosis Paralysis of rear limbs Night blindness Congenital defects	Retarded bone growth Increase in cerebrospinal fluid pressure Degeneration of sciatic and femoral nerves Minimal visual purple Atrophy of epithelial layers of genital tract
Vitamin D	Rickets Osteomalacia Low calcium tetany	Lack of bone calcification and proliferation of epiphyseal cartilage Rib and vertebra fracture Low plasma calcium, magnesium, and inorganic phosphorus levels Elevated serum alkaline phosphatase levels
Vitamin E-Selenium	Edema Sudden death	Generalized edema Liver necrosis (hepatosis dietetica) Microangiopathy Cardiac muscle degeneration (mulberry heart) Pale, dystrophic muscle
Vitamin K	Pale newborn pigs with loss of blood from umbilical cord Sudden death following dicoumarin intake	Increased prothrombin time Increased blood-clotting time Internal hemorrhage Anemia due to blood loss
Thiamin	Poor appetite Poor growth Sudden death	Cardiac hypertrophy Bradycardia First and second degree auriculoventricular block Elevated plasma pyruvate
Riboflavin	Slow growth Seborrhea Impaired sow reproductivity	Lens cataracts Increase in neutrophilic leukocytes Birth of weak pigs with skeletal anomalies

TABLE 43. SIGNS OF NUTRIENT DEFICIENCIES IN SWINE (*Continued*)

Nutrient	Signs of Nutrient Deficiency: Clinical	Signs of Nutrient Deficiency: Subclinical
Niacin	Poor appetite Poor growth Severe diarrhea Dermatitis	Necrotic lesions of intestine
Pantothenic acid	Poor appetite Poor growth Diarrhea Unusual gait (goose-stepping) Impaired sow reproductivity	Inflammation of colon Degeneration of sciatic and peripheral nerves Reduced blood pantothenic acid level Reduced milk-free-pantothenic acid level
Vitamin B_6	Poor growth Epileptic seizures	Microcytic hypochromic anemia Elevated serum iron Fatty infiltration of liver Elevated urinary xanthurenic acid Elevated gamma globulin-like blood protein fraction
Vitamin B_{12}	Depressed growth Hypersensitivity Reduced sow reproductivity	Reduced serum and tissue B_{12} levels
Choline	Slow growth Reduced litter size	Fatty infiltration of liver Reduced conception rate
Biotin	Dermatosis Spasticity of hind legs	Reduced urinary biotin excretion
Folacin	Poor growth Weakness	Normocytic anemia
Calcium	Rickets Osteomalacia Low calcium tetany	Lack of bone calcification Bones easily fractured Low plasma calcium level Elevated serum inorganic phosphorus and alkaline phosphatase
Phosphorus	Poor growth Rickets Osteomalacia	Lack of bone calcification Bones easily fractured Low serum inorganic phosphorus level Elevated serum calcium and alkaline phosphatase Enlarged costochondral junction (beading)
Magnesium	Poor growth Stepping syndrome Weakened carpo-metacarpo-phalangeal and tarso-metatarso-phalangeal joints Tetany	Los serum magnesium and calcium Reduced bone magnesium
Potassium	Anorexia Rough hair coat Emaciation Ataxia	Reduced heart rate Increased PR, QRS, and QT intervals on electrocardiogram Reduced serum potassium

TABLE 43. SIGNS OF NUTRIENT DEFICIENCIES IN SWINE (*Continued*)

	Signs of Nutrient Deficiency	
Nutrient	Clinical	Subclinical
dium	Poor appetite Low water consumption Unthriftiness	Negative sodium balance Elevated serum potassium Elevated plasma urea nitrogen Reduced chlorine retention
lorine	Poor growth	Reduced plasma chlorine Reduced sodium and potassium retention
n	Poor growth Rough hair coat Pallor Anoxia	Hypochromic microcytic anemia Enlarged heart and spleen Enlarged fatty liver Ascites Clumping of erythroblastic cells in bone marrow Reduced serum iron and percent transferrin saturation
pper	Leg weakness Ataxia	Microcytic hypochromic anemia Reduced serum copper and ceruloplasmin Aortic rupture Cardiac hypertrophy
c	Poor growth Poor appetite Parakeratosis	Reduced serum, tissue, and milk zinc Reduced serum albumin-globulin ratio Reduced serum alkaline phosphatase Reduced thymus weight Retarded testicular development Impaired reproductivity of sows
ine	Goiter Myxedema Sows farrow weak, hairless pigs	Enlarged hemorrhagic thyroid Hyperplasia of follicular epithelium of thyroid Reduced plasma protein-bound iodine
nganese	Lameness in growing pigs Increased fat deposition in pregnant gilts with birth of weak pigs with poor sense of balance	Replacement of cancellous bone with fibrous tissue Early closure of distal epiphyseal plate Low serum manganese and alkaline phosphatase Negative manganese balance
ter	Poor appetite Dehydration Loss of body weight Possible salt poisoning Death	Elevated hematocrit Elevated plasma electrolytes Loss of temperature regulation Tissue deyhdration

rom *Nutrient Requirements of Swine*, National Research Council (1979).

PROTEIN

Feeding a suboptimal level of protein to pigs results in reduce gains, fatter carcasses and poorer feed conversion. Protein def ciency may result from a suboptimal feed intake or from an imba ance of one or more of the essential amino acids. For optim utilization of protein, all essential amino acids must be liberate during digestion at rates commensurate with needs. Therefore, pr tein supplement should not be hand-fed at infrequent intervals, bu should be mixed with the grain or be available at all times wit grain on a free-choice basis.

No evidence has been presented to support the theory of "pr tein poisoning." Rations containing as much as 34 to 51% protei have proved laxative, but not harmful and no toxic effects wer noted.

FAT

A semipurified ration containing 0.06% fat produced such def ciency signs as loss of hair, scaly dermatitis, necrotic areas on th skin of the neck and shoulders, and an unthrifty appearance i growing pigs. However, a level of 1.0 to 1.5% fat in the diet ap peared ample to furnish the essential fatty acids required by swine With practical rations, a specific fat deficiency is unknown.

MINERALS

The clinical signs of deficiencies of the more important minera elements are briefly discussed under the headings below.

Calcium and Phosphorus: Deficiencies of calcium and phos phorus result in rickets in growing pigs and osteomalacia in matur swine. Signs include deformity and bending of long bones, an lameness in young swine and fractures and posterior paralysis i older swine. Deficient sows produce weak pigs, and usually show posterior paralysis, sometimes as a result of fractures in the lumba region. Sows with a marginal deficiency often give birth to stron and vigorous pigs that grow normally. However, after nursing th pigs for 3 or more weeks, the sows develop a posterior paralysis. A deficiency of vitamin D also will cause these signs especially if th dietary calcium or phosphorus differs markedly from the recom mended feeding level. (*See* RICKETS, p. 579.)

Sodium and Chlorine: Pigs fed low-salt diets show slow growth reduced appetite and poor hair and skin condition.

Iodine: Bred females fed rations deficient in iodine produce pig that are weak or stillborn, and hairless at birth. With a borderlin deficiency, the newborn pigs may only be weak at birth, but o necropsy, enlarged thyroids are found together with histologic ab normalities of these glands. (*See also* GOITER, p. 203.)

Iron and Copper: Deficiency of these 2 elements reduces the rate of hemoglobin formation and produces typical nutritional anemia. Signs of nutritional anemia in suckling pigs include low hemoglobin and red blood cell count, pale membranes, enlarged heart, an edematous condition of the skin about the neck and shoulders, listlessness and rapid breathing (thumps).

Zinc: A relative lack of this element results in parakeratosis (q.v., p. 935) in growing swine, particularly when diets contain more than the recommended amount of calcium. The exact mode of action of zinc in the prevention of parakeratosis is not known, nor has its role in the support of other life processes yet been fully elucidated.

Selenium/Vitamin E: Sudden death of young rapidly growing swine may be observed due to a deficiency of these nutrients (*see* CARDIAC AND SKELETAL MYOPATHIES AND HEPATOSIS DIAETETICA IN SWINE, p. 597).

VITAMINS

Signs resulting from deficiency of the vitamins of greatest practical importance are briefly discussed below.

Vitamin A: Vitamin A deficiency results in disturbances of the eye and of the epithelial tissues of the respiratory, reproductive, nervous, urinary and digestive systems. Reproduction is impaired in sows and vitamin A-deficient sows may farrow blind, eyeless, weak or malformed pigs. Herniation of the spinal cord in the fetal pigs is reported as a unique sign of vitamin A deficiency in the pregnant sow. Growing pigs, deficient in vitamin A, show incoordinated movements and develop night blindness and respiratory disorders.

Vitamin D: Deficiency signs include rickets, stiffness, weak and bent bones, and posterior paralysis.

Riboflavin: In riboflavin-deficient swine, reproduction is impaired. Deficient sows exhibit anorexia and farrow dead pigs from 4 to 16 days prematurely. The stillborn pigs have very little hair, often are partially resorbed and may have enlarged forelegs. Growing pigs fed low-riboflavin rations gain very slowly, have poor appetite, exhibit a rough haircoat and an exudate on the skin, and may have cataracts.

Niacin: Niacin-deficient pigs have inflammatory lesions of the gastrointestinal tract. The pigs exhibit diarrhea, weight loss, rough skin and haircoat, and a dermatitis on the ears. Enteric conditions may be due to niacin deficiency, bacterial infection, or both. Deficient pigs respond readily to niacin therapy, but infectious enteritis is not benefited. However, adequate dietary niacin probably allows the pig to maintain its resistance to bacterial invasion.

Pantothenic acid: Growing pigs and pregnant sows develop a typical "goose-stepping" gait and show incoordination and a noninfectious bloody diarrhea when maintained on pantothenic acid-defi-

TABLE 44. SIGNS OF DIETARY EXCESS IN SWINE

Nutrient	Toxic Dietary Level[a]	Age	Signs of Dietary Excess
Calcium	1% (with limited zinc)	Immature	Depressed appetite, reduced rate of gain, parakeratosis
	1% (with adequate zinc and limited phosphorus)	Immature	Reduced rate of gain and reduced bone strength
Copper	800-500 mg/kg (in absence of higher levels of dietary iron and zinc)[b]	Immature	Reduced growth, lower hemoglobin, icterus, and death[c]
Iodine	800 mg/kg	Immature	Depressed feed intake and rate of gain, lowered hemoglobin,[d] and eye lesions
Iron	5,000 mg/kg	Immature	Depressed feed intake and rate of gain, reduced serum inorganic phosphorus and femur ash, rickets[e]
Manganese	4,000 mg/kg	Immature	Depressed feed intake, reduced growth rate, stiffness, and stilted gait
Selenium	5-8 mg/kg[f]	Immature	Anorexia, hair loss, separation of hoof and skin at coronary band, degenerative changes in liver and kidney
	10 mg/kg	Breeding (sows)	Reduced conception; pigs small, weak or dead at birth
Sodium chloride and other sodium salts	1-8% (with severe water restriction)	All ages	Nervousness, weakness, staggering, epileptic seizures, paralysis and death
Zinc	2,000 mg/kg	Immature	Growth depression, arthritis, hemorrhage in axillary spaces, gastritis and enteritis
Arsenic	990 mg/kg	Immature	Poor growth, erythema, ataxia, posterior paralysis, quadraplegia and blindness, Myelin degeneration of optic and peripheral nerves
Cadmium	50 mg/kg	Immature	Reduced gain and hematocrit
	150 mg/kg	Immature	Severe depression of gain and hematocrit
	450 mg/kg	Immature	Severe depression of gain and hematocrit and appearance of dermatitis

Cobalt	400 mg/kg	Immature	Anorexia, growth depression, stiff-legged, humped back, incoordination and muscle tremors, anemia[g]
Fluorine:			
Soluble fluorides	100 mg/kg	Mature	Mottled enamel, enamel hypoplasia, softening of teeth, osteomalacia, excessive loss of weight by lactative sows
Rock phosphate F	200 mg/kg	Mature	
Gossypol[h]	200 mg/kg	Immature	Muscular weakness, dyspnea, generalized edema, death; myocarditis, hepatitis, and nephritis
Lead	600 mg/kg	Immature	Squealing as if in pain, diarrhea, salivation, grinding of teeth, depressed appetite, reduced growth rate, muscular tremors, ataxia, increased respiratory rate, decreased heart rate, enlarged carpal joints, impaired vision, clonic seizures, death
Mercury	Single oral dose of 5 to 15 mg methyl mercury dicyandiamide per kilogram of body weight	Immature	Anorexia, bodyweight loss, central nervous system depression, weakness, gagging, vomiting, diarrhea, ataxia, cyanosis, muscular tremors, postural and gait abnormalities, polyuria
Nitrate	1,800 mg NO_2/kg	Immature	Growth depression, dyspnea and cyanosis, elevated methemoglobin, lymphocytosis, reduced serum vitamin A and E levels
Nitrite	400 mg NO_2/kg	Immature	
Urea	2.5%	Immature	Reduced feed intake and growth rate, increased plasma urea nitrogen level

[a] The toxic dietary levels listed are those that have experimentally produced the signs indicated and are not necessarily minimum toxic or maximum tolerant levels.

[b] In a few instances, a dietary level of 250 mg/kg has resulted in signs of excess.

[c] In some instances, 500 mg/kg of copper has been fed without icterus or death occurring.

[d] Anemia of iodine toxicity alleviated with supplemental iron.

[e] Rickets from excessive dietary iron alleviated by increasing dietary phophorus.

[f] Selenium toxicity partially alleviated with arsenic.

[g] Cobalt toxicity alleviated by supplemental methionine, iron, zinc, and manganese.

[h] Gossypol toxicity alleviated by increasing dietary iron to equal the weight of free gossypol.

(From *Nutrient Requirements of Swinc*, National Research Council, 1979.)

cient diets. When the deficiency becomes severe, anorexia develops.

Choline: Choline-deficient pigs exhibit incoordinated movements and an abnormal shoulder conformation. At necropsy, they may have fatty livers and usually show kidney damage (renal glomerular occlusion and tubular epithelial necrosis).

Vitamin B_{12}: Baby pigs fed synthetic diets low in vitamin B_{12} show hyperirritability, voice failure, pain in the hindquarters and posterior incoordination. Histologic examination of the bone marrow reveals an impairment of the hemopoietic system. Fatty livers are also noted upon necropsy. Under farm conditions, weanling pigs fed practical diets low in vitamin B_{12} do not show the above signs, but merely gain more slowly than pigs receiving an adequate allowance of this vitamin.

NUTRITIONAL DEFICIENCIES IN HORSES

Descriptions of uncomplicated nutrient deficiencies in the horse are rare. The natural feeds typically consumed are most likely to be deficient in protein, calcium, phosphorus, sodium, chlorine, iodine and selenium, depending on the age and productive level of the horse and the geographic area. Dried, weathered forages may be very low in carotene and if these are fed for long periods, vitamin A deficiency may develop. Certain anemias have responded to vitamin B_{12} therapy. Thiamin and riboflavin deficiencies have been produced experimentally.

Signs of deficiency are frequently nonspecific and diagnosis may be complicated by a simultaneous shortage of several nutrients. The consequences of increased susceptibility to parasitism and bacterial infections may superimpose still other clinical signs. In the following paragraphs, signs of deficiency noted in the horse will be recorded where these are available. Where they are not, the most likely signs, which might be expected from research with other species, will be described.

ENERGY

Many of the nonspecific changes found in deficient subjects are related to caloric deficiency and result from inadequate intake of a well-balanced diet or from poor utilization of the diet which follows the development of a specific deficiency. In partial or complete starvation most internal organs exhibit some atrophy. The brain is least affected, but the size of the gonads may be strikingly decreased, and estrus may be delayed. Hypoplasia of lymph nodes, spleen and thymus leads to a marked reduction in their size. The adrenal glands are usually enlarged. The young skeleton is extremely sensitive and growth slows or may completely stop. In the adult, the skeleton may become osteoporotic. A decrease in adipose tissue is an early and conspicuous sign, not only in the subcutis, but in the mesentery, around the kidneys, uterus and testes, and in the retroperitoneal area. Low fat content of the marrow in the long bones is a good indicator of prolonged inanition. The ability to perform work is impaired, and endogenous nitrogen losses increase as muscle proteins are metabolized for energy.

PROTEIN

A deficiency of dietary protein may represent either an inadequate intake of high-quality protein or the lack of a specific essential amino acid. It is doubtful that synthesis by microorganisms in the gut plus proteolysis of microbial protein is adequate to meet the essential amino acid needs of the horse. The deficiency effects are generally unspecific and many of the signs differ in no respect from the effects of partial or total caloric restriction. In addition, there may be depressed appetite, decreased formation of hemoglobin, erythrocytes and plasma proteins. Edema is sometimes associated with the hypoproteinemia. Milk production is decreased in lactating mares. Decreased activity of the following liver enzymes has been noted: pyruvic oxidase, succinoxidase, succinic acid dehydrogenase, D-amino acid oxidase, DPN-cytochrome C reductase and uricase. Corneal vascularization and lens degeneration have been noted in some species. Antibody formation is impaired.

MINERALS

Calcium: The young growing horse or the lactating mare being fed on poor-quality grass hay or pasture are most likely to develop calcium deficiencies. Serum calcium levels may be depressed while serum inorganic phosphorus levels may be elevated; however, single samples of blood are generally not diagnostic. Serum alkaline phosphatase activity is usually elevated. Clotting time may be prolonged slightly. Young, growing bone is frequently rachitic and brittle. Fractures may be common and poor healing follows. Adult bone may be osteoporotic.

Phosphorus: A deficiency is most likely in horses being fed poor-quality grass hay or pasture without grain. Serum inorganic phosphorus levels may be depressed and serum alkaline phosphatase activity increased. Occasionally, serum calcium levels may be elevated. An insidious shifting lameness may be seen. Bone changes resemble those described for calcium deficiency.

Sodium and Chlorine: Horses are most likely to develop signs of sodium chloride (salt) deficiency when worked hard in hot weather. Perspiration and urinary losses are appreciable. Horses deprived of salt tire easily, stop sweating and exhibit muscle spasms. Anorexia and pica may be evident. However, pica is not a specific sign of sodium chloride deficiency. The milk production of lactating mares will seriously decline. Hemoconcentration and acidosis may be expected.

Potassium: Deficiency results in decreased rate of growth, anorexia and hypokalemia.

Magnesium: Foals fed a purified diet containing 3.6 mg/lb (8 mg/kg) exhibited hypomagnesemia, nervousness, muscular tremors, and ataxia followed by collapse, with hyperpnea, sweating, convulsive paddling of legs and death.

Iron: Deficiency may be secondary to parasitism and results in microcytic, hypochromic anemia.

Zinc: Deficiency in the foal is accompanied by reduced growth rate, anorexia, cutaneous lesions on the lower extremities, alopecia, lowered blood levels of zinc and reduced plasma alkaline phosphatase activity.

Copper: An apparent relationship between low serum copper levels and bleeding in aged parturient mares suggested reduced copper absorption with age or reduced ability to mobilize copper stores.

Iodine: Deficiency is an endemic problem in many areas (*see* GOITER, p. 203).

Cobalt: Deficiency is apparently rare in horses; they have been known to thrive on pastures so low in cobalt that sheep and cattle dependent upon them wasted and died.

Selenium: Deficiency results in reduced serum selenium, elevated serum glutamic oxalacetic transaminase activity, white muscle disease, alopecia, yellow-brown fat, and numerous small hemorrhages (q.v., p. 591).

VITAMINS

Vitamin A: A deficiency may develop if dried, poor-quality roughage is fed for a prolonged period. If body stores are high, several months may pass before signs appear. The deficiency is characterized by nyctalopia, lacrimation, keratinization of the cornea, susceptibility to pneumonia, abscesses of the sublingual gland, incoordination, impaired reproduction, capricious appetite and progressive weakness. Hooves are frequently deformed, the horny layer unevenly laid down and unusually brittle. Metaplasia of the intestinal mucosa and achlorhydria have been reported. Genitourinary mucosal metaplasia may be expected. Bone remodeling is defective. The foramina do not enlarge properly during growth and skeletal deformities are evident.

Vitamin D: If sun-cured hay is consumed or the horse is exposed to sunlight, it is doubtful that a deficiency of vitamin D will develop. Prolonged confinement of a young, growing horse offered only limited amounts of sun-cured hay may result in reduced bone calcification, stiff and swollen joints, stiffness of gait, irritability and reduction in serum calcium and phosphorus.

Thiamin: The signs of deficiency, which have been produced experimentally in the horse, include anorexia, loss of weight, incoordination, lowered blood thiamin and elevated blood pyruvate. At necropsy the heart is dilated. Similar signs have been observed in bracken fern poisoning (q.v., p. 1015). Under normal circumstances the natural diet plus synthesis by microorganisms in the gut probably meet the thiamin need.

Riboflavin: Although natural feeds plus synthesis within the gut should normally provide adequate riboflavin, limited evidence indicates an occasional deficiency when the diet is of poor quality. The first sign of acute riboflavin deficiency is the appearance of catarrhal conjunctivitis in one or both eyes. This is accompanied by photophobia and lacrimation. There may be a gradual deterioration of the retina, lens and ocular fluids, resulting in impaired vision or blindness. Periodic ophthalmia, which has been linked to riboflavin deficiency, is possibly one of the sequelae of leptospirosis (q.v., p. 384), or of onchocerciasis (q.v., p. 709).

Cyanocobalamin (vitamin B_{12}): The normal feedstuffs of horses generally contain very little vitamin B_{12}. However, the horse can synthesize this vitamin in the gut where it is absorbed. Certain anemias have been reported in horses which responded to vitamin B_{12} therapy.

NUTRITIONAL DEFICIENCIES IN DOGS

Disease of nutritional origin in pet dogs is more often due to dietary imbalance or overfeeding than to a simple nutrient deficiency. Clinical signs are unlikely to conform to the classic descriptions (often based on experimentally induced deficiencies) and the lack of specific signs is often complicated by infectious disease, poor management or parasitism. Diagnosis often depends on a history of a bizarre diet or feeding practice, and recovery follows return to a diet based on sound nutritional principles.

Energy: Although deficiency of energy intake may well be due to underfeeding and neglect, it may also occur under the following conditions: (1) **Low dietary-caloric density of the food** (one designed for obesity control). Even large meals do not meet requirements and most puppies in particular are unable to eat enough at 2 or even 3 meals to maintain energy balance. They may be potbellied, but thin and always hungry, with poor muscle development. Similarly, the lactating bitch is unable to maintain body weight on a diet of low-energy density. (2) **High-energy expenditure.** Police or army dogs, sledge dogs, and lactating bitches may receive insufficient food to compensate for major increases in energy requirement. Cold weather can increase the energy requirements for short-haired dogs in uninsulated houses by as much as 200 to 300%. Feeding frequency, caloric density and palatability must be increased to meet energy requirements, which may be 2 to 3 times maintenance levels.

Protein: Deficiency is most likely in the growing puppy and lactating bitch fed an unpalatable diet of low-protein concentration or quality. Poor growth and condition, potbelly, poor muscle development, anemia, reduced immunity and poor wound healing are characteristic. It may also occur in the lactating bitch receiving inadequate increases in the amount or quality of her dietary protein. A relative deficiency of protein may result from too much fat or carbohydrate in the diet; protein of mixed plant and animal origin should supply not less than 20 to 25% of the total calories.

Fat: A minimum of 2% (as corn oil or its equivalent) of dietary fat is required by the dog. This amount is probably sufficient to supply the essential fatty acids for prostaglandin synthesis among other basic biochemical functions. Deficiency is manifested by loss of hair, scurfy skin, increased susceptibility to infection, and impaired reproduction. Lard, bacon or vegetable fats are useful supplements because of their relatively high linoleic acid content. However, polyunsaturated fatty acids in excess of 1% linoleic acid equivalent serve no beneficial purpose. Rancid fat is readily eaten by dogs, but development of rancidity destroys vitamins E and A and essential fatty acids.

Vitamins: A commercial, mixed diet of a variety of animal, cereal and vegetable matter is unlikely to have major vitamin deficiencies unless subjected to prolonged heating or exposure to air. The losses of heat labile vitamins (particularly thiamin) that occur during processing of proprietary diets are offset by preprocessing supplementation and postprocessing analytical checks to establish adequacy.

Vitamin A: The dog has a much greater tolerance of hypo- and hyper-vitaminosis A than the cat and clinical nutritional abnormalities rarely occur. Unlike the cat, the dog can convert the provitamin carotene found in vegetables to vitamin A in the body. Preformed vitamin A is supplied by milk, fat, liver and to a lesser extent by kidney and the fat of muscle meat. Commercial diets include stabilized vitamin A. Because the vitamin is stored in the body in liver kidney and fat, prolonged dietary deficiency is necessary before clinical signs develop. Hypervitaminosis A is uncommon in the dog.

Vitamin D: Deficiency of this vitamin in association with deficiency of calcium or phosphorus, gives rise to rickets in young dogs and osteomalacia in adults (q.v., p. 579 and 580). Too much fish liver oil or other vitamin D supplements is more likely to cause vitamin-D-associated disease than is dietary insufficiency. Oversupplementation with vitamin D, particularly in the giant breeds, may be associated with bone dystrophies (with severe calcium deficiency or relative phosphorus excess) and calcification of soft tissues (where minerals are liberally supplied). *See also* DYSTROPHIES ASSOCIATED WITH CALCIUM, PHOSPHORUS AND VITAMIN D, p. 576.

Vitamin E: Diets containing rancid fat or excess quantities of polyunsaturated fatty acids, particularly those in fish oils, may provoke vitamin E deficiency after prolonged feeding to dogs. Puppies may be whelped dead or weak and the survivors suffer from muscular dystrophy or cardiac insufficiency. A deficiency of vitamin E is unlikely in dogs fed a commercial diet.

Vitamin K: Although normally not a dietary requirement, as sufficient is synthesized in the gut by bacterial flora, increased clotting time and deaths from massive hemorrhage have occurred in growing pups on synthetic diets that were otherwise nutritionally adequate. Good response to vitamin K administration occurred.

Vitamin B complex: Thiamin (Vitamin B_1)—Clinical deficiencies have been reported in dogs and cats in which low amounts of naturally occurring vitamins were destroyed by heating. Characteristic signs were decreased appetite, constipation, weight loss, weakness, drowsiness, paralysis, chronic convulsions and other nervous signs. Signs resolve readily on parenteral thiamin administration and supplementation of the diet with a thiamin source such as yeast or thiamin tablets. Some raw fish contains the enzyme thiaminase, which destroys thiamin and may be associated with a thiamin deficiency syndrome. Raw fish diets have been associated with paralytic signs in dogs and silver foxes due to the destruction of thiamin by the thermo-labile enzyme thiaminase present in the fish. Cooking the fish and administration of thiamin abolished the syndrome.

Niacin—Black tongue or canine pellagra, a niacin deficiency syndrome, used to occur in farm or shepherd dogs fed a diet primarily of flaked corn (maize) with little or no milk or other material of animal origin. The condition was characterized by reddening of the oral mucosa, emaciation and eventual death.

Vitamin C: Normal dogs do not require a dietary source of vitamin C, and claims that massive supplementation shortens or reduces the severity of various viral diseases in dogs and cats are unsubstantiated. In the condition that has been called Barlow's disease in dogs because of its similarity to infantile scurvy in humans, a specific deficiency of ascorbic acid has not been identified nor have claims been substantiated that vitamin C administration to puppies reduces the severity of hip dysplasia.

Minerals: Disease may result from deficiency, imbalance or an excess of minerals. As with other nutrients the likelihood of deficiency is greatest in the growing or lactating animal. Such deficiency will rarely occur if balanced commercial food is fed, since increased caloric intake will result in a corresponding increase in mineral intake.

Calcium and Phosphorus: The most commonly recognized dietary mineral deficiency is the imbalance of calcium and phosphorus. This is due to a failure to correct the adverse Ca to P ratio in meat supplements (1 to 20). Optimum ratios are between 1.2 and 1.4 parts of calcium to 1 of phosphorus. In the puppy, imbalance or deficiency of calcium and phosphorus leads to bone dystrophies, slow growth and spontaneous fractures. On the other hand excessive calcium nutrition can cause a hypertrophic osteodystrophy in growing dogs of large breeds on a high plane of nutrition. In the adult, primary deficiency signs are rare, but demineralization of bone may occur under extreme conditions. Most commercial diets supply a satisfactory amount and balance of calcium and phosphorus. To bring meat supplements into calcium balance, 2 to 3 gm of calcium carbonate should be mixed with each pound of meat fed. *See also* DYSTROPHIES ASSOCIATED WITH CALCIUM, PHOSPHORUS AND VITAMIN D, p. 576.

Other minerals: Deficiencies of magnesium, potassium, sodium, chlorine and the trace elements iron, copper, cobalt, iodine, manganese, and zinc are unlikely to be encountered in dogs fed all but the most abnormal diets. However, puppies with hookworm infections may be deficient in iron, copper and cobalt, and manganese deficiencies have been reported.

NUTRITIONAL DEFICIENCIES IN CATS

Water

Dehydration is a serious problem in disorders of the alimentary and respiratory tracts and kidneys. During anorexia, 1% glucose-saline or similar solutions, 20 to 30 ml/lb (44 to 66 ml/kg) of body wt per day (30 to 40 ml/lb [66 to 88 ml/kg] in kittens), given orally or parenterally, will help maintain fluid balance and urine flow.

Insufficient fluid intake may precipitate urolithiasis. Fluid intake is increased substantially by adding 1% sodium chloride and mixing additional water in the food. Excessive thirst and frequent urination may indicate diabetes mellitus, diabetes insipidus or kidney damage. The cat with polydipsia, or having salt added to its diet, should never be denied drinking water.

Protein and Energy

Unless there is sufficient energy in a cat's diet, some protein needed for other body functions will be converted to energy. Feedstuffs too low in fat, containing too much indigestible carbohydrate or not enough B-complex vitamins all can result in an energy-deficient diet. Too little high quality protein, too much fat or too much carbohydrate can cause a protein-deficient diet.

The signs produced by an improper protein-calorie ratio coupled with fatty acid deficiency may include any or all of the following: weight loss; dull, unkempt haircoat; anorexia; reproductive problems; persistent, unresponsive parasitism; persistent, unresponsive, low-grade infection; unexplained "breaks" in the vaccination program; rapid, precipitous weight loss after injury or during disease; failure to respond properly to injury or disease—and should suggest modification of the diet.

Fat-Soluble Vitamins

Vitamin A: Liver and fish liver oils and synthetic vitamin A are the principal sources of vitamin A for cats since they cannot utilize carotene. Classical xerophthalmia, follicular hyperkeratosis, and retinal degeneration occur rarely, usually associated with concomitant protein deficiency. Borderline deficiency is more common, especially in chronic ill health. Plasma vitamin A levels below 20 mcg/100 ml indicate deficiency. Hypovitaminosis A affects reproduction, causing stillbirths, congenital anomalies (hydrocephaly, blindness, deafness, ataxia, cerebellar dysplasia, intestinal hernia) and resorption of fetuses. Overdosing with vitamin A must be avoided. Hypervitaminosis A may produce forelimb lameness, with or without hyperesthesia, associated with radiologic evidence of scoliosis, ankylosis and exostosis.

Vitamin D: Classical signs of rickets (q.v., p. 579) are rare in kittens and confined to those born in winter, kept permanently in dark quarters, or from queens fed vitamin D-deficient rations. It is important to avoid hypervitaminosis D through overdosing.

Vitamin E: Steatitis (q.v., p. 596) results from a diet high in polyunsaturated fatty acids, particularly from marine fish oils. Kittens develop anorexia and muscular dystrophy; depot fat becomes discolored by brown or orange pigment. Lesions occur in cardiac and skeletal muscles.

Water-Soluble Vitamins

Apart from thiamin and pyridoxine deficiency, water-soluble vitamin deficiencies are usually the result of disease processes, which limit alimentary synthesis or absorption, or increase metabolic requirements or kidney loss. In such circumstances, oral or parenteral administration of multiple B-vitamin preparations may prevent the onset of "feline pellagra," which is characterized by ulcerative stomatitis, especially of the tongue, and by conjunctivitis.

Thiamin deficiency rarely occurs on a fresh-meat or good commercial diet. Thiaminase from uncooked fish can produce a deficiency. Destruction of thiamin may also result from treatment of food with sulfur dioxide or heating during drying or canning. Cats eating a thiamin-deficient diet develop anorexia, an unkempt coat and a hunched appearance. Convulsions follow, becoming more severe, leading in a few days to prostration and death-signs often described by owners as indicative of "poisoning." Diagnosis can be confirmed in the early stages by giving thiamin orally or IM. Recovery occurs in a matter of hours. If the diet is not supplemented following this treatment, a relapse can be expected. At necropsy, small petechial hemorrhages may be found in the cerebrum and midbrain.

The **pyridoxine**-deficient cat loses weight, becomes anemic and suffers kidney damage due to the accumulation of oxalate. A severe form of calcium oxalate urolithiasis ensues.

Minerals

The requirement for dietary **calcium** is increased in kittens and queens. Insufficient supplies result in nutritional hyperparathyroidism (q.v., p. 577). Signs of irritability, hyperesthesia and loss of muscle tone appear with temporary or permanent paralysis. Rarefaction of the skeleton, particularly the pelvis and vertebral bodies, can be confirmed radiologically, and is a valuable diagnostic aid. There is often a history of diet confined almost wholly to meat. The condition can be corrected by feeding a diet that is known to be capable of supporting kitten growth.

Iodine deficiency may occur on meat diets but rarely on diets containing saltwater fish or on good cat rations. The deficient kitten will show signs of hyperthyroidism in the early stages, with increased excitability, followed later by hypothyroidism and lethargy. The condition can be confirmed by size (over 12 mg/100 gm of body wt) and histopathology of the thyroid gland at necropsy.

Iron and copper in meat can be utilized efficiently by cats. Occasionally deficiencies probably result from alimentary disorders. Excess dietary manganese may darken coat color in partial albinos such as Siamese, and also reduce fertility.

NUTRITIONAL DEFICIENCIES IN POULTRY

A nutritional deficiency may be either simple or multiple, that is, the total feed consumed may not contain an adequate quantity of one or more indispensable nutrients. A given deficiency may be borderline, marked, or absolute. About the only observable result of a borderline deficiency is slightly retarded growth, slightly decreased egg production, or slightly reduced hatchability. An absolute deficiency of any indispensable nutrient causes death. A marked deficiency of one or more indispensable nutrients leads to the development of a deficiency disease.

Many deficiency diseases cause the same general signs, such as retarded growth, poor feathering and weakness. Thus it is not always possible to recognize the cause from the signs. In most instances, a correct diagnosis can be made only by obtaining complete information about the diet and management of the birds, in addition to the signs in the affected living birds and necropsies of at least a few birds soon after death. Because they are difficult to diagnose, chronic deficiencies may be more injurious in the long run than acute ones.

In assessing a diet, it is well to keep in mind that the composition of the individual ingredients is variable and that some nutrients are comparatively unstable and some are unavailable as they occur naturally in feeds. A diet that appears to contain just enough of one or more nutrients may actually be deficient to some degree in those nutrients. Conditions of stress (bacterial, parasitic and viral infections; high or low temperatures; low humidity; drugs) may either interfere with the absorption of a nutrient or increase the quantity required. Thus some chemical compound, toxin, microorganism etc. can destroy, or render unavailable to the bird a particular nutrient that is present in the diet at adequate levels.

Only deficiencies occurring on practical diets in the field are discussed herein.

PROTEIN AND AMINO ACID DEFICIENCIES

Etiology: The optimal level of protein intake for the young growing chick appears to be about 18 to 23% of the diet; for the young growing poult and gallinaceous upland game birds, about 26 to 30% and for young growing ducklings, about 20 to 22%. When the protein content of the diet is reduced below these levels, the birds tend to grow more slowly. Small reductions in the protein content of the diet, however, often may be offset by an increased feed intake unless the diet is unusually bulky.

Even though a diet contains the above specified quantities of protein, satisfactory growth will not result without sufficient amounts of all the indispensable amino acids. A deficiency of protein causes an increased deposition of fat in the bird since productive use cannot be made of the energy consumed if protein intake is suboptimal.

Clinical Findings: Except in the case of lysine, the only apparent indication of amino acid deficiency is retarded growth. In the turkey poult (particularly the bronze variety), a deficiency of lysine inhibits the pigmentation of the feathers; some of the feathers on the wings are white or have a white bar. Normal pigmentation of new feathers takes place as soon as adequate diet is fed, but the unpigmented portion of an already existing feather remains colorless.

MINERAL DEFICIENCIES

Calcium and Phosphorus Deficiencies

A deficiency of either calcium or phosphorus in the diet of young growing birds results in an abnormal development of the skeleton even though the diet contains a fully adequate quantity of vitamin D (*see* VITAMIN D DEFICIENCY, p. 1428). The abnormal development is neither prevented nor stopped by increasing the intake of vitamin D, if the deficiency of either calcium or phosphorus is marked.

This abnormal condition of the skeleton commonly is referred to as rickets, but some writers distinguish between the condition that results from a deficiency of calcium (osteoporosis) and that which results from a deficiency of phosphorus (rickets). Osteoporosis may be observed in adult as well as in young growing birds, whereas rickets is observed only in the latter.

Etiology: The newly hatched bird is essentially osteoporotic as its bones have a much lower calcium:phosphorus ratio than they do later on if the diet is fully adequate. Hence, the newly hatched bird requires an immediate supply of calcium in its diet. If the diet is markedly deficient in either calcium or vitamin D, the osteoporotic condition becomes more pronounced. If, however, the diet contains sufficient calcium, but is deficient in either phosphorus or vitamin D, rickets develops. One means of producing rickets experimentally is to feed a diet high in calcium, but low in phosphorus.

Clinical Findings: The first signs of a deficiency of calcium or phosphorus, or both, in young growing birds are very similar to those of vitamin D deficiency. Typical of all 3 deficiencies (calcium, phosphorus and vitamin D) are a lame, stiff-legged gait, retardation of growth and ruffled feathers. In calcium deficiency, the leg bones are springy, but in phosphorus or in vitamin D deficiency, they are rubbery and the joints tend to be enlarged. In calcium, but not in phosphorus deficiency, some of the birds may become paralyzed.

If a bird in heavy egg production does not obtain enough calcium from its feed, the skeleton is depleted and becomes osteoporotic; a few thin-shelled eggs and also eggs with low hatchability are produced and then production ceases. If there is a very marked deficiency of calcium, a paralytic condition may develop. If calcium is not supplied, death follows within 1 to 3 days after the onset of the paralysis.

Laboratory Findings: In both rickets and osteoporosis, there is a decreased ash content of the bones. The changes in the content of calcium and phosphorus in the blood depend on the content of calcium and phosphorus in the diet. If the dietary calcium level is low, the blood may have an approximately normal calcium and a high phosphorus content. If the diet is deficient in both calcium and phosphorus, the blood may contain less than the normal quantities of these elements.

Prophylaxis and Treatment: For the prevention of calcium and phosphorus deficiencies, it is sufficient to provide diets with adequate quantities of these 2 elements. In the case of the growing bird, it is particularly desirable not to have a gross excess of calcium in the diet because rickets will tend to occur on a diet normally adequate in phosphorus and vitamin D if a gross excess of calcium is added to it. Feeding diets containing more than 2.5% calcium during the growing period produces a high incidence of nephrosis, visceral gout, calcium urate deposits in the ureters and high mortality.

An improvement in egg-shell strength can be achieved by feeding about two-thirds of the calcium supplement in the form of oyster-shell flakes or coarse limestone, with the remaining one-third as ground limestone. At no time should oyster shell or any other form of calcium supplement be added without an equivalent reduction in the amount of limestone as feeding too much calcium reduces shell quality. Offering the coarse supplement permits the birds to pick out their requirements when they need it most.

If paralysis resulting from calcium deficiency should develop, an effective treatment—if started very soon after the paralysis occurs—is to give orally 1 gm of calcium carbonate in a gelatin capsule daily for 2 or 3 days and to feed a fully adequate diet. Treatment of experimental calcium deficiency usually causes disappearance of the paralysis within 48 hours.

Manganese Deficiency

A deficiency of manganese in the diet of young growing chickens is one of the causes—the first to be recognized—of perosis; in the diet of laying chickens, it is one of the causes of thin-shelled eggs and poor hatchability (*see* CALCIUM AND PHOSPHORUS DEFICIENCIES, p. 1422, *also* VITAMIN D DEFICIENCY, p. 1428).

Etiology: Many of the feedstuffs used in feeding poultry do not contain enough manganese to meet the requirement for this element. This is especially true of corn, and diets based on corn usually are deficient in manganese unless they contain a special source, such as manganese sulfate or manganese oxide. Manganese deficiency is now much less common because virtually all commercial feeds contain added manganese. For that reason, it is well to consider the other possible causes when perosis is encountered.

Clinical Findings: Perosis is a malformation of the hock joint. The signs usually found are swelling and flattening of the hock joint, sometimes followed by slipping of the Achilles tendon from its condyles. The tibia and the tarsometatarsus may exhibit bending near the joint and lateral rotation. One or both legs may be affected. A shortening and thickening of the long bones of the legs and wings is also apparent. Perosis caused by manganese deficiency is exacerbated by excessive amounts of calcium and phosphorus in the diet. Birds reared on wire or slatted floors are more susceptible to perosis than those reared on litter.

The signs of perosis in poults, ducklings and goslings are similar to those observed in chicks. Perosis has been observed in various wild birds, including pheasants, grouse, quail and sparrows.

When adult chickens are fed a diet deficient in manganese, no observable changes in their leg joints occur, but the shells of their eggs tend to become thinner and less resistant to breakage. If the deficiency is sufficiently marked, both egg production and hatchability are reduced. The reduced hatchability results from an increase in the embryonic mortality that occurs after the 10th day of incubation. The embryonic mortality reaches its peak at about the 20th and 21st days. The embryos that die after the 10th day usually are chondrodystrophic; they have short, thickened legs, short wings, "parrot beaks," a globular contour of the head, protruding abdomen and, in the most severe cases, retarded development of the down. The few chicks that sometimes hatch usually have very short leg bones (micromelia) and in some cases, the bones may be deformed as in the chicks in which perosis develops after hatching.

Prophylaxis and Treatment: The only way to prevent perosis is to feed a diet adequate in all indispensable nutrients, especially manganese, choline, niacin, biotin and folic acid. After deformities have occurred, they cannot be corrected by feeding an adequate diet. Effects of manganese deficiency on egg production are fully corrected by an adequate diet that contains 30 to 40 mg/kg of manganese, provided that the diet does not contain excessive quantities of calcium and phosphorus. The intake of calcium may be excessive where calcium supplements are provided free choice. When meat scrap or meat-and-bone scrap is used as the principal source of protein, the feed may contain an excessive quantity of phosphorus.

Iron and Copper Deficiencies

A microcytic, hypochromic anemia with no change in the number of red blood cells can be produced by iron or copper deficiency.

Both copper and iron deficiencies will cause depigmentation in the feathers of Rhode Island Red or New Hampshire chickens. Copper deficiency in chicks produces dissecting aneurysms of the aorta and various bone deformities. Copper is needed in elastin formation. Most practical diets for poultry will contain enough iron and copper to prevent deficiencies. Some feed manufacturers add small amounts as an insurance measure.

Iodine Deficiency

Very few cases of goiter, or enlarged thyroids, have been observed in poultry, probably because it is difficult to observe the glands. Goiter has been produced experimentally in chickens by feeding a diet exceedingly low in iodine (about 0.025 ppm) to laying hens. The possibility of an iodine deficiency in poultry may easily be obviated by adding as little as 0.35 mg of iodine per kilogram of feed.

Magnesium Deficiency

Magnesium deficiency does not occur in poultry fed practical diets. It may be produced experimentally by feeding a diet of highly purified feedstuffs. When such a diet is fed to young chicks, one observes poor growth and feathering, decreased muscle tone, ataxia, progressive incoordination and convulsions followed by death.

Potassium Deficiency

A great majority of the natural feedstuffs and many of the by-product feedstuffs used in feeding poultry contain much more potassium than is needed. Deficiencies of this mineral, therefore, are not seen in commercially raised poultry.

Salt Deficiency

The salt requirement of chickens, and presumably other kinds of poultry, is rather low. Of the 2 chemical elements in salt, sodium is required in appreciably larger quantity than chlorine. Diets containing less than 0.15% of sodium retard growth in young chicks and depress egg production and hatchability in laying chickens. A high level of potassium appears to increase the requirement of sodium and a high level of sodium appears to increase the requirement of potassium. Most practical poultry diets require the addition of 0.25 to 0.5% of sodium chloride to prevent a deficiency.

Inasmuch as nearly all feedstuffs contain some salt and a few contain from 1 to 4.5% or more (e.g. whey, fish meal, meat scrap, condensed fish solubles), an excess of salt is possible. An excess causes the droppings to be loose and watery. Chickens may be raised on diets that contain as much as 3% of salt, but growth is retarded and efficiency of feed utilization is reduced. The same percentage—or even less—of salt in the drinking water is very toxic.

Zinc Deficiency

With a diet deficient in zinc, growth is retarded and feather development is poor. The hock joints become enlarged and the long bones are shortened and thickened. Slipping of the tendons does not occur. On occasion the skin on the foot pads becomes dry and thickened with fissures and hyperkeratosis developing.

In mature hens, zinc deficiency reduces egg production and hatchability. Embryos show a wide range of skeletal abnormalities including micromelia, curvature of the spine, and shortened, fused thoracic and lumbar vertebrae. It is usual practice to include a zinc supplement in all practical poultry diets.

Selenium Deficiency

A deficiency of selenium in growing chickens causes exudative diathesis. The early signs (unthriftiness, ruffled feathers) usually occur between 5 and 11 weeks of age. The subcut. edema results in weeping of the skin which is often seen on the inner surface of the thighs and wings. The birds bruise easily, with large scabs often forming on an old bruise. In laying hens, the tissue damage is unusual but egg production and feed conversion are adversely affected.

In many countries it is now legal to add selenium to starter and grower diets. In most cases 0.1 ppm is permitted in chicken diets and 0.2 ppm in turkey diets. The forms of selenium commonly used are sodium selenate and sodium selenite. Feeds grown on high-selenium soils are good sources of selenium and may be used in poultry rations in order to supply a source of selenium. Fish meal and dried brewer's yeast are also good sources. There is considerable variation in availability of selenium in different feedstuffs.

Even in the presence of adequate levels of vitamin E, poultry rations must contain 0.15 to 0.2 mg of selenium per kilogram of feed. As little as 8 to 10 mg/kg is toxic to poultry.

VITAMIN DEFICIENCIES

Vitamin A Deficiency

Vitamin A is required for the normal development and repair of all epithelial structures and for the normal development of the bones. Although vitamin A has not been found to be of value in building immunity, it is of value in maintaining the "first line of defense," the epithelial structures.

Etiology: Vitamin A and its several precursors (α, β, and γ-carotene and cryptoxanthin) are relatively unstable.

Feeds stored for a long time before being fed may contain too little vitamin A activity to meet the requirements of birds to which they are fed, especially if they contain meat scrap or fish meal from particular lots.

Clinical Findings: When young chicks are fed a diet markedly deficient in vitamin A activity, their rate of growth becomes subnormal after about 3 weeks and then declines very rapidly. The first characteristic signs, other than decline in rate of growth, are droopiness, ataxia and a ruffled appearance of the feathers. If the chicks survive more than a week after they become droopy, the eyes may become inflamed and there may be a discharge from the nostrils; in some chicks, there is swelling around the eyes and an accumulation of a sticky exudate beneath the lids. When the diet is not markedly deficient in vitamin A, the first signs may not appear until the chicks are 5 to 6 weeks old, in which case a larger proportion of the chicks eventually develop eye lesions and marked nervousness.

The signs of vitamin A deficiency in the poult are similar to those in the chick, but tend to be more acute.

In mature chickens and other poultry, the signs of vitamin A deficiency develop more slowly than in young birds, but the inflammation of the nose and eyes is much more pronounced. A borderline deficiency of vitamin A results in decreased egg production and reduced hatchability.

Lesions: In mature birds, vitamin A deficiency produces lesions resembling pustules in the mouth, pharynx and esophagus; in young growing birds, these lesions are found less frequently. Often there are white or grayish white deposits of urates in the kidneys and ureters. Such deposits, however, occur more frequently in young chickens than in young turkeys. Sometimes, there are deposits of urates on the surface of the heart, liver and spleen. Usually, urate or urate-like deposits are found in the thickened folds of the bursa of Fabricius.

In general, there is keratinization of the epithelial cells of the olfactory, respiratory, upper alimentary and urinary tracts. In severe cases, especially if the birds are mature, virtually all organs may be affected. Also, there are degenerative changes in both the central and peripheral nervous systems.

In very marked vitamin A deficiency in the chicken, the uric acid content of the blood may increase to 8 or 9 times its normal value. The accumulation of uric acid in the blood and the previously mentioned occurrence of deposits of uric acid in the ureters, kidneys and elsewhere probably are the result of failure of repair of the epithelial structures, especially those of the kidneys.

The nasal structures apparently may be used in diagnosing borderline deficiencies. In all degrees of vitamin A deficiency, there are true squamous metaplasia of the secretory and glandular epithelium, and secondary inflammatory or obstructive changes. In absolute vitamin A deficiency, there are atrophy, squamous metaplasia and hyperkeratinization.

Prophylaxis and Treatment: While the naturally occurring vitamin A precursors tend to be unstable in storage, most feed manufacturers include an antioxidant in feed which is to be stored for an appreciable length of time. This coupled with the fact that stabilized, dry vitamin A supplements are almost universally used today, makes it unlikely that vitamin A deficiency will be encountered in practice.

However, if vitamin A deficiency does develop through inadvertently omitting the vitamin A supplement or because of poor mixing, feed containing 3 to 4 times the normally recommended level can be fed for about 2 weeks. The dry, stabilized forms of vitamin A are the supplements of choice for the feed. There are also water-dispersible forms of vitamin A which can be administered through the drinking water; when feasible, this will usually give faster recovery than medication of the feed.

Vitamin D Deficiency

Abnormal development of the bones has been discussed under calcium and phosphorus deficiencies (p. 1422) and manganese deficiency (p. 1423). Vitamin D is required for the normal absorption and metabolism of calcium and phosphorus. A deficiency of vitamin D always produces rickets in young growing chickens and other poultry, even when the diet contains calcium and phosphorus in adequate quantities.

Etiology: The rickets and osteoporosis encountered in the practical production of poultry most frequently are the result of a deficiency of vitamin D. When poultry are reared in strict confinement, they require more vitamin D, as such, than when they have access to sunshine.

Clinical Findings: The first signs in young growing chickens and turkeys are a tendency to rest frequently in a squatting position, a disinclination to walk and a lame, stiff-legged gait. These are distinguished from the clinical signs of vitamin A deficiency in that birds with a vitamin D deficiency are alert rather than droopy and walk with a lame rather than a staggering gait (ataxia). Other signs, in the usual order of their occurrence, are retardation of growth, enlargement of the hock joints, beading at the ends of the ribs and marked softening of the beak. As in many other nutritional diseases of poultry, the feathers soon become ruffled.

In red or buff color breeds of chickens, a deficiency of vitamin D causes an abnormal black pigmentation of some of the feathers, especially those of the wings. If the deficiency is very marked, the blackening becomes pronounced and nearly all the feathers may be affected. When vitamin D is supplied in adequate quantity, the new feathers and the newer part of the older feathers are normal in color; the discolored portion remains black.

When laying chickens are fed a diet deficient in vitamin D, the first sign of the deficiency is a thinning of the shells of their eggs. If the deficiency is marked, there is a rather prompt reduction of both egg production and hatchability. Embryos frequently die at 18 to 19 days of age. After a time, the breast bones become noticeably less rigid and there may be beading at the ends of the ribs.

Lesions: In young chickens and turkeys, a deficiency of vitamin D produces marked changes in the bones and the parathyroid and thyroid glands, and variable changes in the calcium and phosphorus content of the blood (*see* CALCIUM AND PHOSPHORUS DEFICIENCIES, p. 1422). The bones may be quite soft or only moderately so. The epiphyses of the long bones usually are enlarged. The parathyroid becomes enlarged, sometimes to about 8 times its normal size, as a result of an increase in both the size of the cells and the number of epithelial cells.

In adult chickens, a deficiency of vitamin D eventually produces changes in the parathyroid similar to those produced in young chicks. The bones tend to become rarefied (osteoporotic) rather than soft.

Treatment: Enough extra vitamin D is added to currently used mashes to provide 3 times the normally recommended level for a period of about 3 weeks. Dry, stabilized forms of vitamin D_3 are recommended for feeding to poultry.

VITAMIN E DEFICIENCY

Chicks fed a diet deficient in vitamin E may show one or more of 3 classical deficiency disorders, namely, encephalomalacia, exudative diathesis and muscular dystrophy. Various dietary changes unrelated to the vitamin E content of the diet can completely prevent any one of these diseases without affecting the course of the other two. Thus, synthetic antioxidants can prevent encephalomalacia, inorganic selenium can prevent exudative diathesis while cystine can prevent muscular dystrophy. It would appear that no common metabolic defect can account for all 3 disorders.

Vitamin E is required for normal reproductive performance in the hen and for normal fertility in the mature male.

Etiology: Although both selenium and antioxidants can spare the requirements of vitamin E for certain functions, practical poultry diets must still contain sufficient vitamin E. Encephalomalacia has been a field problem for many years. It occurs with diets borderline in vitamin E that also contain polyunsaturated fats such as cod-liver oil or soybean oil in the process of undergoing oxidative rancidity. Since it is correlated with peroxidation of fats it may be prevented with vitamin E or a suitable antioxidant such as ethoxyquin. Exudative diathesis is a frequent occurrence on corn and soybean meal diets when these are grown on soils deficient in selenium. Both vitamin E and selenium are necessary to prevent the disease. Nutritional muscular dystrophy, not ordinarily a commercial problem, is found only when the diet is deficient in both vitamin E and sulfur amino acids. Because of the importance of sulfur amino acids for growth and feed efficiency they are usually present in adequate levels in practical diets.

Clinical Findings: Signs of encephalomalacia are sudden prostration, with legs outstretched and toes flexed, and retraction of the head. In the early stages the gait is incoordinate. Upon necropsy lesions are found in the cerebellum and sometimes in the cerebrum. In some birds necrotic reddish or brownish areas can be detected on the surface of the cerebellum.

Exudative diathesis is a severe edema produced by a marked increase in capillary permeability (*see* SELENIUM DEFICIENCY, p. 1426). Broilers are often severely downgraded because of the yellow staining inside the thighs caused by leakage of plasma into the subcut. tissues in this area.

Nutritional muscular dystrophy in chicks is characterized by degeneration of the muscle fibers, especially of the breast but also occurring occasionally in the leg muscles. There is perivascular infiltration, with marked accumulation of eosinophils, lymphocytes and histiocytes. These cells, along with the degenerated muscle fibers, present a picture of degeneration, with large numbers of free nuclei in evidence.

In mature chickens no outward signs of vitamin E deficiency are apparent even after a prolonged period. However, degenerative changes in the testes may occur, leading to loss of fertility. Egg production appears not to be affected by a vitamin E deficiency, but hatchability is markedly reduced. During incubation of the eggs growth and differentiation are slow with many embryos dying during the first 2 days of incubation due to circulatory failure.

Vitamin E deficiency in poults causes nutritional myopathy. This disorder is characterized by lesions in the muscular wall of the gizzard which appear as circumscribed gray areas that often are of firmer texture than normal muscle and are not unlike scar tissue.

Prophylaxis and Treatment: Only stabilized fat should be used in feed. Where feed is to be stored for more than 2 weeks a chemical antioxidant should be used. Storage at high environmental temperatures and high humidity accentuates destruction of vitamin E.

Signs of exudative diathesis and muscular dystrophy, when

caused by lack of vitamin E, can be reversed if seen in time, by administration of vitamin E by oral dosing or through the feed. Oral administration of a single dose of 300 IU of vitamin E per bird will usually cause remission of the diseases. Old feed should be removed and replaced by a fresh supply, amply fortified with vitamin E.

VITAMIN K DEFICIENCY

A deficiency of vitamin K causes a reduction in the prothrombin content of the blood and, in the chick, may reduce the quantity in the plasma to less than 2% of normal. Since the prothrombin content of the blood of normal, newly hatched chicks is only about 40% of that of adult birds, very young chicks are readily affected by a deficiency of vitamin K.

Etiology: One of the probable causes of a rise in the incidence of hemorrhagic disease in young growing chickens may lie in changes made in poultry feeds. The disease responds favorably to supplementary vitamin K or vitamin K plus vitamin E, and for a time there was a tendency to reduce the quantity of alfalfa meal, a rich natural source of these vitamins, in poultry feeds. There has also been a trend toward the use of solvent-extracted soybean meal and other seed meals and better quality but less putrefied fish meals, which are lower in vitamin K than the original expeller meals and putrid fish meals. It has been suggested that hemorrhagic syndrome (q.v., p. 1104) is not a vitamin K deficiency, but probably caused by certain toxic substances elaborated by molds normally found on grains and corn and in feeds made from such grains.

Clinical Findings: In very young chicks deficient in vitamin K, blood coagulation time begins to increase after about 5 to 10 days of age and becomes greatly prolonged in 7 to 12 days. After about a week, hemorrhages often occur in any part of the body, either spontaneously or as the result of an injury or bruise. The only external signs are the resulting accumulations of blood under the skin. Postmortem examination usually reveals accumulations of blood in the various parts of the body; sometimes there are petechial hemorrhages in the liver and almost invariably there is erosion of the gizzard lining.

When hemorrhagic disease is encountered under practical conditions, the signs usually are observed after the age of 3 weeks.

Prophylaxis and Treatment: Vitamin K deficiency usually can be prevented by including about 2.5% of alfalfa meal in the feed. The inclusion of menadione at the rate of 1.0 gm/ton of feed is effective and is now a common practice. If signs of vitamin K deficiency are encountered, the level should be doubled to 2 gm/ton.

There are a number of stress factors that increase the requirements for vitamin K. Dicumarol, sulfaquinoxaline and warfarin are antimetabolites of vitamin K. Coccidiosis and other intestinal parasitic diseases also increase the need for this vitamin.

VITAMIN B_{12} DEFICIENCY

The vitamin B_{12} requirement of poultry is exceedingly small; an adequate allowance is only a few mcg/kg of feed. Vitamin B_{12} is produced by many bacteria and, in general, is present in feedstuffs of animal origin and in feces. Vitamin B_{12} is now included in most commercial poultry feeds, thus making a deficiency unlikely. It is required for growth and hatchability.

Marked vitamin B_{12} deficiency is difficult, if not impossible, to produce in birds that have free access to their droppings. However, such birds may not receive optimal vitamin B_{12} levels and may fail to achieve growth at a maximal rate. No truly characteristic signs of vitamin B_{12} deficiency have been reported, except for an increased incidence of gizzard erosion. A deficiency of vitamin B_{12}, however is one of several causes of retarded growth, decreased feed efficiency and reduced hatchability. Vitamin B_{12} deficiency is easily prevented and cured by feeding a diet containing feedstuffs of animal origin or a commercial cobalamin supplement.

CHOLINE DEFICIENCY

Choline has several physiologic functions in poultry. In addition to being necessary for the prevention of perosis, it plays a role in growth, methylation and the regulation of the synthesis and transport of lipids. A deficiency of choline in the diet, even when there are adequate quantities of manganese, biotin, folic acid and niacin, results in the development of perosis (*see* MANGANESE DEFICIENCY, p. 1425) and the retardation of growth. There is some evidence that choline is required for the maintenance of maximal egg production and high hatchability. However, the laying hen has considerable ability to synthesize choline and practical diets may provide sufficient for their needs.

Prophylaxis and Treatment: Diets containing appreciable quantities of soybean meal, wheat bran and wheat middlings are not likely to be deficient in choline because soybean meal is a good source of choline, and wheat bran and middlings are good sources of betaine, which is able to perform the methyl-donor function of choline. Other good sources of choline are distillers' grains, fish meal, liver meal, meat scrap, distillers' solubles and yeast. A number of commercial choline supplements are available and choline is routinely added to a number of poultry feeds.

NIACIN (NICOTINIC ACID) DEFICIENCY

Etiology: There is good evidence that chickens—even chick and turkey embryos—are able to synthesize niacin, but that the rate of synthesis may be too slow for optimal growth. It has been claimed that before there can be a marked deficiency of niacin in the chicken, there must first be a deficiency of tryptophan, a precursor of niacin.

Niacin deficiency has been observed in chicks, ducks, geese and turkey poults when certain practical-type diets were fed. Diets high in corn and soybean meal are particularly amenable to improvement by inclusion of supplementary niacin. Ducks and geese have a considerably higher requirement for niacin than chicks. Most of the niacin present in practical feedstuffs such as corn is unavailable to poultry. Mature birds have considerably more ability to synthesize niacin than young birds.

Clinical Findings: In the case of a borderline deficiency of niacin in the diet of chicks, the only sign is retarded growth. Chicks and turkey poults fed a diet deficient in niacin develop a hock disorder similar in appearance to perosis, with swollen hocks and bowed legs. Both goslings and ducklings develop abnormalities of the legs. The condition in goslings has been referred to as perosis and that in ducklings as bowed legs. When laying chickens are fed a diet deficient in niacin, there is a loss of weight and both egg production and hatchability are reduced. (*See also* MANGANESE DEFICIENCY, p. 1425.)

Prophylaxis and Treatment: Niacin deficiency in chickens may be prevented by feeding a diet that contains about 27 mg/kg, but a number of nutritionists recommend 2 to 2½ times as much. An allowance of 55 to 70 mg of niacin per kilogram of feed appears to be satisfactory for ducks, geese and turkeys. It is good economics to provide ample niacin in poultry diets so that the birds do not have to synthesize it from tryptophan, which is difficult to supply.

PANTOTHENIC ACID DEFICIENCY

Etiology: Although most feedstuffs used in feeding poultry are fairly good sources of pantothenic acid, diets composed largely of cereal grains and containing some meat scrap or fish meal, or both, may not contain enough of this vitamin. Corn that has been kiln-dried tends to have a lowered content and in general, pantothenic acid in feedstuffs is destroyed by dry heat.

Clinical Findings: When chicks are deficient in pantothenic acid, their growth is retarded and their feathers acquire a ragged appearance. Within 12 to 14 days, the margins of the eyelids become granulated and frequently a viscous exudate causes the eyelids to stick together. Crusty scabs appear at the corners of the mouth; the skin on the bottoms of the feet often becomes thickened and cornified. In chronic pantothenic acid deficiency, after a period of 4 to 5 months, there is a loss of feathers from the head and neck. Depigmentation of the feathers has been reported.

The signs of pantothenic acid deficiency in young turkeys are similar to those in young chickens and include general weakness, keratitis and sticking together of the eyelids. Young ducks do not show the usual signs seen in chickens and turkeys, except retarded growth; however, their mortality is very high.

When the diet of laying chickens is deficient in pantothenic acid, the concentration of this vitamin in their eggs decreases and hatchability is greatly reduced. The few chicks that hatch grow slowly and their mortality is high.

Lesions: Lesions of the spinal cord, characterized by myelin degeneration of the medullated fibers, occur in chicks fed a diet deficient in pantothenic acid. Degenerating fibers may be found in all segments of the spinal cord down to the lumbar region. Involution of the thymus, a fatty liver and an acute nephritis have also been reported.

Prophylaxis and Treatment: While it is easy to formulate feed mixtures that are fully adequate in pantothenic acid, it is often more economical to add calcium pantothenate (at the rate of about 5.0 to 5.5 mg/kg of feed).

Sometimes, half-grown chickens fed practical diets develop a scaly condition of the skin. The exact cause of this condition is not known, but it has been treated successfully in some instances by putting both calcium pantothenate and riboflavin in the drinking water (2.0 gm of calcium pantothenate and 0.5 gm of riboflavin in 50 gal. [190 L] of water) for a few days.

Riboflavin Deficiency

Etiology: Only a few of the feedstuffs fed to poultry contain enough riboflavin to meet the requirement of the young growing chick, poult, or duckling. Hence, if the ingredients of a poultry feed are not carefully selected or if a special supplement is not included, it may be deficient. Riboflavin is generally added to practical rations so that its deficiency is now relatively uncommon.

Clinical Findings: The characteristic sign of riboflavin deficiency in the chick is "curled toe" paralysis. It, however, does not develop when there is an absolute deficiency, or when the deficiency is very marked, because the chicks die before it appears. Three degrees of severity of "curled toe" paralysis have been described. The first is characterized by a tendency of the chicks to rest on their hocks and a slight curling of the toes; the second, by marked weakness of the legs and a distinct curling of the toes on one or both feet; and the third, by toes that are completely curled inward or under and a weakened condition of the legs that compels the chicks to walk on their hocks.

Other signs of riboflavin deficiency are stunting, diarrhea after 8 to 10 days and high mortality after about 3 weeks. There is no apparent impairment of the growth of the feathers; on the contrary, the main wing feathers often appear to be disproportionately long.

Signs of riboflavin deficiency in the poult and duckling differ from those in the chick. In the poult, a dermatitis appears in about 8 days, the vent becomes encrusted, inflamed and excoriated, growth is retarded or completely stopped by about the 17th day and deaths begin to occur about the 21st day. In the duckling, there usually is diarrhea and cessation of growth.

When laying hens are fed a diet deficient in riboflavin, egg production is decreased and hatchability reduced, roughly in proportion to the degree of the deficiency. The embryonic mortality has 2 typical peaks and often a third peak. These are, respectively, on the fourth and 20th days and on the 14th day of incubation. Most of the embryos are dwarfed and exhibit pronounced micromelia; some of the embryos are edematous. The down fails to emerge properly, thus resulting in a typical abnormality, termed "clubbed" down, which is most common in the areas of the neck and around the vent.

Lesions: Riboflavin deficiency in young poultry produces specific changes in the main peripheral nerve trunks. In acute cases, there are hypertrophy of the nerve trunks and readily observable changes in their appearance. Degenerative changes also appear in the myelin of the nerves. Congestion and premature atrophy of the lobes of the thymus may also be observed.

Prophylaxis and Treatment: By formulating the diet to contain about 3.6 to 4.0 mg of riboflavin per kilogram, riboflavin deficiency is easily prevented.

THIAMIN (VITAMIN B_1) AND PYRIDOXINE (VITAMIN B_6) DEFICIENCIES

Most of the feedstuffs used in feeding poultry contain more than adequate quantities of thiamin and pyridoxine. Accordingly deficiencies of these vitamins rarely, if ever, occur when practical diets are fed. However, there have been several reports recently of poults and chicks coming down with a thiamin deficiency due to the thiamin in the diet being tied up by certain chemicals.

FOLIC ACID (FOLACIN) DEFICIENCY

Etiology: Until recently it was believed unlikely that folic acid deficiency would occur in chicks or turkeys under field conditions. However, modern solvent-extracted soybean meal appears to be lower in the vitamin than the old expeller meal and today much of the folic acid in alfalfa is destroyed by pelleting. Also, fish meal and meat meal are rather poor sources. While much of the folic acid is present in feedstuffs in conjugated form, the young chick can utilize it well.

Clinical Findings: In young chicks the chief signs are retarded growth, poor feather formation, feather depigmentation in colored breeds and excessive mortality. The outward signs are accompanied by a macrocytic hyperchromic anemia. In turkey poults, growth rate is reduced and a characteristic cervical paralysis develops in which the birds extend their necks and appear to gaze downwards. Since field cases have usually appeared in young poults, it is possible that the breeder hens were fed diets deficient in the vitamin. In breeding chickens, folic acid deficiency reduces egg production and hatchability. Deficient embryos show bending of the tibiotarsus mandible defects, syndactyly and hemorrhages.

Prophylaxis and Treatment: Where fish meal or solvent-extracted soybean meal are used as a major source of protein or the feed is pelleted, it may be advisable to supplement breeder diets with synthetic folic acid. Many feed manufacturers are also supplementing turkey starter diets with folic acid at the rate of about 0.5 to 1.0 gm/ton. Where signs occur in young poults, the vitamin may be added to the drinking water at the rate of 150 to 200 mg/gal. In birds that are down, injection of 150 mg of folic acid per bird usually results in recovery within a few days.

BIOTIN DEFICIENCY

Etiology: The vitamin is necessary to prevent perosis in chicks and poults. Deficiencies have been reported recently in turkey poults and young chicks. While the exact cause of such a deficiency has not been elucidated, there is some evidence that certain disease conditions in poults can increase the requirement for biotin. A deficiency is more likely to occur on diets high in wheat or barley than if corn is being fed, suggesting that the availability of biotin may be low in these cereals. Good sources of biotin include liver, dried brewer's yeast, molasses and green leafy plants. Cereals, meat meal and fish meal are poor sources. Some of the biotin in natural feeds occurs in bound form which is poorly available to the bird. An abnormal intestinal flora can increase the requirement of birds for the vitamin.

Clinical Findings: In poults the typical signs include broken flight feathers, bending of the metatarsus and a dermatitis affecting the bottoms of the feet, the corners of the mouth and the edges of the eyelids. In mature turkeys and chickens, biotin deficiency causes reduced egg hatchability. Signs in embryos include "parrot beak," chondrodystrophy, micromelia and syndactyly. Dermatitis of mature birds similar to that in chicks and poults has not been reported. There is also good evidence that a fatty liver and kidney syndrome reported from some parts of the world is the result of a deficiency of biotin.

Prophylaxis and Treatment: A number of factors increase biotin requirements, including oxidative rancidity of feed fat, competition by intestinal microorganisms and a lack of carry-over into the newly hatched poult. Since the best feed sources of biotin are often expensive or difficult to obtain and not completely available to the bird, it is good practice to add 150 to 200 mg of synthetic biotin to turkey breeder and starter diets. Certain antibiotics added to the feed will spare the need for biotin, presumably by fostering a less competitive intestinal flora.

Raising the feed level of materials such as dried brewer's yeast or adding synthetic biotin to the feed or water are effective means of counteracting existing cases of biotin deficiency.

COMPOSITION OF FEEDSTUFFS

At times, it may be necessary to calculate the nutrient composition of a feed to determine whether the feed is deficient in one or more nutrients. It also may be necessary to formulate a special feed from locally available feedstuffs, or add a supplement which is particularly rich in a specific mineral, vitamin, or amino acid. In view of this, the nutrient composition of a wide variety of grains, concentrates, roughages, silages and other feeds are shown in the following tables.

The trace mineral contents of basic feedstuffs are listed in TABLE 45. For calculation of ruminant diets, the composition of grains, hays, silages, roots and tubers is given in detail in TABLE 46. Because of the unique nutritional requirements of poultry and swine, the composition of feedstuffs commonly used for these species is given in TABLE 47. The amino acid composition of most of these feedstuffs is given in TABLE 48.

The values presented in these tables represent averages, of course, and local conditions may cause certain components to vary considerably. When rations are being calculated, such variation should be determined or a reasonable margin must be allowed in the composition of the particular ration at hand.

TABLE 45. TRACE MINERAL CONTENT OF BASIC FEEDSTUFFS*

Feedstuffs	Chlorine	Cobalt	Copper	Iodine	Iron	Magnesium	Manganese	Potassium	Selenium	Sodium	Zinc
	%	ppm	ppm	ppm	ppm	%	ppm	%	ppm	%	ppm
Alfalfa meal, 17% protein	0.37	0.18	10	0.5	200	0.3	43	1.8	0.05-0.45*	0.18	35
Barley	0.15	0.1	7.5	0.05	50	0.12	16	0.6	0.1-03	0.02	17
Beet pulp, dried	—	0.1	12.5	—	300	0.25	35	0.2	—	—	1
Blood meal	0.27	0.1	9	—	3800	0.2	5	0.9	0.07	0.3	—
Bone meal, steamed	0.02	0.1	16	—	800	0.6	30	0.2	—	0.45	425
Citrus pulp, dried	—	—	6	—	200	0.16	7	0.6	—	—	14
Coconut oil meal	0.03	2.0	19	—	680	0.25	55	1.1	—	0.04	—
Corn, dent, yellow, No. 2	0.05	0.1	4.5	0.05	35	0.12	5	0.3	0.03-0.38	0.01	10
Corn gluten feed	0.22	0.1	50	—	500	0.3	25	0.6	0.2	0.1	—
Corn gluten meal	0.07	0.1	30	—	400	0.05	7	0.03	1.15	0.01	—
Cottonseed meal	0.03	0.1	20	0.12	100	0.55	20	1.3	0.06	0.04	—
Distillers' dried corn grains	0.17	0.1	45	—	200	0.06	19	0.8	—	0.2	—
Distillers' dried corn solubles	0.26	—	80	—	600	0.64	74	1.7	0.50	0.3	85
Fish meal, menhaden	1.20	—	8	—	270	—	36	0.7	1.7	0.3	150
Fish meal, herring	1.00	—	20	1.0	300	0.1	10	0.5	1.5-2.45	0.5	110
Fish solubles, 50% solubles	2.7	—	48	—	300	0.2	25	1.8	1.0	3.0	38
Hominy feed, white or yellow	0.05	0.1	2	—	10	0.24	14	0.2	0.1	0.04	—
Linseed oil meal	0.2	0.2	25	0.07	300	0.6	37	1.3	1.1	0.14	—
Meat and bone scrap, 50% protein	0.75	0.2	12	1.3	500	1.13	19	0.55	0.1-0.8	0.7	100
Milk, cow's	0.1	—	0.3	0.04	2	0.01	0.06	0.14	0.04	0.05	4
Milo	0.07	0.1	14	0.02	50	0.13	13	0.35	—	0.01	17
Molasses, beet	1.3	0.4	18	1.6	100	0.23	5	4.75	—	1.15	—
Molasses, cane	2.8	0.9	60	1.6	100	0.35	42	2.4	—	0.17	—
Oats	0.12	0.06	6	0.06	70	0.17	38	0.37	0.05-0.22	0.06	—
Oyster shell, ground	—	—	—	—	2900	0.3	130	0.1	0.01	0.2	—
Peanut oil meal	0.03	—	30	—	20	0.24	25	1.15	0.28	0.07	20
Rice bran	0.07	—	13	—	190	0.95	200	1.7	—	0.07	30
Rye grain	—	—	6	0.05	45	0.12	35	0.7	0.2	—	35
Sesame meal	0.06	—	—	—	—	0.75	48	1.2	—	0.04	100
Skim milk	0.9	—	3	—	30	0.11	2	1.5	0.08-0.15	0.5	40

Soybean meal, 44% protein	0.04	0.1	20	0.13	150	0.27	35	2.0	0.05-1.0	0.01	27
Soybean meal, dehulled	0.03	0.1	20	0.1	150	0.25	40	2.0	0.05-1.0	0.01	45
Wheat bran	0.08	0.1	12	0.07	150	0.55	115	1.2	0.6	0.06	80
Wheat grain	0.08	0.08	7	0.04	50	0.16	20	0.5	0.05-0.8	0.06	15
Wheat standard middlings	0.03	0.1	22	0.1	100	0.37	118	1.0	0.28-0.88	0.02	150
Whey, dried	0.7	0.1	45	—	7	0.13	5	1.2	0.8	0.5	3
Yeast, dried brewers'	0.12	0.2	30	0.01	50	0.23	6	1.7	0.11-1.1	0.07	40
Yeast, dried torula	0.02	0.04	13	—	90	0.13	13	1.9	0.03-0.05	0.01	100

* The trace element content of most feedstuffs varies over a wide range, depending largely upon the trace element content of the soil upon which the crops were grown. This is especially true of selenium.

TABLE 46. AVERAGE COMPOSITION OF FEEDSTUFFS FOR CATTLE, HORSES AND SHEEP

GRAINS, SEEDS AND BY-PRODUCT CONCENTRATES

Feedsuffs	Dry Matter	Crude Protein	Digest. Protein	TDN	Fat	Fiber	Calcium	Phos-phorus	Carotene
	%	%	%	%	%	%	%	%	mg/lb
Barley	89	11.5	10.0	71	1.9	5.0	0.1	0.4	—
Beet pulp, dried	90	9.0	4.3	62	0.6	19.0	0.68	0.1	—
Blood meal or dried blood	91	80.0	56.5	60	1.5	1.0	0.3	0.22	—
Bone meal, steamed	95	12.0	9.0	10	3.0	2.0	29.0	13.5	—
Brewers' grains, dried	92	25.0	20.7	60	6.2	15.0	0.27	0.5	—
Buttermilk, dried	93	32.0	28.8	83	6.0	0.3	1.35	0.9	—
Citrus pulp, dried	90	6.5	2.9	75	5.4	13.0	2.0	0.1	—
Coconut meal	93	20.0	17.3	77	6.6	12.0	0.2	0.6	—
Corn, dent, yellow, No. 2	86	8.7	6.7	81	3.8	2.0	0.03	0.27	1.3
Corn, flint	89	9.9	7.5	83	4.3	2.0	0.02	0.2	—
Corn gluten feed	90	25.0	21.8	75	2.4	8.0	0.46	0.77	3.8
Corn gluten meal	91	43.0	36.5	80	2.3	4.0	0.15	0.4	7.4
Cottonseed meal	91	41.5	33.0	63	1.6	11.0	0.15	1.1	—
Distillers' dried corn grains	92	27.0	19.8	84	9.0	12.0	0.1	0.4	1.4
Distillers' dried corn grains with solubles	92	27.0	19.8	82	9.0	9.0	0.1	0.4	1.7
Distillers' dried solubles	93	27.0	21.0	78	9.0	4.0	0.35	1.4	0.3
Fish meal, menhaden	92	61.0	50.0	58	7.5	1.0	5.5	2.8	—
Fish meal, sardine	93	65.0	53.5	71	4.5	1.0	4.9	2.8	—
Flaxseed screenings	91	15.8	8.8	56	9.5	12.0	0.37	0.43	—
Hominy feed, white or yellow (y)	91	10.7	7.5	84	6.5	5.0	0.05	0.5	4.0 (y)
Kafir grain	90	11.8	9.5	80	3.0	2.0	0.04	0.33	—
Limestone	—	—	—	—	—	—	30-38	—	—
Linseed meal	91	35.0	30.5	75	4.5	9.0	0.4	0.9	—
Meat and bone scrap, 50% protein	94	53.0	43.8	67	10.0	2.0	10.6	5.1	—
Milk. cow's	12	3.1	2.9	16	3.7	0	0.12	0.09	0.4
Milo	89	11.0	8.6	84	2.8	2.0	0.04	0.29	—
Molasses, beet	77	6.7	3.5	61	—	—	0.15	0.03	—
Molasses, cane	75	3.2	—	72	—	—	0.9	0.1	—
Oats	89	11.8	9.4	60	4.5	11.0	0.1	0.35	—
Oyster shell, ground	—	—	—	—	—	—	38.0	—	—
Peanut meal, solvent-extracted	92	47.5	42.0	77	1.2	13.0	0.2	0.65	—
Phosphate, defluorinated rock	100	—	—	—	—	—	32.0	18.0	—
Phosphate, dicalcium	96	—	—	—	—	—	27.0	19.0	—

Potato meal, or dried potatoes	90	6.0	2.1	70	0.4	2.0	0.07	0.02	—
Oat hay	88	8.0	4.9	57	2.7	27.5	0.25	0.20	40
Oat millfeed	92	4.5	2.7	35	1.8	30.0	0.1	0.2	0.1
Oat straw	90	4.0	0.7	47	2.0	37.0	0.3	0.1	—
Pea hay, field	89	13.5	10.6	55	2.5	25.0	1.2	0.25	—
Peanut hay	91	11.0	7.0	58	5.0	24.5	1.15	0.15	21
Prairie hay, western, moderately green	92	6.3	2.0	50	2.4	29.0	0.5	0.17	13
Prairie hay, western, mature	92	4.2	0.9	44	2.3	31.0	0.35	0.08	4
Reed canarygrass hay	91	8.0	5.0	42	2.0	31.0	0.30	0.25	—
Ryegrass hay	88	8.4	2.8	50	2.2	28.0	0.45	0.28	—
Ryegrass straw	91	3.5	0	50	1.1	36.0	0.28	0.1	—
Sorghum fodder	86	6.8	3.5	49	2.1	22.0	0.35	0.15	8
Soybean hay	89	14.5	9.7	46	2.7	29.0	1.15	0.2	14
Soybean hay, in bloom	90	15.0	12.0	51	3.0	27.0	1.2	0.20	3
Soybean straw	88	4.8	1.4	37	1.2	39.0	1.4	0.05	—
Sudan grass hay	89	11.3	5.5	54	2.0	26.0	0.50	0.30	2
Timothy hay, all analyses	88	6.8	3.1	45	2.3	30.0	0.30	0.17	5
Timothy hay, early bloom	88	7.6	4.2	47	2.3	29.0	0.55	0.23	25
Timothy hay, mature	86	5.1	1.8	35	2.2	31.0	0.15	0.15	2
Vetch hay	88	17.5	13.5	52	2.3	25.0	1.2	0.30	—
Wheat hay	86	6.4	3.4	44	1.7	24.0	0.15	0.18	44
Wheat straw	90	3.2	0.3	43	1.5	37.0	0.15	0.07	—
SILAGES, ROOTS, TUBERS									
Alfalfa silage, wilted	36	6.4	4.4	21	1.2	11.0	0.5	0.1	9
Alfalfa, not wilted, no preservative	26	4.6	2.6	14	1.0	9.2	0.5	0.1	12
Alfalfa silage, molasses added	32	5.6	3.7	18	1.1	9.5	0.6	0.10	14
Beet top silage, sugar	32	3.8	2.5	15	0.6	3.9	0.31	0.07	5
Clover, ladino, silage	25	5.3	3.8	21	1.4	7.5	0.36	0.07	15
Corn silage, well-matured	27	2.2	1.2	20	0.8	7.0	0.1	0.06	2
Corn silage, dough stage	26	2.2	1.0	15	0.8	7.0	0.05	0.05	4
Corn stover silage (ears removed)	27	2.0	0.6	14	0.7	8.5	0.10	0.05	—
Cowpea silage	26	3.7	1.8	13	1.2	7.0	0.4	0.1	—
Mangels	9	1.3	0.9	7	0.1	0.8	0.02	0.02	—
Orchardgrass silage	24	3.4	2.0	20	1.0	7.5	0.3	0.1	18
Potato, tubers	21	2.2	1.3	17	0.1	0.4	0.01	0.05	—
Sorghum silage, sweet	27	2.1	0.8	15	0.7	7.5	0.08	0.05	2

continued on next page

TABLE 46. (*Continued*)

Feedsuffs	Dry Matter	Crude Protein	Digest. Protein	TDN	Fat	Fiber	Calcium	Phos-phorus	Carotene
	%	%	%	%	%	%	%	%	mg/lb
Soybean silage, not wilted	25	4.0	2.9	15	0.7	7.5	0.35	0.18	10
Rice bran	91	13.5	9.2	55	15.0	11.0	0.06	1.82	—
Rice, rough	89	7.3	6.0	70	1.9	9.0	0.04	0.26	—
Rice polishings	90	11.8	9.0	78	13.0	3.0	0.04	1.4	—
Rye	89	11.9	9.4	72	1.6	2.0	0.06	0.35	—
Sesame meal	93	48.0	43.5	71	5.0	5.0	2.0	1.3	—
Skimmed milk, dried	94	33.5	30.0	80	1.0	0.2	1.3	1.0	—
Soybean meal, 44% protein	89	45.8	42.0	73	1.0	6.0	0.3	0.65	—
Soybean meal, dehulled	88	49.5	46.3	78	0.8	3.0	0.25	0.6	—
Wheat, hard, winter	89	13.5	11.5	77	1.8	3.0	0.05	0.4	—
Wheat, soft	89	10.8	8.3	78	1.7	2.3	0.09	0.3	—
Wheat bran	89	16.0	13.0	63	4.1	10.0	0.15	1.15	1.2
Wheat flour middlings	90	18.0	15.4	81	4.2	5.0	0.1	0.75	0.08
Wheat screenings	89	15.0	10.8	65	3.0	7.0	0.08	0.35	—
Wheat standard middlings	90	17.0	14.5	62	4.5	8.0	0.15	0.9	1.4
Whey, dried	94	13.8	11.8	78	0.8	—	0.9	0.8	—
Yeast, dried brewers'	93	45.0	38.5	73	5.0	3.0	0.15	1.4	—
Yeast, dried torula	93	48.0	41.5	70	5.0	2.0	0.55	1.7	—
DRY ROUGHAGES									
Alfalfa hay, average	89	15.5	11.0	50	1.9	28.0	1.48	0.23	20
Alfalfa hay, ¾ to full-bloom	88	14.0	10.0	48	1.6	30.0	1.15	0.15	15
Alfalfa leaf meal, good	89	21.0	16.5	58	2.8	14.6	2.10	0.25	80
Alfalfa meal, dehydrated, 17% Protein	92	17.5	12.2	47	2.6	25.0	1.3	0.3	45
Alfalfa straw	90	9.5	4.9	41	1.2	40.0	0.8	0.2	6
Barley hay	87	7.8	4.3	49	1.8	23.0	0.18	0.25	—
Barley straw	88	3.6	0.7	40	1.6	37.5	0.30	0.1	—
Bromegrass hay, all analyses	90	11.0	5.6	47	2.3	28.5	0.40	0.25	26
Clover hay, alsike, all analyses	88	12.9	8.6	48	2.5	26.0	1.15	0.22	75
Clover hay, crimson	88	14.8	10.2	55	2.0	28.0	1.25	0.15	—

Clover hay, ladino	91	21.0	16.2	60	3.0	17.5	1.25	0.35	67
Clover hay, red	88	13.0	7.9	48	2.6	26.5	1.4	0.2	15
Corn cobs, ground	90	2.5	0	46	0.5	32.5	0.1	0.04	—
Corn fodder, all analyses	82	7.3	3.8	53	2.0	21.0	0.4	0.2	16
Corn stover, all analyses	79	5.0	2.1	51	1.2	27.0	0.38	0.07	1.4
Cowpea hay	91	16.5	12.3	51	2.6	25.0	1.20	0.30	—
Kafir fodder	89	8.2	4.3	50	2.4	25.0	0.35	0.15	8
Kafir stover	82	4.8	1.9	51	1.6	27.0	0.35	0.1	1
Lespedeza hay, all analyses	91	13.0	5.6	45	2.5	28.0	1.0	0.20	19
Lespedeza hay, in bloom	93	12.5	6.1	46	2.9	29.0	1.0	0.20	19
Soybean, silage, wilted	35	6.7	3.7	19	0.9	9.0	0.45	0.12	10
Sudan grass silage	23	2.4	1.5	15	0.7	8.0	0.15	0.05	—
Timothy silage, all analyses	38	3.8	1.9	19	1.2	13.0	0.20	0.10	13

TABLE 47. AVERAGE COMPOSITION OF FEEDSTUFFS FOR POULTRY AND SWINE*

Feedstuffs	Metabolizable Energy	Protein	Fat	Fiber	Calcium	Phosphorus	Niacin	Riboflavin	Pantothenic Acid	Choline
	Kcal/lb	%	%	%	%	%	mg/lb	mg/lb	mg/lb	gm/lb
Alfalfa meal, dehydrated, 17% protein	620	17.5	2.6	25	1.3	0.3	16	5.0	12.0	0.72
Barley, adequate rainfall	1290	11.5	1.9	5	0.1	0.4	26	0.8	3.0	0.45
Blood meal	1300	80	1.5	1	0.3	0.22	14	0.7	0.5	0.13
Bone meal, steamed	—	12	3	2	29.0	13.5	2	0.4	0.45	—
Buttermilk, dried	1240	32	6	0.3	1.35	0.9	4	14.0	13.5	0.80
Citrus pulp, dried	—	6.5	4.5	13	2.0	0.1	10	1.0	6.0	0.42
Corn, dent, yellow	1560	8.7	3.8	2	0.03	0.27	10	0.5	2.2	0.20
Corn gluten meal, 60% protein	1680	60	2.3	2	0	0.4	28	0.85	5.5	0.18
Cottonseed meal, solvent process	920	41	1.6	11	0.15	1.1	20	2.3	8.0	1.3
Crab meal	850	31	1.8	11	15.5	1.6	20	3.0	3.0	0.9
Distillers' dried corn solubles	1320	27	9	4	0.35	1.4	52	7.7	9.5	2.2
Fats:										
Animal tallow	3230	—	100	—	—	—	—	—	—	—
Lard	3980	—	100	—	—	—	—	—	—	—
Vegetable oils	4050	—	100	—	—	—	—	—	—	—
Feather meal	1050	84	2.5	1.3	0.2	0.8	14	1.0	5.0	0.4
Fish meal	1350	61	7.5	1	5.5	2.8	26	2.4	4.0	1.4
Fish oils	3660	100	—	—	—	—	—	—	—	—
Fish solubles, 50% solids	670	30	4	0	0.1	0.7	110	4.5	17.0	1.2
Hominy feed, 5% fat	1300	11	6.5	5	0.05	0.5	23	1.0	3.5	0.45
Liver and glandular meal	1300	65	16	2	0.7	1.1	73	18.0	48.0	4.8
Meat and bone scrap, 50% protein	900	53	10	2	10.6	5.1	18	1.1	1.2	0.75
Molasses, beet	900	6.7	0	0	0.15	0.03	19	1.2	2.1	0.4
Molasses, cane	890	3.2	0	0	0.9	0.1	16	1.5	17.5	0.4
Oats	1190	11.8	4.5	11	0.1	0.35	7	0.7	6.0	0.49
Oatmeal, feeding	1420	16.9	6	3	0.09	0.45	5	0.9	6.6	0.57
Peanut meal	1200	47.5	1.2	13	0.2	0.65	77	5.0	24.0	2.0
Rice bran	740	13	15	11	0.06	1.82	130	1.2	10.5	0.57
Rice polishings	1300	11.8	13	3	0.04	1.4	240	0.8	26.0	0.6
Skimmed milk, dried	1140	33	1	0.2	1.30	1.0	5	9.1	15.0	0.6

Sesame meal	870	48	5	5	2.0	1.3	14	1.7	2.5	0.7
Sorghum kafir	1480**	11.8	3	2	0.04	0.33	18	0.6	5.7	0.2
Sorghum milo	1480	11	2.8	2	0.04	0.29	19	0.5	5.0	0.3
Soybean meal, 44% protein	1020	45	1	6	0.3	0.65	12	1.5	6.6	1.2
Soybean meal, dehulled	1150	49.5	0.8	3	0.25	0.6	10	1.4	6.6	1.2
Sunflower seed meal	900	47	3	11	0.3	1.2	132	3.0	18.0	1.9
Wheat, hard	1480	13.5	1.8	3	0.05	0.4	23	0.5	6.0	0.45
Wheat, soft	1480	10	1.7	2.3	0.09	0.3	27	0.5	5.0	0.45
Wheat bran	590	15	4.1	10	0.15	1.15	95	1.4	13.0	0.46
Wheat shorts	1200	17	4.2	5	0.10	0.75	44	0.9	8.0	0.83
Wheat red dog flour	1240	17	4.5	4	0.07	0.5	24	0.4	6.2	0.8
Wheat middlings	820	17	4.5	8	0.15	0.9	45	0.9	9.0	0.8
Whey, dried	870	13.8	0.8	0	0.9	0.8	5	14.0	22.0	1.1
Yeast, dried brewer's	840	45	5	3	0.15	1.4	200	16.0	50.0	1.75
Yeast, dried torula	840	48	5	2	0.55	1.7	230	20.0	38.0	1.3

* *See* TABLE 48 for amino acids in feedstuffs.
** Estimated value.

TABLE 48. IMPORTANT AMINO ACIDS IN FEEDSTUFFS FOR POULTRY AND SWINE

Feedstuffs	Arginine	Lysine	Methionine	Cystine	Tryptophan	Glycine
	%	%	%	%	%	%
Alfalfa meal, dehydrated, 17% protein	0.8	0.9	0.29	0.32	0.21	0.9
Barley	0.53	0.53	0.18	0.18	0.18	0.36
Blood meal	3.5	6.9	0.9	1.4	1.1	3.4
Buttermilk, dried	1.1	2.4	0.7	0.3	0.5	—
Citrus pulp, dried	0.2	0.2	0.08	0.11	0.06	—
Corn, dent, yellow	0.45	0.2	0.18	0.18	0.1	0.5
Corn gluten meal	1.4	0.8	1.0	0.7	0.2	1.5
Cottonseed meal, solvent process	3.3	1.6	0.5	1.0	0.5	2.4
Crab meal	1.7	1.4	0.5	—	0.3	—
Distillers' dried corn solubles	1.0	0.9	0.6	0.6	0.2	1.1
Feather meal	5.9	2.0	0.6	3.0	0.5	—
Fish meal	4.0	5.3	1.8	0.94	0.6	4.4
Fish solubles, 50% solids	2.4	2.7	1.0	1.7	0.8	4.9
Hominy feed	0.5	0.4	0.18	0.18	0.1	0.5
Liver and glandular meal	4.1	4.8	1.3	1.0	0.6	5.6
Meat and bone scrap, 50% protein	3.5	3.5	0.7	0.6	0.7	7.5
Oats	0.7	0.4	0.18	0.18	0.18	0.5
Oatmeal, feeding	1.0	0.5	0.20	0.20	0.2	0.2
Peanut meal	5.9	2.3	0.4	0.7	0.5	2.5
Rice bran	0.5	0.5	0.2	0.1	0.1	—
Rice polishings	0.5	0.5	0.2	0.1	0.1	—
Skimmed milk, dried	1.2	2.8	0.9	0.4	0.4	0.2
Sesame meal	4.3	1.2	1.2	0.6	0.6	—
Sorghum milo	0.4	0.3	0.16	0.18	0.09	—
Soybean meal, solvent-extracted	3.2	2.9	0.67	0.75	0.60	2.6
Soybean meal, dehulled	3.6	3.2	0.74	0.83	0.65	2.9
Sunflower seed meal	3.2	1.3	0.65	0.4	0.6	—
Wheat, hard	0.8	0.45	0.24	0.24	0.16	0.7
Wheat, soft	0.6	0.3	0.22	0.22	0.14	0.5
Wheat bran	0.8	0.5	0.17	0.2	0.3	0.9
Wheat shorts	0.9	0.7	0.18	0.2	0.19	0.4
Wheat red dog flour	1.0	0.6	0.15	0.2	0.2	0.4
Wheat middlings	0.9	0.6	0.17	0.2	0.2	0.4
Whey, dried	0.5	1.2	0.2	0.4	0.2	0.3
Yeast, dried brewer's	2.3	3.1	0.75	0.55	0.5	1.7
Yeast, dried torula	2.6	3.8	0.8	0.6	0.5	2.7

PART VI
BEHAVIOR

BEHAVIOR

GENERAL

Behavior is the means whereby the animal interacts with its environment, both animate and inanimate. The scientific study of animal behavior is termed Ethology, and Veterinary Ethology is a study of the behavior of domestic species when used as means of appraising health or welfare.

Behavior is an inextricable blend of inherited or species-specific and acquired or learned components. The CNS and the body hormones provide for the expression and maintenance of behavior, and some of the species characteristics are encoded in the genes. In particular, behavior systems closely tied to the survival of the species, reproductive behavior, maternal behavior and fight-flight behavior show precise species-characteristics patterns. Yet domestic animals have a well-developed cerebral cortex and an ability to learn and adopt useful strategies for survival within their particular environment.

A system of behavior classification widely used at present provides 9 behavior categories as follows:

Ingestive: This class includes eating and drinking, the selectivity associated with grazing, and the diurnal patterns of grazing or eating cycles. The specific forms of food prehension, suckling of the young, coprophagia and other behavior of a similar nature fall into this class.

Shelter seeking: Animals are mobile and therefore able to utilize the favorable aspects of their environment to maintain body homeostasis. Sheep tend to seek shelter before lambing especially if they are not in heavy wool. Animals can also find shelter within their herd or flock.

Investigation: The need to explore an environment and be familiar with its features is closely related to survival. It is well developed in the young. In some species like the rat, extreme caution is shown to new objects in the familiar areas—neophobia. Strange animals meeting for the first time investigate visually, by smelling and nibbling to determine the sex, reproductive state and other identifying factors of the stranger. The investigation of other species members can lead to mutual grooming.

Allelomimetic: Sometimes called associative or contagious behavior, the social species come together in groups, flocks, herds or schools. Learning is not necessarily involved, but the early bonds formed between parent and young may be generalized to include other species members. After weaning, animals may form new associative groups. Social dominance hierarchies, precise patterns of leadership-followership and other social associations are characteristic of farm species and have important implications for animal management and welfare.

Agonistic: A class of behavior that involves the response patterns of approach, threat, fight or other display and flight, appeasement and retreat. Agonistic behavior (derived from the Greek term "to struggle") may be shown in a variety of contexts such as defining a territory or home range area, competing for mates or other limited resources such as supplementary feed space.

Eliminative: The expulsion of waste materials, general care of body surfaces and other maintenance activities are important and are often shown in complex species-specific behavior responses. Many of the elimination patterns such as that of the cat, dog or horse are characteristic of the species; cattle avoid their own dung patches when grazing. Grooming or body care occurs as licking, nibbling, rubbing, rolling, scratching, wallowing and preening. Changes in patterns of elimination and general body care may be the first signs of ill-health at the subclinical or clinical levels.

Sexual: It is impossible to generalize or provide a broad definition of sexual behavior that will cover all species. In some species, reproductive behavior includes courtship, copulation, nest-building and incubation, all in one continuous process. In other species, the coital activity may be separated by many months from the preparation of the birth site and parturition. The selection and maintenance of territory may or may not be intimately related to the sexual activities.

Care giving (epimeletic): Many young at birth cannot care for themselves, and maternal or paternal care may be required. Usually coupled with this category is **Care Soliciting (et-epimeletic)** behavior shown by the young, subordinate or helpless animal to attract care.

Play: Play activity is shown most by young animals. Many later adult patterns of behavior are incorporated in play activities (e.g. mounting by calves and lambs), but such play may be poorly directed or break off in the middle of a sequence.

BEHAVIOR, STRESS AND ANIMAL WELFARE

The control exerted by man on domestic animals continues to grow as new phases of intensive farming continue to be developed. Larger numbers of animals are being kept in high density conditions within artificial environments and there is public demand for veterinarians to assess the management conditions with a consideration for the welfare of farm animals.

The factors in such environments that can induce states of stress have been termed **stressors.** In many cases, the condition of stress may be apparent only in the behavior changes of the animal and its strategies to overcome stressor influences. A number of recent attempts have been made to evaluate the various stressors in an environment and to calculate a stressor index. It is clear that: (1) animals require some stimulation to overcome stress or "boredom" in a barren environment, (2) the animal can show an effective adaptive response to normal stressors and (3) beyond a critical level of stress the animal may be unable to adapt and produces abnormal or anomalous responses.

Much of the research focus in the past has been on feeding requirements, health and hygiene, and to some degree, the behavioral requirements of the animals were poorly understood. Overcrowding led to various stressor effects and the resulting behavior patterns have often been labelled **vices.** The issues of animal welfare can be highlighted for the veterinarian by the following question, "What methods of handling, housing and general management can be adopted to impose the least amount of distress (the negative aspects of stress) on the particular animal species under consideration?" Some indices for the assessment of stress such as physiological responses are now available and farm animal behavior studies describing the normal patterns of behavior under acceptable farming conditions are becoming available. Departures from both of these baselines can be used for making veterinary decisions.

The anomalous or abnormal patterns shown by each species in distress will be discussed under the species section as they relate to ways particular species try to cope with imposed hazards.

SOCIAL BEHAVIOR

Certain behavior patterns are seen in animals during social interactions between males, females and the young. Many of these have been studied in detail both in wild and domestic conditions. Castration of either sex modifies social behavior. The domestic animal's social interaction with man varies considerably from species to species depending on the farming system or whether the animal is a companion.

The actions of pet and farm livestock are sometimes poorly understood or even misinterpreted by their owners. Veterinarians have some basic knowledge of the functions of behavior and can make an important contribution in this area. The following brief discussions outline some of the many elements of social behavior in domesticated animals.

Relations Between Man and Animal

The removal of the young animal from its own dam to be raised by hand can lead to social attachments to humans. The optimum time for close relationships to be satisfactorily formed and the timing of this developmental process varies with the species. For example, in altricial species not well developed behaviorally at birth, such as the dog, the optimum time is between 3 and 8 weeks of age. With precocial species, behaviorally competent at birth like the sheep, the corresponding time is from birth to 4 to 6 days. If the attachments to humans have been too exclusive, such hand-raised animals will tend to relate sexually to humans. Some of the charm of caged birds is in their paying courtship to the human owners.

A domestic animal is dependent for some or all of its care and well-being on a human caretaker, and man is thus woven in some way into the social reactions of his animal. A leader-follower relationship may occur in which the animal follows the human for food or companionship. In species that develop a dominance-subordination type of social structure it is important that the caretaker be dominant, particularly when the adult animals are dangerous. The dairy bull asserts increased dominance with maturing and growth. Dominance is best established at the appropriate time for the species, usually early in life when no punishment may be needed. As the social dominance interactions are specific for individuals, the fact the one person dominates an animal is no guarantee that another will be able to do so.

When animals are kept for specific purposes, for companionship or as a child substitute, unexpected social behavior may be encountered, reinforced by the close interaction of the owner. The early and complete isolation of an animal from its own kind not only leads to difficulties in later mating but increases the aggressiveness towards strangers and inhibits good mothering of the young. On the other hand, overcrowding and poor management may lead to a considerable upset in normally expected social behavior and result in vice, injury or unthriftiness. A good stockman or veterinarian can predict these conditions from the social behavior of the animals. Preventive, remedial steps can be taken before stock condition deteriorates due to adverse maintenance.

The basic behavior traits of each species do not alter through domestication, but the normal social behavior is transferred more or less to the human caretaker. Most dogs fit well into families because they react to man as they react to being a member of the pack. The approach to the master with attempts to lick the face is analogous to the normal greeting pattern of a subordinate wolf to its superior.

Social Behavior of Dogs

The social behavior of dogs is similar to that of wolves. Wolves regularly travel over runways or hunting trails and urinate, defecate and scratch the ground as "scent posts" or "marking places." Similarly, free running dogs move over regular routes using "scent posts." Males travel more extensively than females and are more apt to use the posts. The stimulus for marking is the scent of urine or feces of strange animals together with a territorial drive. This "scent post" behavior keeps males informed of the sexual receptivity of females. Bitches in heat secrete a substance in urine which excites males, who then track them to mate. The female is attractive to the male a few days before bleeding begins, but is not receptive until it ends.

In wolves, both parents cooperate to feed the young when the pups are approximately 3 weeks old, by vomiting food. Weaning takes place at 7 to 10 weeks, and young wolves have been seen hunting at about 4 months, although not independently. The same general timing is followed in domestic dogs. Vestiges of wild parental behavior are seen in the tendency for bitches to vomit food for their pups, and all dogs to bury bones and food.

Like the wolf, the dog is basically a pack-hunting animal. Either dogs or humans can satisfy this need for companionship. Isolation of a dog can act as a punishment, e.g. during training. As pack animals, both wolves and dogs develop dominance-subordination relationships that permit them to live in stable groups. A stable social order helps inhibit fighting in competitive situations, such as those relating to food, living space and desire for human attention. Because size, strength and sex largely determine social dominance, these relationships develop effectively among young puppies. Strange dogs of the same breed are more often attacked and rejected from a closed social group than dogs of a different breed, though there are wide breed differences in the tolerance of strangers. There is little evidence that either wolves or dogs develop any strong system of leadership.

Man-Dog Relationship: Man and dog interact on at least 3 planes: (1) With cage-dependency, which begins in early puppyhood. The adult dog, too, depends on his master for food, shelter and companionship, and in relation to man, is a perpetual dependent. (2) Within the social dominance structures, where the human must be dominant or risk being threatened or bitten in competitive situations. Dominance is best established by restraint rather than severe punishment. If a small dog challenges its owner's authority, it can be lifted off its feet by the loose skin of the neck and shaken into submission. (3) In a leader-follower relationship, which requires some training to produce in most dogs.

PUPPY BEHAVIOR

House-Training: The bitch keeps her puppies clean by licking them and swallowing their excreta until they begin to eat solid food at about 3 weeks of age. A puppy avoids soiling its bed and will leave it to defecate and urinate but will not begin to use specific toilet areas until about 8 weeks. It must be kept under constant supervision from 7 weeks to prevent use of the wrong areas. The puppy can be tied on a short leash or kept in a small crate between hourly trips to the yard, and may soon be left loose in a room after being outside. During the day, most puppies cannot be continent for more than 2 hours before 12 weeks of age.

Social Development: A dog's behavior is largely determined by breed and strain; temperament and "trainability" are important in the choice of puppy. As the most impressionable age to develop a strong relationship between dog and master is between 3 and 12 weeks, the new puppy should be selected at about 5 weeks and taken home as soon as possible. Puppies raised in kennels away from much human association will become man-shy unless they are handled frequently from 4 to 5 weeks; if no handling is given until 4 months, they may never be able to adapt themselves to human beings. Patience and careful training may partially overcome this shyness, but both the dog and owner are under a severe handicap. Such dogs frequently develop a "kennel dog" syndrome; they lack confidence, may be aggressive and show fear-biting. These signs may completely disappear if the dog is restored to its original kennel. Dogs kept too long in kennels form their strongest relationships with other dogs and do not make good pets. Dogs reared exclusively with human beings may be difficult to mate. Such bitches often show "frigidity" with estrus.

Fundamentals of Training: All dogs should be taught obedience to commands such as: sit, stay, come, heel and no. A trained dog does willingly what its owner asks. As little as 10 minutes a day can produce a well-trained dog at 16 weeks, if the training is begun at 7 weeks. These lessons should be uninterrupted and should start with simple tasks that the puppy can perform. Moderate repetition, consistency, praise for good performance and firmness towards misbehavior, with a relationship based on mutual trust and affection are the fundamentals of training.

PROTECTIVE AND TERRITORIAL BEHAVIOR

Adult dogs normally guard the territory around their homes and will attempt to keep out strangers by threat or attack. When off the home territory they seldom make trouble, and if moved to a new home, take up to 10 days to establish their new territory. Some control is necessary at this stage to prevent habits of chasing or biting. Dogs are also likely to attack if the master is threatened. If a dog has developed this type of behavior keenly it must be kept under strict control. A well-trained, well-controlled dog will seldom be a behavior problem.

Abnormal Behavior in Dogs: A dog owner must realize that, although he dominates his pet, a passerby may not and may be bitten. If a dog is allowed to fight dogs or people, this becomes a habit making the animal a danger and a nuisance. A severely threatened dog may bite from fear; in the typical "fear biter" this has become a habit. If a young dog is allowed to mount owners' arms or legs, masturbate against objects, or chew shoes or old furniture as seemingly harmless responses, such behavior may finally become a more serious problem to deal with in later adulthood.

SOCIAL BEHAVIOR OF CATS

Although cats are solitary animals, some males form stable groups and roam. Fighting between members is rare once a social order has been established, though newcomers have to fight for a social position. Females and neutered males defend home territories more vigorously than entire males, which may wander extensively.

Mating Behavior in the Cat: Best mating occurs when females are taken to males for the 3 days when the female is receptive. If the female will stand she may be held to aid the male mounting. The presence of a male heightens her sexual receptivity. Sexual behavior begins in females between 6 to 8 months and during her breeding season the estrous cycle is repeated each 3 to 4 weeks. However, receptivity is confined to 4 to 10 days in this cycle. The 8-week breeding period of mature females in temperate zones tends to occur in early spring and early fall, but occurs more often in the tropics. Males mature at about 11 months of age (range 6 to 18 months).

The female can be tested for receptivity by grasping the loose skin of her neck, rubbing her back and gently patting her anogenital area. Spontaneous signs of receptivity consist of the female approaching and crouching before the male, frequently treading and moaning. When fully aroused she twists from side to side, lifting the hind quarters as she crouches showing lordosis, or depression of the back.

The mating act: Some males approach the female with a sharp howl. As the female crouches the male grips the loose skin of the neck with his teeth and mounts. He kneads her sides with his forepaws and because the penis is backward pointing he uses the hind legs to position himself for a series of rapid pelvic thrusts. Penetration is achieved within a few minutes and is signaled by a loud cry from the female. After ejaculation the male releases or is thrown off the female as she turns on her side to roll her mouth, nose and face along the floor. She stops to lick her forelegs, body and genital area and will not allow the male to remount for at least 5 minutes.

Castration: No mating patterns develop in males castrated earlier than 4 months (puberty) and little is shown by mature, castrated and inexperienced males. After castration, experienced adult males show a gradual decline in sexual behavior after the first week or 2, though some may persist for years. Ovariectomy leads to permanent loss of sexual behavior within 24 hours.

Parturition and Maternal Behavior: During birth of her litter, which usually lasts from 1 to 3 hours, the female changes position frequently. By licking each fetus she cleans them of birth membranes and stimulates breathing. The afterbirth is eaten and the first nursing occurs within 2 hours of the birth of the litter. Licking of the anogenital region encourages urination and defecation in the kitten. Similar manual stimulation is required for hand-reared kittens.

Social Development of Kittens: Kittens approach and keep in contact with their mother and huddle at the home or "nest" site. From less than a week of age they are disturbed when separated from mother, litter mates or homesite. They cry and the female retrieves them. Until 3 weeks of age they use contact (thigmotaxis), smell and warmth to locate and grasp a nipple for suckling, though both eyes and ears open earlier. There is little competition for nipples after suckling positions have been adopted.

After the third week, kittens can leave the homesite. Using hearing and sight they follow the mother when she goes to feed, and they begin to eat meat and other foods with her. She periodically permits them to suckle. They can be weaned after the sixth week if they can take milk and meat from dishes.

From the fourth or fifth week, kittens paw, chase, hug and roll together in play with little injury. A social order is formed within the litter. Lone kittens play with objects and their tails but are often frightened of other kittens. Play declines with sexual maturity but may reappear in castrated animals. Mature males play slightly more than females. Single male kittens are usually more aggressive when mature than those reared in a litter. By the fifth week, kittens no longer huddle together but sleep singly or in pairs.

Social Behavior of Farm Animals

Herd or Group Structure: Farm livestock associate together in groups, even under free-range farming systems. Sheep, cattle and horses maintain visual contact. Swine, more a body-contact animal with their poorer vision, keep in auditory communication. If disturbed, sheep and horses first bunch and then run from the source of disturbance while pigs and cattle move in a looser group. Sheep orient themselves to one another at a visual angle of approximately 110°. During the bunching of animal groups in natural or high-density situations, individuals may be forced to violate the personal space of other species members. Social interactions at such close quarters depend on the position of the animals in the dominance order, where one adopts a dominant, and the other a subordinate posture. These orders, which are stable, require: (1) a recognition of individual animals, (2) an initial encounter when the social position is first established and (3) a durable memory that enables each animal to react to the other according to its established social status. Since aggressive behavior is most seen when groups of pigs, cattle or horses are first formed, the frequent changing of group members should be avoided. Production of milk and other physiologic responses can be affected for several days while aggressive social interactions are taking place. Although sheep seldom show overt social dominance, rams compete at the start of each breeding season and sheep may show aggressive butting if intensive husbandry conditions increase competition over food or bedding areas. Butting in cattle and sheep, biting of the mane or withers in the horse, and pushing, biting and side-ripping with the tusks in boars are the common forms of agonistic behavior.

Development of Social Dominance: Piglets show some competitive fighting within a few days of birth for preferred nipples of the sow. Other species do not develop a stable social order until some time after weaning. In semiwild cattle, bull calves stay in the cow herd and dominate the females by about 2½ years of age and then move into the bull group. Social-dominance effects can be very important in cases of high stock densities or poor farm layout. Inadequate trough space, narrow races, inadequate space in indoor housing or lack of feeders can mean that dominant animals command resources at the expense of subordinate animals. The latter will suffer and health and general production can be affected. Documented examples include the higher internal parasite load carried in some subordinate goats and the higher death rate during droughts when scarce food was commandeered by dominant stock. There may be an upper limit to the number of group members that can be recognized or remembered by one individual. This number could be 50 to 70 in cattle and 20 to 30 in pigs.

The horse is very responsive to small changes in stance or skin pressures and these cues used during dominance-subordination interactions are utilized by good horsemen. Sometimes tranquilizers have been used to aid social tolerance when strange pigs have to be penned together or when wild horses have to be broken.

Leader-Follower Relationships: Pigs are reluctant to lead and require to be driven, but cattle and horses are all subjected to leader-follower order in free-range conditions. In naturally constituted flocks of sheep, the oldest ewe may tend to lead; in groups of dairy cows the mid-dominant animals lead. Some use is made by man of the "Judas" animal to lead groups to slaughter, thus using the natural movement patterns of the species concerned. Sheep, cattle and horses can all be trained to lead, and cattle tied in pairs after weaning teach each other to lead. In the dairy cow, the movement order to milking is rather consistent over a season, though the rear animals are more fixed than the "leaders." The milking order is not necessarily the same as the leader-follower order when moving between grazing areas. Under free-range conditions the older stock can transfer information about seasonal pathways, good pasture areas, and watering points to their offspring if this bond is not disrupted before weaning. In this way, home-range areas can be established. Sheep in pastures of 250 acres (100 ha) may establish up to 3 separate home-range areas. To this extent they can be considered territorial, and subgroups of the whole flock work with minimal overlap in these regions. In smaller pastures, dairy bulls set up small territories under set-stocking conditions between the age of 4 and 5 years but not before. The sudden attacks of dairy bulls on known handlers might be caused by this change to territorial behavior.

Sexual Behavior: The presence of the male at the beginning of the breeding season has an influence on the onset of the breeding cycle in sheep. Although the courtship procedures under free-range conditions are not as elaborate as in some wild species, male sheep and cattle spend considerable hours or even days in attendance on the pre-estral female. This interplay between male and female, which aids reproductive success, is not possible with artificial insemination programs. In the Asiatic buffalo, at least one dominant and one subordinate male are required for successful mating. In sheep, ewes at the peak of estrus attend the harem of the dominant male while the subordinate males mate with ewes before and after the maximal heat period. In many management systems the lack of libido or infertility of the most dominant male can greatly reduce the number of fertile matings that occur in the group.

Birth and Maternal Behavior: In feral sheep there is a strong tendency for the ewe to withdraw from the main flock for up to 3 days after giving birth before leading the lamb back into the group.

Imprinting and the mutual social bond are then well established. In domestic conditions where possibilities do not exist for this withdrawal, other ewes a few hours from lambing may steal the newly dropped lambs, being attracted by the presence of the birth fluids. Dominant cows can take calves from subordinate cows, but generally lose interest in them after producing their own young. The uninterrupted formation of the maternal-offspring bond within the first few hours after birth maximizes survival under free-range conditions. Bucket rearing of calves in competitive situations can influence later adult behavior, including mothering ability, and rapid drinking of milk from the bucket may lead to continued sucking of ears, testicles or other parts of fellow calves and establish undesirable habits of inter-suckling in older stock.

Abnormal Behavior in Swine: One of the consequences of sharply increasing population densities (crowding) in penning and housing is tail-biting in fattening pigs. The peck order or social hierarchy can operate satisfactorily in swine groups if they are fairly permanent in their composition and have adequate space for subordinate animals to avoid dominant aggressors. When confined in stalls for extended periods, swine frequently exhibit a stereotyped behavioral vice in the form of habitual mouthing of metal fixtures, and confined sows will engage for long periods in chewing on steel nipple-type waterers and bar-gnawing on pipe railings in the front of their stalls.

Abnormal Behavior in Cattle: In cattle a variety of forms of anomalous behavior taking the form of "stereotypes" are evident in systems of management that feature close confinement. Calves kept under crowded conditions indulge in excessive sucking of the underparts and appendages of their companion animals. Excessive self-grooming can also be observed, sometimes leading to the formation of hair balls in the alimentary canal with possible acute obstruction of the digestive system.

A recently recognized form of anomalous behavior in adult cattle is **tongue-rolling.** This habit involves frequent rolling of the tongue within the usually open mouth; in the course of this the tongue is partially swallowed. This occurs in adult cattle, such as nonlactating cows, which are maintained statically in groups in a confinement system for extended periods of time.

Abnormal Behavior in Sheep: There is a growing trend to maintain sheep in densely housed groups and many breeders now mature young rams in large numbers in small paddocks, both conditions of high population density. Among the densely raised rams there is a considerable amount of homosexual activity at the age of puberty, and many rams may maintain such anomalous behavior for a time when put with ewes. Most eventually adjust to normal breeding activity, but some do not.

For ewes, husbandry systems are being developed in which they are maintained in rows of pens of limited size, within houses of substantial size. Among such sheep **wool-picking** or **wool-pulling** occurs during which some ewes pull with their mouths on the strands of wool on the backs of others around them. Eventually all the sheep in the group may lose most of the long wool from their backs. Bare areas of skin do not develop, but only wool fibres of approximately 3 cm cover the back while fleece of normal length is still carried elsewhere.

Abnormal Behavior in Horses: The stable vices of horses are probably the forms of anomalous behavior that have been longest recognized among domesticated animals. These are understood to be the consequence of boredom due to being stabled for long periods of time without adequate exercise. The commonest forms of behavioral vices are probably **cribbing** and **weaving.** A cribber habitually sets its upper incisor teeth on a firm object such as a manger, and sucks in and swallows air, usually with a characteristic grunting sound. In time, this addiction has an adverse effect on the animal's health. Horses that have learned the vice of cribbing sometimes progress to an associated vice, **wind-sucking** or **aerophagia,** which is cribbing without the need to bite onto an object when the air is being sucked in.

Weaving in horses is also a common stable vice clearly associated with "boredom." The habit, acquired while in the stall, entails rocking from side to side or back and forward in a repetitive way, with a precise type of movement which usually involves stepping actions of the forefeet. This is often sustained for such lengthy periods that deterioration in physical condition results. Another vice associated with inadequate exercising and protracted stall living is **stall-kicking** in which horses kick forcefully with their hind feet against the sides or rear posts of their stalls. This can occur so frequently that the animals acquire chronic injuries to their hind legs.

Polydipsia nervosa is also seen in some horses isolated and confined in stalls with water supplied *ad lib.* Some will consume about 30 gal. (115 L) daily compared with the normal upper limit of 10 gal., and this can precipitate gastric or intestinal volvulus. An associated polyuria may be the first indication of the condition. The habit can be broken by controlling the water supply and increasing exercise.

Social Behavior of Chickens

Development of Social Behavior: The chick shows early social responses while still in the shell: it may give low-pitched distress calls if cooled, or rapid twitterings of contentment if warmed. Chicks hatched at slightly subnormal temperatures give distress calls as their moist down dries and they lose contact with the egg shell. Contact with a broody hen or other warm object prevents these calls. Newly hatched chicks are attracted to the hen by warmth, contact, clucking and body movements. This attraction is greatest on the day of hatching. They learn to eat, roost, drink and avoid enemies in the company of their mother.

In chicks the most sensitive period for imprinting, i.e. fixation upon the mother, is between 9 and 20 hours after hatching and fear is shown by the third day. The attachment to the mother is further strengthened as her voice and appearance are recognized. She rejects the chicks as the down starts to disappear from their heads by pecking at them, and the clutch is dispersed.

Sexual Behavior: The testes secrete testosterone as the cockerel approaches maturity. This stimulates growth of comb and wattles and leads to crowing. Male courtship activities include "tidbiting," a wing flutter and waltzing, which leads to copulation. Crowing, which is rare in capons, advertises the location of the male and his territory to prospective mates and warns off other males. Interference by other males with copulation is common where several males are crowded into small pens with a few females.

In the pullet the ovarian medulla secretes enough male hormone for the growth of wattle and comb and some degree of aggressiveness. The ovarian cortex secretes female hormone which stimulates the growth of oviducts, inhibits male-type plumage and leads to the sex crouch when the cock places one foot on the back prior to mating.

Parental Behavior: Except in "nonbroody" breeds, incubation commences after a number of eggs have been laid. During sittings the eggs are turned, so preventing adhesions within the shell. A warm, defeathered, highly vascular brood-patch develops on each side of the breast. The broody hen clucks and ruffles her feathers if disturbed. Under feral conditions an elaborate approach behavior confuses predators and allows her to return to the nest undetected. During incubation (20 to 22 days), prolactin reduces ovarian activity and sexual behavior so that egg-laying ceases.

The hen uses brief, repetitive, low-pitched vocalizations to lead the chicks and indicate food sources. She warns them about ground or overhead predators, by cackling or by issuing a loud scream.

Flock Behavior: The clutch is the basis of flock organization and even after it has dispersed, chickens need company. A chick reared in isolation tends to stay apart from the flock. Flock birds eat more than birds kept singly. Adult flock formation depends on mutual tolerance. Strangers are attacked and are only gradually integrated into the flock. Newcomers are relegated to positions near the bottom and only active fighting will change it. Hens and cocks have separate peck orders as males in the breeding season do not peck hens. The male order is less stable than the female owing to greater aggressiveness.

The **peck order** is most clearly seen in competition for food or mates, and subordinate hens may obtain so little food that they lay fewer eggs. Dominant hens mate less frequently than subordinate hens but dominant males mate more often than subordinate males. Birds in a flock kept in a state of social disorganization by the removal and replacement of birds eat less, may lose weight or grow poorly, and tend to lay fewer eggs than do birds in stable flocks. Additional feed and water troughs distributed about the pen enable subordinate hens to feed unmolested, and an adequate number of nesting boxes ensures these birds the continuous opportunity to lay. Flocks of over 80 birds tend to separate into 2 distinct groups and at least 2 separate peck orders will be established.

Abnormal Behavior in Poultry: Debeaking does not eliminate aggressive pecking entirely or prevent the development of the peck order, but pecks by debeaked birds are more often ignored by subordinates. Hens kept crowded on wire cannot exercise their normal pecking drive. They often attack other birds and feather pecking may develop. The use of "polypeepers," banned in some countries, reduces the rate of pecking among birds, allows reduced stress levels when weights of the adrenal glands are used as the index of stress, assists a full body cover of plumage to remain on all birds and generally leads to increases in production. *See also* CANNIBALISM, p. 1152.

SOCIAL BEHAVIOR OF DOMESTIC TURKEYS

Social Organization: Domestic and wild turkeys have similar flocking patterns and social organization, but management practices determine the size and composition of domestic groups. Flock groups are organized according to a social dominance order that is less stable than that of chickens. In penned males some changes in rank may occur every few days. Certain varieties of turkeys tend to dominate others; e.g. Black over Bronze over Gray and in mixed sex groups, males dominate females.

The commonest pair encounter is a simple threat, with one bird submitting to the other, otherwise both birds warily circle each other with wing feathers spread, tails fanned, and each emits a high-pitched trill. Then one or both turkeys will leap into the air and attempt to claw the other. The one that can push, pull or press down the head of the other will usually win the encounter. Bouts usually last a few minutes.

Much blood may be shed during a tugging battle since richly vascularized skin areas may be torn, but actual physical damage is slight and birds do not fight to the death. An injured lower ranking bird must be separated from the group, however, until its wounds heal, as others will tend to peck and aggravate the wound.

Sexual Behavior: Turkeys are seasonal breeders with a peak in spring. With the use of artificial light, they can be kept sexually active throughout the year. Turkeys are sexually mature in 8 months and breed the season after hatching. Males initiate an elaborate courtship with postures and movements, but are ignored by all except receptive females. Such females crouch in response to the male's strutting, sitting down quietly with the head drawn in close to the body. The male slowly approaches, mounts, treads and makes cloacal contact with the everted oviduct of the female. The courtship process can take up to 10 minutes. Ejaculation follows swiftly the male dismounts, and the female executes a postcopulatory feather ruffling and brief run. If the male fails to dismount she squirms out from under him. The receptivity of a female lasts for 2 days on average, whether or not insemination has been achieved but males often strut again immediately following copulation, and have been seen to mate with as many as 10 females in 30 minutes. No pair bonds are formed but range males often gather harems which they defend against other males. Only higher ranking males successfully complete a mating. Lower ranking females are mated more often than high ranking females but they lay fewer and smaller eggs. After a single mating, fertile eggs can be laid for 5 or 6 weeks. When eggs are removed routinely, broody behavior is postponed.

Development and Social Behavior: Incubation takes 28 days and the poults move freely shortly after hatching. They become socially attached to the mother during the first day or 2 though occasionally they may imprint with siblings, humans or other objects. Normally imprinted poults form tightly knit groups which may initially cluster for warmth but are cohesive even in fairly warm environments. Birds tend to "tidbit," feed or wander as a group, and if they are with the mother, she is the focus of activity, providing leadership and defense against intruders. Vocal and visual signals are used by both parent and young to stay in contact until the poults are at least 8 weeks old. Fighting is rare prior to 3 months of age, but increases to a peak at 5 months, when social orders are formed. Males fight more vigorously among themselves than do females.

Social Behavior of Ducks

Most domestic ducks have originated from 2 species—the mallard (*Anas platyrhynchos*) and the muscovy (*Cairina moschata*). The muscovy has bare skin on the face of both sexes.

Social Behavior of Muscovies: Muscovies are promiscuous. The adult males, which are twice as heavy as females, are solitary and aggressive towards other males. Their displays are primitive and their calls are simple. The female, when alarmed, utters a weak quack. A hissing noise with tail-shaking, crest-raising and swinging of the head in the males is both a threat to other males and a sexual display towards females. As females generally avoid displaying males, they may be chased to exhaustion before mating is possible. Following fertilization the female retires to her nest site and lays an egg a day. The nest is not continuously occupied until incubation begins with the last or second last egg. Eggs are hatched after 35 days. The male will attack sexually any female he may meet and he plays no part in the selection of the nest, incubation or care of the young.

Social Behavior of Mallards: Wild mallards are monogamous and stay together from midwinter until the beginning of incubation, a period of 5 months. In domestic situations this may not be possible if sex numbers are not balanced.

Social Courtship: Social courtship begins after the summer molt of males. Sexually stimulated males display singly or in groups towards particular females, which in turn incite the males with a rather formalized display alternating between threatening and submissive gestures with a peculiar call. The threat is toward a strange male and submission is shown to the preferred male, who then swims ahead of the female and turns his nape towards her. Aquatic chases turn to aerial courtship flights as other males jockey for this favored position. Other courtship displays by competing males expose specific plumage towards the courting female. Fighting among males is typical but is not crucial to pairing.

Paired birds leave the flock, but in domestic situations females cannot avoid attack by unpaired males and may be drowned or chased to exhaustion. The females are protected by mates until egg-laying is complete, and the male then deserts to molt. Thereafter incubation is disrupted by the sexual attacks of other males. Incubation takes 28 days and the young leave the nest after the first day. The female undergoes her annual molt in the 6 to 8 weeks before the brood can fly.

Growth of Social Bonds: The young normally become firmly attached to their mother during a sensitive period in the first few days after hatching. A second, more gradual kind of "imprinting" helps them respond sexually to their own species mates when mature. Males raised apart from their mothers tend to form homosexual pairs when mature, or when raised with females of another species attempt to mate with them. Female mallards respond sexually only to the visual and vocal stimuli of males of their own species.

PART VII
ADDENDUM

DIAGNOSTIC PROCEDURES FOR THE OFFICE LABORATORY

Procedures suitable for the veterinarian's office are included in this chapter. Emphasis is given to those simple, rapid procedures that give essential information with a minimum of equipment and technical skill. While an enlarging spectrum of packaged kits for clinical chemistry makes it increasingly feasible to perform difficult and cumbersome tests, the time and care that must be devoted to quality control preclude their utilization in many practices. Commercial laboratories that specialize in inexpensive automated chemistry now provide a broad panel of accurate biochemical results.

PARASITOLOGIC EXAMINATIONS

Examination of Feces

Feces should be fresh or refrigerated whenever possible, since the results are more difficult to interpret on samples in which development of embryos or deterioration of oocysts or eggs has occurred. Only fresh feces must be examined for lungworm larvae, since other larvae may be found in older feces. *Strongyloides* are passed as larvae or as eggs that hatch shortly thereafter in dog feces. Specimens of feces to be mailed to a diagnostic laboratory should be fixed in 5% formaldehyde solution (suitable for all parasitologic examinations).

Examination by Flotation: A saturated salt (NaCl) solution is prepared by dissolving as much granulated table salt as possible in water at room temperature. It does not require a preservative, and is neither sticky nor attractive to flies. A saturated sucrose solution containing 50 ml of 5% phenol per liter may be utilized. This solution is capable of floating the eggs of *Dicrocoelium* and is slower to destroy larvae and delicate oocysts. A number of kits for fecal analysis are also available.

About 2 gm of feces are placed in a waxed paper cup and approximately 15 ml of the salt or sugar solution is added. This is stirred with a wooden tongue depressor until the entire sample is in suspension, then strained through a clean gauze square into a test tube, using enough solution to fill it to within 0.25 in. (6 mm) from the top. The tube is placed in a centrifuge and run at low speed (1,000 to 2,000 rpm) for approximately 6 minutes. When centrifugation is completed, a large drop is lifted from the surface film by means of a beaded glass rod and transferred to a microscope slide, covering a circular area approximately 1 cm in diameter.

Drops from several samples may be placed on one slide to achieve economy of effort. The floated debris is examined by means of a compound microscope, using the low-power lens for scanning and the high-dry for further study if necessary for identification. Reduced illumination from a good light source is used so that the relatively transparent eggs and oocysts are well defined. Paper cups, tongue depressors and gauze are discarded after each sample.

Quantitative Examination: This procedure utilizes both flotation and quantitation and requires not only an aliquot of a uniform specimen but also a special counting chamber, the McMaster slide. This is available commercially, and is sold complete with directions for use. The number of eggs per gram of feces, coupled with the presence or absence of clinical signs will indicate the degree of infection and the measures to be taken (but egg counts alone are notoriously unreliable as indicators of degree of infection).

Examination of Blood for Parasites and Microorganisms

Dirofilaria immitis in the dog and occasionally in the cat and other carnivores, and *Dipetalonema reconditum* in the dog and possibly other carnivores, spend part of their life cycles in the blood stream. (*See* Knott's Test, p. 706, or use a commercially available test.) Certain protozoan parasites are also found in the peripheral blood, for example, the nonpathogenic *Trypanosoma theileri* (*americanum*) may be seen occasionally in cattle blood. These protozoa are found free in the plasma. Other parasites, which may be seen on or inside the red blood cells are *Piroplasma* (*Babesia*) in the dog and horse, *Haemobartonella* in the dog and cat, *Eperythrozoon* in pigs, *Anaplasma* in cattle, *Leucocytozoon* in ducks and *Haemoproteus* in pigeons. *Ehrlichia canis* may be found occasionally in mononuclear cells of the peripheral blood in dogs. They may also be found rarely in the neutrophils. Rarely *Toxoplasma gondii* can be found in circulating phagocytes. *Histoplasma capsulatum*, the yeast phase, can also be seen occasionally in peripheral monocytes in the dog and perhaps the cat. *Erysipelothrix rhusiopathiae* and other bacteria may be demonstrated within neutrophils.

Examination of the Erythrocytes for Parasites: Several blood smears (q.v., p. 1473) of varying thicknesses are made on clean slides; the smears are fixed for at least 2 minutes with absolute methanol; stained with Wright's or, perhaps better, with Giemsa stain (q.v., p. 1479) and carefully examined by means of the oil-immersion objective. Confusing artifacts are usually refractive as compared with the parasites. New methylene blue (q.v., p. 1473) may also be used to visualize red cells and contents.

URINALYSIS

Strip-Test and Tablet Procedures: The commercial availability of many strip tests and tablets for urinalysis has simplified the procedures considerably. These test strips have as many as 6 tests on the one plastic strip (glucose, pH, bilirubin, ketone bodies, protein and blood). Test tablets are available for reducing substances, bilirubin and blood. A test strip is also available for urobilinogen. These strips are sufficiently reliable to be most useful, especially in the small laboratory. The rapidity with which the various abnormal constituents can be detected precludes their determination by more cumbersome methods. However, when urine is highly colored due to the presence of hemoglobin, myoglobin, bilirubin or other colored excretory product, the accurate reading of these strips becomes impossible.

Collection of the Specimen: A specimen is obtained as voided or by catheterization. Unless tests can be run within an hour, the urine specimen is placed in the refrigerator. If urine is to be kept longer or sent through the mail, toluene (2 mg/100 ml of urine) is added as a preservative. Other preservatives may be used; however, it is recommended that the preservative be identified as some interfere with subsequent tests.

Specific Gravity: If a Goldberg refractometer is unavailable, the specific gravity may be determined using a urinometer cylinder. The urinometer cylinder is filled approximately two-thirds full with urine and the float is placed into the tube, being careful that it does not adhere to the sides of the cylinder. The specific gravity of the urine is read at the bottom of the meniscus on the stem of the hydrometer float. If the temperature of the urine differs appreciably from that at which the urinometer was standardized, 0.001 is added for each 3°C above the temperature standard or subtracted for each 3°C below it. The approximate normal range (all species) is 1.015 to 1.050. It is a mark of a normal kidney that the specific gravity will vary with the hydration of the animal. Values above and below normal can reflect marked alterations in hydration. Renal disease may occur when the specific gravity falls within the normal range. In such cases a persistent proteinuria is often present along with alterations in the sediment. It is characteristic of widespread tubular damage that the specific gravity remains in the range 1.010 ± 0.002 and urine volume and water intake are increased. (As normal plasma has a specific gravity of about 1.018, the size and shape of red blood cells in urine of similar specific gravity will appear normal. Specific gravities above 1.018 will crenate the cells and below 1.018 will hemolyze or swell them.)

Color: The color of the freshly voided urine is noted in a standard container, either the collection bottle or the urinometer cylinder. The normal color may range from very pale yellow (practically colorless) to dark amber. Abnormal colors of red or green may denote the presence of blood, blood pigments, pigmented drugs or their breakdown products. Urine may change color on standing, especially horse urine, which becomes dark brown.

Transparency: Normal freshly voided urine usually is clear, but may be turbid due to crystalline precipitates. Horse urine is normally turbid due to the presence of calcium carbonate crystals and mucin. A fine, diffuse cloudiness may be due to bacteria. Increased turbidity usually is the result of pus cells.

Reaction: A strip of indicator paper (Nitrazine or pHydrion) is dipped into fresh urine; the color change is noted and the pH is read by comparing it with the color standard included with the paper. The pH of urine of dogs and cats may range from 4.5 to 7.5. The urine of herbivorous farm animals usually is neutral to pH 8.0, becoming more alkaline upon standing. Suckling calves, because of their high-protein diet, will have an acid urine until their rumens develop.

Protein: If the urine is not clear, it should be cleared by centrifugation before performing the test. If the turbidity is due to lipoproteins, clarification can be achieved by adding a gram of talc to 10 ml of urine and filtering. A few drops of 20% sulfosalicylic acid are added to 1 or 2 ml of urine in a test tube. Development of a milky precipitate is a positive reaction. The Bumintest tablets permit detection of protein by the sulfosalicylic acid method. Commercially available indicator-impregnated strips are less reliable for detecting proteinuria; these require only a drop of urine. Highly alkaline urines produce a false-positive reaction. A small amount of protein is filtered normally by the kidney; however, the detection methods are not sensitive enough to indicate its presence. Sexually mature male dogs may show a trace to 1+ reaction due to sexual secretions.

Glucose: A reagent strip (Dextrostix) moistened in fresh well-mixed urine gives a color reaction if glucose is present. The color is checked against the chart provided, at 10 seconds after moistening. Glucosuria usually indicates a blood glucose level exceeding 160 mg/100 ml of blood, although rarely kidney tubular damage will lead to loss at "normal" blood levels.

Ketone Bodies: An approximate level of ketone bodies is easily determined by means of Acetest tablets or powder. Commercially available reagent-impregnated paper strips (or multi-test dip sticks) are possibly more practical for small-animal practice. Ketone determination is of limited practical interest in species other than the cow and sheep (*see* KETOSIS, p. 512). However, in extreme instances of diabetes in any species, a positive reaction may sometimes occur, as it may with starvation, persistent diarrhea or vomiting, or with febrile or cachetic diseases.

Bilirubin (Bile Pigment): A piece of filter paper is soaked in urine, spread out and allowed to dry partially; a drop of concentrated nitric acid is placed on the most discolored portion of the paper. A play of bluish green color indicates the presence of bile pigments and varies from faint green (1+) to very dark green (4+). Alternatively, the Ictotest tablet available commercially detects conjugated bilirubin in a drop of urine. This test is specific and sensitive.

In most species, the detection of conjugated bilirubin in the urine is an indication of impaired biliary excretion, and serves to differentiate obstructive from hemolytic icterus. However, many healthy dogs and possibly 1 in 4 normal cattle have bilirubinuria.

Blood: The presence of blood usually can be detected grossly by the color and turbidity of the specimen. Blood causes the urine to appear red or pink and opaque, whereas hemoglobin yields a red or pink and clear solution. Centrifugation at 1,500 rpm for 5 minutes will differentiate between red blood cells (hematuria) and hemoglobin (hemoglobinuria). Both blood and hemoglobin have a brownish color in very acid urine. Test tablets for blood in urine are available commercially. These tablets will also give a positive reaction for myoglobin.

Microscopic Examination of Urinary Sediment: A sample of whole urine is centrifuged at slow speed (approximately 600 to 1,000 rpm) for about 6 minutes. The supernatant fluid is poured off into another tube to be used for the chemical tests and a small amount of sediment is placed on a slide; a cover glass is applied and the sediment is examined microscopically. The sediment may consist of formed materials (epithelial cells, leukocytes, erythrocytes, tube casts and bacteria) and crystals that vary in amount and variety, according to the reaction and concentration of the urine. In alkaline urines, triple phosphates and carbonates are the most common. In acid urines, oxalates, calcium sulfate and various urate crystals appear. In dogs, other than Dalmatians, crystals of uric acid or other urates seldom appear. Recently the Sternheimer-Malbin staining technique has replaced the examination of unstained urinary sediment. The various constituents stain characteristically with the dye, thus making identification relatively simple. The presence of crystals in the urinary sediment is frequently of little diagnostic significance; however, oxalate crystals suggest oxalate or ethylene glycol poisoning, and quantities of cystine crystals suggest congenital cystinuria. Dogs with portacaval shunts may have ammonium urate crystals in their urine.

HEMATOLOGY

Counting the cellular elements in the blood of animals is valuable in assessing conditions of health and disease. The variation from animal to animal of the same species is considerable and depends in part on the sex, nutrition, age, diurnal and sexual cycles, and stresses such as strenuous exercise and excessive environmental heat or cold. For these reasons, the values given in TABLE 1 must be considered as guides rather than as rigid criteria. With malnutrition, iron deficiency or chronic disease, the animal may develop an anemia expressed as a reduction in the number of circulating red blood cells or in the content of hemoglobin in each cell. (*See* ANEMIA, p. 19.)

The white blood cell count usually rises well above its normal range in acute bacterial infections and also in such conditions as neoplasia, chemical or metabolic intoxication, trauma and tissue necrosis. However, the same conditions can on occasion lead to lowered white cell counts; e.g. overwhelming bacterial septicemias may cause profound neutropenia. In acute viral infections, the white blood cell count usually decreases from its normal level. The response varies depending on the nature of the invading microorganism and the species of animal. With most pus-forming organisms, the number of neutrophils (polymorphonuclear leukocytes) increases markedly. A marked rise also is seen in anthrax, encephalitis and meningitis. An increase in monocytes and lymphocytes usually indicates a more chronic process or the end stage of an acute infectious process. A rise in eosinophils may represent an allergic response, sometimes due to parasitic infection. Abnormal or immature cells in the blood may present evidence for a disease of the blood-forming organs (bone marrow, liver, spleen, lymph nodes) as in leukemia and certain toxic states.

Collection of the Specimen: Blood should be collected by means of venipuncture with a dry needle and syringe. (If the equipment is wet-sterilized, it should be thoroughly rinsed in isotonic saline solution before the venipuncture.) Dogs are usually bled from the cephalic vein, although when large amounts of blood are to be collected, the jugular vein may be employed. Pigs are best bled by puncture of the anterior vena cava, and the larger animals by jugular puncture. Samples for hemoglobin and cell counts may be collected from kittens and other small animals by shaving an ear and nicking the external ear vein, or by clipping a toenail. Blood collected by venipuncture into vials containing KEDTA (potassium ethylenediamine tetraacetic acid) is satisfactory for the various procedures if done within a few hours of collection. The specimen should be mixed thoroughly before taking samples from the container. Ideally, smears for differential cell counts should be made from blood before the use of an anticoagulant; however, this is not always possible. KEDTA is the anticoagulant of choice for most hematologic procedures.

Packed Cell Volume (Hematocrit): One of the easier and more useful tests for the small laboratory, this determination has largely superseded the erythrocyte count and hemoglobin determination as

TABLE 1. SOME NORMAL LEUKOCYTE VALUES*
(Approximate ranges—in 10^3/cu mm)

	Leukocytes	Neutrophils	Immature Neutrophils	Lymphocytes	Eosinophils	Monocytes
Horse	5-15	3-7	0-0.1	1.5-5.5	0-0.5	0-0.8
Ox	5-13	0.6-4	0-0.12	2.5-7.5	0-2.4	0.25-0.84
Sheep	5-13	0.7-6	rare	2-4	0-1	0-0.75
Goat	5-13	1.2-7.2	rare	2-9	0.05-0.65	0-0.55
Pig	7-20	3.2-10	0-0.8	4.5-13	0.5-2	0.25-2
Dog	8-18	3-12	0-0.3	1-4.8	1-1.3	0.15-14
Cat	8-25	2.5-13	0-0.3	1.5-7	0-1.5	0-0.85
Rabbit	6-13	2-6	rare	0.2-0.5	0-0.5	0.1-1
Rat	5-25	0.001-5	rare	7-13	0-1	0-1
Mouse	4-12	0.5-4	rare	3-9	0.05	0-1
Chicken	9-56	3-17	—	10-30	0-0.5	0-5

* For erythrocyte counts, hematocrit values (PCV,%) and hemoglobin levels *see* ANEMIA, p. 19.

a practical means of evaluating the red cell status. The microhematocrit procedure is most suitable. Blood is drawn into the capillary tube (containing an anticoagulant) directly from a venous or capillary puncture, sealed and centrifuged. A reading is obtained by placing the centrifuged tube against a special hematocrit chart.

Leukocyte Count: The Unopette, a system utilizing disposable pipettes, is satisfactory for determination of total leukocyte counts, and also for erythrocyte (*see* PACKED CELL VOLUME, above) and thrombocyte counts. Directions for use are supplied by the manufacturer along with the necessary materials.

Differential Leukocyte Count: New, "electronically clean," dry slides are used for making blood smears. A medium-sized drop of blood is placed near one end of a slide placed horizontally on a table; another slide held at an angle (approximately 30°C) is pulled back until it touches the drop. As the drop spreads along the acute angle so formed, the spreader slide is pushed quickly and smoothly toward the opposite end, spreading a thin film on the slide; the slide is then waved in the air to obtain quick drying of the smear. Rapid drying of the smear prevents crenation and other distortions of the cells. When preparing blood smears in cool or humid stables or kennels or outdoors in winter, the slide should be warmed beforehand and if possible, warm air should be blown over the film to prevent crenation of the erythrocytes. Unstained smears should be stored in a dry dust-free box until staining (never in the refrigerator).

The smears are stained with Wright's, Diff-Quik or Giemsa stain (q.v., p. 1479), washed thoroughly in flowing water and permitted to dry. The smear is scanned with the low-power lens to ascertain adequacy of staining and distribution of the leukocytes. Then the slide is examined by oil-immersion microscopy and 100 or 200 cells are classified and the values expressed as percent. This relative value when multiplied by the total count gives the differential count in absolute values. The absolute values are less subject to error in interpretation than are relative values.

Reticulocyte Count: A few drops of blood are mixed with an equal volume of a solution composed of 1% **new methylene blue** (℞ 661) in isotonic salt solution and permitted to stand in a stoppered tube for 15 minutes or longer at room temperature. A drop of the mixture is placed on a slide, smeared and air-dried. The oil-immersion objective is used, noting the percent of reticulocytes as compared with the total number of erythrocytes seen. Reticulocytes in dogs and cats vary from 0 to 1%, while in hoofed animals they are rarely seen. Counting the number of reticulocytes seen per 1,000 red blood cells is the standard procedure and the value is expressed as a percent.

Platelet Count: While the error in counting platelets is high, the accuracy is usually sufficient to be useful. An estimate may be obtained (1) by using the Unopette system, or (2) in conjunction with a total leukocyte count, by counting the number of platelets per 100 white blood cells in a blood film. From this, the number of platelets per cubic millimeter is obtained by dividing 100 into the number of platelets multiplied by the white cells per cubic millimeter. A count of 5 to 25 may be taken as normal. Because of the likelihood of error, 10 fields should be counted and the results averaged. Counts are elevated following stress, including surgery. The cause of primary thrombocytopenia is unknown. The secondary condition follows disease of the bone marrow or spleen, and in a number of the diseases of the blood and reticuloendothelial systems.

BLOOD CHEMISTRY

Blood-chemical determinations are useful in the diagnosis of animal diseases. They should be used sparingly and wisely chosen. Attention must be given to relatively simple tests that will assist in improved diagnosis and prognosis. Also, the choice of the test should be governed by findings in the clinical examination and in preliminary urine and blood studies. The technique used is not important and may differ according to the facilities of the office laboratory. The easiest and cheapest methods, where only a few types of tests are to be run, are those for which commercial laboratory kits have been prepared containing all the apparatus and reagents necessary for a single test. The tests usually depend on titration or visual colorimetry, by means of blood color standards.

For example, a rapid, simply conducted yet reasonably accurate chromatographic method for the determination of urea nitrogen, the Urograph technique, is obtainable. (If many kinds of procedures are planned, it is more economic to purchase a photoelectric colorimeter that may be used for all the determinations and is adapted to methods of greater accuracy.) The techniques recommended by the distributors of these kits should be followed, since they are adapted to the particular instrument. The recommended reagents should be purchased ready-mixed. Recently many office-laboratory diagnostic systems have become available; some of them include ancillary equipment such as a centrifuge, colorimeter, heating unit, and some are based on prepackaged reagent kits. The various systems are basically similar and have many procedures in common for the more frequently determined blood constituents. The reagents and equipment such as test tubes and pipettes are disposable. Although each differs in some respect, and they are highly competitive, the test results are sufficiently reliable to have practical value in the small laboratory. Very small amounts of serum or plasma are used for the analyses, thus eliminating the necessity of a protein-free filtrate.

TABLE 2. BLOOD CHEMISTRY
SOME NORMAL VALUES (Approx. range)

	Urea Nitrogen	Glucose	Ca^{++}	PO_4^{---}	Mg^{++}	Na^+	K^+	Cl^-
	Values in mg/100 ml				in mEq/L*			
Dog	10-20	70-100	8-12	2-5	2-5	135-150	3.5-5.5	100-115
Cat	20-30	70-100	8-12	4-8	2-5	145-155	3.5-5.5	100-115
Ox	10-20	40-60	8-12	4-8	2-5	130-150	3.5-5.5	100-115
Sheep	8-20	30-60	8-12	4-8	2-5	150-160	3.5-5.5	100-115
Pig	8-20	75-150**	8-12	4-8	2-5	140-160	3.5-5.5	100-115
Horse	10-20	60-110	8-12	3-6	2-5	145-150	3.5-5.5	100-115

* For conversion of mEq/L to mg/L, *see* p. 1523.
** Baby pig.

Procedures must be followed precisely or very variable results will be obtained. Quality control, utilizing control serums, is important.

Blood Glucose: A simple and reliable colorimetric field test (Dextrotest) is available making it possible to estimate blood glucose at 100, 150 or 200 mg/100 ml of blood. In addition Dextrostix can provide an estimate of elevated blood glucose values as in diabetes mellitus. For the detection of hypoglycemia greater accuracy is needed and other methods should be employed. The Acetest tablet may be employed to detect elevated levels of ketones in blood, milk or urine.

LIVER FUNCTION TESTS

Serum Bile Pigments: The quantitative Ehrlich reaction (van den Bergh test) measures both the total bilirubin and the bilirubin glucuronide in the blood. The difference is free bilirubin. High levels of bilirubin glucuronide (direct-reacting pigment) indicate an obstructive lesion either in the liver or in the bile duct system. High levels of mainly free bilirubin (indirect-reacting pigment) suggest a hemolytic process. An exception is the horse, in which nearly all bilirubin in the blood reacts indirectly irrespective of cause. A careful correlation of the clinical and laboratory findings is quite important. Specific clinical tests for bilirubin must be used in the horse.

Urobilinogen: Strip tests are now available commercially for the determination of urobilinogen. The presence of anaerobic bacteria in normal dogs' livers make the interpretations of this test difficult since these organisms are capable of producing urobilinogen in the liver when the bile duct is completely obstructed. The absence of urobilinogen in the urine, when associated with clay-colored feces, indicates obstruction of the bile duct. Increased levels are observed in both hemolytic and hepatocellular diseases.

Fecal Stercobilin and Urobilin: These pigments impart color to the normal feces; clay-colored feces suggest bile-duct obstruction. Light-colored feces also occur following the ingestion of bones and antibiotics, as well as in some pancreatic diseases. Many dietary substances contribute substantially also to the color of feces.

Bromsulfophthalein (BSP) Excretion Test: This dye test is primarily helpful in detecting latent hepatic disease without icterus. BSP is injected IV into dogs at 5 mg/kg. Normal dogs exhibit less than 5% retention at 30 minutes. A BSP clearance test is recommended in large animals. A dose of 1 gm of BSP is administered IV to the horse and cow. A normal mature horse clears ½ of the measured concentration in 2 to 3.7 minutes. A cow's T/2 is 2.5 to 4.1 minutes.

Serum Enzyme Concentration: Hepatocellular damage may be detected by using SGPT (ALT) in small animals because this enzyme is specific for liver damage. SGOT (AST) may be used in large or small animals but also responds to muscle damage. SDH may be used for all species. The enzyme is not stable in storage. OCT may be used for all species. The latter 2 enzymes are specific for liver damage. In biliary obstruction ALP will show an increased activity of 3 to 30× the normal levels. It may rise with hepatocellular damage and the administration of corticosteroids or due to hyperadrenocorticoidism in dogs.

PANCREATIC FUNCTION TESTS (DOG)

Acute Pancreatitis: If it is associated with acute abdominal signs, the finding of an elevated activity of serum lipase, which is liberated from a necrotic pancreas, is usually diagnostic. Serum lipase activity as measured by conventional techniques is usually less than 1 unit in normal dogs. Serum amylase can also be employed. Best results accrue from the use of both tests.

Chronic Pancreatic Fibrosis or Atrophy: Two tests (*see* below) may be used: Test 1 is simple and is tried first but it may yield 25% false negative results. The gelatin emulsion on many modern radiographic films resists digestion by normal feces. Test 2 should be tried if no digestion of film occurs in Test 1.

Test No. 1 (X-ray film test): Nine ml of 5% sodium bicarbonate solution are made up to 10 ml total volume by adding feces and stirred. A drop of the mixture is placed on X-ray film (undeveloped film or dark portion of developed film). This is incubated at 37.5°C for 1 hour or for 2½ hours at room temperature. (**Caution:** if drop dries, test is unreliable.) The material is washed off under a gentle stream of tap water. A cleared area under the drop indicates the presence of trypsin. In the absence of trypsin, the film is only watermarked.

Test No. 2 (gelatin tube test): Nine ml of water are made up to 10 ml total volume by adding feces and mixed. A tube containing 2 ml of 7.5% gelatin is warmed to 37.5°C until the gelatin is liquid, and then 1 ml each of the fecal dilution and 5% sodium bicarbonate are added. This is well mixed and then incubated at 37.5°C for 1 hour or at room temperature for 2½ hours, followed by refrigeration for 20 minutes. Failure of the mixture to gel indicates the presence of trypsin (proteolytic enzyme).

CLINICAL MICROBIOLOGY

Bacteriologic methods adapted to the office laboratory are the study of stained and unstained smears, preparation of simple cultures and antibiotic susceptibility tests. Stains, culture media and test disks for the various antibiotics are available. It is useful to examine smears of urinary sediment (especially if the sample can be obtained without catheterization) or of various exudates stained by Gram's method.

Gram Stain: This technique serves the purpose of indicating the presence of bacteria as well as being a basic differential stain. A moderately thin film is prepared and fixed by heating gently over a flame. The smear is covered with Gram's gentian or crystal violet for 1 minute, washed briefly with water and covered with Gram's iodine for 1 minute. It is decolorized 5 to 10 seconds with acetone-alcohol, immediately flooded with water, drained and counterstained with safranine or basic fuchsin for 1 minute. It is then washed, dried and examined by oil-immersion microscopy. Gram-positive organisms, such as cocci, appear dark-blue or black, and gram-negative organisms, such as the coliforms and pseudomonads, appear pink. The nuclei of leukocytes stain pink. All fungi are gram-positive.

The Cleared, Unstained Smear Method: The technique is employed to demonstrate ringworm fungi, molds and the "ray fungi" of actinomycosis. Mange mites, if present, may also be detected. For ringworm, a recent lesion is selected and hair and skin scales are secured by scraping the periphery of the lesion with a scalpel. If the lesion is dry or scaly the scalpel blade may be moistened with oil or glycerol. Scrape deeply (to blood) when mange mites are suspected. Oil interferes with the examination for ringworm. For actinomycosis or molds growing in tissue, pus or tissue debris must be used. The material is placed on a slide, and a few drops of 10 to 40% sodium hydroxide solution are added. It is allowed to stand for 30 minutes (or heated gently for 5 minutes), and a cover glass is carefully pressed on the preparation. The hairs and epithelial cells must be a single **thin** layer; otherwise the fungal elements will be missed. Examination is with the low- and high-power objectives using reduced illumination, looking for spores within or along the hair shafts or in epidermal cells in the case of ringworm. "Ray fungi" and mycelial segments are diagnostic of actinomycosis or tissue mold infection.

Wright's Stain: Commercial Wright's stain may be purchased in liquid form, and is used with phosphate buffer (℞ 666). The slide is placed on a staining rack and sufficient Wright's stain is added to cover the slide. After 1 minute an equal amount of the phosphate buffer is added and mixed by blowing on the slide until a metallic sheen appears. Time for stain to react must be determined for each batch of stain; 3 minutes is suggested as a trial period. Scum and stain are quickly floated off with neutral distilled water (*see* ℞ 666), and the slide is air-dried.

Giemsa Stain should be purchased in liquid form. The film is fixed in absolute methanol for 3 to 5 minutes and is dried. A Coplin jar is filled with staining solution prepared by adding one drop of the Giemsa stain to each ml of neutral distilled water (*see* ℞ 666). The air-dried slide is left in this for 30 minutes, washed in neutral distilled water and again air-dried.

Diff-Quik stain is a commercially available blood stain for which the manufacturer's directions should be followed.

Cultures: Cultures may be prepared by inoculating media (thioglycollate broth or transport media) in the office or field and sending them to a diagnostic laboratory for identification, or by submitting specimens of aseptically collected exudates and other materials. Appropriate culture media can be purchased in screw-capped vials and kept in the refrigerator until needed. Thioglycollate broth supports both aerobic and anaerobic growth, and may be used for initial culture along with an all purpose medium such as brain-heart-infusion agar, blood agar, and a selective, enteric medium such as MacConkey's agar. This is either submitted to a diagnostic laboratory or incubated for 24 hours at 37°C. If growth occurs, it may be subcultured, stained or spread on blood agar or Mueller-Hinton medium for susceptibility testing.

Susceptibility Testing: Paper disks, impregnated with various antibiotics, are available commercially for detecting sensitivity of organisms. These disks are applied to the surface of blood-agar plates or Mueller-Hinton agar that have been streaked with the suspect organism. After incubation for 24 hours at 37°C the inhibition of growth of the organism is determined by the colony-free zone around the disk. It is the presence or absence of a colony-free zone, not its width, that is significant. For more accurate results, the Kirby-Bauer technique should be employed.

CLINICAL PROTOZOOLOGY

As an office procedure, clinical protozoology is confined to collection of samples and identification of the organism, as culture of protozoa is beyond the capability of most small laboratories.

For the direct examination of fecal or vaginal material for trophozoites of *Entamoeba, Giardia* or trichomonads, the sample must be fresh and kept warm as the trophozoites are very fragile. The specimen may be mixed with warm 0.9% saline solution for ease of examination. The smear can also be stained with an aqueous (1:10) dilution of 1% iodine in 2% potassium iodide. This solution will bring out some of the morphologic features of the protozoa. More satisfactory protozoan stains are demanding in terms of technique, and perhaps best done only in laboratories that handle enough volume to allow reliable competence.

If immediate examination is not possible or necessary, prepared fixed smears may be submitted to a diagnostic laboratory. It is possible to obtain slides with a fixative already on them. It is then only necessary to make a smear on these pre-processed slides and mail them, a procedure suitable for detecting both intestinal and vaginal protozoa.

CLINICAL CYTOLOGY

These techniques may be used to study the cellular character of tumors and tissues from various disease processes to obtain a diagnosis without tissue sectioning. Smears may be prepared from material obtained by punch or aspiration biopsy or by imprinting blocks of tissue. As an example: A fresh surface on a piece of liver tissue is prepared at necropsy and imprints made by touching the cut surface to a slide, stained with Wright's, Giemsa or new methylene blue stain (q.v., p. 1473) and examined for the presence of intranuclear inclusions. These are diagnostic of infectious canine hepatitis (q.v., p. 355); however, the possibility of infection with other organisms, such as bacteria, *Toxoplasma*, or *Histoplasma* should not be overlooked. As another example, *Ehrlichia canis* is more readily detected in impression smears of the lung than in peripheral blood.

SOME PHYSIOLOGIC VALUES

BODY TEMPERATURE

The body temperature is determined by the balances between heat production and heat loss. Normal body function depends upon a relatively constant body temperature. Heat production results from basic metabolic processes, food assimilation and muscular activity. The rate of production is increased by shivering, exertion, food intake and the secretion of norepinephrine and epinephrine. In herbivores, bacterial fermentation in the alimentary tract is an additional source of heat. Heat is lost from the body by radiation, conduction and vaporization of water in the respiratory passages and on the skin; small amounts are removed in the feces and urine. Losses are accelerated by exposing more surface area, cutaneous vasodilatation, increased respiration and sweating. Animals exposed to excessive heat will spontaneously seek a cooler environment where heat losses are accelerated. Since fur reduces the ability to lose heat, fur-coated animals are very vulnerable to high temperatures. Ruminants possess a limited sweating mechanism, hence their evaporative loss is inefficient. The temperature regulating mechanisms are controlled and coordinated from centers in the hypothalamus. In warm-blooded or homoiothermic animals, the actual temperature at which the body is maintained varies from species to species and sometimes between individuals (TABLES 1 and 2 on pp. 1482, 1483). Normal temperature may vary from as low as 95°F (35°C) to as high as 110°F (43°C) depending upon the species. Various parts of the body are at different temperatures due largely to the environmental temperature. The rectal temperature is representative of the temperature at the core of the body and varies least. Basal temperature may be obtained early in the morning after a period of rest, without exciting the animal.

Normal Variation: The body temperature of healthy animals is subject to slight diurnal variations. The temperature rises during the day and falls during the night. Large animals, such as the horse, cow and elephant, show small diurnal variations of about 1°F (0.5°C). Certain animals, such as the camel, which are adapted to large variations in environmental temperature and restricted availability of water, have diurnal fluctuations of body temperature of as much as 11°F (5°C).

Exertion, excitement, or prolonged exposure to warm or humid environments, may cause a rise of several degrees in the body temperature. **Hyperthermia** due to reduced heat loss may seriously affect normal functions. For example, cows subjected to excessively high environmental temperatures reduce their food intake, lose weight and fail in milk production. Heat loss is associated with water loss. Teratogenic effects have been demonstrated in embryos when the dam has been subjected to hyperthermia during pregnancy. When water is not available, dehydration leads to inhibition of sweating and fever may develop. This form of hyperthermia is treated readily by the administration of water.

Seasonal variations in body temperature are related to environmental stresses and to the reproductive cycle. In cold weather, the rectal temperature may be recorded 1 to 2°F (1°C) below the summer levels. Prior to ovulation, the basal temperature may be 1°F below the level of the preceding days. During estrus, the level is somewhat higher. It is slightly above the normal range during the first half of pregnancy.

Young animals have more labile temperature levels than older animals, with somewhat greater diurnal fluctuations; the young respond to infection with a much higher temperature elevation than do older animals. In very old animals, even severe infection may produce little or no change in the body temperature.

A characteristic of **fever** is hyperthermia in which the thermoregulatory mechanisms behave as if adjusted to maintain body temperature above the normal level. In diurnal fever, which may indicate chronic infection, the temperature levels may rise several degrees during the day, returning to normal each night. Many infections

TABLE 1. BASAL BODY TEMPERATURE OF VARIOUS SPECIES, RELATED TO WEIGHT

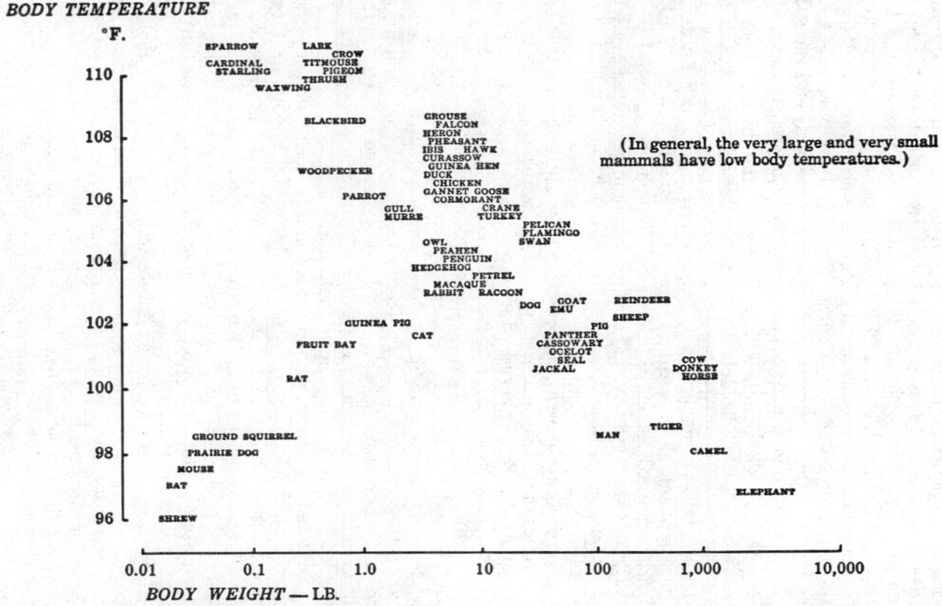

Adapted from *Science* 111:465, 1950.

TABLE 2. RECTAL TEMPERATURES

Animal	°F ± 1°F	°C ± 0.5°C
Horse	100.5	38
Cattle	101.5	38.5
Sheep	103	39.5
Goat	102	39
Pig	102	39
Dog	102	39
Cat	101.5	38.5
Rabbit	102.5	39.3

cause fever by inducing the production of endogenous pyrogen from polymorphonuclear leukocytes in the blood. This fever-producing substance acts on the thermoregulatory centers in the brain to reset them. In acute infections, the temperature may remain several degrees above the normal level for a few days, sometimes with a superimposed diurnal fluctuation. The relapsing fever of some chronic infections (e.g. brucellosis) is characterized by several days of elevated body temperature, followed by several days of normal temperature.

A chill usually heralds a febrile episode. The episode begins with extreme irritability, shivering, the seeking out of a warm environment and the reduction of body surface area from which heat can be lost, as by curling up. At the time of the chill, the body temperature is already above normal; shivering produces more heat and causes the temperature to rise further.

Metabolic disturbances occur as a result of fever. The most striking of these is due to excessive loss of water leading to dehydration. Severe dehydration may produce a rise in body temperature, which is resolved on the administration of fluids. Persistent fever can lead to a loss of sodium chloride and brain damage. Disturbances in acid:base and salt:water balances, associated with prolonged fever or hyperthermia, may lead to acidosis. During hot weather and after fever, horses and cattle should have salt available to replenish losses.

If fever persists, convulsions may ensue. These must be stopped since they lead to excessive heat production. The fever may be treated by cooling the animals with cold soaks or dips, or in smaller animals, alcohol sponge baths. Convulsions may be controlled by sedation or anesthetic doses of barbiturates given by injection, preferably IV. Aspirin stimulates the heat loss centers of the hypothalamus. The maximum body temperature compatible with life is 10°F (5°C) above the normal level of the animal.

Hypothermia: When the skin or the blood is cooled enough to lower the body temperature in nonhibernating animals, metabolic and physiologic processes slow down. Respiration and heart rate are slow, blood pressure is low and consciousness is lost. Below a rectal temperature of 82°F (28°C), the ability to return the temperature to normal is lost, but the animal will continue to survive and if rewarmed using external heat, will return to a normal state. These findings have been adapted and used extensively in heart and brain surgery in man. In hypothermic states the oxygen need of cells, particularly neurons, is greatly reduced and the circulation can be stopped for relatively long periods.

A lowered body temperature is seen in moribund states. It is a poor prognostic sign in infectious diseases. In accidental hypothermia, the animal should be brought into a heated environment and allowed to warm slowly to its normal temperature.

TABLE 3. HEART RATES
beats/minute

Animal	*Avg.*	*Range*	*Animal*	*Avg.*	*Range*
Man	70	(58-104)	Horse	44	(23-70)
Ass	50	(40-56)	Lion	40	
Bat	750	(100-970)	Monkey	192	(165-240)
Camel	30	(25-32)	Mouse	534	(324-858)
Cat	120	(110-140)	Rabbit	205	(123-304)
Cow		(60-70)	Rat	328	(261-600)
Dog		(100-130)	Sheep	75	(60-120)
Elephant	35	(22-53)	Skunk	166	(144-192)
Giraffe	66		Squirrel	249	(96-378)
Goat	90	(70-135)	Swine		(58-86)
Guinea pig	280	(260-400)	Chicken (adult)		(250-300)
Hamster	450	(300-600)	Chicken (baby)		(350-450)

TABLE 4. RESPIRATORY RATES
breaths/min

Animal	*Resp. rate*	*Animal*	*Resp. rate*
Hamster	74	Horse	12
Rat	97	Chicken: Male	12-20
Guinea pig	90	Female	20-36
Rabbit	39	Duck: Male	42
Monkey	40	Female	110
Cat	26	Goose: Male	20
Dog	22	Female	40
Sheep	19	Pigeon	25-30
Man	12	Turkey: Male	28
Cow	30	Female	49

TABLE 5. DAILY URINE VOLUME

Animal	*ml/kg of body wt*
Cat	10-20
Cattle	17-45
Dog	20-100
Goat	10-40
Horse	3-18
Sheep	10-40
Swine	5-30
Man	8.6-28.6

TABLE 6. DAILY FECAL OUTPUT

Animal	*Kilograms*
Horse	13-28
Sheep	1-3
Swine	0.5-3
Dog	0.027-0.041 when fed flesh
	0.13-0.4 moderate amount of bread
	1 large amount of bread
Dairy cow	0.06/kg of body wt
Ox	14-34 maintenance & low production
	35-50 fattening

The data in the above tables, (TABLES 2 through 6), were adapted in part from *Duke's Physiology of Domestic Animals,* 8th ed.; M. J. Swenson, Ed., © 1970, by permission of Cornell University Press, and from other sources.

VETERINARY RADIOLOGY

RADIOGRAPHY

Equipment: The basic equipment for satisfactory veterinary radiography is a diagnostic-type X-ray machine with adequate protective housing. In small animal practice such a machine should have a capacity of 100 kVp (kilovolt peak) and 100 mA (milliamperes). A machine of greater capacity, in a well-planned fixed installation is necessary for use on large domestic animals. However, a light, mobile unit with a highly flexible, well-shielded head, with a capacity of 85 kVp and 30 mA is satisfactory for radiography of the extremities of large animals.

A filter in the useful beam of not less than 2.5 mm of aluminum and an interval timer that can be used at 1/60 of a second with the larger unit and 1/10 of a second with the mobile unit are essential.

All units must be equipped with a coning device to reduce scatter and limit stray primary radiation. A collimator with adjustable lead shutters and an illuminated field effectively limits the primary beam thereby reducing the radiation hazard and improving the technique.

Whenever the part to be radiographed exceeds 10 cm in thickness, the use of a grid markedly improves detail. A grid with a 6:1 ratio and 60 lines per inch is satisfactory for most diagnostic needs in large- and small-animal radiography. Additional equipment should include at least two 10 by 12 in. and two 14 by 17 in. cassettes with par- or high-speed screens, film hangers, a film-marking device, calipers to measure the part thickness, a tape for measuring source to tabletop or focal-film distance, 2 film illuminators and darkroom supplies. Protective aprons and gloves of at least 0.5 mm lead equivalent should be provided for 2 or more persons.

Darkroom: The darkroom must be lightproof and so designed as to provide separate wet and dry working surfaces. The room should be equipped with a 3-compartment tank for developer, water rinse and fixer and with a capacity to handle 14 to 17 in. films. The temperature of the solutions must be maintained between 60 and 74°F (15.5 and 23°C), preferably at 68°F (20°C), by running water or refrigeration. Since the rate of development varies directly with the temperature of the developer, the temperature of the solutions should be checked before use and a time-temperature chart should be consulted at temperatures other than 68°F (20°C). Manufacturer's instructions should be followed, but as a rule the developing time for screen film is 5 min and fixing requires 10 min. Films should be washed for 30 min in running water prior to drying in a dust-free atmosphere.

During processing, films should be removed from the solutions quickly and the excess solution not be permitted to drain back into the tank. This loss is replaced by replenishing from stock solutions, thereby maintaining the strength of the developer and fixer. Replenishing cannot be continued indefinitely, and the solutions should be discarded when the volume of replenisher used equals 3 times the original quantity of developer. In any event, the solutions should be discarded at the end of a 3-month period because of oxidation. Developing solutions must not be replenished while films are being processed.

Automatic processors are available that are compact in size and in a price range within the economic reach of most practices. These small processors can be installed in existing darkrooms. In new construction, the cost of the processor may be offset by reduction in the space normally allocated to the darkroom. These processors reduce the processing time, provide radiographs ready for interpretation and by virtue of their consistent processing technique, eliminate common darkroom errors.

Essential Factors in Radiography: The following factors contribute to the production of a satisfactory radiograph; (1) correct kVp for satisfactory penetration, (2) sufficient milliamperes per second (mAs) to ensure proper density, (3) time of exposure short enough to stop motion, (4) proper target-to-film distance to obtain maximum photographic detail, (5) close approximation of the part radiographed to the film, (6) immobilization of the part, (7) uniform sensitivity of screens and films, (8) standard darkroom technique, (9) standard positions for exposure.

The **kilovolt peak (kVp)** is the crest-value measurement of the pulsating potential generator. It indicates a measurement of the energy level in the X-ray beam and when the value is high the penetrating power of the beam is greater, the contrast on the film is diminished and the quality of the beam is said to be "hard." When he kVp is lower, the beam is said to be "softer" and, because ıbsorption is greater, contrast is improved while penetration is liminished. Good radiologic technique requires the selection of a eam sufficient to penetrate the thickness of the tissue examined vhile providing contrast sufficient for the examination of the various tissues involved.

Milliamperage (mA) is a measurement of current flowing across he X-ray tube. The mAs directly determines the total film exposure r density. Good technique requires the proper selection of time ınd amperage to give the density required under the condition of he examination. The mAs required to produce a given radiographic lensity is directly proportional to the square of the focal-film disance when other factors are constant.

The use of a higher kVp with a reduction in mAs results in less adiation exposure to the patient without significantly detracting rom film quality.

In order to reduce the loss of detail by motion of the patient, short xposure times are desirable. Motion may be further reduced or liminated by sedation or anesthesia. To minimize image distortion aused by divergence of the X-rays, the part to be radiographed hould be in close contact with the cassette. As previously recomnended, par- or high-speed screens increase the photographic effect vith little loss of detail.

To accomplish the best radiography, a **technique chart** should be leveloped using thickness of the part measured in centimeters, elating each change in thickness to a corresponding change in kVp o mAs. A handy rule for determining a technique is as follows: Two imes the thickness of the part in centimeters plus 40 equals the kVp. Using the calculated kVp and 3 mAs with par-speed screens, he films should be of diagnostic quality. For parts exceeding 10 cm, ı 60 line, 6:1 grid should be employed and the mAs must be inreased to 6.

Positioning: Correct positioning of the patient is essential for good adiography, and 2 views should always be taken at right angles to each other. Whenever possible, positioning should be accomplished by the use of foam rubber blocks, leg ties, etc., always striving to reduce human exposure. Rotation of the part is to be avoided, particularly in radiographs of the thorax, skull and canine pelvis.

Whenever a joint is to be examined, the beam should be projected directly across the articular surface so that the intra-articular space and articular facets can be assessed. The beam should be perpendicular to the film to minimize distortion.

Standard lateral projections utilizing a horizontal beam are useful in demonstrating free fluid in the thoracic cavity or the multiple fluid levels and gas caps seen in stasis of the bowel.

Radiographic Interpretation: Immediately following processing, th films should be examined for technical quality and a preliminar diagnosis may be made. A definitive diagnosis should await thorough study of the dried radiograph.

In assessing the image for pathologic changes a systematic ster by-step analysis is made of each anatomic part. Gross pathologi changes usually fall into one or more of the following categories: Alteration in the position of an organ or part. Such alterations ma be the result of a congenital anomaly, inadequate support, passiv displacement by enlargement of adjacent viscera and rotation c viscera as in gastric torsion.

2) Alteration in size. Increase in size of an organ may be indicativ of hypertrophy, hyperplasia, neoplasia, congenital anomaly, etc Reductions in size occur with atrophy, hypoplasia, scarring, mal development, etc.

3) Alterations in contour. Contour changes may affect a localize portion orithe entire organ silhouette. They may result from mal development, trauma, cicatrization, loss of tone, neoplasia, necrosis etc.

4) Alteration in density. Increases in density of tissues that ar normally radiolucent are frequently due to calcification of soft tis sues. Such calcium deposits are commonly indicative of poorl nourished or necrotic tissue, precipitation due to altered tissue pH or around a nidus, and metaplasia or neoplasia. Other dense minera concrements include renal and cystic calculi and fecal concretions Decreases in the density of soft tissues usually are due to th abnormal presence of air or gas in tissues as in gangrene, subcut emphysema or ileus of the small intestine.

In assessing osseous structures with diminished radiographi density, 2 major causes should be considered: disturbance in min aralization and disturbance of osteoid formation. The former in cludes rickets and related nutritional deficiency states, whereas th latter is osteoporosis and may be due to endocrine disturbances disuse atrophy, protein deficiency, etc.

Increases in bone density may be the result of increased minera deposition within the substance of the bone proper or by periostea proliferation. The pattern of periosteal new bone may be classifie as layer-like, lace-like or spiculated and may be indicative of th cause.

On occasion, productive and destructive changes may occur in th same bone, as in osteomyelitis and neoplasia.

5) Alteration in architecture. To determine the presence of archi tectural changes requires familiarity with normal anatomy and it aberrations. When in doubt about a particular radiologic finding comparison with film of a similar part in another patient is ofter helpful.

6) Alterations in alignment or function. Alignment of bones and joints is usually demonstrable in plain films and dynamic phenomena may be studied by means of fluoroscopy.

Contrast Media: Selective delineation of an organ or body cavity may be accomplished by use of contrast media. Basically there are 2 types of contrast media: (1) negative media such as air, CO_2 and O_2 which outline the structure by increasing blackness on the film, and (2) positive media such as insoluble salts of heavy metals or inorganic iodides which are opaque and appear white on the film.

Negative media are commonly used in pneumocystograms, pneumoperitoneums and pneumocolons. Barium sulfate, a positive medium, is ideal for visualization of all parts of the gastrointestinal tract. The urinary bladder can be defined by introduction of 10% sodium iodide and when used in conjunction with air, the double contrast effect is excellent in defining intraluminal lesions. Numerous commercially prepared media with organic soluble iodides as the base are available for urography, cardioangiography, angiography, etc., and the selection of the medium is left to the discretion of the veterinarian. For detailed instructions on the radiographic technique of contrast studies, the reader is referred to texts on radiology.

FLUOROSCOPY

Fluoroscopy is an excellent means of studying the dynamic phenomena of an organ or part, but it must be used judiciously. Unfortunately the diagnostic units in most veterinary hospitals are not designed for safe operation as fluoroscopes and in such cases the technique should be avoided. For details of equipment standards the National Council on Radiation Protection, Publication No. 36, should be consulted.

The eyes of the fluoroscopist should be dark-adapted for 20 minutes before the examination of the patient, and protective aprons and gloves must be worn. Only persons actively participating in the procedure should be in the room, and if possible the patient should be anesthetized or sedated to expedite the procedure.

The inherent disadvantages and hazards of fluoroscopy have been overcome or markedly reduced by image amplification by means of electronic intensification. The image produced on a fluorescent screen is detected by a light sensitive photocathode and the light pattern is converted to low-energy photoelectrons. By accelerating and focusing these photoelectrons against an output phosphor screen, the image so produced is markedly brighter although reduced in size. By means of a system of lenses and mirrors, the image may be viewed directly by the operator or indirectly on a television monitor. This technique permits the added advantage of permanent recording by means of videotape, cine films or spot films.

RADIATION PROTECTION

While it is possible to use X-rays and radioactive material with safety, many private veterinary establishments are not equipped to provide the necessary protection for the veterinarian, his assistants and clients. There are few diagnostic or portable X-ray units used in veterinary practice capable of delivering a dose required for therapy with safety to the tube and operator. Because of the large amounts of radiation required, it is questionable whether the general practitioner should attempt radiation therapy of neoplastic or even inflammatory lesions in his patients. Since radiation therapy centers, with qualified veterinary radiologists, are becoming established, the general practitioner might well refer patients requiring this form of therapy to such specialists.

According to the recommendation of the National Council on Radiation Protection and Measurements, maximum exposure to X-ray or gamma radiation from external sources for radiation workers is 100 milliroentgens per week. All persons using equipment producing such radiation should wear film-badges routinely and the degree of exposure should be checked regularly. Hands and other parts of the body always should be kept out of the primary beam and leaded gloves and aprons should be worn routinely for protection against stray radiation.

Users of ionizing radiation are referred to the National Council on Radiation Protection, Publication No. 36, "Radiation Protection in Veterinary Medicine" and reports numbered 17, 22, 33, 34 and 35.

ROUTES FOR MEDICATION

Selection of a drug and its route of administration is determined by assessment of several factors. The diagnosis of the disease process and the disease status of the patient will dictate the treatment needed. The species or breed of the patient, its size, temperament, tractability and idiosyncrasies will influence the form, frequency and manner in which the drug is administered. The treatment of an out-patient may vary considerably from that of a hospitalized patient. The ability and willingness of an owner to treat the patient often is the ultimate determinant of a treatment regime. With all factors considered, it is essential that the clinician's decision complement the indications, properties and optimal therapeutic efficacy of the drug selected.

Topical medication applies primarily to the treatment of ocular, otic, dermatologic and nasal disorders. Topical preparations are available in ointments, aqueous solutions, aerosols and powders. The use of aqueous forms requires frequent administration (e.g. every 2 hours);

ointments act over a longer period and should be applied in small amounts at longer intervals. Ocular preparations should be limited to ointments and aqueous solutions. Topical treatment of skin lesions can be frustrating in some species, requiring concurrent use of restraint collars or sedatives. Only thin layers of a medicament should be applied, and it should be gently worked into the lesions. Aqueous solutions and aerosols can be used in the nasal passages; oily preparations are generally contraindicated because of the chance of causing lipid pneumonia. Some propellants are also hazardous. Since absorption of topical medication can occur, the toxic potential of any medicament must be respected.

Oral administration of drugs is a popular method of treatment. Its efficacy is dependent on the condition of the gastrointestinal system, and in some instances the tolerance of the system to the drug administered. Vomiting or diarrhea are obvious reasons for unsuccessful attempts to attain therapeutic drug levels. Coated drug preparations (e.g. enteric-coated sodium chloride) have on occasion passed undissolved in fecal material. A patient that has recently eaten may retain medication in the stomach long enough to diminish optimal therapeutic effect.

Oral preparations are available in tablets, pills, capsules, pastes or liquid mixtures. To insure that a particular drug reaches the lower bowel before it disintegrates, it is often coated with a substance that is resistant to the acid medium of the stomach. Depending upon the situation and the type of patient, administration of a drug may be "easier said than done" (e.g. the owner's inability to treat his cat is a common complaint) and requires patience, ingenuity and persistence to be successful. If the patient is reliably consuming food or water, the drug may be administered in either of these. Palatability must be taken into consideration; animals that chew their food (e.g. cats, monkeys) can detect pills readily. Manual administration of pills or capsules allows visual assurance of drug intake in cats and dogs; forceps may be used in difficult patients. "Balling guns" are used in large animals. Liquid preparations should be given carefully to avoid the complication of aspiration pneumonia. Stomach tubes, passed through the mouth or nostril, may be used in most species; the size of tubing depends upon the age, species, purpose and route selected. Many patients can be drenched with special syringes. A convenient pouch for deposition can be created in the dog by drawing the cheek outward at the outer commissure of the mouth. Fortunate is the clinician whose patient voluntarily drinks its medication.

Parenteral administration of drugs implies injection of drugs into a patient's body. With few exceptions (subconjunctival, intrauterine, rectal) this requires preparation of the skin; hair is clipped or parted and the exposed skin is cleansed and an antiseptic applied. The drug container cap is also sterilized. Particular care is exercised in preparing vials containing modified live virus so as not to destroy immunologic properties. The use of sterile needles and syringes is imperative and is accomplished by autoclaving, boiling or antiseptic soaks; disposable sterile units are very popular. A respect for the anatomic relationships of muscle, nerve and vascular channels, and proper restraint of the patient allows correct injection technique. Before deposition of medication, withdrawal of the syringe plunger is important, regardless of the tissue involved; aspiration of blood into the syringe is acceptable only in IV injections.

Injection therapy is not without its complications and the following are a few of the situations that may result: Sterile as well as bacterial abscesses form occasionally. Anaphylactic or allergic reactions occur with biologics and antibiotics. Extravascular spillage of irritant drugs can lead to skin sloughs. The tonicity of drugs (i.e. isotonic, hypertonic) can be a factor abused in the selection of route of administration. Sciatic palsy has resulted from poor injection technique. Arterial administration, instead of by IV routes, while sometimes useful, may be catastrophic in some situations (e.g. tranquilizers in horses). Pyrogen-contaminated fluid units can cause febrile reactions. Transfusions of incompatible blood types can result in severe systemic reactions.

Intravenous (IV) injection offers several advantages. The rapid availability of a drug, or use of larger volume of solutions, is possible. Irritating drugs or hypertonic drugs can be given with fewer problems. Induction anesthesia is controlled effectively by this route. Generally, medication is given slowly; increased rate of flow is indicated in cases of recent blood loss. When large volumes of a solution, or increased rate of flow, are necessary the patient should be monitored closely, particularly cardiovascular patients. Should restraint of a patient be a problem, or if a patient is being monitored in an intensive care situation, the use of indwelling IV catheters of inert plastic tubing is advantageous.

Subcutaneous (subcut.) and intraperitoneal (IP) injections are often referred to as the "pool routes"; depots of fluid in these areas allow slower but sustained absorption benefits. Should a vascular channel not be accessible, blood transfusions can be given IP. However, a very debilitated patient, or a patient in shock, will not pick up these "pool" fluids. Irritating drugs should not be administered by these routes; if given subcut., such drugs should be administered in small amounts at several sites. Dialysis in uremic patients and cases of intoxication has been done by IP lavage techniques.

Intramuscular (IM) injections benefit from good blood supply and rapid absorption. Drugs should be given in small amounts. Pain and lameness may occur with this route of administration. "Kapture" guns loaded with special syringes containing tranquilizers or paralyzing drugs are available for catching or treating untamed large animals.

Other routes of injection include **intradermal** (TB testing); **intraruminal** via the left flank region in cattle and sheep (antifoaming agents in bloat); and **intramammary** (infectious mastitis of cattle and sheep). **Intrathoracic** injection may be used as in cases of exudative pleurisy of cats where enzymes and antibiotics might be helpful. **Rectal** injection has primarily been limited to suppositories and enemas, although its application to fluid therapy and anesthesia is appreciated. **Epidural** injection of local anesthesia is a common technique in obstetrical procedures in cattle, and has been used in other species. **Implantation** is a form of subcut. injection whereby repository pellets of certain substances are slowly absorbed over a given period (e.g. stilbestrol in feeder cattle, desoxycorticosterone acetate in dogs with hypoadrenocorticalism). **Inhalation** administration is practiced with gas anesthetics, nebulization therapy and oxygen therapy (*see* OXYGEN THERAPY, below).

Administration of gases is done by use of masks, specially adapted cages or containers, and endotracheal tubes. Although induction anesthesia can be accomplished with masks or closed containers, the more popular method is to anesthetize the patient with IV administration of an ultrashort-acting anesthetic and then intubate the trachea; the method chosen obviously depends on the species dealt with (e.g. rat, dog, horse). Maintenance anesthesia can be administered by a gas anesthetic machine or a drop method into a cone or mask.

Nebulization therapy is finding more application in veterinary medicine, particularly in situations where oxygen is being given. The procedure can be as simple as adding certain volatile substances to hot water (tincture of benzoin or oil of eucalyptus); the resulting steam carries these vaporized substances into the treatment environment. Certain drugs, such as ephedrine, epinephrine and penicillin can be directly atomized into an oxygen supply line. Sophisticated equipment uses compressed air or oxygen to deliver antifoaming agents (e.g. ethyl alcohol) to patients with pulmonary edema, and detergent materials (Tergemist or Mucomist) to patients with bronchial exudates.

OXYGEN THERAPY (SM. AN.)

Oxygen therapy is a supportive measure rather than a specific treatment. It is designed to prevent **hypoxia** or to limit it so that serious or perhaps irreparable damage does not develop before treatment has become effective. Oxygen therapy bolsters the patient and acts as an adjunct to other treatments in such conditions as pneumonia and heart disease. When hypoxia occurs the inhalation of oxygen-enriched atmospheric air enables blood to absorb and transport increased quantities of oxygen.

Pathologic Physiology of Hypoxia: (1) Decreased arterial PO_2 **(anoxemic anoxia).** This could result from any of: (a) decreased inspired oxygen; (b) uneven distribution of alveolar ventilation-capillary blood flow; (c) right to left vascular shunts. These shunts allow blood to bypass ventilated alveoli so that venous blood mixes with oxygenated blood returning from the lung causing a decrease in arterial PO_2.

(2) Decreased capacity of the blood for oxygen **(anemic anoxia).** Anemia, carbon monoxide inhalation, or abnormal types of hemoglobin could produce this condition.

(3) Reduced blood flow to the tissues **(stagnation anoxia).** A deficiency in circulation is the primary cause of this condition.

(4) Inhibition of the cytochromes of the cell **(histotoxic anoxia).** This is caused by certain chemicals such as cyanide and alcohol.

Clinical Signs Indicating the Need for Oxygen: (1) Cyanosis— blueness of the skin and mucous membranes interpreted clinically as an indication of the presence of an abnormal amount of de-oxygenated hemoglobin in the blood. (2) Dyspnea—difficult breathing, which is generally related to increased mechanical effort. (3) Hyperventilation—rapid breathing as seen in an animal suffering from hyperthermia. (4) Hypoventilation—very slow breathing as seen in an animal in severe shock.

Diseases and conditions of the pulmonary and cardiovascular system in which oxygen therapy is indicated:

(1) Those causing decreased arterial PO_2: (a) airway obstructions—from tumors, trauma, infection, foreign bodies and deformities of the airway, (b) pulmonary edema—from left heart failure, acute smoke inhalation, or electrocution, (c) pneumothorax—from a chest wound or fractured ribs reducing the negative pressure in the pleural space, (d) diaphragmatic hernia—decreases the efficiency of the diaphragm, (e) feline bronchial asthma, (f) atelectasis, consolidation and neoplasms supplied by pulmonary circulation resulting in right-to-left vascular shunts, (g) pulmonary embolus.

(2) Those diseases and conditions causing a decreased affinity of the blood for oxygen: (a) anemia—from a decrease in the number of red blood cells, the amount of hemoglobin perired blood cell, chronic liver disease and iron deficiency, (b) carbon monoxide inhalation—carbon monoxide binds with hemoglobin with more affinity than oxygen, (c) hyperphosphatemia caused by chronic renal failure and the physiologic anemia of the young.

(3) Those conditions and diseases caused by a reduced blood flow to the tissues: (a) any type of shock; peripheral circulatory failure is common to all types, (b) acute heart failure, (c) chronic heart failure.

Equipment Used in Oxygen Therapy: The basic oxygen therapy unit consists of a tank (cylinder), a regulator and a length of tube. To this basic unit can be attached any number of appliances, some fairly simple, some extremely complicated. So many methods and so much equipment have been developed exclusively for veterinary use that almost any required oxygen concentration can be obtained. Information about the various types of standard oxygen equipment available is best obtained from a reliable commercial medical supply house. Oxygen is available in high-pressure cylinders of various sizes. A pressure-reducing valve must be attached to the cylinder valve outlet before such cylinders can be safely used.

Cautions: (1) Although oxygen itself is not explosive it strongly supports combustion. Protection from fire depends on keeping all hazards, such as cigarettes, open flames, electric connections or heating pads away from any concentration of oxygen. (2) Oxygen is explosive in combination with certain other substances such as cyclopropane and oil. Therefore valves or any other threads or equipment through which oxygen is to be passed should not be oiled. (3) Oxygen cylinders contain the gas under high pressure and therefore must be handled with particular care. Obsolete or makeshift regulators should not be used. When a new cylinder is opened, pressure should be released gradually and the valve pointed, as a gun would be, away from persons or animals.

Oxygen Administration: Regardless of the need for oxygen, administration is carried out in a similar way for all conditions. In most cases the administration of 30 to 40% oxygen is more than adequate to treat cases of hypoxia correctable by oxygen therapy. Higher concentrations may be needed for severe circulatory failure. There are 4 basic ways of administering oxygen.

(1) Intratracheal—Insertion of a 14- or 16-gauge plastic catheter percutaneously into the trachea in the ventral midcervical area and affixing this to the neck with tape is a very satisfactory method of administering oxygen. Oxygen should be administered at the rate of 0.5 to 3.0 L/min depending on size of animal and respiratory rate. If oxygen is to be administered longer than 4 hours it must be humidified (by bubbling the oxygen through water) so as not to damage the cilia and dry the mucous membranes of the respiratory tract.

(2) Oxygen Cages—These specially designed cages consist of a sealed compartment, carbon dioxide absorber, humidifier, thermostat and oxygen analyzer. (A pediatric incubator can be used for small dogs and cats.)

(3) Mask—A mask should only be used for initial emergency treatment. The mask is inefficient and requires high oxygen flows.

(4) Nasal Catheters—A rubber catheter coated with an anesthetic ointment and premeasured can be placed in the nasopharynx and then taped into place. An oxygen flow rate of 2 to 4 L/min is needed.

ROUTINE IMMUNOLOGIC PROCEDURES

Vaccination is an important adjunct in the control of many livestock diseases, but the immunity is relative and may be overcome by massive exposure, by moderate contact with a highly virulent strain of the infecting agent or by stress, such as poor environmental conditions. Vaccination should not be considered a panacea in disease control and it should be supplemented with sanitary and management measures designed to prevent the introduction and spread of infection.

When an effective immunizing agent is injected, the tissues react to form immune bodies against the agent. This reaction may be accompanied by signs of distress, and these signs may be exaggerated if the animal is not in a state of good health when vaccinated. If a live vaccine is employed in an unhealthy animal, it may actually produce the disease it was intended to prevent.

Effective active immunization can be accomplished only by vaccines that are high in specific antigen content, or in the case of passive immunization, serum rich in antibody. Improved methods for virus culture have resulted in vaccines that contain a high concentration of antigen. Newer methods of attenuation, particularly by passage through unnatural hosts or tissue culture have further improved the viral vaccines. Employing heterotypic viruses as vaccines has provided cross-protection in some cases without exposing the patient to the actual causal agent.

The following is a description of the various biologics used routinely to immunize livestock including poultry:

Vaccines: In common usage, the term vaccine has come to mean all types of biologic agents used to produce active immunity.

Toxoids: Toxoids are prepared from potent toxin which is detoxified with formalin and the active antigenic fraction precipitated with alum and resuspended in isotonic salt solution. It has the antigenic but not the poisonous properties of the toxin.

Bacterins: These are bacterial suspensions inactivated by physical and chemical means. A formalized whole culture of bacteria is called anaculture. These agents will not produce disease, but their immunizing power usually is lower than that of living agents. The maximum duration of the immunity ordinarily is not more than 12 months.

Live bacterial suspensions: These produce a more solid and lasting immunity than the bacterins. They may, however, cause the disease and should be given either in the form of attenuated strains or at an age when the effects would be the least harmful. Their effectiveness is dependent on the number of viable organisms in the suspension. Careless handling, such as failure to keep under refrigeration and permitting contamination, lowers the viable count and results in ineffective vaccination. Brucellosis vaccine Strain 19 is an example of an attenuated live bacterial suspension.

Spore vaccines: Against anthrax, suspensions of spores are used, the virulence of which has been lowered by cultivation at a higher than optimal temperature. The culture is allowed to sporulate, the cells washed from the media and the resultant suspension heated to destroy vegetative forms. Such a vaccine provides a more solid immunity than the bacterin, but is only good for a year. Because it is living, this vaccine should be used only in areas where anthrax is endemic.

Live unmodified viruses: These confer, if properly handled, an effective and lasting immunity. They must be used with caution and given with antiserum if the virus is one that may cause an acute fatal disease. Otherwise, they may be given at an age when they cause only a mild form of the disease from which animals or birds recover prior to going into production. This type of immunization is called premunizing and the result premunition. Fowl pox vaccine is an example.

Modified viruses: Such viruses are modified by serial passage through unnatural hosts or tissue culture. During these passages, the virus loses virulence for the natural host and becomes adapted to growth on the new host. Although losing virulence, the virus retains its antigenic properties and acts as a vaccine. These are effective and produce lasting and solid immunity. Infectious bovine rhinotracheitis modified virus is a vaccine of this type, as are the viruses that have been adapted to grow in the embryonated egg and are used in the living state.

Inactivated viruses: These have been inactivated by chemicals, usually formalin, phenol, or chloroform. Their effectiveness depends on the quantity of antigen present. Most are grown in the embryonating egg and are rich in antigen. The immunity produced is strong in most instances, but vaccination should be repeated annually. In some cases, 2 injections are recommended with a 2 week interval.

Antisera: These are hyperimmune sera originating from a variety of sources depending on the specific antigen. Some are homologous because the antigen is active in only one species. When other than homologous serum is used, anaphylactic reactions may occur. Included in this group are the antitoxins. Immunity is present immediately following the administration of an antiserum but is of brief duration, approximately 2 weeks. Antisera are used prophylactically and therapeutically in certain viral and bacterial diseases.

HANDLING VACCINES

Biologics produced under license are free from contaminants. Care should be taken to maintain that condition. Containers with multiple doses should be discarded when partially used unless they are opened in an aseptic manner and stored under refrigeration. When lyophilized products are reconstituted with diluent, they should be used immediately or they will deteriorate rapidly. Vaccines have varying expiration dates, depending on the particular product. They should not be used beyond the stated time. This date is based on holding the vaccine under optimum conditions, such as keeping it in a cool place, or preferably refrigerated. Vaccines that are outdated or improperly stored have lost part of their antigenic properties and are ineffective as immunizing agents. Empty live-virus containers should be burned or immersed in strong disinfectant. Carelessly discarded virus bottles can result in outbreaks of disease.

The degree of sanitation practiced during vaccination varies with the extent of the operation. It varies from the vaccination of a single dog where complete asepsis is possible, to the vaccination of a thousand or more head of cattle passing through a chute in a dusty corral. In the latter operation, cleanliness can be obtained without sacrificing efficiency. A liberal supply of disposable needles is advisable. Disease can be transmitted in mass vaccinations when the same needle is used to vaccinate numerous animals.

Biologics should be administered in accordance with the producer's directions; some are given intradermally, others subcut. or IM. In most instances, the material is inoculated in one site. Where the amount is large, as in the case of antiserum in large animals, it is advisable to inject the material in several sites.

Maximum active immunity should not be considered to be established until at least 10 days following vaccination. It is not the purpose of an active immunizing agent to protect an animal that is inoculated while in the incubation stage of a disease. Antiserum should be administered simultaneously with the vaccine if the individual has been recently exposed to the etiologic agent. In some cases such simultaneous administration may interfere with long-term immunity and revaccination should be performed.

When live, unmodified, fully virulent viruses are used, it should be remembered that the vaccinated animal may become a carrier and shed the virus for varying periods. This means that susceptible stock should not have contact with vaccinates until the period of elimination has passed. This varies with each virus.

(Text continues on page 1506.)

FISH

Disease	*Agent*	*Procedure*
1. Enteric redmouth	*Yersinia ruckerii* bacterin	Mass immunize juvenile trout one time.
2. Vibriosis	*Vibrio anguillarum* bacterin	Mass immunize salmon or trout before exposure of fish to agent in saltwater.

CATTLE

1. Anaplasmosis (*Anaplasma marginale, A. centrale*)	Virulent blood that contains the organism (not permitted in the U.S.A.)	Give to calves less than 1 year old during winter months—Premunition.
(*Anaplasma marginale*)	Vaccine, inactivated	Give 2 injections, 4 to 19 weeks apart, with last dose preceding vector season by at least 2 weeks. A booster injection should be given the following year.
2. Anthrax (*Bacillus anthracis*)	Spore vaccine, attenuated	Used each spring where anthrax is endemic.
	Avirulent vaccine	Used each spring where anthrax is endemic.
	Anaculture	Used each spring in areas where the disease is not endemic, but may occur.
3. Blackleg (*Clostridium chauvoei*)	Anaculture	Used on animals 6 to 12 months of age.
4. Botulism (*Clostridium botulinum*)	Toxoid (Types C & D)	Used 2 weeks before turning cattle on pasture in areas where the disease is prevalent.
5. Brucellosis (*Brucella abortus*)	Strain-19 vaccine, lyophilized	Administer to calves at 3 to 8 months of age and adults in infected herds when approved by regulatory agencies.
6. Contagious pleuropneumonia (*Mycoplasma mycoides*)	Vaccine, chick embryo-adapted	Administer to young cattle in infected areas.
7. Dysentery (*Clostridium* (*perfringens*)	Anaculture (Types B & C)	Used to immunize dams before calves are born. Also used to induce active immunity in calves after birth.
	Antiserum (Types B, C & D)	Used for immediate protection of newborn calves.
8. Black disease (*Clostridium novyi* [*oedematiens*], *Cl. sordelli*)	Anaculture	Administer in early spring. Yearly booster doses recommended in problem areas.

CATTLE (*Continued*)

Disease	Agent	Procedure
9. Foot-and-mouth disease (Virus)	Tissue culture vaccine, formalin-treated	Used only in areas where FMD is present.
10. Infectious bovine rhinotracheitis (IBR-IPV virus)	Tissue culture vaccine, modified	Produces active immunity for about 12 months.
	Vaccine, inactivated bovine tissue culture	Two injections at a 14-day interval. Can be used on pregnant cows.
11. Bacillary hemoglobinuria (*Clostridium haemolyticum*)	Anaculture	Protects for a full pasture season.
12. Leptospirosis (*Leptospira pomona, L. canicola, L. hardjo, L. grippotyphosa* and *L. icterohaemorrhagiae*)	Anaculture or chick embryo vaccine, inactivated	Protects for 6 to 12 months.
13. Malignant edema (*Clostridium septicum*)	Anaculture	Usually produces life-long immunity.
14. Pasteurellosis (*Pasteurella multocida*)	Bacterin	Administer 10 to 14 days before animal is to be subjected to a stress.
15. Parainfluenza 3, SF-4 Strain	Vaccine, inactivated virus	Administer 2 doses at least 3 weeks apart prior to stress.
TELC Strain	Intranasal vaccine, porcine tissue origin	Spray nasal cavity 3 weeks prior to stress.
	Antiserum	Used to produce immediate passive immunity.
16. Piroplasmosis (*Babesia bigemina*)	Infected ticks	Place 1 or 2 on calf several weeks before turning out on pasture.
17. Rinderpest (Virus)	Goat-cell culture rabbit measles or egg adapted vaccine or measles vaccine	Protects up to 1 year.
	Antiserum	Produces immediate immunity.
18. Salmonellosis (*Salmonella dublin*)	Bacterin, formalized and alum-precipitated	Administer to cow to protect newborn calf or to the calf.
19. Papillomas (warts) (Virus)	Bovine tissue vaccine	Produces only fair immunity.
20. Bovine virus diarrhea (Mucosal disease) (Virus)	Vaccine, modified, tissue culture origin	Long-term immunity.
21. Staphylococcal mastitis (*S. aureus*)	Toxoid	Administer prior to calving. Protection is questionable.

CATTLE (*Continued*)

Disease	Agent	Procedure
22. Campylobacteriosis (*Campylobacter fetus*)	Bacterin	Administer 2 injections at least 2 weeks apart prior to breeding season.
23. Rabies (Virus)	Modified live virus, porcine tissue culture origin	Can be used in 6 species (dog, cat, horse, cattle, sheep and goat). Long-term immunity.
24. Lungworms (*Dictyocaulus viviparus*)	Irradiated larvae	Administer irradiated larvae twice, with a 6-week interval.
25. Calf scours (Reo-like and coronavirus)	Vaccine modified	Administer orally to calves at birth. Protects during susceptible age.

HORSES

Disease	Agent	Procedure
1. African horse sickness (Virus)	Mouse brain-adapted vaccine	Annual vaccination.
2. Equine encephalomyelitis (Virus)	Chick embryo vaccine, inactivated 1) Eastern 2) Western 3) Mixed	Administer each year in spring using type or types prevalent.
3. Venezuelan equine encephalomyelitis (Virus)	Guinea pig heart-adapted vaccine	Duration of immunity 1 to 3 years.
4. Equine rhinopneumonitis (Equine virus abortion)	Hamster-adapted virus vaccine, equine cell line. All horses 3 mo. of age and older 2 doses IM, 4- to 8-week interval. Pregnant mare should not be vaccinated during the first 2 mo. of pregnancy	Intranasal vaccination during summer and fall of each year — Premunition.
5. Equine influenza	Tissue culture vaccine	Administered to young horses annually before beginning training, or when an epidemic threatens.
6. Malignant edema (*Clostridium septicum*)	(*See* cattle, above)	
7. Strangles (*Streptococcus equi*)	Bacterin, 4- to 5-hour-old culture killed in virulent phase	Administer to foal about 2 weeks before weaning. Be cautious about administering during or immediately following an outbreak.
8. Tetanus (*Clostridium tetani*)	Toxoid	Produces active immunity that can be maintained by yearly booster doses.
	Antitoxin (equine)	Used to produce immediate immunity.

SHEEP

Disease	*Agent*	*Procedure*
1. Anthrax (*Bacillus anthracis*)	(*See* cattle, above)	
2. Black disease (*Clostridium novyi* [*oedematiens*])	Anaculture	Several doses needed to produce solid immunity.
3. Blackleg (*Clostridium chauvoei*)	Anaculture	Vaccinate before turning out to pasture and ewes 3 weeks prior to lambing.
4. Bluetongue (Virus)	Vaccine, chick embryo-adapted	Immunize lambs shortly before weaning and ewes prior to the breeding season.
5. Botulism (*Clostridium botulinum*)	Toxoid (Type C)	Used in areas where the disease is common, before putting animals on pasture.
6. Contagious ecthyma (Virus)	Vaccine, dried scab material.	Vaccinate lambs each spring before pasture season begins.
7. Enterotoxemia (*Clostridium perfringens*)	Anaculture (Type D)	Administer to lambs about 2 weeks before entering feed lot, or to ewes 3 weeks prior to lambing.
8. Enzootic ovine abortion (*Chlamydia* sp.)	Vaccine, oil emulsion of alum-precipitated material from infected fetal membranes	One injection gives adequate protection for 3 pregnancies and possibly for life.
9. Epididymitis (*Brucella ovis*)	*B. abortus* Strain 19 vaccine plus bacterin of formalized *B. ovis* *B. melitensis* (strain Rev 1) if available	Administer to rams at 9 to 12 months of age, or before start of breeding season.
10. Johne's disease (*Mycobacterium paratuberculosis*)	Bacterin, heat-killed suspension in light mineral oil	Lambs are vaccinated subcut. at 6 to 7 months of age with 1 ml of bacterin.
11. Lamb dysentery (*Clostridium perfringens*)	Anaculture (Type B)	Administer to pregnant ewes about 3 weeks prior to lambing.
	Antitoxin	Administer to lambs at birth.
12. Louping ill (Virus)	Vaccine, formalized nerve tissue	Administer to young lambs at weaning time or least 3 weeks prior to the season of active ticks.
13. Malignant edema (*Clostridium septicum*)	(*See* cattle, above)	
14. Pasteurellosis (*Pasteurella multocida*)	(*See* cattle, above)	
15. Rift Valley fever (Virus)	Vaccine, chick embryo-adapted	Administer to nonpregnant ewes.

SHEEP (*Continued*)

Disease	*Agent*	*Procedure*
6. Struck (*Clostridium*) *perfringens*)	Anaculture (Type C)	Administer to lambs at weaning time.
7. Tetanus (*Clostridium*) *tetani*)	(*See* horses, above)	

SWINE

Disease	*Agent*	*Procedure*
1. Hog cholera (Virus)	Vaccine, modified by serial passage in rabbits or tissue culture	Administer with or without serum to produce active immunity.
	Vaccine, inactivated	Used to produce active immunity in swine in areas where disease is not common.
	Antiserum, homologous	Administer at the onset of an outbreak or simultaneously with virus to immunize healthy pigs.
2. Leptospirosis (*Leptospira pomona*)	Bacterin	Protects young swine.
3. Swine erysipelas (*Erysipelothrix rhusiopathiae*)	Vaccine, virulent	Used only in areas where simultaneous method authorized.
	Vaccine, lyophilized	Administer to weanling pigs.
	Bacterin, alum-absorbed, formalized	Administer to weanling pigs.
	Antiserum	Administer at onset of outbreak.
4. Jowl abscesses (Group E *Streptococcus*)	Vaccine, live culture, avirulent (oral vaccine)	Use in healthy swine at least 10 weeks of age. Apply to posterior portion of hard palate and tonsillar area.
5. Transmissible gastroenteritis (Virus)	Vaccine porcine tissue culture IM.	Administer IM to pregnant sows. Two doses with one month interval with lag dose 14 days prior to farrowing.
6. Atrophic rhinitis (Lancefield Group E *Streptococcus*)	Bacterin	Administer to young pigs at 7 and 28 days of age.

FOWL

Disease	*Agent*	*Procedure*
1. Infectious bronchitis (Virus)	Vaccine, chick embryo, lyophilized	Administer to chicks by placing in the drinking water, eye, or nasal passages at 7 to 14 days of age and repeat at 4 to 5 weeks and again at 14 to 16 weeks.
2. Laryngotracheitis (Virus)	Vaccine, chick embryo, or tissue-culture origin	Drop in eye of healthy birds over 6 weeks of age.

FOWL (*Continued*)

Disease	*Agent*	*Procedure*
3. Fowl pox (Virus)	Vaccine, chick embryo, lyophilized	Administer in feather fo licle or skin puncture healthy birds at least month before the sta of egg production.
	Pigeon pox vaccine, chick embryo, lyophilized	Same as fowl pox.
4. Newcastle disease (Virus)	Vaccine, chick embryo	Same as infectious bro chitis.
5. Pasteurellosis (fowl cholera) (*Pasteurella multocida*)	Bacterin	Used to control fowl cho era in birds.
6. *Erysipelothrix* infection	Bacterin, alum-absorbed, formalized	Used especially to vacc nate turkey poults b fore placing on range.
7. Marek's disease	Vaccine, turkey herpesvirus	One day of age. Subcu or IP.
	Live culture	Administer in drinkin water to turkeys.

DOGS

Disease	*Agent*	*Procedure*
1. Canine distemper	Vaccine, chick embryo-modified, lyophilized Vaccine, tissue-culture origin, modified live virus	Pups of unknown immun status should be give a dose of vaccine older than 3 months. younger than 3 month 2 or more doses shoul be administered; th first dose should b given after the pup weaned and the last dos at 12 to 16 weeks of ag Administration of a dos of vaccine at 2-week in tervals more nearly ap proaches the ideal.
	Antiserum and concentrated antiserum	There is increasing evi dence that routine pro phylactic use of agent that will passively im munize against canin distemper in pups ha less merit than multipl doses of attenuated liv virus vaccines. To avoi blocking of active im munization, the use o antiserum or concen trated antiserum fo short-term protection to be discouraged.
		Antiserum or concentrate antiserum is of question able value in the treat ment of dogs with clini cal signs of distemper.

DOGS (*Continued*)

Disease	*Agent*	*Procedure*
2. Infectious canine hepatitis (Virus)	Vaccine, tissue-cultured, modified	Administer to young dogs. (Simultaneous vaccination with modified distemper and infectious canine hepatitis virus is effective.)
3. Rabies (Virus)	*See* p. 280.	

FOXES

1. Canine distemper (Virus)	(*See* dogs, above)	
2. Epizootic fox encephalitis (Infectious canine hepatitis)	(*See* dogs, above)	
	Antiserum	Used to stop outbreaks.

MINK

1. Botulism (*Clostridium botulinum*)	Toxoid (Type C)	Administer to young mink to produce active immunity.
2. Canine distemper (Virus)	(*See* dogs, above)	

CATS

1. Feline panleukopenia (Virus)	Vaccine, formalized tissues of infected cats	Used to immunize healthy kittens.
	Antiserum	Used to protect susceptible kittens.
2. Feline pneumonitis (*Chlamydia psittaci*)	Vaccine, live, modified, egg origin	Vaccinate at 12 to 14 weeks, and every 6 months thereafter.
3. Feline rhinotracheitis and calici virus infection	Vaccines available 1. Modified live virus, feline cell line origin	Innoculate vaccine into nasal passages or one drop into eye and remainder into nasal passages. Vaccinate cats older than 12 weeks of age. Revaccinate annually.
	2. Modified live and killed virus, feline cell line and tissue culture origin.	Administer IM 2 doses 3 or 4 weeks apart if over 12 weeks of age. Revaccinate annually.
4. *Chlamydia* infection	Vaccine, chlamydia chick embryo origin combined with rhinotracheitis-calici vaccine	Inject IM or subcut. at 10 weeks of age and repeat in 3 to 4 weeks. Adult cats require one dose followed by a booster dose in 3 weeks. Revaccinate every 6 months. Do not vaccinate pregnant cats.
5. Rabies (Virus)	*See* RABIES, p. 280.	

FERRETS

Disease	Agent	Procedure
Canine distemper	(*See* dogs, above)	

GUINEA PIGS

Disease	Agent	Procedure
Pseudotuberculosis (*Pasteurella pseudotuberculosis*)	Vaccine, avirulent	Administer to guinea pigs at weaning time.

PASSIVE IMMUNITY IN THE NEWBORN

In certain species, antibodies are transferred to the fetus through the placenta or the yolk sac. In others, such transfer does not occur. The newborn from the latter lack passive immunity. This is compensated for, usually, by high-antibody concentration in the colostrum. Horses, cattle, sheep, goats, pigs and dogs are species in which passive immunity in the newborn is acquired by way of the colostrum. Antibodies from the colostrum are readily absorbed from the intestinal tract of the newborn, in most cases during the first 24 hours of life only. Because it is essential that the newborn animal receive all the passive immunity available to protect it during early life, efforts should be made to provide the necessary colostrum as soon as possible after birth; antibodies are absorbed at a decreasing rate even during the first 24 hours. The newborn animal is subject to infection until the antibodies are absorbed.

COMMON IMMUNIZING AGENTS

The list (p. 1499 *et seq*) includes vaccination procedures commonly carried out on most of the domestic animals in the principal livestock-raising areas of the world. Only those agents and measures are listed which are regarded as producing reliable and effective immunity for specific diseases. Autogenous vaccines and mixed bacterins containing a number of antigens are not included, although both mixed bacterins and autogenous vaccines are known to be effective. Certain of the procedures listed are not practiced in North America because the diseases are unknown or have been eradicated. Nevertheless, they are included in the table for guidance for veterinarians who may find themselves confronted with unusual disease problems in other areas. More detailed instructions regarding each specific agent will be found in the chapter dealing with the disease in question. The directions of the manufacturer, regarding dosage, administration and cautions, should be followed strictly.

RUMEN INOCULATION

Inoculation of rumen contents from a healthy ruminant animal into the rumen of another animal for the purpose of initiating or restoring normal rumen function. The procedure has been used almost exclusively in cattle.

Functions of Rumen Microorganisms: The healthy rumen performs important digestive and nutritional functions because of the presence of enormous numbers of bacteria and ciliated protozoa. These microorganisms collectively produce enzymes capable of digesting cellulose and other plant constituents. They also synthesize many essential amino acids that are made available to the host by the subsequent digestion of the bacteria and protozoa in the abomasum and intestine. In addition, the rumen bacteria synthesize vitamins of the B-group plus vitamin K. Sufficient numbers and balance between species of these microorganisms are, therefore, important for the efficiency of the ruminant animal, and if they are upset by inadequate or abnormal food intake, drugs, poisons, or disease, rumen function is impaired.

Procedure: Rumen inoculum can be obtained at a local abattoir if there is need for a large quantity. For most purposes, however, the inoculum can be taken from a healthy animal by passing a stomach tube and siphoning some of the liquid from the rumen. The administration of approximately 4 gal. (15 L) of lukewarm water will allow removal of greater quantities of rumen juice. One gallon (4 L) of fresh rumen contents usually is sufficient for one inoculation and is given to the recipient animal by stomach tube or drench. To facilitate administration, coarse material can be removed. Fresh rumen material is far superior to frozen or processed products.

Clinical Use: Any disease or condition that alters rumen function is detrimental to the normal flora present and this in turn may delay the return to normal of the convalescent animal. Cattle recovering from any gastrointestinal disorder, or diseases that have required administration of sulfonamides, antibiotics or other drugs may show anorexia due to rumen dysfunction and will benefit from rumen inoculation.

EXAMINATION OF ANIMALS PRIOR TO SALE

This examination is requested of a veterinarian by the prospective buyer of an animal and is welcomed by the honest seller. Occasionally, the seller will request an examination of a limited nature, certifying one or more of the animal's soundness of body, health of udder, stage of pregnancy, semen quality or freedom from evidence of disease as determined by diagnostic tests or clinical examination. The results of these examinations usually are written as certificates and are used to assist in the sale and to serve as a measure of protection to the seller.

When examining an animal for a buyer, however, the examination usually is wider in scope and more complete. Advice is often sought on minor defects or blemishes, conformation, past diseases and injuries to the animal, its recent environment and record as well as precautions to be taken in introducing the animal into the client's herd or flock. The results and findings of all examinations should be recorded and reported accurately, particularly in cases of valuable animals that may be transported long distances. Then, if any disagreement should arise between the buyer and seller, the examination record is available and hopefully complete enough to satisfy both parties. The completeness of the examination may vary with the type and value of the animal. In making the examination, several steps should be taken.

History: It is desirable to get the history as completely as possible by questioning the seller, examining his records and even examining the rest of the herd and conditions under which they are quartered. The animal's breed, sex, age and markings should be noted, its registration papers checked and its identity established. Consideration should also be given to the records of the sire and dam of the animal in question; for example, their breeding ability; the possibility of heritable defects in the strain to which each belongs, particularly if the animal is to be used for breeding; and, if they are dead, the cause of their deaths.

Inquiry or examination of records should be made as to whether the animal has had any previous diseases, injuries, or surgical operations and how severe these conditions were. Any previous preventive inoculations should be noted, as well as their type and time of administration.

If the animal to be sold is to be used for breeding purposes, breeding records should be reviewed to determine whether the animal is fertile, relatively fertile, or infertile. Breeding records of the herd from which the animal came should be examined to obtain evidence of diseases likely to affect reproduction. If the animal is an adult breeding female, the service dates should be noted.

The health of the herd of origin and possible contacts with other animals before the sale should, if possible, be determined as a protection to the purchaser. Animals at the time of sale, if so exposed, could be in the incubation period of the disease. If a complete history cannot be obtained, the client should be advised of the possibility of such diseases either being present, or in the incubative stage. Animals may have been given drugs such as tranquilizers, butazolidin or glucocorticoids that could alter the animals' normal state. A suitable withdrawal period of several days or more may be required for the animal to return to its original state.

Clinical Examination: General examination of the animal consists of noting the signalment including the breed, sex, age and color markings. The physical attitude, condition, conformation and temperature should be observed carefully. Conformation is of importance as certain types may predispose the animal to defects or diseases. The gait, especially in horses, should be observed at various speeds for evidence of lameness. The skin and coat should be examined for evidence of alopecia, ringworm, mange and pediculosis. It is also an indication of general health. The temperature should be taken as this may detect a febrile disease in its early or incubative stage. This general examination should be made carefully as suggestive signs of internal diseases or abnormalities often are found at this time, especially diseases of the nervous system, such as "wobbles," chorea, spastic signs and blindness.

Specific Examination: Any abnormalities in pulse rate, nature or type of pulse or heart sounds should be carefully assessed, particularly in the horse used for heavy work. The size and fullness of the external veins are noted. Any edema of dependent portions of the body or ascites is noted and its cause determined. After examining the animal at rest, it should be exercised and the pulse and heart checked again. This is particularly important with horses. The external lymph nodes are then palpated.

The respiratory system is examined by noting the respiratory rate at rest and after work, as well as by auscultation of the lungs for evidence of bronchitis, heaves or chronic pneumonia. The trachea should be pinched near the larynx to see if a cough can be elicited. Horses may have to be worked vigorously to bring out any evidence of heaves or roaring. In cases of difficult breathing, the nasal passages and sinuses may be examined for evidence of obstruction. Sneezing and bleeding from the nose is common in swine with atrophic rhinitis. Atrophy of the turbinates with distortion of the face and obstruction of the nasolacrimal duct occurs in the more advanced cases. Evidence of any abnormal nasal discharge should be noted and its cause ascertained if possible. External palpation of the pharynx, larynx and trachea may reveal defects or abnormalities.

In examining the digestive system, the animal should be observed while eating and drinking to note abnormalities in appetite, chewing, or swallowing. The teeth should be inspected to check for age and the presence of abnormal teeth. The tongue and mouth should be examined at the same time and the size of the salivary glands noted. In the ruminant, the act of rumination should be observed. Auscultation of the abdominal cavity will reveal the degree of peristalsis of the large and small intestine and rumen activity. The consistency, color and odor of the feces should be observed.

Examination of the urinary system in large animals may be done by rectal examination, palpating the kidneys, ureters and bladder. The urine should be examined for color and evidence of any abnormality, such as the presence of blood, pus, or excessive albumin. If possible, the animal should be observed urinating.

In large animals to be used for breeding, the genital system in the female should be carefully checked by external, vaginal and rectal examination. If the female is not pregnant, abnormalities or infections of the vulva, vagina, cervix, uterus, oviducts and ovaries that might prevent conception should be noted. The mammary glands and teats must be examined and palpated for evidence of disease or defects. If the animal is lactating, the milk should be examined. In young animals, the number and distribution of mammae and teats should be noted. If the female is pregnant, rectal findings should correlate with the breeding history. In the male, the external genital organs, penis, sheath, testicles and epididymides should be inspected and palpated for abnormalities. Rectal examination of the male accessory sex glands and vasa deferentia should be made. (*See* BREEDING SOUNDNESS EXAMINATION IN THE MALE, p. 794.) The male should be observed in the act of copulating to note his libido and ability to mate. Examination of a semen sample is often required (q.v., p. 802).

The sensory organs, especially the eyes, should be carefully examined. Visual examination employing a flashlight in a dark stall or room is necessary to detect certain diseases of the eye that interfere with vision. The ophthalmoscope is useful to locate certain kinds of eye lesions. (*See* VETERINARY OPHTHALMOLOGY, p. 216). The ears should be examined and impairment or lack of hearing noted.

In the horse particularly, further careful examination at various gaits, and while backing and turning, is required to determine abnormalities in coordination and postural reflexes, or lamenesses. Evidence of laminitis or soreness should be noted. The limbs, feet and hoofs or claws should be carefully inspected for any unsoundness or blemish. The severity and possible future importance of such abnormalities should be assessed.

Special or Diagnostic Tests: Certain special diagnostic tests are routinely performed at the time of sale; others may be desired by the buyer. Tests may be indicated by the findings of the clinical examination. If the animal is to be shipped into another state or country after purchase, the required tests or inoculations have either to be performed before the sale or the sale may be subject to the satisfactory passing of these tests by the animals. The regulations of the state or country to which the animal is to be sent must, therefore, be thoroughly understood.

Commonly, serologic tests are carried out for brucellosis and leptospirosis in cattle and swine and equine infectious anemia in horses. Diagnostic inoculations also are usually made to test for the presence of certain diseases, such as tuberculosis and Johne's disease. Fecal examinations may be made for the presence of parasites.

Urine examinations to indicate the presence of blood, albumin, sugar or low specific gravity may be desirable.

Cultural tests may be conducted on samples of milk to determine the presence and type of infection in the udder, on urine specimens for evidence of urinary infection, on cervical or vaginal swabs from mares or cows for the presence of pathogenic organisms causing genital diseases, such as streptococcal and *Klebsiella* infections in mares, and campylobacteriosis or trichomoniasis in cows. For the latter infections in bulls, culturing of the semen or preputial samples, or even test-mating with virgin heifers, may be indicated.

In certain abnormalities or diseases of the circulatory system, hemograms and blood chemistry tests may be employed. In lameness and lesions of the limb, roentgenographs or nerve blocks may be desirable.

It must be emphasized that these special tests merely supplement the information obtained from the history and physical examination. Rarely do they provide data for an absolute statement of freedom from disease. The limitations of each procedure should, therefore, be drawn to the client's attention, so that there is no misunderstanding later. Certificates should be written with the greatest care and in such a fashion that they cannot be misinterpreted and should contain such qualifications as may be necessary.

The exhaustiveness of the examination is usually determined by the wishes of the client and the value of the animal in question. Even after the most elaborate examination and testing, however, the client is well advised to isolate his newly purchased animal from the rest of his stock for a period of 3 weeks.

MEAT INSPECTION

Meat inspection is conducted for the purpose of protecting consumers of meat from the infectious, toxic and physical health hazards that may originate in animals, the environment or in other humans and may be transmitted through meat; and from adulterated or mislabeled meat or meat products. Inspection activities are divided into antemortem, postmortem and processing inspection.

Antemortem Inspection

Antemortem inspection is conducted at the abattoir on the day of slaughter. Its purpose is to detect and condemn animals that are unfit for slaughter and to detect signs or lesions of diuease that may not be apparent after slaughter, such as rabies, listeriosis and heavy metal poisoning. Animals found at antemortem to show signs or lesions of localized conditions or conditions that do not warrant immediate condemnation can be identified as "suspects" so that they can be slaughtered separately and the antemortem data can be considered at the time of postmortem inspection. A third option is to identify and retain certain animals to enable treatment of disease or to allow metabolic depletion of toxic residues.

Animals to be inspected must be in properly lighted pens where they can be observed at rest and in motion. Facilities for segregating abnormal animals, for restraining segregated abnormal animals, for restraining segregated animals for closer examination and for applying identification to "suspects" must be available.

Postmortem Inspection

Postmortem inspection is conducted immediately after slaughter and evisceration to enable detection and evaluation of all signs and lesions relevant to the suitability of the animal for food. It requires the systematic examination of all parts of the carcass, and control of dressing procedures and environmental sanitation to prevent contamination of edible parts. Assurance must also be provided that condemned carcasses and parts are disposed of in a manner that precludes a human or animal health hazard.

The routine postmortem examination should consist of at least the following procedures:

Cattle: Heads—(1) Incise and examine left and right mandibular, parotid, atlantal, and suprapharyngeal lymph nodes. (2) Examine 2 incised layers of both masseter muscles. (3) Examine and palpate tongue. **Viscera**—(1) Examine mesenteric lymph nodes and abdominal viscera. (2) Examine and palpate ruminoreticular junction. (3) Examine esophagus and spleen. (4) Incise and examine anterior, middle and posterior mediastinal and right and left bronchial lymph nodes. (5) Examine and palpate costal and ventral surfaces of the lungs. (6) Incise heart from base to apex through interventricular septum, and examine and cut inner and outer surfaces. (7) Incise and examine hepatic (portal) lymph nodes. (8) Open bile duct in both directions and observe contents. (9) Examine and palpate ventral and dorsal surfaces and renal impression of the liver. **Carcass**—(1) Examine exposed internal and external surfaces. (2) Palpate superficial inguinal or supramammary, and internal iliac lymph nodes. (3) Examine and palpate kidneys and diaphragm.

Calves and Veal: Heads—(1) Incise and examine suprapharyngeal lymph nodes. **Viscera**—(1) Examine and palpate lungs, bronchial and mediastinal lymph nodes and heart. (2) Examine spleen. (3) Examine and palpate dorsal and ventral surfaces of the liver, and palpate portal lymph nodes. (4) Examine abdominal viscera. **Carcass**—(1) Examine exposed inner and outer surfaces. (2) Palpate internal iliac lymph nodes and kidneys.

Sheep and Goats: Viscera—(1) Examine abdominal viscera, esophagus, mesenteric lymph nodes, omental fat and spleen. (2) Examine bile duct and content and express gall bladder. (3) Examine and palpate liver, and costal and ventral surfaces of lungs. (4) Palpate bronchial and mediastinal lymph nodes. (5) Examine and palpate heart. **Carcass and Head**—(1) Examine outer surfaces and body cavities. (2) Examine and palpate kidneys. (3) Palpate prefemoral, superficial inguinal or supramammary, and popliteal lymph nodes. (4) Palpate back and sides of carcass. (5) Palpate prescapular lymph nodes. (6) Examine neck, shoulders and head. (7) Incise lymph nodes when required to rule out caseous lymphadenitis.

Swine: Heads—(1) Examine head and cervical muscles. (2) Incise left and right mandibular lymph nodes. **Viscera**—(1) Examine and palpate spleen and mesenteric lymph nodes. (2) Palpate portal lymph nodes. (3) Examine dorsal and ventral surfaces of the liver. (4) Palpate right and left bronchial and mediastinal lymph nodes. (5) Examine and palpate dorsal and ventral surfaces of the lungs. (6) Examine and palpate heart. **Carcass**—(1) Examine external surface, cut surfaces and body cavities. (2) Examine and palpate kidneys.

Horses: Heads—(1) Examine surfaces. (2) Palpate and incise, as required, mandibular, pharyngeal, and parotid lymph nodes, guttural pouches and tongue. **Viscera**—(1) Examine and palpate lungs, bronchial and mediastinal lymph nodes (incise when abnormal). (2) Examine and palpate spleen, liver and portal lymph nodes. (3) Open hepatic duct. (4) Examine remaining viscera. **Carcass**—Inspect as for cattle. In addition examine and incise when necessary: (1) inner abdominal walls for encysted parasites, (2) spinous process of thoracic vertebrae, supraspinous bursa and first 2 cervical vertebrae for fistulous conditions, (3) axillary and subscapular spaces of white and gray horses for melanosis.

Poultry: (1) Examine external surfaces for dressing defects, bruises or disease lesions. (2) Palpate tibia to detect bone diseases. (3) Examine inner surfaces, lungs and kidneys in place. (4) Examine viscera and palpate liver, heart and spleen. Crush the spleens of mature poultry.

Dispositions—General

Carcasses should be disposed of with the following considerations in mind: (1) Carcasses bearing, throughout the tissues, infectious, toxic or physical agents hazardous to human health should be condemned when a specific determination can be made. (2) Carcasses affected by generalized conditions or disease processes, including malignant tumors, that have so altered the normal characteristics of the meat as to cause it to be inedible or adulterated should be condemned. (3) Carcasses or parts affected by a condition so repugnant, solely from an aesthetic point of view, as to be unfit for food should be condemned. (4) Localized conditions that do not affect the wholesomeness of the entire carcass should be removed by trimming to enable the utilization of the remainder of the carcass for food.

Special Considerations

Tuberculosis: The entire carcass should be condemned when: (1) the lesions are generalized; (2) an antemortem fever is associated with an active lesion; (3) the animal is cachexic; (4) the lesion occurs in muscle, intermuscular tissue, bone, joint, abdominal organ (excluding the gastrointestinal tract) or any lymph node that drains muscle, bone, joint or abdominal organs (excluding the gastrointestinal tract) with the exceptions cited hereafter; (5) there are other indications that the lesions are not localized. **Organs or parts should be condemned** when they contain lesions or the corresponding lymph nodes contain lesions. Bovine, ovine and equine carcasses **may be passed for cooking:** (1) when the number, character and extent of the lesions indicate a localized condition, and if the lesions indicate a localized condition, and if the lesions are calcified or encapsulated provided the affected organ or part is condemned; and (2) when cattle that have reacted to the tuberculin test are found to be free of lesions. **Swine bearing lesions** may be passed without restriction when the lesions are localized and confined to one site of infection, such as the cervical lymph nodes, the mediastinal lymph nodes or the mesenteric lymph nodes after condemnation of the affected parts. **Parts of carcasses may be passed for cooking** when the lesions are more numerous or severe than those described in the preceding paragraph, but not so numerous or severe as those described in the section dealing with condemnation, after condemnation of the affected parts.

Abattoir Sanitation

The buildings, equipment and operating procedures should assure the continued wholesomeness and freedom from adulteration of carcasses and meat. Floors, walls and ceilings should be constructed of materials and in a manner that allows sanitary operations and thorough cleaning. An ample supply of hot and cold water and cleaning materials should be conveniently available for slaughtering, cleaning and personal hygiene. Water at 180°F (82°C) should be available for sterilizing tools and equipment after cleaning. Equipment, knives and other utensils that have contacted diseased carcasses should be cleaned and sterilized before use is resumed. Drainage, with proper trapping and sewage disposal should be adequate to maintain the abattoir in a sanitary condition. Ventilation should ensure that edible product areas are free of obnoxious odors. Flies, rodents and other vermin should be excluded from all departments. Lighting in all departments should be maintained at a level adequate for cleaning and inspection. Equipment should be of such material and so constructed as to be readily and thoroughly cleaned and should be properly maintained. Clean containers for edible and inedible materials should be provided at convenient locations. Tables or racks should be provided for heads. Clean garments should be worn by employees.

DETECTION OF UNWHOLESOME MEAT

Meat for human consumption should be prepared from healthy animals that have died through bleeding. Animals bearing infectious, toxic or physical agents in their tissues that may be hazardous to human health or are otherwise unhealthy should not be used for food. Fitness for food must be determined conclusively by a comprehensive evaluation that includes organoleptic, histologic, microbiologic, chemical and toxicologic examinations.

Meat should be examined, if possible, in good daylight with the help of a binocular loupe or a dissecting microscope. A large microscope lamp may be useful for illumination. Foreign objects on the surface, or visible within the tissue, can be collected for further examination. Items such as feathers, hair, fibers, parasites or insect larvae may provide valuable data on the species, origin and handling of the meat.

Texture, color and odor should be noted. Meat should be firm and cut surfaces should be glossy. Gray or green discolorations may indicate bacterial action. A dark-red color may result from the gravitation of blood after death in animals that have not died by bleeding. A stable bright-red color in old meat is sometimes produced by the addition of sulfite. Rodent urine and substances produced by certain spoilage bacteria will fluoresce under ultraviolet light. Areas of bruising, hemorrhage or inflammation should be readily recognized. Foreign odors from chemicals, urine, fish or other sources may be present. Some of these can be accentuated by boiling or frying the meat.

Histologic examination can often detect characteristic pathologic changes caused by infectious or toxic agents, or the agents themselves. Adulteration of meat with materials such as organ tissue, skin, ground bone and vegetable matter can also be so noted.

Microbiologic examination of meats for spoilage organisms or those capable of causing infectious or toxic illness in the consumer, and serologic examination to determine species should be done by recognized methods. The *Microbiology Laboratory Guidebook*, available from the Meat and Poultry Inspection Program, U.S. Department of Agriculture, Washington, D.C. 20250, is a useful source.

Chemical and toxicologic examinations can be made to detect postmortem change and the presence of adulterative or toxic substances. Recognized testing procedures should be employed. The materials and methods required for specific procedures are available from the Chemistry Division, Science, Food Safety and Quality Service, U.S. Department of Agriculture, Washington, D.C. 20250.

COLLECTION AND SUBMISSION OF SPECIMENS FOR HISTOPATHOLOGIC EXAMINATION

Microscopic examination of routinely prepared histologic sections of tissues from diseased animals is a valuable diagnostic aid. The cellular changes produced in diseased tissues are often characteristic for a specific disease or group of diseases that can be recognized by an experienced veterinary pathologist. The use of this relatively rapid and inexpensive diagnostic technique can often result in substantial savings in time, money and animal life. Every clinician should investigate the existence, location and capacity of facilities for histopathologic diagnosis available to him and make use of this service.

Tissues for histopathologic examination should be collected as soon as possible after death to minimize the effect of autolysis. They should *never be frozen* prior to fixation. Specimens of the various organs should be cut less than one centimeter thick (preferably 7 mm.) and should be placed immediately into at least 10 times their volume of phosphate-buffered 10% formalin solution for fixation. The thin slices or cubes will insure that the fixative will penetrate adequately. The tissues should be allowed to remain in this fixative, with some agitation, for at least 24 hours. Specimens should always be shipped in solid containers and packed in such a way to prevent breakage and spillage during shipment.

For the brain, where the whole organ is often required, the following procedure is recommended. The brain is placed into concentrated formalin (formaldehyde 40%—in which it will float) and water added slowly with mixing until the brain just sinks below the surface but not to the bottom. To allow faster fixation a longitudinal incision is made in the cerebrum to expose the lateral ventricles. It is allowed to remain in this solution for 24 hours or longer after which it may be removed and placed in a solid container in 10% formalin and mailed (suitably packed), or placed into 10% formalin until such time that processing is desired. Often the brain is halved longitudinally and one-half sent unfixed (fresh), properly refrigerated, for microbiologic tests.

The specimen taken for examination should be representative of he lesion and, if possible, should include some of the apparently ormal surrounding tissue. Specimens of all organs should be sent. f the animal exhibited CNS signs, it is imperative to include the rain and portions of the spinal cord. The mucosal surface of specinens from the gastrointestinal track should be exposed before fixaion. Autolytic changes occur very rapidly in the mucosa of the astrointestinal tract. Ideally, sections of stomach and gut should be ixed within 1 to 2 minutes after death.

A covering letter with a detailed case history should be sent sepaately with a copy accompanying the specimens to permit tracing of lelayed or lost samples and to assist the pathologist in arriving at a liagnosis. This report should identify the animal's species, breed including morbidity and mortality), sex, age and owner; describe he clinical signs, gross appearance, size and location of the lesion r lesions; indicate whether the condition had been previously reated and if so, what type of treatment was given and the time of ecurrence.

It is always wise to freeze and hold portions of organ, so that urther tests (virology, bacteriology, toxicology, etc.) may be carried ut pending the results of the histopathologic examination. When ubmitting formalized tissues to the laboratory, indicate whether rozen tissues are being held.

Tissues that are badly autolyzed at the time of necropsy are eldom of value for histopathologic examination.

COLLECTION AND SUBMISSION OF SPECIMENS FOR TOXICOLOGIC EXAMINATION

To diagnose a suspected poisoning in an unexpected death the ppropriate specimens must be submitted. Attention should be iven to a thorough history, signs, treatment, postmortem lesions, ircumstances involved, etc. If a known toxic substance is suspected r probable it should be mentioned so that "tests for all poisons" not e requested. If death losses are large, potential economic loss hould be indicated. Remember that many infectious diseases can timulate poisonings.

Tissues or fluids for chemical and histopathologic examination hould be as fresh as possible and kept in a refrigerator or preserved hemically. The container for packing and transporting specimens hould be chemically clean and prepared beforehand. Plastic conainers, both bags and jars, are ideal. Jars with metal screw caps hould be avoided, especially when metal poison is suspected. Specimens should be packed individually. Containers must be labeled with all information necessary to identify the specimen, and if mailed must conform to postal regulations.

If legal action is a possibility, all containers for shipment should be sealed in a way that tampering can be detected *or* hand carried to the laboratory and a receipt obtained.

It is best to pack the sample(s) with ice or solid carbon dioxide. A polystyrene refrigerator box, metal can, or stout cardboard box may be used for shipment. Packing must withstand breakage if all the ice melts. With dry ice, it is possible to preserve specimens for 72 hours. Packages containing dry ice must be so labeled on the outside and suitably vented to prevent pressure build-up.

For chemical preservation 95% ethyl alcohol, about 1 ml/gm of sample, is satisfactory. Denatured alcohol should not be used because of the contamination introduced by the denaturant. Formaldehyde is undesirable in many instances as it interferes with many tests. In cases of suspected cyanide poisoning, the liver, muscle and stomach contents should be preserved with a solution of 1% mercuric chloride and refrigerated. Adequate refrigeration is of special importance when submitting clean body fluids (readily obtained from an eye) and material for nitrate or nitrite analysis, since these salts are so rapidly metabolized by microorganisms that only low or insignificant levels may be found upon analysis.

In poisonings where a feed or water is suspected, samples of these and any descriptive feed tag should accompany the tissue specimens. It is especially important that a representative composite sample of the feed be submitted from the lot or shipment involved in the poisoning. In many instances the amount of feed involved allows some of it to be fed to experimental animals in an effort to reproduce the signs and lesions observed in the field cases.

To summarize, in collecting and submitting specimens for toxicologic examination the following directions are useful: 1. Supply adequate information regarding the history, signs, postmortem lesions, environment and economic loss. 2. Collect an adequate sample of the proper tissue, feed or other material. 3. Give careful attention to using chemically clean containers and to proper sealing, labeling and preservation of samples. 4. Handle each case as if the evidence accumulated and the diagnosis made were to be used in court if there is any possibility of legal action.

If there is doubt about proper handling, preservation of the specimens, or other essential procedures a telephone call to the laboratory for instructions is prudent.

DEAD-ANIMAL DISPOSAL AND DISINFECTION OF PREMISES

When animals die on farms, other than by slaughter for food, disposal of the carcass and cleaning of the premises should be carried out in a manner that prevents any infectious or toxic health hazard to domestic or wild animals or man. When animal health laws apply, the procedures required for disposal and disinfection should be followed.

General Precautions: Persons handling carcasses and contaminated materials should be clothed, equipped and supervised to prevent hazards to themselves or further contamination of the premises. The handling and disposition should preclude contamination of soil, air or water. Practices such as saving hides from animals that have died from infectious disease should be avoided.

Disposition: Rendering is a safe, rapid, convenient and economical method of disposition when the service is available and the situation permits. Renderers are usually required to use trucks, equipment and practices that prevent health hazards to animals or man.

When disposition on the farm is necessary, burying is the preferred method. In selecting a site it is well to consider the soil depth and the presence of underground cables, water or gas lines, septic tanks, water wells, etc. The trench should be at least 7 ft wide and 9 ft deep (2.3 × 3 m). At this depth, 14 sq ft (3.7 m^2) of floor space is required for each mature bovine carcass, each 5 mature hogs or each 5 mature sheep. Soil conditions may require a deeper trench. For each additional 3 ft (1 m) in depth the number of animals per 14 sq ft of floor space may be doubled. Contaminated bedding, soil, manure, feed, milk or other materials should be placed in the trench with the carcasses and covered with at least 6 ft (2 m) of soil. The trench should not be packed. Decomposition and gas formation causes cracking, bubbling and the leaking of fluids from a packed trench. The trench area should be mounded and neatly graded.

Burning is difficult and expensive in labor and fuel. It should be used only when conditions such as a high water table, excessive rock or public health considerations prevent burial. In selecting a site one should consider the proximity to buildings, stored materials, overhead cables, underground pipes and prevailing winds that may carry smoke and odors. Burning requires the placing of the carcass on a combustible platform that may include oil, wood, coal, straw, tires, etc. The fire burns better if the platform is at right angles to the wind. The fire should be tended until all material is destroyed to keep it burning and to prevent dissemination of contaminated material by animals or birds.

Combustible material required for each cattle carcass (one cattle carcass equals 5 mature hogs or 5 mature sheep) is as follows: Straw—3 bales per carcass; Heavy timbers—24 cu ft (1 cu m) per carcass; Kindling wood—50 lb (22.5 kg) per carcass; Tires—4 per carcass; Coal—500 lb (225 kg) per carcass. These figures should be used to compute the total amount of a combination of fuel materials required in any specific situation.

To prepare the fire: Stake out the area of the firebed allowing 3 ft (1 m) of length for each cattle carcass; Lay 3 rows of straw or hay bales lengthwise along the line of the firebed; Allow 3 ft (1 m) run per cattle carcass with rows 12 in. (30 cm) apart and 12 in. (30 cm) between bales in a row; Place loose straw between bales; Place large timbers lengthwise on each row; Place remaining timbers across rows with 6 to 12 in. (15 to 30 cm) between timbers; Place old tires and kindling on timbers; Spread loose straw over wood and tires; Spread coal at a rate of 500 lb/yd (225 kg/m) over wood and tires to make a level bed; Place carcasses on the firebed on their backs, alternately head to tail; Place loose straw on carcasses and between carcasses; Pour or spray on liquid fuel (**Caution**—do not use gasoline); Start fire along the full length of the firebed.

Under favorable conditions burning should be complete in 48 hours. Additional fuel may be needed. When fire has died out the ashes should be buried and the area cleaned, graded or plowed and prepared for seeding.

Cleaning and disinfection: Cleaning and disinfection should be appropriate for the suspected agent. For infectious agents cleaning should require that: 1. all manure and litter be removed and buried as previously described; 2. dirt floors be scraped down to clean soil; 3. any material—such as wood—that cannot be thoroughly cleaned be removed and buried or burned; 4. buildings be thoroughly cleaned—ceilings, floors, walls and all other surfaces; 5. all equipment used in material removal—such as manure loaders, shovels, brushes and scrapers—be thoroughly cleaned (A cleaning agent must be used in the water. Trisodium phosphate and sodium carbonate are excellent for the purpose. They are readily available, inexpensive, safe to use and do not interfere with the action of disinfectants. Sodium hydroxide causes the precipitation of colloids, which protects organisms from disinfectants and is not recommended); 6. a final rinse be given to all cleaned facilities and equipment with clean water, and liberal application made of an appropriate disinfectant.

Disinfectants recommended for use against both hydrophilic and lipophilic viruses as well as unknown agents are: (1) phenol, 5%; (2) sodium hypochlorite, 1,200 ppm available chlorine; (3) calcium hypochlorite, 1,200 ppm available chlorine.

Disinfectants recommended for use against lipophilic viruses and against many bacteria, rickettsia and protozoans are: (1) cresylic acid, 4%; (2) sodium orthophenylphenate, 2%.

READY REFERENCE GUIDES

WEIGHTS, MEASURES AND EQUIVALENTS

APOTHECARIES' SYSTEM

Weight		Volume	
1 scruple (℈)	= 20 grains (gr.)	1 fluid dram (ʒ)	= 60 minims (♏)
1 dram (ʒ)	= 60 grains	1 fluid ounce (℥)	= 480 minims
	= 3 scruples		= 8 fluid drams
1 ounce (℥)	= 480 grains	1 pint (pt)*	= 7,680 minims
	= 8 drams		= 16 fluid ounces
1 pound (lb)	= 5,760 grains	1 quart (qt)*	= 2 pints
	= 12 ounces	1 gallon (gal.)*	= 4 quarts
(avoir.)	= 16 ounces		

METRIC SYSTEM

Weight		Volume	
1 microgram (mcg)	= 1,000,000 micro-micrograms	1 milliliter	= 1,000 microliters
1 milligram (mg)	= 1,000 micrograms	1 liter (L)	= 1,000 milliliters
1 gram (gm)	= 1,000 milligrams		
1 kilogram (kg)	= 1,000 grams		

EQUIVALENTS (ALL APPROXIMATE)

WEIGHTS

Metric	Apothecaries'	Metric	Apothecaries'
0.2 mg	= 1/300 grain	65.0 mg	= 1 grain
0.3 mg	= 1/200 grain	0.13 gm	= 2 grains
0.4 mg	= 1/150 grain	0.2 gm	= 3 grains
0.5 mg	= 1/120 grain	0.5 gm	= 7½ grains
0.6 mg	= 1/100 grain	0.3 gm	= 5 grains
1.0 mg	= 1/60 grain	0.7 gm	= 10 grains
3.0 mg	= 1/20 grain	1.0 gm	= 15 grains
6.0 mg	= 1/10 grain	4.0 gm	= 60 grains (1 dram)
10.0 mg	= 1/6 grain	6.0 gm	= 90 grains
15.0 mg	= ¼ grain	10.0 gm	= 2½ drams
25.0 mg	= ⅜ grain	15.0 gm	= 4 drams
30.0 mg	= ½ grain	31.0 gm	= 1 ounce

LIQUID MEASURE

Metric	Apothecaries'	Metric	Apothecaries'
0.06 ml	= 1 minim	30 ml	= 1 fl ounce
0.5 ml	= 8 minims	250 ml	= 8 fl ounces +
1.0 ml	= 15 minims	500 ml	= 1 pint +*
4.0 ml	= 1 fl. dram	1,000 ml (1L)	= 1 quart +*
		3.785L	= 1 gal.

HOUSEHOLD MEASURES

(with approximate equivalents)

20 drops	≃	1 ml
1 teaspoon (tsp.)	=	4 ml = 1 fl dr
1 dessertspoon	=	8 ml = 2 fl dr
1 tablespoon (tbsp.)	=	15 ml = ½ fl oz
1 wineglass	=	60 ml = 2 fl oz
1 teacup	=	120 ml = 4 fl oz
1 tumbler	=	240 ml = 8 fl oz

COMPARATIVE APPROXIMATE LINEAR MEASURES

1 millimeter (mm)	= 0.04 inch (in.)	1 inch (in.)	= 2.54 centimeters (cm)
1 centimeter (cm)	= 0.4 inch		
1 decimeter (dm)	= 4.0 inches	1 foot (ft)	= 30.48 cm
1 meter (m)	= 39.37 inches	1 yard (yd)	= 91.44 cm

* In the Imperial System, 1 pint = 20 fluid ounces, 1 quart = 40 fluid ounces, 1 gallon = 160 fluid ounces.

CELCIUS-FAHRENHEIT EQUIVALENTS

Conversion;

To convert degrees F to degrees C subtract 32, then multiply by 5/9.

To convert degrees C to degrees F multiply by 9/5, then add 32.

Celcius°	Fahrenheit°	Celcius°	Fahrenheit°
Freezing (water at sea level):		Clinical Range:	
0	32	36.0	96.8
Boiling (water at sea level):		36.5	97.7
100.0	212.0	37.0	98.6
—40	—40	37.5	99.5
Pasteurization (Holding), 30 min at:		38.0	100.4
61.6	143.0	38.5	101.3
Pasteurization (Flash), 15 sec at:		39.0	102.2
71.1	160.0	39.5	103.1
		40.0	104.0
		40.5	104.9
		41.0	105.8
		41.5	106.7
		42.0	107.6

MILLIGRAM—MILLIEQUIVALENT CONVERSIONS

The unit of measure of electrolytes is the milliequivalent (mEq), which expresses the chemical activity, or combining power, of a substance relative to the acivity of 1 mg of hydrogen. Thus, 1 mEq is represented by 1 mg of hydrogen, 23 mg of Na, 39 mg of K, 20 mg of Ca, and 35 mg of Cl. Conversion equations are as follows:

$$\text{mEq/L} = \frac{(\text{mg/L}) \times \text{Valence}}{\text{Formula Wt}}$$

$$\text{mg/L} = \frac{(\text{mEq/L}) \times \text{Formula Wt}}{\text{Valence}}$$

(*N.B.:* Formula Wt = Atomic or Molecular Wt)

Milliosmols

The mEq is roughly equivalent to the milliosmol (mOsm), the unit of measure of osmolarity or tonicity. Normally, the body fluid compartments each contain about 280 mOsm of solute per liter.

ATOMIC WEIGHTS (APPROXIMATE) OF SOME COMMON ELEMENTS

Hydrogen (H) = 1	Sodium (Na) = 23
Carbon (C) = 12	Magnesium (Mg) = 24
Nitrogen (N) = 14	Chlorine (Cl) = 35.5
Oxygen (O) = 16	Potassium (K) = 39
	Calcium (Ca) = 40

CONVERSION FORMULAS

For Converting Weight

Weight of Additive Per Ton*	Percent in feed	ppm
(grams)		
1	0.00011	1.1
5	0.00055	5.5
10	0.0011	11
100	0.0110	110
(pounds)		
1	0.05	500
2	0.10	1,000

* 2,000 lb (907.2 kg); note that the metric ton (1,000 kg) = 2204.6 lb.

CONVERSION FORMULAS

Gallons into Pounds: Multiply the specific gravity of the liquid by 8.33* (weight in pounds of 1 gallon of water); then multiply this result by the number of gallons, to obtain the weight in pounds.

Pounds into Gallons: Multiply the specific gravity of the liquid by 8.33* (weight in pounds of 1 gallon of water); then divide the number of pounds by the result, to obtain the volume in gallons.

Milliliters into Grams: Multiply the specific gravity of the substance by the number of milliliters, to obtain the weight in grams.

Grams into Milliliters: Divide the number of grams by the specific gravity of the substance, to obtain its volume in milliliters.

Milliliters into Pounds: Multiply the numberiof milliliters by the specific gravity of the substance; then divide the product by 453.59 (equivalent in grams of 1 avoirdupois pound), to obtain its weight in pounds.

Pounds into Milliliters: Multiply the number of pounds by 453.59 (equivalent in grams of 1 avoirdupois pound); then divide the product by the specific gravity of the substance, to obtain the volume in milliliters.

Milliliters into Ounces: Multiply the number of milliliters by the specific gravity of the substance; then divided the product by 28.35 (equivalent in grams of 1 avoirdupois ounce), to obtain its volume in ounces.

Ounces into Milliliters: Multiply the number of ounces by 28.35 (equivalent in grams of 1 avoirdupois ounce); then divide the product by the specific gravity of the substance, to obtain its volume in milliliters.

Grains, Drams and Ounces into Grams (or ml): (1) Divide the number of grains by 15: or (2) multiply the number of drams by 4; or (3) multiply the number of ounces by 30. The result in each case equals the approximate number of grams (or ml).

Kilograms into Pounds: Multiply the number of kilograms by 2.2 or multiply the number of kilograms by 2 and add 10% to the product.

Pounds into Kilograms: Divide the number of pounds by 2.2.

* 10 for Imperial gallons

PART VIII
PRESCRIPTIONS

All the prescriptions referred to throughout the book are contained in this section. They are grouped in several classes, mainly according to their chief pharmacologic or therapeutic effect, but are numbered serially in the order of their listing, irrespective of classification. Thus, any prescription number in the text (e.g. ℞ 123) allows the reader to refer directly to the corresponding prescription in this section.

The drugs listed have been designated by their generic name(s). In those instances in which drug combinations are recommended, as well as with some of the newer drugs, their proprietary names have been included (within quotation marks). Where a drug is sold under 2 or more proprietary names, only the generic name is given. The pharmaceutical preparations set forth are those suggested by the authors of the various chapters. Where only one or a few of a number of possible preparations is given, those shown indicate only the preferences of the authors. Their appearance here does not constitute an implied or expressed warranty regarding specific products, nor does it imply endorsement of any one product over another by MERCK & CO., Inc. Every effort has been made to select representative drugs or preparations, but this should not be construed as restricting in any way the clinical judgment of the veterinarian in choosing related products or substituting other effective remedies at his discretion. Careful attention has also been given to the quantities and doses of the various agents listed, but personal experience, changes in manufacturer's formulations, or unusual conditions may make departures from those given necessary or desirable. Naturally, no guarantees can be made by the Editors regarding these recommendations. In all cases, current labeling directions should be consulted.

Most drugs are now subject to federal regulations. These regulations have as their objective the protection of public health and welfare by establishing the safety and efficacy of drugs and tolerances for safe concentrations of drug residues in edible animal products. The latter requirement has necessitated the definition of specific withdrawal times and other warnings and cautions governing the use of certain compounds. Some products, for example, cannot be used to treat meat-producing livestock, while others cannot be used for poultry. The same precaution applies to such preparations as antibacterial compounds or other pharmaceuticals that may be given to dairy cattle in lactation. However, **since the regulatory status of any specific drug is subject to change at any time, the veterinarian should inform himself in detail regarding the conditions and cautions under which such agents are to be used. The manufacturer's instructions in this regard, which by law are placed conspicuously on the label, should be followed conscientiously and precisely.**

Many of the prescriptions that appear throughout the text refer to various antibacterial agents. A detailed discussion of the uses, doses and administration of these substances is presented in the chapters titled SULFONAMIDE AND TRIMETHOPRIM THERAPY (p. 470), ANTIBIOTIC THERAPY (p. 482) and NITROFURAN THERAPY (p. 505). Reading these chapters will provide the veterinarian with a much more complete picture of the usefulness of current and generally accepted anti-infectious agents than can be gained from the prescriptions alone. **Corticosteroid therapy** is also discussed, in the chapter beginning on p. 603.

In this edition of THE MERCK VETERINARY MANUAL, most doses of drugs or quantities of ingredients in prescriptions are given in U.S. and metric measure. Conversion tables, given under the READY REFERENCE GUIDES (q.v., p. 1521), will quickly provide the reader with proper equivalents, whenever these are necessary.

Antibiotics

1. ℞ Amoxicillin

   Orally: 5 mg/lb (11 mg/kg) body wt b.i.d.

2. ℞ Ampicillin

   Horses: orally: 2 to 4.5 mg/lb (4 to 10 mg/kg) body wt. Subcut. *or* IM: 1 to 3 mg/lb (2 to 7 mg/kg) body wt.

   Dogs: orally: 9 mg/lb (20 mg/kg) body wt, daily in 3 divided doses. IM *or* IV: 2.3 mg/lb (5 mg/kg) daily in 3 divided doses.

3. ℞ Ampicillin

   Orally: 5 mg/lb (11 mg/kg) of body wt, t.i.d.
   or subcut. *or* IM: 3 mg/lb (6.6 mg/kg) b.i.d.

4. ℞ Ampicillin

   IV *or* IM: 4.5 to 9 mg/lb (10 to 20 mg/kg) of body wt, daily for 3 to 6 days.

5. ℞ Ampicillin

   Small animals: orally *or* IV: 9 mg/lb (20 mg/kg) body wt, t.i.d.

6. ℞ Ampicillin

   Cats and dogs: orally, 14 to 27 mg/lb (30 to 60 mg/kg) body wt, daily in divided doses.
   IV *or* IM: 4.5 to 9 mg/lb (10 to 20 mg/kg) daily in divided doses.

7. ℞ Ampicillin

   Orally: 18 to 36 mg/lb (40 to 80 mg/kg) of body wt, in 3 to 4 divided doses.

8. ℞ Ampicillin

   IM: 11.4 mg/lb (25 mg/kg) daily in divided doses.

9. ℞ Ampicillin

   Dogs: orally, 25 to 50 mg/lb (55 to 110 mg/kg) body wt, daily divided into 3 doses.

10. ℞ Ampicillin

    IM: 45 mg/lb (100 mg/kg) body wt daily, divided into 2 or 3 equal doses.

Read introduction to prescriptions, pp. 1526 to 1527. Note all warnings and cautions appearing on drug labels and observe all local laws and regulations pertaining to drug usage.

11. ℞ Benzathine penicillin G
Procaine penicillin G . . . . . āā 150,000 u/ml
Up to 50 lb (23 kg) of body wt: IM, 1 ml; *over 50 lb:* 2 ml. Repeat every 3 to 5 days.

12. ℞ Cephalexin
Dogs and cats: orally; 14 mg/lb (30 mg/kg) body wt, b.i.d.

13. ℞ Cephaloradine
Subcut. *or* IM: 5 mg/lb (11 mg/kg) body wt b.i.d. Treatment should not exceed 7 days without reassessment.

14. ℞ Cephaloridine ("Keflodin")
IM: 12.5 mg once daily for 2 weeks.

15. ℞ Cephalothin
IM: 25 mg/lb (55 mg/kg) body wt daily, divided into 4 equal doses.

16. ℞ Chloramphenicol
Large animals: IM, 2 to 5 mg/lb (4.5 to 11 mg/kg) body wt.
Small animals: Orally, 9 to 22 mg/lb (20 to 50 mg/kg) body wt daily, divided into 3 doses,
or IM, 5 mg/lb (11 mg/kg) body wt, once or twice daily.

17. ℞ Chloramphenicol
Dogs and cats: orally, 9 to 23 mg/lb (20 to 50 mg/kg) body wt, every 8 hours.
or IV: 9 mg/lb (20 mg/kg) every 6 to 8 hr daily for 3 to 6 days.

18. ℞ Chloramphenicol
Large animals: IM *or* IV, 5 to 10 mg/lb (10 to 22 mg/kg) body wt, t.i.d.
Small animals: Orally, 25 to 50 mg/lb (55 to 110 mg/kg) body wt, daily, divided into 3 doses,
or IM, 5 to 15 mg/lb (11 to 33 mg/kg) once or twice daily.

19. ℞ Chloramphenicol
Orally: 9 to 23 mg/lb (20 to 50 mg/kg) body wt, every 8 hours. IM *or* IV: 4.5 mg/lb (10 mg/kg) every 12 hours.

For standard equivalents for measures, see pp. 1521 to 1524.

20. ℞ Chloramphenicol

Orally: 18 to 36.5 mg/lb (40 to 80 mg/kg) body wt, in 3 to 4 divided doses daily,

or IV: 11.5 mg/lb (25 mg/kg) body wt, in divided doses.

21. ℞ Chloramphenicol

Calves: IV *or* IM, 10 mg/lb (22 mg/kg) body wt, repeated every 8 hours.

Foals: IV *or* IM, 10 to 20 mg/lb (22 to 44 mg/kg) body wt, repeated every 8 hours.

Piglets: IM, 15 mg/lb (33 mg/kg) body wt, repeated every 8 to 12 hours.

22. ℞ Chloramphenicol

Orally: 10 to 50 mg/lb (22 to 110 mg/kg) body wt in 3 or 4 divided doses.

IM: 2 to 4.5 mg/lb (5 to 10 mg/kg) in 2 divided doses.

23. ℞ Chloramphenicol

All species: orally, 10 to 25 mg/lb (22 to 55 mg/kg) body wt, t.i.d., daily for 3 to 6 days,

or IM *or* IV: 4.5 to 9 mg/lb (10 to 20 mg/kg) body wt, every 6 to 12 hr for 3 to 6 days.

24. ℞ Chloramphenicol

Small animals: subcut. *or* IM, 15 mg/lb (33 mg/kg) body wt daily, divided into 2 or 3 doses.

25. ℞ Chloramphenicol

Cats and laboratory animals: IV, 23 mg/lb (50 mg/kg) body wt, b.i.d.,

or orally divided into 4 doses.

26. ℞ Chloramphenicol

Fishes: 36 mg/lb (80 mg/kg) in food or by injection. Only to be used with extreme care and in nonfood species.

27. ℞ Chlortetracycline

FOR STANDARD THERAPY: orally, 15 to 50 mg/lb (33 to 110 mg/kg) body wt daily, in divided doses,

or IV, 2 to 5 mg/lb (4 to 9 mg/kg) body wt daily, in 2 equal doses. Administer until temperature has been normal for at least 24 hr after last dose.

Read introduction to prescriptions, pp. 1526 to 1527. Note all warnings and cautions appearing on drug labels and observe all local laws and regulations pertaining to drug usage.

FOR SPECIFIC USES IN BOVINE ANAPLASMOSIS: *Elimination of carrier infection:* parenterally, 5 mg/lb (11 mg/kg) body wt daily, for 10 consecutive days,

or orally at 5 mg/lb daily for 45 to 60 days.

Prevention by low-level feeding: 0.5 mg/lb (1.1 mg/kg) body wt daily, in feed for up to 120 days or until the risk of transmission is over.

Premunition: parenterally, 2.5 mg/lb (5.5 mg/kg) body wt, in single dose when infected animals show first febrile response or approximately 3% of the erythrocytes contain anaplasmas.

FOR SPECIFIC USE IN PREVENTING UROLITHIASIS IN CATTLE AND SHEEP: 10 to 20 mg/lb (22 to 44 mg/kg) daily, *or* mix 20 gm/ton (0.0022%) of feed.

28. ℞ Chlortetracycline

200 to 400 gm/ton (0.022 to 0.044%) of mash for 2 weeks.

29. ℞ Chlortetracycline

For porcine leptospirosis: 400 gm/ton (0.044%) of feed, continued for 14 days.

For jowl abscesses of swine: 100 to 200 gm/ton (0.011 to 0.022%) of feed. Useful only to prevent development of additional abscesses.

30. ℞ Chlortetracycline (capsule)

50 mg per bird daily, orally.

31. ℞ Chlortetracycline boluses (500 mg)

Insert 2 to 4 boluses into uterus.

32. ℞ Chlortetracycline hydrochloride

Add 1 gm to each gal. (0.25 gm/L) of water, for 4 or 5 days.

33. ℞ Cloxacillin

All species: IM, 1 mg/lb (2.2 mg/kg) body wt, b.i.d. or t.i.d.

34. ℞ Dihydrostreptomycin

IM: 5 mg/lb (11 mg/kg) of body wt, b.i.d.

35. ℞ Dihydrostreptomycin

IM: 5 to 10 mg/lb (11 to 22 mg/kg) body wt once or twice daily until at least 24 hours after apparent return to normal. Also intramammary infusion of 1 to 5 gm in aqueous vehicle.

For standard equivalents for measures, see pp. 1521 to 1524.

36. ℞ Dihydrostreptomycin . . . . 1.0 gm
Kaolin . . . . 10.0 gm
Pectin . . . . 0.9 gm
Water . . . . 100 ml
1 tsp every 4 hours.

37. ℞ Erythromycin
In drinking water: 0.5 gm/gal. (3.8 L) for 7 days.
In feed: 92.5 gm/ton (0.0102%) for 7 to 14 days.

38. ℞ Erythromycin solution (200 mg/ml)
IV: 1 to 2 mg/lb (2.2 to 4.4 mg/kg) body wt. Repeat in 12 hours.

39. ℞ Erythromycin
Orally: 2 to 5 mg/lb (4.5 to 11 mg/kg) body wt, t.i.d. or q.i.d.
IM *or* IV: 1 to 2 mg/lb (2 to 4.5 mg/kg) body wt, only until oral medication is possible.

40. ℞ Gentamicin
Subcut. *or* IM: 2 mg/lb (4.4 mg/kg) body wt b.i.d., first day, then once daily thereafter. Treatment should not exceed 7 days without reassessment.

41. ℞ Kanamycin
IM: 2.7 mg/lb (6 mg/kg) body wt, every 12 hours.

42. ℞ Lincomycin
Dogs and cats: orally, 7 mg/lb (15 mg/kg) body wt, t.i.d.
or IM, 4.5 mg/lb (10 mg/kg), b.i.d.

43. ℞ Lincomycin hydrochloride monohydrate
Dogs: subcut. *or* orally, 10 mg/lb (22 mg/kg) body wt, b.i.d.

44. ℞ Lincomycin
Orally: 14 mg/lb (30 mg/kg) body wt, daily divided into 4 equal doses
or IM: 9 mg/lb (20 mg/kg) daily, divided into 2 equal doses.

Read introduction to prescriptions, pp. 1526 to 1527. Note all warnings and cautions appearing on drug labels and observe all local laws and regulations pertaining to drug usage.

45. ℞ Lincomycin

Prophylaxis: 40 gm/ton (0.0044%) of feed as the sole ration.
Treatment: 100 gm/ton (0.011%) of feed as the sole ration for 3 weeks or until signs of disease disappear.

46. ℞ Neomycin sulfate

Neonatal septicemias and diarrhea, all species: IM *or* orally, 5 mg/lb (11 mg/kg) body wt, b.i.d.

47. ℞ Antibiotic solution

Neomycin sulfate	500 mg
Bacitracin	50,000 u
Polymyxin B sulfate	100 mg
Water	q.s. ad 100 ml
or Penicillin G (K or Na)	1,000,000 u
Dihydrostreptomycin	1 gm
Water	q.s. ad 10 to 100 ml

48. ℞ Oxytetracycline

Cattle and horses: IV *or* IM, 2 mg/lb (4.5 mg/kg) body wt, daily for 3 or 4 days, or until recovery.

49. ℞ Oxytetracycline

IM: 2.3 mg/lb (5 mg/kg) body wt, b.i.d.

50. ℞ Oxytetracycline

Large animals: IM *or* IV, 3 to 5 mg/lb (6.6 to 11 mg/kg) body wt, daily.
Small animals: IM, 5 mg/lb (11 mg/kg) body wt, daily, in divided doses at 6- to 12-hr intervals.
Poultry: For spirochetosis: IM, 1 to 5 mg/lb (2 to 11 mg/kg) body wt once.

51. ℞ Oxytetracycline

All species: IV *or* IM, 3.5 mg/lb (8 mg/kg) body wt, daily.

52. ℞ Oxytetracycline

Cattle: IV, 4.5 mg/lb (10 mg/kg) body wt, every 12 to 18 hr for 3 treatments.

53. ℞ Oxytetracycline

Cattle: IV *or* IM, 5 mg/lb (11 mg/kg) of body wt, daily for 3 days.

For standard equivalents for measures, see pp. 1521 to 1524.

54. ℞ Oxytetracycline

IV: 5 to 15 mg/lb (11 to 33 mg/kg) body wt, daily. Orally, 30 to 50 mg/lb (66 to 110 mg/kg) body wt, in 3 to 4 divided doses daily.

55. ℞ Oxytetracycline (oral)

23 mg/lb (50 mg/kg) body wt daily (200 mg/pt [425 mg/L] of drinking water) prepared fresh 3 times weekly.

56. ℞ Oxytetracycline (oral)

25 to 50 mg/lb (55 to 110 mg/kg) body wt in divided doses at 12-hr intervals.
For diarrhea in newborn calves, foals, lambs and piglets: **15 to 50 mg/lb (33 to 110 mg/kg) body wt. (Oral administration limited to small animals and swine, calves, foals or lambs not yet consuming roughage.)**

57. ℞ Oxytetracycline (capsule)

Orally: 50 mg per bird per day.

58. ℞ Oxytetracycline (water-soluble)

3 gm/10 gal. (80 mg/L) drinking water.

59. ℞ Oxytetracycline capsules (250 mg)

Insert 4 to 8 capsules into uterus.

60. ℞ Oxytetracycline

Swine: **400 gm/ton (0.044%) of feed, continued for 14 days.**
For prevention of additional jowl abscesses in swine: **100 to 200 gm/ton (0.011 to 0.022%) of feed.**
Calves: **500 gm/ton (0.055%) of feed. Feed 2-lb mixtura daily for 3 to 5 days.**
Poultry: **200 gm/ton (0.022%) of mash for 2 weeks.**
Fish: **2.5 to 3.5 gm/100 lb (50 to 75 mg/kg) of fish, daily for 10 to 14 days. Incorporate into ration.**

61. ℞ Penethamate hydriodide injection

IM: 3 to 5 million units per animal.

62. ℞ Penicillin G potassium or sodium

IV *or* IM: Initial dose 3,000 to 10,000 u/lb (6,600 to 22,000 u/kg) body wt. Follow at once with a similar IM dose of procaine penicillin in aqueous suspension, and repeat the latter daily.

Read introduction to prescriptions, pp. 1526 to 1527. Note all warnings and cautions appearing on drug labels and observe all local laws and regulations pertaining to drug usage.

63. ℞ Procaine penicillin G aqueous suspension
Large animals: IM, 5,000 to 10,000 u/lb (11,000 to 22,000 u/kg) body wt, daily. *For anthrax use higher dose.*
Small animals: IM, 10,000 to 20,000 u/lb (22,000 to 44,000 u/kg) body wt, daily.

64. ℞ Penicillin G, sodium or potassium
Dogs and cats: orally, 18,000 u/lb (40,000 u/kg) body wt, every 6 hr on an empty stomach.

65. ℞ Procaine penicillin G
Dogs: IM, 20,000 u/lb (44,000 u/kg) body wt, daily.

66. ℞ Procaine penicillin G aqueous suspension
All species: IM, 5,000 to 10,000 u/lb (11,000 to 22,000 u/kg) body wt,
and Streptomycin or Dihydrostreptomycin, aqueous.
All species: IM, 5 to 10 mg/lb (11 to 22 mg/kg) body wt, daily. Mix drugs together and give in 2 or 3 divided doses. Continue until temperature has been normal for at least 24 hours.

67. ℞ Penicillin G potassium . . . . 250,000 u
Sterile water . . . . 10 ml
Inject 2.5 ml into joint space b.i.d. for 3 or 4 days.

68. ℞ Penicillin . . . . 400,000 u/ml
Streptomycin . . . . 0.5 gm/ml
Into bursae: Inject 0.5 to 2.0 ml daily.
Into anal gland: Inject 1.0 ml once or twice weekly.

69. ℞ Procaine penicillin G . . . . . 1,000,000 u
Dihydrostreptomycin . . . . . 1.0 gm
Emulsifying vehicle* . . . . . . q.s. ad 100 ml
Instill 25 to 50 ml into the vagina. May be repeated at daily intervals as indicated.
*May also be used with water-dispersible ointment base, 15 gm.

70. ℞ Potassium penicillin . . . . 5,000,000 u
Dihydrostreptomycin . . . . 2 gm
Isotonic salt solution . . . . 100 ml
Flush into the guttural pouches daily for 7 to 10 days.

For standard equivalents for measures, see pp. 1521 to 1524.

71. ℞ Crystalline penicillin G . . . . 5,000,000 u
Dihydrostreptomycin . . . . 5 gm
Isotonic salt solution . . . . . . 100 ml
Infuse into uterus: Cattle: 20 ml; *Mares:* 100 ml.

72. ℞ Streptomycin
Large animals: IM, 5 mg/lb (11 mg/kg) body wt, b.i.d.

73. ℞ Streptomycin or Dihydrostreptomycin
All species: IM, 5 to 10 mg/lb (11 to 22 mg/kg) body wt, daily in divided doses every 6 to 12 hours.
For leptospirosis: Large animals: IM, 11 mg/lb (25 mg/kg) body wt, in a single dose. May be repeated for 3 daily doses.
Small animals: IM, 5 to 10 mg/lb (11 to 22 mg/kg) body wt, every 12 hours.

74. ℞ Streptomycin
Prophylaxis: 1 gm/gal. (265 mg/L) of drinking water continuously, or 5 to 10 gm/gal. (1.3 to 2.6 gm/L) for several days before and after suspected exposure.
Treatment: Depending on severity, 5 to 15 gm/gal. (1.3 to 4 gm/L) of drinking water for 5 to 10 days, then 1 gm/gal. for 5 days.

75. ℞ Streptomycin *or* Dihydrostreptomycin . 1 gm
Distilled water . . . . 10 ml
Inject 2.5 ml into joint space, b.i.d. for 3 or 4 days.
For bovine campylobacteriosis: Infuse 10 ml of the solution into uterus with a suitable catheter.

76. ℞ Tetracycline
Oral: (large animals) 5 to 10 mg/lb (11 to 22 mg/kg) body wt; *(small animals)* 15 to 50 mg/lb (33 to 110 mg/kg) body wt daily in 3 or 4 divided doses.
IM: 1 to 5 mg/lb (2 to 11 mg/kg) body wt daily.
IV: 1 to 5 mg/lb body wt once or twice daily. Continue treatment until animal has been afebrile for 24 to 48 hours.

77. ℞ Tetracycline
Dog and cats: orally, 7 mg/lb (15 mg/kg) of body wt every 8 hours.

Read introduction to prescriptions, pp. 1526 to 1527. Note all warnings and cautions appearing on drug labels and observe all local laws and regulations pertaining to drug usage.

78. ℞ Tetracycline

Oral: 15 to 50 mg/lb (33 to 110 mg/kg) of body wt daily divided into 2 or 3 doses.
For canine ehrlichiosis: orally, 15 mg/lb (33 mg/kg) body wt b.i.d. for 14 days, *or* 3 mg/lb (6.6 mg/kg) daily for 30 days.
Parenteral: 2 to 5 mg/lb (5 to 11 mg/kg) of body wt daily divided into 2 doses.

79. ℞ Tetracycline

Orally: 25 mg/lb (55 mg/kg) of body wt daily in divided doses every 6 hours.

80. ℞ Tetracycline

Orally: 25 to 50 mg/lb (55 to 110 mg/kg) body wt daily, in 3 or 4 divided doses. *(Oral administration limited to small animals and swine, and calves, colts or lambs not yet consuming roughage.)*
or IV: 3 to 5 mg/lb (7 to 11 mg/kg) body wt, in 2 divided doses.

81. ℞ Tylosin

Dogs: Orally, 5 to 10 mg/lb (11 to 22 mg/kg) of body wt, t.i.d.
Cattle: IM, 1 to 2 mg/lb (2 to 4.5 mg/kg) of body wt.

82. ℞ Tylosin

Prophylaxis: 100 gm/ton (0.011%) of feed for at least 3 weeks followed by 40 gm/ton (0.0044%) of feed until swine reach market weight.
Treatment: 0.25 gm/gal. (65 mg/L) water for 3 to 10 days followed by 40 to 100 gm/ton (0.0044 to 0.011%) of feed for 2 to 6 weeks after drinking water treatment.

83. ℞ Tylosin

IM: 100 to 400 mg/100 lb (2 to 9 mg/kg) body wt, daily for not more than 3 days.

84. ℞ Virginiamycin

Prophylaxis: For swine up to 120 lb: 25 gm/ton (0.0027%) of feed, where signs have not yet occurred.
Treatment and control: For swine up to 120 lb: 120 gm/ton (0.0132%) for 2 wk followed by 50 gm/ton (0.0055%), where signs of dysentery have appeared.

For standard equivalents for measures, see pp. 1521 to 1524.

Sulfonamides

85. ℞ Phthalylsulfathiazole ("Sulfathalidine")

Orally: 70 to 100 mg/lb (150 to 220 mg/kg) body wt, daily for 3 or 4 days.

86. ℞ Salicylazosulfapyridine ("Azulfidine")

Small animals: orally, 27 mg/lb (60 mg/kg) body wt, t.i.d.

87. ℞ Sulfabromomethazine ("Sulfabrom")

100 mg/lb (220 mg/kg) body wt, in the feed daily for 2 consecutive days.

88. ℞ Sulfadiazine

Orally *or* IV: 30 mg/lb (66 mg/kg) body wt, b.i.d.

89. ℞ Sulfadiazine sodium
Sulfamerazine sodium . . . . āā 50 mg

Given in the water or feed, daily per animal for 10 to 14 days.

90. ℞ Sulfadiazine
Sulfamerazine
Sulfathiazole . . . . āā 150 mg

1 tablet per 7.5 lb (3.5 kg) body wt orally, in divided doses, for 4 days.

91. ℞ Sulfadimethoxine

Dogs: IV *or* subcut., 6 to 25 mg/lb (13 to 55 mg/kg) body wt, daily.
Horses: orally, 12.5 to 25 mg/lb (28 to 55 mg/kg) body wt, daily.

92. ℞ Sulfadimethoxine (tablets)

Orally: 12.5 mg/lb (28 mg/kg) body wt, on the first day, then 6.5 mg/lb (14 mg/kg) body wt, for 5 days.

93. ℞ Sulfadimethoxine

Chickens: 95 gm/50 gal. (0.05%), in drinking water, given for 6 days (*for infectious coryza:* for 3 to 5 days).
Turkeys: 95 gm/100 gal. (0.025%), in drinking water, given for 6 days.

Read introduction to prescriptions, pp. 1526 to 1527. Note all warnings and cautions appearing on drug labels and observe all local laws and regulations pertaining to drug usage.

94. ℞ Sulfaguanidine

Cattle: orally, 1.0 to 7.3 gm/lb (2 to 16 gm/kg) body wt, daily for 3 or 4 days.

95. ℞ Sulfaguanidine

Mix with chopped hay or grain at the rate of 1 gm/lb (2.2 gm/kg) feed.

96. ℞ Sulfamerazine sodium

Orally, 60 mg/lb (130 mg/kg) body wt, followed by 30 mg/lb (65 mg/kg) every 24 hr for 4 days.

97. ℞ Sulfamerazine sodium

Poultry: 10 lb/ton (0.5%) in feed, given for 5 to 7 days.

Sulfamerazine

Fish: 8 to 10 gm/100 lb (175 to 220 mg/kg) of trout, daily for 14 days. Incorporate into ration.

98. ℞ Sulfamerazine sodium
Sulfapyridine sodium
Sulfathiazole sodium . . . . āā 20 gm
Sterile water . . . . q.s. ad 500 ml

IV *or* IP: 0.5 to 1.0 ml/lb (1.1 to 2.2 ml/kg) body wt, initially, then half the initial dose every 12 hours.

99. ℞ Sulfamethazine

Mass medication: 45.5 to 68 mg/lb (100 to 150 mg/kg) of body wt daily for 10 days to 2 wk, added to feed or drinking water.

100. ℞ Sulfamethazine sodium

Orally *or* preferably IV: 60 mg/lb (130 mg/kg) body wt, followed by 30 mg/lb (65 mg/kg) orally every 24 hr or 3 or 4 days.

101. ℞ Sulfamethazine or sodium salt

Cattle: orally, IV *or* IP, 91 mg/lb (200 mg/kg) body wt, daily for 3 days.

102. ℞ Sulfamethazine

Orally *or* IV, 100 mg/lb (220 mg/kg) body wt the first day, then 50 mg/lb (110 mg/kg) daily for 3 or 4 days.

103. ℞ Sulfamethazine sodium

8 gm/gal. (0.25%) in drinking water for 5 days,
or orally: 5 to 10 drops of a 25% solution daily.

For standard equivalents for measures, see pp. 1521 to 1524.

104. ℞ Sulfamethazine

In feed: 8 lb/ton (0.4%) of feed for 3 to 5 days.

or Sulfamethazine sodium, 12.5% solution.

In water: 1 fl oz/gal. (8 ml/L) drinking water; medicate for 2 days.

105. ℞ Sulfanilamide

Orally: 60 mg/lb (132 mg/kg) body wt, on the first day, followed by 45 mg/lb (100 mg/kg) on succeeding days, until temperature has been normal for 48 hours.

106. ℞ Sulfapyridine

Orally: 60 mg/lb (132 mg/kg) body wt, followed by 30 mg/lb (66 mg/kg) every 12 hours for 4 days,

or Sulfapyridine sodium IV:

30 mg/lb body wt, daily for 4 days.

107. ℞ Sulfaquinoxaline sodium

For first 2 or 3 days, 0.04% in drinking water,

or 0.1% in the feed. If disease recurs, use 0.025% in the water,

or 0.05% in the feed for 2 days and repeat, if necessary, at 4-day intervals.

108. ℞ Sulfaquinoxaline

1 lb/ton (0.05%) in feed, given for a minimum of 5 days.

109. ℞ Sulfaquinoxaline

6 mg/lb (13 mg/kg) body wt orally, daily for 3 to 5 days.

For therapy in cattle and sheep: 6 mg/lb body wt in the drinking water daily until signs subside.

For prophylaxis in cattle: 0.6 mg/lb (1.3 mg/kg) body wt in the drinking water daily for 30 days, starting when animals are likely to be exposed to clinical infection.

CAUTION: *In dogs:* larger doses may produce hypoprothrombinemia, which may be reversed or prevented by the use of menadione (℞ 570) or vitamin K_1 (℞ 574).

110. ℞ Sulfathiazole

Horses and cats: orally, 90 mg/lb (200 mg/kg) body wt, t.i.d.

Read introduction to prescriptions, pp. 1526 to 1527. Note all warnings and cautions appearing on drug labels and observe all local laws and regulations pertaining to drug usage.

Cattle, sheep, swine, dogs: orally, 120 to 180 mg/lb (265 to 400 mg/kg) body wt, in equal fractional doses every 4 to 6 hours.

111. ℞ Sulfathiazole (5%) and urea (10%) ointment
Topically: b.i.d. until infection subsides.

112. ℞ Sulfisoxazole
Orally: 60 to 120 mg/lb (130 to 265 mg/kg) body wt.

113. ℞ Sulfisoxazole
80 to 100 mg/lb (180 to 220 mg/kg) of trout, daily for 14 days. Incorporate into ration.

114. ℞ Potentiated sulfonamide
Sulfazamet and trimethoprim 20:1
Fish: 100 mg/kg of body wt, in food or by injection.

115. ℞ Trimethoprim-sulfadiazine ("Tribrissen")
Trimethoprim . . . . 20 or 80 mg
Sulfadiazine . . . . 100 or 400 mg
Dogs and cats: orally, 14 mg/lb (30 mg/kg) body wt, daily in divided doses.

116. ℞ Trimethoprim-sulfadoxine ("Trivetrin")
Each milliliter contains: 40 mg trimethoprim and 200 mg sulfadoxine.
IM *or* IV: 1 ml/5 to 7 lb (10 to 15 kg) body wt, daily for 3 to 6 days.

Nitrofurans

117. ℞ Furazolidone
1 gm/lb (2.2 gm/kg) of ration for 2 to 4 weeks.

118. ℞ Furazolidone suspension (100 mg/ml)
Piglets: orally, 2 ml as initial dose and 1 ml every 8 hours. Treatment may be continued for 3 days. Treat all pigs in the litter.

119. ℞ Furazolidone
Prophylaxis: 100 gm/ton (0.011%) in feed (5 wk); 150 gm/ton (0.0165%) in feed (3 wk); 200 gm/ton (0.022%) in feed (2 wk).
Treatment: 300 gm/ton (0.033%) in feed 10 to 14 days.

120. ℞ Nifurpirinol
Expose fish to 1 ppm for 1 hr as a bath.

For standard equivalents for measures, see pp. 1521 to 1524.

121. ℞ Nitrofurantoin

Tracheobronchitis: orally, 2 mg/lb (4.5 mg/kg) body wt, every 8 hr for 4 to 7 days.
Urinary tract infections: orally, 2 mg/lb body wt, every 8 hr for 7 to 14 days.

122. ℞ Nitrofurazone

Orally, 5 mg/lb (11 mg/kg) body wt, for 3 days.

123. ℞ Nitrofurazone

Orally: 9 mg/lb (20 mg/kg) body wt, daily for 6 days.

124. ℞ Nitrofurazone

Swine: 0.055% in feed for 7 days.

125. ℞ Nitrofurazone

Feed mix: 30 to 40 mg/lb (66 to 88 mg/kg) of fish daily
or water mix: 3 to 5 ppm in bath treatment.

126. ℞ Nitrofurazone solution 0.2%

5 to 60 ml/flush.

Biologicals

127. ℞ Anti-distemper, hepatitis and *Leptospira* serum

Subcut.: 0.5 to 1.0 ml/lb (1.1 to 2.2 ml/kg) body wt, repeated at 7- to 10-day intervals if the animal is kept under conditions of exposure to the virus, and every 14 days if kept at home.

128. ℞ *Clostridium botulinum* Type A and Type C antitoxin

IP: 2 to 4 ml, depending on weight of bird.

129. ℞ *Clostridium chauvoei-septicum* bacterin

Cattle, horses: 5 ml subcut.
Sheep, goats: 3 ml subcut.

130. ℞ *Clostridium perfringens* Type D toxoid

5 ml subcut.

131. ℞ "Flea Antigen" (Haver Lockhart)

Intradermally: 3 injections of 0.5 ml at 7-day intervals.

Read introduction to prescriptions, pp. 1526 to 1527. Note all warnings and cautions appearing on drug labels and observe all local laws and regulations pertaining to drug usage.

132. ℞ *Haemophilus gallinarum* bacterin

Requires 2 separate doses of 0.5 ml subcut. at the back of the neck. Second dose to be given 3 to 4 wk later.

133. ℞ Encephalomyelitis vaccine,

Eastern strain
or Western strain
or Eastern- and Western-strain mixture.
Intradermally: 2 doses of 1 ml each at 7- to 10-day intervals.

134. ℞ Equine rhinopneumonitis virus ("Pneumabort") (hamster-adapted live virus)

Immunization against viral rhinopneumonitis of horses: Intranasally: 2-ml dose in July and October to farm horses. Use 2-ml dose once annually for horses in training and racing.

Corticosteroids and Anti-inflammatory Agents

135. ℞ Betamethasone

Betamethasone acetate	3 mg
Betamethasone disodium phosphate	1 mg

Horses: Inject 5 ml of suspension intra-articularly.

136. ℞ Corticotropin (ACTH)

Dogs: IM, 1 u/lb (2.2 u/kg) body wt, once or twice daily. Reduce dosage gradually over a 7-day period.

137. ℞ Corticotropin (ACTH) in gelatin or oil or other delayed-absorption vehicle

Large animals: IM: 200 to 600 u. Repeat after 2 or 3 days if necessary.
Small animals: IM: 1 u/lb (2.2 u/kg) body wt. Repeat after 2 days.

138. ℞ Cortisone acetate (suspension or tablets)

Large animals: IM, 0.5 to 1.5 gm. Repeat on following day if necessary.
Small animals: IM *or* orally, 1 to 5 mg/lb (2 to 11 mg/kg) body wt. Dose must be adjusted to response of animal to treatment.
Poultry: oral: 2.5 mg/bird. IM: 2.0 mg/bird.

139. ℞ Deoxycorticosterone acetate (DOCA)

Dogs: IM, 1 to 2 mg, daily.
Pellet implants: 125 mg, 1 to 2 pellets given each 6 to 12 months.

For standard equivalents for measures, see pp. 1521 to 1524.

140. ℞ Dexamethasone

IV: 1 mg/lb (2.2 mg/kg) body wt.

141. ℞ Dexamethasone

Horses: parenterally, 5 to 10 mg daily in single or divided doses. This dosage should be administered until a therapeutic effect is achieved or for 5 days.

142. ℞ Dexamethasone (tablets or suspension)

Large animals: IM *or* orally, 5 to 20 mg daily.
Small animals: IM *or* orally, 0.125 to 2 mg daily.
Subsequent daily dose to be reduced.

143. ℞ Dexamethasone

Dogs and cats: IV *or* IM, 0.13 to 1.0 mg.
Cattle: IV *or* IM, 5 to 20 mg.
Horses: IV *or* IM, 2.5 to 5 mg.

144. ℞ Dexamethasone

IM: 20 mg, at approximately the time of normal parturition.

145. ℞ Dexamethasone, aspirin and aluminum hydroxide ("Decagesic")

Each table contains:

Dexamethasone	0.25 mg
Aspirin	500 mg
Aluminum hydroxide	75 mg

One or 2 tablets once or twice daily.

146. ℞ Fluoroprednisolone-Neomycin

9-Fluoroprednisolone acetate	2 mg/ml
Neomycin sulfate	5 mg/ml

of aqueous solution for infection.
IM: 10 to 20 ml, according to severity of condition.

147. ℞ Hydrocortisone acetate (tablets or suspension)

Large animals: IM, 0.5 to 1.5 gm. Repeat if necessary.
Small animals: orally *or* IM, 1 to 2 mg/lb (2 to 5 mg/kg) body wt. Divide into 2 to 4 doses if given orally. Adjust dose to patient's response and reduce to minimum effective maintenance dose.

Read introduction to prescriptions, pp. 1526 to 1527. Note all warnings and cautions appearing on drug labels and observe all local laws and regulations pertaining to drug usage.

148. ℞ Hydrocortisone solution (100 mg/ml)

Large animals: IV, 100 to 600 mg given by slow infusion in 500 to 1,000 ml of 10% dextrose or isotonic sodium chloride.
Small animals: 9 to 18 mg/lb (20 to 40 mg/kg) body wt, by slow IV infusion in 25 to 250 ml of 5% dextrose or isotonic sodium chloride.

149. ℞ Methylprednisolone acetate (20 to 40 mg/ml)

Inject into the lesion *or* give parenterally every 2 to 3 weeks.
Dogs: The average dose is 20 mg. In accordance with size and severity of the condition, dose may range from 2 mg in miniature breeds to 40 mg in medium breeds and even as high as 120 mg in the largest breeds or with severe involvement.
Cats: The average dose is 10 mg with a range of up to 20 mg.

150. ℞ Phenylbutazone

Large animals: orally, 2 to 4 mg/lb (4.5 to 9 mg/kg) body wt, for 3 to 5 days.
Small animals: orally, 100 to 250 mg, t.i.d. Dosage can be reduced after the 4th day.

151. ℞ Prednisolone

Orally: 0.25 to 1.0 mg/lb (0.5 to 2.2 mg/kg) body wt, daily *or* as needed—divided in 2 daily doses; long-term every other day.

152. ℞ Prednisolone (tablets or injectable)

0.5 to 0.9 mg/lb (1 to 2 mg/kg) body wt, daily for 3 days, then 1.0 mg daily for 3 days, followed by 0.09 mg/lb (0.2 mg/kg) body wt, daily for 1 to 6 weeks.

153. ℞ Prednisolone

Small animals: orally, 2.5 mg, b.i.d. or t.i.d.

154. ℞ Prednisolone (tablets or suspension)

Cattle and horses: IM, 100 to 400 mg.
Dogs: Orally *or* IM, 0.22 to 0.45 mg/lb (0.5 to 1.0 mg/kg) body wt, b.i.d. for 3 to 5 days.
Adjust dose to patient's response; then reduce gradually to minimum level needed to maintain remission. Alternate-day treatment will minimize side effects of long-term therapy.
For allergy, other immune disorders and thrombocytopenic states: 1 to 2 mg/lb (2 to 4 mg/kg) body wt daily in divided doses

For standard equivalents for measures, see pp. 1521 to 1524.

or twice this dosage every other day until condition is controlled. Adjust dosage downwards, in incremental steps, to minimum maintenance level.

155. ℞ Prednisolone t-butylacetate

Arthritis and synovitis: Aspirate all fluid from cavity and inject 2 to 5 ml.
Curb and sore shins: Inject 0.5 to 1.0 ml in several sites over area of swelling.

156. ℞ Triamcinolone

Orally, IM *or* subcut.: 50 to 100 mcg/lb (110 to 220 mcg/kg) body wt. Oral dosage should be reduced gradually within 2 weeks to maintenance levels of 10 to 20 mcg/lb (22 to 44 mcg/kg) body wt.

157. ℞ Triamcinolone acetonide (2 to 6 mg/ml)

Aspirate all available fluid from the synovial cavity and inject:
Dogs: 1 to 3 mg.
Horses: 6 to 30 mg.
Depending on size of the cavity.

Hormones and Hormone-like Mediators

158. ℞ Chlorpropamide tablet (100 mg)

Orally: 100 to 250 mg daily. Dosage must be adjusted individually.

159. ℞ Chorionic gonadotropin

Large animals: IM, 1,000 to 10,000 IU,
or IV, 2,500 to 5,000 IU.
Dogs: IM *or* subcut., 250 to 500 IU, at weekly intervals for 4 to 8 weeks.
For hyperestrinism in bitches: IM, 100 to 500 IU, daily until bleeding or signs subside.

160. ℞ Cloprostenol ("Estrumate")

Cows: IM, 500 mcg, once.

161. ℞ Cloprostenol sodium

Cows: IM, 530 mcg.

162. ℞ Dexamethasone

Cattle: IM, 20 to 40 mg, once.

Read introduction to prescriptions, pp. 1526 to 1527. Note all warnings and cautions appearing on drug labels and observe all local laws and regulations pertaining to drug usage.

163. ℞ Dexamethasone trimethylacetate

IM: 20 to 30 mg between 240 and 280 days of pregnancy, in cattle induces parturition and lactation with minimal complications from retained fetal membranes. Parturition occurs 11 to 12 days (6 to 25) after injection.

164. ℞ Diethylstilbestrol

IM: 0.5 to 4.0 mg in oil, on the first day, *then* orally, 0.5 to 4.0 mg on the following 5 to 7 days

or IM, repository diethylstilbestrol 0.5 mg/lb (1.1 mg/kg), body wt, within 5 days of mating.

165. ℞ Diethylstilbestrol

Dogs: IM (repository form), 0.1 mg/lb (0.2 mg/kg) body wt, once, to a maximum of 10 mg/animal,

or 1-mg tablet daily for 5 days.

Mares: IM, 2.5 to 10 mg.

166. ℞ Diethylstilbestrol

Cattle and horses: IM, subcut. *or* orally, 15 to 60 mg, daily.

Sheep and swine: IM, subcut. *or* orally, 4 to 5 mg, daily.

Dogs: IM (repository form): 0.2 to 0.9 mg/lb (0.5 to 2 mg/kg) body wt once, with maximum of 25 mg/animal,

or 1-mg tablet daily for 5 days.

167. ℞ Dinoprost tromethamine ("Prostin F2 alpha")

Cows: 3 mg—Administer in the uterine horn ipsilateral to the corpus luteum.

168. ℞ Dinoprost tromethamine ("Prostin F2 alpha")

Cows: 6 mg—Administer in the cervix or anterior vagina.

169. ℞ Dinoprost tromethamine ("Prostin F2 alpha")

Mares: 5 to 10 mg, subcut.

Cows: 20 to 25 mg, IM.

Doe goats and ewes: 15 mg, IM.

170. ℞ Dinoprost tromethamine ("Prostin F2 alpha")

Cows: IM, 25 to 30 mg in a single dose.

Mares: Subcut., 5 mg.

For standard equivalents for measures, see pp. 1521 to 1524.

171. ℞ Estradiol 17-β cypionate

Dogs: IM, 0.5 to 2.0 mg within 5 days of mating. In toy breeds the dose may be reduced to 0.25 mg.
Mares: IM, 1 to 5 mg.

172. ℞ Conjugated estrogens ("Premarin")

Large animals: IV, 20 mg.

173. ℞ Flumethasone

IM: 5 mg at approximately the time of normal parturition.

174. ℞ Fluprostenol ("Equimate")

Mares: IM, 250 mcg.

175. ℞ Gonadotropic hormone (pregnant mare serum)

Cows: IM *or* subcut., 1,000 IU for 2 or 3 consecutive days.
Bulls and stallions: IM *or* subcut., 500 IU weekly. Repeat weekly if necessary.
Ewes: subcut., 500 IU.
Bitches: subcut., 500 IU daily for 9 days.
Dogs: subcut., 375 to 750 IU. Repeat when necessary.

176. ℞ Gonadotropin releasing hormone (GnRH)

Cows: IM, 1 to 2.5 mg at estrus.
Mares: IM, 1 to 2 mg once on day-2 of estrus
or IM, 1 to 2 mg daily or starting from day-2 of estrus.
Sows: IV, 1 to 1.5 mg.

177. ℞ Human chorionic gonadotropin (HCG)

Bitches: IM *or* subcut., 500 to 1,000 IU on day 10.
Cows: IM, IV *or* subcut., 3,000 to 10,000 IU.
Doe goats: IM *or* subcut., 500 to 5,000 IU at estrus.
Mares: IV, 1,500 to 6,000 IU.
Queens: IM *or* subcut., 50 to 500 IU on day 9.
Sows: IM, 200 to 1,000 IU.

178. ℞ Human chorionic gonadotropin (HCG)

Large animals: IM *or* IV, 1,500 to 3,000 IU twice weekly for 4 to 6 weeks.
Small animals: IM *or* IV, 500 IU twice weekly for 4 to 6 weeks.

Read introduction to prescriptions, pp. 1526 to 1527. Note all warnings and cautions appearing on drug labels and observe all local laws and regulations pertaining to drug usage.

79. ℞ Pregnant mare serum gonadotropin (PMSG)

Cows: IM *or* subcut., 1,000 to 2,000 IU followed 2 days later with prostaglandin treatment.
Bitches: IM or subcut., 500 IU daily for 9 days.
Queens: IM or subcut., 100 IU followed by 50 IU daily for 7 days.
Doe goats: IM or subcut., 500 to 1,000 IU, 2 days before removal of tampons.

80. ℞ Pregnant mare serum gonadotropin (PMSG) . . . . 400 IU
Human chorionic gonadotropin (HCG) 200 IU

Give IM, simultaneously.

81. ℞ Pregnant mare serum . . . . 1,500 to 2,000 IU
Human chorionic gonadotropin . . . . 3,000 to 10,000 IU

Administer simultaneously in a single dose by subcut. *or* IM injection.

82. ℞ Insulin (crystalline zinc)

Diabetes mellitus: IM *or* subcut., 0.5 to 2.3 u/lb (1 to 5 u/kg) body wt,
or ½ dose IV in emergencies. Peak activity in 2 to 4 hr, duration 5 to 7 hours.

83. ℞ Insulin (neutral protamine Hagedorn, NPH)

Subcut.: 0.5 to 2.3 u/lb (1 to 5 u/kg) of body wt. Peak activity in 6 to 8 hr, duration of activity is ca. 24 hours.

84. ℞ Insulin (protamine zinc)

Subcut.: 5 to 50 u daily, depending on animal's size and response. Peak activity in 14 to 24 hr; duration is 36 hours.

85. ℞ Luteinizing hormone (LH)

Bitches: 12.5 mg, IM *or* IV on day-10.
Queens: 5 to 12.5 mg, IM *or* IV on day-9.
Cows: 25 to 50 mg, IM *or* IV at estrus.

86. ℞ Pituitary gonadotropin (LH)

Large animals: IV, 25 mg (5 ml). Repeat after 1 to 4 weeks if necessary.
Small animals: IM *or* subcut., 1 mg (0.2 ml) at weekly intervals as indicated.

For standard equivalents for measures, see pp. 1521 to 1524.

187. ℞ Megestrol acetate tablets

Orally: 0.23 mg/lb (0.5 mg/kg) daily for a maximum of 40 days, beginning 7 to 14 days prior to desiring the effect,

or during proestrus: administer 0.9 mg/lb (2 mg/kg) daily for 8 days.

188. ℞ Megestrol acetate

Dogs and cats: for postponement of estrus: (a) *Proestrus treatment:* orally, 1 mg/lb (2.2 mg/kg) body wt, daily for 8 days. (b) *Anestrus treatment:* orally, 0.25 mg/lb (0.55 mg/kg) body wt, daily for 32 days.

189. ℞ Megestrol acetate

Orally: 2.5 to 5 mg every 2nd or 3rd day until lesion regresses, then once weekly.

190. ℞ Methylprednisolone acetate (20 or 40 mg/ml)

Arthritis and related disorders:
Dogs: Aspirate all available fluid from synovial cavity and inject 10 to 20 mg.
Horses: Aspirate all available fluid from synovial cavity and inject 40 to 160 mg depending on size of cavity.
Curb and sore shins: Horses: Inject 10 to 120 mg in several sites over area of swelling.

191. ℞ Methyltestosterone (tablets)

Orally: 0.5 to 1.0 mg/lb (1 to 2.2 mg/kg) body wt, daily for 6 to 10 days.

192. ℞ Mibolerone ("Cheque")

Dogs: Orally or in feed, 1 to 25 lb (0.5 to 11.4 kg) body wt, give 30 mcg.
26 to 50 lb (20 to 22.7 kg) body wt, give 60 mcg.
51 to 100 lb (23 to 45.5 kg) body wt, give 120 mcg.
Over 100 lb (45.5 kg) body wt, give 180 mcg.
German shepherd dog—give 180 mcg.

193. ℞ Oxytocin

Small animals: IM *or* subcut., 5 to 30 u.
Sheep and swine: IM *or* subcut., 30 to 50 u.
Cattle and horses: IM *or* subcut., 40 to 100 u.
Bovine mastitis: IV, 20 to 40 u.
Rabbits: IM *or* subcut., 1 to 2 u.

Read introduction to prescriptions, pp. 1526 to 1527. Note all warnings and cautions appearing on drug labels and observe all local laws and regulations pertaining to drug usage.

194. ℞ Progesterone

Cattle and swine: IM, 50 to 100 mg daily.
Sheep: IM, 10 mg daily.
Dogs: IM, 10 to 50 mg daily, until bleeding or signs subside.

195. ℞ Progesterone in arachis oil

Mares: IM, 0.14 mg/lb (0.3 mg/kg) body wt,
or 100 to 150 mg daily.
Cows: IM, 100 to 125 mg daily for 10 to 14 days.

196. ℞ Prostalene

Cows: 0.5 mg—Administer in the uterine horn ipsilateral to the corpus luteum.

197. ℞ Prostalene

Cows: 1 mg—Administer into the anterior vagina or cervix.

198. ℞ Prostalene

Cows: IM, 2 mg.
Mares: subcut., 2 mg.

199. ℞ Purified posterior pituitary injection (10 or 20 u/ml)

Cattle and horses: IM, IV *or* subcut., 2 to 5 ml.
Sheep and swine: IM, IV *or* subcut., 1 to 2 ml.
Dogs: IM *or* subcut., 0.1 to 0.5 ml.

200. ℞ Testosterone propionate

Large animals: subcut., 50 mg daily for 4 days.
Small animals: IM, 10 to 50 mg.

201. ℞ Thyroprotein (iodinated casein)

Cattle, sheep and goats: 10 to 15 mg/lb (22 to 33 mg/kg) body wt, daily in feed.

202. ℞ L-Thyroxin

Orally, 4.5 to 9 mcg/lb (10 to 20 mcg/kg) body wt b.i.d.

203. ℞ L-Thyroxin (T_4, tetraiodothyronine)

Cattle: IM *or* subcut., 5 to 10 mg, daily
or orally, 50 to 100 mg.
Horses: orally, 7 to 15 mg daily.
Sheep: IM, 1 mg, daily.
Dogs: orally, 0.9 to 9 mcg/lb (2 to 20 mcg/kg) body wt, b.i.d.

For standard equivalents for measures, see pp. 1521 to 1524.

204. ℞ Tolbutamide tablets (500 mg)

Orally, 0.5 to 3.0 gm daily. Dosage must be adjusted individually.

205. ℞ Vasopressin (ADH) tannate in oil

Dogs: IM, 0.25 to 2 u once or twice daily, adjusted to response. Dose should be doubled or tripled for diagnostic test.

Intramammary Infusions

206. ℞ Furaltadone and penicillin ("Altapen")

Infuse into teat canal at 12-hour intervals for 3 or more treatments.

207. ℞ Benzathine cloxacillin

500 mg in 3% aluminum monostearate base. Infuse into each quarter at drying off and leave without milking out.

208. ℞ Procaine penicillin G (slow-release) . (300 mg)

One infusion in each quarter at drying off.

209. ℞ Procaine penicillin G . . . . 300 mg
Novobiocin . . . . 250 mg
in a slow-release base.

Infuse into each quarter at drying off.

210. ℞ Sodium carbenicillin

5 gm as an infusion into the infected quarter. Repeat in 24 hours.

211. ℞ Chlortetracycline mastitis ointment

400 mg infused into the teat canal. Repeat at 24- to 48-hr intervals if necessary.

212. ℞ Sodium cloxacillin, 200 mg in 3% aluminum monostearate base

Infuse 3 times at 48-hr intervals into the infected quarter. Treated quarters may be milked out at normal milking intervals.

213. ℞ Dihydrostreptomycin

0.25 to 1.0 gm in suspension, infused into the teat canal. May be repeated after 24 to 48 hours.

Read introduction to prescriptions, pp. 1526 to 1527. Note all warnings and cautions appearing on drug labels and observe all local laws and regulations pertaining to drug usage.

214. ℞ Erythromycin mastitis infusion (300 mg)

Infuse after each of 3 successive milkings.

215. ℞ Lincomycin hydrochloride mastitis infusion (200 mg)

Infuse 3 times at 12- to 24-hr intervals.

216. ℞ Neomycin mastitis ointment

500 mg of active substance infused into the teat canal. Repeat at 24- to 48-hr intervals if necessary.

217. ℞ Oxytetracycline mastitis ointment

200 to 400 mg of active substance infused into the teat canal. Repeat at 24- to 48-hr. intervals if necessary.

218. ℞ Penicillin mastitis ointment or suspension

Infuse into teat canal: 100,000 u, 2 doses 24 hr apart. (Continue regular milking.)

219. ℞ Penicillin and dihydrostreptomycin sulfate

Intramammary infusion: 100,000 u penicillin and 1 gm dihydrostreptomycin sulfate in emulsion-type vehicle. Repeat daily for 4 doses.

220. ℞ Penicillin-streptomycin dry-cow infusion (slow release)

Procaine penicillin G	1,000,000 u
Dihydrostreptomycin	1 gm

Use as intramammary infusions after the last milking of the lactation.

Caution: Use only in dry cows and not within 14 days of calving.

Anthelmintics

221. ℞ Thiabendazole-piperazine phosphate ("Equizole A")

Each ounce contains: 6.67 gm thiabendazole and 8.33 gm piperazine base.

Horses: orally, 1½ oz/500 lb (227 kg) body wt.

222. ℞ Albendazole

Cattle and sheep: Orally, 3.4 mg/lb (7.5 mg/kg) body wt.

For adult liver flukes: 4.5 mg/lb (10 mg/kg).

For standard equivalents for measures, see pp. 1521 to 1524.

223. ℞ Aracoline acetarsol (tablets)

Dogs: **22 mg/10 lb (5 mg/kg) body wt.**
Cats: **15 mg/10 lb (3.3 mg/kg) body wt. For best results give after a light meal.**

224. ℞ Arecoline hydrobromide

Dogs: **orally, 0.75 to 1.25 mg/lb (1.7 to 2.8 mg/kg) body wt, up to a maximum of 75 mg, after a 12-hr fast. If purgation does not occur within 1½ to 2 hr give a warm soapy enema.**

225. ℞ Arsenamide solution

IV, 0.1 ml/lb (0.22 ml/kg) body wt, b.i.d. for 2 days. Restrict exercise for up to 2 months. If pulmonary reaction occurs, give single dose of 20 mg prednisone IM, followed by daily injections of antibiotics.
NOTE: Avoid perivascular leakage since arsenamide is a sclerosing drug.

226. ℞ Bephenium embonate (*or* hydroxynaphthoate)

Sheep: **drench, 125 mg/lb (275 mg/kg) body wt, in a single dose.**
Dogs: **orally, 15 mg/lb (33 mg/kg) body wt, repeated after 6 to 10 hours.**

227. ℞ Bunamidine hydrochloride

Dogs and cats: **orally, 12.5 mg/lb (25 mg/kg) after 12-hr fast. Repeat in 48 hours. In cases of *Echinococcus* infection double the dose. Vomiting or diarrhea may occur.**

228. ℞ *n*-Butyl chloride

For ascarids and hookworms: **orally, 1 ml/5 lb (2.3 kg) body wt, up to 15 lb (7 kg); 1 ml for each additional 10 lb (4.5 kg). Maximum dose 5 ml.**
For whipworms: **orally, 0.6 to 1.0 ml/lb (0.5 kg) body wt, following 18-hr starvation period.**

229. ℞ Cambendazole paste, bolus, crumbles or pellets

Cattle: **11.5 mg/lb (25 mg/kg) body wt.**
Horses: **9 mg/lb (20 mg/kg) body wt.**
Sheep: **9 to 11.5 mg/lb (20 to 25 mg/kg) body wt.**
Swine: **9 mg/lb (20 mg/kg) body wt.**

Read introduction to prescriptions, pp. 1526 to 1527. Note all warnings and cautions appearing on drug labels and observe all local laws and regulations pertaining to drug usage.

230. ℞ Carbon disulfide

Horses: orally, 2 ml/100 lb (45.5 kg) body wt, not to exceed 20 ml.
Swine: orally, 8 to 10 ml/100 lb body wt, after 36-hr starvation period. Give in capsules or via stomach tube.

231. ℞ Diethylcarbamazine citrate

Dogs: orally, 25 to 50 mg/lb (55 to 110 mg/kg) body wt.

232. ℞ Dichlorophen

Dogs and cats: orally, 90 mg/lb (198 mg/kg) body wt, given immediately before feeding.

233. ℞ Dichlorophene-toluene ("Difolin") capsules

Cats and dogs: Dichlorophene, 100 mg/lb (220 mg/kg) body wt; toluene, 120 mg/lb (264 mg/kg) body wt, orally. Withhold food before treatment. A mild saline cathartic may be desirable.

234. ℞ Dichlorvos

Horses: in feed, 14 to 19 mg/lb (31 to 41 mg/kg) body wt, as a single dose or in a divided dose 8 to 12 hr later.
Swine: Up to 70 lb (32 kg) body wt: 0.0384% medicated feed for 2 days.
70+ lb body wt: 8.4 lb of 0.0384% medicated feed per animal.
For boars, open or bred gilts: Divide above dose in half and feed for 2 days.
Dogs: orally, 15 to 24 mg/lb (33 to 53 mg/kg) body wt.

235. ℞ Diethylcarbamazine

For heartworm prophylaxis: orally, 2.5 mg/lb (5.5 mg/kg) body wt, daily from start of mosquito season until 2 mo. after it ends.
For ascariasis (Sm. An.) and canine strongyloidosis: orally, 13 to 25 mg/lb (29 to 55 mg/kg) body wt. Administer only after feeding.
For lungworms: parenterally, 10 mg/lb (22 mg/kg) body wt, daily for 3 successive days or 20 mg/lb (44 mg/kg) once. Effective against immature but not against adult lungworms.

For standard equivalents for measures, see pp. 1521 to 1524.

236. ℞ Disophenol

For the common hookworm (Ancylostoma caninum) of dogs: subcut., 0.1 ml/lb (0.2 ml/kg) body wt, once.
For Uncinaria stenocephala: subcut., 0.13 ml/lb (0.29 ml/kg) body wt.

237. ℞ Dithiazanine iodide

For large roundworms: orally, 10 mg/lb (22 mg/kg) body wt, for 5 days.
For microfilariae of heartworms and Ancylostoma caninum: orally, 5 mg/lb (11 mg/kg) 7 to 10 days.
For hookworm and whipworm: orally, 10 mg/lb (22 mg/kg) for 10 days.
For intestinal threadworms: orally, 10 mg/lb for 3 weeks.

238. ℞ Fenbendazole

For large and small strongyles and pinworms; horses, sheep, swine: orally, 2.3 mg/lb (5 mg/kg) body wt.
Cattle: orally, 3.4 mg/lb (7.5 mg/kg).

239. ℞ Fenbendazole

For ascarids in horses, sheep, swine: orally, 4.6 mg/lb (10 mg/kg).

240. ℞ Haloxon

Cattle: orally, 20 mg/lb (44 mg/kg) body wt.
Sheep and goats: orally, 16 to 23 mg/lb (35 to 50 mg/kg) body wt.

241. ℞ Hexylresorcinol

Puppies: 0.2 to 0.4 gm.
Adult dogs: 0.6 to 1.0 gm.
Give orally in coated tablets or capsules after 12-hr fast. Follow with saline cathartic after 24 hours.

242. ℞ Hygromycin

12 gm/ton (0.0013%) of complete ration, fed continuously.

243. ℞ Lead arsenate

Calves: 1 gm.
Mature cattle: 2 gm.
Sheep: 0.5 to 1.0 gm.
Given orally and followed by castor oil.

Read introduction to prescriptions, pp. 1526 to 1527. Note all warnings and cautions appearing on drug labels and observe all local laws and regulations pertaining to drug usage.

244. ℞ Levamisole drench, bolus, pellet or water formulation
Cattle, sheep and swine: 2 to 5 mg/lb (4 to 11 mg/kg) body wt.

245. ℞ Mebendazole
Dogs: orally, 10 mg/lb (22 mg/kg) body wt, once daily for 5 days.

246. ℞ Mebendazole
Horses: orally, 4 mg/lb (8.8 mg/kg) body wt.

247. ℞ Oxfendazole
Cattle: orally, 2 mg/lb (4.5 mg/kg) body wt.
Sheep: orally, 2.3 mg/lb (5 mg/kg) body wt.

248. ℞ Niclosamide
Cattle: drench, 22 mg/lb (48 mg/kg) body wt.
Sheep: drench, 35 mg/lb (77 mg/kg) body wt.
Dogs and cats: orally, 50 mg/lb (110 mg/kg) body wt. Effective against large dog and cat tapeworms, but not *Echinococcus* spp. or *Dipylidium* sp.

249. ℞ Niclosamide
90 mg/oz (3 mg/gm) of feed for 24 to 36 hr, to provide 215 mg/lb (450 mg/kg) body wt. Repeat in 8 to 10 days.

250. ℞ Piperazine-carbon disulfide complex ("Parvex")
Horses: Administer via stomach tube, 20 to 40 gm/500 lb (90 to 182 mg/kg) body wt.
Swine: 60 mg/lb (130 mg/kg) body wt, mixed in about one-fourth of the daily ration.

251. ℞ Piperazine-carbon disulfide complex with phenothiazine ("Parvex Plus")
Horses: Administer by stomach tube, 1 fl oz/100 lb (0.7 ml/kg) body wt.

252. ℞ Phenothiazine
Cattle: orally, 10 gm/100 lb (220 mg/kg) body wt, not to exceed 60 gm. *Prophylactically*, feed 2 gm daily for a month following therapeutic dosing.
Sheep: orally, 12.5 gm for lambs under 50 lb (23 kg), 25 gm for adults.
Horses: orally, 3 gm/100 lb (66 mg/kg) body wt. Do not exceed 30 gm.

For standard equivalents for measures, see pp. 1521 to 1524.

253. ℞ Phthalofyne

Orally *or* IV: 100 mg/lb (220 mg/kg) body wt, given once.
Caution: Use IV only when oral treatment is impractical.

254. ℞ Piperazine hexahydrate

Growing pigs: 50 mg of piperazine base per lb (110 mg/kg) body wt in drinking water (withhold all drinking water for the preceding 24 hours).

255. ℞ Piperazine salt of niclosamide ("Mansonil")

Cattle: 28 mg/lb (62 mg/kg) body wt, as a drench.
Sheep: 42 mg/lb (92 mg/kg) body wt, as a drench.
Dog, cats: orally, 55 mg/lb (120 mg/kg).

256. ℞ Piperazine salts

Salt	*% Active Piperazine*
Adipate	37
Chloride	48
Citrate	35
Dihydrochloride	50–53
Hexahydrate	44
Phosphate	42
Sulfate	46

Doses are given in terms of piperazine base (see above). For specific dosages, see product information.
Cattle, sheep, horses, swine, most large zoo animals: orally, 50 mg/lb (110 mg/kg) body wt.
Cats, dogs: orally, 20 to 30 mg/lb (45 to 65 mg/kg) body wt.
Laboratory rats and mice: orally, 400 to 500 mg/100 ml drinking water.

257. ℞ Pyrantel embonate

Horses: orally, 8.7 mg/lb (19 mg/kg) body wt.

258. ℞ Pyrantel pamoate solution

Each ml contains: 2.27 mg of pyrantel base. Orally *or* in feed, 1 ml/lb (2.2 ml/kg) body wt.

259. ℞ Pyrantel pamoate

For hookworms and roundworms in dogs: orally, 7 mg/lb (15 mg/kg) body wt, once.

Read introduction to prescriptions, pp. 1526 to 1527. Note all warnings and cautions appearing on drug labels and observe all local laws and regulations pertaining to drug usage.

260. ℞ Pyrantel tartrate

Horses: 5 gm/100 lb (110 mg/kg) body wt, given in the feed.
Swine: 10 mg/lb (22 mg/kg) body wt, given in the feed.

261. ℞ Sulfadimethoxine-ormetoprim ("Rofenaid 40")

In feed: sulfadimethoxine 0.0125% and ormetoprim 0.0075%.

262. ℞ Styrylpyridinium-diethylcarbamazine ("Styrid/Caricide") tablets

Each tablet contains:

Styrylpyridinium chloride	50 mg
Diethylcarbamazine citrate	60 mg

For *control of hookworms* and the *prevention of heartworms* in dogs: 1 tablet/20 lb (9 kg).

263. ℞ Thenium closylate

For hookworms in dogs: orally, 25 mg/lb (55 mg/kg)
Pups: daily for 2 days;
Adults: 250 mg/animal b.i.d.

264. ℞ Thiabendazole

For migrating strongyle larvae: orally, 200 mg/lb (440 mg/kg) body wt once (10× normal dose).

265. ℞ Thiabendazole

Cattle, routine worming: orally, 3 gm/100 lb (66 mg/kg) body wt.
For severe parasitism and infection with Cooperia: orally, 5 gm/100 lb (110 mg/kg) body wt.
Sheep, routine worming: drench, 2 gm/100 lb (44 mg/kg) body wt.
For severe parasitism: drench, 3 gm/100 lb (66 mg/kg) body wt.
Swine, for Strongyloides ransomi: paste formulation, at 30 to 40 mg/lb (65 to 90 mg/kg) body wt.
Horses: orally, 20 mg/lb (45 mg/kg) body wt. Double the dose when treating for ascarids.
Laboratory animals: orally, 22 to 45 mg/lb (48 to 100 mg/kg) body wt. Repeat after 2 wk if severely infected.

266. ℞ Thiophanate

Cattle, sheep, goats and swine: drench or mix with feed, 22 to 45 mg/lb (50 to 100 mg/kg) body wt.

For standard equivalents for measures, see pp. 1521 to 1524.

267. ℞ Toluene

Cats and dogs: orally, 100 mg/lb (220 mg/kg) body wt.

268. ℞ Trichlorfon 12.3% w/v solution

Horses: Administer by stomach tube, ½ fl oz/100 lb (0.3 ml/kg) body wt.

Insecticides and Acaricides

269. ℞ Benzylbenzoate 25.0%
Lindane 1.0%

In emulsion or ointment base.
Dogs only: Apply thoroughly to affected areas daily on alternate weeks or every third day.

270. ℞ Benzylbenzoate 25 or 50%, emulsion

Dogs only: Apply thoroughly to affected areas.

271. ℞ "Canex" Solution
Chloroform . . . . 7.5 %
Rotenone 0.12%
Other ether extractives of derris . . 0.38%
Inert ingredients 92.00%

Cats and dogs: Thoroughly massage into affected areas.

272. ℞ Caraway oil . . . . 1 part
Petrolatum . . . . 4 parts

Apply to affected areas of skin.

273. ℞ Chlordane 0.5% dip

Bathe animal or sponge on and let dry. Repeat after 7 days if necessary.

274. ℞ Chlorpyrifos 43.2% ("Dursban 44') concentrate solution

Apply to one spot at the top mid-line area of the animal, just behind the shoulder blades and neck junction. Use at the rate of 2 ml/100 lb (45.5 kg) body wt up to 800 lb (364 kg).

275. ℞ "Ciovap" emulsible
Crotoxyphos . . . . 10 %
Dichlorvos 2.3%

Read introduction to prescriptions, pp. 1526 to 1527. Note all warnings and cautions appearing on drug labels and observe all local laws and regulations pertaining to drug usage.

Related compounds to 2.5% dichlorvos 0.2%

Cattle, sheep, goats, swine: Use as spray in dilutions of 0.25, 0.5 or 1.0% on animals or around pen areas.

276. ℞ Coumaphos 0.25% suspension or emulsion (dip or spray)

Agitate dip suspension thoroughly prior to each use to assure uniform suspension during use. Dip animals in standard fashion. Use high-pressure spray to wet skin.

277. ℞ Coumaphos 0.03 to 0.06% suspension or emulsion

For lactating dairy cattle: 0.03%.
Beef cattle, sheep, goats and swine: 0.06%.
Use as spray or dip.

278. ℞ Coumaphos 0.375 to 0.5% suspension or emulsion

Spray cattle: wetting skin thoroughly. Spray pressures of 300 lb or higher recommended. Maintain adequate agitation in spray tank to insure uniform suspension or emulsion during use. The higher concentration needed in northern areas, or for late fall application when long hair coats make thorough wetting of the skin difficult.

279. ℞ Coumaphos 0.5% dust

Use 1 to 2 oz (28 to 57 gm) per animal on sheep or goats.
For control of lice on dogs: dust thoroughly under the hair over the entire body.

280. ℞ Coumaphos 1% oil solution or dust

Cattle: Apply not more than 2 oz (60 ml)/animal.
Swine: For bedding treatment of swine, apply 2 oz/30 sq ft (55 gm/8 sq m) not more than 1 oz/animal.
Caution: Do not treat swine or bedding more often than every 10 days.

281. ℞ Coumaphos 1% oil solution

For saturating back rubbers use 1 gal./20 ft (0.6 L/m) of cable.

For standard equivalents for measures, see pp. 1521 to 1524.

282. ℞ Coumaphos 4% solution (pour-on)

Pour evenly along animal's backline ½ fl oz/100 lb (0.3 ml/kg) body wt.

283. ℞ Crotoxyphos ("Ciodrin") emulsible concentrate

Use in appropriate dilutions (0.25, 0.5, 1.0 or 2.0%) and spray on animals,
or **use 1% in oil solution for back rubbers.**

284. ℞ Diazinon suspension or emulsion

Sheep and dogs: **0.03%.**
For use in fly control, spray appropriate animal quarters using 1% suspension or emulsion.

285. ℞ Dichlorvos 0.5 to 10% oil-base spray (May include pyrethrins and synergist)

Apply by hand or electric atomizer or automatic cattle sprayer at not over 2 fl oz (60 ml) per cow daily.

286. ℞ Dichlorvos 20% resin strip

Hang one strip for every 1,000 cu ft (28 cu m) of enclosed area. Replace in 4 months.

287. ℞ Dimethoate 1% emulsion

Use as residual spray for premises only.

288. ℞ Dioxathion 1.5% oil solution

For saturating back rubbers at 1 gal./20 ft (3.8 L/6 m) of cable.

289. ℞ Famophos 13.2% pour-on concentrate solution

Pour evenly along animal's backline: ½ fl oz/100 lb (0.3 ml/kg) body wt; maximum 4 fl oz (120 ml)/animal.

290. ℞ Fenthion 1 or 3% emulsion

For flies and mosquitoes (1% emulsion): **Use as residual spray for premises spraying only.**
For cattle grubs (3% solution): **Apply pour-on evenly along backline, ½ fl oz/100 lb (0.3 ml/kg) of body wt.**

Read introduction to prescriptions, pp. 1526 to 1527. Note all warnings and cautions appearing on drug labels and observe all local laws and regulations pertaining to drug usage.

291. ℞ Fenthion 8% pour-on

Apply at 0.5 fl oz/100 lb (0.3 ml/kg) body wt. Pour the correct amount of solution along the backline starting just behind the ears and continuing to the rump. Make second application, if needed, no sooner than 35 days after first treatment.

292. ℞ Lime and sulfur solution (30 to 32% calcium polysulfide)

Dilute in ratio of 1:16 of water, and apply as dip or wash.

Large animals: Treatment repeated at 10- to 12-day intervals. Use at 95 to 105°F (35 to 40.5°C) against *Psoroptes ovis.*

Dogs and cats: Treatment repeated at 5-day intervals.

293. ℞ Lindane 0.012, 0.03 or 0.06%

Use as a wash, dip or spray. Repeat as indicated.

294. ℞ Lindane 0.03% emulsion or suspension

For beef cattle, calves and swine.

295. ℞ Lindane 1% emulsion

As a roost paint: Apply 1 pt/150 ft (0.5 L/45 m) of roost. Head lice are not controlled by this method. Effective for a month.

As a litter spray: Apply just enough to wet the surface of the litter. Effective for 3 months.

296. ℞ Malathion 0.5% suspension or emulsion

May be used in a spray, as a dip or in an oil solution.

297. ℞ Malathion 2% emulsion or oil solution

As a roost paint (emulsion): 1 pt/150 ft (11 ml/m) of roost. Repeat after 10 days or as necessary. Head lice are not controlled by this method.

As house spray (emulsion): Apply liberally to walls, ceilings, roosts, litter, nests and adjacent areas. Will control poultry mites as well as lice.

For saturating back rubbers (oil solution) 1 gal./20 ft (0.6 L/m) of cable.

298. ℞ Malathion 4% dust

Liberally dust litter, floor space, nests, roosts, using approximately 1 lb/40 sq ft (125 gm/sq m) or use 2 lb (1 kg) per dusting box. A 2- by 3-ft (0.6 × 1 m) box will care for 100 hens.

Use a shaker can or rotary duster to treat individual

birds—1 lb (450 gm)/160 birds. Repeat after 4 to 8 weeks or when necessary.

299. ℞ Malathion Ultra Low Volume 91% (ULV)

Apply to feedlots and holding pens in dilution containing 6 to 8 oz/acre (415 to 554 gm/ha).

300. ℞ Methoprene 0.02% mineral mix or block

Place medicated feed in diat daily throughout horn-fly season. Place block in pasture. Recommended consumption of medicament 0.25 to 0.5 lb/100 lb (2.4 to 5 gm/kg) of body wt per month.

301. ℞ Methoxychlor 0.5% suspension

For stable fly control by spraying of premises only.

For flies and mosquitoes, or pediculosis: Use 2 or 5 times the concentration, respectively.

302. ℞ Methoxychlor 50% wettable powder

For hornfly control on dairy cattle, use ½ oz (15 gm) per animal, on back only, every 3 weeks. *For sheep keds and lice,* use ½ oz (15 gm) per animal after shearing.

303. ℞ "Mulzyl"

Benzyl benzoate	20 %
Gamma benzene hexachloride . . .	0.9 %
Chlorobutanol (chloral derivative) .	0.5 %
Phenylmercuric borate	0.02%

Give 2 to 3 applications at intervals of 4 to 7 days. Do not get in the eye.

304. ℞ Naled 1% oil solution or emulsion

Spray oil solution around animal areas and housing. Emulsion, at appropriate levels, may be sprayed by aircraft.

305. ℞ Nicotine sulfate 40%

As a roost paint: Use 0.5 lb/100 ft (225 gm/30 m) of perch. Apply just before roosting time and provide adequate ventilation. Repeat after 10 days.

NOTE: Head lice will not be controlled by this method.

306. ℞ Phosmet 0.25% emulsion

Apply as a high-pressure spray; wet the skin thoroughly. Apply about 1 gal. (4 L) per adult animal.

Read introduction to prescriptions, pp. 1526 to 1527. Note all warnings and cautions appearing on drug labels and observe all local laws and regulations pertaining to drug usage.

07. ℞ Phosmet 3.8% emulsion (pour-on)

Pour evenly along backline 1 fl oz/100 lb (0.65 ml/kg) body wt; maximum 8 fl oz (240 ml) per animal.

08. ℞ Pyrethrins 0.025% and Piperonyl butoxide 0.25%, emulsion

2½ gal. (9.5L) of concentrate containing 1% pyrethrins and 10% piperonyl butoxide or MGK 264 in 100 gal. (379 L) of water.
NOTE: *For all birds and mammals.*

09. ℞ Synergized pyrethrum emulsion

Pyrethrins	0.05%
Piperonyl butoxide	0.5 %

For spray: Dilute a 1% pyrethrin concentrate with 9 parts of water and use about 1 qt (1 L) per animal. Repeat application when fly annoyance recommences.
For automatic treadle sprayers: Use concentration to 0.5%, apply 2 ml b.i.d. MGK 264 may be used instead of piperonyl butoxide.
For space spraying against adult mosquitoes, use Microsol Fog machine.

10. ℞ Synergized pyrethrum oil-base spray

Pyrethrins	0.05 to 0.1%
Piperonyl butoxide	0.40 to 0.8%
Cattle spray base oil	99.55 to 99.1%

Apply by hand or electric atomizer at milking time, not exceeding 2 fl oz (60 ml) per cow. Also useful on any mammal to repel and kill flies. May be used in the milk room, or residence at 2 fl oz/1,000 cu ft (2 ml/cu m) of space.

11. ℞ Synergized pyrethrum and repellent spray

Pyrethrins	0.03 to 0.1%
Synergist	0.25 to 1.0%
Repellent	0.2 to 8.0%
Cattle spray base oil	99.52 to 90.9%

The repellent may be Stabilene, MGK 11 or MGK 326. The synergist may be piperonyl butoxide, MGK 264 or sulfoxide.
For use on all mammals including dairy cows. Apply lightly with a hand or electric atomizer, wetting hair ends only, not over 2 fl oz (60 ml) per animal. Repeat as necessary.

For standard equivalents for measures, see pp. 1521 to 1524.

312. ℞ "Ravap" emulsible concentrate

Stirofos	0.35%
Dichlorvos	0.10%

Beef cattle: Use ½ to 1 gal. (2 to 4 L) of spray per animal depending on size and hair coat.

313. ℞ "Ravap" emulsible concentrate

Stirofos	1.0 %
Dichlorvos	0.25%

Use as spray, ½ to 1 gal. (2 to 4 L) of 0.45% solution; or in oil solution for back rubbers at 1 gal./20 ft. (0.6L/m).

314. ℞ Ronnel 0.25, 0.5 or 1% emulsion

As a dip or for sponging animals: 0.25% emulsion.
Sheep or goats: For wool maggots, use as a spray or dip: 0.5% emulsion.
For residual spray for spraying of premises, or for saturated back rubbers (1% emulsion or in oil solution): 1 gal./20 ft (3.8 L/6 m) of cable.
Cats: 0.25% emulsion.
Dogs: 1% emulsion, sponge 3 times at 7- to 10-day intervals.

315. ℞ Ronnel 0.26% in feed

Feed 5 oz of the medicated feed per 100 lb (3 gm/kg) body wt, per day for 14 consecutive days. Mix thoroughly with the daily feed ration. The balance of the daily ration should not include ronnel-medicated feed.

316. ℞ Ronnel 2.5% pressurized spray

Spray infested area liberally, working toward the center of the infestation. Shearing or removing the wool from the infested area is not necessary. Retreat at 5- to 7-day intervals as needed.

317. ℞ Ronnel 5% granules

Apply ½ lb/100 sq ft (25 gm/sq m) of bedding.

318. ℞ Ronnel 5.5% mineral block or granules

Feed continuously free-choice, summer and fall for a period of at least 75 days. Consumption should be 0.25 lb/100 lb (2.5 gm/kg) body wt, per month for effective grub control and throughout horn-fly season.

Read introduction to prescriptions, pp. 1526 to 1527. Note all warnings and cautions appearing on drug labels and observe all local laws and regulations pertaining to drug usage.

319. ℞ Ronnel tablets (250 mg) *or* emulsion (1%)

Demodectic mange: both oral and topical treatment.
Orally: Tablets (in divided doses) at 25 mg/lb (55 mg/kg) body wt, daily.
Topically: Apply over entire body every 4 days. Both oral and topical application continued for a 30-day period.

320. ℞ Rotenone 0.0125% suspension*

***For all animals* except swine: 1 lb (450 gm) cube- or derris-root powder containing 5% rotenone per 100 gal. (379 L) of water; 20 lb (9.1 kg) wettable sulfur may be added per 100 gal. (380 L) of water to increase ease of preparation of the dip and effectiveness.**
***0.5 lb (225 gm) detergent per 100 gal. (380 L) of water facilitates wetting and mixing.**

321. ℞ Rotenone 0.5% suspension*

4 lb cube- or derris-root powder containing 5% rotenone per 5 gal. (2 kg/20 L) of water. For external application. Keep mixture well agitated.
***½ oz (15 gm) detergent per 5 gal. (20 L) of water facilitates emulsification.**

322. ℞ Rotenone 1% dust

Cube- or derris-root powder containing 5% rotenone	20 lb (9.1 kg)
Diluent (talc, clay, sulfur, etc.)	78 lb (35.4 kg)

For range flock sheep ked and louse control.
For birds and mammals, except swine.
***Dust all birds thoroughly:* 1 lb (450 gm) per 100 birds.**

323. ℞ Rotenone powder

Rotenone	1.00%
Other cube extractives	1.66%
Pyrethrins	0.54%

Sprinkle on coat and rub thoroughly. Repeat after 3 days if necessary. Dusting bedding and quarters with this powder is advisable.

324. ℞ "Goodwinol" ointment

Rotenone	1%
Orthophenylphenol, ethylaminobenzoate and lanolins in water-in-oil absorption base	

Apply t.i.d. to affected areas of skin after cleansing.

For standard equivalents for measures, see pp. 1521 to 1524.

325. ℞ Stirofos 0.009% feed mix or mineral block

0.25 lb/100 lb (2.5 gm/kg) body wt per month. Provide one mineral-mix feeder or block for each 15 to 20 head of cattle. Feed throughout the horn-fly season.

326. ℞ Stirofos 0.35% suspension or emulsion

Use ½ to 1 gal. (2 to 4 L) of spray per animal.

327. ℞ Stirofos 1% suspension or emulsion

Apply 1 gal. (3.8 L) of solution per 500 to 1,000 sq ft (45 to 90 sq m) to walls, ceilings, posts, fences, under troughs or other fly-gathering areas.

328. ℞ Stirofos 0.5 or 1% emulsion

Beef cattle: Apply 1% oil emulsion.
Swine: Apply 0.5% emulsion as a coarse spray using 1 to 2 qt (1 to 2 L) per head to thoroughly wet the animal. Repeat in 2 weeks if necessary.

329. ℞ Stirofos 3% dust

Cattle: Apply by hand at 2 oz (60 gm) per animal or by dust bag. Forced use of dust bags is preferred. Free-choice aids in control. For free-choice use, hang one bag per 25 to 30 animals.
Swine: Apply 3 to 4 oz (90 to 120 gm) of dust by conventional hand or power duster to each animal with special attention given to the neck and around the ears. In severe infestations of swine, both individual animals and bedding may be treated. 1 lb (450 gm) of dust should be applied per 150 sq ft (14 sq m) of bedding.

330. ℞

Stirofos	1.0 %
Pyrethrum	0.09%
Piperonyl butoxide	0.18%
Repellent	1.3 %

Horses: As protection from flies (face, house, stable, horse, deer, horn), biting gnats and mosquitoes. Apply solution as wipe-on or spray.

331. ℞ Stirofos 1% and pyrethrins 0.09%

Horses: Apply as spray or wipe-on at 1 to 2 fl oz (30 to 60 ml) per animal. Be sure to apply to inside of ear.

Read introduction to prescriptions, pp. 1526 to 1527. Note all warnings and cautions appearing on drug labels and observe all local laws and regulations pertaining to drug usage.

332. ℞ Stirofos 2% and pyrethrins 0.09%
Apply thin film of gel to head, neck, belly and forelegs. Treat ears well.

333. ℞ Sulfur Ointment USP
Apply thoroughly to affected areas once a day.

334. ℞ "Thionium" shampoo with lindane
Potassium tetrathionate 2.00%
Lindane 0.25%
Use for routine shampooing of dogs.

335. ℞ Toxaphene 0.5% emulsion
For use on beef cattle, horses, sheep or swine.

336. ℞ Toxaphene 5% oil solution
For saturating back rubbers at 1 gal./50 ft (250 ml/m) of cable.

337. ℞ Trichlorfon 1 or 8% (pour-on) solution
Spray cattle, wetting skin thoroughly (1% solution): Spray pressures of 300 lb or higher recommended.
8% Pour-on: Pour evenly along animal's backline, ½ fl oz/100 lb (0.33 ml/kg) body wt.

Antiprotozoan Agents

338. ℞ Amicarbalide diisethionate 50% solution
For babesiosis in cattle: IM, subcut. or slow IV injection, 2.3 mg/lb (5 mg/kg) body wt.
For peracute cases in adult cattle: double the dose. Repeat if hemoglobinuria persists beyond 24 hours.

339. ℞ Amprolium
For avian coccidiosis: 0.024 or 0.012% in drinking water, for 5 to 7 days. Reduce to 0.006% for an additional 2 weeks.

340. ℞ Amprolium
For mammalian coccidiosis: Calves: Prophylactic use: 225 mg/100 lb (5 mg/kg) body wt, daily in feed or drinking water for 21 days.
Therapeutic use: 450 mg/100 lb (10 mg/kg) body wt, in feed or drinking water for 5 days.

For standard equivalents for measures, see pp. 1521 to 1524.

341. ℞ Decoquinate

Cattle: Prophylactic use: orally, 23 mg/100 lb (0.5 mg/kg) body wt, for at least 28 days.

342. ℞ Carbarsone

Turkeys: Prophylaxis: 0.0375% (340 gm/ton) in feed continuously until 5 days before marketing.

343. ℞ Dimetridazole

Prophylaxis: 225 mg/lb (500 mg/kg) of feed, continuously until 5 days before marketing.
Treatment: (soluble powder) 0.05% (1.25 gm/L) in water for 6 days followed by preventive feed medication.

344. ℞ Diminazene aceturate

For babesiosis in cow, horse, sheep and dog, and for Trypanosoma vivax and T. congolense: subcut. or IM, a single dose of 1.4 mg/lb (3.5 mg/kg) body wt will usually relieve clinical signs in 24 hours.
For persistent trypanosome infections: 3.6 mg/lb (8 mg/kg) body wt may be given. Maximum dose is 4 gm. Local reactions at site of infection may be severe in horses.

345. ℞ Ethidium bromide 1% aqueous solution

Active against Trypanosoma congolense and T. vivax; less active against T. brucei; inactive against T. evansi.
Treatment: subcut. *or* preferably IM, 45 mg/100 lb (45.5 kg) body wt.

346. ℞ Furazolidone

Hexamitiasis: Prophylaxis: 0.0055% (25 mg/lb) of ration. Feed continuously.
Treatment: 0.011% (50 mg/lb) of ration. Feed 2 or 3 weeks.
Histomoniasis: Prophylaxis: 0.011% (50 mg/lb) of feed. Feed continuously.
Treatment: 0.0165% (75 mg/lb) of feed. Feed 2 or 3 weeks.

347. ℞ Homidium bromide ("Ethidium")

Horses and cattle: IV, IM *or* subcut., 0.45 to 0.7 mg/lb (1.0 to 1.5 mg/kg) body wt.
Dogs: IV, IM or subcut., 0.45 mg/lb (1.0 mg/kg) body wt.

Read introduction to prescriptions, pp. 1526 to 1527. Note all warnings and cautions appearing on drug labels and observe all local laws and regulations pertaining to drug usage.

348. ℞ Imidocarb dipropionate 10% solution
Horses: IM *or* IV, 1.0 mg/lb (2 mg/kg) of body wt. (Twice for *B. caballi;* 4 times at 72-hour intervals for *B. equi.*)
Dogs: IV *or* IM, 2.0 mg/lb (4 mg/kg) of body wt.

349. ℞ Isometamidium ("Samorin")
Treatment: IM, 0.5 to 1.0 mg/lb (1.0 to 2.0 mg/kg) body wt (½ this dose in dogs).
Prophylaxis: IM, 0.2 to 0.5 mg/lb (0.5 to 1.0 mg/kg).

350. ℞ Lasalocid
Calves: Prophylactic use: 1.4 mg/lb (3 mg/kg) body wt fed continuously.

351. ℞ Nitarsone
0.01875% (164 gm/ton) of feed until 5 days before marketing.

352. ℞ Pamaquine naphthoate
IM: 2.2 to 4.5 mg/lb (5 to 10 mg/kg) body wt, daily.

353. ℞ Phenamidine isethionate 2% solution
Subcut.: 0.25 ml/lb (0.55 ml/kg) body wt.

354. ℞ Phenanthridinium, Pyrimidinium ("Prothidium")
Prophylaxis: 1 mg/lb (2 mg/kg) body wt provides protection for 3 to 5 months.

355. ℞ "Polystat-3"

Butynorate	0.02%
Sulfanitran	0.03%
Dinsed	0.02%
Roxarsone	0.0025 to 0.005%

Use level in feed.
Turkeys: For coccidiosis (E. meleagridis, E. melagrimitis, E. gallopavonis), large roundworms, tapeworms and hexamitiasis.
Chickens: For preventing coccidiosis (E. tenella, E. necatrix, E. acervulina), large roundworms and tapeworms.

356. ℞ Quinacrine hydrochloride
Dogs (large breeds): 200 mg t.i.d. on the 1st day and twice during each of the subsequent 6 days; *(small breeds):* 100 mg, twice on the 1st day and once daily for each of the next 6 days; *(puppies):* 50 mg, twice a day for 6 days.
Concurrent administration of sodium bicarbonate

For standard equivalents for measures, see pp. 1521 to 1524.

aids in preventing vomiting.

357. ℞ Quinacrine hydrochloride . . . . . . 0.9 gm
Diiodohydroxyquin . . . . 0.9 gm
Water . . . . 100 ml

Spray the solution with an atomizer onto the pellets and hay until the food ingredients are slightly damp. Approximately 0.5 ml are used per animal daily for 2 weeks. Fresh mixture should be prepared daily.

358. ℞ Quinapyramine sulfate

Treatment: subcut., 2.0 mg/lb (4.4 mg/kg) body wt in a 10% solution. Careful weight estimation is needed. Animals should be handled quietly at treatment time, and provided with shade and water. *In horses,* divide dose and give in 2 or 3 sites, or better, give ½ dose and then a second half-dose 5 to 6 hours later. There are occasional anaphylactic-type reactions in Equidae.
Prophylaxis: The soluble sulfate is combined (3:2) with the less soluble chloride. Subcut., 0.114 ml/10 lb (0.025 ml/kg) body wt of a solution containing 166 mg of the mixed salts per milliliter. Must be repeated at 2- to 3-month intervals. A hard nodular swelling persists at the injection site for months or years.

359. ℞ Quinuronium sulfate ("Acaprin") 5% solution

Cattle: IM *or* subcut., 1 ml/100 lb (45.5 kg) body wt.
Dogs: IM *or* subcut., 1 ml/45 lb (21 kg) body wt.

360. ℞ Ronidazole

Turkeys: Prophylaxis: 0.006 to 0.012% (60 to 120 ppm) medicated feed, depending on severity of exposure.
Therapy: For severe outbreaks, 0.006% in drinking water for 10 to 14 days (then give in medicated feed at 60 ppm for prophylaxis).

361. ℞ Sulfamethazine

For all species of coccidia in chickens and turkeys: Given either as 30 ml of a 12.5% solution per gal. (3.8 L) of drinking water

Read introduction to prescriptions, pp. 1526 to 1527. Note all warnings and cautions appearing on drug labels and observe all local laws and regulations pertaining to drug usage.

or 0.4% (8 lb/ton of feed) in all-mash ration. Given for 3 days, followed by unmedicated feed or water for 3 days, then an additional 3 days of treatment. After 3 more days on plain feed or water, it may be necessary to repeat treatment for 1 or 2 days.

362. ℞ Sulfaquinoxaline sodium

For coccidiosis in chickens: 0.04% in drinking water *or* 0.1% in the feed, given for the first 48 or 72 hr, followed by 3 days on plain feed or water, then 0.05% in the feed *or* 0.025% in drinking water for two 2-day periods with a 3-day unmedicated interval.

For coccidiosis in turkeys: 0.025%, in the drinking water

or 0.05% in an all-mash ration, given for 3 days, then unmedicated water or feed for 3 days, then repeat treatment for 3 days. An additional 1 or 2 days of treatment following another 3 days' rest may be necessary.

363. ℞ Suramin

For trypanosomiasis: Administer IV as a 10% solution. Special care must be taken in calculating the doses for Equidae.

Treatment: Horses: IV, 320 to 455 mg/100 lb (7 to 10 mg/kg) body wt, 2 or 3 times at weekly intervals.

Cattle: IV, 545 mg/100 lb (12 mg/kg).

Camels: IV, 365 to 545 mg/100 lb (8 to 12 mg/kg).

Prophylaxis: to be repeated at 10-day intervals;

Horses, 2 gm;

Camels, 1 to 2 gm.

Antifungal Agents

364. ℞ Amphotericin B, 0.1% solution in 5% dextrose

IV slowly: at 125 to 250 mcg/lb (275 to 550 mcg/kg) on alternate days or twice weekly. Total cumulative doses in excess of 5 mg/lb (11 mg/kg) are associated with nephrotoxicity. Fever, chilling and nausea may be relieved with aspirin and antihistamines. BUN should be monitored and treatment suspended when levels exceed 75 mg% or when vomiting occurs.

365. ℞ Griseofulvin tablets

25 mg/lb (55 mg/kg) body wt daily until skin or claws are negative for fungi (at least 3 to 4 weeks).

For standard equivalents for measures, see pp. 1521 to 1524.

366. ℞ Griseofulvin

Guinea pigs: Feed in the daily diet at 2.5 mg/100 gm body wt.
Primates: orally, 25 mg/kg body wt, for at least 3 to 4 weeks.

367. ℞ Nystatin oral suspension (100,000 u/ml)

Orally: 1 ml, q.i.d. Continue for 48 hr after clinical recovery.

368. ℞ Nystatin tablets (500,000 u)

1 tablet t.i.d. for 10 or more days.

369. ℞ Nystatin ointment (100,000 u/gm)

Apply to lesions b.i.d. or t.i.d.

370. ℞ "Sporastacin" cream

Chlordantoin 1.00%
Benzalkonium chloride 0.05%

Apply to affected area once or twice daily as required.

371. ℞ Salicylic acid (3%), benzoic acid (6%)

For skin infections: Use topically in ointment or alcoholic solution.

372. ℞ Thiabendazole

57 to 113 gm of thiabendazole per 20 gal. of water per acre (1.8 to 3.6 gm/L/ha). Powder is thoroughly suspended in water and evenly sprayed onto pastures by boom or aerial spray during dry, still weather conditions.

373. ℞ Tolnaftate cream 1%

Apply cream to each lesion and massage gently b.i.d. for 2 to 3 weeks.

Tranquilizers

374. ℞ Acepromazine maleate

Horses: Give IV, IM *or* subcut., 2.0 to 4.0 mg/100 lb (0.044 to 0.088 mg/kg) body wt.
Dogs: 0.25 to 0.5 mg/lb (0.6 to 1.1 mg/kg) body wt.
Cats: 0.5 to 1.0 mg/lb (1.1 to 2.2 mg/kg) body wt.

Read introduction to prescriptions, pp. 1526 to 1527. Note all warnings and cautions appearing on drug labels and observe all local laws and regulations pertaining to drug usage.

375. ℞ Chlormezanone (chlormethazanone) tablets (200 mg)
50 to 200 mg, t.i.d. or q.i.d.

376. ℞ Chlorpromazine
Small animals: orally, 0.9 to 1.8 mg/lb (2 to 4 mg/kg) body wt every 8 hours.

377. ℞ Chlorpromazine
Large animals: IV, 0.09 to 0.23 mg/lb (0.2 to 0.5 mg/kg) body wt,
or IM, 0.5 to 0.9 mg/lb (1 to 2 mg/kg) body wt, 1 to 4 times a day.
Small animals: orally *or* IM, 0.5 to 1.4 mg/lb (1 to 3 mg/kg) body wt, 1 to 4 times a day. Dose and frequency of administration must be adjusted to response of animal.

378. ℞ Etymemazine
Orally *or* IM, 2 to 5 mg/lb (4.4 to 11 mg/kg) body wt,
or IV, 1 to 2 mg/lb (2 to 4.4 mg/kg) body wt.

379. ℞ Mepazine
Orally *or* parenterally: 5 to 15 mg/lb (11 to 33 mg/kg) body wt. Dose depends on degree of tranquilization required and response of patient.

380. ℞ Meperidine hydrochloride
Dogs: IM *or* subcut., 2.5 to 4.5 mg/lb (6 to 10 mg/kg).
Cats: IM *or* subcut., 0.9 to 1.8 mg/lb (2 to 4 mg/kg). The duration of effect is 1 to 2 hours.

381. ℞ Meprobamate
Dogs: orally, 200 to 400 mg, b.i.d. to t.i.d.

382. ℞ Perphenazine
Large animals: IM *or* IV, 10 mg/100 lb (0.22 mg/kg) body wt.
Small animals: orally, 4 mg/10 lb (1 mg/kg) body wt b.i.d.,
or IM *or* IV, 5 mg/20 lb (5.5 mg/10 kg) body wt.

383. ℞ Promazine hydrochloride
Large animals: IM *or* IV, 20 to 50 mg/100 lb (22 to 55 mg/50 kg) body wt.

For standard equivalents for measures, see pp. 1521 to 1524.

Small animals: orally, IM *or* IV, 1 to 2 mg/lb (2 to 4.5 mg/kg) body wt.
Zoo species: IM, 2 to 4 mg/lb (4.5 to 9 mg/kg). Repeat after 4 to 6 hours if necessary.

384. ℞ Propiopromazine hydrochloride

Large animals: IM *or* IV, 0.05 to 0.1 mg/lb (0.11 to 0.22 mg/kg) body wt. The lower dose given IV is preferred in thoroughbred and standardbred horses.

385. ℞ Propionylpromazine hydrochloride

Small animals: IM *or* IV, 0.1 mg/lb (0.22 mg/kg) body wt.

Eye Medications, topical and systemic

386. ℞ Atropine sulfate 0.26 to 4%, ointment or solution

Ointment: Place small ribbon on eye every 2 to 12 hours.
Solution: Place a drop on eye every 1 to 6 hours.

387. ℞ Atropine sulfate 0.5% ophthalmic ointment

Small amount in the conjunctival sac t.i.d.

388. ℞ Bacitracin ophthalmic ointment (500 u/gm)

Large animals: Apply inside lower lid of affected eye b.i.d.
Small animals: Apply inside lower lid of affected eye t.i.d. or q.i.d.

389. ℞ Chloramphenicol 1% ophthalmic ointment

Apply inside lower lid of affected eye 3 to 6 times daily.

390. ℞ Chloramphenicol (0.5%) ophthalmic solution or (1%) ophthalmic ointment

Place a drop on eye every 2 to 12 hours.

391. ℞ Chlortetracycline 1% ointment

Place small ribbon on eye every 4 to 12 hours.

392. ℞ Demecarium bromide 0.125% solution

One drop into conjunctival sac daily.

Read introduction to prescriptions, pp. 1526 to 1527. Note all warnings and cautions appearing on drug labels and observe all local laws and regulations pertaining to drug usage.

393. ℞ Dichlorphenamide tablets
Orally: 0.9 to 1.8 mg/lb (2 to 4 mg/kg) daily.

394. ℞ Diisopropyl fluorophosphate 0.1% solution in peanut oil
1 to 2 drops into affected eye every 8 to 72 hours.

395. ℞ Epinephrine hydrochloride, borate or bitartrate (0.25 to 2.0%) solution
In glaucoma: a drop on eye every 4 to 12 hr during monitoring of intraocular pressure.

396. ℞ Gentamicin and betamethasone solution ("Gentocin Durafilm")
Each ml contains: gentamicin sulfate equivalent to 3 mg gentamicin base; and 1 mg betamethasone acetate equivalent to 0.089 mg betamethasone alcohol. Give every 2 to 6 hours.
Caution: Do not give when cornea is ulcerated.

397. ℞ Glycerin USP
Orally: *For emergency reduction of intraocular pressure:* 0.5 to 1.0 ml/lb (1 to 2.2 ml/kg) body wt.

398. ℞ Mannitol 20% solution
For preoperative or emergency reduction of intraocular pressure: IV, 0.5 gm/lb (1.1 gm/kg) body wt.

399. ℞ Methylcellulose 0.25 to 1.0% solution
Place 1 to 2 drops on eye every 1 to 6 hours.

400. ℞ Methylprednisolone (40 mg/ml)
Subconjunctivally: 0.5 to 1.0 ml.

401. ℞ Methylprednisolone acetate (20, 40 and 80 mg/ml)
Subconjunctivally: 50 to 80 mg once weekly.
Caution: Do not give when cornea is ulcerated.

402. ℞ Neomycin, polymyxin B and flumethasone ophthalmic solution ("Neomycin F")
Each milliliter contains:

Flumethasone	0.10 mg
Neomycin sulfate (3.5 mg neomycin base)	5.0 mg
Polymyxin B sulfate	10,000 u

Apply every 2 to 6 hr, depending on severity. Do not give when cornea is ulcerated.

For standard equivalents for measures, see pp. 1521 to 1524.

403. ℞ Penicillin ophthalmic ointment (1,000 or 2,000 u/gm)

Apply inside lower lid of affected eye t.i.d. or q.i.d.

404. ℞ Phenylephrine 10% solution

Place a drop in the eye every 4 to 12 hours.

405. ℞ Pilocarpine hydrochloride 1 to 4% solution

Place a drop on eye every 4 to 24 hours. In glaucoma therapy, drug concentration and medication frequency vary with evaluation of intraocularipressure.

406. ℞ Polyvinylpyrrolidone 0.55%
Hydroxyethylcellulose 0.44%

Place 1 to 2 drops of solution on eye every 1 to 6 hours.

407. ℞ Prednisolone acetate solution or ointment

0.12 to 1% solution: **Apply every 2 to 6 hours.**
0.25% ointment: **Apply every 4 to 12 hours.**
Caution: Do not give when cornea is ulcerated.

408. ℞ Prednisolone 21-phosphate with neomycin ophthalmic solution and ointment
Prednisolone 21-phosphate . . . . 5 mg/ml
Neomycin . . . . 5 mg/ml

Inflammation or infection of anterior eye: **Apply in conjunctival sac b.i.d. or t.i.d.**
Otitis externa: **Instill into ear canal with gentle massage: solution t.i.d. to q.i.d., ointment once or twice daily.**

409. ℞ Scopolamine hydrobromide 0.25 to 0.5%
or 0.3% Scopolamine hydrobromide and 10% phenylephrine hydrochloride solution

For maximum mydriasis and cycloplegia: **Place a drop on eye every 1 to 12 hours.**

410. ℞ Sulfacetamide 10% and prednisolone 0.25%

Ointment: **Apply every 4 to 12 hours.**
Solution: **Apply every 2 to 6 hours.**

411. ℞ Sulfathiazole 5% ophthalmic ointment

Apply to conjunctival surface b.i.d. or t.i.d.

Read introduction to prescriptions, pp. 1526 to 1527. Note all warnings and cautions appearing on drug labels and observe all local laws and regulations pertaining to drug usage.

412. ℞ Sulfathiazole 5% and sulfanilamide 5% ophthalmic ointment

Apply to conjunctival surface b.i.d. or t.i.d.

413. ℞ Tetracaine hydrochloride 0.5% solution

1 drop into conjunctival sac every 2 to 3 hours.

414. ℞ Tetracycline hydrochloride 0.5% solution or 1% ointment

Solution: Place a drop on eye every 2 to 6 hours. *Ointment:* Place small ribbon on eye every 4 to 12 hours.

415. ℞ Tropicamide 0.5 to 1.0% solution

Primarily for ophthalmoscopic examination: place a drop on the eye; wait 10 to 15 minutes.

Expectorants, Antitussives and Inhalants

416. ℞ Ammonium chloride
Ammonium carbonate . . . . āā 16 gm
Camphor . . . . 4 gm
Fluidextract Belladonna . . . . 30 ml
Syrup . . . . q.s. ad 500 ml

Large animals: orally, 15 to 30 ml every 4 hours.

417. ℞ Compound Benzoin Tincture USP

Given in steam inhalations, 10 to 15 min, several times daily

418. ℞ Codeine

Dogs: orally, 5 mg every 6 to 8 hours.

419. ℞ Cresol

15 to 30 ml in a pail of steaming hot water. Allow animal to inhale vapor for 10 to 12 min, several times daily.

420. ℞ Terpin hydrate elixir with codeine

Orally, 5 mg every 6 to 8 hours.

Topical Dressings and Antiseptics

421. ℞ Acetic acid (glacial)

1:500 in water. Immerse fish for 1 minute.

422. ℞ Bacitracin . . . . 500 u
Neomycin . . . . 5 mg
Polymyxin sulfate . . . . 5,000 u

For standard equivalents for measures, see pp. 1521 to 1524.

Anhydrous lanolin and hydrophilic ointment base.
Apply t.i.d. to affected areas.

423. ℞ Benzalkonium chloride aqueous solution 1:1,000

Flush mouth freely as needed,
or apply to ear canal t.i.d.

424. ℞ Benzalkonium chlorides

A. Alkyl benzalkonium chloride (10 to 50%) 1.0 to 2.0 ppm of active ingredient. For 1 hr for 3 consecutive days for epidemics and 1-hr exposure for prevention.
B. *n*-Alkyl dimethylbenzylammonium chloride (50%). Use in same way as benzalkonium chloride. Effective in hard-water areas.
C. Benzethonium chloride (98.8%). Use in same way as benzalkonium chloride.

425. ℞ Burrow's Solution 1:20 (Aluminum Acetate Solution USP)

Moisten 8 to 10 layers of gauze and wring out drip free. Apply to the affected area for 15 to 20 min, t.i.d. to q.i.d., remoisten when the gauze reaches body temperature.

426. ℞ Calamine Lotion USP

Apply under a bandage.

427. ℞ Calcium oxide

130 to 175 lb/acre (150 to 200 kg/ha)

428. ℞ Chlorhexidine . . . . 15 ml
Water . . . . 2 qt (2 L)

Irrigate uterus with two-way flow catheter.
Topically: apply undiluted as a spray as needed.

429. ℞ Chlortetracycline hydrochloride 3% ointment

Apply to affected areas b.i.d. to q.i.d.

430. ℞ Copper sulfate or acetate

0.2 to 0.5 ppm in the water (depending on hardness of water—very toxic in soft water). Do not use in waters containing less than 50 ppm calcium carbonate.

Read introduction to prescriptions, pp. 1526 to 1527. Note all warnings and cautions appearing on drug labels and observe all local laws and regulations pertaining to drug usage.

431. ℞ "Cortisporin" ointment
Each gm contains:

Polymyxin B sulfate	5,000 u
Zinc bacitracin	400 u
Neomycin sulfate	5 mg
Hydrocortisone	10 mg

Apply b.i.d. to t.i.d. to affected areas.

432. ℞ Di-*n*-butyl tin oxide or tin dilaurate
114 mg/lb (250 mg/kg) of fish daily for 5 days.

433. ℞

DMSO (dimethylsulfoxide)	30 ml
Prednisolone solution	0.5 mg/ml
Nitrofurazone, 0.2% solution	30 ml

Pharyngeal spray for nodular pharyngitis. Apply topically to pharynx as a spray twice daily.

434. ℞ Fibrinolysin-desoxyribonuclease-thimerosal ("Elase") ointment
Each 30-gm tube contains:

Fibrinolysin (bovine origin) . . .	30 u
Desoxyribonuclease (bovine origin)	20,000 u
Thimerosal (mercury derivative) .	120 mcg

Use topically as a debriding agent in a variety of inflammatory and infected lesions.

435. ℞

Formaldehyde solution 37%	200 ml
Water	4 qt (4 L)

Apply locally or use in a foot bath through which the sheep are driven.

436. ℞ Formaldehyde solution (37%)
1:4,000 (250 ppm) to 1:6,000 (167 ppm) as a bath for 1 hr with oxygenation or continuous flow for 1 hour.
Caution: Lower concentration recommended in soft acid waters or at high temp.
Paraformaldehyde or formic acid, both toxic to fish, form on storage at low or high temp., respectively. Formalin storage should be at 64 to 70°F (18 to 21°C).
Always apply to small number of fish in initial trial.

437. ℞ Formaldehyde solution-malachite green
Prepare stock of 14 gm of malachite green in 1 gal. (3.8 L) of formaldehyde solution (37%). Apply mixture at 25 ppm as bath treatment *not to exceed 6 hours.*

For standard equivalents for measures, see pp. 1521 to 1524.

438. ℞ Gentian violet 1:500 aqueous solution

Stomatitis: Apply daily to ulcerated areas.
Vaginitis: Inject into vagina with catheter, or apply to mucosa with swab twice weekly.

439. ℞ Hexachlorophene 3%

Use as a cleanser to wash lesions; rinse well.

440. ℞ Ichthammol
Salicylic acid . . . . āā 10 gm
Zinc oxide ointment . . . . 250 gm

Apply to affected areas once daily.

441. ℞ Tincture of iodine 2%

Apply freely to gums after scaling teeth.

442. ℞ Tincture of iodine 2% . . . . 1 ml
Glycerin . . . . 30 ml

Apply to inflamed mucous membranes with a cotton swab.

443. ℞ Iodochlorhydroxyquin-hydrocortisone cream or ointment
Iodochlorhydroxyquin 3%
Hydrocortisone 1%

Apply to lesions t.i.d.

444. ℞ Malachite green

Eggs: 2 mg/L daily as a flush or bath for 1 hour.
Live fish: 1% soln. as lesion swabs; 67 mg/L as dip for 1 min (maintain aeration); 0.015 mg/L for prolonged immersion.
Caution: Apply at 50°F (10°C). At high temperatures dose should be progressively reduced.
Only oxalate, chloride or sulfate salts are acceptable. Never use zinc salt. Some evidence of carcinogenicity indicated. Use with care.

445. ℞ "Masoten"

Insoluble polymerisate with carboxyl groups of 80% polyacrylic acid and 20% insoluble potassium polyacrylate. Give 0.25 ppm in fish bath.
For copepods: Weekly for 4 weeks.
For monogenetic trematodes: For a week.

Read introduction to prescriptions, pp. 1526 to 1527. Note all warnings and cautions appearing on drug labels and observe all local laws and regulations pertaining to drug usage.

446. ℞ Neomycin 0.5% solution or ointment
Apply locally as wet dressings t.i.d.

447. ℞ Nitrofurazone Ointment NF XIII
Apply topically daily as indicated.

448. ℞ Nystatin . . . . 100,000 u
Neomycin . . . . 2.5 mg
Thiostrepton . . . . 2,500 u
Triamcinolone acetonide . . . . 1.0 mg
In hydrocarbon gel
Apply daily as directed.

449. ℞ Oxytetracycline-hydrocortisone spray
Each 3 oz contains:
Oxytetracycline hydrochloride . . . . 300 mg
Hydrocortisone . . . . 100 mg
Apply b.i.d. to affected areas.

450. ℞ Potassium permanganate 1:4,000 solution
Flush the mouth or sponge the gums as frequently as necessary.

451. ℞ "Pragmatar" ointment
Cetyl alcohol-coal tar distillate 4%
Near-colloidal sulfur 3%
Salicylic acid 3%
Oil-water emulsion . . . . . . q.s. ad 100 gm
Apply daily to affected areas.

452. ℞ Precipitated sulfur . . . . 15 gm
Lanolin . . . . 7 gm
White ointment . . . . q.s. ad 100 gm
Apply locally.

453. ℞ Salt solution
1 tsp table salt in a glass of warm water to be used as mouth wash. Flush mouth as needed.

454. ℞ Selenium sulfide 1% suspension
Dogs: Shampoo the entire body. Flush off residue thoroughly after use.
Cats: Apply only to affected areas.

455. ℞ Sodium bicarbonate
1 tsp in a glass of warm water to be used to flush mouth as needed.

For standard equivalents for measures, see pp. 1521 to 1524.

456. ℞ Sodium chloride
2.5% in the water for 2 to 4 days.

457. ℞ Sulfathiazole 5% ointment
Apply as wound dressing b.i.d. ot t.i.d.

458. ℞ Cephalonium, iodochlorhydroxyquin, polymyxin B, flumethasone, piperocaine hydrochloride ("Toptic" ointment)
Apply b.i.d. to affected areas.

459. ℞ Tyloxapol 0.125% ("Alevaire")
5 to 30 ml/flush.

460. ℞ Tyrothricin cream (0.5 mg/gm)
Apply topically daily as indicated.

461. ℞ Polyalkyleneglycol-iodine ("Weladol") shampoo (1% iodine) *or* cream (2% iodine)
Pyoderma: Shampoo entire body, then massage cream thoroughly into skin. Repeat cream massage daily for 3 to 10 days, depending on degree and duration of infection. May be repeated as necessary.
Otitis externa: Apply cream in ear canal daily.

462. ℞ Zinc chloride solution

Zinc chloride	2 gm
Water	q.s. ad 1 L

Flush mouth with solution as needed.

463. ℞

Zinc oxide	25.0 gm
Precipitated calcium carbonate	25.0 gm
Oleic acid	2.5 gm
Linseed oil	25.0 gm
Limewater	22.5 ml

Apply daily to affected areas.

Ear and Nasal Preparations

464. ℞

Alcohol	10 ml
Glycerin	90 ml
Salicylic acid	q.s. ad saturation
Boric acid	q.s. ad saturation
Tannic acid	q.s. ad saturation

Warm and apply in ear canal as drops, then massage gently.

Read introduction to prescriptions, pp. 1526 to 1527. Note all warnings and cautions appearing on drug labels and observe all local laws and regulations pertaining to drug usage.

465. ℞ Antibiotic-steroid ointment

Neomycin base (as sulfate)	3 mg/gm
Bacitracin	500 u/gm
Polymyxin B sulfate	10,000 u/gm
Hydrocortisone acetate	10 mg/gm
Lanolin-petrolatum base	q.s.

Instill into ear canal with massage 1 to 2 times daily.

466. ℞ "Canex" Solution

Chloroform	7.5 %
Rotenone	0.12%
Other ether extractives of derris . .	0.38%
Inert ingredients	92 %

Mix 1 part with 3 parts mineral oil and instill into external ear as drops or apply with cotton swab at 3-day intervals.

467. ℞ "Cerumenex"

Triethylanolamine polypeptide oleate condensate	10.0%
Chlorobutanol	0.5%
Propylene glycol	89.5%

Partially fill the ear canal, massage for a few minutes and clean.

468. ℞ Ephedrine sulfate 1% solution

2 drops in each nostril every 3 hours.

469. ℞ Hydrocortisone-neomycin ointment or solution

Hydrocortisone acetate	15 mg/gm or ml
Neomycin sulfate	5 mg/gm or ml

Instill 2 to 6 drops into ear canal with gentle massage, t.i.d. to q.i.d. Instill ointment into external ear canal with gentle massage once or twice daily.

470. ℞ "Mercaptocaine Creme"

2-Mercaptobenzothiazole	2 %
Benzocaine	5 %
2-Chloro-4-phenylphenol in emulsion base	0.2%

Apply in ear canal with cotton swab daily.

471. ℞ "Metimyd" ointment with neomycin

Each ⅛-oz tube contains:

Prednisolone acetate	5 mg

For standard equivalents for measures, see pp. 1521 to 1524.

Sodium sulfacetamide	100 mg
Neomycin sulfate	2.5 mg

After cleansing lesion, gently rub on ointment t.i.d. or q.i.d.

472. ℞ "Panalog" dermatologic ointment
Each ml contains:

Nystatin	100,000 u
Neomycin sulfate	2.5 mg
Thiostrepton	2,500 u
Triamcinolone acetonide	1.0 mg

Otitis: Clean ear of impacted cerumen and foreign bodies. Instill 2 to 3 drops of ointment.
For mild cases: once daily to once a week;
For severe cases: as often as b.i.d. or t.i.d.

473. ℞ "Pelene" drops

Resorcinol	5 %
Zinc oxide	4 %
Calamine	2 %
Oil of cade	1 %
Pyroligneous acid purified	0.4%
Zinc hydroxide	8 %

Instill 4 to 6 drops in cleaned ear canal daily.

474. ℞ "Pellitol"

Resorcin	5%
Bismuth subgallate	1%
Bismuth subnitrate	9%
Zinc oxide	17%
Calamine	10%
Oil of cade	1%
Special ointment base	q.s.

Apply in cleaned ear canal with cotton swabs or with special ear applicator tube.

475. ℞ Penicillin G sodium . . . . 100,000 u
Distilled water . . . . 10 ml

Spray into each nostril with suitable atomizer as necessary.

476. ℞ Phenylephrine hydrochloride 0.25% solution

Small animals: nasal drops, use b.i.d. to q.i.d.

Read introduction to prescriptions, pp. 1526 to 1527. Note all warnings and cautions appearing on drug labels and observe all local laws and regulations pertaining to drug usage.

77. ℞ Phenylmercuric nitrate 1:5,000 (alcoholic solution)
Use saturated cotton swab to clean the ear canal.

78. ℞ "Ridamite"

Dimethyl phthalate	24%
Cottonseed oil	76%

Place 1 to 2 ml into the ear canal and massage gently. Also swab the pinnae of the ear and the feet. Repeat every 3 to 4 days until the condition is cleared.

479. ℞

Thymol	0.6 gm
Ethyl alcohol 70%	30.0 ml

3 or 4 drops in ear canal every 2 days.

480. ℞ "Tresaderm" dermatologic solution
Each ml contains:

Thiabendazole	40.0 mg
Neomycin sulfate	3.2 mg
Dexamethasone	1.0 mg

After cleaning the surface of the lesion of ceruminous or other material, apply topically b.i.d. to t.i.d. For otitis externa instill 5 to 15 drops. For surface lesions apply enough to moisten.

Emetics and Antiemetics

481. ℞ Apomorphine hydrochloride
Dogs: 3 to 6 mg subcut. May also be given by dropping a prepared tablet into the conjunctival sac.
Cats: 1 to 2 mg subcut.

482. ℞ Dimenhydrinate tablets
0.5 mg/lb (1.1 mg/kg) body wt.

483. ℞ Meclizine
Orally: 1 mg/lb (2.2 mg/kg) body wt each 24 hours.

484. ℞ Methylatropine nitrate tablets (1 mg)
IM *or* subcut.: 2 to 5 mg, *or* 1 to 2 tablets 30 min before trip.

485. ℞ Metoclopramide
Dogs: 2.5 to 10 mg subcut.

486. ℞ Promethazine hydrochloride
Orally: 0.5 mg/lb (1.1 mg/kg) body wt.

For standard equivalents for measures, see pp. 1521 to 1524.

487. ℞ Dicyclomine hydrochloride and phenobarbital ("Spastyl") capsules
Each capsule contains:

Dicyclomine HCl	10 mg
Phenobarbital	15 mg

Dogs under 20 lb (9 kg): 1 capsule b.i.d.
Dogs over 20 lb: 1 capsule b.i.d. to q.i.d. as indicated.

488. ℞ Trimethobenzamide hydrochloride
Small animals: IV *or* IM: 100 to 200 mg, 1 to 4 times daily.

Antacids and Antidiarrheal Agents

489. ℞ Aluminum Hydroxide Gel USP (suspension)
Orally: 1 to 3 tsp (0.25 to 1.0 gm) t.i.d. or q.i.d.

490. ℞ "Anistat"
Each 8 oz (225 gm) contains:

Chloramphenicol	1.0 gm
Neomycin base (as sulfate)	1.0 gm
Sulfathiazole	6.0 gm
Sulfamethazine	2.0 gm
Absorbent demulcent base	q.s.

Calves and foals: 1st day: orally, 3 oz (85 gm), b.i.d. morning and evening; 2nd day: 2 oz (57 gm), b.i.d.
Pigs and lambs: Initial dose, 1 tsp/5 lb body wt followed in 12 hr by 1 tsp/10 lb body wt. Repeat as required.

491. ℞ Bismuth subnitrate *or* subcarbonate (may be given with kaolin)
Dogs: 1 gm in 1 tbsp milk, t.i.d.
Cows and horses: orally, 30 to 60 gm in capsule t.i.d.
Calves: orally, 10 to 20 gm in capsule.
Lambs: orally, 2 to 4 gm in capsule t.i.d.

492. ℞ Biosol-M
Each ml contains

Neomycin sulfate	50 mg
Methscopolamine bromide	0.25 mg

Dogs and cats: orally, 1 ml/20 lb (1 ml/9 kg) b.i.d.

Read introduction to prescriptions, pp. 1526 to 1527. Note all warnings and cautions appearing on drug labels and observe all local laws and regulations pertaining to drug usage.

93. ℞ Charcoal activated

Orally: 1 to 3 gm.

94. ℞ Nifuraldezone-bismuth ("Entefur")

Calves: 1-gm bolus, b.i.d. for 2 days.

95. ℞

Kaolin	200 gm
Pectin	4 gm
Water	q.s. ad 1 L

Adult cattle and horses: 180 to 300 ml every 3 hours.
Foals and calves: 90 to 120 ml every 2 to 3 hours.
Dogs and cats: 10 to 40 ml every 4 hours.

96. ℞ Diphenoxylate-atropine ("Lomotil")

Diphenoxylate hydrochloride	2.5 mg
Atropine sulfate	0.025 mg

Dogs: 0.7 to 0.9 mg/lb (0.3 to 0.4 mg/kg) body wt in divided doses.

97. ℞

Sodium bicarbonate	15 mEq
Pectin	50 mg
Kaolin	2 gm
Neomycin sulfate	125 mg
Potassium gluconate	23 mEq
Water	50 ml

Dose for 4- to 7-kg monkey; adjust proportionately for smaller or larger animals. Intubate via the nostril. Repeat dose b.i.d. for 3 to 7 days.

98. ℞ Sodium bicarbonate

IV: 3.75 gm/L of water (cannot be autoclaved).
Orally: as powder or tablets.
Horses: up to 60 gm.
Cattle: up to 120 gm.
Dogs and cats: up to 1.5 gm.

99. ℞

Tannic acid	0.6 gm
Water	30.0 ml

Dogs: 5 to 25 ml, orally.
Cats: 2.5 to 20.0 ml, orally.

00. ℞ Calf scour powder

Sodium chloride	117 gm
Potassium chloride	130 gm
Sodium bicarbonate	168 gm
Potassium phosphate (dibasic potassium phosphate)	135 gm

To prepare 1 L of the solution: Add 5.7 gm of the powder to 1 qt (1 L) of water to which may also be added 50 gm of glucose.
For 1 gal.: Add 1 oz (28 gm) powder and 0.5 lb (225 gm) glucose to 1 gal. (3.8 L) of water. Give or feed 1 gal. of solution to a 100-lb calf in divided doses in 24 hours.

Laxatives and Cathartics

501. ℞ Carbachol USP 1:1,000

Subcut.: 2 to 4 ml.

502. ℞ Epsom salt

1 lb (450 gm) mixed with bran in wet mash for 75 to 100 chickens. Withhold other feed until consumed, but provide fresh water.

503. ℞ Milk of Magnesia (Magnesium oxide)

1 pt mixed in 15 lb (0.5 L/7 kg) of wet bran mash for 500 birds; fed on top of the mash. Withhold other feed until consumed. Repeat the next day.

504. ℞ Milk of Magnesia

Magnesium hydroxide	1 to 2 lb (0.5 to 1 kg)
Water	q.s. ad 1 gal. (3.8 L)

Administer in one dose by stomach tube.

505. ℞ Mineral oil

Cattle and horses: Give by stomach tube 2 to 4 qt (2 to 4 L).
Sheep and swine: Give by stomach tube 1 to 2 pt (0.5 to 1 L).
Dogs: 1 to 4 tbsp daily.

506. ℞ Mucilose flakes (purified psyllium)

Small animals: 1 to 2 tsp sprinkled on moist food b.i.d.

507. ℞

Physostigmine salicylate	65 mg
Pilocarpine hydrochloride	130 mg
Strychnine	32 mg

To be dissolved in 20 ml of water for subcut. injection, for 500- to 600-lb (225- to 270-kg) animal. *For cattle 1,000 lb (450 kg) or more:* double the dose. *Sheep:* require ¼ of this dose.

Read introduction to prescriptions, pp. 1526 to 1527. Note all warnings and cautions appearing on drug labels and observe all local laws and regulations pertaining to drug usage.

)8. ℞ Psyllium hydrophilic mucilloid ("Metamucil") flakes

Dogs: orally, 1 tsp t.i.d.

)9. ℞ Dioctyl calcium sulfosuccinate and danthron ("Doxidan")

Small animals: 1 capsule daily until the feces become normal.

ntispasmodics

10. ℞ Aminopropazine furmarate ("Jenotone") (25 mg/ml)

Horses: IV or IM, 0.25 mg/lb (0.55 mg/kg) body wt.

11. ℞ Atropine sulfate

Inject IM *or* subcut., b.i.d. to q.i.d.
Cattle and horses: 0.014 to 0.032 mg/lb (0.03 to 0.07 mg/kg) body wt.
Dogs: 40 to 50 mcg/lb (88 to 110 mcg/kg) body wt.
For pancreatic disease: 9 mcg/lb (20 mcg/kg).
Cats: 20 to 40 mcg/lb (44 to 88 mcg/kg) body wt.

12. ℞ Belladonna Tincture USP . . . . 6 ml
Deodorized Opium
Tincture USP . . . . q.s. ad 30 ml

50 drops in water orally every 4 hours.

13. ℞ Dipyrone 50%

Administer IV, IM or subcut.:
Horses: 10 to 20 ml.
Cattle: 5 to 15 ml.
Swine: 5 to 10 ml.
Dogs: 1 to 5 ml.
Cats: 0.25 to 2 ml.

14. ℞ Methylatropine nitrate solution (5 mg/ml) or tablets (1 mg)

Large animals: IM *or* subcut., 5 to 15 mg.
Small animals: IM *or* subcut., 2 to 5 mg, or 1 or 2 tablets before feeding, or t.i.d. to q.i.d.

15. ℞ Propantheline bromide

Orally: 7.5 to 30 mg every 8 to 12 hours.

Iiscellaneous Digestants, Stomachics and Antiferments

16. ℞ Aromatic spirits of ammonia

Horses: via stomach tube, 30 to 60 ml dissolved in 1 pt (500 ml) of water.

For standard equivalents for measures, see pp. 1521 to 1524.

Cattle: orally, 30 to 120 ml dissolved in 1 qt (1 L) of water.

517. ℞ Magnesium sulfate . . . . 300 gm
Formalin . . . . 30 ml
Water . . . . 12 L

Warm to body temperature and give slowly via stomach tube.

518. ℞ Pancreatin granules or powder

Mix sufficient with each meal to keep stools normal (approximately 1 to 1.5 gm).

519. ℞ Polysorbate 80

Orally: 1 gm, t.i.d.

Hematinics

520. ℞ Injectable iron solution (50 to 100 mg elemental iron per ml)

Prophylaxis: 2 ml per pig at 2 to 4 days of age.
Treatment: 2 ml per pig any time between 7 and 21 days of age.

521. ℞ Iron and ammonium citrate . . . . . 1.2 gm
Copper gluconate . . . . 60.0 mg
Cobalt sulfate . . . . 15.0 mg
Honey or other flavored base . q.s. ad 30.0 ml

Cattle and horses: 15 to 30 ml b.i.d. to t.i.d.
Suckling pigs: Paint on udder of sow t.i.d. Individual pigs can be treated with 5 to 10 drops each daily.
Weaned pigs: 60 ml/100 animals daily, mixed in ration or drinking water.

Cardiovascular Agents

522. ℞ Aminophylline

Dogs and cats: IV slowly, 4.6 mg/lb (10 mg/kg) body wt,
or same dose IM *or* orally every 8 hours.
Horses: IV *or* orally, 0.5 mg/lb (1.1 mg/kg) t.i.d.

523. ℞ Atropine sulfate

Subcut.: 0.05 mg/lb (0.11 mg/kg) body wt every 8 hours,
or orally, 0.5 to 2.0 mg every 8 hours.

Read introduction to prescriptions, pp. 1526 to 1527. Note all warnings and cautions appearing on drug labels and observe all local laws and regulations pertaining to drug usage.

24. ℞ Atropine sulfate

Small animals: subcut., 18 mcg/lb (40 mcg/kg) body wt, b.i.d. to q.i.d.

25. ℞ Digitoxin Injection USP

Cattle: Total digitalization dose: IM, 30 to 40 mcg/lb (66 to 88 mcg/kg) body wt in divided doses over a 24-hour period.
Maintenance dose: 1/10 of the above dose.

26. ℞ Digoxin (*or* Digitoxin Tablets USP *or* Digoxin Elixir USP)

Dogs: IV *(Estimated total dose, intensive)*, 20 mcg/lb (44 mcg/kg) body wt. Give 50% of total dose initially followed by 25% of dose (10 mcg/kg) every 6 hr until toxicity or digitalization.
Total digitalization dose: orally, 32 to 100 mcg/lb (70 to 220 mcg/kg). Large dogs take lower doses. Divide into 6 equal doses and give every 8 hr for 2 days or until digitalization or toxicity occurs.
Maintenance dose: 1/8 to 1/5 of final dose required for digitalization. Approximately 10 mcg/lb (22 mcg/kg) divided into 2 doses b.i.d.
Cats: Oral method only recommended: 3.6 to 5.5 mcg/lb (8 to 12 mcg/kg) body wt in 2 divided doses daily.
Horses: IV, 0.033 mg/kg body wt *estimated total dose.* Give 50% of dose initially followed by 25% every 4 hr until signs of toxicity or ECG changes. Digitalization generally achieved at end of third dose. No oral regime established. *Maintenance dose:* 1/4 of digitalizing dose.

527. ℞ Diphenylhydantoin ("Dilantin")

For digitalis toxicity and ventricular tachycardias:
Dogs: IV slowly, 0.9 to 2.3 mg/lb (2 to 5 mg/kg) body wt until control or a maximum of 4.6 mg/lb (10 mg/kg) given. Follow with tablets at 10 mg/kg daily given orally in divided doses.
Caution: Rapid IV injection may produce death. Use for this purpose is not fully documented in dogs.

528. ℞ Epinephrine Solution 1:1,000 USP

Horses and cattle: IV *or* subcut., 5 to 15 ml.
Sheep and swine: IV *or* subcut., 2 to 4 ml.
Dogs: IM, IV *or* subcut., 0.1 to 0.5 ml.

For standard equivalents for measures, see pp. 1521 to 1524.

529. ℞ Epinephrine Solution 1:1,000 USP

Dilute with 10 parts of isotonic salt solution.

Large animals: intracardially, 3 to 8 ml.
Small animals: intracardially, 0.1 to 0.5 ml.

530. ℞ Epinephrine Solution 1:1,000 USP

Cattle and horses: subcut., 4 to 8 ml.
Sheep and swine: subcut., 1 to 3 ml.
Dogs and cats: subcut., 0.1 to 1.0 ml; *or* IV, 0.01 ml (or more).

531. ℞ Isoproterenol

Dogs: Oral tablets. 15 to 30 mg every 3 to 4 hours. In emergency may be given IV. Use solution containing 0.2 mg isoproterenol in 250 ml of 5% dextrose. Infuse at the rate of 1 ml/kg body wt per min (0.045 to 0.090 mcg/min). Rate of infusion can be adjusted according to desired heart rate. ECG monitoring highly recommended.

532. ℞ Levarterenol Bitartrate Injection USP (2 mg/ml)

4 ml/L of 5% dextrose. IV: 0.5 ml/min.

533. ℞ Ouabain Injection USP (0.25 or 0.5 mg)

Cattle: Total digitalization dose: IV, 6 to 10 mcg/lb (13 to 22 mcg/kg) body wt, divided into 4 doses and given over a 24-hour period.
Maintenance dose: ⅛ to ⅕ the total digitalization dose.

534. ℞ Ouabain Injection USP

Dogs: IV *or* IM, 10 to 15 mcg/lb (22 to 33 mcg/kg) body wt, repeated after 24 to 36 hours. For safety, divide the calculated amount in 2 equal doses and give 3 to 4 hours apart.

535. ℞ Phenylephrine

Dogs: IV, 0.15 to 0.8 mg in diluted solution (with caution),
or subcut., 0.6 to 3.2 mg.

536. ℞ Propranolol

Dogs: IV, 1 to 3 mg; orally, 2 to 40 mg, t.i.d.
Caution: Should not be given in presence of cardiac failure unless animal is fully digitalized. Monitor IV administration with ECG. Excessive bradycardia should be treated with atropine.

Read introduction to prescriptions, pp. 1526 to 1527. Note all warnings and cautions appearing on drug labels and observe all local laws and regulations pertaining to drug usage.

37. ℞ Quinidine sulfate

Horses: Initial dose 10 gm followed by increments of 10 gm daily (2nd day—20 gm, 3rd day—30 gm) until conversion or toxicity occurs. Conversion usually occurs at daily dose of 20 to 40 gm. Toxicity is likely at higher doses, which must be approached with caution. Treatment stopped if there is obstructive swelling of nasal mucosa, laminitis, severe depression, excessive sweating, diarrhea or renal damage.

Other regimes have been used and some prefer to administer 10 gm quinidine sulfate every 2 hr until conversion or toxicity. Some prefer to digitalize the horse prior to conversion.

38. ℞ Quinidine sulfate tablets

Dogs: orally, 2.7 to 10 mg/lb (6 to 22 mg/kg) body wt, every 6 to 8 hours. Dosing every 2 to 4 hr may be necessary for initial control of the arrhythmia.

Diuretics

39. ℞ Acetazolamide

Dogs: orally, 2 to 4.6 mg/lb (5 to 10 mg/kg) body wt, t.i.d.

40. ℞ Acetazolamide

IM, 0.45 mg/lb (1 mg/kg) body wt daily.

41. ℞ Chlorothiazide

Cattle: orally, 8 mg/lb (17.6 mg/kg) body wt daily, preferably in divided doses. (*Calves* may need up to 12 mg/lb [26 mg/kg] body wt.)

Dogs: orally, 5 to 10 mg/lb (11 to 22 mg/kg) body wt preferably in divided doses.

42. ℞ Cyclothiazide

Dogs: Orally, 16 to 35 lb (7 to 16 kg) body wt—0.5 to 1.0 mg; 36 to 55 lb (16 to 25 kg) body wt—1.0 to 1.5 mg; over 56 lb (> 25 kg) body wt—1.5 to 2.0 mg.

43. ℞ Furosemide

Dogs and cats: orally, IM *or* IV, 1 to 2 mg/lb (2 to 5 mg/kg) body wt, once or twice daily for 2 to 3 days.

Horses: orally, IM *or* IV, 250 to 500 mg once or twice daily for 2 to 3 days.

For standard equivalents for measures, see pp. 1521 to 1524.

544. ℞ Hydrochlorothiazide

Cattle: IV *or* IM, up to 1 mg/lb (2.2 mg/kg) body wt daily, preferably in divided doses.

545. ℞ Mannitol 20% solution

Mix conc. soln. in IV fluids to deliver 0.09 to 0.23 gm/lb (0.2 to 0.5 gm/kg) body wt.

546. ℞ Mercurophylline Injection USP

Dogs: IM *or* IV, 0.25 to 2.0 ml (50 to 200 mg). The IM route is somewhat safer and smaller doses should be used first to establish effective level. Use one dose every day for 3 to 6 doses and repeat if necessary after resting for 5 days, or 1 to 3 doses may be given every week as needed.

547. ℞ Trichlormethiazide 200 mg and dexamethasone 5 mg ("Naquasone")

Cattle: b.i.d. for 1 to 3 days. Use only after calving; if used earlier premature birth and retained placenta may result.

Sedatives and Anticonvulsants

548. ℞ Chloral hydrate

For ketosis in cattle: 30 gm in capsule or dissolved in water and given via stomach tube, daily.
For myopathies and related conditions: IV, 30 gm in 500 ml sterile water *or* orally, 45 gm in 500 ml of water.

549. ℞ Diphenylhydantoin sodium

Orally: 2 mg/lb (4.4 mg/kg) body wt every 6 to 8 hours.

550. ℞ Mephenesin solution or tablets

Cattle: IV, 400 to 600 ml of a 2% solution (single injection),
or orally, 10 gm, t.i.d. for 2 to 3 days.
Small animals: orally, 0.5 to 1.0 gm t.i.d.

551. ℞ Pentobarbital sodium

Small animals: IV, slowly to effect (anesthetic dose 10 mg/lb [22 mg/kg] body wt).

552. ℞ Phenobarbital tablets

Orally: 0.5 to 1.0 mg/lb (1 to 2.2 mg/kg) body wt, every 6 to 8 hours.

Read introduction to prescriptions, pp. 1526 to 1527. Note all warnings and cautions appearing on drug labels and observe all local laws and regulations pertaining to drug usage.

53. ℞ Primidone tablets (125 mg)

Increase gradually from ½ tablet daily to 2 tablets daily over a 2-week period. *Maintenance dose:* 2 tablets daily.

54. ℞ Xylazine

Horses: IV, 0.5 mg/lb (1.1 mg/kg) body wt,
or IM, 0.01 mg/lb (0.022 mg/kg).

ntihistaminics

55. ℞ Chlorpheniramine maleate

Adult cats: orally, 8 mg every 12 hours.
Kittens: orally, 4 mg every 12 hours.

56. ℞ Diphenhydramine capsules or solution

Orally *or* IV: 0.2 to 1.0 mg/lb (0.5 to 2.2 mg/kg) body wt, 1 to 3 times daily.

57. ℞ Promethazine hydrochloride ("Phenergan") solution (25 mg/ml),
or tablets (12.5, 25 or 50 mg)

0.1 to 0.5 mg/lb (0.2 to 1.1 mg/kg) body wt, t.i.d.

58. ℞ "Antiphrine"

Each ml contains:

Pyrilamine maleate	25 mg
Ephedrine hydrochloride	10 mg
Chlorobutanol (chloral derivative)	0.35%

Administer slowly, IM, IV *or* subcut.: *Cattle, horses, sheep & swine:* 2 ml/100 lb (46 kg) body wt. *Dogs and cats (do not administer IV):* 0.5 ml/20 to 25 lb (9 to 11 kg) body wt.

59. ℞ Pyrilamine maleate solution (2.5%)
or tablets (12.5, 25 or 50 mg)

Large animals: IM *or* subcut., 2 ml/100 lb (45 kg) body wt.

60. ℞ Tripelennamine

Cattle and horses: IM *or* subcut., 20 to 40 mg/100 lb (0.4 to 0.8 mg/kg) body wt. May be repeated after 2 hr if necessary.
Dogs: orally, 0.9 mg/lb (2 mg/kg) body wt. Divide the total daily dose into 3 or 4 parts and give at 6-to 8-hr intervals.

For standard equivalents for measures, see pp. 1521 to 1524.

561. ℞ Tripelennamine citrate . . . . 150 mg
Ammonium chloride . . . . 400 mg
Ephedrine sulfate . . . . 50 mg
Syrup . . . . q.s. ad 20 ml

1 tsp every 4 hours.

Urinary Antiseptics and Acidifiers

562. ℞ Ammonium chloride

Dogs: Orally, 0.3 to 1.2 gm freely diluted with water t.i.d. to q.i.d.
Cattle and sheep: 4 to 30 gm daily.

563. ℞ Ethylenediamine dihydrochloride tablets (90 mg)

1 tablet t.i.d. Increase dosage if necessary to make urine acid to litmus paper.

564. ℞ Methenamine Mandelate USP

Dogs: orally, 0.25 to 1.0 gm 1 to 4 times daily.

Hemostatics

565. ℞ Adrenochrome isonicotinic acid hydrazone

Large animals: IM, 5 ml.
Small animals: IM, 0.25 to 1.0 ml.

566. ℞ Carbazochrome salicylate

Large animals: IM, 25 mg.
Small animals: orally or IM, 1 mg/6 lb (3.7 mg/10 kg) body wt.

567. ℞ "Gelfoam"

Saturate a small square of Gelfoam in isotonic salt solution or in thrombin solution and apply to bleeding areas, using mild pressure or leave in wound as a pack.

568. ℞ Hemostatic solution (aqueous emulsion of cephalin and lecithin)

Large animals: preferably IV, 10 ml.
Small animals: IV *or* IM, 1 to 5 ml.

569. ℞ Protamine sulfate 1 to 2% solution

IV: no greater than 50 mg over a 10-min period.

Read introduction to prescriptions, pp. 1526 to 1527. Note all warnings and cautions appearing on drug labels and observe all local laws and regulations pertaining to drug usage.

570. ℞ Menadione Sodium Bisulfite Injection USP (2.5 mg/0.5 ml)

IV: 0.5 to 1.0 ml. Repeat after 12 hr if needed. As much as 5 mg/lb (11 mg/kg) body wt may be necessary when profound hypoprothrombinemia occurs (e.g. sulfaquinoxaline overdose).

571. ℞ Protamine Sulfate Injection USP

IV: 25 to 50 mg in 10 to 20 ml isotonic saline.

572. ℞ Thrombin NF Bovine Topical XIII (solution)

Apply topically as lyophilized material or dilute to 100 to 1000 u/ml with isotonic saline solution.

573. ℞ Tolonium chloride

IV, IM *or* subcut.: 1 ml/10 lb (4.5 kg) body wt. Dosage may be repeated as needed.

574. ℞ Vitamin K_1 injection

IV: 90 to 275 mcg/lb (200 to 600 mcg/kg) body wt, IV for 1 to 2 days, followed by 5 to 10 mg orally for 5 to 7 days.

Solutions, parenteral

575. ℞ Dalton's oral electrolyte solution

Sodium chloride	117 gm
Potassium chloride	150 gm
Sodium bicarbonate	168 gm
Potassium phosphate (dibasic)	135 gm

Add 1 oz/gal. (30 gm/4 L) of water.
For calves: Feed as warm solution or give by stomach tube an amount equivalent to 10% of body weight daily divided into 2 or 3 feeds.
For horses: In drinking water: Use ½ oz/gal. (15 gm/4 L). Most horses will readily drink this concentration; however, the palatability should be confirmed for each individual animal.

576. ℞ Dextran 70, 6%

IV: 500 ml for 2 days then on alternate days for 2 weeks.

577. ℞ Dextrose 5% and isotonic sodium chloride solution

Large animals: IV, 250 to 1,000 ml daily.
Dogs: slow IV drip, 5 to 10 ml/lb (11 to 22 ml/kg) body wt.

For standard equivalents for measures, see pp. 1521 to 1524.

578. ℞ 5% Dextrose in lactated Ringer's solution

Dogs: slow IV drip, 15 to 35 ml/lb (30 to 75 ml/kg) body wt.

579. ℞ Electrolyte solution

Sodium chloride	5.50 gm
Calcium chloride	0.30 gm
Magnesium chloride	0.30 gm
Sodium acetate	6.10 gm
Potassium acetate	1.00 gm
Water for injections	q.s. ad 1 L

Calves: Administer IV by continuous drip at the following rate:
(A) Moderately dehydrated calves:
(1) 25 ml/lb (55 ml/kg) body wt in first 4 to 6 hours;
(2) continue treatment for 20 hr at 70 ml/lb (154 ml/kg) body wt.
Severely dehydrated calves:
(1) 50 ml/lb (110 ml/kg) body wt in first 4 to 6 hours;
(2) continue treatment for 20 hr at 70 ml/lb wt.
Mature cattle: Give 25 to 50 ml/lb (50 to 110 ml/kg) body wt in first 4 to 6 hr and continue for next 20 hr as required (e.g. at approximately 25 ml/lb for severe grain overload).

580. ℞ Electrolyte solution ("Multisol R")
Replacement electrolytes in water
Each 100 ml contains:

Sodium chloride	526 mg
Sodium acetate	222 mg
Sodium gluconate	502 mg
Potassium chloride	37 mg
Magnesium chloride	14 mg

pH adjusted with hydrochloric acid (approx. 1 mEq/L)

Small animals: Moderate dehydration—6 to 8% of body wt of water is deficit. Severe dehydration—8 to 10% of body wt of water is deficit. Administer appropriate amount by slow IV infusion over 8- to 16-hr period.

581. ℞ "Eltras"
Each milliliter contains:

Dextrose . . . . 5 gm

Read introduction to prescriptions, pp. 1526 to 1527. Note all warnings and cautions appearing on drug labels and observe all local laws and regulations pertaining to drug usage.

Sodium chloride . . . . 0.5 gm
Sodium acetate . . . . 0.75 gm
Potassium chloride . . . . 0.075 gm
Calcium chloride . . . . 0.04 gm
Magnesium chloride hexahydrate . 0.03 gm

Dogs and cats: IV, 50 to 250 ml.
Puppies: IV, 25 ml/lb (55 ml/kg) body wt.

582. ℞ Fluorescein 10% solution
Fluorescein, soluble . . . . 3 gm
Isotonic salt solution . . . . 30 ml

Dissolve, autoclave and use IV in one dose as the fluorescein test. The animal should be placed in a stall away from the sunlight.

583. ℞ Fresh horse blood plasma
Horses: IV, 40 to 60 ml/min or more in a case of severe shock.

584. ℞ Glucose 5% solution
Subcut. *or* IV: 10 ml/lb (22 ml/kg) body wt daily, preferably in divided doses.

585. ℞ Glucose 50% solution
IV: 500 ml.

586. ℞ Magnesium sulfate 25% solution
Cattle: Subcut., 400 ml.

587. ℞ Parenterin
IM *or* subcut.: 10 to 20 ml.

588. ℞ Lactated Ringer's solution
For maintenance: 18 to 27 ml/lb (40 to 60 ml/kg) body wt, daily.
For dehydration: 5 to 10% body wt.

589. ℞ Ringer's solution
Sodium chloride . . . . 90 mg
Potassium chloride . . . . 30 mg
Calcium chloride . . . . 30 mg
Water for injections . . . . . q.s. ad 100 ml

Via slow IV drip: 9 to 18 ml/lb (20 to 40 ml/kg) body wt.

590. ℞ Saline-bicarbonate solution
Sodium chloride . . . . 8.5 gm/L
Sodium bicarbonate . . . . 13.0 gm/L

For standard equivalents for measures, see pp. 1521 to 1524.

For parenteral administration: mix equal volumes of each together.
Dosage: 10% of body wt over 24 hr; initially 1 L of solution may be given IV over 2 hours.

591. ℞ Isotonic saline with dextrose 6%
Piglets: orally, 2 fl oz (60 ml) every 4 hours
or subcut. 15 ml every 6 hours.

592. ℞ Saline and dextrose solution

Sodium chloride	0.425 gm
Glucose	2.5 gm
Distilled water	q.s. ad 100 ml

IV or subcut.: 10 ml/lb (22 ml/kg) body wt, daily, preferably in divided doses, or as required.

Parenteral Enzyme Preparations

593. ℞ Chymotrypsin
2,000 to 5,000 u in a suitable volume of sterile water.

594. ℞ Streptokinase-streptodornase mixture ("Varidase")
All animals (except cattle): Dissolve 5,000 to 10,000 u in sterile water. Inject into pleural cavity or IM every 24 hours.

Iodine Preparations

595. ℞ Ethylenediamine dihydriodide
1 oz (28 gm), b.i.d. in feed or capsule for 8 days, starting 10 days after estrus.

596. ℞ Ethylenediamine dihydriodide (20 grains per oz)
Cattle: ½ oz (15 gm) b.i.d. for 8 to 10 days.
Calves: 6 months old, 1 lb (450 gm)/300 head daily for 7 days, then 1 lb/500 head daily.
Adults: 1 lb/100 head daily for 7 days, then 1 lb/300 head daily.

597. ℞

Lugol's iodine 5%	1 ml
Isotonic salt solution	9 ml

Using a fine gauge needle, make several 0.5 ml injections into the affected muscles.

Read introduction to prescriptions, pp. 1526 to 1527. Note all warnings and cautions appearing on drug labels and observe all local laws and regulations pertaining to drug usage.

598. ℞ Iodochlorhydroxyquin

Orally: 15 gm daily. As feces become firm reduce by 1 gm daily until daily dose of 2 gm. Maintain at 2 gm for a week.

599. ℞ Lugol's solution 5%

Dilute with equal parts of distilled water and inject 2 ml into bursa.

600. ℞ Potassium Iodide Solution NF XIII

2 to 5 drops in water, daily for 2 or 3 days.

601. ℞ Potassium or sodium iodide

Horses: orally, 4 to 10 gm.
Cattle: orally, 10 mg/lb (22 mg/kg) body wt. Daily doses for 2 to 4 weeks. Discontinue medication if signs of iodism appear.

602. ℞ Povidone-iodine 1% ("Betadine")

Use as a soap to wash lesions; rinse well.

603. ℞ Povidone-iodine solution, titratable iodine, 0.5% ("Betadine")

5 to 60 ml/flush.

604. ℞ Sodium iodide

IV: 7.5 mg/lb (16.5 mg/kg) body wt, repeated every 4 or 5 days. Discontinue medication if signs of iodism appear.

605. ℞ Sodium iodide 5 to 20% solution

IV, inject slowly: 30 mg/lb (66 mg/kg) body wt. Repeat after 7 to 10 days.

606. ℞ Strong Iodine Solution USP (Lugol's solution)

10 to 20 drops in water daily for 2 or 3 days.

Calcium Preparations

607. ℞ Calcium borogluconate 25% solution

Cattle: IV *or* IP, 250 to 500 ml.
Sheep: IV *or* IP, 100 ml.
Horses: IV, 200 to 500 ml.
Small animals: subcut., IM *or* IV, slowly to effect, 5 to 20 ml.

608. ℞ Calcium borogluconate . . . . 250 gm
Magnesium borogluconate or sulfate . 50 gm
Distilled water . . . . q.s. ad 1 L

For standard equivalents for measures, see pp. 1521 to 1524.

Cattle: IV, subcut. or IP, 400 to 800 ml.
Sheep: IV, subcut. or IP, 100 ml.
Horses: IV, 100 to 850 ml.

609. ℞ Calcium gluconate

Cattle and horses: IV, 250 to 500 ml, 20% solution, or half the dose IV and half subcut.
Sheep: IV, 50 ml of a 20% solution.
Dogs: IV, 5 to 20 ml of a 10% solution.
Cats: IV, 2 to 5 ml of a 10% solution.

610. ℞ Calcium lactate
Sodium lactate . . . . āā 250 gm
Water . . . . 500 ml

Orally: 250 gm b.i.d. for 10 days.

611. ℞ Calcium-vitamin D_2 ("Calpho-D")
Each tablet contains:
Calcium gluconate . . . . 160 mg
Calcium lactate . . . . 90 mg
Dicalcium phosphate . . . . 230 mg
Vitamin D_2 . . . . 400 IU

Dogs and cats: 1 or more tablets t.i.d.

Analgesics and Local Anesthetics

612. ℞ Aspirin

Orally: 5 to 18 mg/lb (10 to 40 mg/kg) body wt daily, or every 8 to 12 hours.
Caution: Some cats are sensitive. Use with care in this species.

613. ℞ Aspirin

For DIC in dogs: orally, 150 to 300 mg daily,
or every other day up to 10 days.
For DIC in cats (some are sensitive): orally, 50 to 100 mg.

614. ℞ Benzocaine

Light anesthesia: 20 to 30 ppm.
Deep anesthesia: 50 ppm.
Dissolve benzocaine in small volume of acetone before adding to water.

615. ℞ Dibucaine ointment

Apply to rectum and anus every 4 hours.

Read introduction to prescriptions, pp. 1526 to 1527. Note all warnings and cautions appearing on drug labels and observe all local laws and regulations pertaining to drug usage.

616. ℞ Lidocaine

IV: 0.9 to 1.8 mg/lb (2 to 4 mg/kg) body wt. IV infusion of a 2% solution (1 to 2 ml/22 lb [10 kg]) body wt, over 1- to 2-min period. Effect lasts from 10 to 20 minutes.

617. ℞ Meperidine hydrochloride

***All species:* IM, 1 to 2.3 mg/lb (3 to 5 mg/kg) body wt, as well as orally in small animals. Repeat every 8 to 12 hours.**

618. ℞ Methampyrone

***Horses:* IV, IM or subcut., 10 to 20 ml.**
***Cattle:* IV, IM *or* subcut., 5 to 15 ml.**

619. ℞ Morphine sulfate

***Horses:* subcut., 60 to 90 mg.**
***Dogs:* subcut., 15 mg repeated at 4- to 8-hr intervals if necessary.**

620. ℞ Pentazocine lactate

***Horses:* IV *or* IM, 0.3 mg/lb (0.66 mg/kg) body wt.**

621. ℞ Phenylbutazone Tablets NF XIII (100 mg)

***Horses:* 2 to 4 mg/lb (4 to 9 mg/kg) body wt, not to exceed 4 gm daily.**
***Dogs:* 20 mg/lb (44 mg/kg) body wt in 3 divided doses daily.**

Dietary Supplements

622. ℞ Ascorbic acid

***Dogs:* orally, 250 mg, t.i.d.**

623. ℞ Brewer's yeast dried

***Cattle and horses:* 120 to 150 gm daily.**
***Sheep and swine:* 30 to 60 gm daily. Mix thoroughly with grain or ground feed.**
***Dogs:* 1 to 3 gm daily, as tablets or in food.**

624. ℞ Choline chloride

0.5 to 2.5 gm added to diet daily.

625. ℞ DL-Methionine

***Cats:* orally, 200 mg, b.i.d. *or* t.i.d.**
***Dogs:* orally, 1 gm every 8 hours.**

For standard equivalents for measures, see pp. 1521 to 1524.

Detoxifying Agents

626. ℞ Calcium disodium edetate (CaEDTA)

Cattle and horses: IV, 50 mg/lb (110 mg/kg) body wt, 2 doses 6 hr apart, every other day for 3 treatments.
Dogs: subcut., 50 mg/lb (110 mg/kg) body wt of a 1% solution (dilute with 0.9% saline solution or 5% dextrose solution), divided into 4 doses, every other day for 3 treatments.

627. ℞ Dicalcium-phosphogluconate ("C.G.P.")

Cattle and horses: IV, 250 to 500 ml.
Sheep and swine: IV, 50 to 100 ml. Repeat after several hours.

628. ℞ Dimercaprol (BAL)

IM: 1.4 mg/lb (3 mg/kg) body wt, every 4 hr for the first 2 days; every 6 hr on the third day; and every 12 hr for the next 10 days, or until recovery is complete.

629. ℞ Diphenylthiocarbazone (Dithizone)

For acute thallium poisoning in dogs: orally, 32 mg/lb (70 mg/kg) body wt.
For chronic thallium poisoning in dogs: orally, 2.3 to 3.2 mg/lb (5 to 7 mg/kg) body wt, b.i.d. (Larger doses may release sufficient thallium from the tissues to precipitate acute poisoning.)

630. ℞ DL-Batyl alcohol . . . . 5 gm
Olive oil . . . . 50 ml

Subcut.: 10 ml daily for 5 days.

631. ℞ DL-Batyl alcohol 2% solution in 1% saline (brought into solution with 5% "Tween 80")

IV slowly: 25 to 50 ml daily.

632. ℞ Magnesium sulfate

Horses and cattle: orally, 500 to 1,000 gm.
Swine: orally, 50 to 200 gm.
Sheep: orally, 20 to 50 gm.

633. ℞ Methylene blue . . . . 10 gm
Water . . . . 500 ml

IV: 20 ml/100 lb (45 kg) body wt. Repeat if necessary.

Read introduction to prescriptions, pp. 1526 to 1527. Note all warnings and cautions appearing on drug labels and observe all local laws and regulations pertaining to drug usage.

634. ℞ Methylene blue 20% solution

IV: 10 ml/500 lb (225 kg) body wt. Repeat if necessary.

635. ℞ Pralidoxime chloride (2-PAM chloride)

All species: IV, 11 to 23 mg/lb (25 to 50 mg/kg) body wt. Therapy is most effective in the presence of atropine (℞ 511).

636. ℞ Sodium iodide 10% solution

IV: 30 to 45 mg/lb (65 to 100 mg/kg)

637. ℞ Sodium nitrite . . . . 20 gm
Sodium thiosulfate . . . . 30 gm
Sterile water . . . . q.s. ad 500 ml

IV: 20 ml/100 lb (45 kg) body wt. To be given slowly and repeated once only if necessary.

638. ℞ Sodium thiosulfate 20% solution

IV: 10 ml/100 lb (45 kg) body wt. Repeat if necessary.

Astringents, Counterirritants and Escharotics

639. ℞ Alum . . . . 5 gm
Water . . . . q.s. ad 100 ml

Apply topically to mucosa.

640. ℞ Ferrous sulfate dried
Copper sulfate dried
Zinc sulfate dried . . . . āā 10 gm

Thrush: Apply to bottom of affected sulcus and retain with pledget of cotton or oakum.
Canker: Apply to affected area and retain with bandage and foot pack.

641. ℞ Mandl's solution
Iodine . . . . 0.60 gm
Potassium iodide . . . . 1.20 gm
Peppermint oil . . . . 0.25 gm
Glycerin . . . . q.s. ad 30 ml

For topical application.

642. ℞ Silver nitrate 2% solution

Pharyngitis: Apply to inflamed mucous membranes with a cotton swab.
Nonfunctional quarter: Infuse into teat canal and milk out after 7 days. Repeat treatment after 2 or 3 weeks if necessary.
NOTE: The total amount of chemical used should

not exceed 1 gm (50 ml of a 2% solution) to avoid severe toxic reactions.

643. ℞ Silver nitrate 5% solution

For topical use in cauterizing cysts, fistulas and mucosal lesions.

644. ℞ Tannic acid . . . . 1 ml
Glycerin . . . . 30 ml

Apply to inflamed mucous membranes with a cotton swab.

645. ℞ Tannic acid
Salicylic acid . . . . āā 5 gm
Alcohol 70% . . . . q.s. ad 100 ml

Apply b.i.d. to the affected areas of the skin after cleansing.

646. ℞ Zinc sulfate
Lead acetate
Copper sulfate . . . . āā 60 gm
Water . . . . q.s. ad 600 ml

Apply b.i.d. after washing the leg.

647. ℞ Red mercuric iodide . . . . 20 gm
Petrolatum . . . . 80 gm

Mix thoroughly, clip hair from area to be blistered and rub in well for 5 to 10 minutes. Cover with sheet cotton and bandage. Remove dressing after 4 days.

648. ℞ Tincture of iodine 2%

Dilute with equal parts of distilled water and inject 2 ml into bursa.

649. ℞ Tincture of iodine 2.5% . . . . 60 ml
Pine tar . . . . 240 gm
Soft soap . . . . 90 gm

Apply locally.

650. ℞ Tincture of iodine 5%

Rub well into coronet with brush. Repeat daily for 4 or 5 days.

Read introduction to prescriptions, pp. 1526 to 1527. Note all warnings and cautions appearing on drug labels and observe all local laws and regulations pertaining to drug usage.

Semen Diluters

651. ℞ Citrate buffer solution

Sodium citrate	3 gm
Water distilled over glass and heated to 100°C	100 ml

Sterilize and store in darkness.

Diluter

Buffer solution	
Yolk from fresh eggs āā	
Penicillin	1,000 u/ml
Streptomycin	1 mg/ml

Mix on the day it is to be used to dilute semen.

652. ℞ For milk and glycerin diluter

Place 500 ml of milk in double boiler and heat to 200°F (93°C) for 10 minutes. Remove scum from top of milk. Cool and measure out 450 ml of milk in sterile flask. Add 500,000 u of penicillin and 500 mg of streptomycin. Measure out 200 ml of milk and add 50 ml of glycerol.

Add semen to unglycerolated milk and cool to 40°F (4.5°C) over a 3- or 4-hour period. Add similarly cooled glycerolated milk to semen-milk mixture in three equal portions at 10-minute intervals.

653. ℞ Phosphate buffer solution

Potassium phosphate monobasic (KH_2PO_4)	0.2 gm
Sodium phosphate dibasic dodecahydrate ($Na_2HPO_4 \cdot 12H_2O$)	2.0 gm
Water distilled over glass and heated to 100°C	100 ml

Sterilize and store in darkness.

Diluter

Buffer solution	
Yolk from fresh eggs āā	
Penicillin	1,000 u/ml
Streptomycin	1 mg/ml

Mix on the day it is to be used to dilute semen.

Miscellaneous

654. ℞ Amphetamine sulfate

Cattle and horses: subcut., 0.1 to 0.3 gm.
Dogs: orally *or* subcut., 0.5 to 2.0 mg/lb (1 to 4.5 mg/kg) body wt.

For standard equivalents for measures, see pp. 1521 to 1524.

655. ℞ Bethanechol chloride

Dogs: orally, 5 to 15 mg, t.i.d. to q.i.d.

656. ℞ Cyclophosphamide tablets or powder for injectable solution

For immunosuppression: orally *or* IV, 0.9 to 1.4 mg/lb (2 to 3 mg/kg) body wt for 6 days.
For lymphoma: 13.6 mg/lb (30 mg/kg) body wt, once.

657. ℞ Cyclophosphamide

Dogs: orally, 10 to 25 mg/day divided b.i.d. Administer 7 to 10 days; repeat if neoplasia recurs.

658. ℞ Iodine agglutination test (IAT) for Aleutian disease

The iodine test solution is unstable and must be prepared for each testing period. It is stored refrigerated in amber bottles. Avoid contact with metal or rubber.

Iodine crystals	2 gm
Potassium iodide	4 gm
Distilled water	30 ml

Blood from a clipped toenail is collected in a nonheparinized capillary tube and centrifuged. The serum is mixed on a glass slide with fresh solution and stirred with a wooden applicator stick. Clumping or precipitation within a few seconds constitutes a positive reaction.

659. ℞

Lobelia fluid extract	60 ml
Belladonna fluid extract	30 ml
Fowler's solution	q.s. ad 500 ml

1 tbsp on feed, t.i.d.

660. ℞ Sterile milk

Large animals: IM *or* subcut., 5 to 25 ml. Repeat at intervals of 1 to 5 days if indicated.
Small animals: IM *or* subcut., 0.5 to 1.0 ml, as an initial dose. Subsequent doses depend upon response and sensitivity of the patient.

661. ℞ New methylene blue stain

New methylene blue	0.5 gm
Potassium oxalate	1.6 gm
Distilled watter	100 ml

Filter before use.

Read introduction to prescriptions, pp. 1526 to 1527. Note all warnings and cautions appearing on drug labels and observe all local laws and regulations pertaining to drug usage.

662. ℞ Mitotane (*o,p'* DDD)

Dogs: orally, 25 mg/lb (50 mg/kg) body wt, once daily until response or side effects produced—usually about 7 days. Thereafter, once a week.

663. ℞ Oxymetholone tablets

Orally: 5 to 25 mg daily for 6 to 10 days.

664. ℞ D-Penicillamine tablets

Dogs: 15 mg/lb (30 mg/kg) body wt in divided doses. Reduce dose if vomiting occurs.

665. ℞ Pentylenetetrazole injection (100 mg/ml)

IV slowly: 0.05 to 0.1 ml (May also be given in electrolyte or dextrose infusion).

666. ℞ Phosphate buffer

Disodium hydrogen phosphate	3.80 gm
Potassium dihydrogen phosphate	5.47 gm

Dissolve in 500 ml of distilled water and bring volume to 1 liter. The distilled water *must be neutralized* using hematoxylin as the indicator. Rinse clean test tube, add 5 ml of the distilled water and a few crystals of hematoxylin:
neutral—pale lavender in 10 seconds;
acid—becomes yellow and remains so for over 5 minutes;
alkaline—becomes red-purple at once or within a minute.
Adjust pH with 1% potassium hydroxide or 1% hydrochloric acid as necessary. Prepare neutral water daily or as necessary.

667. ℞ Pilocarpine hydrochloride

Orally: 1 mg/10 lb (1 mg/5 kg) body wt; mix with feed b.i.d., and increase every 2 or 3 days by 1 mg until signs of excessive lacrimation noted. The highest level possible without producing toxicity should be maintained.

668. ℞ Vitamin A and D

Vitamin A	500,000 IU/ml
Vitamin D_2	75,000 IU/ml

Horses (yearlings): 1 to 2 ml/head.

669. ℞ Propylene Glycol USP

Orally: 250 gm mixed with an equal volume of water b.i.d. for 5 days.

For standard equivalents for measures, see pp. 1521 to 1524.

670. ℞ Sodium morrhuate 5% solution
0.5 ml injected at 1-in. intervals into the tendon.

671. ℞ Sodium propionate
Orally: 120 gm b.i.d. for 10 days.

672. ℞ Glycobiarsol
Orally: 100 mg/lb (220 mg/kg) body wt, once daily, for 5 consecutive days.

673. ℞ Monensin
Calves: Prophylactic use: 0.9 mg/lb (2 mg/kg) body wt, fed continuously.

674. ℞ Sodium arsanilate or arsanilic acid
Prophylaxis: 0.01% (90 gm/ton) in feed.
Treatment: 0.025 to 0.4% in feed for 5 to 6 days for control of swine dysentery.

675. ℞ Heparin Sodium USP
Dogs: IV, 68 u/lb (150 u/kg) body wt every 4 to 6 hours.

676. ℞ Ethoxyzolamide
Dogs: orally, 2.1 mg/lb (4.6 mg/kg) body wt b.i.d.

INDEX

(Throughout the index, page numbers appearing in roman type indicate that the subject is identified in the text either as a heading or by boldface or italic type or by quotation marks. Page numbers in *italics* signify that the term occurs in the text merely as part of the discussion, without typographical emphasis.)

A

B

C

D

G

H

I

J

K

L

N

O

P

Q

R

U

V

W

X

Y

Z